Nutrition
ACROSS LIFE STAGES

Melissa Bernstein, PhD, RD, LD, FAND
Rosalind Franklin University of Medicine and Science

Kimberley McMahon, MDA, RD
Logan University

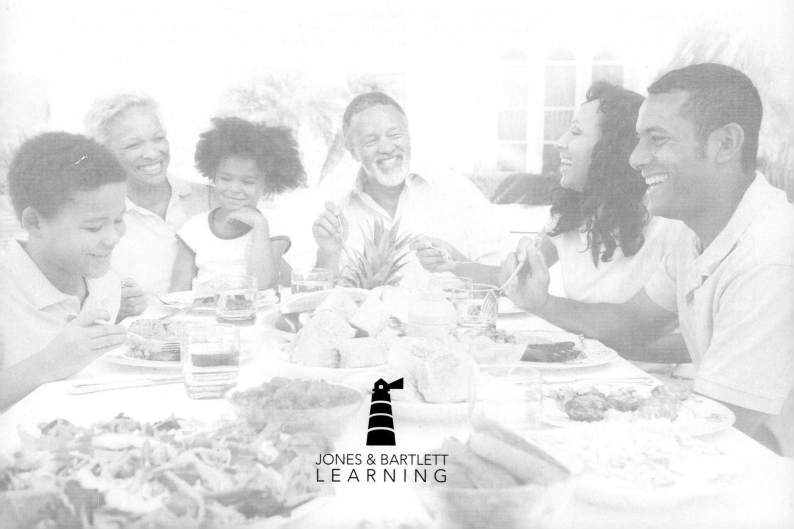

JONES & BARTLETT
LEARNING

World Headquarters
Jones & Bartlett Learning
5 Wall Street
Burlington, MA 01803
978-443-5000
info@jblearning.com
www.jblearning.com

Jones & Bartlett Learning books and products are available through most bookstores and online booksellers. To contact Jones & Bartlett Learning directly, call 800-832-0034, fax 978-443-8000, or visit our website, www.jblearning.com.

Substantial discounts on bulk quantities of Jones & Bartlett Learning publications are available to corporations, professional associations, and other qualified organizations. For details and specific discount information, contact the special sales department at Jones & Bartlett Learning via the above contact information or send an email to specialsales@jblearning.com.

10223-9

Production Credits
VP, Executive Publisher: David D. Cella
Acquisitions Editor: Sean Fabery
Associate Editor: Taylor Maurice
Director of Production: Jenny L. Corriveau
Associate Production Editor: Alex Schab
Director of Marketing: Andrea DeFronzo
VP, Manufacturing and Inventory Control: Therese Connell

Composition: Integra Software Services Pvt. Ltd.
Cover Design: Theresa Manley
Rights & Media Specialist: Merideth Tumasz
Media Development Editor: Shannon Sheehan
Cover Image and Title Page: © Monkey Business Images/Getty Images
Printing and Binding: LSC Communications
Cover Printing: LSC Communications

Library of Congress Cataloging-in-Publication Data
Names: Bernstein, Melissa, author. | McMahon, Kimberley, author.
Title: Nutrition across life stages / Melissa Bernstein and Kimberley McMahon.
Description: First edition. | Burlington, Massachusetts : Jones & Bartlett
Learning, [2018] | Includes bibliographical references.
Identifiers: LCCN 2016054750 | ISBN 9781284102161
Subjects: | MESH: Nutritional Physiological Phenomena | Diet
Classification: LCC RA776.75 | NLM QU 145 | DDC 613.2--dc23
LC record available at https://lccn.loc.gov/2016054750

6048

Printed in the United States of America
21 20 19 18 17   10 9 8 7 6 5 4 3 2

CONTENTS

CHAPTER 4   Nutrition Needs During Lactation 91

CHAPTER **14**   **Older Adult Nutrition 451**

CHAPTER **15**   **Geriatric Nutrition 493**

DEDICATION

Nutrition Across Life Stages is dedicated to my grandmother, Cherie Fine, who passed away at the age of 95 as we were nearing the completion of this edition. She had a special gift of connecting with people of all ages. Everyone who was fortunate to be a part of her life experienced her warmth, generosity, and wisdom. May her memory be a blessing.

—Melissa Bernstein

Nutrition Across Life Stages is dedicated to my three children. May they always see the value in making good choices for their health and well–being, and that they set good examples for others.

—Kimberley McMahon

FOREWORD

In *Nutrition Across Life Stages*, Melissa Bernstein and Kimberly McMahon take us across the life cycle with scientific clarity, covering the intersection between nutrition and health from preconception to adolescence to older adulthood. Over the course of this whirlwind trip, the authors raise insightful questions vital to the study of life cycle nutrition. What are the benefits and disadvantages of iron supplements? Can being underweight affect a pregnancy? Why is it important for a woman to take folic acid before she becomes pregnant? The authors discuss which substances found in the home or workplace can make it more difficult for a woman to become pregnant or to provide a healthy environment for her baby. Has she been exposed to toxic substances such as lead, mercury, pesticides, solvents, or radiation? These conditions are reviewed in detail.

Bernstein and McMahon are particularly good at citing the latest studies to show the consequences of dietary decisions. Vitamin D deficiency, for example, is a major, unrecognized epidemic in adult women of childbearing age and can result in significant health problems in children born to these women. What about women who are strict vegetarians? Can they meet all their nutritional needs?

A very strong and compelling part of the book is the material related to the older adult and geriatric population. The authors expertly discuss the role of nutrition in the management of acute or chronic conditions specific to mature adults, such as drug–nutrient interactions, depression, anorexia of aging, arthritis, osteoporosis, overweight and obesity, and Alzheimer's disease. Given the increased role registered dietitian nutritionists now play in healthcare for older adults, the latter part of the book becomes a veritable page turner.

Paul Insel, PhD
Stanford University

PREFACE

Welcome to *Nutrition Across Life Stages*! This text covers topics applicable and relevant for entry-level Nutrition and Dietetics students who are focusing their study on nutritional requirements and challenges during each life stage. As such, *Nutrition Across Life Stages* includes chapters highlighting clinical-, health-, and disease-related topics specific to each age group that provide students with a knowledge and understanding of prevalent nutritional concerns from preconception to advanced age. Throughout, we as authors have strived to incorporate topics of special interest and to break down complex topics into key components to improve student understanding and build their practical knowledge base.

In writing this text, we kept in mind the needs of undergraduate students enrolled in an introductory life cycle nutrition course. As such, our aim has been to map to the way these courses are taught in a Nutrition and Dietetics program; however, we hope Nursing programs and programs that offer nutrition certification will also find this book a good fit.

The Goal of this Text

Good nutrition is a critical component at every stage of life, from preconception to end-of-life care. The maintenance of good health for all ages requires approaches that recognize multiple levels of influence on the individual and the impact of social, cultural, environmental, organizational, and medical factors. At any given age, there are significant challenges to healthy eating, especially for those affected by chronic conditions, physical limitations, and financial constraints; those who are racial and ethnic minorities; and those who reside in potentially challenging environments. More attention, resources, and nutrition expertise are needed to meet the food and nutrition requirements of vulnerable populations so that they can live healthfully with a good quality of life at every stage of life. Healthcare providers have opportunities to develop care plans that can help individuals of all ages promote personal well-being. Providing targeted and personalized nutrition guidance, services, and programs is vital to making a positive impact in the lives of all people.

As authors on two well-established introductory nutrition texts—*Nutrition* and *Discovering Nutrition*—we aim to keep our texts current and engaging for instructors and students alike. Having taught Life Cycle Nutrition ourselves, we saw a need for a fresh approach to

this material. Learning about the varying needs and challenges of different age groups begins with a solid foundation in nutrition basics, before then applying that knowledge to different ages, environments, challenges, and medical conditions. By using an approach that begins with normal nutrition and then considers alterations in nutritional needs and challenges resulting from common diseases and conditions that affect individuals at various ages, *Nutrition Across Life Stages* strives to keep students engaged and thinking critically in order to creatively apply their knowledge to problem-solving challenging real-life scenarios. Our aim is to make learning the material approachable, interesting, relevant, and fun without feeling overwhelming. We believe *Nutrition Across Life Stages* accomplishes this by presenting fresh pedagogy and engaging, student-centered learning activities that appeal to various learning styles.

Nutrition Across Life Stages facilitates active and participatory learning by providing many opportunities for classroom discussion and active engagement, presenting students with a multidimensional approach to the material. Discussion prompts and learning activities embedded throughout the text are designed to facilitate personalized teacher interaction with students. In lieu of rote lecturing, these endeavor to create a dynamic learning experience, whether they're used in a traditional classroom, as part of an online curriculum, or some hybrid of the two.

In crafting this text, we wanted to avoid categorizing older adults by chronological age. As a result, this is the first life cycle nutrition text to break out coverage of older adults across three unique chapters. Chapter 14, "Older Adult Nutrition," discusses normal nutrition for otherwise healthy older adults, while Chapter 15, "Geriatric Nutrition," highlights topics relevant to those who are frail, ill, and whose health is failing. Finally, Chapter 16, "Nutrition for Health and Disease in Older Adults and Geriatrics," addresses common health-related situations that require additional nutrition consideration.

Organization of the Text

We wrote *Nutrition Across Life Stages* with the typical Life Cycle Nutrition course in mind—that is, one focused on normal nutrition. *Nutrition Across Life Stages* begins in Chapter 1 with an overview of normal nutrition, national nutrition guidelines, and recommendations. Subsequent chapters then follow a consistent pattern: first, normal nutritional needs at two to three life stages are presented, followed by a chapter discussing the nutritional implications of health and common conditions and diseases, their consequences, and treatment for those life stages. The text reviews the life cycle progressively by breaking it into the following stages:

- Preconception
- Pregnancy
- Lactation
- Infancy
- Early childhood
- Preadolescence
- Adolescence
- Adulthood
- Older adulthood
- Geriatrics

The last two categories aren't necessarily chronological but rather more categorically based on health status in old age, an organizing principle unique to this text.

Features and Benefits

Nutrition Across Life Stages incorporates a strong array of pedagogical features, including several that contain a strong visual component. These are deployed consistently across chapters, ensuring a uniform learning experience for the student.

Each chapter begins with a brief Chapter Outline, along with a series of Learning Objectives that establish what the chapter seeks to convey to the reader. Toward the beginning of each chapter, a Case Study is also introduced that is directly relevant to the content being discussed. These case studies are progressive and revisited throughout the chapter; questions tied to each Case Study have been included that can be used for self-study or as part of a classroom assignment. Additionally, each section within each chapter begins with a *Preview* statement and ends with a summarizing *Recap* that includes questions that allow the reader the opportunity to identify key concepts.

Within the chapters, several boxed features appear. These include the following:

- *The Big Picture* is an enhanced visual feature that incorporates key photos, diagrams, graphs, and illustrations to help visual learners by highlighting key concepts and breaking down tough concepts to their constituent components.
- *News You Can Use* presents topics of special interest to students, usually tied to current research in nutritional science.
- *Let's Discuss* provides topics that are meant to trigger engaging and insightful conversations in the classroom.

Each chapter concludes with a Learning Portfolio that contains the following:

- Visual Chapter Summary
- Key Terms
- Discussion Questions
- Activities
- Study Questions
- Weblinks

The Complete Learning Package

Nutrition Across the Life Stages provides instructors with a full suite of resources, including:

- Test Bank, containing more than 500 questions
- Slides in PowerPoint format, featuring more than 350 slides
- Image Bank, collecting photographs and illustrations that appear in the text
- Instructor's Manual, including an array of useful instructor tools:
  - Learning Objectives
  - Chapter Outlines
  - Answers to in-text Case Study questions
  - Answers to in-text Study Questions
  - Answers to in-text Discussion Questions
  - Nursing Notes, highlighting content especially relevant to Nursing students

Melissa Bernstein
Kimberley McMahon

THE PEDAGOGY

Nutrition Across Life Stages incorporates an array of pedagogical features in order to facilitate active student engagement and class discussion.

The **Chapter Outline** at the beginning of each chapter gives students a preview of topics that will be covered.

Learning Objectives focus students on the key concepts of each chapter and the material they will learn.

A **Case Study** is introduced at the beginning of each chapter, illustrating how topics discussed in the text might appear in real-life. These case studies are revisited throughout the chapter, building in concert with the foundational material. As the case study progresses, questions are incorporated to encourage active student engagement with the scenarios.

Key Terms are in boldface type the first time they are mentioned, with definitions appearing in the end-of-chapter Learning Portfolio.

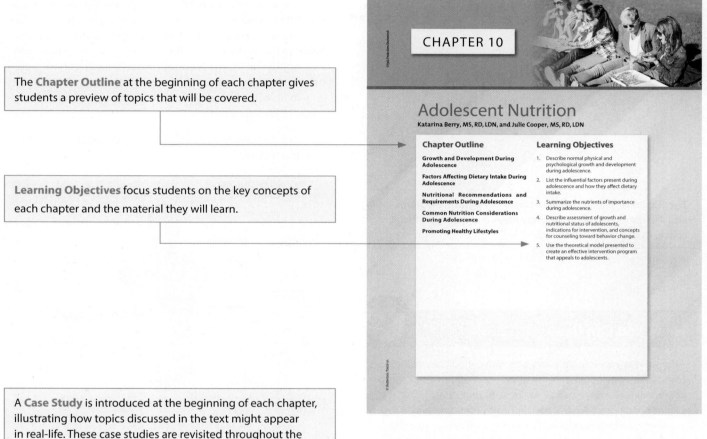

CHAPTER 10

Adolescent Nutrition

Katarina Berry, MS, RD, LDN, and Julie Cooper, MS, RD, LDN

Chapter Outline

Growth and Development During Adolescence

Factors Affecting Dietary Intake During Adolescence

Nutritional Recommendations and Requirements During Adolescence

Common Nutrition Considerations During Adolescence

Promoting Healthy Lifestyles

Learning Objectives

1. Describe normal physical and psychological growth and development during adolescence.

2. List the influential factors present during adolescence and how they affect dietary intake.

3. Summarize the nutrients of importance during adolescence.

4. Describe assessment of growth and nutritional status of adolescents, indications for intervention, and concepts for counseling toward behavior change.

5. Use the theoretical model presented to create an effective intervention program that appeals to adolescents.

Case Study

©KateStone/Shutterstock

Carla is a 14-year-old girl who lives with her mom and 17-year-old brother. She has had annual preventive health care from birth and has grown along average height and weight trends. Her medical history includes only seasonal allergies. Carla's parents divorced when she was very young, and she does not see her dad. Her mom has a full-time job and is comfortably able to provide food for the family. Carla is a strong student at her public middle school and has enjoyed participating in team sports for the past several years.

Adolescence is a period of great physical, psychological, and emotional development that spans ages 10 to 19 years.[1] Perhaps the simplest way to define its endpoints is the entrance of a child and emergence of a young adult. Changes over this near decade of life are constant, with internal influences such as hormonal shifts and external factors such as family, school, media, and daily social interactions. Adequate nutrition is necessary for adolescents to achieve their growth potential, and with this period of development comes increased and unique nutrient needs. The American Academy of Pediatrics (AAP) recommends discussion of nutrition and physical activity with during annual preventive care appointments.[2] The role for registered dietitian nutritionists and other healthcare providers in supporting healthy adolescent development is increasingly vital.

is a well-accepted method of evaluation in adolescent health care.[4,5] A child with an SMR of stage 1 has no visual signs of change, which indicates prepuberty, whereas SMR stage 5 is reached once adult characteristics have developed. Secondary sexual characteristics at each stage are outlined in **TABLE 10.1**.[4,5] Gonadarche is the first visual sign of puberty and heralds the child's transition from stage 1 to stage 2. Boys generally reach this milestone about 2 years behind girls. Gonadarche in girls is marked by breast budding, also called thelarche, and usually occurs between 9 and 13 years of age.[6] In boys, gonadarche is marked by an increase in testicular size. On average for boys, this occurs at 11.5 to 12 years of age,[7] with the vast majority of boys beginning pubertal genital development by age 13.[3]

During normal development of both boys and girls, changes associated with progression through SMR stages appear in a specific sequence and do not vary. This sequence is shown in **TABLE 10.2**.[8] The pace, or tempo, at which an adolescent moves through these stages is unique to each person. On average, it takes 4 years for a girl to progress from breast budding (SMR stage 2) to adult breast development (SMR stage 5). Boys, on average, take 3 years to move from SMR stage 2 to stage 5.[6] Total time of puberty, however, can range from these averages and can take as little as 1.5 years to as long as 8 years in girls, and from 2 to 5 years in boys.[9] Varied tempo of puberty is important to keep in mind because nutritional needs change during progression through SMR stages, and age itself is therefore not a good determinant of dietary requirements.[6]

Each section begins with a **Preview** statement, giving the reader a sense of what content to expect.

Preview Human milk is a unique, bioactive substance derived by the body to further the biological development of the human infant. Use of human milk enhances the immune, gastrointestinal, and metabolic health of infants.

Recap boxes summarize each section and provide open-ended questions, encouraging students to reflect on what they've just read.

Recap The structure of the breast allows for its function of providing nutrients to an infant. Hormones enhance development of the mammary gland and prepare the mammary system for milk production. For the initial stage of milk production, the mother's body produces colostrum, the first secretion from the mammary glands of the mother after giving birth. Colostrum is uniquely nutritive and significantly important, because this is the first feedings for an infant who has been well nourished by the maternal blood supply during pregnancy. The composition of breastmilk changes through the course of lactation, providing the vast majority of nutrients required for infant growth.

1. Explain how prolactin and oxytocin influence human milk production.

The Big Picture feature incorporates key photos, diagrams, and illustrations, highlighting key ideas and making difficult concepts easier to understand.

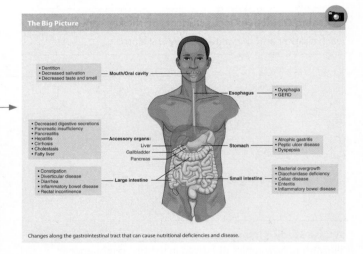

The Big Picture

Changes along the gastrointestinal tract that can cause nutritional deficiencies and disease.

News You Can Use

Adults use complementary and alternative medicine, including taking dietary supplements, for a few main reasons, such as to prevent illness and for overall wellness, to reduce pain and treat painful conditions, to treat a specific health condition, and to supplement conventional medical treatments. More than two-thirds of adults do not discuss their supplement use with a healthcare provider, often because they do not consider herbs or dietary supplements medications.[a] This is alarming because some dietary supplements can affect the absorption of other nutrients, interfere with the absorption and metabolism of prescription medications, contribute to polypharmacy, and, in large amounts, have toxic or other negative effects on health. St. John's wort, for example, an herb used in the treatment of mild to moderate depression, can interfere with the action of many prescription medications.[a]

References

a. National Center for Complementary and Integrative Health, National Institutes of Health, U.S. Department of Health and Human Services. Complementary and alternative medicine: what people aged 50 and older discuss with their health care providers. Bethesda, MD: National Center for Complementary and Integrative Health; updated December 15, 2015. Retrieved from: https://nccih.nih.gov/research/statistics/2010. Accessed May 18, 2016.

The **News You Can Use** feature presents topics of special interest to students, usually anchored in current nutritional science research.

The **Let's Discuss** feature provides prompts for class discussion.

Let's Discuss

What are students' personal experiences related to breastfeeding? Have any perceptions of breastfeeding been affected after reading about the benefits of breastfeeding? Do you know if you were breastfed, and if so, for how long?

Each chapter concludes with a **Learning Portfolio**, assembling an array of student-centered resources and activities.

The **Visual Chapter Summary** summarizes the chapter content in bullet form, complemented by important illustrations and photos found in the chapter.

Learning Portfolio

Visual Chapter Summary

Introduction

- As we study nutrition needs and recommendations throughout life, we must keep in mind these basic principles that are important for healthy eating regardless of age:
  - Poor nutrition status can result from either inadequate or excessive nutrition intake and can contribute to the development of certain chronic diseases.

©Hartphotography/Shutterstock

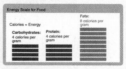
Energy Scale for Food

- Energy produced by the body, which is needed for a variety of functions, is provided by food and drink in the form of carbohydrates, proteins, and fats

©Syda Productions/Shutterstock

(macronutrients). Each macronutrient provides a specific amount of energy measured in calories.
- Energy needs vary from person to person and depend on such factors as basal metabolic rate (BMR) and activity level.

©ifong/Shutterstock

- There are many components of healthy eating, with adequacy, balance, moderation, and variety in food choices being key characteristics.

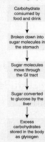

Carbohydrate consumed by food and drink
↓
Broken down into sugar molecules in the stomach
↓
Sugar molecules move through the GI tract
↓
Sugar converted to glucose by the liver
↓
Excess carbohydrates stored in the body as glycogen

Process by which carbohydrates are converted to glucose for energy, or glycogen for storage.

Learning Portfolio (continued)

Each chapter ends with an inventory of **Key Terms** and their definitions; all terms and definitions are also found in the end-of-text Glossary.

Key Terms

activities of daily living (ADLs): Daily activities that people tend to do every day without needing assistance, such as eating, bathing, dressing, toileting, transferring (walking), and continence (holding their bowels and bladder).
andropause: A gradual but progressive decline in testosterone levels with age.
energy balance: When calories consumed equal calories burned.
functional fibers: Isolated, nondigestible forms of carbohydrate that have been extracted from starchy foods or manufactured from starches or sugars. They may have some of the benefits of naturally occurring dietary fiber, such as helping to prevent constipation or lowering blood glucose levels after meals.
menopause: A natural biological process in women that involves a decline in estrogen production. It typically occurs 12 months after the last menstrual period and marks the end of menstrual cycles.
orthorexia nervosa: An obsession with eating foods that one considers healthy and pure; a fixation on righteous eating.

resting metabolic rate (RMR): The number of calories needed to support basic functions, including breathing and circulation.
sarcopenia: Age-associated loss of skeletal muscle mass (lean body mass) and function. The causes of sarcopenia are multifactorial and can include disuse, altered endocrine function, chronic diseases, inflammation, insulin resistance, and nutritional deficiencies. Sarcopenia is associated with muscle weakness, functional limitations, and disability, as well as impairments in cardiovascular capacity and metabolic health.
senescence: The inevitable decline in organ function and physiological function that occurs over time in the absence of injury, illness, or poor lifestyle choices. The process of growing old; senescence involves the accumulation of deleterious changes in cells that cause them to die more rapidly than they are replaced.
thermic effect of food (TEF): The increase in energy expenditure in response to the digestion, absorption, and storage of food.

Discussion Questions encourage students to probe deeper into the chapter content, making connections and gaining new insights.

Discussion Questions

1. The physiological changes that occur during adulthood are inevitable. Choose one physiological change discussed in the chapter, and discuss healthy lifestyle habits that can help prevent or slow the decline in physical health that often accompanies aging.
2. Discuss the many factors contributing to obesity. By what means is *Healthy People 2020* aiming to promote healthy nutrition and weight?

3. Outline a healthy adult's macro- and micronutrient needs and discuss how Estimated Energy Requirements can be calculated.
4. You've just been hired as an intern with the Department of Public Health. Your manager asks you to write an overview of healthy eating and physical activity recommendations. What key recommendations would you include?

Suggested **Activities** encourage students to put theory into practice.

Activities

1. **Health Promotion: Create Your Own Awareness Program.** Based on the needs of your community, create plans for an awareness program that promotes healthy habits. Create a slideshow presentation using the following items to guide your presentation.

   a. The name of your program (be creative!)
   b. Why this program is needed (what are the issues?)
   c. What will this program aim to do (how can the issues be solved/helped?)
   d. What activities/programming will this program provide?

   e. How will you measure the outcomes of the program?
   f. What barriers might you face?

2. **Fad Diets: Debunking Bad Advice!** Find a fad diet or herbal/nutritional supplement of interest to you, and be prepared to answer the following questions:
   a. What is product/diet, and what benefits does it claim to have?
   b. What does the scientific evidence say about this product/diet? Is there any scientific evidence?
   c. What possible harm can this product/diet cause?

Study Questions provide multiple-choice and true/false questions at the end of each chapter, testing students' knowledge of the information covered in the text. These can be utilized for student self-assessment or as homework material.

Study Questions

1. Physiological functions begin to deteriorate increasingly after which age?
   a. 25 years
   b. 30 years
   c. 35 years
   d. 40 years
2. Senescence is a term that refers to a decline in organ function and physiological function caused by injury, illness, or poor lifestyle choices.
   a. True
   b. False
3. Which physiological changes occur with aging?
   a. Increase in LBM and increase in fat mass
   b. Decrease in LBM and decrease in bone mass
   c. Increase in bone mass and increase in estrogen
   d. Increase in fat mass and increase in testosterone
4. What is bone mass affected by?
   a. Dietary micronutrient intake
   b. The body's micronutrient stores
   c. Level of physical activity
   d. All of the above
5. Factors that contribute to the obesogenic environment include all of the following except which one?
   a. Lack of sidewalks
   b. Expensive gym memberships
   c. Reduced portion sizes at restaurants
   d. Long commutes to and from work
6. Healthy People has established benchmarks and monitored progress over time to help encourage community collaboration and empower individuals to make good health decisions.
   a. True
   b. False
7. A "superfood" can help you lose weight.
   a. True
   b. False
8. What is a characteristic of people who struggle with orthorexia nervosa?
   a. They are focused on eating only vegan food.
   b. They want to lose weight and be thin.
   c. They vomit when they eat unhealthy foods.
   d. They can feel superior to others in regard to their food habits.
9. What is the Estimated Energy Requirement?
   a. The additional calories needed by the body to support weight gain
   b. The needed dietary energy intake to sustain energy balance
   c. The number of calories needed to promote weight loss in obese adults
   d. The energy required to promote health
10. What is the basal metabolic rate?
    a. The energy needed to support main body functions
    b. The energy required to support activities of daily living
    c. The energy required daily to support an exercise program
    d. The energy required to metabolize the food consumed
11. What is the thermic effect of food?
    a. The energy required to facilitate exercise
    b. The reaction that occurs when food is consumed
    c. The energy required for the ingestion, digestion, and absorption of food
    d. The energy required for the synthesis and secretion of hormones
12. What are macronutrients?
    a. Substances that provide vitamins and minerals to the body
    b. Substances such as vitamin B_6, B_{12}, and zinc
    c. Substances such as carbohydrates, protein, and fat
    d. Substances that help the body preserve body temperature and cardiac output
13. What is a function of carbohydrates?
    a. Help repair cells in the body
    b. Supply energy to the cells in the body
    c. Maintain proper GI tract functioning
    d. Promote heart function
14. What are amino acids?
    a. The basic structures of proteins
    b. The basic structures of carbohydrates
    c. The basic structures of fat
    d. Substances needed for vitamin absorption
15. What are micronutrients?
    a. Substances such as carbohydrates, protein, and fat
    b. Vitamins and minerals
    c. Substances essential for the absorption of fat-soluble vitamins and carotenoids
    d. Structural components of all the cells in humans
16. Mrs. Jones is a 24-year-old woman who is breastfeeding her 2-month-old child. What are her caloric needs?
    a. The same as the calorie needs of other 24-year-old females with the same level of activity, height, and weight.

Weblinks direct students to online resources relevant to the chapter content.

Weblinks

- **Minnesota Public Radio, "The Salt": Fad Diets Will Seem Even Crazier After You See This**
  http://www.npr.org/sections/thesalt/2013/08/23/214912007/fad-diets-will-seem-even-crazier-after-you-see-this
  Visit this provoking website to see a unique photo series visually representing fad diets!

- **Baylor College of Medicine Calorie Needs Calculator**
  https://www.bcm.edu/cnrc-apps/caloriesneed.cfm
  Use this tool to estimate how many calories you need.

- **Choose MyPlate Interactive Tools: SuperTracker**
  http://www.choosemyplate.gov/supertracker-other-tools

  Do you want to plan a healthy diet and track your physical activity? Use the Chose MyPlate SuperTracker to help you achieve your health and fitness goals.

- **USDA Choose MyPlate: Pregnancy and Lactation**
  http://www.choosemyplate.gov/moms-pregnancy-breastfeeding
  Learn more about nutrition needs during pregnancy and lactation.

- **Interactive DRI Tool for Healthcare Professionals**
  http://fnic.nal.usda.gov/fnic/interactiveDRI/
  Use this tool to calculate daily nutrient recommendations to assist you with planning your diet based on the Dietary Reference Intakes (DRIs).

ABOUT THE AUTHORS

Dr. Melissa Bernstein is a registered dietitian, licensed dietitian, and Fellow of the Academy of Nutrition and Dietetics. She received her doctoral degree from the Gerald J. and Dorothy R. Friedman School of Nutrition Science and Policy at Tufts University (Boston, MA). As an assistant professor in the Department of Nutrition at Rosalind Franklin University of Medicine and Science (North Chicago, IL), Dr. Bernstein is innovative in creating engaging and challenging nutrition courses. Her interests include introductory nutrition, health and wellness, geriatric nutrition, physical activity, and nutritional biochemistry. In addition to co-authoring leading nutrition textbooks—including *Nutrition*, *Discovering Nutrition*, and *Nutrition for the Older Adult*—Dr. Bernstein has reviewed and authored textbook chapters, position statements, and peer-reviewed journal publications on the topics of nutrition and nutrition for older adults. She is the co-author of the *Position of the Academy of Nutrition and Dietetics: Food and Nutrition for Older Adults: Promoting Health and Wellness*. She has served on review and advisory committees for the Academy's Evidence Analysis Library and as a reviewer for upcoming position statements.

Kimberley McMahon is a registered dietitian, licensed dietitian, and university instructor. She received her undergraduate degree from Montana State University and master's degree from Utah State University. She has taught nutrition courses in both traditional and online settings. She currently teaches in the Master of Science in Nutrition and Human Performance program at Logan University (Chesterfield, MO). In addition to co-authoring leading nutrition textbooks—including *Nutrition* and *Discovering Nutrition*—she has contributed to and authored textbook chapters on a variety of nutrition topics. Her interests and experiences are in the areas of wellness, weight management, sports nutrition, and eating disorders.

ACKNOWLEDGEMENTS

The completion of this edition of *Nutrition Across Life Stages* would not have been possible without the guidance, contributions, and support of so many people. We are grateful for the dedication and tremendous hard work of Elizabeth Peck, MS, RD, LD, our go-to for everything. We are fortunate to have Elizabeth's expertise in creating a robust instructor's package to accompany this edition.

To our mentor, advisor, and colleague, Paul Insel, we are deeply grateful to you for giving us the opportunity to work with you on numerous texts. Thank you for guiding us and encouraging us to pursue our passion.

We would like to thank our awesome team at Jones & Bartlett Learning for partnering with us on this undertaking. Sean, Taylor, Merideth, Alex, and Shannon: You guys are *the best*. Thank you for believing in us and supporting us. Your advice, guidance, and dedication make it a pleasure to be working with you all. To all our contributors who put their expertise into this manuscript, we thank every one of you. Thank you to our reviewers who contributed thoughtful feedback and knowledge to this edition.

Thank you to our colleagues for their guidance, support, and contributions to our academic growth. We also want to express our sincere thanks to our past, present, and future students from whom we continually learn.

Finally to our families, we are genuinely appreciative of all the love, support, encouragement, and patience you give us.

CONTRIBUTORS

Katarina Berry, MS, RD, LDN
Inpatient Clinical Dietitian II
Children's Hospital of Philadelphia
Philadelphia, PA
Chapter 10

Sukhada Bhatte-Paralkar, RD, CDE
Assistant Professor
Nirmala Niketan College of Home Science
University of Mumbai
Mumbai, India
Chapter 5

Julia Buckley, MS, RD
Clinical Dietitian
Valley Health System
Ridgewood, NJ
Chapter 5

Susan Casey, RDN, CD
Pediatric Pulmonary Dietitian
Division of Pulmonary and Sleep Medicine
Seattle Children's Hospital
Seattle, WA
Chapter 8

Rebecca Charlton, MPH, RDN
Director, Coordinated Program in Dietetics
Assistant Professor
Nutrition, Dietetics, and Food Sciences Department
Utah State University
Logan, UT
Chapter 4

Julie A. Cooper, MS, RD, LDN
Clinical Dietitian
Children's Hospital of Philadelphia
Philadelphia, PA
Chapter 10

Melissa Edwards, MS, RDN, CNSC
Clinical Pediatric Dietitian
Biochemical Genetics Program
Seattle Children's Hospital
Seattle, WA
Chapter 8

Rachel Fine, MS, RD, CSSD, CDN
Owner and Chief Executive Officer
To The Pointe Nutrition
New York City, NY
Chapter 11

Roschelle A. Heuberger, PhD, RD
Director of Graduate Programs in Nutrition and Dietetics
Professor of Nutrition and Dietetics
Department of Human Environmental Studies
Central Michigan University
Mt. Pleasant, MI
Chapter 15

Kathryn Hillstrom, EdD, MPH, RDN
Associate Professor
Coordinator, Graduate Program in Nutritional Science
School of Kinesiology and Nutritional Science
California State University, Los Angeles
Los Angeles, CA
Chapter 2

Kathryn L. Hunt, RDN, CD, CSO
Pediatric Oncology Dietitian
Cancer and Blood Disorders Center
Seattle Children's Hospital
Seattle, WA
Chapter 8

Stephanie Lakinger, MS, RD
Pediatric Dietitian
Children's Hospital Colorado
Denver, CO
Chapter 9

Camille L. Lanier, RDN, CD
Clinical Pediatric Dietitian
Craniofacial Center
Rehabilitation Medicine
Seattle Children's Hospital
Seattle, WA
Chapter 8

April Litchford, MS, RD
Instructor
Utah State University
Logan, UT
Chapter 6

Nancy Munoz, DCN, MHA, RDN, FAND
Lecturer
University of Massachusetts, Amherst
Amherst, MA
Assistant Chief, Nutrition and Food Service
Southern Nevada VA Healthcare System
Las Vegas, NV
Chapters 12 and 16

Regina Nagy-Steinert, RDN, CD
Pediatric Dietitian
Seattle Children's Hospital
Seattle, WA
Chapter 8

Shelly Ben Harush Negari, MD
Head of the Center for Adolescent Medicine
Wilf Children's Hospital
Shaare Zedek Medical Center
Hebrew University Medical School
Jerusalem, Israel
Chapter 11

Kim Nowak-Cooperman, MS, RDN, CD
Clinical Pediatric Dietitian
Growth and Feeding Dynamics Clinic
Seattle Children's Hospital
Seattle, WA
Chapter 8

Elizabeth Peck, MS, RD, LD
Renal Dietitian
DaVita
Arden Hills, MN
Chapter 12

Kimberly Powell, PhD, MS, RD
Assistant Professor
Department of Human Sciences
North Carolina Central University
Durham, NC
Chapter 7

Mateja R. Savoie Roskos, PhD, MPH, RD, CD, CNP
Professional Practice Assistant Professor
Nutrition, Dietetics and Food Sciences Department
Utah State University
Logan, UT
Chapter 3 and 5

Sushila Sharangdhar, RD
Consultant Dietitian
Wockhardt Hospitals
BFY Sports & Fitness
Mumbai, India
Chapter 5

Christina Stella, MS, RDN, CDN, CDE
Clinical Outpatient Adult and Pediatric Dietitian/
   Nutritionist
Certified Diabetes Educator

Memorial Sloan Kettering Cancer Center
New York City, NY
Chapter 9

Mary Verbovski, MS, RDN, CD, CSO
Pediatric Oncology Dietitian
Cancer and Blood Disorders Center
Seattle Children's Hospital
Seattle, WA
Chapter 8

Chris Wellington, RD, MS, BSc
Adjunct Professor of Medicine
Schulich School of Medicine and Dentistry
London, ON
Sessional Instructor
University of Windsor
Windsor, ON
Lecturer
Rosalind Franklin University of Medicine and Science
North Chicago, IL
Registered Dietitian
VON Nurse Practitioner-Led Clinic
Belle River, ON
Chapter 13

Nila Williamson, MPH, RDN, CNSC
Pediatric GI Dietitian
Seattle Children's Hospital
Seattle, WA
Chapter 8

Barb York, MS, RDN, CD
Pediatric Dietitian (Avoidant Restrictive Feeding
   Disorders—Autism)
Seattle Children's Pediatric Feeding Program at the
   Autism Center
Seattle Children's Hospital
Seattle, WA
Chapter 8

Sigalit Cohen Zabar, RD
Clinical Dietitian
Center for Adolescent Medicine
Wilf Children's Hospital
Shaare Zedek Medical Center
Hebrew University Medical School
Jerusalem, Israel
Chapter 11

REVIEWERS

Sandra Baker, EdD, RDN, LDN
Assistant Professor
Behavioral Health and Nutrition
College of Health Sciences
University of Delaware
Newark, DE

Janet Colson, PhD, RD
Professor
Department of Human Sciences
Middle Tennessee State University
Murfreesboro, TN

Lisa Hesse, MPH, RDN
Instructor
Food & Nutrition
Orange Coast College
Costa Mesa, CA

Samantha Hutson, MS, RDN, LDN
Lecturer
School of Human Ecology
Tennessee Technological University
Cookeville, TN

Teresa W. Johnson, DCN, RD
Professor
Department of Kinesiology and Health Promotion
Troy University
Troy, AL

Jean Maxwell, MS, RD
Adjunct Instructor
Food Science and Nutrition Program
Norfolk State University
Suffolk, VA

Keri Stoner-Davis, MS, RDN/LD
Visiting Assistant Clinical Professor
Nutrition and Food Sciences Department
Texas Woman's University
Denton, TX

Rachel Vollmer, PhD, RDN
Assistant Professor
Department of Family and Consumer Sciences
Illinois State University
Normal, IL

JoAnne Whelan, MS, RD
Adjunct Professor
School of Health and Rehabilitation Sciences
Indiana University—Purdue University Indianapolis
Indianapolis, IN

CHAPTER 1

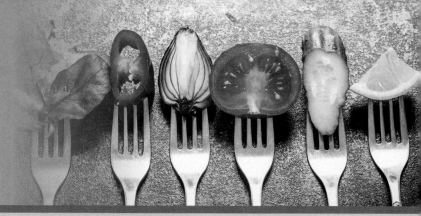

Nutrition Overview

Kimberley McMahon, MDA, RD

Chapter Outline

The Science of Nutrition

Micronutrients

Nutrition Assessment

The Dietary Guidelines for Americans 2015–2020

Physical Activity Guidelines

The Obesity Epidemic May Be Decreasing Life Expectancy

Learning Objectives

1. Describe four basic principles of healthy eating.

2. Describe how Dietary Reference Intakes are used to help determine needs of healthy individuals.

3. Describe each macronutrient, its function in the body, and food sources.

4. List primary functions and common food sources of major and trace minerals.

5. List the various functions of water in your body.

6. List and define what is considered the ABCDs of nutrition assessment.

7. List the five overarching guidelines and the key recommendations outlined in the *Dietary Guidelines for Americans 2015–2020*.

8. List the key guidelines included in the *Physical Activity Guidelines* for Americans.

9. Explain how the current obesity epidemic may be decreasing life expectancy in the United States.

Case Study

Consider your own lifestyle and nutrition choices. Do you make healthy food and activity choices most of the time? What components of your lifestyle could use some adjustments? What components of your lifestyle are you proud of because you know these are steps to being healthy? Through the chapter, you will have the opportunity to evaluate components of your lifestyle, which will help you to establish nutrition and activity goals.

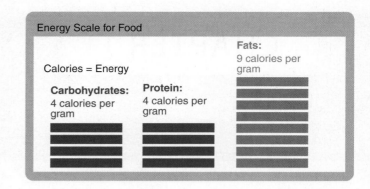

Energy Scale for Food

Calories = Energy

Carbohydrates:
4 calories per gram

Protein:
4 calories per gram

Fats:
9 calories per gram

The human body has varying nutrition requirements as it moves through different stages of life; however, regardless of which life stage an individual is in, the same fundamental concepts build the foundation for adequate nutrition. As we study nutrition needs and recommendations throughout life, we can keep in mind these basic principles, which are important for healthy eating regardless of age:

- An individual's poor nutrition status can result from either inadequate or excessive levels of nutrition intake, contributing to the possibility of poor nutrition influencing the development of certain chronic diseases.

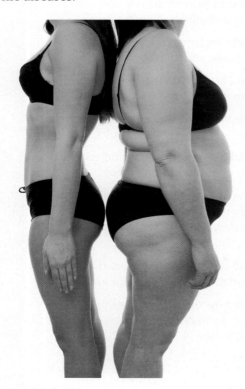

©Hartphotography/Shutterstock

- Energy produced by the body, which is needed for a variety of functions, is provided by food and drink in the form of carbohydrate, protein, and fats (macronutrients), with each macronutrient providing a specific amount of energy measured in calories.

- Energy needs vary from person to person and depend on such factors as basal metabolic rate (BMR) and level of activity.

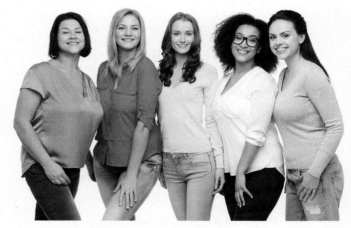

©Syda Productions/Shutterstock

- There are many components of healthy eating, with adequacy, balance, variety, and moderation in food choices being key characteristics.

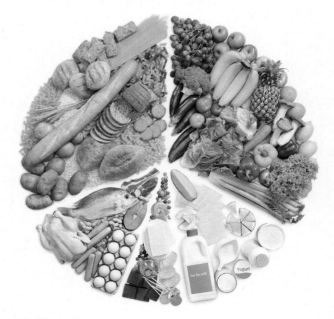

©Ifong/Shutterstock

From the time of conception to the time of death, to maintain life the body relies on nutrients provided by foods we eat and drink. Food provides information to the body, signaling basic biological functions and normalizing physiological processes.[1] During early life, growth, development, and maintenance of the body depend on a correct supply of all the necessary nutrients. Later in life, when growth and development are complete, the body depends on its food supply more for maintenance and repair. Additionally, food habits established during childhood and those that carry into adolescence and adulthood affect overall health and well-being throughout life. Food is considered a primary treatment for health promotion, risk reduction, and generally improved well-being. The absence or existence of chronic disease develops over time; therefore, what we eat today affects not only how we feel today but also our overall health.

Case Study

Think about how you eat. Do you usually select the same foods each day, or do you include a variety of foods and drinks? Challenge yourself to try one new protein and one new fruit or vegetable this week. Consider adding more variety to your overall diet.

The Science of Nutrition

Preview Human physical survival depends on an intake of nutrients provided by both food and water. These nutrients are varied and plentiful, offering both advantages and disadvantages to individual health and well-being. Optimal nutrition is obtained by giving ourselves the best possible intake of nutrients to aid the body in being as healthy and free of illness as possible. Human growth and health rely on not only nutrients and other dietary factors (such as phytochemicals, carotenoids, fiber, and lignans) but also the calories that food and drink provide.

Essential and Nonessential Nutrients

Nutrients are categorized as either essential or nonessential according to whether the body must obtain them through diet or can synthesize them. Essential nutrients are required for normal physiological function and cannot be synthesized by the body; therefore, they must be obtained from the diet. Essential nutrients include water; minerals; certain vitamins, amino acids, and fats; and carbohydrates. See **TABLE 1.1** . Nonessential nutrients are required by the body for supporting bodily processes;

Table 1.1

Essential Nutrients and Their Functions

Essential Nutrient	Function
Carbohydrates	Provide energy and are the main source of fuel needed for physical activity, brain function, and operation of the organs.
Protein • Essential amino acids include arginine, histidine, isoleucine, leucine, lysine, methionine, phenylalanine, threonine, tryptophan, valine	The major structural component of cells and responsible for the building and repair of body tissues. Proteins are broken down into amino acids. Nine of the 20 amino acids are essential.
Fat	An energy source; increases the absorption of fat-soluble vitamins; helps to maintain core body temperature.
Vitamins and Minerals	
• Vitamin A	• Helps to maintain healthy skin, teeth, skeletal and soft tissue, mucous membranes, and skin; promotes vision.
• B vitamins	• Energy production, immune function, and iron absorption.
• Vitamin C	• Strengthens blood vessels and gives skin its elasticity; antioxidant function and iron absorption.
• Vitamin D	• Bone health.
• Vitamin E	• Blood circulation and protection from free radicals.
• Vitamin K	• Blood coagulation.
• Folic acid	• Cell renewal and preventing birth defects during pregnancy.
• Calcium	• Promotes healthy teeth and bones.
• Iron	• Maintains healthy blood.
• Zinc	• Immunity, growth, and fertility.
• Chromium	• Helps glucose enter cells.
• Chloride	• Needed for proper fluid balance, and a component of stomach acid.
• Copper	• Part of many enzymes; needed for iron metabolism.
• Iodine	• Found in thyroid hormone, which helps regulate growth, development, and metabolism.
• Magnesium	• Found in bones; needed for making protein, muscle contraction, nerve transmission, immune system health.
• Manganese	• Part of many enzymes.
• Molybdenum	• Part of many enzymes.
• Phosphorus	• Important for healthy bones and teeth; found in every cell; part of the system that maintains acid–base balance.
• Potassium	• Needed for proper fluid balance, nerve transmission, and muscle contraction.
• Selenium	• Antioxidant.
• Sodium	• Needed for proper fluid balance, nerve transmission, and muscle contraction.
Water	Used to regulate body temperature and maintain other body functions.

however, the body can manufacture these nutrients (although some nutrients such as vitamin D can also come from food sources) and therefore they do not have to be obtained from foods that we eat. Examples of nonessential nutrients include vitamin D and the amino acids alanine, arginine, and glutamine. See (**TABLE 1.2**). Additionally, **phytochemicals**, which are substances found in plants, are not considered essential, yet they play important roles in maintaining health and well-being.

Table 1.2

Nonessential Amino Acids

• Alanine	• Glutamic acid	• Proline
• Arginine	• Glutamine	• Selenocysteine
• Asparagine	• Glycone	• Serine
• Aspartic acid	• Histidine	• Taurine
• L-cysteine	• Ornithine	• Tyrosine

News You Can Use

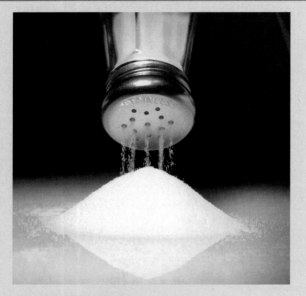

©Element Photo/StockFood/age fotostock

Sodium is necessary for proper fluid balance, nerve transmission, and muscle contraction. In general, Americans should limit their intake of sodium to no more than 2,300 mg per day. The current American lifestyle makes it difficult *not* to consume too much sodium. The average intake for Americans is 3,400 mg per day, and it's not just adults who are eating too much sodium; children and teens consume more than is recommended. Limit sodium intake by eating less fast food; do not add salt while cooking or to food after it has been prepared; be aware of the amount of sodium in canned foods, restaurant foods, and drinks.

Dietary Reference Intakes

Estimated needs of all nutrients are not the same for every individual. **Dietary Reference Intakes (DRIs)** are developed and published by the Institute of Medicine and represent the most current scientific knowledge on nutrient needs of healthy individuals. These suggested nutrient intake values are intended to serve as a guide for good nutrition and are specific based on age, gender, and life stage. DRIs cover more than 40 nutrient substances and include the following specific recommendations: **Recommended Dietary Allowance (RDA)**, **Adequate Intake (AI)**, **Estimated Average Requirement (EAR)**, and **Tolerable Upper Intake Level (UL)**.[2] (See **FIGURE 1.1**.)

- *Recommended Dietary Allowance (RDA):* Average daily intake level that is sufficient to meet the nutrient requirements of nearly all (97–98%) healthy individuals in a group.
- *Adequate Intake (AI):* A value based on observed or experimentally determined approximations of nutrient intake by a group of healthy people and used when an RDA cannot be determined.
- *Estimated Average Requirements (EARs):* Nutrient intake values that are estimated to meet the requirements of half of the healthy individuals in a group.
- *Tolerable Upper Intake Level (UL):* The highest level of daily nutrient intake that is likely to pose no risk of adverse side effects to almost all individuals in the general population. As intake increases above the UL, the risk of adverse effects increases.

All values given for the DRIs represent the quantity of the nutrient or food component supplied from a diet similar to those consumed in Canada and the United States, and the values apply to a healthy population. Reference intakes are expressed for different life stage groups, and reference weights and heights are used.

Macronutrients Provide Calories (Energy)

A **calorie**, defined as the energy needed to raise the temperature of 1 g of water 1°C, is the unit used to measure the potential energy in food as it is transferred from its source to the body. The macronutrients carbohydrate, protein, and fat all contribute to the calorie content of food.

Carbohydrates

Carbohydrates are organic compounds that occur in food. These compounds contain carbon, oxygen, and hydrogen and can be broken down to release energy in the body. (See **FIGURE 1.2**.)

Carbohydrates are the body's preferred source of energy, providing energy to the brain, muscles, and nervous system. In addition, carbohydrates facilitate the

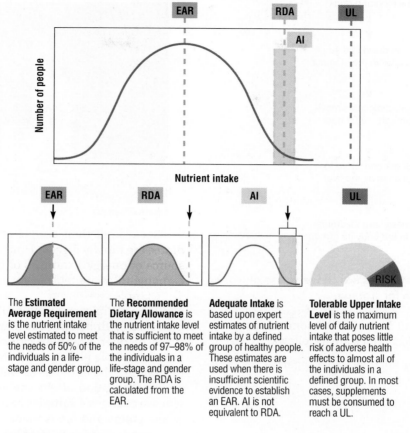

All DRI values refer to intakes averaged over time
EAR
RDA
UL
AI
Number of people
Nutrient intake
EAR
RDA
AI
UL
RISK
The **Estimated Average Requirement** is the nutrient intake level estimated to meet the needs of 50% of the individuals in a life-stage and gender group.
The **Recommended Dietary Allowance** is the nutrient intake level that is sufficient to meet the needs of 97–98% of the individuals in a life-stage and gender group. The RDA is calculated from the EAR.
Adequate Intake is based upon expert estimates of nutrient intake by a defined group of healthy people. These estimates are used when there is insufficient scientific evidence to establish an EAR. AI is not equivalent to RDA.
Tolerable Upper Intake Level is the maximum level of daily nutrient intake that poses little risk of adverse health effects to almost all of the individuals in a defined group. In most cases, supplements must be consumed to reach a UL.

Figure 1.1
Dietary Reference Intakes and average requirements.

metabolism of fat and, when in sufficient supply, ensure that the protein in your muscles is not broken down as an energy source. Carbohydrates consumed from food and drinks are broken down into small sugar molecules in the mouth and the small intestine, which then move through the digestive tract and are converted into glucose by the liver to make a usable form of energy for the brain and muscles. Excess carbohydrates are stored by the body in the form of glycogen. The liver and the muscles are storage sites for glycogen. (See FIGURE 1.3.)

The structure of a carbohydrate determines whether it is a simple or complex carbohydrate. **Simple carbohydrates** are monosaccharides (one simple sugar molecule) and disaccharides (two simple sugar molecules linked together). The most common monosaccharides are glucose, fructose, and galactose. The most common disaccharides

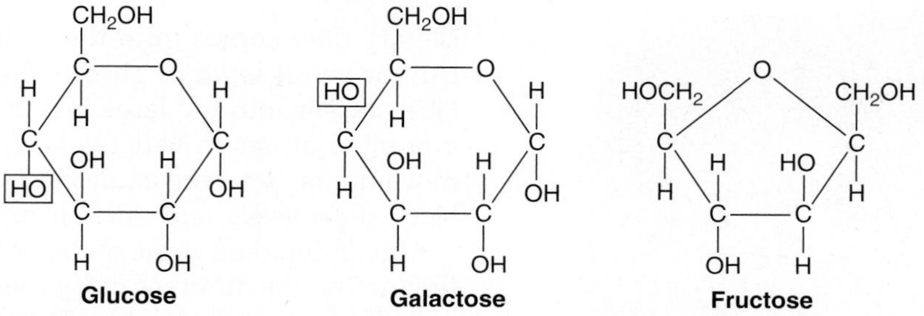

Glucose
Galactose
Fructose

The structures of glucose and galactose differ only by the location of the OH on carbon number 4.

Figure 1.2
Chemical structure of the carbohydrates glucose, fructose, and galactose.

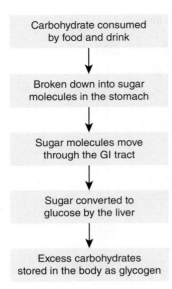

Figure 1.3
Process by which carbohydrates are converted to glucose for energy or to glycogen for storage.

are sucrose, maltose, and lactose. The monosaccharides that make up these disaccharides are as follows:

- Glucose + Fructose = Sucrose (table sugar) →

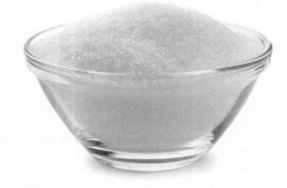

©Coprid/Shutterstock

- Glucose + Glucose = Maltose (malt sugar) →

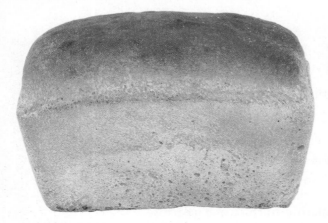

©Donikz/Shutterstock

- Glucose + Galactose = Lactose (milk sugar) →

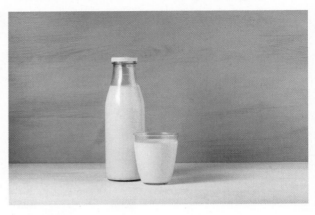

©Iprachenko/Shutterstock

Because of their simple structure, simple carbohydrates are rapidly digested and are therefore the quickest source of energy. Examples of foods that contain simple carbohydrates are table sugar, corn syrup, and honey.

Complex carbohydrates are called polysaccharides and are multiple sugar molecules linked together. Complex carbohydrates include starches, glycogen, and most types of fiber. Complex carbohydrates are commonly found in whole plant foods, which are also good sources of vitamins and minerals as well as fiber, which slows the body's absorption of glucose and limits dramatic blood glucose changes. Examples of complex carbohydrates are whole grains and foods made from them, such as pasta and bread; starchy vegetables, such as potatoes, sweet potatoes, and corn; and beans, lentils, and peas.

Overall, carbohydrates are present in a variety of foods such as fruits, vegetables, grains, legumes (beans, peas, lentils), milk and milk products, and foods containing added sugar in the form of starch, sugar, or fiber. With the exception of fiber, each gram of carbohydrate provides 4 calories. Although in general fiber is *not* broken down in the digestive tract, some types of fiber can be broken down in the gut and do release energy; however, energy production is minimal and we do not view energy production as a main function of fiber.

Dietary Fiber

Dietary fiber comes from the edible parts of plants and cannot be digested or absorbed in the small intestine. Fiber passes into the large intestine intact, contributing a number of health benefits such as normalizing bowel movements, lowering cholesterol levels, helping control blood sugar levels, and aiding in achieving healthy weight.

To understand some of the benefits of fiber, we must first define the different categories of fiber: **soluble fiber** and **insoluble fiber**. Soluble fiber attracts water and turns to a gel during digestion. This characteristic helps a person feel full longer, and possibly slows the digestion and absorption of carbohydrates, which prevents spikes in blood glucose following a meal. Food sources of soluble fiber include oat bran, barley, nuts, seeds, beans, peas,

The Big Picture

A fiber-rich meal adds bulk and volume to stomach contents, slowing the digestion of food and the absorption of nutrients, delaying the rise in blood glucose that occurs after a meal. In a low-fiber meal, nutrients are concentrated, causing digestion and absorption to occur more rapidly and thus a sharper rise in blood glucose.

Fiber-rich meal

Low-fiber meal

Blood glucose change over time

— Fiber-rich meal
— Low-fiber meal

Blood glucose / Time after eating

and some fruits and vegetables. Soluble fiber is associated with lowering the risk of heart disease.

Insoluble fiber adds bulk to stool and appears to help food pass through the stomach and intestines, serving to prevent constipation by increasing stool weight and decreasing gut transit time, which in turn can reduce the risk of diseases and disorders such as diverticular disease and hemorrhoids. Insoluble fiber is found in foods such as wheat bran, vegetables, and whole grains. Fiber is also associated with possible prevention of coronary heart disease by improving the blood lipid profile.[3]

The Institute of Medicine sets the DRI for carbohydrates as 45% to 65% of daily calories. The RDA for fiber is 38 g per day for adult men and 25 g per day for adult women up to age 50 years. The RDA for fiber in men older than age 50 years is 30 g per day, and for women older than age 50 years, the RDA for fiber is 21 g per day.

Protein

A **protein** is any group of organic molecules that contain carbon, hydrogen, oxygen, and nitrogen and one or more chains of amino acids. Protein is in every cell in the body and functions to build, repair, and maintain bones, muscles, and skin. For example, proteins make up collagen for supportive tissue, hemoglobin for transport, antibodies for immune defense, and enzymes for metabolism.

Proteins are made of individual amino acids linked together by peptide bonds. Amino acids consist of a central carbon atom connected to an amino group, a carboxyl group, a hydrogen atom, and a variable component called a side chain. Proteins are built from a set of 20 amino acids, each of which has a unique side chain. See **FIGURE 1.4**.

Proteins provide 4 calories per gram, and food sources include meat, fish, eggs, milk, and legumes. It is important to eat protein every day because your body does not store protein the same way that it stores carbohydrates. The protein we eat is broken into individual amino acids used to build body proteins, is reconfigured into glucose to be used as energy, or is reconfigured into fat and is stored. The DRI for protein is 0.8 g per kilogram of body weight, or 0.36 g per pound of body weight. A typical American diet provides enough protein each day.

Fat

Fat is a macronutrient that not only provides energy but also helps your body absorb the fat-soluble vitamins (vitamins A, D, E, and K), keeps your skin and hair healthy, and offers the sensation of satiety after eating it. Fat also is a source of two essential (cannot be manufactured by the body) fatty acids: linoleic acid and alpha-linolenic acid. The body needs these fatty acids for brain development, inflammation control, and blood clotting.

Linoleic Acid

Linoleic acid is an essential, polyunsaturated, omega-6 fatty acid that is necessary for healthy brain function, skin and hair growth, bone density, energy production, and reproductive health. Your body can convert linoleic acid into two forms: arachidonic acid and gamma linolenic acid, or GLA. Arachidonic acid is an omega-6 fatty acid that supports brain and muscle function and promotes and resolves inflammation.[4] GLA has been found to be an anti-inflammatory agent as well and may benefit conditions such as diabetic neuropathy, rheumatoid arthritis, allergies, and menopausal disorders.[5] Food sources of linoleic acid include safflower and sunflower seeds, soybean oil, corn oil, pine nuts, and pecans.

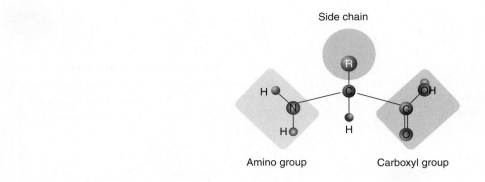

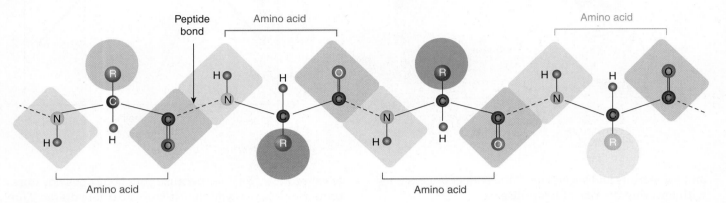

Figure 1.4
Protein configuration.

Alpha-Linolenic Acid

Alpha-linolenic acid is an essential, polyunsaturated, omega-3 fatty acid essential to the body for formation of prostaglandins. Alpha-linolenic acid is a precursor to the omega-3 fatty acids eicosapentaenoic acid (EPA) and docosahexaenoic acid (DHA), both of which are found in fish oil and are known to be important during fetal development.[6] EPA and DHA have also been shown to reduce inflammation and may help prevent chronic diseases such as heart disease and arthritis.[7] The body can convert small amounts of EPA and DHA from alpha-linolenic acid. Food sources of alpha-linolenic acid include flaxseed oil, canola oil, soy oil, walnut oil, and the eggs from chickens fed arachidonic acid. Food sources of EPA and DHA include fish and specialty egg and dairy products. The body stores small amounts of DHA and EPA.

Classification of Fats

Whether a fatty acid has single or double bonds between the carbon atoms determines its classification as either **saturated** or **unsaturated**. If the carbon atoms in the fatty acid are linked by single bonds, the fat is classified as saturated. Unsaturated fatty acids have one or more double bonds between the carbon atoms. (See **FIGURE 1.5**.) Unsaturated fatty acids are further classified by the number of double bonds that exist between the carbon atoms. Fatty acids with one double bond are referred to as monounsaturated fats, whereas fatty acids with more than one double bond between carbon atoms are considered polyunsaturated.

Figure 1.5
Saturated and unsaturated fatty acids.

Most foods contain both saturated and unsaturated fats; however, we generally identify them according to the type of the largest amount of fat in them. Animal products tend to contain more saturated fats than unsaturated fats, and plant foods tend to include more unsaturated fats than saturated fats. Saturated fats are associated with raising low-density lipoprotein (LDL) cholesterol, putting a person at risk for heart attack, stroke, and other major health problems. Food sources of saturated fats include those made from animal products such as butter, cheese, whole milk, ice cream, cream, and fatty meats, and some vegetable oils (those that are solid at room temperature). Unsaturated fats can help lower LDL cholesterol. Food sources of unsaturated fats include olive, canola, safflower, sunflower, corn, and soy oils.

A type of unsaturated fat that is created by adding hydrogen to the double bonds between carbon atoms is called a **trans fat**. This process, which converts liquid oils

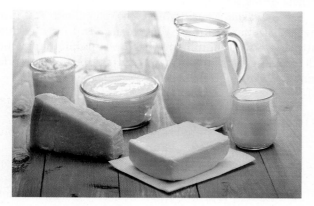

Sources of saturated fats.
©Silberkorn/Shutterstock

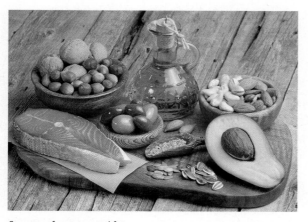

Sources of unsaturated fats.
©Craevschii Family/Shutterstock

into solids, is referred to as hydrogenation, and it creates products such as the oils foods are fried in, and margarine. Trans fats are used in commercial products because they tend to keep some food fresh for a longer period of time. When consumed, trans fats are associated with increasing LDL cholesterol and lowering high-density lipoprotein (HDL) cholesterol levels.

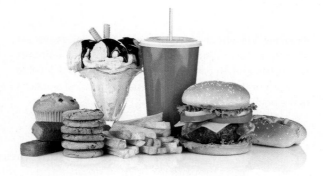

Foods high in trans fat.
©Fcafotodigital/iStock /Getty

Omega-6 and Omega-3 Fatty Acids

Omega-3 fatty acids and **omega-6 fatty acids** are two polyunsaturated fatty acids, both required for the body to function. Each of these fatty acid types has been shown to play a critical role in brain function and normal growth and development. These two fatty acids may have opposite effects when it comes to the inflammatory response and cardiovascular health.

Omega-3 fatty acids (also called n-3 fatty acids) have been shown to decrease the production of inflammatory mediators, having a positive effect in obesity and type 2 diabetes mellitus, whereas there is controversy about whether omega-6 fatty acids have a pro- or anti-inflammatory effect.[8] Omega-3 fatty acids are thought to provide a wide range of health benefits, including lowering the risk of coronary heart disease and improving cholesterol profiles. In addition, omega-3 fatty acids have been associated with improvements in cancer risk, depression treatment and prevention, and attention-deficit hyperactivity disorder (ADHD) treatment, with some of these mentioned health benefits resulting in part from positive changes in gut bacteria brought about by the intake of omega-3 fatty acids.[9]

Omega-6 fatty acids (also called n-6 fatty acids) are believed to play an important role in cell growth, production of hormone-like messengers, and transmission of nerve impulses. Other benefits of omega-6 fatty acid intake include stimulation of skin and hair growth, maintenance of bone health, regulation of metabolism, and maintenance of the reproductive system.

At the onset of the industrial revolution (about 250 years ago), there was a marked shift in the ratio of n-6 to n-3 fatty acids in the typical diet. Consumption of n-6 fats increased at the expense of n-3 fats. This change resulted from both the development of the modern vegetable oil industry and the increased use of cereal grains to feed domestic livestock. Prior to these shifts, the ratio of n-6 to n-3 fatty acids was 1:1, whereas studies now

Fatty Acids in Different Foods

Oil	Omega-6 Content	Omega-3 Content	n-6 to n-3 Ratio
Safflower	75%	25%	3:1
Sunflower	65%	35%	1.9:1
Corn	54%	46%	1.2:1
Walnut	52%	48%	1.1:1
Soybean	51%	49%	1:1
Cottonseed	50%	50%	1:1
Sesame	42%	58%	0.7:1
Peanut	32%	68%	0.5:1
Canola	20%	80%	0.25:1
Flaxseed	14%	86%	0.2:1
Olive	10%	< 1%	10:1

United States Department of Agriculture. Where can I find how much omega-3 and omega-6 fatty acids are in different foods? https://fnic.nal.usda.gov/where-can-i-find-how-much-omega-3-and-omega-6-fatty-acids-are-different-foods

indicate a ratio ranging from 20:1 or higher among U.S. diets.[10] A balance of omega-6 to omega-3 fats in the diet has been shown to be of benefit in the prevention and management of obesity, and most experts agree that the omega-6:omega-3 ratio should range from 1:1 to 5:1.[10] The following chart lists the omega-6 and omega-3 fatty acid profiles of common cooking and seasoning oils.

Cholesterol

Cholesterol is a waxy, fat-like substance found in every cell of the body. Your body needs cholesterol to produce the hormones estrogen and testosterone. Cholesterol is also a precursor of vitamin D. Our bodies produce cholesterol and we obtain cholesterol through various foods that we eat. Sources of cholesterol include eggs, fish, butter, bacon, red meat, cheese, and milk and other dairy products.

Cholesterol travels through the bloodstream packaged in carriers called lipoproteins. There are two kinds of lipoproteins: low-density lipoproteins (LDLs) and high-density lipoproteins (HDLs). LDLs are often referred to as "bad" cholesterol because high LDL levels lead to a buildup of cholesterol in arteries. HDLs are often referred to as "good" cholesterol because these lipoproteins carry cholesterol from other parts of the body to the liver, where it can then be removed.

Having high levels of blood cholesterol is associated with a greater chance of developing coronary heart disease, which results from plaque buildup inside the coronary arteries. Over time, plaque hardens and narrows the coronary arteries, limiting the flow of blood to the heart, which can lead to a heart attack. (See **FIGURE 1.6** .) Although genetics play a role in blood cholesterol levels, for healthy cardiac function, it is advised you limit dietary cholesterol intake.

Dietary fat, regardless of its type, provides 9 calories per gram. The DRI for fat is 20–35% of overall calories (for adults) and 25–40% of overall calorie intake for children. Most experts agree that the omega-6:omega-3 ratio should range from 1:1 to 5:1. The current daily value for cholesterol is 300 mg/day.

Your Guide to Lowering Your Cholesterol with TLC from the U.S. Department of Health and Human Services (https://www.nhlbi.nih.gov/files/docs/public/heart/chol_tlc.pdf) suggests the following nutrition recommendations for lowering serum cholesterol levels:

1. Decrease consumption of saturated fat, trans fat, and cholesterol.
2. Add plant stanols and sterols and increase soluble fiber in your diet.
3. Try to get at least 30 minutes of moderate-intensity exercise most days of the week.
4. If you are overweight, lose the extra weight to help reduce the risks associated with high cholesterol.

> **Recap** Knowing the basic principles of healthy eating can help guide you to healthy nutrition choices. Our diets are made up of a combination of essential and nonessential nutrients, each with a recommended intake level for optimal nutrition. The macronutrients carbohydrate, protein, and fat provide our bodies with calories and essential nutrients. Carbohydrates are the body's preferred source of energy, providing energy to the brain, muscles, and nervous system. Protein exists in every cell of the body and functions to build, repair, and maintain bones, muscles, and skin. Fat provides calories, helps our bodies absorb fat-soluble vitamins, and keeps our skin and hair healthy.
>
> 1. List the nutrients that contribute to the calorie content of food.
> 2. Identify benefits of eating a high-fiber diet.
> 3. Describe two differences between saturated and unsaturated fatty acids.
> 4. Describe the role of LDL and HDL cholesterol in heart disease.

Micronutrients

> **Preview** We obtain micronutrients from foods we eat and drink. Micronutrients are required in small amounts for normal growth and development; they do not provide energy, but they are required to enable chemical reactions in the body.

Micronutrients are chemical elements or substances required in small amounts for normal growth and development of all living organisms. These include vitamins and minerals. Compared with macronutrients, the body

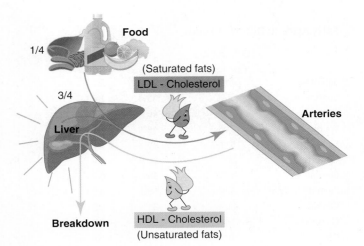

Figure 1.6
The role of LDL and HDL cholesterol in moving fat between the liver and the arteries.

needs only small amounts of the micronutrients; however, both types of nutrients are required. Unlike the macronutrients carbohydrates, protein, and fat, micronutrients do not function to provide energy, but they are required to enable the many chemical reactions that occur throughout the body, including the process of producing energy.

Vitamins

Vitamins are a group of organic substances that are essential for proper functioning of the body. Vitamins are found in food but can also be obtained through vitamin supplements. There are 13 nutrients classified as vitamins. These are further categorized based on their solubility: 4 are fat soluble and 9 are water soluble. (See **TABLE 1.3** .) All of these nutrients are essential to maintain healthy homeostasis and metabolic function.

The fat-soluble vitamins are vitamins A, D, E, and K. Because these are soluble in fat, they are absorbed in fat globules (called chylomicrons) that travel through the lymphatic system of the small intestines and into the general blood circulation of the body. Fat-soluble vitamins can be stored in body fat tissue and in the liver, with stores lasting for months to years.

The water-soluble vitamins are the B-complex vitamins and vitamin C. With few exceptions, they are not stored in the body and, if intake is inadequate over time, the availability of these nutrients can run out within a few weeks to a few months. Water-soluble vitamins are eliminated in the urine and tend to be excreted from the body more quickly than fat-soluble vitamins.

Initially thought to be just one vitamin, the eight vitamins that make up the B complex have different characteristics. The B-complex vitamins are thiamine, riboflavin, niacin, pantothenic acid, pyridoxine, biotin, folate, and cobalamin. The B-complex vitamins are necessary for the body to produce energy because they convert potential energy from the nutrients that we eat into adenosine triphosphate (ATP), which is the energy carrier in the cells of all known organisms. Our bodies produce energy through the production of ATP.

Water-soluble vitamins are generally not stored in the body, and the body adjusts absorption based on needs. However, caution still needs to be exercised because toxicity is possible. Consuming too little or too much of some vitamins can cause a nutritional disorder.

Vit A and D are needed for normal growth and development

Vit A, B$_6$, C, D, and folate are needed for healthy immune function, and help protect from infection

Folate, vitamins B$_6$ and B$_{12}$ are essential for protein and amino acid metabolism

Vit C and E are antioxidants that help to protect from molecules that cause oxidative damage

Vit A, D, K and C are needed for bone health

Vitamins are needed to produce energy from carbohydrates, protein, and fat

Benefits of vitamins

Table 1.3

Vitamins Based on Solubility

Water-Soluble Vitamins	Fat-Soluble Vitamins
B-complex vitamins	Vitamin A (retinol, beta-carotene)
• Thiamin (B$_1$)	Vitamin D (1, 25 dihydroxy-cholecalciferol)
• Riboflavin (B$_2$)	
• Niacin (B$_3$)	Vitamin E (alpha-tocopherol)
• Vitamin B$_6$	Vitamin K
• Folate	
• Vitamin B$_{12}$	
• Biotin	
• Pantothenic acid	
• Choline	
Vitamin C	

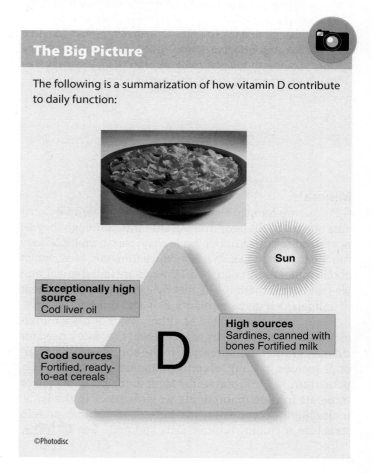

The Big Picture

The following is a summarization of how vitamin D contribute to daily function:

Sun

Exceptionally high source
Cod liver oil

High sources
Sardines, canned with bones Fortified milk

D

Good sources
Fortified, ready-to-eat cereals

©Photodisc

News You Can Use

For decades the message that direct sun exposure is bad for you has been heard loud and clear. The American Academy of Dermatology recommends we never expose bare skin to the sun without sunscreen, and the U.S. Food and Drug Administration calls ultraviolet radiation a carcinogen. This message has been heard so well that it has created paranoia about sunlight, especially among parents who religiously apply sun protection to their children.

Although it is certainly a good idea to avoid the things that research tells us will increase our risk of skin cancer, the sun is also a very reliable way to get vitamin D, especially for those individuals who avoid cow's milk, eggs, tuna fish, salmon, fortified cereal, pork, and mushrooms and who are diligent about using sunscreen. These individuals should use caution in regard to sun exposure in consideration of their vitamin D status.

How much sun exposure is enough? If you're fair skinned, experts say going outside for 10 minutes in the midday sun wearing shorts and a tank top with no sunscreen will give you enough radiation to produce about 10,000 international units (IU) of vitamin D. The RDA for vitamin D is 400 IU for ages birth to 12 months, 600 IU for ages 1 year to 70 years, and 800 IU for those older than 70 years.

The message that direct sun exposure of the skin can increase the risk of cancer is relevant; however, like many topics in nutrition, a little goes a long way. Be cautious about your time in the sun, but also be realistic. After all, deficiencies of vitamin D can be detrimental, and the sunshine vitamin may protect against a host of diseases, including osteoporosis, heart disease, and some forms of cancer. In addition, some exposure to sunlight has benefits such as protecting against depression, insomnia, and an overactive immune system.

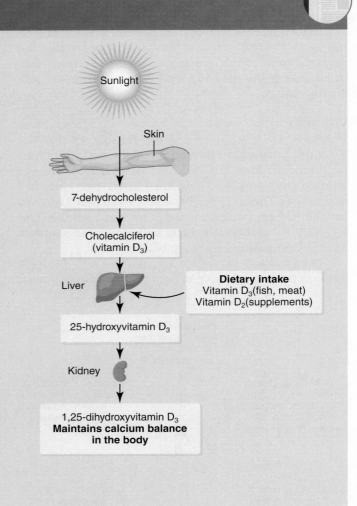

Minerals

Minerals are inorganic substances that are essential nutrients needed by the body in small amounts. Although they do not provide calories, minerals play key roles in multiple body functions. Our bodies do not produce minerals, so we must obtain minerals through food. Minerals are found in soil, and we can obtain them in the diet by eating plants, the meat of animals that graze on plants, fish, and drinking water.

Minerals are classified as either major or trace minerals. This designation does not represent the body's need for them but rather their presence in the body. The major minerals include calcium, chloride, magnesium, phosphorus, potassium, sodium, and sulfur. Main functions of the major minerals include maintaining water balance in the body; maintaining bone health; and helping to stabilize protein structure, including for hair, skin, and nails. See **TABLE 1.4**.

The trace minerals include chromium, copper, fluoride, iodine, iron, manganese, molybdenum, selenium, and zinc. With the exception of chromium, which helps the body keep blood sugar levels normal, trace minerals are incorporated into enzymes or hormones required for metabolism and therefore serve a variety of functions within the body. See **TABLE 1.5**.

Although not as prevalent in the United States, deficiencies in trace minerals are a major global health problem that can impair growth and mental development and can lead to illness or even death. People who consume a balanced diet containing a variety of foods are unlikely to develop either a mineral toxicity or deficiency; however, people who follow strict diets that eliminate certain food groups or overemphasize others can be at risk for nutrition disorders.

Table 1.4

Major Minerals: Functions and Common Food Sources

Nutrient	Primary Function in the Body	Common Food Sources
Calcium	Provides rigidity to bone; 99% of calcium in the body is found in bone and teeth.	Milk, yogurt, fortified orange juice, canned salmon, fortified cereals
Chloride	Travels primarily with sodium and water and helps generate the osmotic pressure of body fluids. Is an essential part of the stomach acid (HCl) that aids in digestion.	A component of table salt or sea salt as sodium chloride, many vegetables, and salt substitutes
Magnesium	Promotes resistance to tooth decay by holding calcium in tooth enamel; stored in bone; component in forming blood clots; necessary for enzyme reactions.	Dark green leafy vegetables, peanut butter, beans and peas, bananas, almonds
Phosphorus	Component of hydroxyapatite crystals in bone.	Yogurt, almonds, milk, cheese, salmon, meat, eggs
Potassium	Maintains alkaline blood pH, which prevents withdrawal of bone minerals.	Spinach, squash, bananas, orange juice, milk, meat, legumes, whole grains
Sodium	Regulates body fluid balance, maintains acid–base balance, aids muscle contractions and nerve impulse transmission.	Table salt
Sulfur	A component of four different amino acids, performs functions in enzyme reactions and protein synthesis.	Meat, fish, poultry, eggs, milk, legumes

Table 1.5

Minor Minerals: Functions and Common Food Sources

Nutrient	Primary Function in the Body	Common Food Sources
Chromium	Important in the metabolism of fats and carbohydrates; stimulates fatty acid and cholesterol synthesis; important in the breakdown of insulin.	Beef, liver, eggs, chicken, oysters, wheat germ, green peppers, apples, bananas, spinach
Copper	Contributes to collagen synthesis.	Liver, cocoa, beans, nuts, whole grains, dried fruit
Fluoride	Strengthens bones and teeth; stimulates osteoblasts.	Seafood, tea, fluoridated water
Iodine	A component of hormones produced by the thyroid gland that are responsible for a number of functions in the body, including growth, metabolism, reproduction, nerve and muscle function, regulation of body temperature, and blood cell production.	Iodized table salt, seafood, dairy products, plants grown in iodine-rich soil
Iron	Cofactor in vitamin D activation; contributes to collagen synthesis.	Meat, seafood, broccoli, peas, bran, enriched bread
Manganese	Cofactor for bone-remodeling enzymes.	Nuts, oats, beans, tea
Molybdenum	A cofactor for four enzymes and necessary for the metabolism of sulfur-containing amino acids.	Legumes, grain products, and nuts
Selenium	A component of the amino acid found in at least 25 different proteins.	Organ meats and seafood
Zinc	Needed for catalytic, structural, and regulatory functions in the body.	Oysters, beef, crab, pork

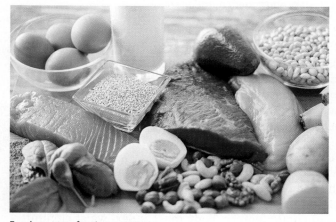

Food sources of various nutrients.
©Syda Productions/Shutterstock

Water

Water makes up more than two-thirds of the weight of the human body, and without it human survival is not possible. All cells, organs, and tissues in the body need water to help regulate temperature and to maintain other body functions. Our bodies are constantly losing water through the processes of respiration, perspiration, and digestion; therefore, keeping the body hydrated through adequate fluid intake is important.

Water serves vital functions in the body, including the following (FIGURE 1.7):

1. Water distributes essential nutrients to cells throughout the body and helps deliver oxygen throughout the body.

What Does Water Do for You?

Forms saliva (digestion)

Needed by the brain to manufacture hormones and neurotransmitters

Keeps mucosal membranes moist

Regulates body temperature (sweating and respiration)

Allows body's cells to grow, reproduce, and survive

Acts as a shock absorber for brain and spinal cord

Flushes body waste, mainly in urine

Converts food to components needed for survival - digestion

Lubricates joints

Water is the major component of most body parts

Helps deliver oxygen all over the body

Figure 1.7
Various functions of water.

2. Water helps to remove waste products, including toxins, through urine and feces.
3. Water is a component of nutrient breakdown and nutrient metabolism, including formation of saliva. For example, water allows the chemical reactions to occur that result in protein and carbohydrates being absorbable and usable by the body.
4. Water helps to regulate body temperature through the process of perspiration. When water evaporates from the skin surface, body temperature is lowered.
5. Water lubricates joints and acts as a shock absorber for the eyes, brain, spinal cord, and in the form of amniotic fluid.
6. Water keeps mucosal membranes moist.

Water is the major component of most body parts.

Intake of water comes from foods we eat and fluids we drink. In addition, the body produces water during the process of metabolism. If water intake is not adequate, body fluids can become out of balance, causing dehydration. The DRI for water is between 91 and 125 fluid ounces (2.7 to 3.5 L) of water per day for adults. However, individual needs depend on weight, age, and activity level. **TABLE 1.6** gives examples of how to calculate fluid needs.

Table 1.6

Various Methods for Calculating Fluid Needs

Method	Calculation
1	Weight (kg) × 30 mL = milliliters of fluid required daily
2	1 mL/kcal of intake = milliliters of fluid required daily
3	(kg body weight – 20) × 15 + 1,500 = milliliters of fluid required daily

Recap Adequate vitamin, mineral, and water intake is essential for life. Our body can produce some of the vitamins it needs; others must come from the diet. Minerals are elements that originate in the earth and cannot be made by human bodies. Plants obtain minerals from the soil, providing us with dietary sources of minerals when we consume the plants directly or indirectly through animal sources that have fed on mineral-rich food sources. Minerals may also be present in the water we drink. Water makes up more than two-thirds of the weight of the human body, and without it human survival is not possible.

1. Describe the difference between how fat-soluble and water-soluble vitamins are stored in the body.
2. List three vital functions of water in the body.
3. Identify the daily requirements for water intake.

Nutrition Assessment

Preview Nutrition assessment is a comprehensive evaluation in which the clinician observes, interprets, analyzes, and infers data in an effort to appraise an individual's nutrition history and current nutrition status.

There are multiple indicators of nutrition health and, therefore, measures of nutrition status should include a number of factors. Typically, these factors are anthropometric measures, biochemical tests, clinical observations, and dietary intake—generally referred to as the ABCDs of nutrition assessment. See **TABLE 1.7**.

Anthropometric Measures

Anthropometric measures are physical measurements of the body. For nutrition assessment purposes, anthropometric measurements generally include height, weight, head circumference, body mass index, waist circumference, and percent body fat. These measurements can be compared with standard values or they can be used to

Table 1.7

The ABCDs of Nutrition Assessment

Assessment Method	What It Measures
Anthropometric measures	Measure growth and show changes in weight, height, and percent body fat over time.
Biochemical tests	Measure blood, urine, and feces for nutrients or metabolites that indicate infection or disease.
Clinical observations	Assess changes in skin color and health, hair.
Dietary intake	Tracks an individual's food intake over time.

assess weight loss or gain in an individual over time. To be effective, anthropometric measurement procedures should follow measurement standards with regard to technique and equipment.

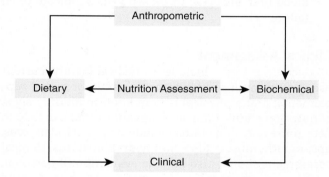

Height, Weight, and Head Circumference

Techniques for measuring height and weight should follow age standards, because infants and children are measured differently than adults. Weight in a nutrition assessment represents various factors because it can be used to assess growth, predict energy expenditure and protein needs, and determine body mass index.

For infants and children, another anthropometric measurement, head circumference, is used in the nutrition assessment. Head circumference is a useful measure of normal growth and development, especially from birth to age 3 years when growth is rapid.

Body Mass Index

Body mass index (BMI) is a number calculated from a person's weight and height, with the result providing a reliable indicator of body fatness. Additionally, this number provides a good gauge of risk for various diseases associated with increased body fat. The higher the BMI, the higher the individual's risk for certain diseases such as heart disease, high blood pressure, type 2 diabetes, gallstones, breathing problems, and certain forms of cancer.[11]

BMI can be used for both males and females; however, this measurement has two known limitations: (1) it may overestimate body fat in athletes and others who have a

Table 1.8

BMI Classifications

Class	BMI
Underweight	Below 18.5
Normal weight	18.5–24.9
Overweight	25.0–29.9
Obesity	30.0 and above

muscular build; and (2) it may underestimate body fat in older persons and others who have lost muscle.[12] Calculating BMI allows comparison of an individual to population standards. The formula for calculating BMI is: BMI = (Weight in kilograms) / (Height in meters)^2. See **TABLE 1.8** for BMI weight classifications.

Waist Circumference

Waist circumference measurements tend to be a good indicator of abdominal fat and therefore a predictor of chronic disease in adults. A high waist circumference is associated with an increased risk for type 2 diabetes, dyslipidemia, hypertension, and cardiovascular disease in patients with a BMI in the range between 25 and 34.9.[13] See **TABLE 1.9**. To correctly measure waist circumference, place a flexible tape measure around the waist just above the hipbone of an individual who is standing.

Percent Body Fat Measurements

Body fat percentages represent fat including essential body fat and storage body fat. Essential body fat is necessary to maintain life and for reproductive functions. Storage body fat consists of fat accumulation in adipose tissue, part of which protects the internal organs. **TABLE 1.10** shows how average percentages of body fat differ according to specified groups.

A number of different methods are used to measure percent body fat. It is essential for the clinician and the individual to employ accurate and consistent techniques to take measurements. Hydrostatic weighing, which requires the individual to be submerged entirely in water, is generally considered the gold standard because of its accuracy in measuring percent body fat. Other methods tend to be less invasive but have slightly higher variances.

Table 1.9

Waist Circumference and Associated Health Risk

Health Risk	Women	Men
Low risk	Below 31.5 inches	Below 37 inches
Moderate risk	31.5 to 35 inches	37 to 40 inches
High risk	35 inches or more	40.2 inches or more

Data from National Institutes of Health, National Heart, Lung, and Blood Institute. Assessing Your Weight and Health Risk. http://www.nhlbi.nih.gov/health/educational/lose_wt/risk.htm. Accessed August 13, 2016.

Table 1.10		
Average Percentage of Body Fat According to Group		
Category	Females	Males
Essential fat	10–13%	2–5%
Competitive athlete	14–20%	6–13%
Individual who exercises regularly, but not competitively	21–24%	14–17%
Average	25–31%	18–24%
Obese	32%+	25%+

A dual-energy X-ray absorptiometry (DEXA) scan is primarily used for measuring bone density by taking a full-body X-ray, and it can provide percent body fat measurements as well. The BOD POD is a costly machine that works by measuring the volume of air that is displaced inside the pod, which then equates to a body fat measurement. The Bod Pod is considered accurate; however, only special facilities have the equipment.

Hand-held devices and body fat scales use bioelectrical impedance to gauge the amount of lean mass, water, and fat in the body by sending an electric current from the metal plates under the feet or the palms of the hands of the individual through the body. Although these methods are generally inexpensive and easy to use, without proper hydration and consistent measurements over time, they tend to be less reliable than others. Calipers are another tool that a person skilled in their use can employ to assess percent body fat. Calipers measure the thickness of skinfolds at certain points on the body. The numbers are tallied and used in a formula to estimate percent body fat. Although calipers are generally considered an accurate method, results can vary widely depending on who is administering the test and whether the calipers themselves are reliable.

The InBody is a machine that combines the ease of use of a bioelectrical impedance analysis (BIA) device with the accuracy of hydrostatic weighing. InBody requires the individual stand on a metal platform and hold on to two handles for about a minute. The InBody uses technology that is fairly new, and the machines tend to be expensive and generally are found in only some health clubs.

Biochemical Data

Biochemical data use laboratory measurements obtained through blood, urine, or stool samples as indicators of nutritional status. Although not all nutrients can or should be assessed by laboratory methods, the following are examples of some of the more likely serum laboratory values used to help assess nutrition status:

- Albumin and prealbumin: Transport proteins used to assess protein status.
- C-reactive protein: Decreased value correlates with end of acute phase and beginning of anabolic phase response when nutrition repletion is possible.

- Insulin-like growth factor 1: Responds to growth hormone stimulation with decreased concentrations seen in protein-energy malnutrition.
- Creatinine height index: Estimates lean body mass.
- Iron, folate, ferritin, hemoglobin, hematocrit, mean corpuscular hemoglobin: Blood-forming nutrients.
- Total lymphocyte count: Affected by conditions such as cancer, inflammation, infection, stress, sepsis, and certain drugs and chemotherapeutic agents.
- Thiamine, riboflavin, niacin, and vitamin C: The water-soluble vitamins.
- Vitamin A, D, E, and K: The fat-soluble vitamins.
- Calcium, iron, iodine, and other trace elements: Minerals.
- Cholesterol, triglycerides, LDL, HDL: Blood lipid levels.
- Glucose (fasting) or glycated hemoglobin (HbA$_{1c}$): Current blood glucose level and average blood glucose level over the past 3 months.
- Blood urea nitrogen: Increased values indicate renal failure.

Clinical Assessment

Clinical assessment includes a medical history; current use of medications or vitamins, minerals, or herbal supplements; and a physical examination to identify signs of nutrition status. Clinical observations that can help to determine nutrition status include hair, nails, skin, eyes, lips, mouth, muscle tone, and hydration status. Clinical assessment should also include evaluation of personal, social, environmental, and lifestyle factors that could affect access to healthy food and nutritional well-being.

Dietary Data

Dietary data is the component of nutrition assessment that looks at food intake over time. There are many ways to document dietary intake; however, obtaining accurate data tends to be challenging because collecting good dietary data relies on the expertise of the clinician in conducting the data collection interview as well as the accuracy and honesty of the information provided by the individual.

Examples of methods used to assess dietary intake include the 24-hour recall for which the clinician asks the individual what he or she has eaten over the past 24 hours, the 3-day food diary for which the individual keeps track of everything ingested over 3 days, and food frequency questionnaires when an individual indicates how often particular foods on a list are eaten over a specific period of time (such as a week or month).

Accurate information regarding portion sizes and how food is prepared are important components of dietary intake records. Estimating portion sizes may be difficult, and the use of food models or photographs of food, or various plate and bowl sizes, can make this process more accurate. Information regarding food allergies or intolerances, food avoidance, and caffeine and alcohol use should also be collected.

Estimated Calorie Needs

An additional component of nutrition assessment is to determine calorie needs. Various methods exist for estimating calorie needs, from simple equations using an individual's height and weight, to more complicated equations, to machines or scales similar to those used to determine percent body fat. Indirect calorimetry and direct calorimetry are two accurate methods for determining estimated energy needs. Indirect calorimetry measures carbon dioxide produced and oxygen consumed. This non-invasive and generally accurate method can determine energy requirements. (See FIGURE 1.8 .) Direct calorimetry measures the amount of heat produced by a subject who is enclosed in a small chamber. (See FIGURE 1.9 .)

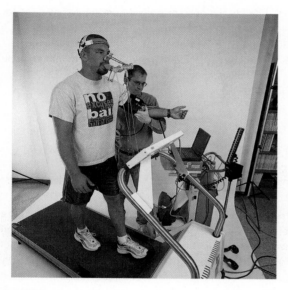

Figure 1.8
Indirect calorimetry.

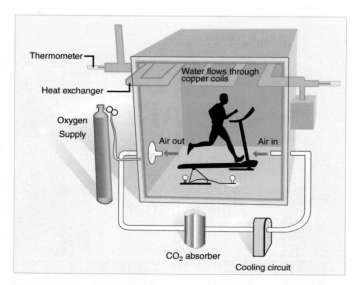

Figure 1.9
Direct calorimetry.

For the purposes of nutrition assessment, and when equipment is not available, mathematical calculations can help estimate daily calorie needs. Various websites provide simple and quick calculations for determining estimated energy expenditure. The following are two familiar calculation methods that can be used.

Method 1

Step 1:

Define the following information:

a. Age
b. Usual physical activity during the day as indicated in the following table
c. Weight in kilograms, which equals your weight in pounds divided by 2.2
d. Height in meters, which equals your height in inches divided by 39.4

Physical Activity Factors for Men and Women

Physical Activity Level	Physical Activity Factor for	
	Men	Women
Sedentary—little or no daily activity	1.0	1.0
Low activity—sedentary for most of the day and light activity, such as walking, for no more than 2 hours daily	1.11	1.12
Moderate activity—equivalent to walking about 1.5 to 3 miles per day at 3 to 4 miles per hour, on most days of the week in addition to light physical activity associated with typical day-to-day life	1.25	1.27
Vigorous activity—activity that requires a lot of effort and causes rapid breathing and a substantial increase in heart rate on most days of the week	1.48	1.45

Step 2:

Using your answers from above (a, b, c, and d), complete the following calculations (EER stands for estimated energy requirement):

For males, 19+ years old

$$EER = 662 - (9.53 \times \underline{\quad}) + \underline{\quad} \times [(15.91 \times \underline{\quad}) + (539.6 \times \underline{\quad})]$$
$$\quad\quad\quad\quad (a)\quad\quad (b)\quad\quad\quad\quad (c)\quad\quad\quad\quad (d)$$

For females, 19+ years old

$$EER = 354 - (6.91 \times \underline{\quad}) + \underline{\quad} \times [(9.36 \times \underline{\quad}) + (726 \times \underline{\quad})]$$
$$\quad\quad\quad\quad (a)\quad\quad (b)\quad\quad\quad (c)\quad\quad\quad\quad (d)$$

Method 2

The *Harris–Benedict equation* is a popular method for calculating estimated calorie needs. This equation uses known variables such as height, weight, age, and activity level. Basal metabolic rate (BMR) is a component of the

Harris–Benedict equation. BMR is the amount of energy (calories) that the body needs during a 24-hour period to perform daily, life-sustaining functions.

To calculate estimated daily calorie needs using the Harris–Benedict equation, first calculate BMR using either of the following equations:

- For females: BMR = (10 × Weight in kilograms) + (6.25 × Height in centimeters) – (5 × Age in years) – 161
- For males: BMR = (10 × Weight in kilograms) + (6.25 × Height in centimeters) – (5 × Age in years) + 5

Next, multiply BMR by one of the following activity levels:

- Little to no exercise: 1.2
- Light exercise (1–3 days per week): 1.375
- Moderate exercise (3–5 days per week): 1.55
- Heavy exercise (6–7 days per week): 1.725
- Very heavy exercise (twice per day, extra heavy workouts): 1.9

Therefore, Estimated energy requirement = BMR × Activity factor.

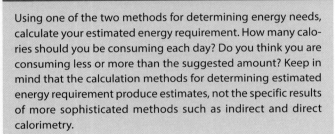

Case Study

Using one of the two methods for determining energy needs, calculate your estimated energy requirement. How many calories should you be consuming each day? Do you think you are consuming less or more than the suggested amount? Keep in mind that the calculation methods for determining estimated energy requirement produce estimates, not the specific results of more sophisticated methods such as indirect and direct calorimetry.

Methods of Evaluating Dietary Intake

Once the nutrient content of the diet has been collected, and estimated energy requirements are established, evaluation of the information should follow. Various methods for evaluating nutrition intake are available. Common methods are computer programs such as the U.S. Department of Agriculture (USDA) food tracker called SuperTracker on the ChooseMyPlate.com website and various telephone and computer applications. If accurate nutrient intake is recorded, these various programs provide a good estimate of the average energy intake and can help individuals determine where nutrition intake can be improved.

Outcomes of Nutrition Assessment

After information for a nutrition assessment is gathered and evaluated, all components should be considered collectively to create an accurate overall assessment. When considered together, anthropometric measures, biochemical tests, clinical exams, and dietary evaluations can give a complete picture of an individual's nutritional health. A complete nutrition assessment can lead to recommendations for diet changes as necessary.

Recap A nutrition assessment is an in-depth evaluation of both objective and subjective data as they relate to an individual's food and nutrient intake, lifestyle, and medical history. Once all of the information that makes up a nutrition assessment is obtained and evaluated, appropriate recommendations for dietary improvements can be made. Overall the nutrition assessment is intended to help people either maintain or attain a healthier nutrition status.

1. Identify the percent body fat considered average for adult females and adult males.
2. Identify each component of a nutrition assessment.
3. Describe two different methods of determining an individual's estimated energy requirements.

The Dietary Guidelines for Americans 2015–2020

Preview The Dietary Guidelines for Americans are a set of guidelines released jointly by the U.S. Department of Health and Human Services (HHS) and the U.S. Department of Agriculture (USDA). The most current guidelines, *The Dietary Guidelines for Americans 2015–2020*, provide science-based advice suggesting how nutrition and physical activity can help promote health across the life span and help reduce the risk for major chronic diseases among the U.S. population ages 2 years and older.[15]

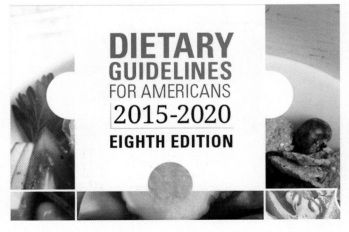

Reproduced from Health.gov. 2015–2020 Dietary Guidelines for Americans. Retrieved from: https://health.gov/dietaryguidelines/2015/

Recommendations within the *Dietary Guidelines for Americans 2015–2020* are what experts have determined to be the best nutrition advice for Americans to reduce the risk of chronic diseases brought about by poor dietary patterns. More and more is being learned about the impact of not only individual eating habits during adulthood but also lifestyle habits created during childhood. Lifestyle choices that include poor diet and low levels of physical activity are among the most important factors contributing to the high rates of overweight and obesity among men, women, and children throughout the United States. In an effort to address this growing problem, the *Dietary Guidelines for Americans 2015-2020* focuses on government, agriculture, health care, business, educators, and communities working together to encourage individuals to make healthy lifestyle changes.[14] These guidelines emphasize a total diet approach by encouraging a holistic approach to what we eat. *The Dietary Guidelines for Americans 2015–2020* provides five overarching guidelines:

- Follow a healthy eating pattern across the life span. All food and beverage choices matter; therefore, choose a healthy eating pattern at an appropriate calorie level during all stages of life to help achieve and maintain a healthy body weight, to support nutrient adequacy, and to reduce the risk of chronic disease.
- Focus on variety, nutrient density, and amount. To meet nutrient needs within calorie limits, choose a variety of nutrient-dense foods across and within all food groups.
- Limit calories from added sugars and saturated fats and reduce sodium intake. Consume an eating pattern low in added sugars, saturated fats, and sodium.
- Shift to healthier food and beverage choices. Choose nutrient-dense foods and beverages across and within all food groups in place of less healthy choices.
- Support healthy eating patterns for all. Everyone has a role in helping to create and support healthy eating patterns in multiple settings nationwide, from home to school, workplace to communities.

Key recommendations from the *Dietary Guidelines for Americans 2015–2020* provide further guidance on how individuals can follow the five guidelines.

Dietary Guidelines for Americans 2015–2020 Key Recommendations

- Consume a healthy eating pattern that accounts for all foods and beverages within an appropriate calorie level.
- Consume less than 10% of calories per day from added sugars.
- Consume less than 10% of calories per day from saturated fats.
- Consume less than 2,300 mg per day of sodium.
- If alcohol is consumed, it should be consumed in moderation—up to one drink per day for women and up to two drinks per day for men—and only by adults of legal drinking age.
- Meet the *Physical Activity Guidelines for Americans*.

Unlike previous editions of the *Dietary Guidelines for Americans*, particular meal patterns and suggested servings are eliminated; instead, eating patterns and the characteristics of foods and beverages as they make up a person's usual eating patterns are emphasized. Examples of suggested eating patterns for various calorie levels are provided. These guidelines offer practical tips for how people can change their diet to integrate healthier choices. See TABLE 1.11.

Adequacy, Balance, Moderation, and Variety

As basic principles for healthy eating, the concepts of adequacy, balance, moderation, and variety within an individual's eating pattern are important. Each of these principles introduces an important component to overall health.

Adequacy

Adequacy as it relates to healthy eating means that the foods you choose to eat provide all of the essential nutrients, fiber, and energy in amounts sufficient to support

---

Table 1.11

Dietary Guidelines for Americans 2015–2020: Benefits, Behaviors, and Tips

	Dietary Guideline Recommendation Benefits to Your Health	Goals or Behaviors that Could Make You Healthier	How-to Tips
Follow a healthy eating pattern across the life span.	• Individuals throughout all stages of life should adopt eating patterns that promote overall health and help prevent chronic disease. • Choose a healthy eating pattern at an appropriate calorie level to help achieve and maintain a healthy body weight, support nutrient adequacy, and reduce the risk of chronic disease.	• Consume foods and drinks to meet, not exceed, calorie needs. • Plan ahead to make healthy food choices. • Track food and calorie intake. • Reduce portion sizes, especially of high-calorie foods. • Choose healthy food options when eating away from home.	• Know your calorie needs. • Prepare and pack healthy snacks at home to be eaten at school or at work.

	Dietary Guideline Recommendation Benefits to Your Health	Goals or Behaviors that Could Make You Healthier	How-to Tips
Focus on variety, nutrient density, and amount.	• Choose a variety of nutrient-dense foods across and within all food groups in recommended amounts.	• Eat five or more servings of vegetables and fruits daily; make up of a variety of choices. • Choose foods that contain nutrients and other beneficial substances that have not been "diluted" by the addition of calories from added solid fats, sugars, or refined starches or by the solid fats naturally present in food.	• Add dark green, red, and orange vegetables to soups, stews, casseroles, stir-fries, and other main and side dishes. • Add beans or peas to salads, soups, and side dishes, or them serve as a main dish. • Have raw, cut-up vegetables and fruit handy for quick side dishes, snacks, salads, and desserts. • When eating out, choose a vegetable as a side dish.
Limit calories from added sugars and saturated fats and reduce sodium intake.	• Cut back on foods and beverages high in added sugars, saturated fats, and sodium to amounts that fit within healthy eating patterns. • Limit added sugars to less than 10% of calories per day. • Limit saturated fat intake to less than 10% of calories per day. • Limit sodium to less than 2,300 mg per day (adults). • Eating a diet that includes saturated fat, trans fat, and dietary cholesterol raises low-density lipoprotein (LDL), or "bad" cholesterol levels, which increases the risk of coronary heart disease (CHD).	• Replace saturated fats with polyunsaturated fats. • Be aware of the most likely sources of trans fat in your diet, such as pastry items and donuts, deep-fried foods, snack chips, cookies, and crackers.	• Eat less cake, cookies, ice cream, other desserts, and candy. • Include foods that provide monounsaturated and polyunsaturated fats, such as olive oil and nuts, in your diet. • Limit intake of foods high in saturated and trans fats such as ground beef and full-fat dairy products.
Shift to healthier food and beverage choices.	• Choose nutrient-dense foods and beverages across and within all food groups. • Excessive alcohol consumption has no benefits, and the health and social hazards of heavy alcohol intake are numerous and well known.	• Drink an adequate amount of water each day. • Choose foods and drinks with added sugars or caloric sweeteners (sugar-sweetened beverages) less frequently. • If you are of legal drinking age and you consume alcohol, do so in moderation. • Mixing alcohol and caffeine is not recognized as safe by the U.S. Food and Drug Administration.	• Drink few or no regular sodas, sports drinks, energy drinks, and fruit drinks. • Choose water, fat-free milk, 100% fruit juice, or unsweetened tea or coffee as drinks. • If alcohol is consumed, limit to no more than one drink per day for women and two drinks per day for men. • Avoid excessive (heavy or binge) drinking. • Avoid alcohol if you are pregnant or may become pregnant.
Support healthy eating patterns for all.	Everyone has a role in helping to create and support healthy eating patterns in multiple settings.	Systems, organizations, and businesses and industries all have important roles in helping individuals make healthy choices. Professionals can work with individuals in a variety of settings to adapt their choices to develop a healthy eating pattern tailored to accommodate physical health; cultural, ethnic, traditional, and personal preferences; as well as personal food budgets and other issues of accessibility.	• Make healthy food choices at home and away from home.

Modified from US Department of Health and Human Services and US Department of Agriculture. *2015–2020 Dietary Guidelines for Americans.* 8th ed. Washington, DC: US Department of Health and Human Services and US Department of Agriculture; December 2015. http://health.gov/dietaryguidelines/2015/guidelines/. Accessed August 13, 2016.

growth and maintain health.[15] Adequacy goes beyond calorie intake. In fact, many Americans eat adequate calories each day but are still considered undernourished. This is because the foods that they choose to eat are high in calories and low in nutrients. Take, for example, a meal of hamburger, french fries, and soda. This meal can provide adequate calories for a single meal; however, because it is high in fat and low in vitamins and minerals, it is therefore low in nutrient density and does not meet the criteria for adequacy. Choosing meals and snacks that are high in vitamins and minerals but low to moderate in calorie content offers important benefits such as normal growth and development for children, health promotion for people of all ages, and reduction of risk for a number of chronic diseases that are major public health problems of today.[15]

Balance and Moderation

Eating healthfully requires having *balance*, or *moderation*, in all food groups, energy sources, and other nutrients such as vitamins and minerals. One challenge when it comes to balance is to consume enough but not too much from all the different food groups. This principle is also where the concept that "all food can fit into a healthy diet" comes into play. Choosing low-nutrient foods occasionally does not classify an individual's diet as unbalanced or unhealthy; rather, eating a balance of high- and low-nutrient-density foods helps to create an overall healthy eating pattern. Like balance, moderation means not taking anything to extremes. Food graphics convey the message of balance and moderation by suggesting amounts of different food groups.

Variety

Variety refers to including a lot of different foods in the diet. This means eating foods from different food groups and different foods within each of those food groups. For example, if apples are the only fruit a person eats, although this individual is including fruit, the diet lacks variety. Variety is important for a number of reasons. Eating different vegetables, for example, provides a mix of different vitamins, minerals, and other nutrients such as phytochemicals. Having variety in the diet helps ensure that individuals are getting all of the nutrients they need. Studies show that people who eat a varied diet are more likely to meet their overall nutrient needs compared with those who eat a less-varied diet.[16]

> **Recap** *Dietary Guidelines for Americans 2015–2020* reflects the current body of nutrition science and provides recommendations to help Americans make healthy food and beverage choices. These guidelines serve as the foundation for vital nutrition policies and programs across the United States. The nutrition principles of adequacy, balance, moderation, and variety can help maintain or improve the overall health of individuals at all stages of life.
>
> 1. List the key recommendations in the *Dietary Guidelines for Americans 2015–2020*.
> 2. Define and describe what *adequacy* refers to in regard to healthy eating.
> 3. Explain the difference between having variety in your diet and eating in moderation.

Physical Activity Guidelines

> **Preview** The *Physical Activity Guidelines for Americans* are based on the latest science and provide guidance on how children and adults can improve their health through physical activity. Being physically active is an important step for individuals of all ages. The HHS, along with the USDA, provides the *Physical Activity Guidelines for Americans.*

The *Physical Activity Guidelines for Americans* complement the *Dietary Guidelines for Americans* and provide science-based guidance to help Americans ages 6 and older improve their health through physical activity. The key guidelines in the *Physical Activity Guidelines* are the following.[16]

Key Guidelines for Children and Adolescents

- Children and adolescents should engage in 60 minutes (1 hour) or more of physical activity daily.

  - Most of the 60 minutes should be either moderate- or vigorous-intensity aerobic physical activity and should include vigorous-intensity activity at least 3 days a week.
  - The 60 minutes should also include muscle-strengthening and bone-strengthening activities at least 3 days a week.

- It is important to encourage young people to participate in physical activities that are appropriate for their age, that are enjoyable, and that offer variety.

Key Guidelines for Adults

- All adults should avoid inactivity. Some physical activity is better than none, and adults who participate in any amount of physical activity gain some health benefits.
- For substantial health benefits, adults should do at least 150 minutes (2 hours and 30 minutes) a week of moderate-intensity or 75 minutes (1 hour and 15 minutes) a week of vigorous-intensity aerobic physical activity or an equivalent combination of moderate- and vigorous-intensity aerobic activity. Aerobic activity should be performed in episodes of at least 10 minutes, and, preferably, it should be spread throughout the week.
- Adults should also do muscle-strengthening activities that are moderate or high intensity and that involve all major muscle groups on two or more days a week, because these activities provide additional health benefits.

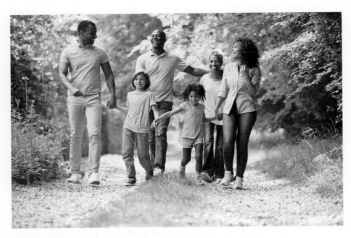

©Monkey Business Images/Shutterstock

The key guidelines for adults also apply to older adults. In addition, the following guidelines are just for older adults:

Key Guidelines for Older Adults

- When older adults cannot do 150 minutes of moderate-intensity aerobic activity a week because of chronic conditions, they should be as physically active as their abilities and conditions allow.
- Older adults should do exercises that maintain or improve balance if they are at risk of falling.
- Older adults should determine their level of effort for physical activity relative to their level of fitness.
- Older adults with chronic conditions should understand whether and how their conditions affect their ability to do regular physical activity safely.

Recap For a healthy lifestyle, it is important to understand the benefits of physical activity and how to make activity a part of your regular routine.

1. What is the daily suggested activity level for children and adolescents?
2. What are the daily suggested activity guidelines for adults to achieve substantial health benefits?
3. What are suggested activity guidelines for older adults who cannot do 150 minutes of moderate-intensity aerobic activity in a week?

The Obesity Epidemic May Be Decreasing Life Expectancy

Preview Rapid changes in the modern lifestyle have introduced many factors that may decrease the life expectancy of the latest generation.

Since the end of the Civil War until the late twentieth century, life span increased rapidly in the United States, a tremendous public health triumph brought about by a more dependable food supply, improved sanitation, and advances in medical care.[17] During the late 1970s, what we now refer to as the obesity epidemic started, and with it a change in U.S. death rates. Rapid changes in today's lifestyle have introduced many factors that have a negative impact on life expectancy. According to the Centers for Disease Control and Prevention (CDC), a quarter of American children today are classified as obese. Childhood obesity can lead to the development of significant health problems at earlier ages—health problems that can contribute to death well before the current U.S. life expectancy of 78 years is reached.

Death rates increased significantly from the year 2015 to the year 2016, most notably involving causes of death related to obesity such as heart disease, diabetes, chronic liver disease, stroke, and Alzheimer disease.[18] CDC reports from 2014 indicate that 34.3% of adult men and 38.3% of adult women are obese. This trend seems likely to accelerate as the current generation of children reaches adulthood because the prevalence of childhood obesity is higher than it has been in the past. Additionally, research suggests that the parents of today's young will actually outlive their children as overall life expectancy declines.

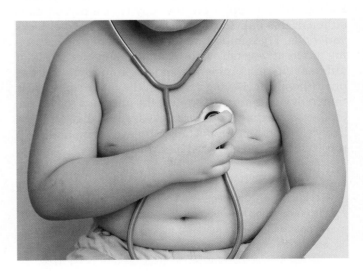

©kwanchai.c/Shutterstock

The formula for achieving and maintaining a healthy weight throughout the life span is multifactorial and even a bit complicated, with suggested factors ranging from genetics, to energy balance, to environmental factors. Recent studies suggest that body weight might have less to do with the body's ability to burn excess calories consumed by increasing activity level and more to do with the type of foods that make up an individual's diet on a regular basis.

As suggested by such sources as the *Dietary Guidelines for Americans*, the public health approach to obesity remains focused on advising people to choose appropriate calorie levels and engage in enough physical activity to achieve or maintain a healthy body weight. At the same time, current trends in the American diet suggest that added sugars and other highly processed carbohydrates comprise the most harmful components of individual diets. Because of this, it may be that national policies must shift away from low-quality commodities such as corn and wheat and instead encourage production of high-quality proteins, fruits and vegetables, legumes, nuts, and other whole foods by offering incentives.[18] Additional action plans from health advocacy groups include taxing sugary beverages, limiting advertising of unhealthy foods targeted to children, and encouraging Congress to increase spending on obesity-related research. Learning and maintaining healthy eating habits early in life can go a long way in preventing deaths resulting from causes brought about by obesity.

Recap As overweight and obesity among the U.S. population continues to increase, in overall numbers and in younger children, the advice to choose appropriate calorie levels and engage in enough physical activity to achieve or maintain a healthy body weight are paramount.

1. Identify the most harmful components of an individual's diet with regard to contributions to obesity.
2. The formula for achieving and maintaining a healthy weight is multifactorial. Identify some factors that may be contributing to unhealthy weight in both children and adults.

Let's Discuss

Consider that the current obesity epidemic may be decreasing life expectancy. Discuss possible changes and phenomena in the modern lifestyle and factors that negatively affect life expectancy. Describe different ways in which social media, cell phones, and video games contribute to childhood obesity.

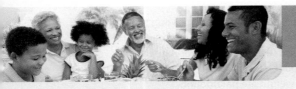

Learning Portfolio

Visual Chapter Summary

Introduction

- As we study nutrition needs and recommendations throughout life, we must keep in mind these basic principles that are important for healthy eating regardless of age:
  - Poor nutrition status can result from either inadequate or excessive nutrition intake and can contribute to the development of certain chronic diseases.

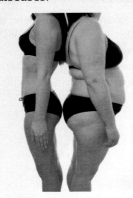

©Hartphotography/Shutterstock

Energy Scale for Food

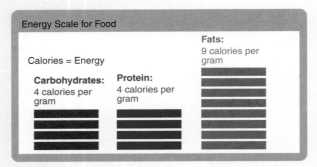

Calories = Energy

Fats:
9 calories per gram

Carbohydrates:
4 calories per gram

Protein:
4 calories per gram

- Energy produced by the body, which is needed for a variety of functions, is provided by food and drink in the form of carbohydrates, proteins, and fats

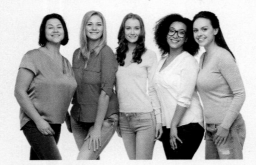

©Syda Productions/Shutterstock

(macronutrients). Each macronutrient provides a specific amount of energy measured in calories.
- Energy needs vary from person to person and depend on such factors as basal metabolic rate (BMR) and activity level.

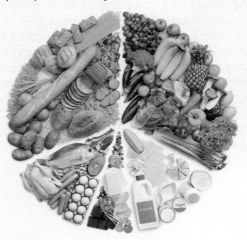

©ifong/Shutterstock

- There are many components of healthy eating, with adequacy, balance, moderation, and variety in food choices being key characteristics.

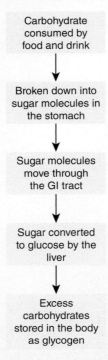

Carbohydrate consumed by food and drink

↓

Broken down into sugar molecules in the stomach

↓

Sugar molecules move through the GI tract

↓

Sugar converted to glucose by the liver

↓

Excess carbohydrates stored in the body as glycogen

Process by which carbohydrates are converted to glucose for energy, or glycogen for storage.

The Science of Nutrition

- Basic principles of healthy eating can help guide healthy nutrition choices.
- Our diets are made up of a combination of essential and nonessential nutrients, each with suggested recommended intake levels for optimal nutrition.
- The macronutrients carbohydrate, protein, and fat provide our bodies with calories and essential nutrients. Carbohydrates are the body's preferred source of energy, providing energy to the brain, muscles, and nervous system. Protein exists in every cell of the body and functions to build, repair, and maintain bones, muscles, and skin. Fat not only provides calories but also helps our bodies absorb fat-soluble vitamins and keeps our skin and hair healthy.

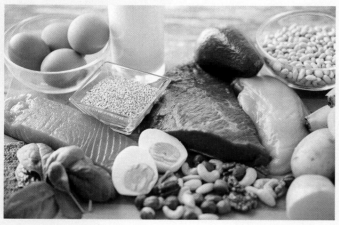

©Syda Productions/Shutterstock

Micronutrients

- Adequate vitamin, mineral, and water intake is essential for life.
- Our body can produce some of the vitamins that it needs; others must come from the diet.
- Minerals are elements that originate in the earth and cannot be made by human bodies. Plants obtain minerals from the soil, providing humans dietary sources of a number of minerals either directly through the consumption of plants or indirectly through the consumption of animal sources that feed on mineral-rich food sources. Minerals may also be present in the water we drink.

What Does Water Do for You?

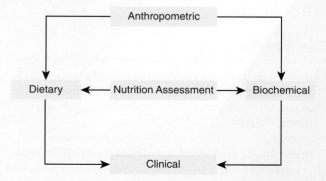

Forms saliva (digestion)

Keeps mucosal membranes moist

Allows body's cells to grow, reproduce, and survive

Flushes body waste, mainly in urine

Lubricates joints

Water is the major component of most body parts

Needed by the brain to manufacture hormones and neurotransmitters

Regulates body temperature (sweating and respiration)

Acts as a shock absorber for brain and spinal cord

Converts food to components needed for survival - digestion

Helps deliver oxygen all over the body

Various functions of water.

Nutrition Assessment

- A nutrition assessment is an in-depth evaluation of both objective and subjective data as they relate to an individual's food and nutrient intake, lifestyle, and medical history. Once all of the information that makes up a nutrition assessment is obtained and evaluated, appropriate recommendations for dietary improvements can be made. Overall, the nutrition assessment is intended to help people either maintain a healthy or attain a healthier nutrition status.

Anthropometric

Dietary ← Nutrition Assessment → Biochemical

Clinical

The Dietary Guidelines for Americans 2015–2020

- *Dietary Guidelines for Americans 2015–2020* reflects the current body of nutrition science. The guidelines provide recommendations that help Americans

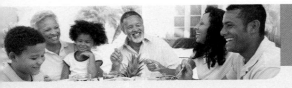

Learning Portfolio (continued)

make healthy food and beverage choices and serve as the foundation for vital nutrition policies and programs across the United States.

■ The nutrition principles of adequacy, balance, moderation, and variety can help individuals maintain or improve their overall health at all stages of life.

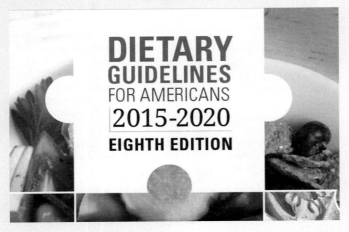

Reproduced from Health.gov. 2015–2020 Dietary Guidelines for Americans. Retrieved from: https://health.gov/dietaryguidelines/2015/

Physical Activity Guidelines

■ It is important to encourage young people to participate in physical activities that are appropriate for their age, that are enjoyable, and that offer variety.

■ Adults should do muscle-strengthening activities that are moderate or high intensity and that involve all major muscle groups on two or more days a

week, because these activities provide additional health benefits.

■ Older adults should do exercises that maintain or improve balance if they are at risk of falling. They should determine their level of effort for physical activity relative to their level of fitness.

The Obesity Epidemic May Be Decreasing Life Expectancy

■ As overweight and obesity among the U.S. population continues to increase, in overall numbers and in younger children, the advice to choose appropriate calorie levels and engage in enough physical activity to achieve or maintain a healthy body weight is paramount.

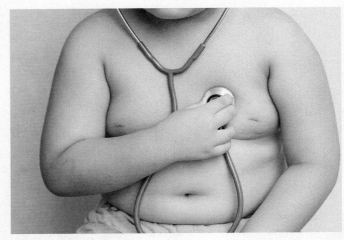

©kwanchai.c/Shutterstock

Key Terms

adequacy As it relates to healthy eating means that the foods you choose to eat provide all of the essential nutrients, fiber, and energy in amounts sufficient to support growth and maintain health.

Adequate Intake (AI) A value based on observed or experimentally determined approximations of nutrient intake by a group of healthy people and used when a Recommended Dietary Allowance (RDA) cannot be determined.

alpha-linolenic acid: A polyunsaturated omega-3 fatty acid essential to the body for the formation of prostaglandins.

anthropometric measures: Physical measurements of the body, including data on height, weight, body composition, that can be used to help develop a nutrition assessment.

biochemical data: Laboratory measurements obtained through blood, urine, or stool samples as indicators of nutritional status.

body mass index (BMI): A measure of body fat that is the ratio of the weight of the body in kilograms to the square of its height in meters. It is a reliable indicator of body fatness.

calorie: The energy needed to raise the temperature of 1 g of water 1°C, and the unit used to measure the potential energy in food as it is transferred from its source to the body.

carbohydrates: Organic compounds that occur in food that contain carbon, oxygen, and hydrogen and that can be broken down to release energy in the body.

cholesterol: A waxy, fat-like substance found in all of the cells of the body that is a precursor of other steroid compounds;

high concentrations of cholesterol in the blood is thought to promote atherosclerosis.

clinical assessment: The component of nutrition assessment that includes a medical history, inventory of currently used medications, vitamins, minerals, and herbal supplements, and a physical examination to identify signs of nutrition status.

complex carbohydrates: A form of carbohydrate made up of multiple sugar molecules (polysaccharides) linked together. Examples include starches, glycogen, and most types of fiber.

dietary data: The component of nutrition assessment that looks at food intake over time.

Dietary Guidelines for Americans: A set of guidelines published every 5 years and released jointly by the U.S. Department of Health and Human Services and the U.S. Department of Agriculture that provide science-based advice suggesting how nutrition and physical activity can help to promote health across the life span and help to reduce the risk of major chronic diseases among the U.S. population ages 2 years and older.

Dietary Reference Intakes (DRIs): Suggested nutrient intake values intended to serve as a guide for good nutrition for healthy people. These dietary standards include Estimated Average Requirement (EAR), Recommended Dietary Allowance (RDA), Adequate Intake (AI), and Tolerable Upper Intake Limit (UL).

direct calorimetry: Measurement of the heat produced by a reaction, as distinguished from indirect methods, which involve measurement of something other than heat production itself.

essential nutrients: Nutrients (vitamins, minerals, fatty acids, and amino acids) required for normal physiological function that cannot be synthesized by the body and that, therefore, must be obtained from the diet.

Estimated Average Requirement (EAR): A nutrient intake value that is estimated to meet the requirement of half the healthy individuals in a group.

fat: A macronutrient that provides an energy source and that helps the body absorb fat-soluble vitamins, keeps skin and hair healthy, and offers the sensation of satiety after eating. Fat is the source of two essential fatty acids and is used by the body during brain development, for controlling inflammation, and in blood clotting.

indirect calorimetry: Calculates heat that living organisms produce by measuring either their production of carbon dioxide and nitrogen waste (frequently ammonia in aquatic organisms, or urea in terrestrial ones) or their consumption of oxygen; a way of determining metabolic rate in critically ill patients.

insoluble fiber: A type of fiber that adds bulk to stool and appears to help food pass more quickly through the stomach and intestines, helping to prevent constipation by increasing stool weight and decreasing gut transit time, which in turn can reduce the risk of diseases and disorders such as diverticular disease and hemorrhoids.

linoleic acid: An essential, polyunsaturated, omega-6 fatty acid that is necessary for healthy brain function, skin and hair growth, bone density, energy production, and reproductive health.

micronutrients: Chemical elements or substances required in small amounts for normal growth and development of all living organisms.

minerals: Inorganic and essential nutrients that are needed by the body in small amounts and that play key roles in several body functions.

nonessential nutrients: Nutrients required by the body for supporting processes. These can be made by the body and therefore do not need to be obtained from the diet.

omega-3 fatty acids: Polyunsaturated fatty acids that have been shown to be beneficial for the heart as well as play a critical role in brain function and normal growth and development.

omega-6 fatty acids: Polyunsaturated fatty acids that have been shown to play a critical role in brain function and normal growth and development. Omega-6 fatty acids may interfere with the health benefits brought about by omega-3 fatty acids.

phytochemicals: Substances found in plants that are not considered essential but that play important roles in maintaining health and well-being.

protein: Any group of organic molecules that contain carbon, hydrogen, oxygen, and nitrogen, and one or more chains of amino acids. Proteins are in every cell in the body and function to build, repair, and maintain bones, muscles, and skin.

Recommended Dietary Allowance (RDA): The average dietary intake level that is sufficient to meet the nutrient requirements of nearly all (97% to 98%) healthy individuals in a group.

saturated fats: A type of fat where the carbon atoms in the fatty acid component are linked by single bonds. Saturated fats are found in meat and other animal products such as butter, cheese, and milk. This type of fat is associated with increased blood cholesterol levels.

simple carbohydrates: Carbohydrates made up of either one (monosaccharide) or two (disaccharide) simple sugar molecules. Examples include sucrose, maltose, and lactose.

soluble fiber: Fiber that attracts water and turns to a gel during digestion, a characteristic that slows down digestion, keeping a person feeling full longer and possibly slowing the digestion and absorption of carbohydrates, which prevents a spike in blood glucose following a meal. Soluble fiber can help lower blood cholesterol and blood glucose levels.

Tolerable Upper Intake Level (UL): The highest level of daily nutrient intake that is likely to pose no risk of adverse side effects to almost all individuals in the general population.

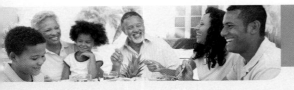

Learning Portfolio (continued)

As intake increases above the UL, the risk of adverse effects increases.

trans fat: A type of unsaturated fat that occurs naturally in some products. The main dietary trans fats are created in an industrial process that adds hydrogen to liquid vegetable oils to make them more solid. Trans fats are used in margarine and many commercial fried products. Like saturated fats, trans fats are associated with increasing blood cholesterol levels. Trans fats on food labels can be referred to as "partially hydrogenated" oils on the ingredient list.

unsaturated fat: A type of fat that has one or more double bonds between the carbon atoms and that is found in plant foods and in fish. This type of fat is associated with being beneficial to heart health.

vitamins: A group of organic substances that are essential for proper functioning of the body.

Discussion Questions

1. Describe the difference between essential and nonessential nutrients.
2. Name and define the four main Dietary Reference Intake categories.
3. Summarize the different health benefits of soluble and insoluble fiber.
4. How do saturated, unsaturated and trans fats differ in relationship to how they function within the body?
5. List functions of water in the body.
6. State and describe the components of nutrition assessment.
7. Identify the Key Recommendations for *the Dietary Guidelines for Americans 2015-2020.*

Activities

1. Identify three foods that you have never tasted before and, with an open mind, prepare each food and taste it.
2. Using a diet analysis program, input three days of your food intake and activity. Run reports to identify the nutrients (macronutrients and micronutrients) for which you have both sufficient and insufficient intake. Write three goals to improve your nutrition status.
3. Interview a child between the ages of 7 and 13 years. Discuss with the child his or her usual food intake and physical activity level.

Study Questions

1. Which type of fat is associated with raising low-density lipoprotein cholesterol levels, which puts a person at risk for heart attack, stroke, and other major health problems?
   a. Saturated fat
   b. Unsaturated fat
   c. Complex carbohydrate
   d. Plant protein
2. Which of the following transport cholesterol molecules from arteries to the liver, where they can be excreted?
   a. Trans fatty acids
   b. Omega-3 fatty acids
   c. Low-density lipoproteins
   d. High-density lipoproteins
3. Vitamins and minerals are included in the classification of elements called micronutrients.
   a. True
   b. False
4. Functions of water in the body include all of the following *except* which one?
   a. Acts as a shock absorber for eyes, brain, and spinal cord and is a component of amniotic fluid.
   b. Lubricates joints.
   c. Helps to regulate body temperature.
   d. Supplies macronutrients to the body.
5. Which of the following are examples of anthropometric measurements taken for nutrition assessment?
   a. Lab values
   b. Assessment of hair and nails
   c. Suggested dietary intake
   d. Height, weight, BMI, percent body fat
6. A body fat measurement of 16% for an adult male suggests that he is:
   a. in the category of underweight.
   b. in the category of being fit.
   c. in the category of being average.
   d. in the category of being obese.

7. Obtaining personal information that includes an individual's medical history, current use of medications or vitamins, and physical examination identifying signs of nutrition status are all examples of which step in nutrition assessment?
   a. Anthropometric measurement
   b. Biochemical measurement
   c. Clinical data
   d. Dietary intake

8. Which health risk category is a female with a waist circumference of 34 inches in?
   a. Low risk
   b. Moderate risk
   c. High risk
   d. Cannot be determined

9. Using the following information, determine the estimated energy requirements for a 20-year-old male who is 5 feet 10 inches tall and weighs 170 pounds. His activity level is considered moderate. Round your answer to the nearest calorie.

   EER = 662 − (9.53 × Age) + [Activity factor × (15.91 × Weight in kilograms) + (539.6 × Height in meters)]

   a. 1,800 calories
   b. 2,345 calories
   c. 2,656 calories
   d. 2,965 calories

   Answer calculation:
   EER = 662 − (9.53 × 20) + [1.25 × (15.91 × 77.27) + (539.6 × 1.77)]
   EER = 662 − 190.6 + (1.25 × 2,184.45)
   EER = 662 − 190.6 + 1,730.56
   EER = 2,655.85 *calories*

10. Which diet principle refers to including a lot of different foods in the diet?
    a. Adequacy
    b. Balance
    c. Moderation
    d. Variety

11. A physical activity guideline for adults is to do muscle-strengthening activities that are moderate or high intensity on two or more days a week.
    a. True
    b. False

Weblinks

- **USDA SuperTracker: My foods. My fitness. My health**
  https://www.supertracker.usda.gov

- **Estimated Energy Requirement**
  https://moritzcycling.com/eer.cgi

- **Academy of Nutrition and Dietetics**
  http://www.eatright.org

References

1. Sandquist L. Food first: nutrition as the foundation for health. *Creat Nurs*. 2015;21(4):213–221.
2. National Institutes of Health. Nutrient recommendations: Dietary Reference Intakes (DRI). https://ods.od.nih.gov/Health_Information/Dietary_Reference_Intakes.aspx. Accessed April 26, 2016.
3. Femades J, Arts J, Dimond E, Hirshberg S, Lofgren IE. Dietary factors are associated with coronary heart disease risk factors in college students. *Nutr Res*. August 2013;33(8): 647–652.
4. Hadley KB, Ryan AS, Forsyth S, et al. The essentiality of arachidonic acid in infant development. *Nutrients*. April 12, 2016;8(4):216.
5. Sergeant S, Rahbar E, Chilton FH. Gamma-linolenic acid, dihommo-gamma linolenic, eicosanoids and inflammatory processes [published online April 12, 2016]. *Eur J Pharmacol*. Aug. 15 2016;785:77–86. doi: 10.1016/j.ejphar.2016.04.020.
6. Leikin-Frenkel AL. Is there a role for alpha-linolenic acid in the fetal programming of health? *J Clin Med*. March 23, 2016;5(4):40.
7. Ito MK. A comparative overview of prescription omega-3 fatty acid products. *P T*. December 2015;40(12):826–857.
8. Tortosa-Caparros E, Navas-Carrillo D, Marin F, Orenes-Pinero E. Anti-inflammatory effects of omega 3 and omega 6 polyunsaturated fatty acids in cardiovascular disease and metabolic syndrome [published online January 8, 2016]. *Crit Rev Food Sci Nutr*. 2016.
9. Noriega BS, Sanchez-Gonzalez MA, Salyakina D, Coffman J. Understanding the impact of omega-3 rich diet on the gut microbiota [published online March 14, 2016]. *Case Rep Med*. 2016. doi:http://dx.doi.org/10.1155/2016/3089303.
10. Simopoulos AP. An increase in the omega-6/omega-3 fatty acid ratio increases the risk for obesity. *Nutrients*. March 2, 2016;8(3):128.

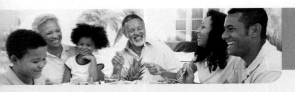

Learning Portfolio (continued)

11. Han TS, Lean ME. A clinical perspective of obesity, metabolic syndrome and cardiovascular disease. *JRSM Cardiovasc Dis.* February 25, 2016;5:2048004016633371.

12. National Heart, Lung, and Blood Institute. Assessing your weight and health risk. https://www.nhlbi.nih.gov/health/educational/lose_wt/risk.htm. Accessed April 30, 2016.

13. Ellulu MS, Khaza'ai H, Rhmat A, et al. Obesity can predict and promote systemic inflammation in healthy adults. *Int J Cardiol.* April 14, 2016;215:318–324.

14. U.S. Department of Agriculture and U.S. Department of Health and Human Services. Scientific report of the 2015 Dietary Guidelines Advisory Committee. http://www.health.gov/dietaryguidelines/2015-scientific-report/04-integration.asp. Accessed May 3, 2016.

15. U.S. Department of Agriculture and U.S. Department of Health and Human Services. *Dietary Guidelines for Americans, 2010.* 7th ed. Washington, DC: US Government Printing Office; December 2010.

16. Office of Disease Prevention and Health Promotion. *2008 Physical Activity Guidelines for Americans Summary.* http://health.gov/paguidelines/guidelines/summary.aspx. Accessed August 13, 2016.

17. Mennella JA, Reiter AR, Daniels LM. Vegetable and fruit acceptance during infancy: impact of ontogeny, genetics, and early experiences. *Adv Nutr.* January 15, 2016;7(1):211S–219S.

18. Ludwig D. Lifespan weighted down by diet [published online April 4, 2016]. JAMA. 2016. doi:10.1001/jama.2016.3829.

CHAPTER 2

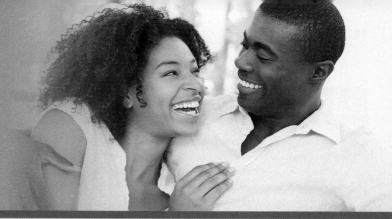

Nutrition Needs During Preconception

Kathryn Hillstrom, EdD, MPH, RDN

Chapter Outline

Preconception Period

The Physiology of Reproduction

Infertility, Subfertility, and Assisted Reproductive Technology

Common Health Conditions

Nutrition Recommendations During Preconception

Lifestyle Habits During Preconception

Learning Objectives

1. Describe the preconception periods for men and women.

2. Summarize the reproductive process, including critical hormones and their roles.

3. Explain subfertility and infertility.

4. List preexisting diseases and conditions that may contribute to infertility or a poor pregnancy outcome.

5. List the common nutrients, including their recommended intake levels, for the preconception period.

6. Describe the role of body weight and lifestyle habits in preconception health.

7. List resources to promote a healthy preconception period.

8. List suggested steps of the Nutrition Care Process.

Case Study

Meet Suzanne, a 35-year-old woman who married 2 years ago. Suzanne works at a busy law firm, and her husband is an engineer. They enjoy outdoor activities as well as spending quiet time at home. Suzanne and her husband have been talking a lot about the right time to start a family.

Do you know someone who is trying to become pregnant? Perhaps you have noticed that, compared to your mother's and her mother's generations, many women are getting pregnant at a later age. Healthy habits used to begin once a woman discovered she was pregnant. Preconception health and lifestyle for women and their partners is a topic being discussed now more than ever before, as more women and men delay having babies or are struggling to conceive. New evidence points to the preconception period as being increasingly important in contributing to a healthy pregnancy outcome for both the woman and child.

Conception outcomes have a wide range, from women struggling to conceive, to women having twins, triplets, and multiples. **Assisted reproductive technology (ART)**, such as the use of fertility medication, artificial insemination, in vitro fertilization, and surrogacy, has been successful at assisting women who are otherwise unable to become pregnant. The health status and lifestyle of both the mother and her partner prior to conception are key factors in a healthy pregnancy and delivering a healthy baby. Pregnancy for a woman with various health conditions or for women older than age 35 years can often bring multiple health challenges for both the mother and the baby, not to mention a deal of ethical considerations.

The preconception period is a critical, and often overlooked, stage of the reproductive cycle. In this chapter, we will explore the journey to conception, identifying important steps a couple should take to ensure the healthiest pregnancy possible. An unhealthy lifestyle prior to conception may result in infertility and poor outcomes during the pregnancy and may result in persistent health issues that impact the baby for his or her entire life. We will review the physiology of reproduction and discuss the topics of infertility, subfertility, and assisted reproductive technology. Preexisting diseases, such as diabetes, celiac disease, and high blood pressure, as possible contributors to infertility and poor pregnancy outcomes will be discussed. Nutrition recommendations that both men and women should follow during the preconception period are outlined, along with recommendations for supplements. How body weight and lifestyle habits during pregnancy help to determine the health of a pregnancy and pregnancy outcomes are described. Finally, resources that exist to promote a healthy preconception period will be reviewed.

Preconception Period

> **Preview** The preconception period is the time prior to or between pregnancies, and it is an important time for women of childbearing age to be in good health.

Today, many women of childbearing age spend the preconception period in less than optimal health, and therefore they start pregnancies as such. For example, about 31% of pregnant women are obese, about 69% do not take folic acid, and an estimated 3% take medications that are known to cause birth defects.[1] If conception occurs during a time of poor maternal nutrition or health status, the health of the expecting mother, the growth and development of the fetus, and the future health of the offspring may all be compromised. In extreme cases, suboptimal health prior to pregnancy can lead to pregnancy-related complications, such as gestational diabetes and high blood pressure, and may result in infant death or premature birth, with associated birth defects and disability.[2]

The Importance of Having a Plan

The importance of preconception nutrition is validated by the fact that the U.S. Department of Health and Human Services (HHS) has included recommendations on this topic in the Healthy People 2020 goals. One recommendation is that all men and women of reproductive age be encouraged to develop a reproductive life plan. Individuals and couples are encouraged to analyze their overall health, their health habits, their social support, and their mental health prior to making the decision to conceive. The eight main recommendations for a healthy pregnancy are presented in TABLE 2.1 . The overarching goal among these recommendations is to improve the woman's and child's health. Men should also be included in the preconception plan and receive care, because they too are integral to ensuring a healthy pregnancy.

Preconception Care

Within about 8 to 10 days after an ovum is fertilized, it implants into the uterine wall and embryo development begins. The time prior to conception represents an important and critical period when nutrition and other exposures can affect conception, maintenance of the pregnancy, and development, growth, and future health of the offspring.[4] The Centers for Disease Control and Prevention (CDC) identifies **preconception health care** as the medical care a woman or man receives from the doctor or other health professionals that focuses on the parts

Table 2.1

Recommendations to Improve Preconception Health[3]

1. Individual Responsibility Across the Life Span	Adult men and women should have a reproductive life plan.
2. Consumer Awareness	Increase public awareness of the importance of preconception health behaviors and preconception care services available.
3. Preventive Visits	Provide risk assessment and health promotion education to all women of childbearing age.
4. Interconception Care	Use the time between pregnancies to provide additional interventions and education to women who have had a previous pregnancy that ended in an adverse outcome.
5. Prepregnancy Checkup	Offer, as a component of maternity care, one prepregnancy visit for couples and persons planning pregnancy.
6. Health Insurance Coverage for Women with Low Income	Increase health insurance coverage for women with low incomes to improve access to preventive women's health and preconception and interconception care.
7. Public Health Programs and Strategies	Integrate components of preconception health into existing local public health and related programs.
8. Monitoring Improvements	Maximize research mechanisms to monitor preconception health.

Modified from Healthy People 2020 Recommendations to Improve Preconception Health

of health that have been shown to increase the chance of having a healthy baby. This care encompasses the biomedical, behavioral, and social health interventions provided to women and couples prior to conception. Because of individual and unique needs, preconception health care differs for every person. A doctor or other healthcare professional should suggest a course of treatment or follow-up care as needed. Research shows that women who receive care prior to pregnancy have improvements in many significant areas, including increased folic acid intake, being current on important vaccinations, less weight gain at the beginning of their pregnancy, and fewer complications for both mother and baby.[5]

In the past, nutrition during preconception and interconception periods has been overlooked. However, today healthcare professionals use a framework that has been developed to counsel, provide care, and monitor the mother so that the health of the mother and the child in the short and long terms will be improved. Research suggests that if medical, behavioral, and social health issues are addressed prior to conception, all of society will feel the benefits. Ideally, preconception care should begin at least 3 months before a woman becomes pregnant. Such care can help individuals be in the best health possible prior to pregnancy. Optimal health before pregnancy results in fewer pregnancy complications and fewer babies born preterm or with low birth weight.

The Academy of Nutrition and Dietetics asserts "Women of childbearing age should adopt a lifestyle optimizing health and reducing risk of birth defects, suboptimal fetal development and chronic health problems in both mother and child."*

---

* Kaiser LL, Campbell CG; Academy Positions Committee Workgroup. Practice paper of the Academy of Nutrition and Dietetics abstract: nutrition and lifestyle for a healthy pregnancy outcome. S J Acad Nutr Diet. 2014 Sep;114(9):1447.

Let's Discuss

Research on general practitioners reveals that they face multiple barriers to providing preconception care. Some are time constraints, lack of preconception visits, competing priorities when women and couples do come in for a visit, cost of care, and lack of resources. How could practitioners encourage more women and couples to attend preconception visits?

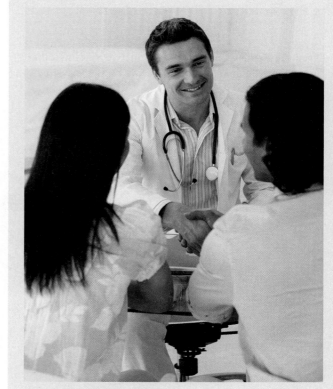

©Wavebreakmedia/Shutterstock

Case Study

Suzanne and her husband have decided that they want to start a family as soon as possible. She is aware that with older age comes increased risk of complications in pregnancy. Additionally, Suzanne really wants to have at least three children.

Questions

1. Would you recommend Suzanne visit her doctor for a preconception appointment?
2. List at least five different areas her health practitioner should assess as part of Suzanne's preconception care.

Recap Women and men of childbearing age should have a reproductive plan to ensure their health and the health of their babies are optimal. Entering pregnancy in optimal health has been shown to reduce poor pregnancy outcomes for both woman and child. Practitioners should be thorough in their assessment of men and women of childbearing age, as the benefits of improved maternal and infant health benefit all of society.

1. List two reasons preconception care is recommended for women who are of childbearing age.
2. Describe the three components of preconception care.

The Physiology of Reproduction

Preview Female and male reproductive systems differ greatly. A woman is born with all the eggs she will ever have—between 1 and 2 million eggs—and she will release about 500 during her reproductive life. Males, on the other hand, can generate millions of new sperm daily. Hormones that play roles in reproduction differ between the sexes as well.

Female Reproductive System and Hormones

The main components of female reproductive anatomy include ovaries, fallopian tubes, cervix, uterus, and vagina. Ovaries are the two small reproductive glands on either side of the uterus that produce hormones that regulate female secondary sex characteristics as well as house the ova (eggs). The fallopian tubes are a pair of long, slender ducts in the female abdomen that transport ova from the ovary to the uterus and, in fertilization, transport sperm cells from the uterus to the released ova. The cervix is the lower part of the uterus that is connected to the vagina. The uterus is the organ where a fetus develops; the upper part is called the corpus and the lower part, the cervix. The vagina is the canal that connects the cervix to the outside of the body and is the site for the delivery of the baby. See **FIGURE 2.1** for an image of the female reproductive system.

The menstrual cycle, which typically lasts about 28 days, is divided into two distinct phases. The first half is called the follicular stage, and the second is the luteal stage. Four major hormones are involved in the female menstrual cycle: follicle-stimulating hormone (FSH), luteinizing hormone (LH), estrogen, and progesterone. How the hormones vary during the cycle is presented in **FIGURE 2.2**.

During the follicular phase, the brain releases FSH and LH, which travel to the ovaries. In the ovaries, they stimulate 15 to 20 eggs to grow, each in its own follicle. Estrogen levels also rise in response to the increase in FSH and LH, and once enough estrogen is released, FSH

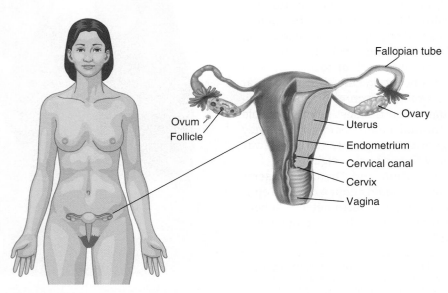

Figure 2.1
The female reproductive system.

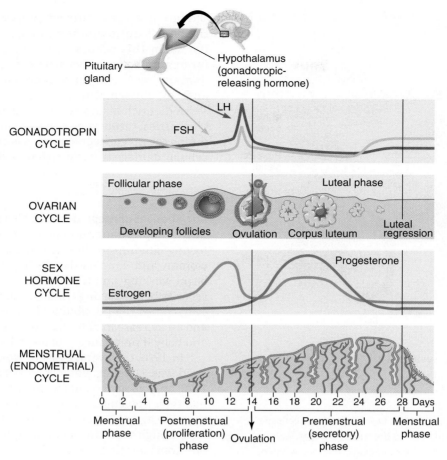

Figure 2.2
Female menstrual cycle hormones.

is turned off, limiting the number of follicles that mature. One follicle becomes dominant and continues to mature, and eventually the others die.

The luteal phase typically begins halfway through the 28-day cycle, or 14 days after the follicular phase began. Estrogen from the dominant follicle stimulates the release of LH by the brain, which causes the follicle to release its egg from the ovary. The egg is captured by the fallopian tubes in the process known as ovulation. The empty follicle becomes the corpus luteum, which secretes progesterone. The progesterone readies the uterus for a fertilized egg if one has been fertilized by sperm. If the egg is not fertilized, the egg passes through the uterus, and the lining of the uterus breaks down and is released, a process known as menstruation.

Male Reproductive System and Hormones
The male reproductive system differs in many ways from the female system. To begin with, the main structures, including the penis, scrotum, and testes, are outside of the body. The penis is the organ used in intercourse and is the site of the release of semen. The scrotum is a small

sack behind the penis that houses the testes. The testes have two roles: to produce testosterone and to create sperm. The sperm move into the epididymis, where they remain until they mature. Millions of sperm can be generated each day, but they take roughly 70 days to reach maturity. Once sperm mature, they move into the vas deferens until they are released into the urethra via the ejaculatory ducts. The urethra also carries urine from the bladder; however, when a man ejaculates, only sperm is secreted. Other important structures include the seminal vesicles, which attach to the vas deferens and provide fructose and fluid to feed and make the sperm mobile, and the prostate gland, which also provides a source of fluid to help the sperm move. **FIGURE 2.3** presents a diagram of the male reproductive system.

Three major hormones are involved in the male reproductive system: follicle-stimulating hormone (FSH), luteinizing hormone (LH), and testosterone. FSH makes sperm in a process called spermatogenesis. LH is responsible for making testosterone, which is also necessary for forming sperm. Finally, testosterone is necessary for the development of male characteristics.

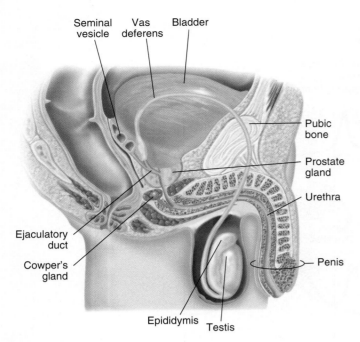

Figure 2.3
The male reproductive system.

Recap In human reproduction, two kinds of sex cells are involved: the egg in females, and the sperm in males. Various hormones control aspects of reproduction in men and women.

1. How do male and female reproductive systems differ?
2. Taking into account how long it takes for sperm to mature, if a man was trying to get healthy prior to conceiving, how many months should he wait to conceive to ensure the healthiest sperm?

Infertility, Subfertility, and Assisted Reproductive Technology

Preview According to the American Society of Reproductive Medicine, infertility in the United States affects about 10–15% of couples. Although couples cannot control all of the causes of infertility, causes related to preconception nutrition can be minimized or avoided. With emphasis on maintaining a healthy weight and choosing foods that create a safe and supportive environment in which a baby can develop and grow, couples may improve their chances of conception.

Antioxidants

Antioxidants protect the cells of the reproductive system from oxidative stress and therefore play an important role in the fertility of both men and women.

Oxidative stress occurs when free radicals outnumber the body's antioxidant defenses. In relation to fertility, when this occurs in the testicular environment, for example, oxidative stress may lead to sperm DNA damage, resulting in a decrease in sperm mobility and cell abnormalities.[6]

A diet rich in antioxidants, such as one that includes blueberries, raspberries, nuts, and dark green vegetables, during the preconception period is critical to help ward off cellular damage resulting from oxidative stress.

Age

Age at onset of pregnancy can also have an effect on fertility and pregnancy outcomes. In our society, instead of having children in their late teens and early 20s, many women and couples decide to finish their education, begin working, and try to achieve some type of financial security before having children. Along with waiting, however, comes the possibility of difficulty getting pregnant and an increase in potential adverse outcomes for mother and baby if pregnancy is achieved.

In 1970, the average age of women having their first child was 21 years, whereas in 2013, it was 26 years.[7] In 1970, only about 1 in 100 women older than the age of 30 had their first child. Currently, about 20% of women older than the age of 35 conceive their first child.[8]

Though there are advantages to delaying conception, one consideration is the risk of infertility or subfertility and possibly fewer offspring than desired. Infertility is defined as the inability to get pregnant after 12 or more months of regular unprotected sexual intercourse. Subfertility is any period of reduced fertility when conception is desired. Delaying childbearing increases the risk of conception problems such as fewer and lower-quality eggs, eggs not released, increase in health conditions that affect female fertility, and increased risk of miscarriage.[9]

There are a variety of non-nutrition-related ways to increase fertility. Using medication to improve the quality of ovulation and therefore pregnancy rate is one popular choice.

A very sophisticated response to the challenges of infertility has been the increased use of assisted reproductive technology (ART). **FIGURE 2.4** describes ART. ART is any treatment or procedure that uses in vitro technology with oocytes (immature ova or egg cells from the female), sperm, or embryos.

In ART, the ovaries are stimulated through medications to produce multiple eggs, then the eggs are surgically removed and fertilized in a lab, and, finally, the embryo is transferred back into the woman. Since 1978, when the first baby was born through in vitro fertilization, the use of ART has risen dramatically. Babies born through ART comprise 1.5% of all babies born in the United States.[10] Although this technology is miraculous for couples who otherwise would not be able to conceive, there is concern

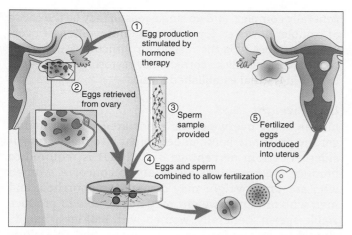

Figure 2.4
Assisted reproductive technology (ART) as seen in in vitro fertilization.

① Egg production stimulated by hormone therapy

② Eggs retrieved from ovary

③ Sperm sample provided

④ Eggs and sperm combined to allow fertilization

⑤ Fertilized eggs introduced into uterus

that ART pregnancies that result in twin and multiple fetuses put the woman and offspring at greater risk of adverse outcomes.[11]

Let's Discuss

Many women and couples are waiting longer to conceive. As we've discussed, this puts the woman and baby at increased risk of health problems during the pregnancy, and even after the birth. One solution that has been identified is harvesting a woman's eggs when she is younger and freezing them for later fertilization and implantation. The process is costly and there is no guarantee of the quality of the eggs after the freezing process. A couple of questions to consider: do you think women who are approaching 35 years of age, the age at which the risks to the woman and baby drastically increase in pregnancy, should be encouraged to get pregnant sooner to reduce potential health problems? Or should they be encouraged to freeze their eggs if they are not yet ready to conceive?

Recap Women today are conceiving later in life, which contributes to lower fertility rates. As a response, ART is one solution. ART works for many women but may put women and babies at risk for adverse outcomes.

1. Give one example of how oxidative stress can contribute to infertility.
2. Describe three ways being older affects a woman's ability to become pregnant.
3. What is the definition of infertility?

Common Health Conditions

Preview A variety of preexisting health conditions and environmental issues may impair fertility in both males and females. These conditions may also cause issues once a woman becomes pregnant. It is advisable for women and men with prior health conditions to be under a physician's care when trying to become pregnant. Fortunately, for many conditions, helpful interventions have been found.

Endometriosis

Endometriosis is a condition found in 5–10% of women. This condition occurs when the lining of the uterus, called the endometrium, grows outside of the uterine cavity. The tissue often grows on the ovaries and fallopian tubes. It can be painful for some women, and others are unaware that they even have the condition. When a woman menstruates, the endometrial tissues grows and bleeds but is unable to be released, which often results in the formation of scar tissue and development of cysts. Endometriosis can only be diagnosed through laparoscopy. Treatment for this condition varies but generally includes pain medication, hormones such as those found in contraceptives, removal of the endometrial tissues through surgery, or, in severe cases, a hysterectomy. It is likely that endometriosis leads to infertility because the endometrium may block the egg or not allow the egg and sperm to unite.

Body Weight and Fertility

There is wide agreement that body weight affects fertility and health. Epidemiological data confirm that both obesity and low body weight each accounts for 6% of primary infertility; that is, 12% of primary infertility results from deviations in body weight (either high or low body weight) from established norms.[12] Infertility caused by weight extremes is generally a result of altered hormone levels that negatively affect ovulation.

Overweight

Given the detrimental influence of maternal overweight and obesity on reproductive and pregnancy outcomes for the mother and child, the position of the Academy of Nutrition and Dietetics is that all overweight and obese women of reproductive age should receive counseling on the roles of diet and physical activity in reproductive health prior to pregnancy, during pregnancy, and in between pregnancies.[13] Weight is often measured and defined as body mass index, or BMI. BMI is a mathematical formula determined by dividing a person's weight in kilograms by his or her height in meters squared. There are four main categories of BMI: underweight, normal weight, overweight, and obese (see TABLE 2.2).

Table 2.2	
BMI Categories	
BMI	**Weight Status**
Below 18.5	Underweight
18.5 – 24.9	Normal or Healthy Weight
25.0 – 29.9	Overweight
30.0 and Above	Obese

Reproduced from CDC. About Adult BMI. Retrieved from: https://www.cdc.gov/healthyweight/assessing/bmi/adult_bmi/. Accessed on 9/27/16.

Although, in some instances, being overweight or obese has no negative effects on fertility, it is associated with contributing to a variety of fertility issues and can have a negative impact on the baby once conception is achieved.

BMI in the obese range may lead to irregular menstrual cycles and irregular ovulation, causing conception to be difficult or delayed.[14] There also seems to be a strong association between obesity and insulin resistance, which is thought to reduce fertility.[15] Obesity is a strong risk factor for polycystic ovary syndrome, which results in menstrual irregularities and chronic anovulation,[16] or failure of the ovary to release an egg over time, usually 3 months or longer. The central distribution of fat, as measured by waist-to-hip ratio, is also related to reproductive functioning, with higher rates of infertility associated with higher waist-to-hip ratios.[17] In addition, obese women have a higher chance of delivering by cesarean section, increased risk of some birth defects, and higher chance of having a high-birth weight baby.[18]

There is some evidence of an association between maternal overweight or obesity and decreased rates of breastfeeding. Specifically, a high BMI before conception has been shown to be inversely related to the successful initiation of breastfeeding, the duration of lactation, and the amount of milk produced.[19] Such results show the importance of encouraging women to start pregnancy with a healthy BMI in an effort to increase the chances of successful breastfeeding.[20]

Obesity affects male fertility as well. Evidence suggests that obesity reduces sperm quality, in particular, altering the physical and molecular structure of germ cells in the testes and ultimately mature sperm.[21] Also concerning is evidence that shows that male obesity impairs offspring metabolic and reproductive health, suggesting that paternal health cues are transmitted to the next generation with sperm as the mediator.[21] The good news is that studies also show that simple diet and exercise interventions can be used to reverse the damaging effects of obesity on sperm function.

How much weight loss is necessary to improve the possibility of conception? Studies suggest that even a modest loss of 5–10% of body weight can restore ovulation, and therefore increase fertility.[22] Fertility issues are generally complex, and no single reason may be the cause of trouble; however, for both men and women, if overweight or obesity is the reason for difficulties with conception, it can likely be corrected by restoring body weight to within normal established limits.

Underweight

Just as being overweight is associated with difficulty getting pregnant, being underweight also has its downsides. A certain percentage of body fat is required to produce the hormones necessary to conceive. Women who are underweight may develop amenorrhea, and men who are underweight may not be able to produce viable sperm. Generally, women with BMI less than 19 should be encouraged to gain weight, and this alone often increases fertility or makes hormone therapy more successful.

Let's Discuss

The rates of obesity among men and women have been discussed. Being obese makes it harder to get pregnant, and research suggests even small amounts of weight loss can help increase the odds of becoming pregnant. Should a woman or couple seeking fertility treatment through a clinic be asked first to try to lose weight rather than beginning more invasive and costly treatments?

Eating Disorders

Bulimia nervosa, anorexia nervosa, and binge eating disorder are common eating disorders that can affect many women during their childbearing years. One side effect of eating disorders, particularly of anorexia nervosa, is fertility problems. **TABLE 2.3** reviews common eating disorders and their characteristics. Some studies indicate a higher prevalence of eating disorders in women undergoing fertility treatment.[23]

Amenorrhea as a consequence of an eating disorder may lead to the belief that pregnancy is not possible, therefore increasing risk for unplanned pregnancy. Women with a past or current eating disorder are more likely to report having unplanned pregnancies.

Women with an active eating disorder or a history of eating disorders would likely benefit from psychological counseling prior to becoming pregnant. Counseling may also help address possible depression and feelings about how the body will change as a result of being pregnant.

Polycystic Ovary Syndrome

Polycystic ovary syndrome (PCOS) is a hormonal imbalance that affects women, making it difficult for them to become pregnant. PCOS is the most common endocrine

Table 2.3

Comparing Characteristics of Eating Disorders

	Body weight	Eating tendency	View of body image	Physical indications	Emotional expression	Interactions with others
Anorexia	Underweight with BMI < 17.5	Limited calorie intake, may have unusual food rituals and limit variety of foods eaten	Obsessed with weight and appearance, viewing the body as overweight	Extreme weight loss, low blood pressure, heart problems, kidney problems, hair loss, fine and thin hair over parts of the body, weakness, fatigue, nutritional deficiencies, cessation of menstruation	Depression, anxiety, obsessive-compulsive behaviors, denial of a problem, fear of gaining weight	Withdrawn, may refuse to eat in front of others
Bulimia	Generally normal weight or overweight	Eats a large amount of food in a short period of time, followed by purging by vomiting and/or using laxatives	Obsessed with weight and appearance	Changes in weight, ulcers, sores in the mouth, core throat, dehydration, dental problems, weakness, fatigue	Depression, anxiety, feeling of guilt, self-destructive behavior	May be withdrawn, but able to develop relationships with others
Binge Eating Disorder	Usually overweight	Eats a large amount of food in a short period of time. Does not purge, however, may restrict food in between binges	Generally is overly focused on weight and appearance	Excessive weight gain, high blood pressure, diabetes, joint pain, fatigue	Depression, feeling of guilt or self-hatred	May be withdrawn, may seem overly sensitive

disorder in women: nearly 1 in 8 women worldwide suffers from it.[24] PCOS is also the number one reason a woman may have trouble achieving conception. When a woman with PCOS does become pregnant, she is at higher risk for gestational diabetes, high blood pressure during her pregnancy, and babies born smaller than typical for their gestational age.[25]

Why a woman gets PCOS is not fully understood, but almost all women with the condition have cysts on their ovaries. In addition, women with PCOS begin to produce the male sex hormones, called androgens. The result is anovulation, facial hair growth, and acne. **TABLE 2.4** shows the common symptoms of PCOS. Insulin is also affected, with the body producing increased amounts of insulin that it may not be able to use. Over time, this increase in insulin can cause diabetes. Because it is a syndrome, and not a disease, women do not need to have all the symptoms of PCOS to be diagnosed. Diagnosis involves having amenorrhea, or the abnormal absence of menstruation, having high levels of androgens, and having cysts on the ovaries.

Taking a medication commonly prescribed for diabetes treatment called metformin (also known as Glucophage) appears to help women with PCOS, especially obese women, to become pregnant; however, use of metformin has been related to the risk of malabsorption of vitamin B_{12}, which may result in anemia. One suggested dietary treatment of PCOS, which also addresses a factor of obesity, is a decrease in consumption of foods that cause insulin to increase, such as carbohydrates, including dairy. However, whether changing diet to reduce carbohydrates and other foods that cause insulin spikes increases fertility rates has not yet been determined.

Table 2.4

Common Symptoms of Polycystic Ovary Syndrome

Menstrual problems	Hair loss from the scalp	Fertility problems or repeat miscarriages	Depression or mood swings
Acne, oily skin, or dandruff	Hair growth on the face, chest, back, stomach, thumbs, or toes	Insulin resistance and too much insulin, which can contribute to obesity	Breathing problems while sleeping
Cysts on the ovaries	Weight gain or obesity, especially around the waist	Skin tags	Pelvic pain

Reproduced from Office on Women's Health, U.S. Department of Health and Human Services. Polycystic ovary syndrome (PCOS). Retrieved from: http://www.womenshealth.gov/publications/our-publications/fact-sheet/polycystic-ovary-syndrome.html#d. Accessed: January 12, 2016.

Case Study

When she was a teenager, Suzanne was told that she had polycystic ovary syndrome and may have trouble getting pregnant. Sure enough, after trying for a year, Suzanne is disappointed that she is unable to conceive. She is contemplating using assisted reproductive therapy (ART) but knows that it is expensive and doesn't guarantee she will get pregnant.

Questions

1. Why might she have trouble getting pregnant?
2. What medications may be helpful to her in getting pregnant?
3. What lifestyle modifications may be helpful to her?

Diabetes

Diabetes rates have increased dramatically in the United States and in women of childbearing age. There are two types of diabetes, type 1 and type 2. **TABLE 2.5** describes the types of diabetes; elsewhere in the text, gestational diabetes, which can occur during pregnancy, is discussed. Diabetes that is poorly controlled can contribute to a host of health problems, including infertility, in both men and women. Glucose control is important for successful fertility because chronic high blood glucose levels affect hormone levels, including levels of estrogen, progesterone, and testosterone.

Studies suggest that men with diabetes are twice as likely to suffer from low testosterone than are men without diabetes. Less testosterone means fewer healthy sperm. Men with diabetes benefit from having their blood sugar under control prior to attempting to conceive.

Table 2.5

Comparison of Type 1 and Type 2 Diabetes Mellitus

Feature	Type 1 Diabetes	Type 2 Diabetes
Onset	Sudden	Gradual
Age at onset	Any age, but mostly in young children up to teenage years	Most common in adults
Body type	Generally thin or normal	Often obese
Presence of endogenous insulin	Low or absent	Normal, decreased, or increased
Prevalence	~10% of all individuals with diabetes in the United States	~90–95% of all individuals with diabetes in the United States

Data from American Diabetes Association. Retrieved from: http://www.diabetes.org

Following dietary recommendations is key to diabetes management for both men and women. The type of diabetes dictates the best diet prescription. However, carbohydrate counting tends to be a generally effective strategy regardless of diabetes type. Carbohydrate counting is a menu-planning strategy for which a person is allotted a specific number of grams of carbohydrates per day, which are divided into meals and snacks. Proteins and healthy fats are encouraged, and consumption of specific rates of the three macronutrients is designed to keep blood sugar within a healthy range.

Individuals with existing diabetes who are trying to conceive should be made aware that tightly regulating their blood sugar is critically important in assisting with becoming pregnant and for their future health and the health of their baby. Seeing a registered dietitian to help formulate a diet during the preconception period is highly recommended.

Celiac Disease

Celiac disease is an autoimmune disorder that occurs when the body is unable to absorb the protein gluten, which is found in wheat, barley, rye, and sometimes oats. If wheat, barley, and rye are consumed, damage is done to the intestinal lining, putting a person at risk for many issues, including anemia, bone problems, and cancer. Because of the damaged small intestine, a number of critical nutrients may not be well absorbed. Celiac disease has also been linked to infertility.[26] In addition, some studies indicate that in celiac patients, the risk of miscarriage, low birth weight, and preterm delivery is significantly higher compared with that in nonceliac patients.[27]

It is hypothesized that fertility may be affected among men and women with celiac disease because of poor absorption of key nutrients, but the exact mechanism is not known. In addition, women with celiac often suffer increased spontaneous abortion and premature delivery.[28] Successful treatment for a person with celiac disease, or any gluten sensitivity, is to eliminate foods that contain gluten. **FIGURE 2.5** shows how the U.S. Department of Agriculture's (USDA) MyPlate can be used for those who choose to eliminate gluten from their diet.

Treatment with a gluten-free diet in those with celiac disease reduces the risks of infertility and all other negative outcomes to the same level as seen in individuals without celiac disease.[27] Because women with celiac disease may not absorb a number of critical nutrients well, it is important that prior to becoming pregnant, blood levels of vitamins and minerals be tested and supplementation began if necessary. Some physicians also believe that in women who suffer from infertility, checking for undiagnosed celiac disease is a reasonable strategy.

Hypertension

Along with obesity rates, the rates of high blood pressure, or hypertension, have also increased. In the United States, an estimated 7.3% of women of childbearing age have high blood pressure.[29] If a woman enters a

The Gluten-Free Diet Plate

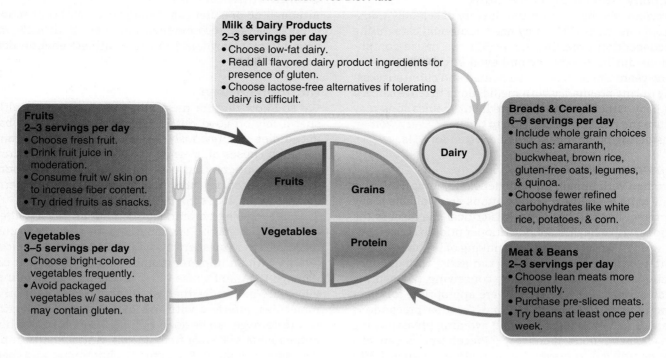

Milk & Dairy Products
2–3 servings per day
- Choose low-fat dairy.
- Read all flavored dairy product ingredients for presence of gluten.
- Choose lactose-free alternatives if tolerating dairy is difficult.

Fruits
2–3 servings per day
- Choose fresh fruit.
- Drink fruit juice in moderation.
- Consume fruit w/ skin on to increase fiber content.
- Try dried fruits as snacks.

Vegetables
3–5 servings per day
- Choose bright-colored vegetables frequently.
- Avoid packaged vegetables w/ sauces that may contain gluten.

Breads & Cereals
6–9 servings per day
- Include whole grain choices such as: amaranth, buckwheat, brown rice, gluten-free oats, legumes, & quinoa.
- Choose fewer refined carbohydrates like white rice, potatoes, & corn.

Meat & Beans
2–3 servings per day
- Choose lean meats more frequently.
- Purchase pre-sliced meats.
- Try beans at least once per week.

Figure 2.5
MyPlate gluten-free diet plate.
Reproduced from ChooseMyPlate.gov.

News You Can Use

Many people today are eliminating gluten from their diets for a variety of reasons. Some have celiac disease, and gluten must be eliminated or else they will suffer from a variety of health issues. People are also experimenting with eliminating gluten for other reasons, including suspected gluten intolerance. For those who are trying to see whether they have issues with gluten, removing it from their diet may be a good idea. For people who have caught on to the gluten-free craze as a way to be healthier, removing gluten from the diet actually may backfire. Research suggests that for the majority of people, eating gluten free can mean a less healthy overall diet with lower amounts of vitamins, minerals, and fiber than is ideal. Gluten-free products can also cost more. It is important not to get swept up with current nutrition trends and to, instead, check websites that offer unbiased information to ensure a healthy approach to eating.

pregnancy with hypertension, her frequency of experiencing preeclampsia is 17% to 25% while she is pregnant compared with a rate of 3% to 5% in women without prior high blood pressure.[30] Preeclampsia is a condition in which high blood pressure and protein in the urine occur and can lead to fetal growth restriction. This will be discussed in more detail in Chapter 3.

Fortunately, if a woman adopts a healthy diet with lower sodium and ample fruits and vegetables following the recommended DASH diet (Dietary Approaches to Stop Hypertension), her blood pressure can be lowered and the likelihood of future problems reduced. TABLE 2.6 shows the DASH diet foods and recommended amounts that are helpful in reducing blood pressure.

Table 2.6

Daily and Weekly DASH Eating Plan Goals for a 2,000-Calorie-a-Day Diet

Food Group	Daily Servings
Grains	6–8
Meats, poultry, and fish	6 or less
Vegetables	4–5
Fruit	4–5
Low-fat or fat-free dairy products	2–3
Fats and oils	2–3
Sodium	2,300 mg*
	Weekly Servings
Nuts, seeds, dry beans, and peas	4–5
Sweets	5 or less

*1,500 milligrams (mg) sodium lowers blood pressure even further than 2,300 mg sodium daily.

Reproduced from National Heart, Lung, and Blood Institute. Description of the DASH eating plan. Retrieved from: https://www.nhlbi.nih.gov/health/health-topics/topics/dash. Accessed January 12, 2016.

Sexually Transmitted Infections

A woman who has a current or history of sexually transmitted infections (STIs) may need additional care during preconception time. Having an STI can cause complications during pregnancy and even affect the baby for many years. Some STIs can be treated and cured successfully during pregnancy with medications that are safe for the baby. Others cannot be cured, but medications may reduce the risk of transmission to the baby. Every woman considering pregnancy should be tested for STIs.

Human Immunodeficiency Virus

A woman with human immunodeficiency virus (HIV) may want to have children. Many options are available today to protect her and her child. It is critical she discuss the options with a healthcare practitioner prior to conceiving. For women with HIV who are thinking of becoming pregnant, preconception counseling can assist with: (1) optimizing maternal health prior to conceiving, (2) ensuring medications taken to treat HIV are appropriate for pregnancy, and (3) alerting the woman to other precautions she will need to take, including avoiding breastfeeding and choosing mode of delivery.[31] Preconception care can also be utilized to prevent unplanned pregnancies. HIV testing should be recommended to all women as part of preconception care.

> **Recap** A wide variety of health conditions can make it harder for a woman to get pregnant and have a healthy pregnancy. Some of these chronic conditions can also affect men. What is most important to remember is that having a chronic condition does not mean that pregnancy is not achievable or that the outcome will be poor. However, people may need to take steps before trying to conceive to decrease the risks that may result from specific conditions.
>
> 1. How do body weight extremes such as being underweight or obese generally affect fertility?
> 2. How common is celiac disease? How does having celiac impair fertility and cause trouble during pregnancy?
> 3. What steps should a man or woman with an STI or HIV take prior to becoming pregnant?

Nutrition Recommendations During Preconception

> **Preview** The nutrition recommendations for women and men trying to conceive are similar in many ways to the Dietary Guidelines for Americans for healthy adults, with a few notable exceptions. In general, women need extra folate, iron, and DHA (an omega-3 fatty acid), and, for men, zinc and antioxidants are important micronutrients to focus on during the preconception period.

Overall Nutrition Plan

Although no one diet can ensure successful conception, general dietary recommendations help both men and women enter pregnancy in the healthiest environment possible.

Nutrition for Men

We do know that for men, a healthy body and healthy sperm rely on good nutrition choices, including a balanced diet. As previously discussed, some of the most common causes of sperm-related infertility result from health conditions that contribute to low sperm count, slow-moving sperm, abnormal shape and size of sperm, and problems with semen.

Unfavorable environmental conditions can also affect the quality of sperm. The environment alone can cause oxidative stress on sperm. Oxidation creates free radicals (atoms with an unpaired number of electrons) that can damage DNA and cause other problems. **Antioxidants**, which are molecules that inhibit the oxidation of other molecules, interfere with this oxidative chain reaction before damage can be done. **FIGURE 2.6** demonstrates how antioxidants scavenge free radicals. Antioxidants in the diet, such as vitamin E, vitamin C, glutathione, and coenzyme Q10, can boost fertility.[32]

In addition, identifying any environmental and occupational factors that are harming sperm is warranted. Studies suggest that exposure to heavy metals, pesticides, heat, and radiation can damage and diminish sperm production. The mineral zinc is an important component of sperm development and number. Men with infertility have been found to have reduced amounts of zinc compared with those men free of infertility issues.[33] Zinc is a powerful antioxidant, and taken in supplement form, not to exceed the U.S. Department of Agriculture (USDA) Tolerable Upper Intake Level (UL), appears to be safe and may support increasing fertility in men.

Folate status may affect male fertility as well, and higher levels of dietary folate intake are related to fewer chromosomally abnormal sperm compared with the sperm of men with lower intakes of folate.[34] Another interesting but controversial nutrient for men is soy. Soy contains

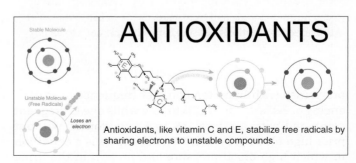

Antioxidants, like vitamin C and E, stabilize free radicals by sharing electrons to unstable compounds.

Figure 2.6
Antioxidants can help scavenge free radicals.

isoflavones, which are similar in structure and function to estrogens and may disrupt the body's natural hormonal balance. More research needs to be conducted before advising men to avoid soy products; however, like for all foods, a moderate soy intake appears to be a good strategy. In addition, alcohol consumption in males prior to pregnancy may cause infertility by affecting male reproductive hormones and impairing sperm.[35] In men, smoking can cause impotence and erectile dysfunction in addition to harming sperm.[36]

See TABLE 2.7 for nutrition and lifestyle guidelines for males to ensure optimal sperm health.

For a number of years, research has focused on how age and lifestyle can affect molecules that control gene function in women, which ultimately can affect pregnancy outcomes; however, research also links some of these same effects with males. For instance, there is evidence that advanced paternal age permanently changes the socialization patterns of offspring in an animal study; [37] this association has been seen among older men resulting in higher risk of their children being born with schizophrenia and autism. Paternal obesity has been associated with enlarged fat cells, diabetes, and obesity among offspring.[38] In addition, fathers' alcohol use is also linked to lower birth weight and brain size and reduced cognitive function, all of which are symptoms of fetal alcohol spectrum disorder (FASD).[39] More research must be conducted before the link between fathers and birth defects can be translated into practical advice; however, it seems reasonable that

personal choices of males can affect offspring just as those of females do.

Nutrition for Women

Even though one way of eating may not work for everyone, some dietary practices in general can help or harm a woman's chances of becoming pregnant. An interesting study using data from nurses found that certain dietary practices, such as eating a high-carbohydrate diet, eating foods with high glycemic index, or eating a diet high in saturated fat, were associated with difficulty getting pregnant. Women in this study who consumed a multivitamin and iron supplement and plant protein rather than animal protein had a lower risk of ovulatory infertility.[40]

Folic Acid

One of the most important nutrients for a woman to consume prior to becoming pregnant is folic acid. Folic acid, which is also called folate, is a B vitamin that helps to produce and maintain each cell in the body, including red blood cells. Folate also supports DNA synthesis. Folate is necessary for the neural tube to develop into the brain and spinal cord. The critical time for this development is from days 17 to 30 after conception, a time when many women may not even be aware that they are pregnant. Furthermore, nearly half of pregnancies in the United States are unplanned, leaving these women at greater risk of adverse effects related to low folic acid intake. Each year, about 3,000 women deliver babies with neural tube defects. The two most common include anencephaly, which occurs when the upper end of the neural tube does not close, so no brain develops, and spina bifida, which occurs when the spinal cord fails to close.

Fortunately, ample folic acid intake in the early days of pregnancy and during the first trimester can prevent many neural tube defects. Folic acid is so important that, in 1998, the U.S. government mandated folate be added to commonly consumed grain foods, such as breakfast cereals, grits, noodles, and breads. Fortification has resulted in an overall decline in the percentage of children born with neural tube defects; however, a recent U.S.-based study indicates that the previous prediction of a 28% decline in neural tube defects since fortification began may actually be more modest.[41]

How much folic acid is enough? The folic acid that is found in foods is referred to as folate. See TABLE 2.8 for a list of foods that contain folate.

How can a woman ensure she is getting enough folic acid? All women should be advised to maintain a folate-rich diet. Women can generally meet 100% of estimated folic acid needs by consuming a basic diet that includes foods fortified with folate, such as breakfast cereal, and by eating 6 to 8 servings of refined grain products each day. However, even if a woman consumes a healthy diet, all women of reproductive age in whom pregnancy is

---

Table 2.7

Eating and Lifestyle Recommendations to Improve the Health of Sperm

Eating	Lifestyle Choices
Consume 2½ cups of vegetables and 2 cups of fruit each day.	If you drink alcohol, do so in moderation—no more than two drinks per day.
Eat at least half of all grains as whole grains each day (choose whole wheat bread, oatmeal).	Avoid cigarettes and marijuana.
Consume at least 3 servings of low-fat dairy each day.	Obtain or maintain a healthy weight.
Evaluate your red meat intake and cut back as able. Choose leaner protein sources: fish, turkey, chicken, pork. Include vegetable proteins such as beans, nuts, seeds, and tofu.	Exercise 5 days a week for at 30 minutes—extreme exercise has been shown to decrease testosterone, which can lower sperm count.
Limit saturated fats from meats, full-fat dairy products, and fried foods. Replace these with healthy fats such as almonds and avocado.	

Data from Sharol Denny, Academy of Nutrition and Dietetics. How a Man's Diet Affects Fertility Too. November 19, 2014. http://www.eatright.org/resource/health/pregnancy/fertility-and-reproduction/how-a-mans-diet-affects-fertility-too..

Table 2.8

Food Sources of Folic Acid

Fortified cereal	Broccoli	Enriched pasta and bread
Cooked lentils and beans	Great Northern beans	Cantaloupe
Spinach	Asparagus	Eggs
Lettuce (cos, or romaine)	Avocado	Tropical fruits

possible should be advised of folic acid/multivitamin supplementation benefits and should supplement at least 2 to 3 months before conception with 0.4–1.0 mg of folic acid daily as part of a multivitamin.[42]

Supplementation should continue throughout pregnancy and during breastfeeding. This guideline applies to all women who may become pregnant because so many pregnancies are unplanned. Folic acid/multivitamin supplementation is needed to achieve the red blood cell folate levels associated with maximal protection against neural tube defects. If a woman has had a child with a neural tube defect in a prior pregnancy, she should talk to her doctor because her recommended intake of folic acid will likely be higher.

Iron

An iron-rich diet may lower the risk of ovulatory infertility, which is when a woman ovulates rarely or not at all, a cause of infertility that affects 25% of infertile couples.[43] Iron deficiency is a very common nutritional

The Big Picture

Adequate folate intake is crucial during specific stages of embryonic development, including the following:

1. Fertilization of an egg (ovum) with sperm creates a zygote, whose cells divide rapidly. The zygote enters and attaches to the uterus (implantation), becoming a hollow ball of cells called a blastocyst.
2. After implantation, the blastocyst starts to develop the placenta and the amniotic sac that will house the

embryo. This stage of embryo development is when most internal organs and external body structures are formed. Within about 16 days of fertilization, the heart and the major blood vessels begin to develop. Most other organs begin to form about 3 weeks after fertilization. The embryo elongates, and the area that will become the brain and spinal cord (neural tube) begin to develop.

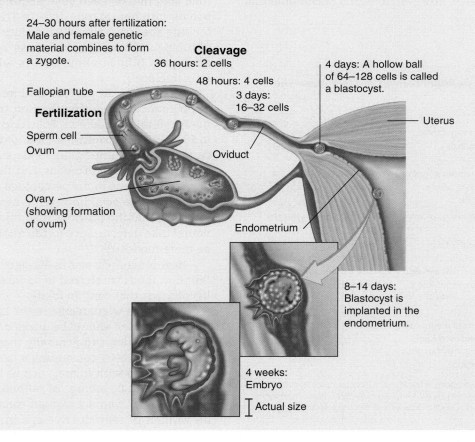

24–30 hours after fertilization: Male and female genetic material combines to form a zygote.

Cleavage
36 hours: 2 cells
48 hours: 4 cells
3 days: 16–32 cells

4 days: A hollow ball of 64–128 cells is called a blastocyst.

Fallopian tube

Fertilization

Sperm cell
Ovum

Oviduct

Uterus

Ovary (showing formation of ovum)

Endometrium

8–14 days: Blastocyst is implanted in the endometrium.

4 weeks: Embryo

Actual size

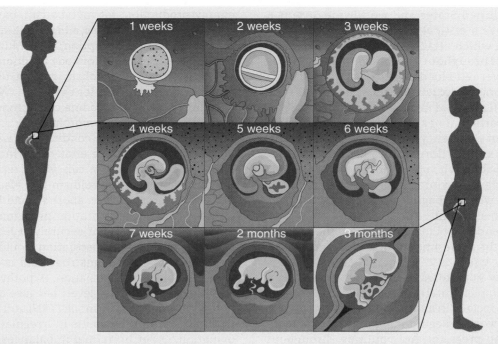

Most birth defects occur during the period when organs are forming. At this time the embryo is most vulnerable to the effects of too little nutrients, such as folic acid, which is essential for spinal cord and brain development. The effects of drugs, radiation, and viruses can also be detrimental during this stage.

3. By the 8th week after fertilization, the embryo is considered a fetus. Structures that have formed grow and develop. By week 12, the fetus fills the entire uterus; by week 14, the sex can be identified; by weeks 16–20, the pregnant woman can feel the fetus move; and by week 24, the fetus has a chance of survival outside of the uterus.

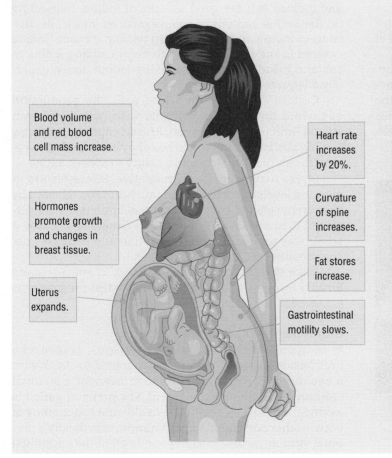

Blood volume and red blood cell mass increase.

Hormones promote growth and changes in breast tissue.

Uterus expands.

Heart rate increases by 20%.

Curvature of spine increases.

Fat stores increase.

Gastrointestinal motility slows.

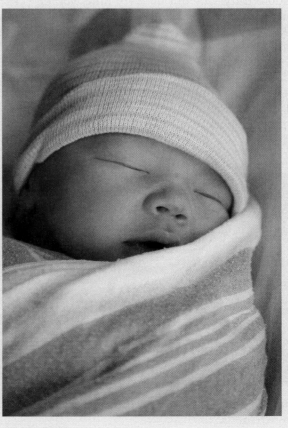

©Steven Blandin/Shutterstock

problem in the United States and worldwide. Iron is a mineral that plays a critical role in creating the protein hemoglobin, which attaches to red blood cells and delivers oxygen throughout the body. In individuals with anemia, fewer red blood cells exist. Although different types of anemia exist, the most common type occurs from a deficiency of iron. Whereas the degree of deficiency is important, it has recently been established that the timing of deficiency is even more important. Women who are anemic during their first trimester of pregnancy have babies who show more delays in development and have behavioral and learning issues.[44] Ensuring that a woman begins pregnancy with adequate iron stores is critical.

The recommended intake of iron during the preconception period is the same amount that is recommended during pregnancy, which is 27 mg per day. If a woman is found to have low iron stores or is already anemic, she may need more supplemental iron. Although iron is found in many foods, especially in animal proteins, it is still recommended that women begin taking iron supplements prior to becoming pregnant and continue throughout pregnancy. Adding vitamin C such as from citrus fruits, bell peppers, or berries to meals enhances iron absorption. **FIGURE 2.7** identifies iron-rich foods.

Iodine

It is widely known that thyroid dysfunction may result in subfertility. One out of every nine women (11%) has thyroid function tests consistent with hypothyroidism,[45] making thyroid dysfunction prevalent among women of reproductive age.

The trace mineral iodine is necessary for proper thyroid function. The thyroid gland needs iodine to manufacture the hormones thyroxine (T_4) and triiodothyronime (T_3). Every cell in the body depends on thyroid hormones for proper regulation of metabolism, blood calcium levels,

energy production, fat metabolism, oxygen utilization, balance among hormones, and weight maintenance. During the time of preconception, proper function of the thyroid gland is necessary for body functions such as proper cell division, cell metabolism, growth, development, and repair of the body and for ovulation. When the thyroid does not have enough iodine owing to iodine deficiency, thyroid functions are compromised.

Hypothyroidism, a condition in which the thyroid gland does not produce enough hormones to keep the body running normally, can affect fertility by inhibiting ovulation. Hypothyroidism can also result in luteal phase problems, such as short second half of the menstrual cycle and implantation problems. When a fertilized egg cannot implant securely, it leaves the body at the same time that menstruation would normally occur, and this passage of menstrual fluid is sometimes mistaken as normal menstruation. Hypothyroidism can also result in high prolactin levels because of elevated levels of thyroid-releasing hormone (TRH) and low levels of thyroxine (T_4), and this results in irregular ovulation or no ovulation. Other hormonal imbalances can result from hypothyroidism, including reduced sex hormone binding globulin (SHBG), estrogen dominance, and progesterone deficiency, all of which interfere with proper reproduction hormone balance.

Iodine may be obtained from drinking water and from foods. In the United States and Canada, seafood and iodized salt are good sources of iodine. Depending on the iodine content of soil, vegetables and fruits also contain iodine. In the United States and Canada, iodine content in the soil is low, and therefore adding iodine to salt and bread is common, making iodine intake generally adequate.

Certain foods can interfere with the production of thyroid hormone. Individuals with hypothyroidism should limit intake of broccoli, Brussels sprouts, cabbage, cauliflower, kale, turnips, and bok choy because these vegetables can block the thyroid's ability to absorb iodine.

Stress management is imperative. Stress results in elevated levels of cortisol, the main hormone released by the adrenal glands. Increased cortisol inhibits the conversion of T_4 to the active T_3. Exercise is beneficial because it stimulates thyroid hormone secretion and increases tissue sensitivity to thyroid hormones.

Once thyroid issues are improved, in some women fertility issues are resolved and successful pregnancy is achieved.

Multivitamins

In addition to eating foods rich in nutrients, women who are considering pregnancy are encouraged to check with a healthcare provider to assess their need for a prenatal vitamin and mineral supplement. The prenatal period is a critical window for the future health and functioning of both mother and child. A multivitamin, specifically a prenatal vitamin, is designed to provide all of the additional

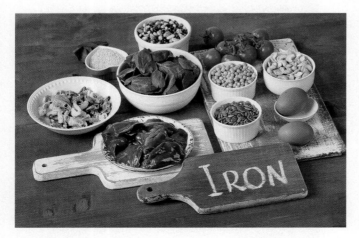

Figure 2.7
Iron-rich foods.

vitamins and minerals a developing baby may need. In general, prenatal vitamins contain many of the same micronutrients found in daily multivitamins, but they usually contain higher levels of folic acid and iron. Many vital organs of a developing fetus are formed by week 10 of pregnancy, so it is important to have all of the essential vitamins and minerals available in advance of conception.

> **Recap** No one eating plan is recommended for all individuals who want to conceive. Women of childbearing age should consider taking supplemental folic acid and iron. Men benefit from a healthy diet and supplementing with zinc and other antioxidants while eliminating environmental exposures that could damage their fertility.
>
> 1. What two nutrients may be important for optimal male fertility?
> 2. Why is it important for women of childbearing age to take a folic acid supplement?
> 3. Describe the importance of iron in pregnancy and why it is important to start out a pregnancy with adequate iron stores.

Lifestyle Habits During Preconception

> **Preview** During the preconception period, it is important for both men and women to avoid certain lifestyle choices. Caffeine consumption, alcohol and recreational drug use, smoking, and use of birth control are all factors that can possibly delay fertility.

Coffee

Coffee and other caffeinated beverages are a common part of many people's daily routines. It was believed that caffeine contributed to miscarriages and low birth weight, but data remain mixed. Today, recommendations on caffeine are for no more than 200 mg per day for women who are pregnant, and this is believed to be a safe recommendation for women who are trying to get pregnant.[46] **FIGURE 2.8** reviews the amount of caffeine in common beverages; it is easy to bypass the 200-mg daily recommendation.

Alcohol and Other Recreational Drugs

Alcohol is a commonly consumed beverage in the United States. In a study, women of childbearing age were asked whether they had consumed alcohol in the 3 months prior to getting pregnant and 50.1% reported that they had.[47] Women who were older than 35 years of age and Caucasian were the most likely to consume alcohol before becoming pregnant.

Alcohol is a known **teratogen** during pregnancy and intake can cause stillbirth, preterm birth, and miscarriage. No amount of alcohol is recommended during pregnancy. For women, no definitive association has been found between moderate drinking and fertility, but there appears to be some evidence to suggest binge or excessive drinking affects fertility. The danger is that many women get pregnant unexpectedly and often are 4–6 weeks into their pregnancy before they realize they are pregnant.

Other recreational drugs, including marijuana, have been found to be teratogenic during pregnancy. It is advised, therefore, for women who are actively trying to conceive to stop using alcohol and other recreational drugs.

Case Study

Suzanne works full time, and at the end of the day she often doesn't feel like cooking. She and her husband eat fast food 3–4 times a week, they hike about 60 minutes once during the weekend, both drink wine 4–5 times a week (Suzanne limits herself to 1 glass, but her husband often consumes up to 3 glasses per occasion), and both consume 2–3 large cups of coffee a day.

Medications: None currently
Supplements: None currently
Biochemical values: Glucose: 105 (high); cholesterol: 210 (high); LDL: 155 (high); HDL: 39 (low); triglycerides: 155 (high)
Blood pressure: 125/80 mm Hg (high)
Anthropometrics: Height: 167.64 cm/66 inches; weight: 90.7 kg/200 lb
Body mass index: 32.3

Questions

1. What diagnoses can be made based on Suzanne's labs?
2. What lifestyle modifications would you recommend for Suzanne prior to her becoming pregnant?
3. What medications may be helpful to her in getting pregnant?
4. Would you recommend a supplement to Suzanne, and if so, what should she make sure it contains?
5. Would you recommend her husband make any modifications to his lifestyle? If yes, which?
6. Should they consider waiting for a while before trying to conceive? If yes, why and for how long?

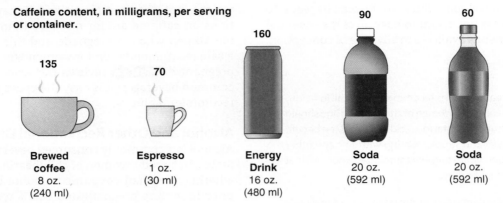

Over the limit on caffeine

Moderate daily intake of caffeine (200 to 300 mg) normally is not harmful, but too much can cause negative helath side effects.

Caffeine content, in milligrams, per serving or container.

135	70	160	90	60
Brewed coffee 8 oz. (240 ml)	**Espresso** 1 oz. (30 ml)	**Energy Drink** 16 oz. (480 ml)	**Soda** 20 oz. (592 ml)	**Soda** 20 oz. (592 ml)

Figure 2.8
Caffeine content of common beverages.

Smoking

A surprising 23.3% of women reported smoking in the 3 months prior to pregnancy.[48] Those who smoked were typically younger than 20 years of age, Caucasian, and their pregnancy was unintended. Smoking is known to be dangerous when a woman is pregnant, because it limits the amount of oxygen available to the baby and can cause tissue damage. This can lead to fewer nutrients being delivered and less waste being removed, an outcome that may eventually lead to birth complications and low birth weight. Smoking can also make it harder for a woman to get pregnant.[49] It is advisable that women stop smoking when they are trying to get pregnant.

Birth Control

About 62% of women of childbearing age use hormonal contraceptives, with the birth control pill the most common method.[50] There is some concern and debate about whether birth control pills and other hormones used to prevent pregnancy impair or delay fertility. Although there is no consensus, birth control pills can cause other issues such as increased cholesterol levels, higher blood pressure, and higher triglycerides, depending on the type of contraceptive used. Birth control is a central component of preconception care and discussion about its use and possible side effects should be included in a preconception visit.

> 1. What are the recommendations for caffeine intake for those trying to become pregnant?
> 2. Describe possible consequences of alcohol use prior to pregnancy.
> 3. How does smoking negatively affect preconception in both men and women?

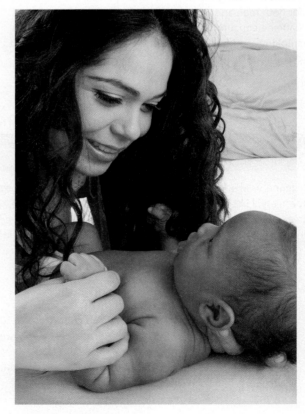

©OLJ Studio/Shutterstock

> **Recap** A number of different lifestyle habits, or choices, during the preconception period for both men and women can hinder chances for successful conception. Caution should be used and guidelines followed to ensure that the health of both baby and mother are protected prior to conception.

Learning Portfolio

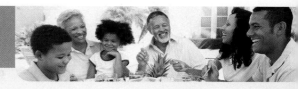

Visual Chapter Summary

Preconception Period

- The preconception period is the time prior to when a woman becomes pregnant.
- Addressing her and her partner's health prior to conception can reduce risks for the mother and child.
- All women and couples should have a reproductive life plan.
- Preconception care encompasses the biomedical, behavioral, and social health interventions provided to women and couples prior to conception.

Table 2.1

Recommendations to Improve Preconception Health[3]

1. Individual Responsibility Across the Life Span	Adult men and women should have a reproductive life plan.
2. Consumer Awareness	Increase public awareness of the importance of preconception health behaviors and preconception care services available.
3. Preventive Visits	Provide risk assessment and health promotion education to all women of childbearing age.
4. Interconception Care	Use the time between pregnancies to provide additional interventions and education to women who have had a previous pregnancy that ended in an adverse outcome.
5. Prepregnancy Checkup	Offer, as a component of maternity care, one prepregnancy visit for couples and persons planning pregnancy.
6. Health Insurance Coverage for Women with Low Income	Increase health insurance coverage for women with low incomes to improve access to preventive women's health and preconception and interconception care.
7. Public Health Programs and Strategies	Integrate components of preconception health into existing local public health and related programs.
8. Monitoring Improvements	Maximize research mechanisms to monitor preconception health.

Modified from Healthy People 2020 Recommendations to Improve Preconception Health

The Physiology of Reproduction

- Preconception care can improve healthy habits and decrease adverse health problems for the mother, child, and society.
- A woman is born with 1 to 2 million eggs and releases about 500 in her lifetime.
- Males can generate millions of new sperm daily.

- The female reproductive system is made up of the ovaries, uterus, fallopian tubes, cervix, and vagina.
- Four main hormones are responsible for the monthly menstrual cycle: FSH, LH, estrogen, and progesterone.
- Men have many structures in their reproductive system, including the penis, scrotum, testes, epididymis, vas deferens, urethra, seminal vesicles, and prostate gland.
- Sperm are produced in the scrotum and move to the epididymis to mature; they are released via the urethra with fluid from the seminal vesicles and prostate gland.

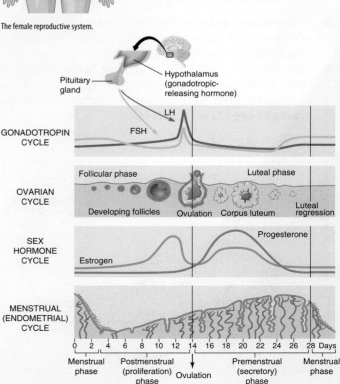

The female reproductive system.

Female menstrual cycle hormones.

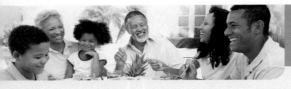

Learning Portfolio (continued)

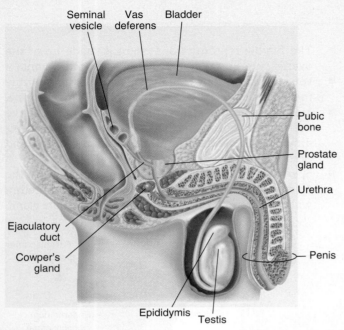

Seminal vesicle · Vas deferens · Bladder · Pubic bone · Prostate gland · Urethra · Penis · Epididymis · Testis · Ejaculatory duct · Cowper's gland

The male reproductive system.

Infertility, Subfertility, and Assisted Reproductive Technology

- The average age for women to conceive has increased.
- Many women and couples delay starting their families until they are 30 years or older.
- Infertility is the inability to achieve conception after 12 or more months of unprotected sex.
- Delaying childbearing can cause reproductive delays owing to egg or sperm issues.

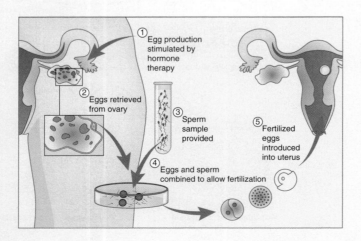

① Egg production stimulated by hormone therapy
② Eggs retrieved from ovary
③ Sperm sample provided
④ Eggs and sperm combined to allow fertilization
⑤ Fertilized eggs introduced into uterus

- ART is one strategy for assisting conception and is gaining popularity.
- ART contributes to a higher number of high-risk birth outcomes because of increased chances of twins and higher-order multiples.

Common Health Conditions

- PCOS is a common condition that affects fertility and is characterized by cysts on the ovaries, high androgen levels, and possibly amenorrhea and anovulation.
- PCOS can be treated with medications and potentially a low-carbohydrate diet.
- Many women are at risk of diabetes.
- Type 1 and type 2 diabetes are different, and women with uncontrolled blood sugar from either type are at risk of poor pregnancy outcomes for themselves and the baby.
- Men with diabetes have lower testosterone levels, which can lead to less healthy sperm.
- Carbohydrate counting is a promising meal-planning strategy that may be helpful prior to pregnancy.
- Many women enter pregnancy with hypertension, which puts them at risk of preeclampsia.
- The DASH diet can help improve outcomes.
- Celiac disease is an autoimmune disease in which people are unable to consume wheat, barley, and rye without damaging their intestines and causing other adverse health outcomes.

Table 2.4

Common Symptoms of Polycystic Ovary Syndrome

Menstrual problems	Hair loss from the scalp	Fertility problems or repeat miscarriages	Depression or mood swings
Acne, oily skin, or dandruff	Hair growth on the face, chest, back, stomach, thumbs, or toes	Insulin resistance and too much insulin, which can contribute to obesity	Breathing problems while sleeping
Cysts on the ovaries	Weight gain or obesity, especially around the waist	Skin tags	Pelvic pain

Reproduced from Office on Women's Health, U.S. Department of Health and Human Services. Polycystic ovary syndrome (PCOS). Retrieved from: http://www.womenshealth.gov/publications/our-publications/fact-sheet/polycystic-ovary-syndrome.html#d. Accessed: January 12, 2016.

<table>
<tr><th colspan="3">Table 2.5</th></tr>
</table>

Comparison of Type 1 and Type 2 Diabetes Mellitus

Feature	Type 1 Diabetes	Type 2 Diabetes
Onset	Sudden	Gradual
Age at onset	Any age, but mostly in young children up to teenage years	Most common in adults
Body type	Generally thin or normal	Often obese
Presence of endogenous insulin	Low or absent	Normal, decreased, or increased
Prevalence	~10% of all individuals with diabetes in the United States	~90–95% of all individuals with diabetes in the United States

Data from American Diabetes Association. Retrieved from: http://www.diabetes.org

<table>
<tr><th>Table 2.6</th></tr>
</table>

Daily and Weekly DASH Eating Plan Goals for a 2,000-Calorie-a-Day Diet

Food Group	Daily Servings
Grains	6–8
Meats, poultry, and fish	6 or less
Vegetables	4–5
Fruit	4–5
Low-fat or fat-free dairy products	2–3
Fats and oils	2–3
Sodium	2,300 mg*
Weekly Servings	
Nuts, seeds, dry beans, and peas	4–5
Sweets	5 or less

*1,500 milligrams (mg) sodium lowers blood pressure even further than 2,300 mg sodium daily.

Reproduced from National Heart, Lung, and Blood Institute. Description of the DASH eating plan. Retrieved from: https://www.nhlbi.nih.gov/health/health-topics/topics/dash. Accessed January 12, 2016.

- Celiac disease can lead to infertility and poor pregnancy outcomes.
- Getting a proper diagnosis and avoiding wheat, barley, rye, and oats have been shown to improve outcomes.
- Individuals with a history of STIs or a current STI should see a healthcare practitioner for treatment; many STIs can be treated prior to pregnancy.
- Women and couples with HIV may have options for conception; alerting their healthcare provider prior to conceiving is critically important.

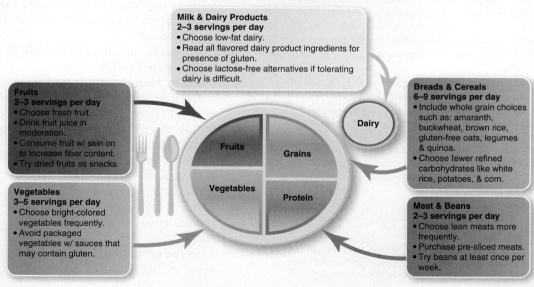

The Gluten-Free Diet Plate

Milk & Dairy Products
2–3 servings per day
- Choose low-fat dairy.
- Read all flavored dairy product ingredients for presence of gluten.
- Choose lactose-free alternatives if tolerating dairy is difficult.

Fruits
2–3 servings per day
- Choose fresh fruit.
- Drink fruit juice in moderation.
- Consume fruit w/ skin on to increase fiber content.
- Try dried fruits as snacks.

Vegetables
3–5 servings per day
- Choose bright-colored vegetables frequently.
- Avoid packaged vegetables w/ sauces that may contain gluten.

Breads & Cereals
6–9 servings per day
- Include whole grain choices such as: amaranth, buckwheat, brown rice, gluten-free oats, legumes & quinoa.
- Choose fewer refined carbohydrates like white rice, potatoes, & corn.

Meat & Beans
2–3 servings per day
- Choose lean meats more frequently.
- Purchase pre-sliced meats.
- Try beans at least once per week.

MyPlate gluten-free diet plate.
Reproduced from ChooseMyPlate.gov.

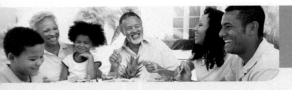

Learning Portfolio (continued)

Nutrition Recommendations During Preconception

- There is no recommended preconception diet other than an overall healthy diet, such as the meal plan found on USDA's ChooseMyPlate.
- A diet high in carbohydrates (especially carbohydrates with a high glycemic index), saturated fat, and animal protein and low in multivitamins and iron may impair fertility.
- Folic acid is an important B vitamin needed to make DNA and produce and maintain cells.
- Insufficient folic acid at critical times of development can lead to neural tube defects.
- Women of childbearing age are recommended to consume 400–800 mcg of folic acid daily in the form of supplements, fortified food, and food.
- Iron is a critical mineral needed to make hemoglobin, which delivers oxygen in the body.
- Low iron and anemia contribute to delayed development and behavioral and learning issues.

- Women are recommended to consume 27 mg of supplemental iron during the preconception period but may need more if stores are low or women are anemic.
- Women should consume 300 mg of DHA in a supplemental form because it helps with brain and eye development and is associated with fewer low-birth-weight and preterm deliveries.
- Multivitamins may be warranted during the preconception period.

Table 2.8

Food Sources of Folic Acid

Fortified cereal	Broccoli	Enriched pasta and bread
Cooked lentils and beans	Great Northern beans	Cantaloupe
Spinach	Asparagus	Eggs
Lettuce (cos, or romaine)	Avocado	Tropical fruits

Table 2.7

Eating and Lifestyle Recommendations to Improve the Health of Sperm

Eating	Lifestyle Choices
Consume 2½ cups of vegetables and 2 cups of fruit each day.	If you drink alcohol, do so in moderation—no more than two drinks per day.
Eat at least half of all grains as whole grains each day (choose whole wheat bread, oatmeal).	Avoid cigarettes and marijuana.
Consume at least 3 servings of low-fat dairy each day.	Obtain or maintain a healthy weight.
Evaluate your red meat intake and cut back as able. Choose leaner protein sources: fish, turkey, chicken, pork. Include vegetable proteins such as beans, nuts, seeds, and tofu.	Exercise 5 days a week for at 30 minutes—extreme exercise has been shown to decrease testosterone, which can lower sperm count.
Limit saturated fats from meats, full-fat dairy products, and fried foods. Replace these with healthy fats such as almonds and avocado.	

Data from Sharol Denny, Academy of Nutrition and Dietetics. How a Man's Diet Affects Fertility Too. November 19, 2014. http://www.eatright.org/resource/health/pregnancy/fertility-and-reproduction/how-a-mans-diet-affects-fertility-too..

Lifestyle Habits During Preconception

- For men, ensuring enough zinc and antioxidants in the daily diet can help produce healthier and larger supplies of sperm.
- For men, occupational and environmental factors such as exposure to heat, heavy metals, and pesticides should be addressed because they may impair sperm health.
- Overweight and obesity rates are at an all-time high in the United States.
- Many women begin pregnancy overweight or obese; a BMI over 25 puts a woman at risk for reduced fertility and pregnancy-related issues.
- Losing 10% of body weight can improve fertility rates among women.
- Bariatric surgery can improve fertility among men and women.
- A BMI of less than 19 can impair fertility.
- Being underweight among men and women disrupts reproductive capabilities.
- Eating disorders are common in the United States, with the most common being bulimia, anorexia nervosa, and binge eating disorder.

- Caffeine can harm the developing baby; recommended amounts are less than 200 mg per day.
- Alcohol and recreational drugs are known teratogens during pregnancy; their use may also reduce fertility and should be eliminated among women and couples actively trying to conceive.

- Smoking during pregnancy limits the oxygen available for the developing baby.
- Smoking can decrease fertility among women and men and should be decreased and ideally stopped prior to conception.
- Birth control has its benefits to prevent unwanted conception; however, the pill can cause increased cholesterol, triglycerides, and blood pressure among some women.

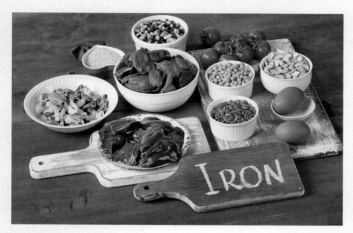

Iron-rich foods
©bitt24/Shutterstock

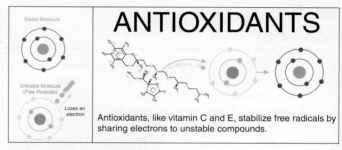

Antioxidants, like vitamin C and E, stabilize free radicals by sharing electrons to unstable compounds.

Antioxidants can help scavenge free radicals.

Key Terms

amenorrhea: The absence of menstruation.

anovulation: Failure of the ovary to release an egg over time, usually 3 months or longer.

antioxidant: A synthetic or natural substance that inhibits the oxidation of another molecule, especially one used to counteract the deterioration of stored food products.

assisted reproductive technology (ART): Any treatment or procedure that uses in vitro technology with oocytes (immature ova or egg cells from the female), sperm, or embryos.

hypothyroidism: A condition caused by an underactive thyroid or inadequate maternal iodine intake during pregnancy that is characterized by intellectual disabilities, growth impairment, and deafness in the infant.

infertility: Inability to get pregnant after 12 or more months of regular unprotected sexual intercourse.

ovulation: When the mature egg is released from the ovary into the fallopian tube and becomes available for fertilization.

preconception health care: A type of health care that identifies medical, behavioral, and social risks and modifies them prior to conception.

preconception period: The time prior to or between conceptions.

preeclampsia: Hypertension with onset following 20 weeks of pregnancy that is characterized by a sudden rise in blood pressure, excessive weight gain, generalized edema, proteinuria, severe headache, and visual disturbances and that may result in eclampsia if untreated. It can lead to fetal growth restriction.

subfertility: Diminished fertility but still able to become pregnant; hypofertility.

teratogen: Something in the environment of the embryo that can cause birth defects`.

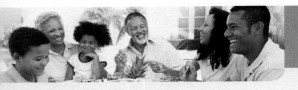

Learning Portfolio (continued)

Discussion Questions

1. If a friend tells you she is having trouble getting pregnant and wants to try ART, what steps would you suggest she take prior to her first appointment?
2. What are the advantages and disadvantages of waiting to have children?
3. In 1998, the U.S. government made the decision to fortify all cereals and many grains with folic acid to prevent neural tube defects. It has worked, and rates of neural tube defects are down. However, research has begun to suggest that there is a surge in cancers that may be related to the increased amount of folic acid being consumed. What do you think? Should we be encouraging *all* members of society, including those at low risk (like men who are not of reproductive age and older adults), to consume folic acid?

Activities

1. Think about yourself right now. Do you have a preconception plan? What steps do you need to take to put a plan into action? What are you doing that is helpful or hurtful if you plan on conceiving in the future?
2. Visit the website http://www.mothertobaby.org/. Look on the Resources tab for fact sheets. Find at least one fact sheet that interests you or that you've never heard about before. Open it and see whether you agree with the information or whether it's what you've always believed. Write a paragraph about the fact sheet to share with the class.

Study Questions

1. What are components of preconception care that should be addressed to improve outcomes for the mother and child?
   a. Medical, behavioral, and social
   b. Social, financial, and medical
   c. Social, financial, and religious
   d. Medical, financial, and behavioral
2. What are the roles of FSH and LH in the follicular phase of the menstrual cycle?
   a. Stimulate estrogen and progesterone production.
   b. Stimulate eggs to grow in the ovaries.
   c. Release the eggs from the ovaries.
   d. FSH and LH are not released during the follicular phase.
3. Which of the following best describes the steps of ovulation?
   a. The follicular phase allows stimulation of egg growth into follicles, allowing one to mature, which is then released from the ovary during the luteal phase.
   b. The luteal phase allows a surge of LH, which stimulates the ovaries to release an egg from the ovary into the fallopian tubes.
   c. Ovulation is when the empty follicle becomes the corpus luteum.
   d. Ovulation is when the egg passes through the uterus and the lining breaks down.
4. How long does it take for sperm to mature?
   a. 30 days
   b. 50 days
   c. 70 days
   d. 90 days
5. What is the trend in age for women having children in the United States?
   a. More teens are having children than ever before.
   b. More women are waiting until they are 35 years and older to have children.
   c. Women are having children at the same age today as they were 40 years ago.
   d. Women older than 40 are not trying to have children.
6. What is the danger in delaying childbearing for women?
   a. There are no risks.
   b. The woman is financially more secure.
   c. There are fewer health risks for a woman and her baby if she is older.
   d. Infertility and increased health risks for her and her baby.

7. What is a possible reason that women with PCOS have trouble getting pregnant?
   a. They produce androgens that interfere with the monthly menstrual cycle because they cause anovulation.
   b. They have low circulating levels of insulin.
   c. They are overweight.
   d. They eat a high-carbohydrate diet.
8. What are the possible negative outcomes for the mother and baby when a woman enters a pregnancy with uncontrolled blood sugar?
   a. Low and high blood sugar
   b. Large babies
   c. Fetal death
   d. High blood pressure for the mother
   e. All of the above
9. What foods should a woman with celiac disease eliminate from her diet?
   a. Only wheat products
   b. All carbohydrates
   c. Wheat, barley, rye, and oats
   d. Lactose
10. Women who have had an STI should not have children because STIs are incurable and may hurt her baby.
    a. True
    b. False
11. In one study of thousands of nurses, certain dietary practices were found to be helpful for women with infertility. Which, from the following list, was *not* helpful?
    a. Low saturated fat
    b. Foods with a high glycemic index
    c. Low supplemental iron intake
    d. High plant protein
    e. Low animal protein
12. Why is folic acid intake so important and recommended to all women of childbearing age prior to conception?
    a. Many women do not know they are pregnant at the time when the folic acid is most needed to close the neural tube.
    b. Up to half of all pregnancies are unplanned.
    c. It is possible to get enough folic acid in food, but you would have to eat a lot of fruit.
    d. Folic acid is so important we fortify cereals and other grains with it.
13. _____ are caused by oxygen and can damage DNA, while _____ can stop the chain reaction.
    a. Antioxidants, free radicals
    b. Free radicals, antioxidants
    c. Free radicals, DHA
    d. Oxygenation, antioxidants
14. What BMI range is found to result in the best chances of getting pregnant?
    a. Lower than 19 and higher than 25
    b. Lower than 19 and higher than 30
    c. Higher than 19 and lower than 30
    d. Higher than 19 and lower than 25
15. Eating disorders can result in amenorrhea, contributing to impaired fertility.
    a. True
    b. False
16. What amount of alcohol has been found to be safe prior to conception?
    a. 1–2 servings a day
    b. 1–2 servings per week
    c. 3–5 servings per week
    d. The data are not clear, but alcohol should be avoided to increase fertility and decrease risks if a woman becomes pregnant accidentally.

Weblinks

- **Show Your Love**
  http://www.cdc.gov/preconception/showyourlove/
  Show Your Love is a national campaign set up through the CDC that is designed to improve the health of women and babies by promoting preconception health and health care.

- **Before, Between & Beyond Pregnancy**
  http://beforeandbeyond.org/toolkit/about-this-toolkit/

The National Preconception Curriculum and Resources Guide for Clinicians from **Before, Between & Beyond Pregnancy** provides information and toolkits to help clinicians build care plans for women seeking pregnancy.

- **Midwifery Obstetrical Nursing**
  http://obgnursing.blogspot.com/2012/07/preconception-care-and-counseling.html

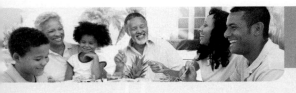

Learning Portfolio (continued)

A website designed for nursing students. Includes a comprehensive checklist of the different areas that should be assessed during a preconception visit.

■ **March of Dimes**
https://www.marchofdimes.org/catalog/category.aspx?categoryid=195&
The March of Dimes has three research-based books for nurses that address a variety of topics related to preconception care. The books are: *Challenges and Management of Infertility, Including ART; Preconception Nursing Care*; and *Preconception Health Promotion*.

■ **Best Start Preconception Health Resources**
http://www.beststart.org/cgi-bin/commerce.cgi?search=action&category=F00E&advanced=yes&sortkey=sku&sortorder=descending
Best Start is an education resource for preconception health developed by the charitable organization Health Nexus. The education provided focuses on the importance of women's and men's health before conception.

References

1. Centers for Disease Control and Prevention; April 6, 2006. Recommendations to Improve Preconception Health and Health Care—United States: A Report of the CDC/ATSDR Preconception Care Work Group and the Select Panel on Preconception Care. http://www.cdc.gov/mmwr/preview/mmwrhtml/rr5506a1.htm. Accessed September 17, 2015.
2. Ramirez-Velez R. In utero fetal programming and its impact on health in adulthood. *Endocrinol Nutr*. June–July 2012;59(6):383–393.
3. Centers for Disease Control and Prevention; August 25, 2014. Preconception Health and Health-Care: Reproductive Life Plan Tool for Health Professionals. http://www.cdc.gov/preconception/rlptool.html. Accessed September 17, 2015.
4. Kauffman AS, Bojkowska K, Rissman EF. Critical periods of susceptibility to short-term energy challenge during pregnancy: impact on fertility and offspring development. *Physiol Behav*. 2010;99:100–108.
5. Beckmann MM, Widmer T, Bolton E. Does preconception care work? *Aust N Z J Obstet Gynaecol*. 2014;54(6):510–514.
6. Efremov EA, Kasatonova EV, Mel'nik JI. Male preconception care. *Urologiia*. May–June 2015;(3):97–100.
7. Centers for Disease Control and Prevention; June 13, 2016. Births and Natality. http://www.cdc.gov/nchs/fastats/births.htm. Accessed September 20, 2015.
8. Centers for Disease Control and Prevention; April 14, 2016. Infertility FAQs. http://www.cdc.gov/reproductivehealth/Infertility/index.htm#e. Accessed September 17, 2015.
9. Schmidt L, Sobotka T, Bentzen JG, Nyboe Andersen A; ESHRE Reproduction and Society Task Force. Demographic and medical consequences of the postponement of parenthood. *Hum Reprod Update*. 2012;18(1):29–43.
10. Zegers-Hochschild F, Adamson GD, de Mouzon J, et al. International Committee for Monitoring Assisted Reproductive Technology (ICMART) and the World Health Organization (WHO) revised glossary of ART terminology, 2009. *Fertil Steril*. 2009;92(5):1520–1524.
11. Gnoth C, Godehardt E, Frank-Herrmann P, et al. Definition and prevalence of subfertility and infertility. *Hum Reprod*. 2005;20(5):1144–1147.
12. American Society for Reproductive Medicine. Abnormal body weight: a preventable cause of infertility. https://www.asrm.org/Abnormal_Body_Weight/. Accessed December 22, 2015.
13. Academy of Nutrition and Dietetics. Position of the American Dietetic Association and American Society for Nutrition: obesity, reproduction, and pregnancy outcomes. *J Am Dietet Assn*. May 2009;109(5):918–927.
14. Hassan MA, Killick SR. Negative lifestyle is associated with a significant reduction in fecundity. *Fertil Steril*. 2004;81(2):384–392.
15. Mouzon SH, Lassance L. Endocrine and metabolic adaptations to pregnancy; impact of obesity. *Horm Mol Biol Clin Investig*. October 1, 2015;24(1):65–72.
16. Barber TM, Dimitriadis GK, Andreou A, Franks S. Polycystic ovary syndrome: insight into pathogenesis and a common association with insulin resistance. *Clin Med*. December 2015;15(Suppl 6):s72–76.
17. Kayatas S, Boza A, Api M, Kurt D, Eroglu M, Annkan SA. Body composition: a predictive factor of cycle fecundity. *Clin Exp Reprod Med*. June 2014;41(2):75–79.
18. Maier JT, Schalinski E, Gauger U, Hellmeyer L. Antenatal body mass index (BMI) and weight gain in pregnancy—its association with pregnancy and birthing complications. *J Perinat Med*. 2016;44(4):397–404.
19. Thompson LA, Zhang S, Black E, et al. The association of maternal pre-pregnancy body mass index with breastfeeding initiation. *Matern Child Health J*. December 2013;17(10):1842–1851.
20. Winkvist A, Brantsaeter A, Brandhagen M. Maternal prepregnant body mass index and gestational weight gain are associated with initiation and duration of breastfeeding among Norwegian mothers. *J Nutr*. June 2015;145(6):1263–1270.
21. Palmer N, Bakos H, Fullston T, Lane M. Impact of obesity on male fertility, sperm function and molecular composition. *Spermatogenesis*. October 1, 2012;2(4):253–263.
22. Duval K, Langlois MF, Carranza-Mamane B, et al. The Obesity-Fertility Protocol: a randomized controlled trial assessing clinical outcomes and costs of a transferable interdisciplinary lifestyle intervention before and during pregnancy, in obese infertile women. *BMC Obes*. December 1, 2015;2:47.
23. Boyles S. Eating disorders affect fertility, pregnancy. WebMD; August 5, 2011. http://www.webmd.com/mental-health/eating-disorders/news/20110805/eating-disorders-affect-fertility-pregnancy. Accessed September 19, 2015.
24. Teede H, Deeks A, Moran L. Polycystic ovary syndrome: a complex condition with psychological, reproductive and

metabolic manifestations that impacts on health across the lifespan. *BMC Med.* 2010;8:41.

25. Fauser BCJM, Tarlatzis BC, Rebar RW, et al. Consensus on women's health aspects of polycystic ovary syndrome (PCOS): the Amsterdam ESHRE/ASRM-Sponsored 3rd PCOS Consensus Workshop Group. *Fertil Steril.* 2011;97(1):28–38.e25.

26. Lebwohi B, Ludvigsson JF, Green PH. Celiac disease and non-celiac gluten sensitivity. *BMJ.* October 5, 2015;351:h4347.

27. Tersigni C, Castellani R, de Waure C, et al. Celiac disease and reproductive disorders: meta-analysis of epidemiologic associations and potential pathogenic mechanisms. *Hum Reprod Update.* July–August 2014;20(4):582–593.

28. Moleski SM, Lindenmeyer CC, Veloski JJ, et al. Increased rates of pregnancy complications in women with celiac disease. *Ann Gastroenterol.* April–June 2015;28(2):236–240.

29. Nwankwo T, Yoon SS, Burt V, Gu Q. Hypertension among adults in the United States: National Health and Nutrition Examination Survey, 2011–2012. *Data Briefs.* October 31, 2013;133. http://www.cdc.gov/nchs/data/databriefs/db133.htm. Accessed September 18, 2015.

30. Seely EW, Ecker J. Chronic hypertension in pregnancy. *N Engl J Med.* 2011;365(5):439–446.

31. New York State Department of Health AIDS Institute; July 2010. Preconception care for HIV-infected women. http://www.hivguidelines.org/wp-content/uploads/2013/07/preconception-care-for-hiv-infected-women-06-17-2013.pdf. Accessed May 10, 2016.

32. Sheweita SA, Tilmisany AM, Al-Sawaf H. Mechanisms of male infertility: role of antioxidants. *Curr Drug Metab.* 2005;6(5):495–501.

33. Young SS, Eskenazi B, Marchetti FM, Block G, Wyrobek AJ. The association of folate, zinc and antioxidant intake with sperm aneuploidy in healthy non-smoking men. *Hum Reprod.* 2008;23:1014–1022.

34. Chavarro JE, Rich-Edwards JW, Rosner BA, et al. Diet and lifestyle in the prevention of ovulatory disorder infertility. *Obstet Gynecol.* 2007,110(5):1050–1058.

35. Muthusami KR, Chinnaswamy P. Effect of chronic alcoholism on male fertility hormones and semen quality. *Fertil Steril.* October 2005;84(4):919–924.

36. Centers for Disease Control and Prevention; July 15, 2016. Contraceptive Use. http://www.cdc.gov/nchs/fastats/contraceptive.htm. Accessed September 20, 2015.

37. Janecka M, Manduca A, Servadio M, et al. Effects of advanced paternal age on trajectories of social behavior in offspring. *Genes Brain Behav.* July 2015;14(6):443–453.

38. Slyvka Y, Zhang Y, Nowak FV. Epigenetic effects of paternal diet on offspring: emphasis on obesity. *Endocrine.* February 2015;48(1):36–46.

39. Finegersh A, Rompala GR, Martin DI, Homanics GE. Drinking beyond a lifetime: new and emerging insights into paternal alcohol exposure on subsequent generations. *Alcohol.* August 2015;49(5):461–470.

40. Wise LA, Rothman KJ, Mikkelsen EM, et al. A prospective cohort study of physical activity and time to pregnancy. *Fertil Steril.* 2012;97:1136–1142.

41. Chitayat D, Matsui D, Amitai Y, et al. Folic acid supplementation for pregnant women and those planning pregnancy: 2015 update. *J Clin Pharmacol.* 2016;56(2):170–175.

42. Wilson RD, Genetics Committee, Wildon RD, et al. Preconception folic acid and multivitamin supplementation for the primary and secondary prevention of neural tube defects and other folic acid-sensitive congenital anomalies. *J Obstet Gynaecol Can.* June 2015;37(6):534–552.

43. Kaufman C, Fertility foods. Academy of Nutrition and Dietetics; June 28, 2016. http://www.eatright.org/resource/health/pregnancy/fertility-and-reproduction/fertility-foods. Accessed August 23, 2016.

44. Mihaila C, Schramm J, Strathmann FG, et al. Identifying a window of vulnerability during fetal development in a maternal iron restriction model. *PloS One.* 2011;6(3):e17483.

45. Stagnaro-Green A, Dogo-Isonaige E, Pearce EN, Spencer C, Gaba ND. Marginal iodine status and high rate of subclinical hypothyroidism in Washington DC women planning conception. *Thyroid.* September 2015;25(10):1151–1154.

46. American College of Obstetricians and Gynecologists. *Moderate caffeine consumption during pregnancy.* Washington, DC: American College of Obstetricians and Gynecologists; 2010, updated 2015. http://www.acog.org/Resources-And-Publications/Committee-Opinions/Committee-on-Obstetric-Practice/Moderate-Caffeine-Consumption-During-Pregnancy. Accessed September 19, 2015.

47. March of Dimes Alcohol during pregnancy. http://www.marchofdimes.org/pregnancy/alcohol-during-pregnancy.aspx. Accessed September 19, 2015.

48. US Department of Health and Human Services. *Highlights: overview of finding regarding reproductive health.* Atlanta: US Dept of Health and Human Services, Centers for Disease Control and Prevention, National Center for Chronic Disease Prevention and Health Promotion, Office on Smoking and Health; 2010. https://www.cdc.gov/tobacco/data_statistics/sgr/2010/highlight_sheets/pdfs/overview_reproductive.pdf. Accessed August 23, 2016.

49. US Department of Health and Human Services. *Let's make the next generation tobacco-free: your guide to the 50th anniversary Surgeon General's report on smoking and health.* Atlanta: US Dept of Health and Human Services, Centers for Disease Control and Prevention, National Center for Chronic Disease Prevention and Health Promotion, Office on Smoking and Health; 2014. http://www.surgeongeneral.gov/library/reports/50-years-of-progress/consumer-guide.pdf. Accessed August 23, 2016.

50. Preconception Care and Health Care: Show Your Love campaign. Centers for Disease Control and Prevention; February 1, 2013. http://www.cdc.gov/preconception/showyourlove/index.html. Accessed September 20, 2015.

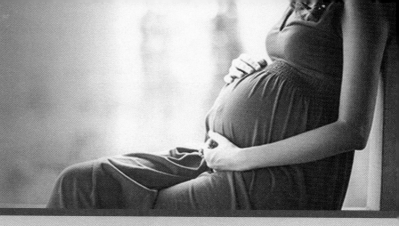

CHAPTER 3

Nutrition Needs During Pregnancy

Mateja R. Savoie Roskos, PhD, MPH, RD, CD, CNP

Chapter Outline

The Physiology of Pregnancy and Factors That Affect Dietary Intake During Pregnancy

Pregnancy Weight Gain

Nutrition Recommendations and Requirements During Pregnancy

Common Nutrition Considerations During Pregnancy

Promoting Healthy Lifestyles

Learning Objectives

1. List 10 normal physiological changes that occur during a healthy pregnancy.

2. Summarize the recommended weight gain ranges for women in all BMI categories and explain why prepregnancy weight influences recommended weight gain during pregnancy.

3. Describe how the nutritional requirements of three macronutrients and three micronutrients change during pregnancy.

4. Explain how physical activity, food insecurity, and mental health can influence pregnancy outcomes.

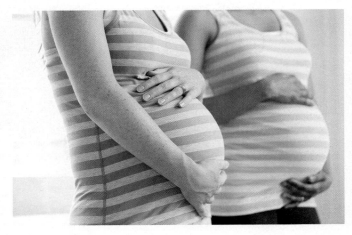

©kate_sept2004/ iStock/Getty

Case Study

Anna is a 28-year-old female entering her second trimester of her first pregnancy. She is a Seventh Day Adventist and has informed her doctor that she follows a strict vegan diet as a result of her religious beliefs. Anna is 5 foot 7 inches with a prepregnancy weight of 130 pounds and a current weight of 142 pounds. Anna does aerobic-type exercise for at least 1 hour each day. She currently takes a prenatal multivitamin, tries to eat three meals and two to three snacks but complains that generally her appetite is low and nothing sounds good to her. Anna has expressed some concerns about advice that her well-meaning grandmother has suggested. Although she does not follow all of the advice given to her, Anna respects the wisdom and knowledge of her grandmother.

Think of someone close to you who has been pregnant. Consider the nutrition recommendations she was provided and from where or from whom the individual received those recommendations. What types of foods did she eat, and did she avoid specific foods? Perhaps there were cultural beliefs behind the food choices. For example, in some cultures women avoid strawberries and black-eyed peas during pregnancy owing to the belief that either may cause distinct birthmarks on the infant. Another culture avoids meat during pregnancy because people believe that the infant will obtain characteristics of the type of animal the mother consumes. In some cultures, pregnant women avoid eating black foods to avoid the birth of an infant with a dark skin tone. Nutritional intake during pregnancy is influenced by many internal, cultural, and environmental factors. However, it is widely believed that eating a healthy, well-balanced diet during pregnancy not only is good for a developing fetus but also can have positive health effects for the infant that extend into adulthood.

At no other time is human growth more rapid than during the fetal development that occurs during the nine months of pregnancy. Many environmental, genetic, and social factors influence the growth and development of the fetus. Some of these factors are choices that can be controlled, while others cannot. The quality of daily food selections of an expecting mother is a controllable factor, and one of the most important factors in determining pregnancy outcomes. The placenta is continuously remodeling, giving the expecting mother the ability to improve fetal nutrition throughout pregnancy. Attention to diet and lifestyle choices has the potential to optimize pregnancy outcomes. In the absence of chromosomal issues, the health of a fetus is strongly determined by the woman's diet, exercise, and lifestyle choices.[1] In fact, the benefits of adequate nutrition during this time are unlike at any other time in life.

This chapter discusses normal physiological changes that occur during pregnancy and how nutrients play a role. Appropriate weight gain during pregnancy is discussed in addition to nutritional needs and how specific nutrients support growth of maternal tissue. This chapter also addresses lifestyle choices during pregnancy.

The Physiology of Pregnancy and Factors That Affect Dietary Intake During Pregnancy

Preview Physiological changes occur during pregnancy to allow for adequate growth and development of the fetal and maternal tissues.

Maternal Physiology

Women experience significant physiological changes during pregnancy, some of which concerned clinicians for many years. Historically, clinicians had recommended limited weight gain, low-sodium diets, and intakes of numerous supplements as intervention strategies to improve pregnancy outcomes and prevent complications. After decades of research, we now know that practices like these were unnecessary and likely harmful to the mother and fetus. Changes in the mother's body during pregnancy are necessary to help protect the woman's normal physiological functioning and to help meet nutrient needs for the developing fetus. Most physiological changes during pregnancy occur as a result of changes in hormones produced by the placenta, such as the steroid hormones estrogen and progesterone.

The human body changes as needs for the mother and fetus change throughout the course of pregnancy. Normal physiological changes include those in maternal tissues, fetal growth, and development of the placenta. The fetus requires nutrients, oxygen, and energy, all of which are delivered through the placenta, making this the first physiological change to occur in the woman's body. Placental growth also occurs rapidly to ensure that it is prepared for fetal weight gain, especially during the second and third trimesters. The fetus relies on these constant physiological changes for proper functioning and development of the placenta and maternal tissues. Any abnormalities can cause severe problems with growth and development resulting in disability or death of the infant.

Normal Physiological Changes During Pregnancy

Two phases of physiological changes occur during pregnancy. The first phase is referred to as the *maternal anabolic phase* and occurs in the first 20 weeks of pregnancy. During this phase, the mother's body builds capacity to deliver all of the blood, oxygen, and nutrients the fetus will require during the second half of pregnancy. Increased appetite, increase in anabolic hormones, and decreased exercise tolerance are all common for the expecting mother during this time. The *catabolic phase* occurs during the last 20 weeks of pregnancy, supporting fetal development by mobilization of stored nutrients to the developing fetus. During this time, the expecting mother experiences an increase in catabolic hormones and increased exercise tolerance. Approximately 10% of fetal growth occurs during the first 20 weeks of pregnancy, and about 90% occurs in the second half.

Physiological changes occur in every organ and system in the body at various rates during pregnancy. These changes allow for proper nutrient and energy availability for the fetus, preparation for labor and delivery, and maternal homeostasis.

The Big Picture

TABLE 3.1 shows normal physiological changes that occur during pregnancy.

Table 3.1

Physiological Changes During Pregnancy

Cardiovascular system

- 20% increase in heart rate by the third trimester.
- 10% reduction in systolic and diastolic blood pressure by 8 weeks of pregnancy with a further decrease until 24 weeks followed by a return to prepregnancy values around term.
- Cardiac output increases 30–50%.

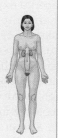

Hematological system

- Plasma volume increases by 10% by 7 weeks of pregnancy and continues to increase by 45–50% by 32 weeks, followed by a decline until term.
- Red blood cell mass increases by 18–25% during early pregnancy as a result of increased demands for oxygen transport; after delivery red blood cell mass returns to normal.

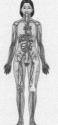

Respiratory system

- An 8% increase in thoracic circumference.
- Looser ligaments allow for lower ribs to "flare".
- An increase of 30–50 mL/min of oxygen consumption, resulting in a 40% increase in ventilation.

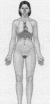

Renal system

- Length of kidneys increase by 1 cm to account for higher blood volume.
- Increased size of the pelvis, ureters, and calyces as a result of increased levels of progesterone.
- Glomerular filtration rate (GFR) increases by 40–50% until 36 weeks.
- Loss of glucose through the kidneys, which can increase the risk for infection.
- Increase in sodium retention.
- Increase in extracellular water volume.

Gastrointestinal system

- Progesterone lowers esophageal sphincter tone, resulting in an increased risk of heartburn and acid reflux.
- Lower intestinal motility transit times, causing bloating and constipation.
- Nausea and vomiting.

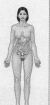

Endocrine system

- Increased production of insulin and increased insulin resistance.
- Pituitary gland increases by 135%.

Postural changes

- Change in the center of gravity
- Forward head position
- Increased cervical lordosis
- Increased base of support in standing©Mathom/Shutterstock

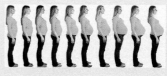

©Mathom/Shutterstock

Data from Carlin A, Alfirevic Z. Physiological changes of pregnancy and monitoring. *Best Pract Clin Obstet Gynaecol.* 2008;22(5):801–823.

Development of the Placenta

The placenta is an endocrine organ that develops in the uterus within the first several weeks of conception and prior to fetal development. The placenta is large, approximately 1 pound, which is larger than the fetus for the first several months of pregnancy (FIGURE 3.1). The placenta is responsible for various functions, including the following:

- Secreting vital hormones such as human chorionic gonadotropin (hCG), estrogen, and progesterone, which are necessary for appropriate nutrient metabolism and fetal growth
- Fighting internal infections by passing immunoglobulin G (IgG) antibodies to the fetus
- Exchanging nutrients and oxygen from the mother to the fetus during the last 20 weeks of pregnancy, fully nourishing the developing fetus
- Removing waste products such as carbon dioxide, uric acid, urea, and creatinine from the fetus to the mother's blood supply

The placenta also acts as a barrier to substances such as bacteria, large proteins, and maternal red blood cells, all of which could be harmful to the fetus. Benefits of the placenta expand to managing the rate that nutrients and other compounds pass from the mother to the fetus. A reservoir of blood is maintained in the placenta for the fetus in case hypotension occurs. Although the placenta assists with protecting and developing the fetus, it is not able to prevent the transport of many harmful substances such as alcohol, illicit drugs, certain medications, and excessive amounts of vitamins. Many infectious agents can also cross the placenta such as measles, polio, and encephalitis, to name a few.

Many different cultural beliefs and values surround the use of the placenta after birth. For example, many cultures bury the placenta for a variety of reasons. The Tahitians, an indigenous Polynesian group from New Zealand, bury the placenta at the base of a fruit tree as a symbol of the relationship between earth and humans.[2] In some cultures, the placenta is eaten after childbirth, a practice known as *placentophagy*. In the United States and other Western countries, the placenta is most commonly incinerated after birth.

Changes in Hormones

Women experience numerous changes to their endocrine system during pregnancy. The many physiological changes previously discussed often occur as a result of increased secretion of hormones by the placenta. What do hormones do? Hormones function by carrying information from one cell to another. Because of this, hormones influence nearly every cell, organ, and body function. During pregnancy, an expecting mother relies on specific hormones such as the steroid hormones progesterone, estrogen, human chorionic gonadotropin (hCG), leptin, and human chorionic somatomammotropin. The functions of each hormone are listed in TABLE 3.2.

Changes in Body Water

Body water significantly increases during pregnancy as a result of increased extracellular fluid, plasma volume, and development of amniotic fluid. On average, a woman's body water increases 7–10 L during pregnancy, most of which goes toward building blood and tissues during the first trimester. Plasma volume, which is the liquid in which blood cells are suspended, starts to increase within the first few weeks of pregnancy and continues until the 34th week, increasing from about 50 mL during the 10th week of gestation to about 800 mL during the 20th week of gestation.[1] Although red blood cells also increase during pregnancy, they do not increase as much as plasma, which makes the blood seem more

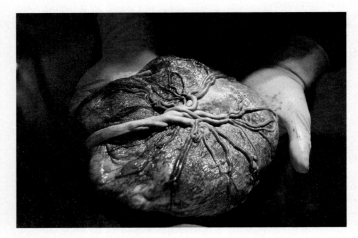

Figure 3.1
Placenta.
©Noctiluxx/E+/Getty

Table 3.2
Hormone Functions During Pregnancy
Estrogen—Promotes growth of the uterus and breast tissues, increases blood circulation, and increases protein synthesis, lipid formation and storage.
Progesterone—Stimulates breast tissue growth, smooths uterine and gastrointestinal muscles, maintains proper functioning of the placenta, promotes lipid accumulation, promotes growth of endometrium, and loosens joints and ligaments.
Human chorionic gonadotropin (hCG)—Used to indicate pregnancy after conception; initiates production of estrogen and progesterone, and stimulates growth of the endometrium.
Human chorionic somatomammotropin (hCS)—Mobilizes free fatty acids to promote glucose conservation, regulates protein metabolism to ensure nutrients are delivered to the fetus for growth, and increases insulin resistance in the mother; responsible for diabetogenic effects that occur during pregnancy.
Leptin—Regulates appetite, mobilizes fat stores, and assists with nutrient transportation; may deliver amino acids to the fetus.

diluted. This "dilution effect" is generally a good sign that the body fluids are adjusting properly to support a healthy pregnancy. The increase in plasma volume during the first trimester of pregnancy may be the primary reason women report fatigue during this time; however, as pregnancy progresses, the body compensates and generally less fatigue is experienced.

The amount of fluid volume gained during pregnancy varies. Women with high gains in fluid experience more edema, excess fluid collecting in body tissues, and greater weight gain. Edema is considered an indicator of a healthy expansion of plasma volume during pregnancy unless it is combined with hypertension, which can cause preterm birth and other complications.[3] Plasma volume is often a good indicator of birth weight, with greater increases in plasma volume leading to larger birth weights.

Maternal Nutrient Metabolism During Pregnancy

Fetal nutrient needs occur primarily in the last half of pregnancy when 90% of fetal growth occurs; however, changes in maternal nutrient metabolism occurs within the first few weeks of pregnancy.[1] For example, calcium metabolism occurs with bone turnover and reformation; increased levels of body water and tissue synthesis require additional sodium and other minerals.

Protein Metabolism During Pregnancy

During pregnancy, maternal protein accumulates in various tissues, including the blood, uterus, breasts, fetus, placenta, and amniotic fluid. Proteins support rapid growth of both maternal and fetal tissues and are required in high amounts, particularly during the second and third trimesters of pregnancy.

Nitrogen, a compound unique to protein, can provide a direct measure of a person's protein status. During pregnancy, there is a natural decline in total nitrogen excretion, which likely contributes to meeting the increased protein needs and suggests that amino acids are conserved for tissue synthesis later in pregnancy. Plasma amino acids decrease during pregnancy. The use of branched-chain amino acids also decreases during the last weeks of pregnancy to allow for additional energy for the fetus. Meeting protein needs during pregnancy is of upmost importance because of how much the developing fetus relies on maternal intake of protein.

Carbohydrate Metabolism During Pregnancy

Between 50% and 80% of fetal energy needs are provided by glucose. Changes in carbohydrate metabolism occurs throughout pregnancy to ensure the fetus receives adequate glucose even if maternal glucose intake is not adequate. As the primary energy source, glucose crosses the placenta more readily than other macronutrients. GLUT 1 and GLUT4 are the glucose transporters that are responsible for transferring a constant supply of glucose from the mother across the placenta to the fetus. During times of hypoglycemia (low blood glucose levels), glucose transporter cells respond by increasing cellular components to ensure sufficient glucose reaches the fetus. During times of hyperglycemia, these transporters adjust to help regulate blood glucose levels. The fetus is able to store glucose just as adults do. Once glucose crosses the placenta, it is converted by the liver to glycogen and stored there. The fetus can also obtain energy from fat if glucose is low. To meet the increased demands of the fetus, maternal glucose production must increase later in pregnancy.

During the first months of pregnancy, maternal cells are more responsive to insulin, causing synthesis of glycogen and limited use of plasma glucose and fatty acids for energy. Insulin secretion often decreases by 50–70% in the later months of pregnancy, causing insulin resistance in the expecting mother.[4] During this time, fat stores become mobilized for energy, glycogen synthesis is diminished, and blood glucose levels rise as indicated in **TABLE 3.3**. This is often referred to as the *diabetogenic effect* of pregnancy, making women slightly intolerant to carbohydrates during the third trimester of pregnancy. This condition is increased by both maternal obesity and repeated pregnancy.

Lipid Metabolism During Pregnancy

Lipid metabolism changes throughout the course of pregnancy. Increases in fat accumulation during the first part of pregnancy, followed by the mobilization of fat during the end of pregnancy, are the two main changes. As a result, the development of hyperlipidemia and increased lipid blood levels are common among pregnant women, with increases in both serum cholesterol and triglyceride levels as pregnancy progresses.[5] High serum cholesterol and triglycerides are common among normal pregnancies, although similar levels among nonpregnant women would be concerning. Increased lipid levels that result during pregnancy do not increase the mother's or fetus's risk for atherosclerosis later in life, and recommendations for cholesterol intake do not change during pregnancy. **TABLE 3.4** shows a comparison of cholesterol and triglyceride levels in pregnant and nonpregnant women.[6]

Table 3.3
Insulin-Related Physiological Changes in Early and Late Pregnancy

Early Pregnancy	Late Pregnancy
The body is in an anabolic phase.	The body is in a catabolic phase.
Increased insulin sensitivity.	Increased insulin resistance.
Accumulation of glycogen stores.	Glycogen stores utilized.
Accumulation of fat and protein stores.	Fat and protein stores are mobilized.

Data from Catalano PM. Obesity, insulin resistance, and pregnancy outcome. *Reproduction.* 2010;140(3):365–371.

Table 3.4

Approximate Serum Cholesterol and Triglyceride Values During Pregnancy and in Nonpregnant Women

Trimester	Cholesterol (mg/dL)	Triglycerides (mg/dL)
1	175 mg/dL	105 mg/dL
2	200 mg/dL	117 mg/dL
3	240 mg/dL	228 mg/dL
Nonpregnant women	165 mg/dL	93 mg/dL

Table 3.5

Weight Gain Recommendations for Women Pregnant with One Baby

If before pregnancy, you were ….	You should gain …
Underweight	
BMI less than 18.5	28–40pounds
Normal weight	
BMI 18.5–24.9	25–35pounds
Overweight	
BMI25.0–29.9	15–25pounds
Obese	
BMI greater than or equal to 30.0	11–20pounds

Reproduced from CDC. Weight gain during pregnancy. Retrieved from: http://www.cdc.gov/reproductivehealth/maternalinfanthealth/pregnancy-weight-gain.htm.

During pregnancy, lipid production increases and lipid enzyme activity decreases. This change supports fetal development by supplying the placenta with cholesterol for steroid hormone synthesis, development of cell membranes, cell proliferation, cell-to-cell communication, and fetal growth. During the early part of pregnancy, the fetus receives cholesterol from the mother. Toward the end of pregnancy, the fetus synthesizes cholesterol on its own.

Recap Women go through numerous physiological changes during pregnancy to assist with the development of the fetal and maternal tissues. Metabolism of macronutrients, protein, carbohydrates, and fat change throughout pregnancy as a result of increased nutrient requirements. Hormones such as progesterone, estrogen, hCG, leptin, and hCS are responsible for many of the physiological changes that occur.

1. Describe the normal physiological changes that occur during pregnancy in the various body systems.
2. List the functions of the placenta during pregnancy.
3. Discuss the changes in protein, carbohydrate, and fat metabolism that occur during pregnancy.

Pregnancy Weight Gain

Preview Appropriate weight gain during pregnancy is a vital component to a healthy mother and fetus.

Weight Gain Recommendations

Current weight gain recommendations during pregnancy are based on the prepregnancy weight status and body mass index (BMI) of the mother. Historically, 15 pounds was the general weight gain recommendation for women of any prepregnancy weight status. In the 1970s, an association was found between restricted weight gain during pregnancy and low birth weight as well as inadequate growth in infants. As a result, weight gain recommendations were increased.

Weight gain recommendations as established by the Institute of Medicine (IOM) can be found in TABLE 3.5 . These guidelines provide clinicians with a basis for practice. Individualized care and clinical judgment are necessary for the most successful weight gain outcomes in all pregnancies.

Used from the beginning of pregnancy, IOM pregnancy weight gain charts can be an effective tool for evaluating and monitoring gestational weight change (see FIGURE 3.2). Such weight gain charts can be useful when counseling and educating women because points

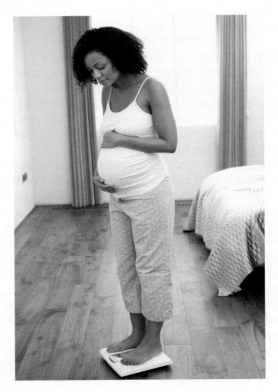

Figure 3.2
Weight gain in pregnancy. Suggested weight gain for a woman with a normal pre-pregnancy weight:
1st trimester 1 to 4.5 pounds
2nd trimester 1 to 2 pounds per week
3rd trimester 1-2 pounds per week

©Monkey Business Images/Shutterstock

on the chart can demonstrate the actual and the expected pattern of weight gain throughout pregnancy. Issues of either too rapid or not sufficient weight change can be easily determined and addressed when maternal weight is charted each week of pregnancy. Lifestyle interventions such as diet and exercise that are influencing maternal weight can be discussed.

Rate of Pregnancy Weight Gain

The rate of weight gain during pregnancy does not seem to be as important to the health outcomes of mother and infant as does the total amount of weight gained throughout pregnancy. Typically, most weight gain for the mother occurs during the second and third trimesters; however, it is important for some weight gain to occur in the first trimester as well. Weight gain often slows down in the last few weeks of pregnancy, but weight loss should not occur until after delivery. Recommendations for weight gain during each trimester are listed in TABLE 3.6.

Some women have a difficult time gaining weight during pregnancy. This can be a result of a number of circumstances such as entering pregnancy underweight, having health issues that prevent adequate weight gain, or being unable to tolerate food because of nausea and vomiting. There are many psychological and physiological reasons why women may experience slow rates of weight gain and possibly weight loss throughout pregnancy. TABLE 3.7 lists reasons for slow weight gain during pregnancy. It is vital for clinicians to determine what is causing slow weight gain to ensure appropriate intervention and management. Babies born to mothers who have had less than a 20-lb weight gain during pregnancy are more likely to be born premature or be small for gestational age.[7]

Composition of Weight Gain

Where does the extra weight go during pregnancy? Only about one-third of the weight gained in a normal-weight woman goes to the fetus. TABLE 3.8 breaks down the composition of weight gain during pregnancy. FIGURE 3.3 demonstrates the composition of weight gain during each week of pregnancy. Increased body fat is essential during pregnancy to meet the nutritional needs of the mother and the fetus. It also ensures that the mother has enough energy to meet her increased energy needs. Specifically, body fat stores provide an average reserve of 30,000 calories for pregnancy and lactation. Fat storage increases

Table 3.6

Weight Gain Recommendations by Trimester

Prepregnancy BMI	Total First-Trimester Weight Gain	Second- and Third-Trimester Gains per Week
Underweight (<18.5 kg/m²)	2.2–6.6 lb (1–3 kg)	1.0–1.3 lb (0.44–0.58 kg)
Normal weight (18.5–24.9 kg/m²)	2.2–6.6 lb (1–3 kg)	0.8–1.1 lb (0.35–0.5 kg)
Overweight (25–29.9 kg/m²)	2.2–6.6 lb (1–3 kg)	0.5–0.7 lb (0.23–0.33 kg)
Obese (≥30 kg/m²)	0.5–4.4 lb (0.2–2 kg)	0.4–0.6 lb (0.17–0.27 kg)

Table 3.7

Reasons for Slow Weight Gain or Weight Loss During Pregnancy

Nausea and vomiting or more severe hyperemesis gravidarum

Poor fetal growth

Resolved edema

Psychosocial problems such as poor appetite, concern about gaining weight, restricted dietary intake, or eating disorders

Medical problems or serious infection

Excess energy expenditure without increased dietary consumption

Limited access to adequate food

Table 3.8

Composition of Weight Gain During Pregnancy

Fetus	8 lb
Placenta	2–3 lb
Amniotic fluid	2–3 lb
Breast tissue	2–3 lb
Blood supply	4 lb
Fat stores	5–9 lb
Uterus growth	2–5 lb

Reproduced from National Institutes of Health. Managing your weight gain during pregnancy. National Institute of Health. https://www.nlm.nih.gov/medlineplus/ency/patientinstructions/000603.htm

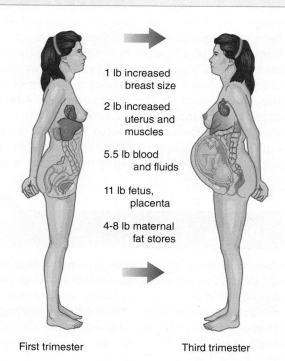

1 lb increased breast size

2 lb increased uterus and muscles

5.5 lb blood and fluids

11 lb fetus, placenta

4-8 lb maternal fat stores

First trimester   Third trimester

Figure 3.3
Average weight distribution during pregnancy.

most significantly during the first several weeks of the second trimester. When energy needs of the fetus increase later in pregnancy, fat stores tend to decrease.

Postpartum Weight Retention

Postpartum weight retention (PPWR), which refers to the amount of weight retained from that gained during pregnancy, is a contributing factor to long-term obesity and associated health risks.[8] On average, women retain 6–7 lb 12 months after delivery, and approximately 10–15% of women experience a long-term weight gain as a result of pregnancy-related weight gain.[9] Postpartum weight retention often occurs in the abdomen, which is also the most harmful location for weight gain because of increased risk for obesity-related chronic diseases and complications in future pregnancies.[10]

Many behavioral and social factors influence weight retention following pregnancy. Long-term weight retention is most common among low-income mothers, women consuming a traditional Western diet, women who have experienced births of twins or mulitples, women who do not exercise, and women who breastfeed for less than 20 weeks.[9]

Interventions to Prevent Excess Weight Gain

Many women have a difficult time gaining appropriate weight during pregnancy, and to a large extent this may be a result of the environment in which they live. Many Americans live in what is referred to as an "obesogenic" environment—an environment that promotes weight gain and makes weight maintenance and weight loss challenging. Numerous lifestyle interventions have been created and are encouraged to reduce excessive weight gain during pregnancy as well as to encourage weight maintenance after pregnancy, including nutrition counseling and education, increased physical activity, and improved diets.

Women who participated in multicomponent interventions (such as physical activity and improved diet) gained 2.6–3.1 lb less during pregnancy than their nonparticipating counterparts.[11] The most current IOM recommendations advise individualized care for women during preconception, prenatal, and postpartum care to assist them in gaining the appropriate amount of weight during pregnancy followed by a healthy postpartum weight.

Let's Discuss

An obesogenic environment is an environment that promotes weight gain and makes weight maintenance and weight loss challenging. What are some of the factors that contribute to an obesogenic environment in the United States? How might pregnant women overcome the challenges associated with gaining a healthy amount of weight during pregnancy while living in an obesogenic environment?

Recap Adequate weight gain is a vital component of a healthy pregnancy and a healthy infant. Weight gain recommendations vary according to prepregnancy weight and twin or multiple pregnancies. Clinicians should monitor weight trends at each appointment and provide counseling on weight gain accordingly.

1. Describe the composition of weight gain during pregnancy.
2. Discuss intervention strategies to prevent excess weight gain during pregnancy.

Nutrition Recommendations and Requirements During Pregnancy

Preview Nutrient needs increase during pregnancy to foster growth and development of the mother and fetus.

Adequate nutrition during pregnancy has a noteworthy impact on the health of the mother and the fetus. Appropriate macronutrient and micronutrient intake influences the growth and development of the fetus and can have positive and long-term effects on the infant. Adequate nutrition intake during this time is essential, and both undernutrition and overnutrition during pregnancy can contribute to long-term consequences. Malnutrition during pregnancy, especially during the first trimester when critical fetal development occurs, has been shown to contribute to various adverse health outcomes, including predisposition to many chronic diseases as infants grow to be children and, later, adults.[12] In addition, fetal exposure to excessive levels of saturated fatty acids, sucrose, fructose, salt, and high-glycemic-index foods may also contribute to later enhanced cardiometabolic risk.[13] Dietary Reference Intakes (DRIs), including the Recommended Dietary Allowance (RDA), Adequate Intake (AI), and Estimated Average Requirement (EAR), continue to be used during pregnancy to determine recommended levels of energy and nutrient needs.

Many factors affect nutrient needs among pregnant women, including the trimester of pregnancy, nutrition status prior to pregnancy, body weight and composition, physical activity level, and overall health status. Most women can meet nutritional needs through a well-balanced diet that incorporates optimal calories, protein, and other essential nutrients.

Energy Needs

Energy needs increase as pregnancy progresses, especially during the second and third trimesters because of the energy necessary for generating maternal and fetal tissues and increased basal metabolism. Basal metabolism increases as a result of the higher requirements for energy from the respiratory system, cardiovascular system, and renal system. The rates of fat synthesis, basal metabolism, and protein synthesis change as maternal and fetal tissues develop throughout pregnancy.

A gross increase of about 80,000 calories is required during pregnancy for proper growth and development of the maternal and fetal tissues. Considering the approximately 250 days that follow the first month of pregnancy, this ends up being about 300 kcal a day. The DRIs to increased energy intake during pregnancy is 340 kcal per day in the second trimester and 452 kcal per day in the third trimester. This is consistent with various studies that have found increased energy needs of 350 kcal and 500 kcal per day in the second and third trimesters,

respectively.[14] **FIGURE 3.4** demonstrates how much food is equal to about 300 kcal.

Energy intake during pregnancy is commonly assessed through weight gain. Independent of edema, steady weight gain over the second and third trimesters of pregnancy is a good indicator of an appropriate caloric balance.

Carbohydrates

The most essential role of carbohydrates is providing energy for the body. Carbohydrate recommendations for adults, including pregnant women, are approximately 45–65% of total caloric intake. According to the RDAs, pregnant women should consume at least 175 g of carbohydrates a day to provide adequate glucose for the brains of the mother and the fetus. A variety

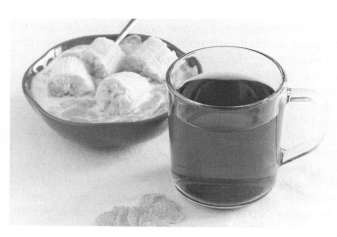

1 cup of cereal; 8 oz 2% milk; 1 medium-size banana; 1 cup of tea

©Petr Malyshev/Shutterstock

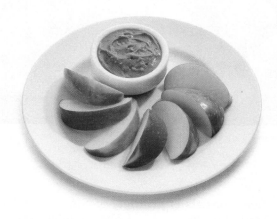

Apple slices and peanut butter

©AbbieImages/iStock/Getty Images Plus/Getty

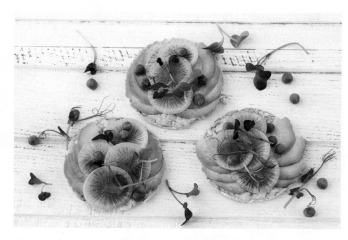

Quinoa cakes with avocado and watermelon radish

©sarsmis/Shutterstock

Figure 3.4
Examples of 300-kcal meals and snacks.

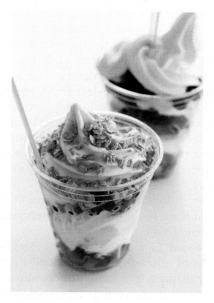

Frozen yogurt with fruit and nuts

©Rick Poon/Moment/Getty

of nutrient-dense foods contain carbohydrates, such as whole grains, fruit, vegetables, and cereal, and other products with grains and fiber are suggested. In addition to providing carbohydrates, these foods provide a variety of nutrients such as antioxidants, phytochemicals, fiber, vitamins, and minerals. Choosing carbohydrates that are not highly processed allows for greatest intake of nutrients and can assist with appropriate weight gain efforts.

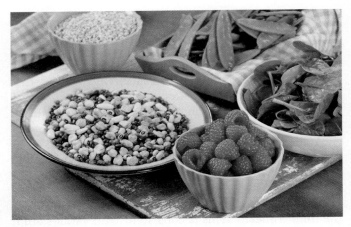

©bitt24/Shutterstock

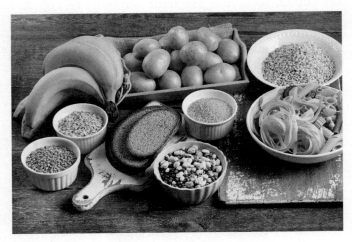

©bitt24/Shutterstock

Fiber

Dietary fiber consists of a variety of complex carbohydrates. There are two types of fiber, soluble fiber and insoluble fiber, both of which offer different benefits for the body. Soluble fiber is found in pectins, gels, and gums. This type of fiber slows the transit time of food in the gastrointestinal tract, allowing for optimal absorption of nutrients. Soluble fiber also binds to cholesterol, which then decreases cholesterol absorption and improves cholesterol levels in the blood. Foods rich in soluble fiber include oats, barley, legumes, and select fruits and vegetables. Insoluble fiber is found in cellulose, hemicellulose, and lignin. This type of fiber increases water-holding capacity, therefore increasing fecal volume and improving the rate of gastric transit. Foods rich in insoluble fiber include whole grains, high-fiber cereals, and the skin of fruits and vegetables.

The fiber RDA for individuals who are pregnant is 28 g per day, which is at the upper end of recommendations for the general public. In a typical American diet, average intake is only about 16 g per day;[15] therefore, fiber should be one focus of a healthy diet, particularly during pregnancy. Fiber is important to reduce constipation, a common symptom of pregnancy. Furthermore, high-fiber diets provide a feeling of fullness, helping to achieve appropriate caloric intake during pregnancy.

Protein

Adequate protein intake is essential during pregnancy to meet additional growth requirements for the development of tissues for the mother and the fetus. The average pregnant woman consumes 82 g per day of protein during pregnancy, which exceeds the DRI recommendations of 71 g per day to support biological changes.[16] Pregnancy recommendations are 25 g higher than recommendations for nonpregnant women. Owing to the increased need for protein synthesis, which occurs when new proteins are formed from free amino acids, less protein is used for energy and more is put toward development of new tissue. Other functions of protein during pregnancy include placenta and uterine growth, extracellular fluid volume increases, and maternal blood increases. Continued intake of protein allows for maintenance of protein tissues during and after pregnancy.

Protein supplementation during pregnancy is inconclusive. Many studies suggest that protein supplementation during pregnancy does not provide any additional benefit for women who are well nourished.[16] Women who consume a well-balanced diet likely meet protein recommendations through diet alone and do not benefit

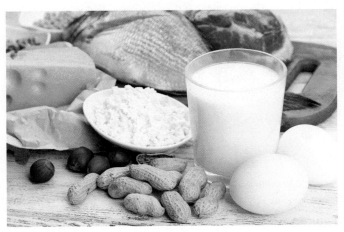

©Africa Studio/Shutterstock

from protein supplementation. However, benefits have been found among women with protein-energy malnutrition.[16] Pregnant women should be encouraged to consume protein from a variety sources such as legumes, eggs, cheese, milk, and lean meats to ensure intake of all essential amino acids. Women who follow vegan diets should be monitored carefully during pregnancy to ensure they meet their protein needs. Clinicians should assist vegan mothers in finding protein-rich foods.

Fat

Adequate fat intake is necessary during pregnancy to assist with fetal growth and development. Additionally, fat is important for cellular signaling, protein function, gene expression, and for the absorbption of fat-soluble vitamins.[17] The main types of fat in the diet are saturated, monounsaturated, polyunsaturated, and trans fats, all of which are classified based on the number and type of double bonds located on the carbon chain. Fat provides essential fatty acids, including omega-6 fatty acids and omega-3 fatty acids. Recommendations for omega-6 and omega-3 fatty acids are 13 and 1.4 g per day, respectively. Most women easily meet recommendations for omega-6 fatty acids but generally fail to meet recommendations for omega-3 fats. The Centers for Disease Control and Prevention (CDC) and American Heart Association specify that omega-3 fats are required for a heart-healthy diet.[18]

The body can produce all of the fatty acids that it needs except for two: linoleic acid, which is an omega-6 fatty acid, and alpha-linolenic acid, which is an omega-3 fatty acids. Linoleic acid and linolenic acid serve as precursors to **eicosanoids** that are used as signaling molecules required for growth after inflammation, physical activity, and ingestion of toxic pathogens. Eicosanoids, derived from linoleic and linolenic acids, regulate organ functions and many bodily systems. They also act as messenger molecules for the central nervous system. Both linoleic acid and alpha-linolenic acid are needed for growth and repair; however, they can also be used to make other fatty acids, such as eicosapentaenoic acid (EPA) and docosahexaenoic acid (DHA). EPA and DHA work together in the body, with each providing its own benefits. EPA supports the immune system, heart, and inflammatory response; DHA supports the eyes, brain, and central nervous system.[19] The conversion to EPA and DHA is limited and therefore sources of these fatty acids should be included in the diet. During pregnancy, EPA and DHA are especially vital for the development of the brain, retina, and neural tissues of the fetus, and they may also play a role in determining the length of gestation and in preventing perinatal depression.[17] DHA is sensitive to light, oxygen, and heat, which make the double bonds break down and create a fishy odor.

Good food sources of EPA and DHA include fish such as salmon, tuna, sardines, anchovies, and herring. Other sources of omega-3 fatty acids such as vegetable oils and flaxseed oil need to be converted to longer-chain EPA and DHA to become biologically useful; therefore, these are not considered to be the best sources. DHA-enriched eggs are another source of omega-3 fatty acids. Many women do not consume fish during pregnancy because of the high mercury content and other pollutants found in some types of fish. The U.S. Food and Drug Administration (FDA) advises pregnant women to avoid fish that are high in mercury content such as tilefish, shark, swordfish, and king mackerel and suggests consumption of 8–12 ounces of fish per week, including salmon, pollock, squid, sardines, and oysters, because they contain the lowest levels of mercury but have the highest amounts of EPA and DHA.[19]

Recommendations also include limiting the consumption of albacore tuna to 6 ounces per week; however, other types of tuna can be consumed more regularly.[20] Because shrimp does not contain mercury, it is considered a very good source of omega-3 fats. Studies also show a link between eating fish or seafood during pregnancy and fewer symptoms of depression or anxiety than in those who ate no fish while pregnant.[21] Pregnancy-related and postpartum depression have been shown to affect child attachment, cognitive development, and behavior. Research has demonstrated that increased intake of long-chain polyunsaturated fatty acids (PUFAs) during pregnancy has reduced the risk of depressive symptoms in the postpartum period.[22] **TABLE 3.9** lists the omega-3 fatty acid content and mercury content in various types of fish. Other sources of linoleic and linolenic acids are listed in **TABLE 3.10**. For pregnant women, the recommendation is to take 200–300 mg of DHA daily.

Omega-3 fatty acid supplements are available to consume during pregnancy; however, the FDA states that consumption of fish, rather than fish oil supplements, is recommended owing to the additional nutritional benefits for mother and fetus. Numerous studies investigating omega-3 supplementation have supported this idea.

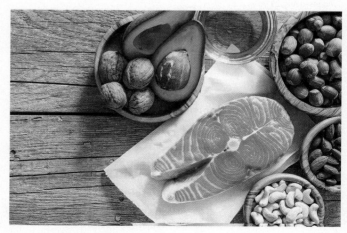

©Oleksandra Naumenko/Shutterstock

Table 3.9

Omega-3 Fatty Acid Content and Mercury Content in Various Fish

Common Varieties	Milligrams of Omega-3 Fatty Acids (Eicosapentaenoic [EPA] and Docosahexaenoic [DHA]) per 4 Ounces of Cooked Fish	Micrograms of Mercury per 4 Ounces of Cooked Fish
Salmon: Atlantic, chinook, coho	1,200–2,400	2
Anchovies, herring, and shad	2,300–2,400	5–10
Mackerel: Atlantic and Pacific (not king)	1,350–2,100	8–13
Tuna: bluefin and albacore	1,700	54–58
Sardines: Atlantic and Pacific	1,100–1,600	2
Oyster: Pacific	1,550	2
Trout: Freshwater	1,000–1,100	11
Tuna: white (albacore) canned	1,000	40
Mussels: blue	900	NA
Salmon: pink and sockeye	700–900	2
Squid	750	11
Pollock: Atlantic and walleye	600	6
Marlin	250–1,030	69
Crab: blue, king, snow, queen, and Dungeness	200–550	9
Tuna: skipjack and yellowfin	150–350	31–49
Flounder, plaice, and sole (flatfish)	350	7
Clams	200–300	<1
Tuna: light canned	150–300	13
Catfish	100–250	7
Cod: Atlantic and Pacific	200	14
Scallops: bay and sea	200	8
Haddock and hake	200	2–5
Lobster: American	200	47
Crayfish	200	5
Tilapia	150	2
Shrimp	100	<1
Orange roughy	42	80
Varieties that should not be consumed by women who are pregnant or breastfeeding or by young children		
Shark	1,250	151
Tilefish: Gulf of Mexico	1,000	219
Swordfish	1,000	147
Mackerel: king	450	110

Reproduced from the U.S. Department of Agriculture, U.S. Department of Human Services; 2010. *Dietary guidelines for Americans*. Retrieved from: https://health.gov/dietaryguidelines/2010/. Accessed Aug. 29, 2014.

Table 3.10

Common Sources of Linoleic and Linolenic Acids

Linoleic Acid	Linolenic Acid
Safflower oil	Chia seeds
Grapeseed oil	Flax seeds and flaxseed oil
Sunflower oil	Walnuts and walnut oil
Hemp oil	Canola (rapeseed) oil
Corn oil	Soybeans and soybean oil
	Leafy-green vegetables
	Fish oil and fatty fish

A review of 48 trials and approximately 37,000 participants found that omega-3 supplementation did not reduce the risk of preeclampsia, postpartum depression, or intrauterine growth restriction, and provided only a slight improvement in birth weight and length.[23] The process of stripping contaminants such as mercury and pesticides from fish oil in the production of supplements also removes antioxidants. It is likely that the additional nutrients found in food sources of fish are what make the health benefits of omega-3 consumption from whole food sources more pronounced than that of supplements.

EPA and DHA are transferred through the placenta to the fetus. During the third trimester, DHA and EPA are accumulated in the tissues of the fetus, making concentrations of DHA higher in the fetus than in the mother. Because this occurs in the third trimester, premature infants are at increased risk for limited stores of DHA and EPA. Mothers that carry until term are at risk for depleting DHA and EPA stores. Some studies have suggested that low DHA and EPA after pregnancy result in postpartum depression among mothers; however, results are inconclusive.[20] Maternal intake of oily fish, such as salmon, mackerel, herring, and albacore tuna (up to 340 g) during pregnancy has been shown to improve fine motor coordination, child IQ stores, communication skills, and social skills.[20]

Because EPA and DHA cross the placenta, the amount that the fetus receives depends on the amount the mother consumes during pregnancy. The amount of EPA and DHA that can be derived from linolenic acid in the body is limited. Less than 10% of linolenic acid is converted to EPA and DHA in pregnant women. Even with high intakes of linolenic acid, most women are unable to consume adequate EPA and DHA. Because the body is unable to make EPA and DHA, women must consume foods high in EPA and DHA or take supplements. The FDA considers supplementation of 500 mg per day of EPA and DHA to be safe for pregnant women. Currently, there are no FDA-established daily requirements for DHA and EPA.

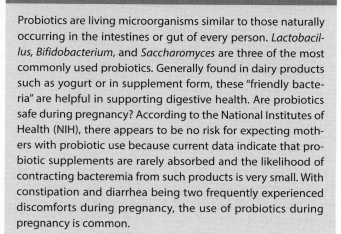

News You Can Use

Probiotics are living microorganisms similar to those naturally occurring in the intestines or gut of every person. *Lactobacillus, Bifidobacterium*, and *Saccharomyces* are three of the most commonly used probiotics. Generally found in dairy products such as yogurt or in supplement form, these "friendly bacteria" are helpful in supporting digestive health. Are probiotics safe during pregnancy? According to the National Institutes of Health (NIH), there appears to be no risk for expecting mothers with probiotic use because current data indicate that probiotic supplements are rarely absorbed and the likelihood of contracting bacteremia from such products is very small. With constipation and diarrhea being two frequently experienced discomforts during pregnancy, the use of probiotics during pregnancy is common.

Vitamins and Minerals

Vitamin A

Vitamin A is an essential nutrient that is especially important for normal cellular function, including reproduction and development. Both deficiency and toxicity of vitamin A can be harmful for a developing fetus. Deficiency of this vitamin is not common in developed countries because vitamin A stores in the liver are usually high enough to supply enough vitamin A during periods of low intake. However, an estimated 8–15% of pregnant women around the globe, most of whom come from developing countries such as Africa and Southeast Asia, experience vitamin A deficiency during pregnancy.[24] This vitamin deficiency during pregnancy can increase the risk of poor pregnancy outcomes such as malformations of the heart and lungs of the infant and night blindness and anemia among mothers. Vitamin A deficiency is typically caused by inadequate intake of vitamin A, with contributing factors such as lack of access to vitamin A–rich foods, poverty, cultural beliefs, and limited education on the importance of vitamin A during pregnancy.[25] Vitamin A supplementation has been provided in many developing countries as an inexpensive, efficient, and quick way to improve health outcomes of mothers and infants.

In the United States, toxicity of vitamin A is much more common than deficiency. Excessive levels of vitamin A occur through medications and supplementation. Specifically, acne and wrinkle medications such as Accutane and Retin-A provide excessive amounts of two forms of vitamin A, retinol and retinoic acid, which increase the risk of fetal abnormalities if taken during pregnancy. Other medications used for psoriasis and some cancer treatments also contain high amounts of retinol. These medications are especially harmful to the fetus when taken during the first trimester of pregnancy, causing retinoic acid syndrome. Infants with this syndrome typically have high foreheads, ear malformations, flat nasal bridges, heart defects, and malformations of the brain.

To prevent excessive levels of vitamin A in the blood, women who are pregnant or who may become pregnant should limit vitamin A intake to 5,000 IU per day, an amount that can be obtained from the typical American diet. Pregnant women should consult with a clinician before taking supplements with high levels of vitamin A during pregnancy. Many supplements on the market use beta-carotene in place of retinol. Beta-carotene is not associated with harmful effects on the fetus; therefore, supplements with beta-carotene are a better option for pregnant mothers.

Good food sources of vitamin A include sweet potatoes, carrots, dark leafy greens such as kale, butternut squash, romaine lettuce, dried apricots, cantaloupe, and sweet red peppers.

Vitamin D

Approximately 40–60% of the adult population in the United States is vitamin D deficient.[26] Adequate vitamin D levels during pregnancy support bone health, immune function, and cell division. Vitamin D assists with the absorption and metabolism of calcium and phosphorus, which are vital for proper bone and tooth formation. At the time of birth, vitamin D levels in the infant are

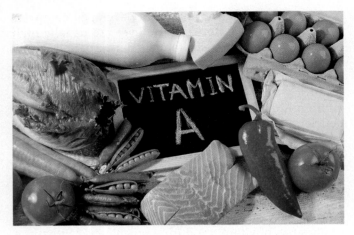

©Bitt24/Shutterstock

around 60–70% of the maternal level; therefore, if maternal vitamin D stores are low, the infant will be born with low levels of vitamin D.[27] Low vitamin D levels during pregnancy can result in a number of negative outcomes for both baby and mother. Examples of possible negative outcomes for the infant include: low birth weight, rickets, and poor bone mineralization. Examples of possible negative outcomes for mother include: osteomalacia, infectious diseases, cardiovascular disease, and preeclampsia.

Very few foods have naturally high levels of vitamin D. In fact, only 10% of vitamin D is obtained through nutritional sources; the rest comes from vitamin D synthesis in the skin.[28] It is estimated that 50–65% of pregnant women are vitamin D deficient.[29] Foods that contain vitamin D include egg yolk, salmon, and cod liver oil. Many dairy products such as milk and yogurt are fortified with vitamin D. Some cereals and orange juices are also fortified with vitamin D. Even with adequate intakes of vitamin D, several factors influence proper vitamin D absorption during pregnancy, including obesity, sun exposure, use of sunscreen, and skin pigmentation. Obesity increases the risk for vitamin D deficiency because of decreased bioavailability as a result of vitamin D deposits in body fat.[30] Limited sun exposure or sun exposure with consistent use of sunblock prevents vitamin D absorption in the skin, increasing the risk for deficiency. Women who consume vegan diets are also at risk for vitamin D deficiency because vitamin D is typically found in animal products. Women with dark skin pigmentation are at higher risk for deficiency of vitamin D because dark skin tones block sunlight that is necessary for catalyzing the production of vitamin D, therefore providing less vitamin D to the mother and fetus.

Pregnant women should be especially careful about meeting vitamin D recommendations of 600 IU per day to prevent symptoms of deficiency. Recommendations can be met through food and sunlight exposure. For example, 2 cups of vitamin D–fortified milk and 1 cup of vitamin

D–fortified yogurt each day provides adequate vitamin D. Sun exposure of 15 minutes twice a week generates 50,000 IU of vitamin D. This short period of time is enough to provide vitamin D benefits without a high risk for sunburn or skin cancer. Geographical location and time of year influence vitamin D absorption. Women in northern climates will not absorb adequate amounts of vitamin D in winter months because of limited and weak sun exposure. Excessive sun exposure is not linked to toxic amounts of vitamin D; however, excessive sun exposure may cause other health problems such as skin cancer. The American College of Obstetricians and Gynecologists recommends 600–2,000 IU of vitamin D each day.[31] Vitamin D supplements can be found in the form of D_3 (cholecalciferol) and D_2 (ergocalciferol). Cholecalciferol is the preferred vitamin D supplementation because of its ability to increase blood levels of vitamin D at higher rates than ergocalciferol can.

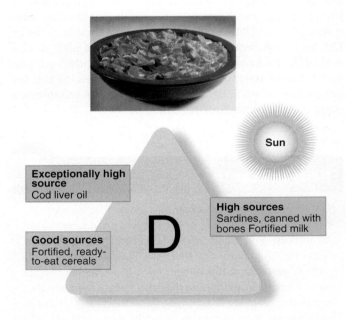

©Photodisc

Calcium

Calcium is essential during pregnancy for a number of reasons. Calcium is needed to build teeth and bones, it allows blood to clot normally, and it allows for muscles, nerves, and the heart to function properly. The skeleton of the fetus requires an average of 30 g of calcium during pregnancy, most of which is accumulated during the third trimester.[32] The absorption of calcium increases from 57% in the second trimester to 72% in the third trimester, when maternal bone turnover is highest.[32] Because calcium absorption increases during pregnancy, calcium needs for pregnant women are the same as those for nonpregnant women. Inadequate intake of calcium during pregnancy can cause negative health outcomes for the mother and fetus. Although deficiency is rare, low calcium can cause pregnancy-induced hypertension (PIH) and pre-eclampsia, which can result in preterm birth.[33]

Good sources of calcium include milk and dairy products, fortified cereal, soy beverages, collard greens, almonds, salmon, tofu, broccoli, and avocado.

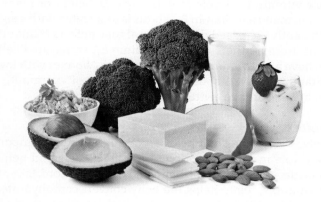

©Robyn Mackenzie/Shutterstock

Iron

Iron is an exceptionally important nutrient during pregnancy, which is why recommendations for iron increases from 18 mg per day in nonpregnant women to 27 mg per day for pregnant women.[34] Iron is necessary to make hemoglobin, an erythrocyte protein that carries oxygen throughout the body to all the tissues and organs. Low hemoglobin levels caused by lack of iron in the blood results in anemia. **TABLE 3.11** lists the hemoglobin and hematocrit levels during each trimester of pregnancy that indicate anemia. Ideally, women should have adequate iron stores prior to conception to ensure additional iron needs are met during pregnancy. During pregnancy, increased iron is necessary to ensure the fetus is receiving adequate oxygen and to increase red blood cell count

necessary for production of fetal blood. Iron is also necessary for metabolism, growth, normal cellular functioning, and synthesis of some hormones.[35] After delivery, iron stores increase as a result of the naturally occurring recycling process of red blood cells.

The Dietary Guidelines for Americans recommend that all women who are pregnant should take an iron supplement.[36] Iron supplementation varies depending on trimester of pregnancy and iron stores in the body. For women who have iron-deficiency anemia during pregnancy, recommendations for iron supplements increase to 60–120 mg per day.[37] Randomized clinical trials have demonstrated significant reductions in iron-deficiency anemia and improvements in health outcomes for mother and infant when iron supplements are taken during pregnancy.[38] Iron supplementation can cause a variety of gastrointestinal side effects such as constipation, abdominal pain, vomiting, and nausea. Taking iron supplements with food can reduce the amount of gastrointestinal discomfort and improve absorption. **TABLE 3.12** suggests action for supplementation that should be taken at various serum ferritin levels.[38]

Absorption of iron varies based on trimester of pregnancy, iron stores, and intake of other nutrients. Iron absorption is especially low during the first trimester, with absorption increasing as the pregnancy continues. Eating a diet that is well balanced and that includes foods high in iron can help ensure adequate intake. The best sources of iron include enriched grain products, lean meat, poultry, fish, and leafy-green vegetables.

Iodine

Iodine is a micronutrient that is vital during pregnancy for thyroid function, brain development of the fetus, and maternal energy production. Pregnancy has a significant impact on the function of the thyroid gland, which affects the health of both the mother and fetus. Iodine needs increase by 50% during pregnancy owing to greater production of thyroid hormones as well as its use in normal fetal brain development and growth.[39] Low iodine intake and low iodine stores in the body can lead to in the mother

Table 3.11

Hemoglobin and Hematocrit Values Defining Anemia During Pregnancy

Pregnancy Trimester	Hemoglobin (g/dL)	Hematocrit (g/dL)
First	<11.0	33.0
Second	<10.5	32.0
Third	<11.0	33.0

Reproduced from Centers for Disease Control and Prevention. Pediatric and Pregnancy Nutrition Surveillance System. What is PedNSS/PNSS? Retrieved from: http://www.cdc.gov/pednss/what_is/pnss_health_indicators.htm#Maternal%20 Health%20Indicators. Accessed September 9, 2016.

Table 3.12

Serum Ferritin Levels at First Prenatal Visit Determining Iron Supplementation Needs

Serum Ferritin (mcg/L)	Action for Supplementation
>60	No supplementation.
20–60	Iron supplementation from 20 weeks gestation.
15–19	Iron supplementation from 12 weeks gestation.
<15	Admit and treat patient.

Data from Mei ZG, Cogswell ME, Looker AC, et al. Assessment of iron status in US pregnant women from the National Health and Nutrition Examination Survey (NHANES), 1999–2006. Am J Clin Nutr. 2011;93(6):1312–1320.

and the fetus. Iodine deficiency in the fetus results in improper neurocognitive development and problems with hearing, speech, and growth. Furthermore, severe deficiency of iodine has been associated with preterm delivery, stillbirth, miscarriage, and congenital abnormalities.[40] **Hypothyroidism** and other pregnancy-related problems resulting from iodine deficiency are rare in the United States; however, they are common in countries in Africa, Asia, and Europe.

Because some soil is richer in iodine than others, the iodine content in foods varies. In the United States, iodized salt is the most common source of iodine. One teaspoon of iodized salt contains 400 mcg of iodine. Most women who consume iodized salt are able to meet dietary requirements of this nutrient. Other foods with iodine include seafood, meat, eggs, dairy products, and some breads. Seaweed and kelp are also natural sources of iodine; however, the amount of iodine found in these foods varies widely and they should not be used to meet iodine recommendations.

It can be difficult to determine how much iodine is consumed because food companies are not required to indicate iodine amounts on the Nutrition Facts label. Approximately half of the multivitamin and mineral supplements available in the United States do not contain iodine. The RDA for iodine for pregnant women is 220 mcg/day. Consistent intake of too much iodine can cause serious health problems; therefore, pregnant women should not consume more than 1,100 mcg of iodine daily.[41]

Sodium

Sodium is required for proper water balance and blood pressure. Sodium requirements significantly increase during pregnancy as a result of an increase in blood volume. Historically, women were advised to reduce salt intake during pregnancy to prevent high blood pressure and to reduce edema.[42] What was later learned is that a low-sodium diet during pregnancy may increase the risk of low blood pressure for the expecting mother because her sodium reserves can be depleted during the pregnancy.[42] Consequently, pregnant women should be advised to consume salt "to taste" and should not be advised to limit salt intake during pregnancy unless otherwise indicated by a physician.

B-Complex Vitamins

B vitamins such as biotin, niacin, folate, thiamine, riboflavin, pantothenic acid, and vitamins B_6 and B_{12} are among the most widely recognized B vitamins. These vitamins are involved with energy metabolism through numerous metabolic pathways, DNA synthesis, cell growth, and homocysteine metabolism. Deficiencies in many of the B vitamins during pregnancy, including vitamin B_6 and B_{12}, riboflavin, and folate, can cause an increase in homocysteine levels in the blood. High levels of homocysteine

cause adverse health outcomes during pregnancy such as low-birth weight infants, stillbirths, preeclampsia, and preterm deliveries.[43] Vitamin B_6 and vitamin B_{12} supplements are sometimes used to improve morning sickness during pregnancy; however, the results are not consistent with all women.

Vitamin B_{12} intake is directly related to serum levels of vitamin B_{12}. Because vitamin B_{12} is found primarily in meats, vegetarians and vegans are at the greatest risk for low vitamin B_{12} levels or deficiency. Deficient or inadequate maternal vitamin B_{12} status is associated with a significantly increased risk for neural tube defects.[44] Infants born from mothers with low vitamin B_{12} stores are likely to have a low vitamin B_{12} status at birth. Women with low vitamin B_{12} levels should increase intake of vitamin B_{12}–rich foods or take a vitamin B_{12} supplement.

Folate

Folate, also called folic acid or vitamin B_9, plays an important role in the production of red blood cells and helps fetal development of the brain and the spinal cord. Like all B vitamins, folate helps the body convert carbohydrates into glucose, which can then be used for energy production. Folate also functions to help the body use fats and protein. Folate is used to make DNA and other genetic material and is needed for body cells to divide.

Folate is a nutrient that cannot be produced in the human body; therefore, it must be consumed through food or supplementation. It is naturally present in many foods and is a mandatory fortification for some common food products such as bread, flour, cornmeal, rice, pasta, and other grain products. Folate needs increase substantially during pregnancy as a result of increased cell division, rapid cell growth, and increased metabolism from fetal development, expansion of maternal blood volume, and uterine growth.[45]

Folic acid fortification has been one of the most effective public health interventions. In 1998, the U.S. Department of Health and Human Services implemented folic acid fortification in refined grain products to reduce the incidence of neural tube defects (NTDs) among infants and to improve folate blood levels among consumers.[45] This mandatory fortification program requires 140 mg of folic acid be added to every 100 g of enriched grain cereals.[46] It was projected that folate fortification would increase average folate intakes by 100 mcg/day; however, since mandatory fortification was implemented in the United States, blood folate levels have increased 150% and the prevalence of NTDs has decreased by 19–32%.[47] As a result of program success, 76 other countries have since adopted flour fortification programs. **FIGURE 3.5** summarizes fortification of folic acid and how this has increased women's intake over time.

Folate can be found in many fruits and vegetables such as spinach, asparagus, brussels sprouts, legumes, eggs, seafood, grains, and meat; however, only a few of

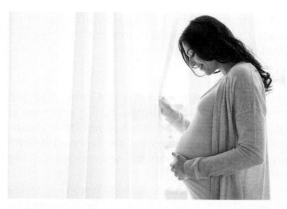

Adequate intake of folate is important for women who are pregnant, and for those who may become pregnant.

©Syda Productions/Shutterstock

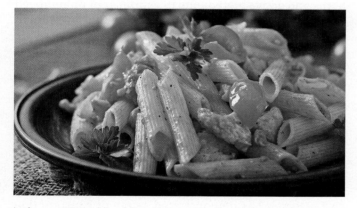

In the year 1998, adding folic acid to cereal and grain products became a requirement by the Food and Drug Administration.

©Timolina/Shutterstock

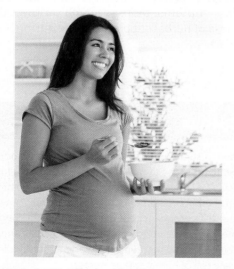

As a result of Folic Acid Fortification, blood folate levels in women has increased over time, and the prevalence of neural tube defects has decreased.

©wavebreakmedia/Shutterstock

Figure 3.5
The success of folic acid fortification.

these provide folate that is highly bioavailable. Foods that are fortified with folic acid such as pasta, breads, cereal, and rice provide approximately twice the dietary folate equivalents as compared with folate naturally found in foods. It is important to check the food labels with whole grain products such as oatmeal, bread, pasta, tortillas, and rice because manufacturers are not required to fortify these products with folic acid.

The IOM recommends that women who are pregnant or who may become pregnant should consume at least 400 mcg of folate a day in either food or supplement form. Folate recommendations for women who have experienced a pregnancy affected by a NTD such as spina bifida need a higher intake of folic acid. It is recommended that these women take 10 times the amount of folate suggested for other women.[48] Some studies show that folic acid supplementation has reduced the risk of oral facial clefts, limb defects, and hydrocephalus.

Bioavailability of folate, measured as dietary folate equivalents, varies depending on the source. Folic acid, the form of folate that is used for fortification and supplementation, is more readily absorbed than folate, which naturally occurs in foods. Folic acid is nearly 100% bioavailable when taken on an empty stomach and 85% bioavailable when taken with food.[49] This is considerably better than the bioavailability of folate, which is roughly 50%.[46]

Initially, adequate folate intake during pregnancy was encouraged to reduce anemia and improve fetal growth. In the past 30 years, extensive research has been conducted regarding low folate blood levels during pregnancy and neural tube defects. The first 28 days after conception are among the most vital for adequate folate intake. If folate intake is inadequate during this time, the neural tube can fail to close, resulting in neural tissues being exposed. Because the onset of NTDs is so early in pregnancy, a complete recovery can be limited. Depending on the severity, these birth defects can cause significant morbidity and even mortality.

The RDAs for folate and other nutrients are found in **TABLE 3.13**.

Supplement Use

Supplements are commonly consumed during pregnancy to help reach the RDA for vitamins and minerals. Ideally, a well-balanced diet provides adequate protein, carbohydrates, and fat to meet the macronutrient needs of the mother and fetus. A general multivitamin and mineral supplement can be taken to provide nutrients that may not be adequately met in the diet. Many women of childbearing age consume inadequate amounts of folic acid, vitamin D, iron, potassium, magnesium, EPA, and DHA.[50] Supplement intake during pregnancy can help some women meet their needs for these nutrients, which are vital to the growth and development of the fetus. Women who benefit from a multivitamin and mineral supplement

Table 3.13

Recommended Dietary Allowances and Upper Limits for Pregnant Adult Women

Nutrient	RDA	Upper Limit
Energy		
1st trimester	0	—
2nd trimester	+350 kcal	—
3rd trimester	+452 kcal	—
Protein	71 g	—
Linoleic acid	13 g	—
Alpha-linolenic acid	1.4 g	—
Vitamin A	770 mcg	3,000 mcg
Vitamin C	85 mg	2,000 mg
Vitamin D	15 mcg	100 mcg
Vitamin E	15 mg	1,000 mcg
Vitamin K	1.4 mcg	—
B vitamins		
Riboflavin	1.5 mg	—
Niacin	18 mg	35 mg
Pantothenic acid	6 mcg	—
Vitamin B_6	1.9 mcg	200 mcg
Biotin	30 mcg	—
Folate	600 mcg	1,000 mcg
Vitamin B_{12}	2.6 mcg	—
Choline	450 mg	3,500 mg
Calcium	1,000 mg	2,500 mg
Chromium	30 mcg	—
Copper	1 mg	10 mg
Fluoride	3 mg	10 mg
Iodine	220 mcg	1,100 mcg
Iron	27 mg	45 mg
Magnesium	350 mg	350 mg
Manganese	2 mg	11 mg
Molybdenum	50 mcg	2,000 mcg
Phosphorus	700 mg	3,500 mg
Potassium	4,700 mg	—
Selenium	60 mcg	400 mcg
Zinc	11 mg	40 mg

Data from Dietary Recommended Intakes (DRIs): http://www.tidyforms.com/download/pregnancy-weight-gain-chart-in-pounds.html

during pregnancy include those who do not consume a well-balanced diet regularly, are vegan, have anemia or another diagnosed deficiency, have a multifetal pregnancy, or consume harmful substances such as tobacco, alcohol, or illicit drugs.[51]

Vitamin and mineral supplements are generally prescribed by a healthcare provider, but they can also be purchased over the counter. The FDA does not regulate the contents of all supplements on the market. Some prenatal supplements contain amounts of vitamins and minerals that exceed the Tolerable Upper Intake Levels. Women should be advised to read the labels on supplements prior to consumption to be sure they do not contain excessive amounts of nutrients. Supplements appropriate during pregnancy should contain no more than the recommended intakes of nutrients.

Herbs

A number of herbal supplements and remedies are generally recognized as safe for use during pregnancy; however, safety of herbal products has not been established through extensive research, so many clinicians recommend that herbal products be avoided during pregnancy.

Unlike prescription medications, herbal supplements and remedies are not required to be approved by the FDA nor are the manufacturers required to indicate the safety of their products if used during pregnancy. Studies have shown inconsistency in the amount of herbs and active ingredients in a number of unapproved FDA products.[52] The FDA recommends that all women who are pregnant consult with a clinician before using herbal products. Women may not be aware of the limitations associated with the disclosure of herbal product safety, which may lead them to use supplements that are unsafe for use during pregnancy. Some commonly used herbs that are unsafe to use during pregnancy include aloe vera, comfrey, ephedra ginkgo, ginseng, kava, and licorice.

A multinational study found that ginger, raspberry, cranberry, and valerian are the most commonly used herbs.[53] Ginger is one of the only herbs in which extensive research has demonstrated safety of consumption during pregnancy.[54] Peppermint tea to help reduce nausea and vomiting also appears to be safe for consumption during pregnancy; however, peppermint can exacerbate heartburn symptoms. More research on the safety and effectiveness of herbal supplement use during pregnancy is warranted.

Let's Discuss

Use of herbal supplements has become very common in the United States as a way to prevent and treat various ailments. It is a clinician's responsibility to determine whether patients are taking any herbal supplements during pregnancy. How should you respond if a pregnant patient tells you she is taking herbal supplements that are not considered safe for use during pregnancy? Where would you send the woman for more information on safe use of herbal supplements?

Water

Pregnant women are vulnerable to dehydration as a result of increased water needs from increased blood volume and formation of amniotic fluid. Women who experience severe nausea and vomiting during pregnancy are at the highest risk for dehydration. Most pregnant women are advised to increase their caloric consumption by about 300 calories, and because water needs can be calculated based on food consumption, an increase of at least 300 mL of additional fluid is also recommended.[55] Many women experience increased levels of thirst during pregnancy, which typically helps meet the increase fluid needs. A variety of fluids count toward daily fluid intake such as water, milk, diluted fruit juice, and unsweetened beverages such as tea. Some women are afraid of retaining water during pregnancy and therefore limit fluid consumption. Contrary to popular belief, drinking adequate fluids during pregnancy actually helps reduce the amount of fluid retention in areas such as the feet and ankles. Pregnant women who are physical active and those who live in hot climates should further increase fluid intake. Light-colored urine at normal volume is an easy way to identify whether adequate fluids are consumed on a regular basis. Dehydration can cause negative health outcomes for the mother and fetus during pregnancy such as miscarriage and preterm birth.[55]

Sweeteners

FDA-approved artificial sweeteners and nonnutritive sweeteners (such as acesulfame K, aspartame, saccharin, sucralose) are considered safe to consume under the conditions of intended use during pregnancy or otherwise.[56] Although they are considered safe to consume during pregnancy, the FDA recommends consumption of artificial sweeteners be in moderation. Artificial sweeteners can be found in a variety of foods such as desserts, candies, pastries, and soft drinks, making them difficult to avoid entirely throughout the course of pregnancy. Beverages containing these sweeteners are typically low in essential nutrients, and therefore use of these beverages should be thoughtful. Nutritive sweeteners such as honey, molasses, maple syrup, and agave nectar should be consumed in moderation owing to their high calorie content and minimal additional nutritional value. Based on recent research, the Academy of Nutrition and Dietetics considers artificial and nonnutritive sweeteners safe to consume during pregnancy.

> **Recap** Nutritional needs change as a result of the growth and development that occurs during pregnancy. High intakes of nutrients such as iron, EPA, DHA, and folate are especially important to improve pregnancy outcomes for the mother and the fetus. Clinicians should encourage a well-balanced diet that supports nutrient needs during pregnancy.
>
> 1. Discuss carbohydrate, fat, and protein needs during pregnancy and explain why EPA and DHA are essential to consume during pregnancy.
> 2. Explain the needs for vitamin A, vitamin D, calcium, and iron during pregnancy and discuss the complications that can occur in the mother and the fetus from inadequate intakes of these nutrients.

Case Study

Anna's physician is concerned that Anna may not be getting enough essential nutrients, specifically protein and iron, to meet maternal and fetal needs. The physician has referred Anna to a dietitian to determine whether nutrient needs are being met and to provide nutritional recommendations accordingly.

Prior to the appointment, the dietitian asked Anna to keep a food record by writing down everything she ate and drank for 3 days to get a sense of her nutrient intake. In her food record, Anna indicated that she takes 400 mg folic acid daily and 500 mg vitamin C daily. She did not report taking any herbal supplements. The dietitian reviews her chart and finds that Anna has gained 2 lb since her first prenatal appointment and has no significant medical history except that her recent labs indicated ferritin 17 mcg. Her chart indicates that she is not taking any medications.

When Anna met with the dietitian, she mentioned that she uses her acne medication, Accutane, once to twice a week. She mentioned that she spends time outside in the summer working in her vegetable garden; however, she always wears sunscreen with a sun protection factor of at least 30. She mentioned that her 3-day food record is a fairly accurate representation of her usual dietary intake. She abstains from alcohol, tobacco, illicit drugs, and caffeine as a result of her religious beliefs.

The results of her 3-day food diary indicate the following:

Kcal: 2,036
Protein: 64 g
Alpha-linolenic acid: 0.61 g
Linoleic acid: 18 g
Vitamin A: 760 mcg
Vitamin D: 4 mcg
Vitamin B$_{12}$: 2.0 mcg
Zinc: 12 mg

Questions

1. Which nutrients, both high and low, are concerning? Why?
2. What other concerns are there from the meeting with Anna?
3. Provide detailed nutrition recommendations for Anna that are suitable for her religious beliefs.

Common Nutrition Considerations During Pregnancy

Preview During pregnancy, nausea and vomiting may need to be managed, caffeine consumption should be limited, and lead exposure prevented. Managing symptoms that may result from gastroesophageal reflux disease (GERD) as well as preventing constipation and taking steps to ensure food safety are all important during pregnancy. Managing common nutrition considerations during pregnancy supports growth and development of the fetus as well as the health of the mother.

Nausea and Vomiting

Nausea and vomiting during pregnancy are common. Although these can occur any time during the day, the condition is often referred to as "morning sickness." The cause of nausea and vomiting during pregnancy is not clear, but generally starts around the 6th week of pregnancy and stops around the 12th week. Unless the nausea and vomiting becomes severe, it is generally not harmful for the expecting mother or for her baby. The American Pregnancy Association provides the following suggestions for how to help prevent and treat nausea during pregnancy: avoid foods and smells that trigger nausea; keep soda crackers by the bed and eat one or two before getting up in the morning; eat small meals more frequently throughout the day instead of three larger meals; drink less water or fluids with meals, but rather drink fluids between meals; consume more dry, plain foods such as white rice, dry toast, or plain baked potato instead of foods that include cream sauce; keep rooms well ventilated or use a fan to keep air flow around you; get plenty of rest; eat foods that contain ginger and lemons, as these may help ease the feeing of nausea; and discuss the particular prenatal vitamin you are taking and/or consider vitamin B_6 supplementation with your doctor.[57] Although nausea and vomiting during pregnancy can be normal, if the condition does not improve, additional treatments may be necessary.

Caffeine

Caffeine is the most commonly consumed pharmacologically active substance in the world.[58] It is also a substance that passes from the mother's blood to the fetus. Limiting caffeine intake during pregnancy has long been recommended because of concerns related to increased risk for preterm birth, low birth weight, gestational diabetes, miscarriage, congenital malformations, and growth retardations.[59] Caffeine acts as a diuretic and increases heart rate, which can be a concern for women during pregnancy.

Caffeine is naturally and artificially found in many foods and beverages consumed in the typical diet. Current recommendations of 200 mg per day is considered a safe dose in nonpregnant women. This amount is also considered safe for pregnant women on the basis of studies that evaluate the effects of caffeine on birth rate, whereas other research indicates that amounts both above and below 200 mg per occasion are considered safe intake levels during pregnancy.[60] Recent research has found associations between caffeine intake during pregnancy and risk of adverse birth outcomes, preterm birth, and increased risk for childhood obesity; other studies have found contradictory results.[61]

Lead Exposure

The metal lead is used for a variety of commercial purposes and has contributed to a contaminated environment. Studies have shown a definite relationship between low-level lead exposure during early brain development and deficits in children's cognitive functions, with the period during pregnancy being more sensitive compared to prenatal exposure.[62] Elevated blood lead levels can be toxic to the developing brain, interfere with calcium and iron absorption, and bring about slowed growth and shorter stature.[63] Animal studies suggest that if results are applicable to women, an increase in dietary calcium during pregnancy can reduce the transfer of lead from prepregnancy maternal exposures to the fetus.[64]

Heartburn

Heartburn is a common symptom that occurs in a number of pregnant women. During pregnancy, the muscles of the gastrointestinal tract relax as a result of an increase in the hormones estrogen and progesterone.[63] The relaxation of the lower esophageal sphincter, located at the top of the stomach, allows for the stomach contents to be moved into the esophagus, causing heartburn, or more severely gastroesophageal reflux disease (GERD). As the pregnancy advances, pressure from the uterus and fetus can also cause heartburn. Heartburn can be managed through several approaches.[63]

- Eat five or six small meals each day.
- Try drinking only small amounts of liquids with meals.
- Drink more of your juice, milk, or water about 1 hour after eating.
- Eat less fatty foods. Fried foods, ice cream, pizza, chips, sausage, pastries, salad dressing, butter, and margarine are examples of fatty foods that can cause or aggravate heartburn.
- Drink less coffee and soda pop.
- Be aware of foods that cause you heartburn. Spicy foods, chocolate, spearmint, and peppermint bother some people.
- Relax, eat slowly, and chew well.

Constipation

Constipation is another common symptom during pregnancy, often becoming a problem in the third trimester. The primary reason for constipation is thought to be from the relaxed muscle tone of the gastrointestinal tract. Constipation can likely be reduced by increasing fiber intake to approximately 30 g per day and by increasing fluid intake to 6 to 8 glasses per day. Soluble fiber products, such as Metamucil and Citrucel, can be consumed during pregnancy to reduce constipation. Laxatives are generally not recommended during pregnancy because they can cause dehydration and nutrient deficiencies.

Food Safety

A critical aspect of proper nutritional intake during pregnancy is consumption of safe food. Pregnant women are more susceptible to foodborne infections owing to their increased progesterone levels, which decrease their ability to fight off infections. **Listeriosis** is a foodborne illness that can be especially harmful during pregnancy. Listeriosis is nearly 20 times more prevalent in pregnant women as compared with the nonpregnant population.[65] This bacteria can spread through ready-to-eat foods, smoked fish, soft cheese made from unpasteurized milk, and refrigerated luncheon meats. It can cause flu-like symptoms such as fever, backache, headache, muscle pains, nausea, and vomiting. *Listeria* crosses into the placenta, increasing the risk for spontaneous abortion and stillbirth of the fetus and potential infection in the mother. **TABLE 3.14** lists ways to prevent listeriosis.

Campylobacter is another bacteria that can spread through unpasteurized milk. It may cause fever and diarrhea and may spread to the blood, causing a life-threatening condition. It is therefore important to eat foods cooked at the right temperatures to minimize the risk of foodborne illnesses.

Toxoplasma gondii is a protozoan that is especially harmful during pregnancy. If consumed, this protozoan is transferred to the fetus via the placenta and can cause mental retardation, blindness, and death.[66] *Toxoplasma gondii* can be found on the surfaces of fruits and vegetables, in undercooked meats, and in cat litter. To avoid this protozoan, pregnant women should wash fruits and vegetables, cook meat thoroughly, and avoid handling cat litter.

Mercury contamination has become an additional food safety concern for pregnant women. Most fish and seafood contain trace amounts of mercury. Mercury is accumulated in fish and seafood when waters are contaminated by industrial pollution. Microorganisms in the water turn mercury into methylmercury, which accumulates in their bodies. Then larger fish consume these smaller organisms, accumulating mercury in their tissues. Mercury crosses the placenta and can cause serious harm to the nervous system of the fetus.[67] Infants who were exposed to large amounts of mercury can develop learning disabilities, seizures, and hearing loss. The Environmental Protection Agency (EPA) recommends that women who are pregnant or those who may become pregnant avoid consuming long-living predatory fish that are known to contain high mercury levels, including swordfish, shark, mackerel, walleye, albacore tuna, bass, and tilefish. There are safe options to help pregnant women meet the recommendation of 12 ounces of fish per week. Fish and seafood with low mercury content include canned light tuna, salmon, cod, tilapia, pollock, and haddock.

Proper hygiene and sanitation must be practiced during food preparation and handling for women who are pregnant to minimize the risk of foodborne illnesses. Some important points to ensure food safety for pregnant women are as follows: [68]

- Adequate hand washing before handling food
- Proper food handling and storage
- Proper cooking and reheating of food

It is important for pregnant women to read labels and identify high-risk ingredients. According to the FDA, consumption of swordfish, tilefish, king mackerel, and shark during pregnancy is inadvisable because of high methylmercury content. In addition, pregnant women should not consume more than 12 ounces of low-mercury fish per week.

TABLE 3.15 provides an overview of some commonly implicated pathogens that cause foodborne illnesses during pregnancy. Every year 2,500 cases of listeriosis are reported in the United States, a third of which occur in pregnant women in whom it can be quite severe.[69]

Four simple steps can help keep individuals safe from food poisoning at home. These steps include clean, separate, cook, and chill:

1. *Clean*: Wash hands and surfaces often. Hands should be washed for 20 seconds with soap and running water. Wash surfaces and utensils after

---

Table 3.14

Suggestions for Preventing Listeriosis

Avoid unpasteurized milk, cheese, or juice or any foods that contain unpasteurized products.

Avoid refrigerated smoked fish or seafood. Canned versions can be safely consumed.

Avoid raw or undercooked meat.

Avoid luncheon meats or hotdogs. If cooked until steaming hot, they can be safely consumed.

Avoid soft cheeses. Hard cheese and processed cheeses are safe.

Rinse, scrub, and dry raw produce before consumption.

Separate poultry and uncooked meats from other foods.

Maintain refrigerator temperature at 40°F or lower

Reproduced from Centers for Disease Control and Prevention; November 20, 2014. *Listeria (listeriosis)* Prevention. Retrieved from: http://www.cdc.gov/listeria/prevention.html. Accessed on July 23, 2015.

Table 3.15

Commonly Implicated Pathogens That Cause Foodborne Illnesses During Pregnancy

Bacteria/Illness	Found in	Symptoms	Effect on Pregnancy
Listeria monocytogenes	Grows at refrigeration temperatures: luncheon meats, cheese, unpasteurized milk	Listeriosis, fever, chills, diarrhea	Miscarriage, fetal death, or severe illness or death in newborns
Toxoplasma gondii	Raw meat, cat litter	Flu-like symptoms, weak immune system	Miscarriage and birth defects
Salmonella	Unpasteurized milk/juice, raw or undercooked meat, eggs, fresh fruits and vegetables (salads)	Bloody diarrhea, nausea, stomach pain	Severe in pregnancy and may cause complications, including death
Escherichia coli	Undercooked beef, contaminated bean sprouts, fresh leafy greens, unpasteurized milk and juice	Abdominal cramps, bloody diarrhea, vomiting	May develop hemolytic-uremic syndrome (HUS)

Data from: FDA.GOV. Food Safety for Pregnant Women. 2016. Available at: http://www.fda.gov/Food/FoodborneIllnessContaminants/PeopleAtRisk/ucm312704.htm. Accessed February 14, 2016; Ward E. Maternal Nutrition. 1st ed. Mead Johnson; 2012. Available at: https://www.meadjohnson.com/pediatrics/us-en/sites/hcp-usa/files/LB2882-Maternal-Nutrition-Monograph-2.pdf. Accessed February 14, 2016.

each use, and wash fruits and vegetables prior to cooking and/or eating.

2. *Separate:* To prevent cross-contamination, use separate cutting boards and plates for produce and for meat, poultry, seafood, and eggs, and keep these foods separate from all other foods when transporting and storing.

3. *Cook:* The "danger zone" temperatures for food is between 40°F and 140°F. Cook food to safe temperatures and keep food hot after cooking.

4. *Chill:* Refrigerate food promptly and properly. Do not allow perishable foods to be in a temperature range of 90°F or warmer for longer than 1–2 hours.

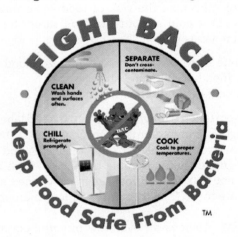

Clean: Wash hands and surfaces often
Separate: Don't cross-contaminate
Cook: Cook to proper temperatures
Chill: Refrigerate properly

Courtesy of Partnership for Food Safety Education, http://fightbac.org.

Changes in Smell and Taste

There are many different beliefs about how food cravings in pregnant women influence the infant. For example, some people believe that excessive intakes of certain foods explain physical outcomes, such as birth marks, or behavioral outcomes of the infant. Others believe that avoiding certain foods, typically foods high in protein, will ease delivery and reduce maternal weight gain. Food cravings and food aversions are very common during pregnancy owing to changes in sense of smell and sense of taste. Every woman is unique in the foods she craves and avoids throughout pregnancy. In general, many women have a preference for fruits, dairy products, and foods that are sweet or salty. Two-thirds of pregnant women report they experienced a heightened sense of smell, with commonly reported stronger smells including cigarette smoke, spices, spoiled food, perfumes, gasoline, cooking odors (especially meat), and coffee.[70] Cravings and aversions are hypothesized to be associated with natural changes in hormones during pregnancy; however, the biological reasoning is not fully understood. Women may become concerned about food cravings that lead to consumption of foods high in fat, sugar, and sodium. Clinicians should help women meet nutrient needs in consideration of the food cravings and aversions each woman experiences.

Recap Women should be aware of numerous nutritional considerations during pregnancy. Nausea and vomiting, excess caffeine intake, and lead exposure can have consequences for the fetus. Pregnant women are at particular high risk for foodborne illness, and proper food handling and storage are necessary to ensure a safe eating environment. During pregnancy, women often experience gastrointestinal symptoms such as nausea, vomiting, heartburn, and constipation, which can be minimized with appropriate nutritional interventions.

1. Discuss the maternal and fetal complications that can occur as a result of exposure to lead during pregnancy.
2. Name the management techniques for preventing or treating symptoms of heartburn and constipation during pregnancy.
3. List and discuss the four steps to ensure food safety.

Promoting Healthy Lifestyles

Preview Nutrition assistance programs, exercise recommendations, food insecurity and hunger, and mental health status should all be discussed with women during pregnancy to promote general health. Healthy nutrition and lifestyle choices influence both the mother and the fetus.

The Special Supplemental Nutrition Program for Women, Infants, and Children

The Special Supplemental Nutrition Program for Women, Infants, and Children (WIC) serves low-income pregnant, postpartum, and breastfeeding women, infants, and children up to age 5 years who are at nutritional risk. WIC is an excellent example of a federally funded nutrition program that improves public health by serving at-risk populations. WIC provides nutrition education and counseling, vouchers for nutritious foods, nutritional assessments, and referrals to other healthcare professionals. See TABLE 3.16 for WIC-approved foods that can be purchased with WIC vouchers.

The WIC program began in 1974, serving only 88,000 people. Currently, WIC serves over 8.6 million women, infants, and children each month in all 50 states, 34 Indian Tribal Organizations, and 6 territories.[71] Pregnant women who are eligible based on the U.S. Poverty Income Guidelines can receive benefits through WIC if they are considered at nutritional risk because of anemia, history of pregnancy complications, poor pregnancy outcomes, overweight or underweight, or they have the inability to meet the Dietary Guidelines for Americans. Participating in WIC is associated with improved birth outcomes such as appropriate infant birth weight.

Participants of WIC and Supplemental Nutrition Assistance Program (SNAP) are further encouraged to use federal nutrition assistance benefits at farmers' markets through newly established matching programs. Matching programs provide a dollar-for-dollar match on each dollar spent at a farmers' market with federal nutrition assistance benefits. Markets all around the country are offering matching programs through federal and private grants. These programs provide incentive to low-income individuals to spend more of their benefits on locally grown foods such as fruits and vegetables. Furthermore, matching programs increase the purchasing power and monthly food dollars of participants of federal nutrition assistance programs.[72]

News You Can Use

Use of Federal Nutrition Assistance at Farmers' Markets

Farmers' markets around the country accept WIC vouchers as a way to increase fruit and vegetable intake, decrease food insecurity, and improve overall diet of WIC participants. Congress established the WIC Farmers' Market Nutrition Program (FMNP) in 1992 as an intervention strategy to allow WIC participants to use vouchers at local farm stands and farmers' markets. In 2013, 46 states, territories, and Indian Tribal Organizations operated this program, and over 1.5 million WIC participants received WIC FMNP benefits. Participants can receive anywhere from $10 to $30 per year to use for locally grown WIC-approved foods. Over 17,000 farmers, 3,300 farmers' markets, and 2,750 roadside stands were authorized to accept WIC FMNP benefits, resulting in over $13.2 million in revenue among local farmers in 2013. Low-income mothers may also be eligible to participate in the Supplemental Nutrition Assistance Program (SNAP), which allows for the purchase of SNAP-approved items at numerous farmers' markets across the country.

Data from U.S. Department of Agriculture Food and Nutrition Service; updated January 13, 2016. Food Buying Guide for Child Nutrition Programs. http://www.fns.usda.gov/tn/food-buying-guide-for-child-nutrition-programs.

Table 3.16

Foods that Can Be Purchased Using WIC Vouchers

Iron-fortified cereal	Peanut butter
Infant cereal	Fruits
Eggs	Vegetables
Milk	Whole wheat bread
Cheese	Tofu
Vitamin C–rich fruit or vegetable juice	Soy-based beverages
Dried or canned beans and peas	Baby food
Canned fish	

Data from U.S. Department of Agriculture Food and Nutrition Service; updated January 13, 2016. Food Buying Guide for Child Nutrition Programs. http://www.fns.usda.gov/tn/food-buying-guide-for-child-nutrition-programs.

Exercise Recommendations

The majority of evidence suggests that moderate to vigorous exercise among healthy women during pregnancy is mentally and physically beneficial for both the mother and the fetus. Weight-bearing exercises have been associated with improved maternal fitness, appropriate weight gain for adequate growth of the fetus, and fostering postpartum recovery.[73] Exercise during pregnancy is also associated with reduced risk of gestational diabetes, preeclampsia, and preterm birth; assistance with appropriate gestational weight gain; improvements in glucose tolerance; and prevention of low back pain.[74] Women who exercise during pregnancy also report less musculoskeletal pain and depression while also experiencing improvements in quality of life and improved self-image.[69] Exercise should be accompanied by a well-balanced diet, proper hydration, and adequate rest to achieve maximum benefits.

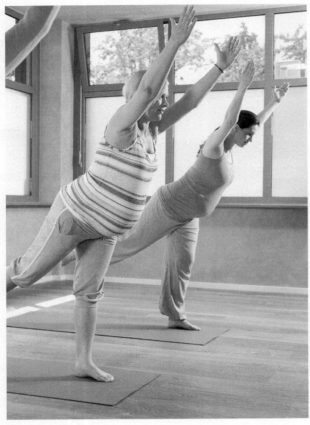

©MITO images/Alamy Stock Photo

Most women, who exercise regularly before pregnancy may continue the same exercise regime during pregnancy. Women with some high-risk pregnancies may be prohibited from vigorous exercise during for a duration of pregnancy. Some physicians may restrict physical activity in women at high risk for miscarriage, preterm delivery, musculoskeletal injury, or poor fetal growth.

Some contraindications for exercise during pregnancy are as follows:[75]

- Low placenta level
- Severe anemia
- Persistent second- or third-trimester bleeding
- Preeclampsia
- Multiple gestation at risk for preterm labor
- Previous history of miscarriage
- Premature labor during current pregnancy

Exercise recommendations for women with uncomplicated pregnancies are for moderate aerobic and strength-conditioning exercises. Heavy weight lifting and similar strenuous activities are discouraged during pregnancy, especially in the second and third trimesters, and exercise in the supine or prone position should be avoided after the first trimester. Unless medically contraindicated, women who are pregnant should be encouraged to exercise with aerobic and strength-training activities for at least 30 minutes five times each week, or for a total of 150 minutes a week.[76] Women who were sedentary prior to pregnancy should begin with 15 minutes of exercise at least three times per week and gradually increase to the amounts recommended for pregnancy in general. Women who were active prior to pregnancy can safely continue to perform their usual routine unless contraindications are present. Female athletes or women with intense exercise routines should consult with a clinician during the early stages of pregnancy. Recommended activities during pregnancy include walking, swimming, water aerobics, cycling, dancing, jogging, and yoga. Each period of exercise should begin with a short warm-up and end with a cooldown.

Physical activity among pregnant women tends to decrease as pregnancy progresses, resulting in few women meeting physical activity guidelines during pregnancy.[77] There are several predictors to increased physical activity during pregnancy, including being white, having higher education and income, being physically active prior to pregnancy, and not having any children in the house.[78] Numerous barriers prevent pregnant women from meeting physical activity recommendations. Clinicians should consider barriers to exercise when providing physical activity recommendations during pregnancy.

Food Insecurity and Hunger

Food insecurity, which is defined as the inability to obtain nutritious and safe foods in socially acceptable ways, and hunger have affected pregnant women for many centuries. Nearly 49.1 million people experienced food insecurity in 2013.[79] Low-income pregnant women are more likely to experience food insecurity and therefore to have less-than-desirable intakes of essential vitamins and minerals during their pregnancy. Food insecurity during pregnancy has been shown to increase the risk of low birth weights and certain birth defects such as spina bifida, cleft palate, and anencephaly.[80]

Mental Health

Anxiety and depression are the most common mental health problems that occur during pregnancy. Approximately 13% of pregnant women experience depression and 27% experience anxiety at some point throughout pregnancy.[81] Anxiety and depression during pregnancy can cause poor health outcomes for the mother and fetus such as preterm delivery, preeclampsia, and low birth weight.[82]

Several vitamins and minerals, such as folate, vitamin B_{12}, and vitamin D, have been linked to improving depression and other mood disorders in the general public because of the relationship these nutrients have with neurotransmitters such as dopamine, serotonin, and norepinephrine. Few studies have been conducted to determine the effect of low nutrient levels on maternal depression; however, owing to increased nutritional needs during pregnancy, it is likely that some women are not consuming enough of these particular nutrients to meet the needs of mother and fetus.[83] When providing counseling and education to pregnant women, it is important that clinicians assist women in selecting foods and beverages that are nutrient dense to avoid nutrient deficiencies.

Recap Nutrition assistance programs such as WIC provide nutritious foods for low-income women to reduce the risk of nutritional deficiencies among this population. This program reduces food insecurity, which has historically caused severe malnutrition among pregnant women. Mental health can also be influenced by poor diet and should be monitored carefully.

1. Explain the benefits of participating in WIC and exercising during pregnancy, and list safe exercises for pregnant women.
2. Discuss how food insecurity and common mental health problems can influence the health of the mother and infant.

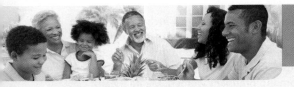

Learning Portfolio

Visual Chapter Summary

The Physiology of Pregnancy and Factors Affecting Dietary Intake During Pregnancy

- Nutritional status of the mother during pregnancy has a significant effect on the current and future health of the mother and the infant.
- Improved nutrition during pregnancy could improve the short- and long-term health of infants in the United States.

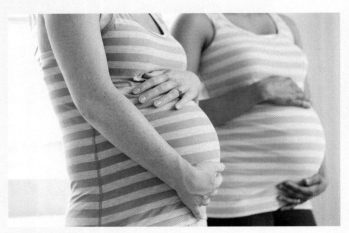

©Weekend Images Inc/iStock /Getty Images Plus/Getty

- Many normal physiological changes occur during pregnancy as a result of increased hormone levels and increased need for nutrients, oxygen, and plasma volume.
- The placenta has many responsibilities, including secreting hormones, fighting infections, exchanging nutrients and oxygen, and removing waste products.
- Hormones such as estrogen, progesterone, hCG, hCS, and leptin play vital roles in developing maternal and fetal tissues, ensuring nutrients are delivered to the fetus, and synthesizing, storing, and mobilizing nutrients.
- Metabolism of macronutrients change during pregnancy to ensure the fetus receives adequate nutrients for growth and development.

Pregnancy Weight Gain

- Pregnancy weight gain recommendations are based on prepregnancy BMI. Appropriate weight gain during pregnancy can improve short- and long-term health outcomes of the infant.
- Postpartum weight retention is most commonly a result of excessive weight gain during pregnancy.

- The rate of weight gain during pregnancy does not seem to be as important to the health outcomes of mother and infant as does the total amount of weight gained throughout pregnancy.

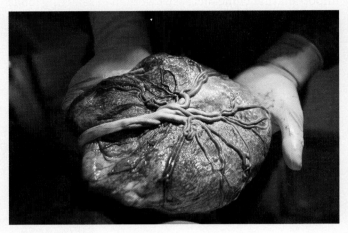

©Noctiluxx/E+/Getty

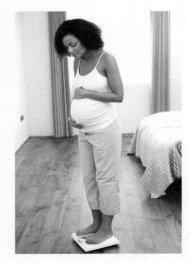

©Monkey Business Images/Shutterstock

- Only about one-third of the weight gained by a normal-weight woman actually goes to the fetus. The rest of the weight supports maternal tissue development that are necessary for pregnancy, delivery, and lactation.

Nutrition Recommendations and Requirements During Pregnancy

- Adequate intakes of calories, fat, and protein are essential for proper growth and development of the fetal and maternal tissues.

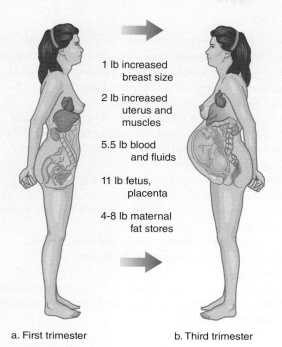

1 lb increased
breast size

2 lb increased
uterus and
muscles

5.5 lb blood
and fluids

11 lb fetus,
placenta

4-8 lb maternal
fat stores

a. First trimester   b. Third trimester

Average weight distribution during pregnancy.

- Linoleic and linolenic acids are vital for the development of the brain, retina, and neural tissues of the fetus. They must be consumed by the mother for the fetus to receive adequate amounts because they cannot be produced in the body.
- Adequate folate during the first 21–28 days after conception has been found to significantly reduce the likelihood of NTDs.

Common Nutrition Considerations During Pregnancy

- Gastrointestinal discomforts such as heartburn and constipation are common during pregnancy and can be reduced through nutrition and lifestyle changes.
- Certain foodborne illnesses such as listeriosis and toxoplasmosis (caused by *Toxoplasma gondii*) can be especially harmful to the fetus during pregnancy. Women should avoid foods during pregnancy that may cause these foodborne illnesses.
- Four simple steps can help keep individuals safe from food poisoning at home. These steps include clean, separate, cook, and chill.
- Women should be cautious when taking herbal supplements during pregnancy because supplements do not go through an extensive review process with the FDA.

Promoting Healthy Lifestyles

- WIC provides nutrition education and counseling, food vouchers, nutritional assessments, and referrals to low-income pregnant women to improve nutrition and health status.
- Food insecurity during pregnancy can result in long-term complications for the mother and infant, including low birth weights and certain birth defects such as spina bifida, cleft palate, and anencephaly.
- Anxiety and depression during pregnancy can cause poor health outcomes for the mother and fetus such as preterm delivery, preeclampsia, and low birth weight.

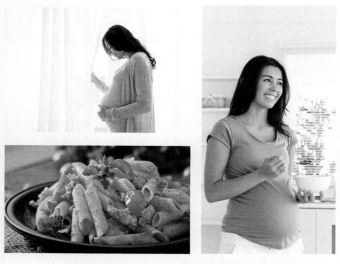

The success of folic acid fortification.

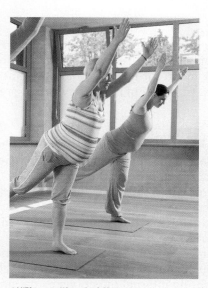

©MITO images/Alamy Stock Photo

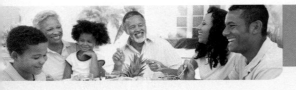

Learning Portfolio (continued)

Key Terms

Campylobacter: Bacteria that can spread through unpasteurized milk, may cause fever and diarrhea, and may spread to the blood, causing a life-threatening condition.

eicosanoids: Signal molecules synthesized by fatty acids that exert control over many systems in the body, including inflammation and immunity. They also act as messengers for the central nervous system.

edema: Excessive extracellular fluid collected usually in the legs and feet, causing swelling.

food insecurity: Limited or uncertain availability of nutritionally adequate and safe foods or limited or uncertain ability to acquire acceptable foods in socially acceptable ways, such as when a person lacks the money or the resources to acquire food. Food insecurity manifests as difficulty providing enough food for all family members at some time during the year as a result of a lack of resources.

gastroesophageal reflux disease (GERD): A highly variable chronic digestive condition that is characterized by periodic episodes of gastroesophageal reflux, when stomach contents flow back up the esophagus, and usually accompanied by heartburn. It may result in histopathologic changes in the esophagus.

hypothyroidism: A condition caused by an underactive thyroid or inadequate maternal iodine intake during pregnancy that is characterized by intellectual disabilities, growth impairment, and deafness in the infant.

listeriosis: A serious infection caused by eating foods contaminated with *Listeria monocytogenes*.

mercury A heavy silvery-white metal that is liquid at ordinary temperatures.

placenta: A disk-shaped organ that connects the fetus to the uterine wall, allowing for nutrient and gas interchange.

Toxoplasma gondii: A parasite found in contaminated and undercooked meats and contaminated water that causes the disease toxoplasmosis.

Discussion Questions

1. Discuss the normal physiological changes that occur during pregnancy and explain how hormones, nutrients, and the placenta play a role.
2. Describe the typical body weight distribution during pregnancy.
3. Discuss why macronutrient and micronutrient needs change during pregnancy and examine the complications associated with inadequate intake of specific nutrients.
4. Discuss the causes of gastrointestinal discomforts most commonly occurring during pregnancy. What are the nutrition and lifestyle interventions aimed to improve these GI problems?
5. Summarize the history of food insecurity among pregnant women. Explain the nutrition and public health programs in the United State that exist to reduce food insecurity in this population.

Activities

1. Develop nutrition recommendations and a 3-day sample menu for a 28-year-old pregnant woman in her first trimester of pregnancy with a prepregnancy BMI of 30. She is experiencing daily heartburn and constipation.

Study Questions

1. The placenta is responsible for all of the following functions *except* which one?
   a. Eliminating hormones such as hCG, estrogen, and progesterone
   b. Transferring nutrients and oxygen from the mother to the fetus
   c. Removing waste products such as uric acid, carbon dioxide, and creatinine from the fetus
   d. Fighting internal infections by passing IgG antibodies to the fetus

2. Which of the following physiological changes is *not* normal during pregnancy?
   a. Increased plasma volume
   b. Decreased production of insulin
   c. Increased sodium retention
   d. Lowered esophageal sphincter tone

3. Which of the following statements about nutrient metabolism occurs in a normal pregnancy?
   a. Cholesterol and triglycerides increase.
   b. Total nitrogen excretion increases.

c. Insulin secretion in the later months of pregnancy increases.
d. Serum albumin increases in the early months of pregnancy.

4. Which of the following is not a recommended weight gain for the associated BMI classification?
    a. Obese: 11–20 lb
    b. Underweight: 28–40 lb
    c. Overweight: 20–30 lb
    d. Normal weight: 25–35 lb

5. Which of the following is *not true* regarding weight gain during pregnancy?
    a. The majority of women do not gain the proper amount of weight during pregnancy.
    b. As BMI increases in prepregnancy, the weight gain required to produce a healthy baby decreases.
    c. The rate of weight gain during pregnancy is more important to the health outcomes of mother and infant than is the total amount of weight gained throughout pregnancy.
    d. Excessive weight gain during pregnancy in a normal-weight woman is associated with a six-fold increase in having a child that is large for gestational age.

6. Which of the following is not a reason for slow weight gain during pregnancy?
    a. Severe nausea and vomiting
    b. Edema
    c. Limited access to adequate food
    d. Poor fetal growth

7. Which of the following statements includes the DRIs of increased energy intake during each trimester of pregnancy?
    a. First trimester: 340 kcal; second trimester: 340 kcal; third trimester: 452 kcal
    b. First trimester: 0 kcal; second trimester: 340 kcal; third trimester: 452 kcal

c. First trimester: 340 kcal; second trimester: 452 kcal; third trimester: 452 kcal
d. First trimester: 0 kcal; second trimester: 452 kcal; third trimester: 452 kcal

8. Which of the following is not a nutrient recommendation for pregnancy?
    a. Protein—71 g per day
    b. Fiber—28 g per day
    c. Carbohydrates—less than 175 g per day
    d. Linoleic acid—14 g per day, and linolenic acid—1.4 g per day

9. Why are linoleic and linolenic acids important to consume during pregnancy?
    a. Reduce likelihood of infection and inflammation.
    b. Assist with appropriate weight gain.
    c. Support the absorption of water-soluble vitamins.
    d. Assist development of the brain, retina, and neural tissues of the fetus.

10. Which of the following is a protozoan that is transferred to the fetus via the placenta and that can cause mental retardation, blindness, and death?
    a. Pica
    b. Mercury
    c. Listeriosis
    d. *Toxoplasma gondii*

11. Which vitamins and minerals have been linked to depression and other mood disorders?
    a. Folate, vitamin B_{12}, and vitamin D
    b. Vitamin A, iron, and vitamin E
    c. Calcium, folate, iron
    d. Vitamin B_6, iodine, vitamin A

12. Physical activity has been shown to reduce the risk of all of the following *except* which one?
    a. Gestational diabetes
    b. Preterm birth
    c. Glucose intolerance
    d. Birth defects

Weblinks

- **Healthy People 2020**
  https://www.healthypeople.gov/2020/topics-objectives/topic/maternal-infant-and-child-health
  Healthy People 2020 provides pregnancy-related objectives, interventions, and resources for mothers and professionals to help reach maternal, infant, and child health objectives.
- **Body Changes During Pregnancy**
  http://www.healthline.com/health/pregnancy/body-changes-infographic

- **Dietary Supplement Label Database**
  http://www.dsld.nlm.nih.gov/dsld/index.jsp
  The National Institutes of Health created a database for consumers that can be used to help identify which prenatal vitamins are safe for consumption during pregnancy.
- **EatRight.org: Pregnancy**
  http://www.eatright.org/resources/health/pregnancy
  The Academy of Nutrition and Dietetics provides research-based information on dietary intake, weight gain, physical activity, and food safety recommendations for pregnant women.

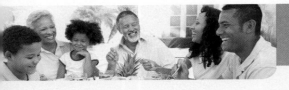

Learning Portfolio (continued)

References

1. Cohain JS. The latest research on preconception and prenatal nutrition. *Midwifery Today Int Midwife.* Summer 2013;(106):52–54.

2. Saura B. Continuity of bodies: the infant's placenta and the island's navel in eastern Polynesia. *J Polyn Soc.* 2002;111(2):127–145.

3. Lind T. Fluid balance during labour: a review. *J R Soc Med.* 1983;76:870–875.

4. Catalano PM. Obesity, insulin resistance, and pregnancy outcome. *Reproduction.* 2010;140(3):365–371.

5. Herrera E, Ortega-Senovilla H. Lipid metabolism during pregnancy and its implications for fetal growth. *Curr Pharm Biotechnol.* 2014;15(1):24–31.

6. Pusukuru R, Shenoi AS, Kyada, PK, et al. Evaluation of lipid profile in second and third trimester of pregnancy. *J Clin Diagn Res. March* 2016;10(3):QC12–16.

7. Wen T, Lv Y. Inadequate gestational weight gain and adverse pregnancy outcomes among normal weight women in China. *Int J Clin Exp Med.* February 15, 2015;8(2):2881–2886.

8. National Library of Medicine; updated November 19, 2014 Managing your weight gain during pregnancy. Retrieved from: http://www.nlm.nih.gov/medlineplus/ency/patientinstructions/000603.htm. Accessed July 24, 2015.

9. He XJ, Hu CL, Chen L, Wang QW, Qin FY. The association between gestational weight gain and substantial weight retention 1-year postpartum. *Arch Gynecol Obstet.* 2014;290(3):493–499.

10. Ma DF, Szeto IMY, Yu K, et al. Association between gestational weight gain according to prepregnancy body mass index and short postpartum weight retention in postpartum women. *Clin Nutr.* 2015;34(2):291–295.

11. Kaiser LL, Campbell CG; Academy Positions Committee Workgroup. Practice paper of the Academy of Nutrition and Dietetics abstract: nutrition and lifestyle for a healthy pregnancy outcome. *J Acad Nutr Diet.* September 2014;114(9):1447.

12. Lopez-Jaramillo P, Gomez-Arbelaez D, Sotomayer-Rubio A. Maternal undernutrition and cardiometabolic disease: A Latin American perspective. *BMC Med.* March 2, 2015;13:41.

13. Szostak-Wegierek D. Intrauterine nutrition: long-term consequences for vascular health. *Int J Womens Health.* July 11, 2014;6:647–656.

14. van der Pligt P, Willcox J, Hesketh KD, et al. Systematic review of lifestyle interventions to limit postpartum weight retention: implications for future opportunities to prevent maternal overweight and obesity following childbirth. *Obes Rev.* 2013;14(10):792–805.

15. King DE, Mainous AG, Lambourne CA. Trends in dietary fiber intake in the United States, 1999–2008. *J Acad Nutr Diet.* 2012;112(5):642–648.

16. Liberato SC, Singh G, Mulholland K. Effects of protein energy supplementation during pregnancy on fetal growth: a review of the literature focusing on contextual factors. *Food Nutr Res.* 2013;57:14.

17. Coletta JM, Bell SJ, Roman AS. Omega-3 fatty acids and pregnancy. *Rev Obstet Gynecol.* 2010;3(4):163–171.

18. Carlson SJ, Fallon EM, Kalish BT, Gura KM, Puder M. The role of the omega-3 fatty acid DHA in the human life cycle. *J Parenter Enteral Nutr.* 2013;37(1):15–22.

19. Wenstrom KD. The FDA's new advice on fish: it's complicated. *Am J Obstet Gynecol.* 2014;211(5):475–478:e1.

20. Swanson D, Block R, Mousa SA. Omega-3 fatty acids EPA and DHA: health benefits throughout life. *Adv Nutr.* 2012;3(1):1–7.

21. Emmett P, Jones L, Golding J. Pregnancy diet and associated outcomes in the Avon Longitudinal Study of Parents and Children [published online September 22, 2015]. *Nutr Rev.* doi:http://dx.doi.org/10.1093/nutrit/nuv053.

22. Makrides M, Gibson RA, McPhee AJ, et al. Effect of DHA supplementation during pregnancy on maternal depression and neurodevelopment of young children: a randomized controlled trial. *JAMA.* 2010;304:1675–1683.

23. Sallis H, Steer C, Patemoster L, et al. Perinatal depression and omega-3 fatty acids: a Mendelian randomization study. *J Affect Disord.* September 2014;166:124–131.

24. Azais-Braesco V, Pascal G. Vitamin A in pregnancy: requirements and safety limits. *Am J Clin Nutr.* 2000;71(5):1325S–1333S.

25. Sauvant P, Feart C, Atgie C. Vitamin A supply to mothers and children: challenges and opportunities. *Curr Opin Clin Nutr Metab Care.* 2012;15(3):310–314.

26. Forrest KYZ, Stuhldreher WL. Prevalence and correlates of vitamin D deficiency in US adults. *Nutr Res.* 2011;31(1):48–54.

27. Karras SN, Anagnostis P, Annweiler C, et al. Maternal vitamin D status during pregnancy: the Mediterranean reality. *Euro J Clin Nutr.* 2014;68(8):864–869.

28. McAree T, Jacobs B, Manickavasagar T, et al. Vitamin D deficiency in pregnancy—still a public health issue. *Matern Child Nutr.* 2013;9(1):23–30.

29. Pereira-Santos M, Costa PRF, Assis AMO, Santos C, Santos DB. Obesity and vitamin D deficiency: a systematic review and meta-analysis. *Obes Rev.* 2015;16(4):341–349.

30. Royal College of Obstetricians and Gynaecologists; June 2014. Vitamin D in pregnancy. Retrieved from: https://www.rcog.org.uk/globalassets/documents/guidelines/scientific-impact-papers/vitamin_d_sip43_june14.pdf. Scientific Impact paper no. 43. Accessed August 24, 2016.

31. Kovacs CS. Maternal vitamin D deficiency: fetal and neonatal implications. *Semin Fetal Neonatal Med.* 2013;18(3):129–135.

32. Hacker AN, Fung EB, King JC. Role of calcium during pregnancy: maternal and fetal needs. *Nutr Rev.* 2012;70(7):397–409.

33. Imdad A, Bhutta ZA. Effects of calcium supplementation during pregnancy on maternal, fetal and birth outcomes. *Paediatr Perinat Epidemiol.* 2012;26:138–152.

34. Goonewardene M, Shehata M, Hamad A. Anaemia in pregnancy. *Best Pract Res Clin Obstet Gynaecol.* 2012;26(1):3–24.

35. National Institutes of Health; updated February 11, 2016. Iron dietary supplement fact sheet. Retrieved from: http://ods.od.nih.gov/factsheets/Iron-HealthProfessional/. Accessed August 23, 2016.

36. US Department of Health and Human Services and US Department of Agriculture. *2015–2020 Dietary Guidelines for Americans.* 8th ed. Washington, DC: US Department of Health and Human Services and US Department of Agriculture; December 2015. Retrieved from: http://health.gov/dietaryguidelines/2015/guidelines/. Accessed January 20, 2016.

37. Berger J, Wieringa FT, Lacroux A, Dijkhuizen MA. Strategies to prevent iron deficiency and improve reproductive health. *Nutr Rev.* 2011;69:S78–S86.

38. Mei ZG, Cogswell ME, Looker AC, et al. Assessment of iron status in US pregnant women from the National Health and Nutrition Examination Survey (NHANES), 1999–2006. *Am J Clin Nutr.* 2011;93(6):1312–1320.

39. Amouzegar A, Khazan M, Hedayati M, Azizi F. An assessment of the iodine status and the correlation between iodine nutrition and thyroid function during pregnancy in an iodine sufficient area. *Euro J Clin Nutr.* 2014;68(3):397–400.

40. Stagnaro-Green A, Abalovich M, Alexander E, et al. Guidelines of the American Thyroid Association for the diagnosis and management of thyroid disease during pregnancy and postpartum. *Thyroid.* 2011;21(10):1081–1125.

41. National Institutes of Health; updated June 24, 2011. Iodine factsheet for health professionals. Retrieved from: https://ods.od.nih.gov/factsheets/Iodine-HealthProfessional/. Accessed July 27, 2015.

42. Villar J, Merialdi M, Gulmezoglu AM, et al. Nutritional interventions during pregnancy for the prevention or treatment of maternal morbidity and preterm delivery: An overview of randomized controlled trials. *J Nutr.* 2003;133(5):1606S–1625S.

43. Molloy AM, Kirke PN, Troendle JF, et al. Maternal vitamin B12 status and risk of neural tube defects in a population with high neural tube defect prevalence and no folic acid fortification. *Pediatrics.* March 2009;123(3):917–923.

44. National Institutes of Health; updated April 20, 2016. Folate dietary supplement fact sheet. Retrieved from: http://ods.od.nih.gov/factsheets/Folate-HealthProfessional/. Accessed August 23, 2016.

45. Crider KS, Bailey LB, Berry RJ. Folic acid food fortification—its history, effect, concerns, and future directions. *Nutrients.* 2011;3(3):370–384.

46. Czeizel AE, Dudas I, Vereczkey A, Banhidy F. Folate deficiency and folic acid supplementation: the prevention of neural-tube defects and congenital heart defects. *Nutrients.* 2013;5(11):4760–4775.

47. Centers for Disease Control and Prevention; updated April 21, 2016. Folic acid: recommendations. Retrieved from: http://www.cdc.gov/ncbddd/folicacid/recommendations.html. Accessed August 24, 2016.

48. Winkels RM, Rouwer IA, Siebelink E, Katan MB, Verhoef P. Bioavailability of food folates is 80% of that of folic acid. *Am J Clin Nutr.* February 2007;85(2):465–473.

49. Canfield MA, Ramadhani TA, Shaw GM, et al. Anencephaly and spina bifida among Hispanics: maternal, sociodemographic, and acculturation factors in the national birth defects prevention study. *Birth Defects Res A Clin Mol Teratol.* 2009;85(7):637–646.

50. Berti C, Biesalski HK, Gartner R, et al. Micronutrients in pregnancy: current knowledge and unresolved questions. *Clin Nutr.* 2011;30(6):689–701.

51. Zerfu TA, Ayele HT. Micronutrients and pregnancy; effect of supplementation on pregnancy and pregnancy outcomes: a systemic review. Nutrition Journal. 2013;12:5

52. Facchinetti F, Pedrielli G, Benoni G, et al. Herbal supplements in pregnancy: unexpected results from a multicentre study. *Hum Reprod.* 2012;27(11):3161–3167.

53. Schweitzer A. Dietary supplements during pregnancy. *J Perinat Educ.* 2006;15:44–45.

54. Ding MS, Leach M, Bradley H. The effectiveness and safety of ginger for pregnancy-induced nausea and vomiting: a systematic review. *Women Birth.* 2013;26(1):E26–E30.

55. Malisova O, Protopappas A, Nyktari A, et al. Estimations of water balance after validating and administering the water balance questionnaire in pregnant women. *Int J Food Sci Nutr.* 2014;65(3):280–285.

56. Fitch C, Keim KS; Academy of Nutrition and Dietetics. Position of the Academy of Nutrition and Dietetics: use of nutritive and nonnutritive sweeteners. *J Acad Nutr Diet.* 2012;112:739–758.

57. American Pregnancy Association. Nausea during pregnancy. Retrieved from: http://americanpregnancy.org/pregnancy-health/nausea-during-pregnancy/. Accessed September 1, 2016

58. Kuczkowski KM. Caffeine in pregnancy. *Arch Gynecol Obstet.* 2009;280(5):695–698.

59. Savitz DA, Chan RL, Herring AH, Howards PP, Hartmann KE. Caffeine and miscarriage risk. *Epidemiology.* 2008; 19(1):55–62.

60. Partosch F, Mielke H, Stahlmann R, et al. Caffeine intake in pregnancy: relationship between internal intake and effect on birth weight. *Food Chem Toxicol.* December 2015;86:291–297.

61. Jarosz M, Wierzejska R, Siuba M. Maternal caffeine intake and its effect on pregnancy outcomes [published online ahead of print December 3, 2011]. *Eur J Obstet Gynecol Reprod Biol.* February 2012;160(2):156–160. doi:10.1016/j.ejogrb.2011.11.021.

62. Rao Barkur R, Bairy LK. Evaluation of passive avoidance learning and spatial memory in rats exposed to low levels of lead during specific periods of early brain development. *Int J Occup Med Environ Health.* 2015;28(3):533–544.

63. Batshaw ML. Genetics and developmental disabilities. In Batshaw ML, Pellegrino I, Roizen NJ, eds. *Children with disabilities.* 6th ed. Baltimore, MD: Paul H. Brookes; 2007:3–21.

64. Law R, Maltepe C, Bozzo P, Einarson A. Treatment of heartburn and acid reflux associated with nausea and vomiting during pregnancy. *Can Fam Physician.* 2010;56(2):143–144.

65. Lamont RF, Sobel J, Mazaki-Tovi S, et al. Listeriosis in human pregnancy: a systematic review. *J Perinat Med.* 2011;39(3):227–236.

66. Centers for Disease Control and Prevention; updated January 10, 2013. Toxoplasmosis frequently asked questions (FAQs). Retrieved from: http://www.cdc.gov/parasites/toxoplasmosis/gen_info/faqs.html. Accessed July 23, 2015.

67. Mahaffey KR, Sunderland EM, Chan HM, et al. Balancing the benefits of n-3 polyunsaturated fatty acids and the risks of methylmercury exposure from fish consumption. *Nutr Rev.* 2011;69(9):493–508.

68. Ward E. *Maternal nutrition.* Siega-Riz AM, ed., with Boettcher J, London E, Drone B. Glenview, IL: Mead Johnson Nutrition; 2012. https://www.meadjohnson.com/pediatrics/us-en/sites/hcp-usa/files/LB2882-Maternal-Nutrition-Monograph-2.pdf. Accessed February 14, 2016.

69. Nascimento SL, Surita FG, Cecatti JG. Physical exercise during pregnancy: a systematic review. *Curr Opin Obstet Gynecol.* 2012;24(6):387–394.

70. Cameron EL. Pregnancy and olfaction: a review. *Front Psychol.* 2014;5:11.

71. US Department of Agriculture; August 3, 2016. Women, Infants, and Children (WIC). Retrieved from: http://www.fns.usda.gov/wic/women-infants-and-children-wic. Accessed August 23, 2016.

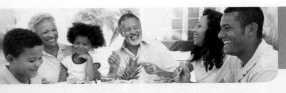

Learning Portfolio (continued)

72. Savoie-Roskos M, Durward C, Jeweks M, LeBlanc H. Reducing food insecurity and improving fruit and vegetable intake among farmers' market incentive program participants. *J Nutr Educ Behav.* 2016;48(1):70–76.

73. Muktabhant B, Lawrie TA, Lumbiganon P, Laopalboon M. Diet or exercise, or both, for preventing excessive weight gain in pregnancy. *Cochrane Database Syst Rev.* June 15, 2015;(6):CD007145. doi:10.1002/14651858.CD007145.pub3.

74. Charlesworth S, Foulds HJA, Burr JF, Bredin SSD. Evidence-based risk assessment and recommendations for physical activity clearance: pregnancy. *Appl Physiol Nutr Metab.* 2011;36:S33–S48.

75. Committee on Obstetric Practice ; December 2015. Physical activity and exercise during pregnancy and the postpartum period. Retrieved from: http://www.acog.org/Resources -And-Publications/Committee-Opinions/Committee-on -Obstetric-Practice/Physical-Activity-and-Exercise-During -Pregnancy-and-the-Postpartum-Period. American College of Obstetricians and Gynecologists Committee Opinion no. 650. Accessed February 14, 2016.

76. National Heart, Lung, and Blood Institute; June 22, 2016. Recommendations for physical activity. Retrieved from: https://www.nhlbi.nih.gov/health/health-topics/topics/phys /recommend. Accessed August 24, 2016.

77. Gaston A, Cramp A. Exercise during pregnancy: a review of patterns and determinants. *J Sport Health Sci.* 2011;14(4):299–305.

78. Krans EE, Chang JC. A will without a way: barriers and facilitators to exercise during pregnancy of low-income, African American women. *Women Health.* 2011;51(8):777–794.

79. US Department of Agriculture; updated January 12, 2015. Food Security in the U.S. Retrieved from: http://www.ers. usda.gov/topics/food-nutrition-assistance/food-security-in-the-us/key-statistics-graphics.aspx. Accessed on July 23, 2015.

80. Carmichael SL, Yang W, Herring A, Abrams B, Shaw GM. Maternal food insecurity is associated with increased risk of certain birth defects. *J Nutr.* 2007;137(9):2087–2092.

81. Brunton RJ, Dryer R, Saliba A, Kohlhoff J. Pregnancy anxiety: a systematic review of current scales. *J Affect Disord.* 2015;176:24–34.

82. Alder J, Fink N, Bitzer J, Hosli I, Holzgreve W. Depression and anxiety during pregnancy: a risk factor for obstetric, fetal and neonatal outcome? A critical review of the literature. *J Matern Fetal Neonatal Med.* 2007;20(3):189–209.

83. Leung BMY, Kaplan BJ. Perinatal depression: prevalence, risks, and the nutrition link—a review of the literature. *J Am Diet Assoc.* 2009;109(9):1566–1575.

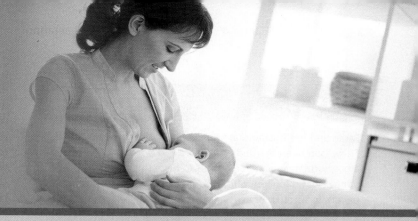

CHAPTER 4

Nutrition Needs During Lactation

Rebecca Charlton, BS, MPH, RDN

Chapter Outline

Benefits of Breastfeeding

The Physiology of Lactation

Human Milk Composition

Nutrition Recommendations and Requirements During Lactation

Feeding in Early Infancy

Nutrition and Lactation Outcomes

Support and Education for Breastfeeding

Pumping and Breastfeeding Interruption

Learning Objectives

1. List the benefits of breastfeeding.

2. Describe the hormonal processes involved in milk production.

3. Describe how latch and infant position work together to release breastmilk and encourage adequate breastmilk supply.

4. List conditions that may limit breastfeeding success.

5. List resources available to nursing mothers to support and promote breastfeeding.

6. Describe the appropriate methods for expression and storage of breastmilk.

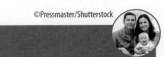

Case Study

Farah and her husband are 26 years old with their first child. They have been married for 4 years and both participated in a prepregnancy plan in an effort to have the healthiest pregnancy possible. Throughout her pregnancy, Farah has been uncertain whether or not she wants to breastfeed.

Breastfeeding was the primary method of infant feeding until advancements in chemistry, hygiene, and food preservation led to the development of appropriate artificial human milk substitutes (also known as infant formula). In the mid-1900s, infant formula marketing campaigns changed public opinion to favor milk substitutes over breastfeeding. Breastfeeding was viewed as being dirty and inadequate, largely because of its use among less affluent groups that could not afford to purchase infant formula.[1]

By the 1970s, human milk feeding was rare. In 1972, only 22% of women had ever breastfed an infant. At that time, a renaissance movement among women interested in "natural" mothering practices renewed interest in biological feedings of infants. Research followed the interest and revealed positive roles of breastmilk in infant intestinal development, immune health, growth, and maturation. Mothers benefit, too, through reduced cancer rates and improved weight management.

In the 1980s, programs and organizations such as La Leche League International, the Special Supplemental Nutrition Program for Women, Infants, and Children (WIC), the World Health Organization (WHO), and the United Nations Children's Fund (UNICEF) began to rapidly change professional practice with respect to breastfeeding.[2]

Lactation consultants, paraprofessionals, and peer counselors engaged the public through marketing campaigns, public health outreach, primary health care, and community grassroots efforts to encourage women to attempt breastfeeding. Breastfeeding trends began to reverse. By 2009, the number of breastfeeding mothers at hospital discharge had increased to 74%.[3] The World Health Organization predicts that, if breastfeeding could replace artificial baby milk as the exclusive route of infant feeding, 800,000 infant deaths could be avoided during the first 5 years of life. In addition, 20,000 maternal lives could be saved through reduction in breast cancer.[4] A recent meta-analysis of infant deaths studies demonstrated that children breastfed from ages 2 to 23 months are two times less likely to die than those who are not.[5]

Breastfeeding rates vary widely by region and country. The country with the highest rate of breastfeeding is Norway, wherein 99% of infants are breastfed at birth with 70% still exclusively breastfed at 6 months.[6] Many factors contribute to this extraordinary success rate. Norway mothers receive one of the most generous parental leave policies in the developing world. The culture supports breastfeeding, and laws protect mothers by providing adequate home time after birth and protection of breastfeeding in the workplace. Both mothers and fathers have access to leave, providing Norwegian infants with adequate home and bonding time during the crucial first year.[6]

Unfortunately, women in the United States face a much less friendly childbearing situation. Many barriers to breastfeeding exist, including separation from the infant at birth and for work, societal and financial pressure to spend more time at work than at home, cultural trends minimizing the role of motherhood in a woman's life, overemphasis on individual choice that limits pro-breastfeeding messages, and a lack of societal support for nonsexualized presentations of the breast. (See FIGURE 4.1 .) In addition, the United States is the only affluent nation that does not provide paid family leave in the first year.[6] Perceived lack of support for public breastfeeding is a significant barrier for many women, especially those who are younger or less economically advantaged, leading to increased use of infant formula.[7] Recently, in-roads to this issue have been made by mothers, including some celebrities, by posting breastfeeding photos on social media and speaking out about the need to support lactation efforts in public and in private.[8]

Despite significant gains in initiation of breastmilk feeding at birth, only 22% of infants in the United States are still being fed breast milk at 1 year of age.[3] Rates of breastfeeding at 1 year vary by state from 11.8% in Alabama to 42.5% in Alaska.[9] The reasons for the dramatic decline are varied and have become the focus of several public health initiatives.

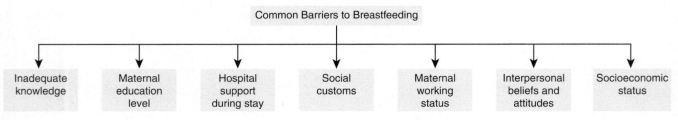

Figure 4.1
Common barriers to breastfeeding.

Benefits of Breastfeeding

Preview Human milk is a unique, bioactive substance derived by the body to further the biological development of the human infant. Use of human milk enhances the immune, gastrointestinal, and metabolic health of infants.

From a nutrition standpoint, human milk is bioactive and bioavailable, meaning that these nutrients are readily available for immediate use. But breastmilk is much more than a mode of nutrition. Scientific analysis demonstrates that stem cells transfer from mother to infant via breastmilk. These cells help to mature and fortify the infant intestines, brain, and immune system to ensure the infant is protected from microbes and toxins in the environment. Milk produced by a mother varies from day to day, and from child to child, meaning that the composition of the same mother's breastmilk changes within a feeding and is uniquely produced for each lactation cycle. Early research into breastmilk revealed that no two samples of breastmilk are alike.[10] Wild variation exists from mother to mother and for an individual mother at different times of day and life cycle of the infant. Simple nutrient levels may shift in response to maternal diet, but the antibody and stem cells in the milk vary constantly in response to biological and environmental triggers.[10]

Breastfeeding Benefit 1: Reduced Death and Illness Rates

In general, mothers and infants who breastfeed are noted to be healthier over a wide variety of wellness indicators.[11] At present, it's estimated that exclusive breastfeeding for the first 6 months of life would reduce the infant death rate by 13% based on the findings that breastfed infants have a significant decrease in the risk of sudden infant death syndrome.[11]

Multiple studies indicate that infants who are given breastmilk have improved long-term immunological function over those who are fed artificial baby milk. Breastmilk enhances **passive immunity** by passing antibodies from the mother to the infant. The antibodies stimulate the infant's immune system to recognize and attack foreign substances.[12] In general, passive immunity is most useful in protecting an infant against bacterial infections, including common respiratory tract, urinary tract, and community-acquired ear infections.[12–14] Breastmilk is not as effective as vaccination at preventing viral disease, so human infants should be immunized per recommended schedules even if exclusively breastfed.[15] Breastmilk feeding, however, may enhance the effectiveness of vaccines and decrease the severity of illness if the baby becomes infected by a virus.[16] Breastfeeding is also associated with decreased risk of a variety of other conditions such as otitis media, upper respiratory tract infections, IBD, diabetes, and SIDS.[17]

Breastmilk Benefit 2: Improved Intestinal Function

One theory for breastmilk's impact on immunity focuses on the role of the intestines in immune function. Healthy intestines are populated by bacterial flora that compete with disease-causing bacteria, aid digestion, and play a role in the development and maturation of the infant intestinal system.[18] The beneficial flora passes from mother to infant through vaginal exposure at birth and through breastmilk. Breastmilk itself nourishes the probiotic flora so that the flora rapidly multiply and colonize the infant's system. Studies indicate that infants fed breastmilk exclusively for 6 months have half the rate of hospitalization for diarrhea as that seen in infants fed infant formula.[12]

Premature infants, in particular, are at risk of damage to the intestinal system after birth. One of the most common and the most serious intestinal diseases among preemies is **necrotizing enterocolitis**. (See **FIGURE 4.2**.) This occurs when tissue in the small or large intestine is injured or dies, causing the intestine to become inflamed. When this happens, the intestine can no longer contain biological waste products, allowing bacteria to pass through the intestine and enter the baby's bloodstream or abdominal cavity. The risk of necrotizing enterocolitis in preterm infants is reduced when infants are breastfed rather than provided specialized premature or regular infant formula.[19] Many neonatal intensive care centers provide stored breastmilk ("donor milk") to at-risk premature infants.[20]

Influence over passive immunity and fortification of the intestines may contribute to a reduced incidence of allergy in children fed breastmilk as the primary feeding source.[21] Exclusive breastfeeding for 4–6 months demonstrates the strongest potential of risk reduction for infants born to parents with known sensitivities or allergies.[22] Children born

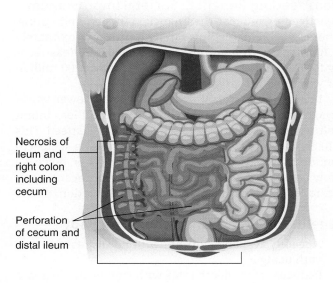

Necrosis of ileum and right colon including cecum

Perforation of cecum and distal ileum

Figure 4.2
Necrotizing enterocolitis.

to parents with no allergy show no difference in allergic response whether fed breastmilk or artificial baby milk.[5]

Breastmilk Benefit 3: Reduced Metabolic Disease

Breastfeeding may have a protective effect on child overweight and obesity by inducing lower plasma insulin levels, thereby decreasing fat storage and preventing excessive early adipocyte development.[23] Breastfed infants, regardless of weight or obesity, are less likely to develop cardiovascular disease or experience the metabolic disturbances common in obesity later in life.[24]

Breastfeeding Benefit 4: Psychosocial Response to Environmental Stress

Breastfeeding enhances the infant's comfort and stability in a new environment as well. Studies of newborn pain relief demonstrated that for routine procedures not requiring full anesthesia, breastfeeding with skin-to-skin contact is superior to all other methods of pain control, including pacifier use, skin-to-skin contact alone, sugar water, and analgesics.[25]

Breastfeeding Benefit 5: Decreased Disease Burden for Mothers

Mothers who provide breastmilk as a primary feeding source for at least 6 months are more likely to return to their prepregnancy weight, and women who provide breastmilk for a year have a significant reduction in ovarian and breast cancers.[12,26] Research indicates that women who feed breastmilk for a total of 2 years or more throughout their lifetime, and who carry the BRCA-1 gene associated with breast cancer, have a significant reduction in lifetime risk of developing breast cancer that is similar to the risk associated with development of breast cancer in women who have had a mastectomy.[26]

Breastfeeding Benefit 6: Societal Improvement

Breastfeeding reduces the financial burden of parenting. Whereas a breastfeeding family saves approximately $1,700.00 per year in formula costs, exclusive breastfeeding for 6 months could save each U.S. state $200 million per year in social service monies.[27]

Mothers who breastfeed tend to miss fewer workdays, have increased productivity, and report less infant maltreatment over mothers who do not breastfeed. This is likely a complex phenomenon that reflects socioeconomic status and education level of the mother; however, many benefits of breastfeeding remain significant when controlled for external factors, such as education.[28]

Benefits for Mother and Benefits for Baby

A readily available nutrient with no cost associated with using it.
Reduces infant death rates with significant decrease in sudden infant death syndrome.
More likely to return to prepregnancy weight

Improved intestinal function.
Possibly reduces risk of cancer development.
Reduce metabolic disease such as overweight and obesity.
Mothers tend to miss fewer workdays, have increased productivity, and report less infant maltreatment.
Enhances infant's comfort and stability in a new environment.

Healthy People 2020 Goals for Breastfeeding

Owing to the many benefits of breastfeeding, goals for initiation and extension of breastfeeding have been included in the United States Healthy People 2020 public health goals. These goals organize national dialogue and create collaboration among health professionals nationwide in high-priority matters of public welfare. Current rates and target values are presented in **TABLE 4.1** .

The data collected for Healthy People 2020 reveal significant trends for breastmilk feeding in the United States. Initiation rates continue to climb. However, those rates drop at 6 months and drop steeply by 1 year of age.

Table 4.1

Healthy People 2020 Breastfeeding Objectives

Objective (MICH-21)	Baseline (%)	Goal (%)
Rate of infants who have ever been breastfed	74	81.9
Proportion of infants fed some breastmilk at 6 months of age	43.5	60.6
Proportion of infants fed some breastmilk at 1 year of age	22.7	34.1
Proportion of infants fed breastmilk exclusively to 3 months of age	33.6	46.2
Percentage of worksites providing lactation programs for employees	25	38
Percentage of infants provided formula in first 2 days of life	24.2	14.2
Babies born in facilities with adequate lactation care	2.9	8.1

Reproduced from Healthy People 2020. Retrieved from: https://www.healthypeople.gov/2020/topics-objectives/topic/maternal-infant-and-child-health/objectives

Case Study

Prior to becoming pregnant, Farah was certain that she would not breastfeed. Neither her grandmother, her mother, or her older sister breastfed any of their children, and she did not feel like she would have their support. During her pregnancy, Farah started to form a positive opinion about breastfeeding because of the many benefits she had been learning about. As a healthcare provider, how would you discuss the pros and cons of breastfeeding with Farah?

Recap Benefits of breastfeeding stretch well beyond basic nutrition. Breastfeeding can protect an infant from certain diseases, both in childhood and as an adult. It decreases the risk of infant death and disease and enhances comfort and stability for infants. Breastfeeding decreases cancer rates among mothers and reduces the likelihood of metabolic disease. Individual and societal benefits to breastfeeding are significant enough that breastfeeding rates are included in Healthy People 2020.

1. Describe how human breastmilk may enhance infant immunity.
2. Name five benefits of breastfeeding.
3. List the Healthy People 2020 goals for breastfeeding.

The Physiology of Lactation

Preview Breastfeeding provides for a dynamic and ever-changing feeding experience for a growing infant. The female body is uniquely designed to create breastmilk for a human infant. The breast adapts to environmental and hormonal stimuli, as well as the infant's stage of development, to prepare the appropriate nutrition and biofactors to aid the growth and development of the baby.

Anatomy of the Female Breast

The structure of the female breast consists of many different and connected parts, including fat and connective tissue, lobes, lobules, ducts, and lymph nodes. Each breast has a number of lobules that are made up of small hollow sacs called alveoli. The lobules are connected by a network of ducts, or thin tubes, which group together at the areola, which is the dark circle around the nipple. During breastfeeding, ducts carry milk from the alveoli toward the areola, where they join into larger ducts ending at the nipple, creating a number of different openings for milk to flow. The space around the lobules and ducts are filled with fat, ligaments, and connective tissue. Breast size is largely determined by the amount of fat within the breast; however, the milk-producing structures are nearly the same in all women, regardless of breast size. Muscle tissue separates the breast from the ribs. Blood vessels carry oxygen and nutrients to breast tissue; lymph nodes under the armpit, behind the breast, and along the collar bone produce lymphocytes that help defend the body against microorganisms and against harmful particles FIGURE 4.3.

Hormone Control and Breastmilk Production

During pregnancy, the placenta releases two key hormones, prolactin and oxytocin, which enhance development of the mammary gland and prepare the mammary system for milk production. The hormone prolactin surges in the expecting mother during the third trimester of pregnancy. This important hormone, released by the pituitary gland as the fetus develops, causing enlargement of the mammary glands of the breast, which helps prepare for the production of milk.

Once the placenta separates from the mother, milk production responds based on supply and demand. An

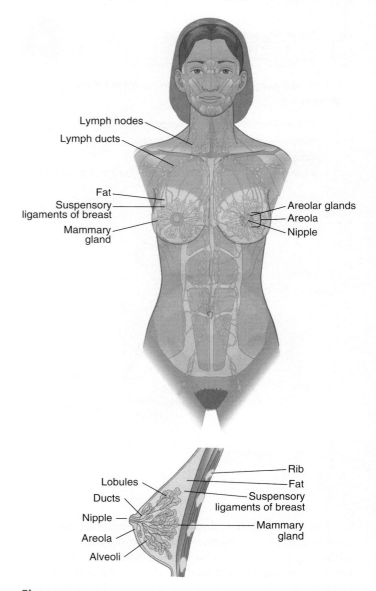

Figure 4.3
Anatomy of the female breast.

infant's suckling stimulates the nerve endings in the nipple and areola, which signal the pituitary gland in the brain to release prolactin and oxytocin. Prolactin causes the alveoli to take nutrients from the blood supply and convert them into breastmilk. Oxytocin, which is associated with contraction of the uterus, also causes the cells around the alveoli to contract and eject the milk down into the milk ducts. A contracting uterus during breastfeeding helps the uterus return to its prepregnancy size more quickly than with not breastfeeding. This passing of the milk down the ducts is called the let-down reflex. Some breastfeeding women experience slow or inhibited let-down, which may result from a number of different factors such as embarrassment, pain, stress, anxiety, cold, smoking, excessive caffeine use, or use of some medications.

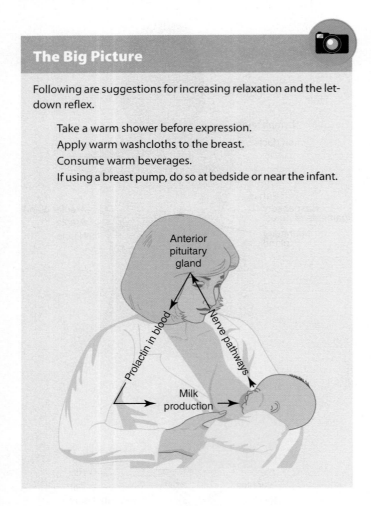

The Big Picture

Following are suggestions for increasing relaxation and the let-down reflex.

Take a warm shower before expression.
Apply warm washcloths to the breast.
Consume warm beverages.
If using a breast pump, do so at bedside or near the infant.

For the first few days after birth, referred to as lactogenesis I, the mother's body produces colostrum. Although not essential to human babies, colostrum is considered the perfect first food because it meets the nutritional needs of the newborn before the mother can start producing breastmilk and it contains important immune factors that newborn infants cannot receive from any other source. Colostrum is rich in immunologic properties, including secretory immunoglobulin A (IgA), lactoferrin, leukocytes, and epidermal growth factor. As such, it's often referred to as the baby's "first vaccine," though the term is somewhat misleading. Colostrum gives a boost to the infant's newly established immune system rather than teaching the infant to resist specific pathogens.

Colostrum is uniquely nutritive and significantly important. The infant is born well nourished by the maternal blood supply during pregnancy and, in the first few days, has little need for nutrients, other than carbohydrate and protein. Colostrum provides this carbohydrate and protein for fuel and growth as well as electrolytes and magnesium for hemodynamic stability, but most other nutrients are absent. (See FIGURE 4.4.) Colostrum comes in small but appropriate amounts for a newborn. The baby will feed approximately every 2 hours during this stage.

Lactogenesis II begins 2–5 days after birth and is commonly referred to as transitional milk or the milk "coming in." Changes in breast tissue over the first 72 hours of life signal the body to increase lactose concentration, which is the sugar present in milk. Lactose concentrations continue to build until 2 weeks after birth. Protein concentrations will vary, and the sodium concentration decreases as other nutrients become more prominent. The baby may decrease feeding frequency to every 3 hours as the milk supply and fat content achieve normal levels.

Lactogenesis III (mature milk) generally occurs 2–5 weeks after birth. By week 6, milk stabilizes in composition and volume unless the infant shows a marked increase or decrease in suckling patterns. (See FIGURE 4.5.) The amount of milk consumed at this stage is typically the amount that the infant will consume throughout the first year of life. The mother has fewer episodes of feeling that her breasts are full or uncomfortable between feeds. Some mothers interpret this lack of fullness as running out of milk, but it's actually a stabilization of consumption and supply.

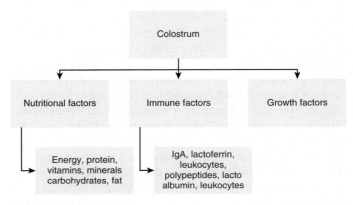

Figure 4.4
Components of colostrum.

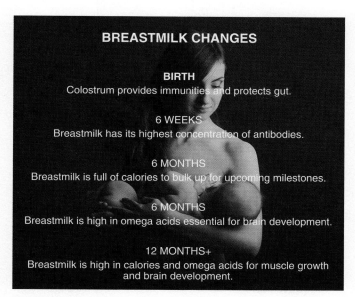

BREASTMILK CHANGES

BIRTH
Colostrum provides immunities and protects gut.

6 WEEKS
Breastmilk has its highest concentration of antibodies.

6 MONTHS
Breastmilk is full of calories to bulk up for upcoming milestones.

6 MONTHS
Breastmilk is high in omega acids essential for brain development.

12 MONTHS+
Breastmilk is high in calories and omega acids for muscle growth and brain development.

©AlohaHawaii/Shutterstock

Figure 4.5
Changes in breastmilk during the first year postpartum.
Used with permission from Lactation Connection, http://www.lactationconnection.com/

Recap The structure of the breast allows for its function of providing nutrients to an infant. Hormones enhance development of the mammary gland and prepare the mammary system for milk production. For the initial stage of milk production, the mother's body produces colostrum, the first secretion from the mammary glands of the mother after giving birth. Colostrum is uniquely nutritive and significantly important, because this is the first feedings for an infant who has been well nourished by the maternal blood supply during pregnancy. The composition of breastmilk changes through the course of lactation, providing the vast majority of nutrients required for infant growth.

1. Explain how prolactin and oxytocin influence human milk production.
2. What are the three factors present in colostrum?
3. How does breastmilk produced during lactogenesis II and lactogenesis III differ?

Human Milk Composition

Preview Overall, the nutritional quality of human milk is maintained at a level and concentration appropriate to infant growth. Maternal diet influences type and quantity of fat, as does duration of feeding and time between feeds. Vitamin D and iron are present in low levels, and most healthcare providers recommend supplementation of these nutrients to prevent deficiency.

Breastmilk and Essential Nutrients
Water
Breastmilk satisfies a baby's fluid needs under normal environmental conditions, and therefore additional fluids are not necessary to meet baby's hydration needs. Mothers should, however, be instructed to monitor the newborn for signs of dehydration, especially in hot, dry climates. Signs of dehydration include sleepiness, irritability, less elasticity in the skin, when the eyes and soft spot on the head appear sunken, a decrease or absence of tears, and decreased number of wet diapers.

Macronutrients
Macronutrient composition differs between preterm and term milk, with preterm milk being higher in protein and fat.[29] The mean macronutrient composition of mature, term breastmilk is estimated to be 0.9–1.2 g/dL for protein, 3.2–3.6 g/dL for fat, and 6.7–7.8 g/dL for lactose.[30] Energy estimates range from 65 to 70 kcal/dL, depending on the fat and protein content. Studies show that mothers who produce higher quantities of milk tend to have lower milk concentrations of fat and protein but higher concentrations of lactose.[30]

Fats: Lipids, DHA, Trans Fats, Cholesterol
Fat is the most highly variable macronutrient of breastmilk. In addition, the concentration of fat in breastmilk changes throughout a feeding. Milk expressed at the end of a feeding has a higher fat content than the milk expressed at the beginning of that particular feeding. The type and quantity of fat is dependent on the maternal diet, therefore, not only does the quantity of fat vary but also the fatty acid profile of human milk varies. Particularly, the long-chain polyunsaturated fatty acid (LCPUFA) profile. The most biologically active form of LCPUFAs are the omega-3 polyunsaturated fatty acids: docosahexanoic acid (DHA), eicosapentaenoic acid (EPA), and arachidonic acid (AA). These fatty acids are involved in several brain and retinal maturation processes, and recent research indicates that the anti-inflammatory properties of LCPUFAs may be of equal significance.[31] Recommended maternal intake of DHA during pregnancy and lactation is 200 mg per day.[32] This amount can be achieved by eating 1–2 portions of fish per week or by taking fish oil supplements. Because the dietary intake and maternal stores of DHA during pregnancy are known to be key determinants of infant blood DHA concentration at birth, low DHA consumption by women eating Western diets has promoted some concern for the neurological and neurocognitive development of their offspring.[31] The DHA and AA that accumulates in the fetal brain during the last trimester of pregnancy continue at very high rates up to the end of the second year of life. Although not mandatory, it is common for infant formula to be supplemented with DHA and EPA. At present, there is no recommended supplementation of DHA and EPA for nursing women or their infants, but supplements do exist in the market for both infant and mother. The need can be met through diet, and dietary sources are preferred over supplements.

Protein: Casein, Whey, Nonprotein Nitrogen

The concentration of protein in breastmilk does not change much, even if the mother's intake of protein does not meet estimated needs.[33] The primary change in protein is biologic. The protein content of milk obtained from mothers who deliver preterm is significantly higher than that of mothers who deliver at term.[29]

Carbohydrates

Lactose is the primary carbohydrate in breastmilk, which also contains a high concentration of oligosaccharides. Human milk oligosaccharides (HMOs) are highly abundant in human milk but do not exist in infant formula. The oligosaccharides in milk are not digestible by human infants. They serve as prebiotics—a form of indigestible carbohydrate that reaches the colon intact and is selectively fermented by desirable gut microflora.[34] HMOs reach the colon intact, where their prebiotic effects promote healthy gut colonization.

Fat-Soluble Vitamins

Vitamin A: Infants need vitamin A for optimal health, growth, and development. Colostrum and transitional breastmilk generally contain high levels of vitamin A, antibodies, and other protective factors. A well-nourished mother provides sufficient vitamin A for the infant for the duration of breastfeeding.

Vitamin D: Vitamin D levels in breastmilk vary with maternal diet and with maternal exposure to sunlight. Breastfed infants can synthesize additional vitamin D through routine sunlight exposure; however, partly because of efforts to decrease the risk of skin cancer, the American Academy of Pediatrics recommends a supplement of 400 IU per day of vitamin D for all breastfed infants in lieu of sun exposure.[35] Vitamin D supplements are given as drops in the baby's mouth. Research indicates that vitamin D may be administered to the mother in high doses to increase the amount of vitamin D in the milk.[36]

Vitamin E: Breastmilk contains antioxidant properties, such as vitamin E, known to protect against the potentially harmful effects of oxidative stress. The level of vitamin E in human milk is adequate to meet the needs of full-term infants. Vitamin E contributes to muscle integrity of infants and prevents the rupture of red blood cells.[37]

Vitamin K: Regardless of maternal diet, vitamin K is extremely low in human milk. The American Academy of Pediatrics recommends an intramuscular injection at birth to avoid hemorrhagic disease of the newborn.[30]

Water-Soluble Vitamins: Thiamine, Riboflavin, Vitamin B₆, Vitamin B₁₂, and Choline

Maternal deficiencies of some micronutrients during lactation can result in low concentrations in breastmilk; however, clinical problems related to water-soluble vitamins are rare, even in infants nursed by mothers with inadequate diets.[38]

TABLE 4.2 shows a comparison of colostrum and mature milk.

Table 4.2

Composition of 100 mL colostrum

Components	Mean Value for colostrum(Days 1-5 Postpartum)	Mean value for mature milk (Day 15 Postpartum)
Vitamin A (retinol equivalents)	151	75
Vitamin B1 (ug)	2	14
Vitamin B2 (ug)	30	40
Vitamin C (ug)	6	5
Total protein (g)	2	0.9-1.2
Calcium (mg)	28	35
Sodium (mg)	48	15
Calories (kcal)	55	65-70
Fat (g)	2.9	3.2-3.6
Lactose (g)	5.3	6.7-7.8

Data from Ballard O, Morrow A L. Human milk composition: nutrients and bioactive factors. *Pediatr Clin North Am.* 2013 Feb;60(1):49–74.

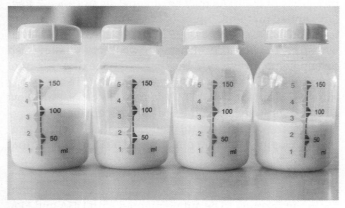

Figure 4.6
Milk protein concentrations, comparing milk from mothers who delivered preterm and term, by gestational age at delivery and weeks postpartum.
©JGI/Jamie Grill/Getty Images

Recap Human milk is a dynamic fluid containing factors and nutrients needed for infant health and development. Human milk composition varies depending on stage of lactation as well as differs between preterm and term deliveries. Most nutrients in breastmilk are stable throughout the first year of life. Maternal diet can impact the type of fat and the fat-soluble vitamin quantity in breastmilk. A satisfactory gain in the infant's weight is the best way to judge the adequacy of the diet of the infant.

1. What makes colostrum different from mature breastmilk?
2. What components of fat in breastmilk are associated with infant brain development?
3. List and describe characteristics of the type of carbohydrate that exists in breastmilk but not in infant formula.

Nutrition Recommendations and Requirements During Lactation

Preview The diet of a women who is breastfeeding influences some properties of breastmilk. A baby who is growing well, coupled with a mother who is eating well, will likely not experience manor nutrient deficiency in the first year of life. Breastfeeding women have slightly higher nutrition needs than women who are not pregnant or breastfeeding.

Maternal nutrition status has minimal impact on macronutrient content of human milk. In extreme conditions, the fat and protein content of breastmilk can be compromised. Examples of situations that may decrease fat and protein content include low maternal muscle and fat mass, inadequate protein intake, return of menstruation, and frequency of infant intake.[11] Therefore, a well-nourished mother is the basis for a healthy breastfed infant. The mother's intake and the infant's growth pattern should be assessed together to determine nourishment of the breastfed infant.

There are no specific foods mothers should eat or avoid during lactation. A general healthful diet with adequate macronutrients is appropriate. Along with nutrients, many flavorings pass through the maternal system and into breastmilk, exposing infants to varied flavor profiles while preparing them for the foods available once breastfeeding is stopped. Research indicates that mothers who consume diets rich in healthy foods are introducing healthy eating to their infant because these flavors are transmitted from the maternal diet to amniotic fluid and to mother's milk, making breastfed infants more accepting of the low-sugar, low-sodium, vegetable-rich diet.[39] In contrast, infants fed formula learn to prefer its unique flavor profile and may have more difficulty initially accepting flavors not found in formula, such as those of fruit and vegetables.[39] Avoidance of allergens, including milk, during pregnancy or lactation is not recommended and may increase likelihood of later food allergy in nonallergic infants.[22]

Daily Food Plans

Breastfeeding women have slightly higher nutrition needs than women who are not pregnant or breastfeeding. The U.S. Department of Agriculture's MyPlate Daily Food Guide has been adapted for pregnant and breastfeeding women, providing intake guidelines to meet the higher needs for some vitamins and minerals. By using the MyPlate Daily Checklist on the ChooseMyPlate.gov website, a suggested food list including an overall calorie level and food group breakdown will show users the foods and amounts that are right for them. An example is provided in **FIGURE 4.7**.

Energy and Nutrient Needs

The Dietary Reference Intakes (DRIs) for normal-weight breastfeeding women are established under the assumption that energy spent for milk production is 500 calories per day in the first 6 months and 400 calories per day afterward.

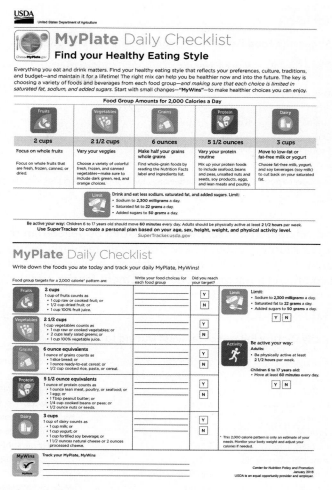

Figure 4.7
MyPlate Daily Checklist

Reproduced from USDA Center for Nutrition Policy and Promotion; January 2016. MyPlate Daily Checklist. Retrieved from: http://www.choosemyplate.gov/sites/default/files/myplate/checklists/MyPlateDailyChecklist_2400cals_Age14plus.pdf.

Breastfeeding mothers should not take in fewer than 1,800 calories per day, even when attempting to lose weight.[40] Determining the amount of kilocalories needed to meet the lactating mother's needs, as well as assist the mother in returning to her prepregnancy weight, is multifactorial and difficult to do based on calculations alone. One reliable measure of adequate energy intake during lactation can be determined by proper infant growth and development.

Micronutrient Considerations Among Lactating Women

Nursing mothers need a diet consisting of whole grains, fruits, and vegetables to ensure adequate micronutrient intake. Most practitioners recommend continuing prenatal vitamin supplementation while breastfeeding, including vitamin D supplementation used during pregnancy (10 mcg/d).[12] Additional nutrients are of particular concern. Cobalamin and folate levels tend to fall during pregnancy, and deficiency can result in the infant. Women who are strict vegans should be monitored regularly and supplemented if needed to prevent anemia due to low iron

Table 4.3

Suggested Food Patterns for Women Who Are Breastfeeding

Food Group	If Breastfeeding Only	If Breastfeeding and Feeding Some Formula	What Counts as 1 Cup or 1 Oz
Vegetables	3 cups	2½ cups	1 cup raw or ½ cup cooked vegetables; 1 cup raw leafy vegetables
Fruits	2 cups	2 cups	1 cup fruit or ⅓ cup 100% fruit juice
Grains	8 oz	6 oz	1 slice of bread, 1 oz of ready-to-eat cereal, ½ cup cooked pasta or rice
Dairy	3 cups	3 cups	1 cup milk, 8 oz yogurt, 1½ oz cheese
Protein	6½ oz	5½ oz	1 oz lean meat, poultry, or seafood; ¼ cup cooked beans; ½ oz of nuts; 1 egg; 1 tbs peanut butter

Reproduced from USDA Tips for Breastfeeding Moms. https://wicworks.fns.usda.gov/wicworks//Topics/BreastfeedingFactSheet.pdf

and cobalamin intake. Infants breastfed by vegetarian or vegan mothers should have iron levels regularly monitored.[41] In these cases, most healthcare practitioners will recommend a micronutrient supplement for the infant.

TABLE 4.3 provides a suggested food pattern for breastfeeding women.

TABLE 4.4 outlines the DRI recommendations during lactation.

Table 4.4

Daily Dietary Reference Intakes* During Lactation

Nutrient	Suggested Intake/Day for Lactating Mother	Some Food Sources
Water	3.8 L	Tap or bottled water, juices, tea, milk, soup
Carbohydrates	210 g	Bread, pasta, rice, fruit
Protein	71 g	Chicken, beef, pork, fish, turkey, dairy products
Total fiber	29 g	Barley, bulgur, beans, peas, artichokes, dates
Linoleic acid	13 g	Safflower oil, sunflower seeds, corn oil, soy oil, pine nuts, pecans
Alpha-linolenic acid	1.3 g	Flaxseed oil, walnuts, canola oil, fatty fish
Vitamin A	1,300 mcg RAE**	Carrots, pumpkin, sweet potato, spinach, collards, kale, cantaloupe
Vitamin E	19 mg	Ready-to-eat cereal, tomato, sunflower seeds, nuts, spinach
Vitamin K	90 mcg	Kale, collards, spinach, turnip greens, beets, broccoli
Vitamin C	120 mg	Oranges, grapefruit, sweet red peppers, cranberries, strawberries, broccoli
Vitamin B_1 (thiamine)	1.4 mg	Ready-to-eat cereal, enriched white rice, wheat flour, oat bran
Vitamin B_2 (riboflavin)	1.6 mg	Milk, ready-to-eat cereal, yogurt, soybeans, spinach
Niacin	17 mg	Chicken, fish, wheat flour, barley, ready-to-eat cereal, tomatoes
Vitamin B_6 (pyridoxine)	2 mg	Ready-to-eat cereal, chickpeas, fish, turkey, enriched white rice, potatoes
Folate	500 mcg	Enriched white rice, ready-to-eat cereal, wheat flour, lentils
Vitamin B_{12} (cyanocobalamin)	2.8 mcg	Cooked clams, cooked oysters, cooked crab, fish, ready-to-eat cereal
Iron	9 mg	Beef, turkey, chicken, soybeans, fortified cereals, lentils, spinach, beans
Iodine	290 mcg	Cheese, bread, milk, salt, cooked seafood
Vitamin D	5 mcg	Salmon, tuna, fortified milk, ready-to-eat cereal
Biotin	35 mcg	Cooked egg, cheddar cheese, whole wheat, cooked salmon, pork, avocado
Choline	550 mg	Eggs, salmon, turkey, beef, soybeans, baked beans, kidney beans
Pantothenic acid	7 mg	Ready-to-eat cereal, beef, mushrooms, milk
Calcium	1,000 mg	Ready-to-eat cereal, milk, cheese, yogurt, collards, spinach
Phosphorous	700 mg	Cornmeal, ricotta cheese, soybeans
Magnesium	320 mg	Buckwheat flour, bulgur, oat bran, semisweet chocolate, tomato products, nuts, sunflower seeds
Zinc	12 mg	Ready-to-eat cereal, baked beans, turkey, beef, chicken, pork
Chromium	45 mcg	Broccoli, grape juice, orange juice, potatoes
Manganese	2.6 mg	Wheat, bulgur, pineapple, nuts, ready-to-eat cereal, white rice
Molybdenum	50 mcg	Beans, lentils, peas, nuts, cereal, broccoli
Selenium	70 mcg	Nuts, fish, turkey, wheat flour, enriched rice
Fluoride	3 mg	Fluoridated drinking water, cooked seafood

* Recommended Dietary Allowances and Adequate Intakes.

** RAE = retinol activity equivalents; 3.33 IU Vitamin A = 1 mcg RAE; 6.66 IU beta carotene from supplement = 1 mcg RAE.

Modified from: Focus Information Technology. Dietary Reference Intakes during lactation. Retrieved from: http://perinatology.com/Reference/RDAlactation.htm.

<table>
<tr><td>

Table 4.5

USDA Nutrition Tips for Lactating Women

- Avoid foods that are low in nutrients and high in calories, such as pastries, soda, and candy.
- Use unsaturated oil in place of solid fats, such as butter or margarine, as much as possible.
- Include a variety of protein food choices such as seafood, lean meat and poultry, eggs, beans and peas, seeds, and nuts.
- Choose fat-free or low-fat dairy products such as milk, yogurt, and cheese.
- Eat whole grains in place of refined grains.
- Eat plenty of fruits and vegetables, filing half of your plate with a variety of fruits and vegetables.

Reproduced from USDA Food and Nutrition Service: February 2013. Tips for Breastfeeding Moms. Retrieved from: https://wicworks.fns.usda.gov/wicworks//Topics/BreastfeedingFactSheet.pdf. Accessed August 24, 2016.
</td></tr>
</table>

TABLE 4.5 provides additional tips on nutrition intake for breastfeeding mothers.

Breastmilk of Vegetarian Mothers

Vegetarian diets include several variations, and care should be taken when a breastfeeding mother avoids any particular food or food groups. For any degree of vegetarianism, the nutrients protein (essential amino acids), omega-3 essential fatty acids, iron, and calcium, as well as vitamin D and vitamin B_{12} should be monitored closely.[42] Vegetarian diets that contain no animal protein require vitamin B_{12} and vitamin D supplementation to avoid a deficiency in the mother and the baby. Mothers should supplement appropriately, and in turn their breastmilk will contain adequate levels of these vitamins.

Case Study

At 37 weeks gestation, Farah delivered a healthy baby girl who weighed 6 lb 1 oz and was 19 inches long. Breastfeeding was successfully established prior to discharge. Farah comes to you with concerns of getting back to her prepregnancy weight as soon as possible while maintaining adequate nutrition intake to support continued breastfeeding. During her pregnancy, Farah gained a total of 35 lb. She is 5 foot 7 inches and currently weighs 150 lb. She reports that she plans to start exercising within the next few weeks. A diet recall indicates that she is eating about 2,300 kcal with limited fruits and vegetables and one serving of milk and has a high carbohydrate intake.

Questions

1. Using either the MyPlate.gov website or the form provided in Figure 4.7, write a sample daily menu that will support Farah in breastfeeding the baby as well as work toward a goal of getting back to her prepregnancy weight.

2. What is the lowest amount of kilocalorie intake that you would recommend any lactating mother to have each day?
3. How could Farah's diet composition and her overall kilocalorie intake affect her milk production?
4. Explain which factor or factors should be used to evaluate whether Farah's daily kilocalorie intake is adequate.

Recap During lactation, nutritional requirements increase to support the increased maternal metabolism associated with breastmilk production and fetal and infant growth. Although the quantity of breastmilk is greatly determined by demand from the breastfeeding infant, inadequate protein and calorie intake of the lactating woman may contribute to milk quality; therefore, it is essential lactating women maintain an adequate and a well-balanced diet throughout the course of lactation.

1. What factors may influence the macronutrient profile of breastmilk?
2. How many servings of protein per week are recommended for lactating women? Give examples of foods that satisfy these recommendations.
3. How many extra calories per day are recommended for nursing mothers per the Dietary Guidelines?

Feeding in Early Infancy

Preview Although instinctive, breastfeeding is something that both the mother and the newborn need to learn.

An infant is born with the ability to feed within hours after birth. The suckling instinct is inherent, as well as the **rooting reflex**, both which help with successful breastfeeding. The rooting reflex is seen when the newborn baby's cheek or lip is touched, causing the face to turn toward the stimulus and make sucking (rooting) motions with the mouth. By using small motions and repeated actions, newborns are also able to communicate hunger. These actions, or **cues**, help the parent understand the needs of the baby. Infant cues begin when the baby is just starting to feel hunger. Babies stir out of a sleep and open their mouth. As their hunger begins to escalate, the cues become more persistent. Babies stretch and move more, arms flail, and legs kick. They also bring their hand to their mouth and suck on it in an attempt to soothe the hunger pains.

At this point the baby is in need of a feeding. Babies continue to become more agitated if their need is not met. Waiting beyond this point to feed the baby can create difficulties for the parent. When the hunger need becomes severe, babies cry and create more agitated movements; they may even turn red in the face. The parent needs to calm the baby before attempting to feed because in this state the baby will gulp the food or fail to latch to the breast properly.

The best time to feed infants is right before they begin to manifest the middle stages of hunger. (See FIGURE 4.8 .) This is especially true for breastfeeding infants; to breastfeed successfully, an infant must be able to latch correctly and suck at a calm, even rate. An agitated baby creates an unsuccessful and frustrating breastfeeding experience.

Breastfeeding Positions and Latch

Although breastfeeding is natural, both babies and mothers need to learn how to nurse. The infant is equipped with several feeding instincts to aid the process; for example, babies are born with the sucking reflex, but they have to learn the mechanics of breastfeeding. To feed the infant, position the baby so that mom and baby are navel to navel. Most infants feed best when skin to skin with the mother. Several things are necessary for appropriate feeding; for example, the mother's nipple should be in line with the center of the baby's lower lip, the mother and baby should have eye contact, and the baby should have a wide mouth latch so that chin and nose are in contact with the breast.[43]

There are many proper positions for infant feeding. Mothers should be encouraged to experiment with various traditional and nontraditional holds until they find a position wherein mother and baby are relaxed and comfortable with maximum eye and skin contact. There is no single right way to feed, and practitioners should avoid being too strict about positioning. Relaxation and comfort are important components of oxytocin release and should be the first considerations in placing a baby to breast FIGURE 4.9 .

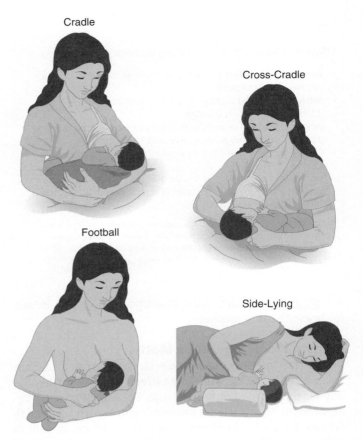

Cradle

Cross-Cradle

Football

Side-Lying

Figure 4.9
Breastfeeding positions.

Latch is the process whereby the infant creates the right type of contact for positive pressure to initiate the flow of milk from ducts. The infant's mouth must close around the small circular area surrounding the nipple called the areola, and it pulls most of the areola and nipple inside the mouth. The nipple touches the back of the mouth. The infant's upper and lower lips fold outward so that maximum lip and gum tissue contact the breast. Compression of the breast happens at the midareola, not at the nipple. A shallow latch that compresses the nipple results in pain and inefficient milk transfer. (See FIGURE 4.10 .)

TABLE 4.6 identifies the steps used in assessing adequacy of an infant's latch during breastfeeding.

A well-latched infant creates the right amount of compression and suction to remove milk effectively from the milk ducts. The average infant will suckle for 10–30 minutes per session, removing 80–90% of existing milk within the breast. Suckling stimulates prolactin, so the body quickly replenishes depleted milk supply. The average infant eats 8–12 times per day and should be fed when showing signs of readiness, regardless of how much time has passed. The baby should empty one breast and self-detach before the second breast is offered. Both breasts should be offered at each feeding. Until breastfeeding

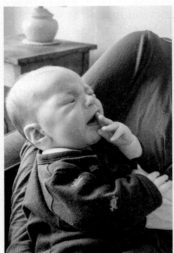
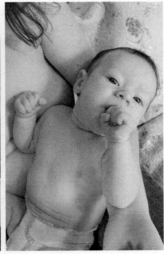

Figure 4.8
Hunger cues of an infant.

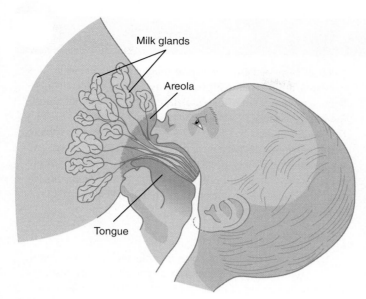

Figure 4.10
Basic latch of infant who is breastfeeding.

Milk glands

Areola

Tongue

is well established, the use of artificial nipples or pacifiers should be discouraged because they will limit the infant's suckling at the breast and potentially reduce supply. Nipple confusion can occur if an infant has difficulty achieving the correct oral configuration, latching technique, and suckling pattern necessary for successful breastfeeding after bottle feeding or other exposure to an artificial nipple. However, after the first month of breastfeeding, use of pacifiers does not correlate with nipple confusion, decreased supply, or a decrease in breastfeeding success.[11]

The only way for the infant to increase the amount of milk available at a feeding is by increased suckling at the breast. As infants age, most settle into a pattern of feeding with 3- to 4-hour breaks between feeds. However,

even in later months, babies vary intake based on availability, growth, and need for comfort. For example, a 4- to 6-month-old infant of a working mother may lessen intake of expressed milk during the day when mom is not available but feed more often during the evening hours. In studies of responsive feedings, many professionals believe that the infant is the best judge of his or her needs. Caregivers should be encouraged to check the diaper every 2–3 hours to verify that the infant is stooling and voiding as anticipated. A well-fed infant urinates at least six times per day and stools at least three times per day by day 4 of life.[44] If stool, void frequency, and growth are normal, a mother should be reassured that she has an adequate and nutritious milk supply.

Recap Although breastfeeding is a natural thing, both baby and mother need to learn how to nurse. A well-latched infant creates the right amount of compression and suction to remove milk effectively from the milk ducts.

1. List the five components of a breastfeeding assessment.
2. Why is it important for the baby to create an appropriate latch when breastfeeding, and what are consequences if the baby feeds without an appropriate latch?
3. In what way can the baby contribute to increased breast-milk production of the mother?

Nutrition and Lactation Outcomes

Preview Adequacy of infant feeds can be determined by assessing growth over time. It is not uncommon, especially for new mothers, to experience some level of difficulty when learning to breastfeed. To ensure adequate feeding, any breast discomfort and issues should be evaluated promptly.

Table 4.6

Breastfeeding Assessment

Good	Significant pain; mom flinches or cries
At risk	Infant behavior
Needs assistance	Roots when breast presented; relaxed during feed
The breast	Sleepy or disinterested
Supple; milk beads when breast squeezed	Arches, pulls from breast, makes high-pitched cry
Breast is hard or milk does not express	Effective milk transfer
Inverted or damaged nipples; mom reports poor or no supply	Chin rocks forward and back; rhythmic, audible swallow
The areola	Non-rhythmic suck with pauses between swallows
Infant latched over nipple with areola drawn into mouth	Infant does not latch or suckle enough to feed
Lips close around nipple	Bonding
Infant not able to latch	Maternal-infant eye contact; spontaneous touch
Maternal Comfort	Mom distracted; infant does not curl into mom
Gentle tug at breast; no pain	Minimal physical contact; mom irritable with infant
Tug with some pain	

News You Can Use

It is well accepted that exclusive breastfeeding is of benefit to both infant and mother. Studies have examined the impact of breastfeeding on maternal body composition, and research supports that breastfeeding can help mothers lose weight during the postpartum period. Women gain visceral fat, body fat that is stored within the abdominal cavity, during pregnancy. Over time, some women have more difficulty returning to their pre-pregnancy visceral fat stores level. A number of factors can contribute to this, and one interesting finding is revealed in a sample of U.S. women aged 45–58 years. In this study, women who breastfed all of their children until 3 months of age or older exhibited significantly greater amounts of metabolically active visceral fat than mothers who had not breastfed all of their children for 3 months. The women who never breastfed had greater visceral adiposity, greater waist-to-hip ratio, and greater waist circumference, all supporting the idea that even years after breastfeeding has ceased, benefits to the mother continue to exist. Long-term benefits to the mother can be seen as a result of breastfeeding as well. For each of the first 2 years a mother breastfeeds throughout her life, she sees a 6% lower risk of breast cancer as well as reduced risk of ovarian cancer.

It has recently been estimated that when mothers around the world decide not to breastfeed, it equates to about $300 billion annually in added costs. One of the largest factors in determining these added costs relates to child deaths that might be prevented each year by improving breastfeeding rates. Breastfeeding can improve infant mortality in a number of ways, notably, researchers have found that breastfeeding prevents about half of all cases of diarrhea and one-third of respiratory infections in infants. Breastfeeding is positively associated with child intelligence independent of parental IQ, and each month of breastfeeding is associated with an increase in IQ points. The effect that breastfeeding has on IQ scores is thought to translate to better academic performance, greater long-term earnings, and improved productivity. Breastfeeding rates at 12 months in the United States were about 27% in 2011, with 79% of infants breastfed immediately after they were born, and 49% breastfed at 6 months.

References

1. Kanazawa S. Breastfeeding is positively associated with child intelligence even net of parental IQ [published online ahead of print September 2, 2015]. *Dev Psychol.* 2015;51(12):1683–1689.
2. López-Olmedo N, Hernández-Cordero S, Neufeld LM, García-Guerra A, Mejía-Rodríguez F, Méndez Gómez-Humarán I. The associations of maternal weight change with breastfeeding, diet and physical activity during the postpartum period. *Matern Child Health J.* November 2, 2016;20(2):270–280.
3. McClure CK, Schwarz EB, Conroy MB, et al. Breastfeeding and subsequent maternal visceral adiposity. *Obesity.* 2011;19(11):2205–2213.
4. Rollins N, Bhandari N, Hajeebhoy N, et al. Why invest, and what it will take to improve breastfeeding practices? *Lancet.* 2016;387(10017):491–504.

Infant Growth Patterns

Breastfed infants have different growth patterns from those of infants fed formula. They generally gain weight faster initially but slow in weight gain for the second half of the first year. Breastfed infants have less visible fat and faster rates of brain growth. As a result, historically, breastfed infants compared to growth standards based on formula-fed infants have been incorrectly considered underweight or failure to thrive.[45] Breastfeeding infants should only be compared to breastfed infant standards, such as the WHO growth charts. These charts were based on infants fed for 4 months exclusively on breast-milk and still breastfed at 12 months. The charts were created based on an international, multiethnic standard and thus are considered appropriate for use with babies in any area of the world. To assess infant growth, standardized procedures and equipment should be used. Infants must be measured lying flat using a length board with stops on both ends. Infants should be weighed regularly on a calibrated, digital scale, naked at a similar time of day.[12] Small changes in procedure can produce large changes in measurement.

Once an accurate length and weight are obtained, the results should be plotted on an appropriate growth standard or chart. These charts demonstrate how well a child is growing based on 100 age- and feeding-matched peers. Therefore, if a child is in the 97th percentile, that child is larger than the average child. This may or may not be important. Instead of aiming for a specific percentile, practitioners should ensure that the infant is growing along a growth channel, or specific percentile line, without large variations up or down.[12] (See FIGURE 4.11.)

Actual and Perceived Barriers to Breastfeeding

Most women in the United State are aware that, under normal circumstances, breastfeeding is the best source of nutrition for their infant, but at the same time, these women lack knowledge about specific benefits of breastfeeding and they are unable to cite the risks associated with not breastfeeding.[46] In general, first-time mothers tend to be uncertain about what to expect with breastfeeding, and the incongruity between expectations about breastfeeding and the reality of the mother's early experiences has been identified as a key reason that many

**Birth to 24 months: Boys
Head circumference-for-age and
Weight-for-length percentiles**

NAME _____

RECORD # _____

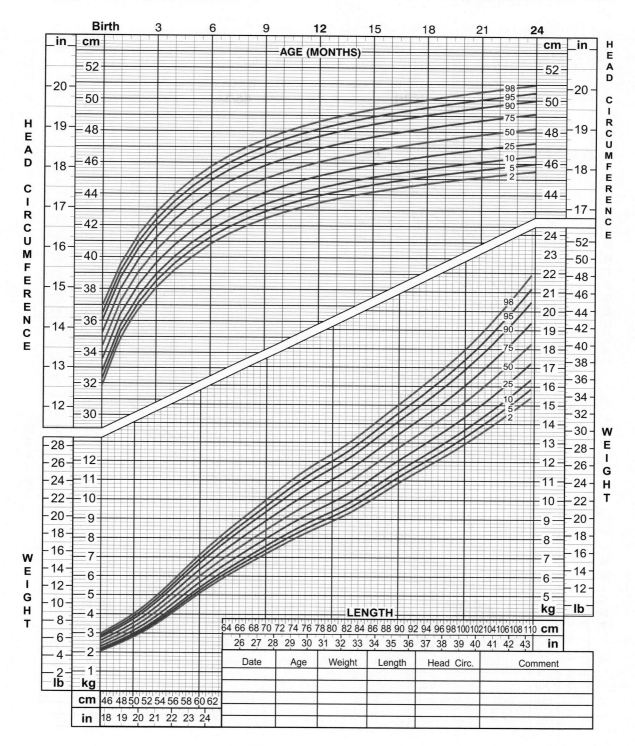

**Birth to 24 months: Girls
Head circumference-for-age and
Weight-for-length percentiles**

NAME _____

RECORD # _____

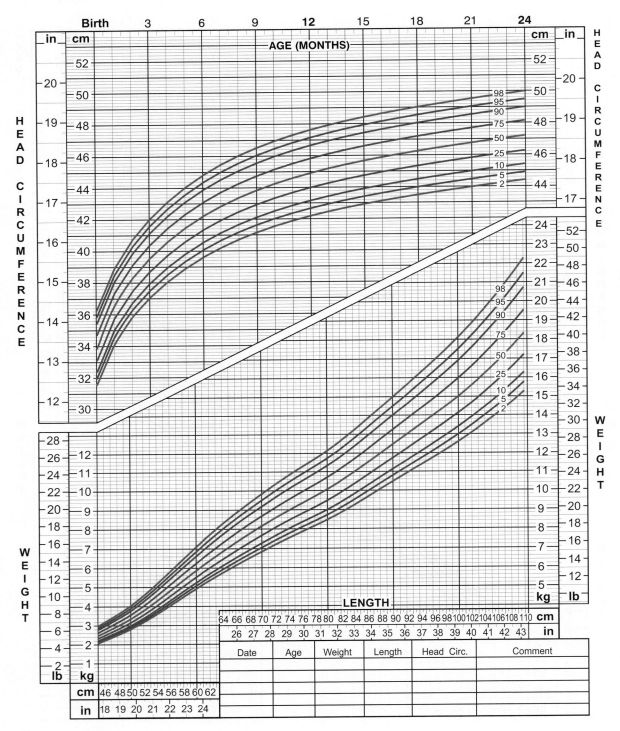

Figure 4.11
CDC growth charts for breastfed infants.

mothers stop breastfeeding within the first 2 weeks post-partum. The perceived inconvenience of breastfeeding may be an issue as well as difficulties in establishing breastfeeding.[46] Another barrier to breastfeeding can occur if the mother's support system verbalizes a negative attitude toward breastfeeding. Family and friends, as well as the attitude of the baby's father, all play significant roles in a mother's decision of whether or not to breastfeed. For many women, feeling embarrassed about breastfeeding either in public or otherwise can also be a barrier. This idea likely stems from within the American culture, where breasts have often been regarded primarily as sexual objects, while the function of nurturing has been downplayed. Other barriers to continued breastfeeding are sore nipples, engorged breasts, mastitis, pain, or the baby's failure to latch. Women who encounter these problems early on are less likely to continue to breastfeed unless they get professional assistance.[46] Concerns about insufficient milk supply and conflicting advice from clinicians may also be viewed as barriers to breastfeeding. Mothers who return to work tend to find this as a barrier to continued breastfeeding. Studies indicate that overall it is the clinicians' knowledge and attitudes about breastfeeding that tend to have a significant impact on whether a mother chooses to breastfeed and chooses to continue to breastfeed after some initial time.[47] See **TABLE 4.7** for common barriers to breastfeeding and possible solutions.

An infant not latching properly can result in nipple discomfort, plugged ducts, **mastitis**, and decreased milk supply. Mastitis is inflammation of the mammary gland in the breast, typically due to bacterial infection because of damage to the nipple **FIGURE 4.12**. When an infant has a shallow or poor latch, milk removal from the breast is

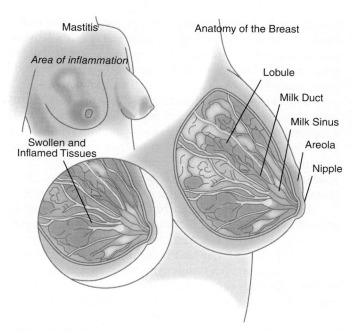

Figure 4.12
Mastitis, an infection in the breast.

incomplete and the nipple can be damaged by contact with the baby's gums and palate. The damaged nipple permits backflow of bacteria that may result in infection. Infections resulting in mastitis are not harmful to the infant but can spread quickly throughout the mother's body. In early stages the mother should be encouraged to rest and apply warm compresses to the breast after feedings. The mother should express a small amount of breastmilk to leave on the nipples after feeds. If this is insufficient for healing, 100% lanolin cream may be applied to maintain the moist environment that is best for nipple healing. Mastitis may worsen rapidly and result in widespread pain and fever, which may require treatment with antibiotics. Pain will inhibit let-down and frustrate the infant. An improper latch puts a mother at risk of stopping breastfeeding.

Mastitis can happen different ways. Bacteria can enter the breast tissue, causing inflammation. Plugged ducts, which can result from poor milk removal or a bra or clothing that restricts the flow of milk through the breast, can damage the inside breast tissue, which allows bacteria to grow. Latch assessment is recommended when a mom complains of a plugged duct. A good latch positions the baby for effective milk removal. The mother should be encouraged to massage her breasts as the baby feeds to encourage milk removal. Between feeds, she can apply warm compresses to relieve pain. Frequent, effective milk removal is the best treatment for plugged ducts.

A baby who tires easily, or one who has poor muscle tone, can be of concern to mothers and health

Table 4.7	
Barriers to Breastfeeding and Possible Solutions	
Barriers to Breastfeeding	Possible Solutions
Lack of support	Learn about breastfeeding before the baby is born; for example, enroll in a breastfeeding class or attend information sessions.
Social or cultural issues	Don't be too concerned about others' opinions regarding breastfeeding, and accept that others may have reservations or be embarrassed no matter what you say or do when it comes to breastfeeding your baby.
Returning to work	Consider using a breast pump and schedule your breaks around your needs for pumping. Pumped breastmilk storage can be portable and discreet.
Breast pain or soreness and/or poor latch	Position the baby to get the best possible latch. Experiment with different holds (Figure 4.9).

practitioners. A sleepy baby may not remove milk effectively or may exhaust easily and end the feeding session prematurely. Poor growth can be common with babies who are not effective at milk removal. Good breastfeeding management of an infant who tires easily or who has poor muscle tone includes: (1) limit sessions to 30 minutes; (2) increase frequency of feeds to every 2 hours; (3) supplement with 10–30 mL of expressed breastmilk after breastfeeding, if needed; and (4) refer to a lactation consultant for ongoing aid and management.[48] With good guidance, most sleepy babies can breastfeed and grow. Most infants gain strength and endurance as they age.

Any mother that reports problems with feeding should be referred to a lactation consultant for assessment. Lactation consultants receive formal education in physiology, lactation, infant care, and counseling strategies through a certification program that requires working side by side with experts for 1,200 hours prior to becoming certified for practice. Lactation consultants work with mothers to optimize latch, reduce pain, and increase milk transfer to the infant. It's important to emphasize unrestricted feeding and discourage nipple shields, feeding schedules, sleep training, infant formula supplementation, and any other practice that limits the infant's ability to feed.

Engorgement, or swelling of the breast, generally occurs in the early periods of breastfeeding when the baby may not be able to remove milk at the rate the body produces the milk. The baby may pull off the breast frequently, spit up excessively, bite the nipple to slow the flow, or gag or cough while feeding. If this happens, mothers should be encouraged to relieve the excess supply by hand-expressing to the point of relief. Mothers may place cold green cabbage leaves or frozen peas on the swollen breast for additional relief. Mothers should be discouraged from overpumping because this can worsen the problem. The milk supply will balance itself within a few days.[49]

After the initial period when the "milk comes in," oversupply is commonly caused by following strict feeding guidelines, such as feeding by the clock or forcing the baby to take each breast or nurse longer than baby desires. Mothers must be retaught to follow the baby's cues so that the supply matches the child's needs. For example, in a mother with a naturally high supply, the infant may nurse for 5–10 minutes on one side only. Although the mother should still offer the second breast, the baby should be allowed to refuse. As long as the infant is growing well, there is no need to force a longer session.[50]

Breastfeeding Considerations and Contraindications

Mothers are naturally very concerned about the safety of the milk provided to the infant. Most women produce milk that is safe for infant consumption. Many mothers falsely believe that conditions in their life prevent them from safely breastfeeding their infant. Contraindications to breastfeeding are rare, but misconceptions are many. The following perceived and actual contraindications should be considered on an individual basis to determine how best to manage breastfeeding.

Galactosemia is a disorder that affects how the body processes the sugar galactose. Galactosemia is a rare metabolic disorder that occurs in 1 in 50,000 births in the United States.[51] Galactose is a by-product of lactose metabolism. In galactosemia, the body cannot process galactose because of a missing enzyme. Harmful by-products accumulate in the blood and damage the liver, brain, and other soft tissue.[52] The only known treatment for galactosemia is the immediate removal of all food products containing lactose or galactose, including breastmilk, in which case the infant must be fed a specialized medical formula.[52]

Human immunodeficiency virus (HIV) can be transmitted from mother to infant as a consequence of breastfeeding. All pregnant and breastfeeding mothers should be encouraged to undergo HIV testing. HIV-positive mothers require treatment and education on infant feeding options. In areas without safe water, the risk of non-HIV mortality from diarrheal and infectious causes is greater than the risk of death from HIV and HIV-related illness. Breastfeeding is the safer and more economical solution to infant feeding in these areas regardless of HIV status. Mothers should be provided with appropriate therapy to decrease viral loads and infants should be regularly tested for HIV throughout the first year of life.[53] Mothers in areas with a safe water supply and low infant mortality rate should discuss breastfeeding options with their medical care team. In mothers with low and controlled viral loads, who take medications as instructed, breastfeeding is not automatically contraindicated. Research indicates that mothers with very low viral loads on appropriate therapy for HIV have minimal risk for passing on the infection. Mothers should undergo frequent CD4 testing to determine viral load and medication adherence. For infants known to be HIV positive at birth, breastfeeding should be the feeding of choice as per recommendations.[54]

HIV is a contraindication to breastfeeding if the viral load is high, maternal adherence to medical regimen is low, or availability of appropriate medical treatment to control viral load is inadequate or unpredictable. In these cases, women should be advised to provide an appropriate human milk substitute. Heat-treated breastmilk purchased from human milk banks could be encouraged if financially feasible for the family.

Neonatal jaundice presents as a yellow appearance of the skin and whites of the eyes of an affected newborn whose liver is not mature enough to get rid of bilirubin that is in the bloodstream. Bilirubin is a natural by-product of protein metabolism but becomes toxic if not removed from the blood. In the immature neonate, the process for removal of bilirubin is inefficient and failure of bilirubin excretion results in a buildup of bilirubin in the blood, causing a yellowish color in skin and eyes. This condition is more likely to occur in babies born before 38 weeks of gestation, and it generally appears between the second and fourth day after birth. Risk factors for neonatal jaundice include: (1) maternal health issues (diabetes, Rh factor); (2) prematurity or low birth weight; (3) neonatal bruising; and (4) excessive weight loss as early neonate.[55] Once thought to be a contraindication to breastfeeding, an infant with jaundice can be safely and effectively breastfed.

Infants who are adequately breastfed can effectively remove bilirubin from blood circulation through regular stooling and voiding. In cases that could not be prevented, treatment options are available that permit breastfeeding to continue without interruption. Infants can be placed in phototherapy booths, usually referred to as "bili lights," at home or in the patient care setting. (See FIGURE 4.13 .)

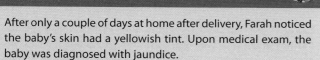

Case Study

After only a couple of days at home after delivery, Farah noticed the baby's skin had a yellowish tint. Upon medical exam, the baby was diagnosed with jaundice.

Questions

1. What is the underlying cause of jaundice in an infant?
2. Which organ is responsible for removing bilirubin from the bloodstream?
3. What causes the yellowish color of skin and eyes in an infant with jaundice?

Other than for feedings, bili light treatment requires that the infant stay inside of the phototherapy booth until blood levels of bilirubin reach acceptable levels. During this phototherapy, the baby may be lethargic and require prompted feedings every 2 hours.

Sleepy or lethargic infants may benefit from a supplemental nursing system (SNS) (see FIGURE 4.14) to ensure adequate intake and hydration. This system consists of a container filled with either pumped breastmilk or infant formula and a capillary tube that leads from the container to the mother's nipple. The SNS is attached to the mother's shoulder with removable tape so that the system remains in place. When the baby suckles at the breast, the latch includes the SNS capillary tube, therefore providing additional nourishment from the SNS. This allows the baby to receive adequate quantities of milk if the mother's milk supply alone is not meeting the infant's needs. Use of the SNS is generally discontinued over time as the mother's milk supply rises in response to the infant suckling. The infant should be breastfed every 2 hours, and the supplemental nursing system will ensure that the infant becomes and remains adequately hydrated throughout the light therapy. Frequent feeding prevents dehydration and increases the rate of bilirubin removal. Infants can be lethargic while bilirubin levels are high; therefore, mothers should be instructed to wake an infant for feeding and should be guided in what to do if the infant struggles to maintain a proper latch for adequate milk transfer.[53]

Mental illness may or may not provide a significant barrier to breastfeeding. All mental illness must be managed well for breastfeeding success. Medical planning should begin in late pregnancy and every mother should have an emergency contact plan that includes what to do with the infant if safety is a concern. Many medications used to treat mental illness can be used safely during

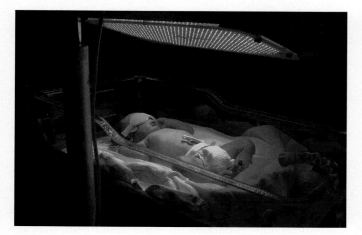

Figure 4.13
Bili light therapy for a newborn.
©Paul Hakimata Photography/Shutterstock

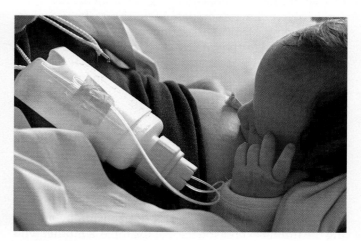

Figure 4.14
Use of a supplemental nursing system.
©Michelle Del Guercio/Science Source/Getty

Table 4.8

Common Medications and Implications for Breastfeeding

Condition	Implications for Breastfeeding
Pain management	• All nonopioids (acetaminophen, ibuprofen) are safe.
Diabetes	• Both oral and injectable treatments are safe.
Bacterial infection	• Penicillin, cephalosporins, macrolides, tetracyclines, and aminoglycosides are all safe and cover most infections.
Hypertension	• Most medications used during pregnancy are safe for use during lactation. Diuretics and medications that reduce heart rate are inappropriate during lactation.
High cholesterol	• Statins to decrease cholesterol should not be used because of their ability to block fat in milk. Because of the utilization of fat in milk, most mothers will not see a rapid increase in cholesterol as a result of not taking these medications. However, if a doctor is concerned, lifestyle modifications should be made.
Seizure disorders	• Seizure medications in usual doses are safe to use while breastfeeding. Mothers with severe disorders may need to consider alternative therapy options for seizure control.
Vaccinations	• Most vaccines are safe. Vaccines used for rare conditions that use live virus (i.e., smallpox, yellow fever) should not be used except in rare circumstances.

Data from National Collaborating Centre for Women's and Children's Health. Intrapartum care: care of healthy women and their babies during childbirth. London (UK): National Institute for Health and Care Excellence (NICE); December 2014. Blumer I, Hadar E, Hadden DR, et al. Diabetes and pregnancy: an Endocrine Society clinical practice guideline.J Clin Endocrinol Metab. 2013 Nov;98(11):4227-49. National Collaborating Centre for Women's and Children's Health. Hypertension in pregnancy. The management of hypertensive disorders during pregnancy. London (UK): National Institute for Health and Clinical Excellence (NICE); August 2010. National Clinical Guideline Centre. Lipidmodification: cardiovascular risk assessment and the modification of blood lipids for the primary and secondary prevention of cardiovascular disease. London (UK): National Institute for Health and Care Excellence (NICE); July 2014. National Institute for Health and Clinical Excellence (NICE). The epilepsies: the diagnosis and management of the epilepsies in adults and children in primary and secondary care. London (UK): National Institute for Health and Clinical Excellence (NICE); January 2012. National Center for Immunization and Respiratory Diseases. General recommendations on immunization. Recommendations of the Advisory Committee on Immunization Practices (ACIP). MMWRSurveillSumm. 2011 Jan 28;60(2):1-64.

breastfeeding.[56,57] Particular care should be taken in patients who experience **psychosis**. Psychosis is a symptom of mental illness in which thought and emotions disconnect from external reality. Infant safety could be at risk, and many antipsychotic drugs are incompatible to breastfeeding.[57] Treatment of the mental illness is a top priority. Mothers should be reassured if they need to provide artificial baby milk or donor milk. Protection of mother and baby is the first concern.

Concerns over the use of medications or herbal remedies can lead to women receiving inappropriate advice to stop or interrupt breastfeeding. Most medications are compatible, or have a compatible substitute, for use when breastfeeding. Medical practitioners should consider the consequences to the infant when weighing the risks of certain medical treatment in the mothers. See **TABLE 4.8** for a list of commonly used medications and their implications for breastfeeding.

Drug and alcohol abuse is a contraindication for providing breastmilk. Infants are at risk of dependence on opioids, heroin, and morphine. If exposure to these drugs has been likely, the infant should be medically managed during detoxification. Alcohol can cause damage during pregnancy, but mild to moderate use postpartum has unknown effects. Healthcare professionals should work with mothers to reduce the risk of exposure by adjusting the timing of breastfeeds. For example, a mother who occasionally drinks alcohol can reduce transmission to the infant by waiting 2–8 hours to feed, depending on quantity of alcohol consumed.

Recap Common breastfeeding issues and concerns include mastitis, and a baby who tires early during feedings. If necessary, medications can be used safely and effectively to help women increase milk supply. Few contraindications for breastfeeding exist; however, management of such conditions should be considered on an individual basis. Galactosemia, HIV, neonatal jaundice, and use of various prescription medications can all be successfully managed with continued breastfeeding.

1. Describe the treatment for perceived or actual low milk supply by a breastfeeding mother.
2. Why might a supplemental nursing system be used for a breastfeeding infant who has jaundice?
3. Summarize the role of a lactation consultant.

Support and Education for Breastfeeding

Preview Most child advocate groups recommend breastmilk as the preferred infant food for the first year of life. Many factors influence a society's breastfeeding rate. Organizations have created pathways to help societies build a more successful breastfeeding culture.

Current recommendations for breastfeeding are that an infant be fed breastmilk exclusively until 6 months of age and then as a supplement to developmentally appropriate solid foods up to age 24 months.[45]

In societies where families and communities work together to promote breastfeeding, the goals for duration and exclusivity have been achieved. When breastfeeding is well incorporated into the family dynamic and within social environments, healthful relationships with food and family are promoted as well.[12] Research points to several avenues that help to increase overall breastfeeding rates. These include: (1) peer support for breastfeeding, (2) adequate professional education before and during breastfeeding, and (3) society-level support in the form of laws, worksite programs, and protections for the breastfeeding pair.

Breastfeeding Success

Breastfeeding rates continue to rise in the United States; however, breastfeeding does not continue in these infants for as long as recommended. Boston University School of Public Health conducts a survey on the reasons breastfeeding rates decline after birth. Findings from the most recent survey can be found in TABLE 4.9 .

Poor lactation support among hospital and healthcare facilities continues to be a significant concern. In the Boston University study, over half of the cited problems could have been resolved with adequate access to lactation support services.

Of infants born in 2011, 49% were still breastfeeding at 6 months and 27% at 12 months.[9] As previously discussed, the first step toward improvement in breastfeeding rates is to provide adequate healthcare support. Professional lactation support at the time of delivery can help mothers initiate and continue breastfeeding successfully.

Breastfeeding Support While in the Hospital

Most women benefit from breastfeeding intervention that begins before birth and continues after birth through peer counselors and one-on-one discussions with medical providers. The combination of prenatal and postnatal promotion activities has been shown to provide the most increase in exclusive breastfeeding.[11,59] Many U.S. hospitals use a program that earns them a "Baby-Friendly" designation. Following the 10 Steps to Successful Breastfeeding, which were developed by a team of global experts and that consist of evidence-based practices that have been shown to increase breastfeeding initiation and duration, allows hospitals and birthing facilities to receive and retain a Baby-Friendly designation.[60] (See TABLE 4.10 .)

Baby-Friendly facilities require that all clinicians who have potential to work with mothers or babies receive education in breastfeeding promotion and support. Suggested topics for this type of education include growth expectations, feeding and sleep patterns, management of growth spurts, hanger and satiety cues, sore nipples, mastitis/blocked ducts, low supply/engorgement, normal stool/voiding in infant, maintaining supply when separated from infant, breastfeeding in public, postpartum depression, and managing breastfeeding during illnesss.[45] FIGURE 4.15 demonstrates an image that promotes breastfeeding.

Breastfeeding Support After Discharge

Peer counselors can be effective assistants in promoting breastfeeding after discharge from the hospital. Peer counselors are generally trained in lactation through formal

Table 4.9

Why Women Stopped Breastfeeding

Reasons Cited by 8% or More Mothers for Not Breastfeeding at 1 Week[a]		Reasons Cited by 8% or More Mothers for Not Breastfeeding at Time of Survey[b]	
My baby had difficulty nursing.	31%	I had trouble getting breastfeeding going well.	39%
It was too hard to get breastfeeding going.	23%	Formula or solid food was more convenient.	22%
Formula was more convenient.	23%	I fed my baby breastmilk as long as I had planned.	22%
I didn't get enough support to get breastfeeding going.	17%	My baby stopped nursing; it was the baby's decision.	18%
I didn't plan to breastfeed much anyway, as I planned to go back to my paying job soon.	13%	I was working at a paying job or school, and other people were feeding the baby.	9%
I had to take medicine and didn't want my baby to get it through breastmilk.	12%	I did not have enough help to work through the challenges.	8%
I tried breastfeeding and didn't like it.	12%	I had to take medicine and didn't want my baby to get it through breastmilk.	8%
It was too hard with my own health challenges.	12%		
After the birth, I changed my mind about wanting to breastfeed.	9%		

[b] Base: breastfeeding at 1 week among follow-up LTM III mothers, n = 551.

Reproduced from National Partnership for Woman & Families. Retrieved from: http://www.nationalpartnership.org/research-library/maternal-health/listening-to-mothers-iii -new-mothers-speak-out-2013.pdf

Table 4.10

The 10 Steps to Successful Breastfeeding

1. Have a written breastfeeding policy that is routinely communicated to all healthcare staff.
2. Train all healthcare staff in the skills necessary to implement this policy.
3. Inform all pregnant women about the benefits and management of breastfeeding.
4. Help mothers initiate breastfeeding within 1 hour of birth.
5. Show mothers how to breastfeed and how to maintain lactation, even if they are separated from their infants.
6. Give infants no food or drink other than breastmilk, unless medically indicated.
7. Practice rooming-in—allow mothers and infants to remain together 24 hours a day.
8. Encourage breastfeeding on demand.
9. Give no pacifiers or artificial nipples to breastfeeding infants.
10. Foster the establishment of breastfeeding support groups and refer mothers to them at discharge from the hospital or birth center.

Data from Baby-Friendly USA. The ten steps to successful breastfeeding. Retrieved from: http://www.babyfriendlyusa.org/about-us/baby-friendly-hospital-initiative/the-ten-steps/. Accessed March 14, 2016.

education and experience. The most effective peer counselors have breastfed and have empathy for the mother during the learning period. Peer counselors may provide in-home support or telephone-based support, and they often provide community events such as breastfeeding cafes, nurse-ins, and education days.[12] Peer counselors can help to identify postpartum depression as well as verify that the baby is receiving safe and adequate care.[12]

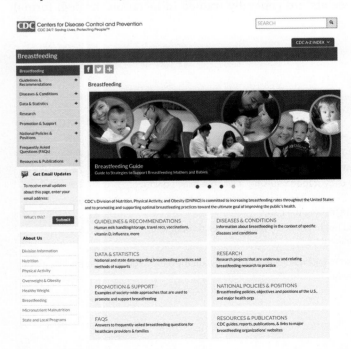

Figure 4.15
Suggested image for promoting breastfeeding.

Courtesy of Centers for Disease Control and Prevention

Peer counselor programs such as La Leche League (http://www.llli.org) were largely responsible for the modern-day resurgence of breastfeeding after rates had plummeted to all-time lows in the 1950s. La Leche League is one of the world's largest sources of breastfeeding support and information, providing information and education from one mother to another.

Societal Support

Societal pressures contribute significantly to breastfeeding failure and use of artificial baby milk supplements. Common societal pressures mothers face include concerns regarding sexuality and poor worksite support for breastfeeding. Convenience, comfort, family pressure, abuse history, and desire for independence and individuality contribute to low breastfeeding rates as well.

In many cultures, breasts are sexualized portions of the female anatomy, and many women are uncomfortable using their breasts in both sexual and nonsexual ways. In these instances, it is helpful for health and nutrition professionals to discuss such concerns openly and without judgment to maximize breastmilk feeding while respecting a woman's sexual identity.[61] Public breastfeeding can be more difficult in these cultures. Women may feel pressure to breastfeed in bathrooms or private areas, leave social gatherings, or wear cover-ups rather than expose the breast for feeding. Mothers in cultures where public breastfeeding is taboo tend to supplement with artificial baby milk when in public rather than face public shame.[62]

Mothers who work face additional difficulties. Only 12% of worksites in the United States provide support or assistance to breastfeeding mothers, such as private pumping space and refrigeration for use by lactating women. Mothers who breastfeed generally miss less work in the first year of their baby's life than those who do not, and businesses with lactation programs report higher work productivity than those who do not support breastfeeding. Several organizations work with businesses to create worksite lactation plans that include onsite day care, pumping facilities, refrigeration, and adequate break time.[17]

Breastfeeding advocates, including men, should encourage workplace policy and laws that promote breastfeeding and breastfeeding support. These policies should include job protection for pregnancy and pumping, adequate maternity leave, sick leave that includes time off for caring for children, access to quality child care, elimination of laws that limit public breastfeeding, and access to healthy foods. As societies move toward acceptance of breastfeeding as the norm for infants, breastfeeding duration rates will improve.[12]

From personal decisions, to society views, a number of factors play a role in the decision to breastfeed. (See **FIGURE 4.16**.) Scientific evidence supports the claim that breastmilk is the most beneficial feeding choice for infants, but some women may face barriers that limit their ability to provide breastmilk to their child. These

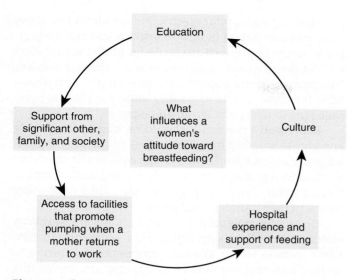

Figure 4.16
Possible factors that contribute to the decision of whether to breastfeed.

barriers can be medical, physical, or psychological, or they may arise from a lack of support from work or from family. When a mother is unable to provide maternal breastmilk, pasteurized donor milk or infant formula are the recommended alternatives. While these options don't provide the full biological impact of the maternal breastmilk, they can provide the nutrients necessary for infant growth and development.

> **Recap** The combination of prenatal and postnatal promotion activities provides the most increase in exclusive breastfeeding. There are a number of support and assistance programs available to breastfeeding mothers. Every level of society plays a role in the promotion of breastfeeding.
>
> 1. Name one lactation assistance and support group.
> 2. Describe possible barriers to breastfeeding for a mother who returns to work.

Pumping and Breastfeeding Interruption

Breastfeeding interruption can happen for a variety of reasons. Children with special healthcare needs, including those born at low weight or premature and those who are ill at birth, may interrupt breastfeeding. Maternal medical issues can also affect breastfeeding. When breastfeeding is interrupted, mothers may require support to meet breastfeeding goals under special circumstances.

A common cause of feed interruption is delivery of preterm infants or those born before 37 weeks of gestation. Infants born before 34 weeks will likely be hospitalized for weeks to months as they mature. Many neonatal care centers provide high-risk infants with pasteurized donor milk if the mother's milk is not sufficient

or available. This provides an alternative to feeding with infant formula while providing the benefits of breastmilk. Breastmilk's immunological components such as secretory immunoglobulin A, lactoferrin, and cytokines provide a framework of immunity that, in conjunction with nutritional support, significantly improves preterm infant health.[62]

Mothers with early preterm infants should be taught to use a hospital-grade pump intended for long-term pumping. Hand pumps do not provide adequate stimulation for establishment of long-term supply. Mothers should pump at least four times per day and once overnight. If the supply begins to wane, additional pump sessions may be necessary. Inhibited let-down is common. Some mothers find that photos of their baby or pumping while skin to skin with the infant encourages milk release.

Late preterm infants (born at 34–37 weeks) and small-for-gestational-age (SGA) infants often have both immature feeding reflexes and low birth weight. These infants are at particular risk for hypoglycemia, hypothermia, hyperbilirubinemia, dehydration, excessive weight loss, and failure to thrive. They require lactation support and frequent evaluation of breastfeeding to ensure latch, milk transfer, and adequate weight gain and instruction in how to manage interruptions in breastfeeding.[12] During breastfeeding, late preterm infants benefit from extended skin-to-skin contact during and between nursing sessions, waking if they nod off before milk transfer is complete, and careful monitoring for signs of readiness to feed. Late preterm infants must be fed in early wakefulness during early stages of feeding readiness. If a mother waits too long, the infant will likely tire during feeding and fail to intake adequate nutrients for appropriate growth. Under these circumstances, mothers should ensure that no longer than 3 hours elapses between feeding sessions.[63, 64]

If low-birth weight or late preterm infants fail to meet growth milestones, mothers should be encouraged to pump after feeds to stimulate an increase in supply. Infants with low birth weight often require supplementation or fortified feedings to obtain adequate nutrition intake.

Fortification can be accomplished by feeding **hind milk** or adding a **human milk–based fortifier** to breastmilk that has been pumped. If the infant is too lethargic to continue suckling at the breast for an entire feeding, hind milk, which is that milk available at the end of a feeding, should be extracted either by a breast pump or by hand and offered to the infant. It is important to provide the hind milk to infants because this milk is higher in fat content than the milk provided at the beginning of that particular feeding. (See **FIGURE 4.17** .) Human milk fortifiers are powders or liquids added to breastmilk to increase the amount of calories and protein in the milk.

Infant weights can be used to determine the exact amount of supplementation needed for infant growth.

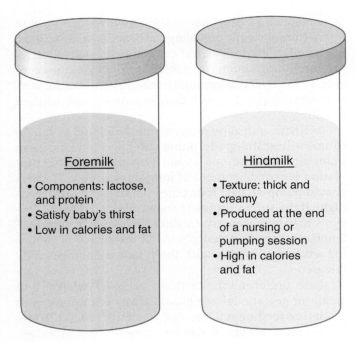

Figure 4.17
Visual comparison of breastmilk from the beginning of a feeding with hindmilk.

Foremilk

- Components: lactose, and protein
- Satisfy baby's thirst
- Low in calories and fat

Hindmilk

- Texture: thick and creamy
- Produced at the end of a nursing or pumping session
- High in calories and fat

Weighing the baby before and after a feeding can give a general idea of how much milk transferred from mother to baby. If the intake is below expectations for age, the missing amount of milk can be provided. In general, this amount will be 10–30 mL of fortified expressed breastmilk.

For short-term breastfeeding interruption, such as time away, mothers should be taught skills to help maintain milk supply. These skills include use of an electric breast pump or hand expression. (See FIGURE 4.18.) Hand expression can be as effective at milk removal as electric pumps are.

Mothers who prefer electric pumps should be given adequate instruction in how to operate and clean equipment. Encourage breast massage for breast stimulation and let-down at the initiation of the pumping session. Pumping sessions should continue for 15–30 minutes until the flow of milk stops and additional breast massage fails to provoke a let-down response.

Expressed breastmilk should be handled in a safe and sterile way, but breastmilk does not require universal precautions. Pumps and storage equipment should be washed in hot, soapy water or by placing pump parts in boiling water. Good hand hygiene should be used every time a person handles breastmilk.

Glass and polypropylene containers are similarly effective as milk storage containers. Most infants consume milk in 60- to 120-mL increments, so storing in similar size containers is most appropriate. Breastmilk may be stored in a refrigerator or a freezer. Fresh milk should always be the preferred milk for feeding. However, refrigerator and freezer storage is safe and milk will be nutritious if properly stored. See TABLE 4.11 for breastmilk storage guidelines.[18]

Table 4.11

Breastmilk Storage Guidelines

1. 3–4 hours at room temperature (50°F–85°F or 10°C–30°C).
2. Up to 5 days at temperatures <39.2°F (4°C) (refrigerator).
3. Up to 6 months at <–0.4°F (–18°C) (freezer).
4. Refrigerating preserves better than freezing.
5. Do not refreeze after thawing.
6. Never use microwave to thaw or heat.

Data from National Institute for Health and Clinical Excellence (NICE). Improving the nutrition of pregnant and breastfeeding mothers and children in low-income households. London (UK): National Institute for Health and Clinical Excellence (NICE); March 2008. (Public Health Guidance; no. 11).

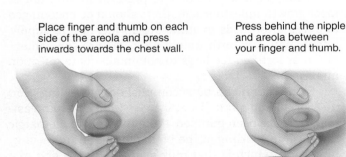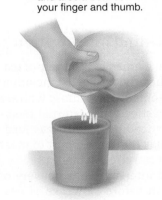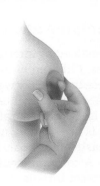

Place finger and thumb on each side of the areola and press inwards towards the chest wall.

Press behind the nipple and areola between your finger and thumb.

Press behind the nipple and areola between your finger and thumb.

Move fingers around to release milk from different areas of the breast.

Figure 4.18
Hand expression of breastmilk.

Freezing breastmilk preserves fat, protein, vitamins A, E, and B, enzymes, lactose, zinc, immunoglobulins, lysozyme, and lactoferrin activity but may decrease vitamin C availability. Some change in flavor or smell is a normal part of the freezing process and does not affect the nutrition of the milk or safety for the infant. To preserve the most antimicrobial and nutrient function, feed the most recently frozen milk first.

Milk should be maintained at a temperature below 40°F. It can be heated up to 95°F–100°F for feeding. The best methods for reheating are to place milk in a warm water bath or under warm running water (FIGURE 4.19). When heating milk, do so slowly by running the bottle under warm water or setting it in a container of warm water, and monitor that the temperature does not go above 140°F to protect the infant and avoid destroying enzymatic activity. Milk should never be warmed in a microwave owing to the potential for superheated hot spots that could burn the baby. Never add warm milk to previously cooled or frozen milk. Do not allow previously frozen milk to remain at room temperature for more than 2 hours.

Galactagogues are medications used to increase milk supply. Common medical regimens include etoclopramide, domperidone, and sulpiride. These drugs work by blocking dopamine, which allows prolactin levels to rise.[65] When a mother has low prolactin levels, milk supply may be affected. Natural galactogogues include fenugreek, blessed thistle, and alfalfa. The method of action for these remedies is less well known but seems to influence the hormones responsible for milk production. Natural galactogogues may provoke an allergic response. Mothers should be warned of this risk and advised how to proceed if an allergic reaction occurs. All of these mentioned substances, whether natural or medicinal, should be used under the care of a trained healthcare practitioner.

Case Study

Low Milk Supply and Breastfeeding

When her baby was 8 weeks old, Farah returned to work. She tried to maintain a regular pumping schedule while at work. Farah comes to you with her baby for evaluation of low milk supply. Her baby has gained weight well until the past 2 weeks. Farah has noticed fewer wet diapers and a decrease in the volume of breastmilk that she has been able to pump. About a week ago, a lactation consultant visited Farah in her home. The evaluation indicated low transfer of milk based on pre- and postfeeding weights, but no nipple trauma. Baby seems to have good coordination with suck and swallow and a good latch.

Questions

1. What factors might contribute to the change in milk supply?
2. What suggestions do you have for Farah to increase her milk supply, particularly with her return to work?

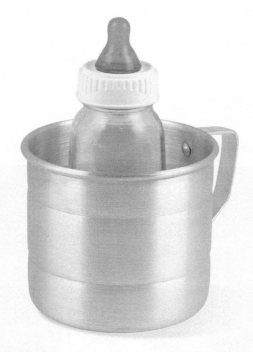

Figure 4.19
Proper technique for warming breastmilk prior to feeding.
©Tcort/iStock/Getty

Recap Premature birth, time away, illness, or other factors can also cause interruptions in breastfeeding. When breastfeeding is interrupted, support for the breastfeeding mother can help keep her milk supply. Proper handling and storage of breastmilk are essential to keep breastmilk safe for infant consumption.

1. If breastfeeding is interrupted, what methods can a mother use to extract her breastmilk?
2. How long is it safe for breastmilk to remain at room temperature?
3. When breastmilk is frozen, what nutrient(s) may be reduced?

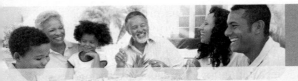

Learning Portfolio

Visual Chapter Summary

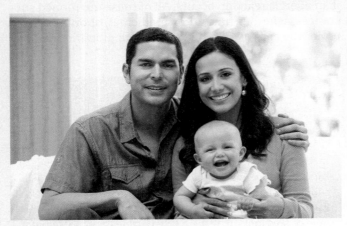

©Pressmaster/Shutterstock

Benefits of Breastfeeding

- Benefits of breastfeeding stretch well beyond basic nutrition.
- Breastfeeding can protect an infant from certain diseases, both in childhood and as an adult.
- Breastfeeding decreases the risk of infant death and disease and enhances comfort and stability for infants.
- Breastfeeding decreases cancer rates among mothers and reduces the likelihood of metabolic disease.

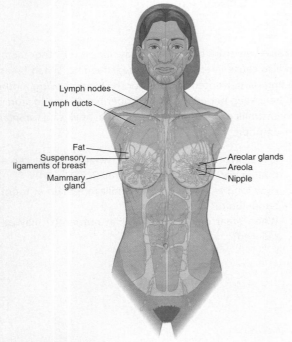

Anatomy of the female breast.

- Individual and societal benefits of breastfeeding are significant enough that breastfeeding rates are included in Healthy People 2020.

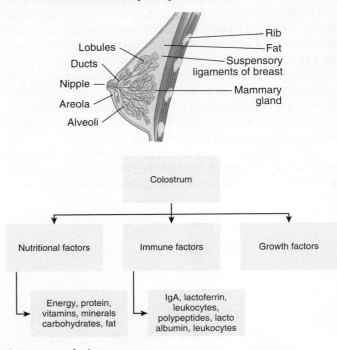

Components of colostrum.

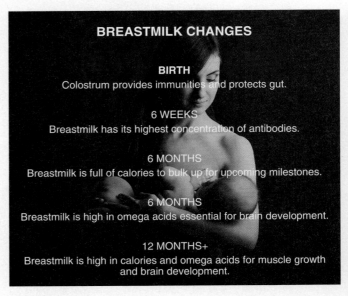

©AlohaHawaii/Shutterstock

Changes in breast milk during the first year postpartum.

Used with permission from Lactation Connection, http://www.lactationconnection.com/

The Physiology of Lactation

- The structure of the breast allows for its function of providing nutrients to an infant.
- Hormones enhance development of the mammary gland and prepare the mammary system for milk production.
- For the initial stage of milk production, the mother's body produces colostrum, the first secretion from the mammary glands of the mother after giving birth. Colostrum is uniquely nutritive and significantly important; it is the first feedings for an infant who has been well nourished by the maternal blood supply during pregnancy.

Human Milk Composition

- Human milk is a dynamic fluid that contains factors and nutrients needed for infant health and development.
- The composition of breastmilk changes through the course of lactation, providing the vast majority of nutrients required for infant growth.

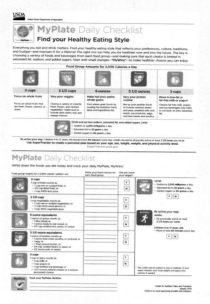

MyPlate Daily Checklist.

Reproduced from USDA Center for Nutrition Policy and Promotion; January 2016. MyPlate Daily Checklist. Retrieved from: http://www.choosemyplate.gov/sites/default/files/myplate/checklists/MyPlateDailyChecklist_2400cals_Age14plus.pdf.

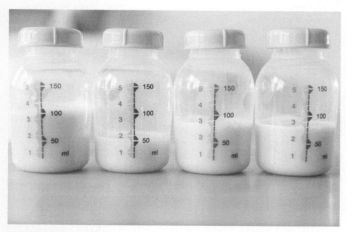

©JGI/Jamie Grill/Getty Images

Milk protein concentrations, comparing milk from mothers who delivered preterm and term, by gestational age at delivery and weeks postpartum.

Nutrition Recommendations and Requirements During Lactation

- Human milk composition varies depending on stage of lactation and it differs between preterm and term deliveries.

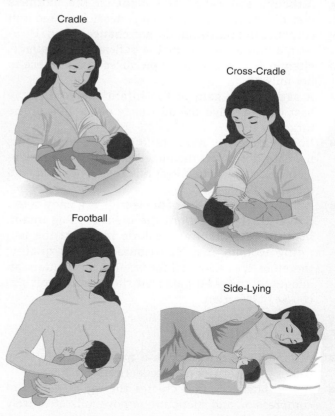

Breastfeeding positions.

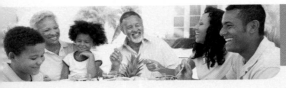

Learning Portfolio (continued)

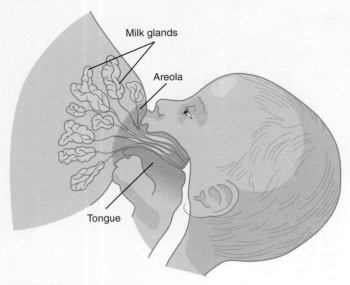

Basic latch of infant who is breastfeeding.

- Although somewhat dependent on the mother's diet, the carbohydrate, protein, fat, calcium, and iron contents in breastmilk do not change much. However, a mother whose diet is deficient in thiamine, vitamin A, and vitamin D produces less of these in her milk.
- A satisfactory gain in the infant's weight is the best way to judge the adequacy of the diet of the infant.
- During lactation, mothers' nutrition requirements increase to support the increased maternal metabolism associated with breastmilk production and fetal and infant growth.
- Although the quantity of breastmilk is greatly determined by demand from the breastfeeding infant, inadequate protein and calorie intake of the lactating woman may contribute to milk quality; therefore, it is essential for women to maintain an adequate and well-balanced diet throughout the course of lactation.

Feeding In Early Infancy

- Although breastfeeding is a natural activity, both babies and mothers need to learn how to nurse.
- A well-latched infant creates the right amount of compression and suction to remove milk effectively from the milk ducts.

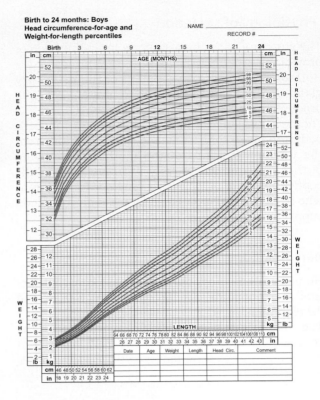

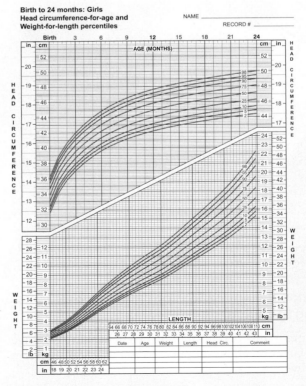

CDC growth charts for breastfed infants.

Reproduced from the Centers for Disease Control.

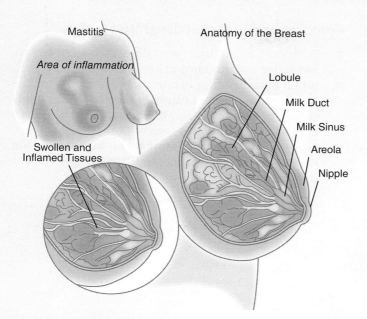

Mastitis

Area of inflammation

Swollen and
Inflamed Tissues

Anatomy of the Breast

Lobule

Milk Duct

Milk Sinus

Areola

Nipple

Mastitis, an infection in the breast.

Nutrition and Lactation Outcomes

■ Common breastfeeding issues and concerns include mastitis, a baby who tires early during feedings, and gastroesophageal reflux.

■ If necessary, medications can be used safely and effectively to help women increase milk supply.

■ Few contraindications for breastfeeding exist; however, management of conditions that do contraindicate breastfeeding should be considered on an individual basis. Galactosemia, HIV, neonatal jaundice, and use of various prescription medications can all be successfully managed with continued breastfeeding.

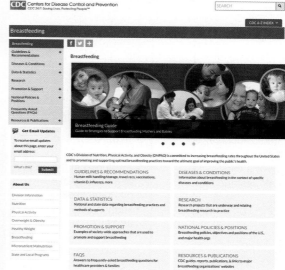

Suggested image for promoting breastfeeding.
Courtesy of Centers for Disease Control and Prevention

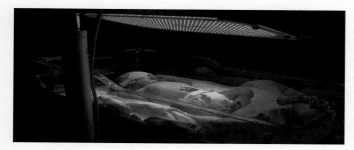

Bili light therapy for a newborn.
©Paul Hakimata Photography/Shutterstock

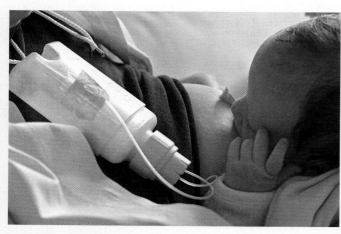

Use of a supplemental nursing system.
©Michelle Del Guercio/Science Source/Getty

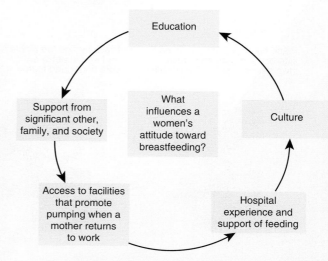

Education

Support from significant other, family, and society

What influences a women's attitude toward breastfeeding?

Culture

Access to facilities that promote pumping when a mother returns to work

Hospital experience and support of feeding

Possible factors that contribute to the decision of whether to breastfeed.
Courtesy of Centers for Disease Control and Prevention

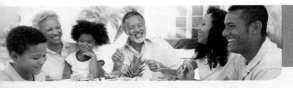

Learning Portfolio (continued)

Support and Education For Breastfeeding

- The combination of prenatal and postnatal promotion activities provides the most increase in exclusive breastfeeding.
- If a new mother decides to breastfeed, a number of support and assistance programs are available to her.
- Barriers to breastfeeding may be difficult to overcome without the support of the community, family, and even friends.

Pumping and Breastfeeding Interruption

- Premature birth, time away, illness, or other factors can cause interruptions in breastfeeding.
- When breastfeeding is interrupted, support for the breastfeeding mother can help keep her milk supply sufficient so that regular breastfeeding can resume once the interruption is resolved.
- Proper handling and storage of breastmilk are essential to keep breastmilk safe for infant consumption.

Foremilk

- Components: lactose, and protein
- Satisfy baby's thirst
- Low in calories and fat

Hindmilk

- Texture: thick and creamy
- Produced at the end of a nursing or pumping session
- High in calories and fat

Visual comparison of breastmilk from the beginning of a feeding with hind milk.

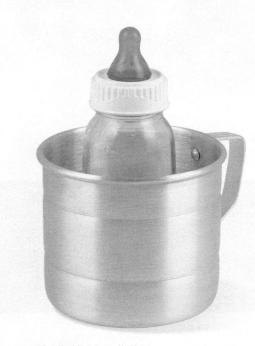

©Tcort/iStock/Getty Images Plus/Getty

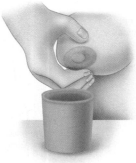
Place finger and thumb on each side of the areola and press inwards towards the chest wall.

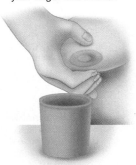
Press behind the nipple and areola between your finger and thumb.

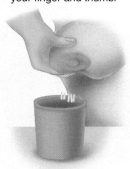
Press behind the nipple and areola between your finger and thumb.

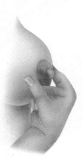
Move fingers around to release milk from different areas of the breast.

Hand expression of breastmilk.

Key Terms

areola: The small circular area surrounding the nipple.

colostrum: The first secretion from the mammary glands of the mother after giving birth. This fluid is rich in immunologic properties.

cues: Help the parent understand the needs of the baby.

engorgement: Swelling of the breast.

galactagogues: Medications used to increase milk supply.

galactosemia: A genetic disorder that creates an inability to metabolize galactose, a common carbohydrate found in milk and a by-product of lactose metabolism. It results in an inability to use galactose to produce energy.

hind milk: The breastmilk available at the end of a feeding that is higher in fat content than milk provided at the beginning of the feeding.

human immunodeficiency virus (HIV): An incurable retrovirus that attacks the immune system, making it difficult for the body to fight off disease.

human milk-based fortifier: Powders or liquids added to breastmilk to increase the amount of calories and protein in the milk.

lactation consultant: Allied health professional who commonly works in hospitals, physician or midwife practices, public health programs, or private practice and who specializes in the clinical management of breastfeeding. Trained professionals are able to help mothers in overcoming common breastfeeding problems.

lactogenesis I: The initial stage of milk production for a postpartum woman.

lactogenesis II: The stage of lactation that begins 2–5 days after birth and is commonly referred to as transitional milk or the milk "coming in."

lactogenesis III: The stage of lactation that generally occurs 2–5 weeks after birth, producing fluid referred to as "mature milk."

lactose: The sugar present in milk.

Le Leche League: An international organization that helps and supports breastfeeding mothers with advice, ideas, and both legal and medical advocacy.

latch: The process whereby the infant creates the right type of contact for positive pressure to initiate the flow of milk from ducts.

let-down reflex: An involuntary reflex during the period of time when a woman is breastfeeding that causes the milk to flow freely.

lymphocyte: A form of small leukocyte (white blood cell) with a single round nucleus that occurs especially in the lymphatic system.

mastitis: Inflammation of the mammary gland in the breast, typically due to bacterial infection of a damaged nipple.

necrotizing enterocolitis: When tissue in the small or large intestine is injured or dies, causing the intestine to become inflamed.

neonatal jaundice: Presents as a yellow discoloration in the skin and eyes of an affected newborn whose liver is not mature enough to get rid of bilirubin that is in the bloodstream.

nipple confusion: Can occur if an infant has difficulty achieving the correct oral configuration, latching technique, and suckling pattern necessary for successful breastfeeding after bottle feeding or other exposure to an artificial nipple.

oxytocin: A hormone associated with contraction of the uterus during labor and that stimulates the ejection of milk into the milk gland.

paraprofessional: Trained aide who assists fully qualified professionals.

passive immunity: Immunity that results from the injection of antibodies passed from the mother to the infant through breastmilk, which actively stimulates the infant's immune system.

peer counselor: Person considered equal to another and who provides knowledge, experience, emotional, social, or practical help.

prolactin: A hormone that helps to produce breastmilk and that is released by the pituitary gland as the fetus develops, causing enlargement of the mammary glands of the breast, which helps prepare for the production of milk.

psychosis: Mental disorder in which thought and emotions are so impaired that contact is lost with external reality.

Rooting Reflex: A reflex that is seen in normal newborn babies who automatically turn the face toward the stimulus and make a sucking or rooting motion with the mouth when the cheek or lip is touched.

Special Supplemental Nutrition Program for Women, Infants, and Children (WIC): A federal assistance program of the Food and Nutrition Service of the U.S. Department of Agriculture. The service provides health care, nutrition education, and financial support for low-income pregnant women, breastfeeding women, and infants and children younger than 5 years.

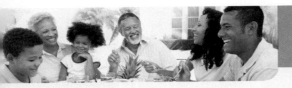

Learning Portfolio (continued)

Discussion Questions

1. Nutrients come in many different forms. Each impacts the digestion and utilization to some extent, and some forms can be more beneficial than others. Using breastmilk as an example, name a few examples of this phenomena.

2. Despite the clear health benefits of breastfeeding, breastfeeding advocates are often encouraged to place personal choice above health in discussions of breastfeeding. Can you name any other health message that places personal choice above health outcome? Why do you think breastfeeding receives this treatment? How do you think healthcare officials should respond to this pressure?

3. Given the many health benefits, how can you be a better advocate for breastfeeding and maternal health? What ways might you, or others you know, be sending negative messages?

4. In what ways do the mother's and infant's bodies work together to ensure infant survival?

5. Mothers of newborns are often overwhelmed. If you were counseling a new mother, how could you simplify messages about maternal diet to ensure adequate intake without contributing to stress?

6. Society benefits when mothers breastfeed, but what to extent does an individual have responsibility to improve the society in which they live? Do you think it is right or wrong to promote a practice to individuals with the aim of improving society as a whole, even if there is no guarantee that the individual child or mother will benefit?

7. Despite very clear science, personal discussions about breastfeeding are often derailed by testimonials claiming that not breastfeeding did no harm to an individual infant. How do you respond to these testimonials? What does it mean to be "at risk" of something due to health decisions?

Activities

1. Interview a breastfeeding mother and a mother who is bottle feeding about the decision they made. Be sure to discuss whether the mothers received prenatal education and lactation support, when they decided whether to breastfeed or bottle feed, how hospital staff reacted, and perceived societal support for breastfeeding.

2. Discuss two to three aspects of your culture that prevent women from breastfeeding or that limit the amount of time a mother might choose to breastfeed.

3. A common misconception is that women with small breasts cannot produce sufficient milk to support infant growth and development. What factors determine how much milk a woman can produce? If a lactating woman is having difficulty with the let-down reflex, what strategies can you provide to enhance the let-down reflex?

Study Questions

1. What is the passing of antibodies from mother to infant through breastmilk called?
   a. Passive immunity
   b. Lactogenesis I
   c. Ankyloglossia
   d. Galactosemia

2. Which of the following choices is the most likely reason breastmilk reduces incidence of allergies?
   a. Breastmilk offers a number of nutrients that formula does not.
   b. Breastmilk composition stays consistent over the course of a feeding.
   c. Breastmilk composition changes over time, offering the infant a variety of different substances.
   d. Breastmilk may enhance passive immunity and fortify the infant's intestines.

3. Which of the following is not considered a benefit of breastfeeding?
   a. Helps the mother's uterus return to normal size sooner.
   b. May help the mother lose weight more quickly.
   c. Reduces the risk of sudden infant death syndrome.
   d. Reduces mothers maltreatment of infants.
   e. All of the above are considered benefits of breastfeeding.

4. As indicated by the Healthy People 2020 breastfeeding objectives, what is the goal rate of infants who are breastfed at 6 months of age?
   a. 33.3%
   b. 50%
   c. 60.6%
   d. 75%

5. Which structure's function is to help defend the body against microorganisms and harmful particles?
   a. Areola
   b. Lymphocyte
   c. Carcinogen
   d. Prolactin

6. The release of which two hormones enhances development of the mammary gland during puberty and prepares the mammary system for milk production?
   a. Oxytocin and insulin
   b. Estrogen and prolactin
   c. Oxytocin and prolactin
   d. Oxytocin and estrogen

7. Which hormone is responsible for allowing let-down of breastmilk?
   a. Prolactin
   b. Estrogen
   c. Progesterone
   d. Oxytocin

8. The concentration of which nutrient relies heavily on maternal dietary intake, and therefore it is the most highly variable component of breastmilk?
   a. Water
   b. Simple carbohydrates
   c. Protein
   d. Fat

9. The concentration of which nutrient in breastmilk does not change much based on maternal intake of the same nutrient? However, its content in breastmilk of mothers who deliver preterm is significantly higher than in milk of mothers who deliver at term.
   a. Water
   b. Simple carbohydrates
   c. Protein
   d. Fat

10. It is unhealthy for breastfeeding mothers to consume fewer than how many calories during breastfeeding?
    a. 2,500
    b. 2,200
    c. 2,000
    d. 1,800

11. Breastfed infants have different growth patterns than infants fed formula, and they tend to gain weight faster initially but slow in weight gain for the second half of the first year.
    a. True
    b. False

12. The only known treatment for which condition is to remove all food products containing lactose or galactose from the diet?
    a. Galactagogues
    b. Galactosemia
    c. Infant diabetes
    d. Jaundice

13. Which of the following is not considered a risk factor for neonatal jaundice?
    a. Maternal health issues such as diabetes mellitus
    b. Prematurity or low birth weight
    c. Neonatal bruising
    d. Excessive weight loss during the first few days of life
    e. All of the above are considered risk factors for neonatal jaundice

14. Breastmilk from which stage of a feeding tends to be higher in fat content?
    a. Breastmilk at the beginning of a feeding
    b. Breastmilk extracted once the feeding has been established (about 2 minutes into the feeding)
    c. Breastmilk extracted once the baby latches on to the second breast during a feeding
    d. Breastmilk at the end of a feeding

15. Which of the following is *not* considered a safe breastmilk storage guideline?
    a. Breastmilk can be held at room temperature for 3–4 hours.
    b. Breastmilk is refrozen after thawing.
    c. Breastmilk can be frozen for up to 2 weeks.
    d. All of the above are considered safe breastmilk storage guidelines.

Weblinks

- **Ameda Breastfeeding** http://ameda.com/breastfeeding
  Provider of breast pumps and breastfeeding supplies as well as education on how to breastfeed under normal and special circumstances.

- **Galactosemia Foundation**
  http://www.galactosemia.org/
  Research organization and education resources for infants with galactosemia.

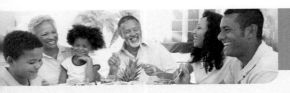

Learning Portfolio (continued)

- **International Lactation Consultant Association**
  http://www.ilca.org/home
  Provides links to lactation care providers by geographical area as well as up-to-date statistics, education, and advice on breastfeeding.

- **LactMed**
  http://toxnet.nlm.nih.gov/newtoxnet/lactmed.htm
  Provides information on medication interactions with breastfeeding.

- **La Leche League International**
  http://www.llli.org/
  A member-based organization that provides peer support and free resources for nursing mothers.

- **Medela Breastfeeding University**
  http://www.medelabreastfeedingus.com/breastfeeding-guidance
  Provider of breast pumps and breastfeeding supplies as well as education on how to breastfeed under normal and special circumstances.

- **Stanford Breastfeeding support videos**
  http://med.stanford.edu/newborns/professional-education/breastfeeding.html

Provide instruction on how to breastfeed under normal and special circumstances.

- **State of the World's Mothers Annual Report**
  https://www.savethechildren.net/state-worlds-mothers-2015
  This annual report discusses trends in maternal and child health, including breastfeeding rates.

- **USDA Food and Nutrition Service**
  http://www.fns.usda.gov/
  Main site for food assistance in the United States. Includes links to WIC and other peer support programs for breastfeeding mothers.

- **WHO Baby-Friendly Hospital Initiative**
  http://www.who.int/nutrition/topics/bfhi/en/
  Discusses healthcare factors related to breastfeeding success and provides training and step-wise direction into how to improve lactation services in healthcare facilities.

- **WHO Growth Standards for Breastfed Infants**
  http://www.cdc.gov/growthcharts/who_charts.htm
  Growth charts derived for breastfed infants only. These charts reflect the unique growth patterns discussed in the chapter.

References

1. Stevens EE, Patrick TE, Pickler R. A history of infant feeding. *J Perinat Educ.* Spring 2009;18(2):32–39.
2. Wright AL, Schanler RJ. The resurgence of breastfeeding at the end of the second millennium. *J Nutr.* 2001;131(2):4215–4255.
3. U.S. Department of Health and Human Services. Healthy People 2020: maternal, infant, and child health. Retrieved from: http://www.healthypeople.gov/2020/topics-objectives/topic/maternal-infant-and-child-health/objectives. Accessed August 12, 2015.
4. World Health Organization; updated July 2015. 10 facts on breastfeeding. Retrieved from: http://www.who.int/features/factfiles/breastfeeding/en/. Accessed July 27, 2016.
5. Sankar MJ, Sinha B, Chowdhury R. Optimal breastfeeding practices and infant and child mortality: a systematic review and meta-analysis. *Acta Paediatr.* 2015;104:3–13.
6. Save the Children; 2012. *Nutrition in the first 1,000 days: state of the world's mothers 2012.* London, England: Retrieved from: http://www.savethechildren.org/atf/cf/%7B9def2ebe-10ae-432c-9bd0-df91d2eba74a%7D/STATE-OF-THE-WORLDS-MOTHERS-REPORT-2012-FINAL.PDF. Accessed August 24, 2016.
7. US Department of Health and Human Services. Executive summary. The Surgeon General's call to action to support breastfeeding. *Breastfeed Med.* 2011; 6(1):3–9.
8. Normalize Breastfeeding. http://normalizebreastfeeding.org/#. Accessed August 24, 2016.
9. National Center for Chronic Disease Prevention and Health Promotion, Division of Nutrition, Physical Activity, and Obesity.

Breastfeeding report card: United States/2014. Atlanta, GA: Centers for Disease Control and Prevention; July 2014. http://www.cdc.gov/breastfeeding/pdf/2014breastfeedingreportcard.pdf. Accessed September 30, 2015.
10. Hibberd CM, Brooke OG, Carter ND, Haug M, Harzer G. Variation in the composition of breast milk in the first 5 weeks: implications for the feeding of pre-term infants. *Arch Dis Child.* 1982;57:658–662.
11. Wilkinson J, Bass C, Diem S, et al. *Preventive services for children and adolescents.* Bloomington, MN: Institute for Clinical Systems Improvement; September 2013.
12. National Institute for Health and Clinical Excellence. *Improving the nutrition of pregnant and breastfeeding mothers and children in low-income households.* London, England: National Institute for Health and Clinical Excellence; March 2008. Public Health Guidance no. 11.
13. Working Group of the Clinical Practice Guidelines for Urinary Tract Infection in Children. *Clinical practice guideline for urinary tract infection in children.* Madrid, Spain: Ministry of Health National Health Service Quality Plan, Social and Equality Policy, Aragon Health Sciences Institute; 2011.
14. Lieberthal AS, Carroll AE, Chonmaitree T, et al. The diagnosis and management of acute otitis media. *Pediatrics.* March 2013;131(3):e964–999.
15. National Center for Immunization and Respiratory Diseases. General recommendations on immunization—recommendations of the Advisory Committee on Immunization Practices (ACIP). *MMWR Recomm Rep.* January 28, 2011;60(2):1–64.

16. Silfverdal SA, Ekholm L, Bodin L. Breastfeeding enhances the antibody response to Hib and pneumococcal serotype 6B and 14 after vaccination with conjugate vaccines. *Vaccine*. 2007;25(8):1497–1502.

17. American Academy of Pediatrics. Policy statement: breast-feeding and the use of human milk. *Pediatrics*. March 2012;129(3):e627–e841. Retrieved from: http://pediatrics.aappublications.org/content/129/3/e827.full#content-block. Accessed July 28, 2016.

18. Academy of Breastfeeding Medicine Protocol Committee. ABM clinical protocol 8: human milk storage information for home use for full-term infants (original protocol March 2004; revision 1 March 2010). *Breastfeed Med*. June 2010;5(3): 127–130.

19. Cincinnati Children's Hospital Medical Center. *Evidence-based care guideline for necrotizing enterocolitis (NEC) among very low birth weight infants*. Cincinnati, OH: Cincinnati Children's Hospital Medical Center; October 7, 2010.

20. Underwood MA, Scoble JA. Human milk and the premature infant: focus on use of pasteurized donor human milk in the NICU. *Diet Nutr Crit Care*. May 29,2015;(part IV): 795–806.

21. Muraro A, Halken S, Arshad SH, et al. EAACI food allergy and anaphylaxis guidelines. Primary prevention of food allergy. *Allergy*. May 2014;69(5):590–601.

22. Singapore Ministry of Health. *Management of food allergy*. Singapore: Singapore Ministry of Health; June 2010.

23. Oddy WH. Infant feeding and obesity risk in the child. *Breastfeed Rev*. July 2012;20(2):7–12.

24. Registered Nurses' Association of Ontario. *Primary prevention of childhood obesity*. 2nd ed. Toronto, ON: Registered Nurses' Association of Ontario; May 2014.

25. Academy of Breastfeeding Medicine Protocol Committee. ABM clinical protocol 23: non-pharmacologic management of procedure-related pain in the breastfeeding infant. *Breastfeed Med*. December 2010;5(6):315–319.

26. National Collaborating Centre for Cancer. *Familial breast cancer. Classification and care of people at risk of familial breast cancer and management of breast cancer and related risks in people with a family history of breast cancer*. London, England: National Institute for Health and Care Excellence; June 2013.

27. Ma P, Brewer-Asling M, Magnus JH. A case study on the economic impact of optimal breastfeeding. *Matern Child Health J*. 2013;17(1):9–13.

28. McKinney CO, Hahn-Holbrook J, Chase-Lansdale PL, et al. Racial and ethnic differences in breastfeeding. *Pediatrics*. July 2016. Retrieved from: http://pediatrics.aappublications.org/content/early/2016/07/11/peds.2015-2388. Accessed July 28, 2016.

29. Butte NF, Garza C, Johnson CA, et al. Longitudinal changes in milk composition of mothers delivering preterm and term infants. *Early Hum Dev*. February 1984;9(2):153–162.

30. Ballard O, Morrow A. Human milk composition: nutrients and bioactive factors. *Pediatr Clin North Am*. February 2013;60(1):49–74.

31. Rogers L, Valentine C, Keim S. DHA supplementation: current implications in pregnancy and childhood. *Pharmacol Res*. April 2013;70(1):13–19.

32. Jia X, Pakseresht M, Wattar N, et at. Women who take n-3 long-chain polyunsaturated fatty acid supplements during pregnancy and lactation meet the recommended intake. *Appl Physiol Nutr Metab*. May 2015;40(5):474–481.

33. Ares SS, Ansótegui J A, Diaz-Gómez NM; en representación del Comité de Lactancia Materna de la Asociación Española de Pediatría. The importance of maternal nutrition during breastfeeding: do breastfeeding mothers need nutritional supplements? [article in Spanish] [published online ahead of print September 14, 2015]. *An Pediatr (Barc)*. June 2016;84(6):347.e1–7.

34. Jantscher-Krenn E, Bode L. Human milk oligosaccharides and their potential benefits for the breast-fed neonate. *Minerva Pediatr*. 2012;64(1):83–99.

35. Centers for Disease Control and Prevention; updated June 17, 2015. Vitamin D supplementation. Retrieved from: http://www.cdc.gov/breastfeeding/recommendations/vitamin_d.htm. Accessed August 24, 2016.

36. Hollis BW, Wagner CL, Howard CR, et al. Maternal versus infant vitamin D supplementation during lactation: a randomized controlled trial. *Pediatrics*. October 1, 2015;136(4):625–634.

37. Zarban A, Toroghi MM, Asli M, et al. Effect of vitamin C and E supplementation on total antioxidant content of human breastmilk and infant urine. *Breastfeed Med*. 2015;10(4):214–217.

38. Allen LH. B vitamins in breast milk: relative importance of maternal status and intake, and effects on infant status and function. *Adv Nutr*. May 2012;3(3):362–369.

39. Mennella JA. Ontogeny of taste preferences: basic biology and implications for health. *Am J Clin Nutr*. 2014;99(3):704S–711S.

40. Segura A, Ansolegui A, Diaz-Gomez, et al. The importance of maternal nutrient during breastfeeding: do breastfeeding mothers need nutritional supplements? *An Pediatr (Barc)*. September 14, 2015.

41. Devalia V, Hamilton MS, Molloy AM; the British Committee for Standards in Haematology. Guidelines for the diagnosis and treatment of cobalamin and folate disorders. *Br J Haematol*. 2014;166(4):496–513.

42. Brzezinska M, Kucharska A, Sinska B. Vegetarian diets in the nutrition of pregnant and breastfeeding women. *Pol Merkur Lekarski*. April 29, 2016;40(238):264–268.

43. Eastman A. The mother-baby dance: positioning and latch-on. *Leaven*. August–September 2000;36(4): 63–68.

44. Philipp BL; Academy of Breastfeeding Medicine Protocol Committee. ABM clinical protocol 7: model breastfeeding policy (revision 2010). *Breastfeed Med*. 2010;5(4):173–177.

45. Grawey AE, Marinelli KA, Holmes AV; Academy of Breast-feeding Medicine. ABM clinical protocol 14: breastfeeding-friendly physician's office: optimizing care for infants and children, revised 2013. *Breastfeed Med*. 2013;8(2):237–242.

46. Office of the Surgeon General; Centers for Disease Control and Prevention; Office on Women's Health. *The Surgeon General's call to action to support breastfeeding*. Rockville, MD: Office of the Surgeon General; 2011. Retrieved from: http://www.ncbi.nlm.nih.gov/books/NBK52688/. Accessed August 24, 2016.

47. Demirci JR, Bogen DL, Holland C, et al. Characteristics of breastfeeding discussions at the initial prenatal visit. *Obstet Gynecol*. 2013;122(6):263–270.

48. Academy of Breastfeeding Medicine. ABM clinical protocol #10: breastfeeding the late preterm infant (34(0/7) to 36 (6/7) weeks gestation). *Breastfeed Med*. 2011 Jun;6(3):151-6

49. West D. Am I making too much milk? La Leche League International; updated July 31, 2008. Retrieved from: http://www.llli.org/faq/oversupply.html. Accessed October 10, 2015.

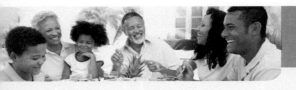

Learning Portfolio (continued)

50. Berry GT. Classic galactosemia and clinical variant galactosemia. Boston, MA: *Boston Children's Hospital,* Harvard Medical School. Published February 4, 2000. Updated April 3, 2014.

51. Shaw KA, Mulle JG, Epstein MP, Fridovich-Kell JL. Gastrointestinal health in classic galactosemia. JIMD Rep. 2016. Jul 1.

52. The galactosemias. Galactosemia Foundation. Retrieved from: http://www.galactosemia.org/understanding-galactosemia/. Accessed October 10, 2015.

53. World Health Organization. *Guidelines on HIV and infant feeding.* Geneva, Switzerland: World Health Organization; 2010.

54. World Health Organization. *Antiretroviral drugs for treating pregnant women and preventing HIV infection in infants.* Geneva, Switzerland: World Health Organization; 2010.

55. Scottish Intercollegiate Guidelines Network (SIGN). *Management of perinatal mood disorders. A national clinical guideline.* Edinburgh, Scotland: Scottish Intercollegiate Guidelines Network (SIGN); March 2012.

56. Kaiser Permanente Care Management Institute. *Diagnosis and treatment of depression in adults: 2012 clinical practice guideline.* Oakland, CA: Kaiser Permanente Care Management Institute; June 2012, 73

57. Academy of Breastfeeding Medicine Protocol Committee. ABM clinical protocol 22: guidelines for management of jaundice in the breastfeeding infant equal to or greater than 35 weeks' gestation. *Breastfeed Med.* 2010;5(2):87–93.

58. Scottish Intercollegiate Guidelines Network. *Management of schizophrenia.* Edinburgh, Scotland: Scottish Intercollegiate Guidelines Network; March 2013.

59. Michigan Quality Improvement Consortium. *Routine prenatal and postnatal care.* Southfield, MI: Michigan Quality Improvement Consortium; June 2012.

60. Baby-Friendly USA. The ten steps to successful breastfeeding. Retrieved from: http://www.babyfriendlyusa.org/about-us/baby-friendly-hospital-initiative/the-ten-steps/. Accessed March 14, 2016.

61. Lamont J, Bajzak K, Bouchard C, et al. Female sexual health consensus clinical guidelines. *J Obstet Gynaecol Can.* 2012;34(8):S1–56.

62. Acker M. Breast is best, but not everywhere. *Sex Roles.* 2009;61:476–490.

63. Thibeau S, DApolito K. Review of the relationships between maternal characteristics and preterm breastmilk immune components. *Biol Res Nurs.* 2012;14(2):207–216.

64. Association of Women's Health, Obstetric and Neonatal Nurses (AWHONN). Assessment and care of the late preterm infant. Evidence-based clinical practice guideline. Washington (DC): *Association of Women's Health, Obstetric and Neonatal Nurses (AWHONN);* 2010. 57 p.

65. Academy of Breastfeeding Medicine. ABM clinical protocol 10: breastfeeding the late preterm infant (34(0/7) to 36 (6/7) weeks gestation). *Breastfeed Med.* 2011;6(3):151–156.

66. Bonyata K. Prescription drugs for increasing milk supply. KellyMom, updated March 16, 2016. Retrieved from: http://kellymom.com/bf/can-i-breastfeed/meds/prescript_galactagogue/. Accessed October 10, 2015.

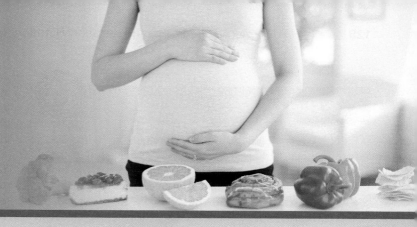

CHAPTER 5

Pregnancy and Lactation: Nutrition-Related Conditions and Diseases

Julia Buckley, MS, RD, **Mateja R. Savoie Roskos**, PhD, MPH, RD, CD, CNP, **Sushila Sharangdhar**, RD **and Sukhada Bhatte-Paralkar**, RD, CDE

Chapter Outline

Gastrointestinal Conditions

Obesity and Malnutrition

Endocrine and Metabolic Conditions

Cardiovascular Conditions

Psychosocial Stressors

Lifestyle Management

Learning Objectives

1. List common gastrointestinal issues among women during pregnancy and lactation and the nutritional implications of these conditions as well as treatment methods.

2. Explain the prevalence of malnutrition and obesity as well as common nutrient deficiencies during pregnancy and lactation and their impact on health outcomes for the mother and fetus.

3. Summarize the metabolic changes that take place during pregnancy and lactation and describe the strategies to enhance proper growth and development in the fetus.

4. Describe nutrition therapy in preeclampsia and perinatal hypertension, including risks and consequences for the fetus and mother.

5. Explain the importance of cognitive health and well-being in addition to physical health during pregnancy and lactation for both mother and child.

6. Explain the impact of substance abuse on nutritional status of the mother and fetus.

Case Study

Rosa received a marriage proposal from her long-term boy-friend on her 23rd birthday. Rosa and her boyfriend would like to adopt healthy lifestyle behaviors the best that they can prior to starting a family of their own. She has recently joined a health club and intends to lose weight before her upcoming wedding. Her mother had gestational diabetes during her pregnancies, and has recently undergone an angioplasty. Rosa took multivitamin supplements as an adolescent but has been inconsistent with supplementation since about age 16 years. During high school, Rosa experienced disordered eating patterns, which included occasional binging and purging. She has not had a binge/purge episode in about a year but is also no longer receiving help or support, and she is still confronted with the urge to binge/purge in moments of stress. Rosa is 5 feet 4 inches tall and weighs 170 pounds, with a body mass index (BMI) of 29. Her hemoglobin was 13 mg/dL and hematocrit was 40% last month. She has been taking oral contraceptives for the past year. She used to be a chain smoker and has continued to smoke on occasion (~1 pack every 2 weeks), and she has an occasional drink or two every weekend.

Questions

1. Discuss Rosa's risk factors that could potentially cause harm to a fetus.
2. Provide a lifestyle and dietary regime for Rosa to minimize the effect of those risk factors on the healthy outcomes for her and her baby during and after pregnancy.

Pregnancy and lactation are critical periods of development during which nutrition and lifestyle needs of women change considerably. During this time, a woman's personal choices greatly influence not only her health but also the health and well-being of the child. According to the Centers for Disease Control and Prevention, 1 in 33 births are complicated by a birth defect.[1] Further, between 2012 and 2014, over 8% of babies were born at a low birth weight (LBW; <2,500 g or 5 pounds, 8 ounces).[2] Unfortunately, birth defects and LBW are among the leading causes of infant deaths in the United States;[3] survivors with birth defects or LBW are at increased risk for a wide variety of complications and health problems.

The health of the mother and her nutritional status at preconception, during pregnancy, and in the postnatal stage have a significant effect on fetal health because of the transfer of nutrients in the womb and during lactation. Consequently, some causes of birth defects or of LBW infants are a direct result of unhealthy choices. Maternal nutrition has been shown to affect the neurological development of the child and may even affect the body composition of a child in later stages of life.[4] Failure of the pregnant woman to meet increased requirements for micronutrients may lead to deficiencies that can cause maternal and fetal complications, decreased physical and mental capacity of the child, birth defects, neural tube defects, and maternal or fetal death or both.[5] Therefore, it is of utmost importance for health practitioners to encourage proper maternal health to ensure adequate fetal growth and development. In this chapter, various nutrition-related conditions and diseases that may pre exist or that occur as a result of pregnancy are discussed, including the potential impact on the health of mother and child as well as treatment recommendations.

Gastrointestinal Conditions

Preview Pregnant and lactating women are susceptible to a host of gastrointestinal (GI) conditions similar to those of the general population. Disturbances may range from common issues such as nausea, vomiting, diarrhea, and constipation to more severe complications, including hyperemesis gravidarum, gastroesophageal reflux disease (GERD), gallstones, peptic ulcers, and inflammatory bowel diseases.

Normal physiological changes during pregnancy may cause dramatic modifications in the GI tract as the body adjusts to accommodate uterine growth.[6] Additionally, hormonal fluctuations have been shown to alter esophageal sphincter pressure and relax smooth muscle, which may decrease GI motility and gallbladder contractility. Therefore, the stress that pregnancy places on the GI tract puts the mother at risk for exacerbation of existing or development of new GI disorders.[6] The following sections outline some of the most common GI complications seen during pregnancy, the prevalence and risk factors for each, as well as nutrition implications and appropriate treatment interventions.

Common Gastrointestinal Disturbances

Similar to the general population, pregnant women are susceptible to common GI disturbances including nausea, vomiting, diarrhea, and constipation. Evidence suggests that physiological, hormonal, and structural changes during pregnancy may result in these bowel function alterations.[7]

Nausea and Vomiting

Symptoms such as nausea and vomiting are common, especially during the early trimesters of pregnancy, usually starting at about 9 weeks of gestation. Nausea and vomiting are commonly referred to as "morning sickness"; however, these symptoms can occur at any time of day or night. It is speculated that changes in hormones, including estrogen and progesterone, early in pregnancy cause nausea and vomiting, but the cause remains unclear. Another theory is that vitamin B deficiency causes nausea and

The Big Picture

Normal anatomy versus anatomy during various stages of pregnancy. A woman's body changes as the developing fetus grows throughout pregnancy.

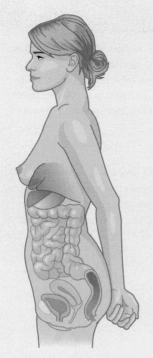
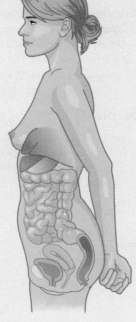
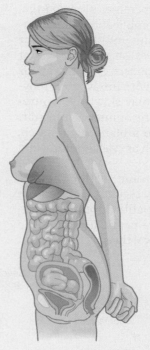
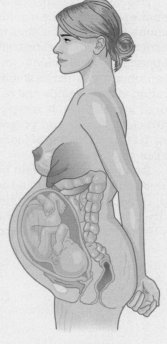

| Anatomy before pregnancy. | First trimester. | Second trimester. | Third trimester. |

vomiting, a likely circumstance because nausea and vomiting decrease in some women who are vitamin B–deficient when they supplement with a multivitamin.[8]

Management of mild nausea and vomiting through dietary interventions can include drinking small amounts of water between and with meals, avoiding foods that are spicy and high in fat, selecting foods that are tolerable, and avoiding foods with strong odors. High-carbohydrate foods such as crackers, popcorn, yogurt, and chips are more likely tolerable. Recommendations for women should be individualized. Nausea and vomiting may be exacerbated from iron supplements, particularly during the first trimester of pregnancy. Taking iron supplements with food as opposed to taking them on an empty stomach can reduce this side effect. Supplements have been found to reduce nausea and vomiting during pregnancy, with suggestions including a multivitamin supplement taken prior and during pregnancy, 10–35 mg of vitamin B_6 (pyridoxine) every 8 hours, or 1 g of ginger every day for several days.[9]

Hyperemesis gravidarum (HG), commonly called hyperemesis, is severe nausea and vomiting throughout much of a pregnancy. Hyperemesis can cause electrolyte imbalances, weight loss, and dehydration. This high-risk condition may require hospitalization, rehydration therapy, and nutrition support to reduce the risk of low birth weight and pregnancy weight loss. Hyperemesis gravidarum occurs in up to 2% of pregnancies, and its etiology is poorly understood.[10]

The symptoms help distinguish between morning sickness and hyperemesis gravidarum. Morning sickness includes nausea that subsides at 12 weeks of gestation or sooner and sometimes is accompanied by vomiting. In addition, morning sickness does not cause severe dehydration, and some food tolerance exists. With hyperemesis gravidarum, vomiting that accompanies nausea does not subside, severe dehydration results, and food tolerance is minimal to none.

Although little is known about the causes of hyperemesis gravidarum, one study found that the condition is three times higher in women whose mothers experienced hyperemesis during their own pregnancies than in those whose mothers did not, suggesting that a genetic component may predispose some women to the condition.[11]

Other risk factors may include multiple pregnancies and the psychology of the patient.

How to prevent hyperemesis gravidarum is not known, and treating complications tends to be how this condition is managed. (See **FIGURE 5.1** for possible complications of hyperemesis gravidarum.)

Possible methods of treating hyperemesis gravidarum, or more specifically the resulting complications, are intravenous (IV) hydration that includes multivitamins for nutrient repletion, bed rest, acupressure, use of ginger or peppermint, medications, and hypnosis. If IV therapy is used, once the patient is stabilized with intravenous rehydration efforts, liquids and solids may slowly be reintroduced into the diet. It is typically recommended to start with clear liquids and progress to a bland high-starch, low-fat diet consisting of foods such as crackers and plain baked potatoes.

Patients with persistent nausea and vomiting beyond the second trimester should be assessed for gastroenteritis, cholecystitis, pancreatitis, hepatitis, pyelonephritis, fatty liver of pregnancy, and active peptic ulcers caused by *Helicobacter pylori*. Pharmacological therapy in pregnant women is similar to that used in nonpregnant women but should always be discussed with medical professionals for possible contraindications in pregnancy.

Case Study

Rosa is starting her 10th week of pregnancy and continues to complain of nausea with persistent vomiting. She is able to tolerate Gatorade, Sprite, soda crackers, mild cheese, some soups, and soft cooked meat. Her current weight is the same as her pre-pregnancy weight. She complains that she is tired most of the time and has headaches often.

Questions

1. What other information would you like to gather from Rosa to better understand whether she is suffering from morning sickness or hyperemesis gravidarum?
2. In an effort to increase her food intake, what suggestions do you have for Rosa?

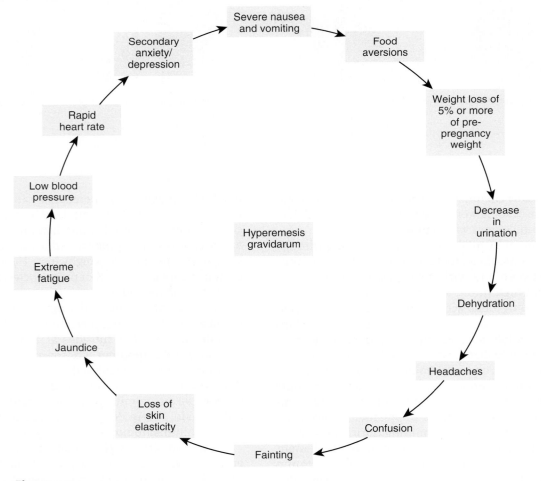

Figure 5.1
Possible complications of hyperemesis gravidarum.

Data from American Pregnancy Association. Promoting Pregnancy Wellness. Hyperemesis Gravidarum. Retrieved from: http://americanpregnancy.org/pregnancy-complications/hyperemesis-gravidarum/

Diarrhea

Few studies have investigated the prevalence or etiology of diarrhea in pregnancy; however, its causes likely mirror causes in the nonpregnant state. Theoretically, the increase in prostaglandins seen in pregnancy may induce contraction of smooth muscle and therefore stimulate propulsive forces and diarrhea.[12] However, the most common causes include infectious agents (*Salmonella* species, *Shigella* species, *Campylobacter* species, *Escherichia coli*, protozoans, viruses); medications; food poisoning and intolerances; lactose, fructose, sorbitol, and mannitol intolerances; inflammatory bowel disease (IBD); and irritable bowel syndrome (IBS).

Although some risk factors, such as IBD, cannot be avoided, pregnant women should be sure to follow food safety protocols closely to prevent bacterial infection and food poisoning. Foods known to cause discomfort and intolerances should also be avoided. If acute diarrhea persists and leads to dehydration, weight loss, or malnutrition, bloody stools, or fever exceeding 100.94°F, further evaluation should be conducted. Stool collection should be assessed and analyzed for bacteria, parasites, and *Clostridium difficile* toxin.

In general, treatment is similar to that of nonpregnant cases of diarrhea. The first lines of treatment are oral rehydration and correction of any electrolyte imbalances (potassium, sodium) with items such as orange juice and bananas, salted crackers, and broth. Small, frequent meals that contain little fat, caffeine, and artificial sweeteners are recommended. In treating cases of IBS during pregnancy, high-fiber diets and stool-bulking agents as well as adequate fluid intake should be effective at correcting diarrhea.

Constipation

Constipation is defined as difficulty emptying the bowels, usually associated with hardened feces and two or fewer bowel movements in a week. Constipation occurs in about 10–40% of pregnancies.[13] Although a clear etiology and incidence rate have not been determined, it is suspected that constipation may arise as a result of physiological and hormonal changes in the GI system, decreased maternal activity, or iron supplementation during pregnancy. As with other GI conditions, constipation can start from the beginning of pregnancy, or it can increase in severity over time, particularly if chronic constipation was an issue prior to pregnancy.

All pregnant women are susceptible to constipation as a result of normal slowed gastrointestinal transit with hormonal shifts (increased progesterone and estrogen, decreased motilin) in pregnancy. Those at increased risk include any pregnant women with anemia who are required to take iron supplementation, those with poor fluid and fiber intake, those with decreased physical activity, and those with psychosocial stress. Women should be encouraged to consume adequate fluids and fiber and maintain moderate levels of safe physical activity to prevent the onset of constipation.

There is limited evidence on the effectiveness of constipation management strategies in pregnancy. However, constipation is rarely severe and can often be treated with the same methods utilized by nonpregnant adults. The expecting mother should ensure fluid intake is at least 3 L per day, and intake of fiber should be a minimum of 28 g per day. High-fiber foods that help to relieve constipation include bran cereals, whole grains, and fresh fruits and vegetables. Physical activity in accordance with medical approval should also be encouraged because it can help stimulate the digestive tract.

If diet and lifestyle modifications do not provide relief, meal supplementation with bran (4 to 6 tablespoons) or other bulk-forming agents such as psyllium, methylcellulose, and polycarbophil may help achieve desired results in 1–3 days. Daily use of these agents with 1 to 2 glasses of water relieves constipation by increasing fecal water content and stool weight while decreasing transit time. In some cases, probiotic supplements containing "healthy bacteria" can alter the gut and colonic flora and thus improve bowel function. Studies on their efficacy in pregnancy are limited, but these supplements pose little to no harm to users.[14] Laxatives, both osmotic and stimulant, should be considered only if the bulk-forming agents mentioned above do not provide symptomatic relief. Fecal impaction as a result of constipation in pregnancy is rare, and mechanical relief is not commonly needed. However, if the situation arises, relief is accomplished in the same way as for a nonpregnant patient with gentle force and fluid enemas.

News You Can Use

We have known for years that fruit has been a significant and important part of the human diet and some studies indicate that certain foods (including fruits) can even give your brain a boost, possibly resulting in increased intelligence. Studies are now uncovering an unknown benefit of fruit consumption in expecting mothers. Can eating fruit during pregnancy make children smarter? One study found that mothers who consumed more fruit during pregnancy gave birth to children who performed better on developmental testing at 1 year of age.

Reference

Bolduc FV, Lau A, Rosenfelt CS, et al. Cognitive enhancement in infants associated with increased materal fruit intake during pregnancy: results from a birth cohort study with validation in an animal model. *EioMedicine*. 8:331-340. Retrieved from: http://www.ebiomedicine.com/article/S2352-3964(16)30161-X/abstract.

Gastroesophageal Reflux Disease

Gastroesophageal reflux disease (GERD) is a digestive disorder that affects the lower esophageal sphincter (LES), which are the muscles between the esophagus and the stomach. GERD symptoms are the same for pregnant and nonpregnant women and include heartburn, regurgitation, indigestion, epigastric pain, nausea, and vomiting. GERD is typically new onset in pregnancy triggered by the impact of fluctuating hormones on the function of the LES. Similar to other mild GI disorders seen in pregnancy, lifestyle modifications are successful at easing symptoms.

GERD can occur as an exacerbation of the preexisting condition or as a result of mechanical factors and hormonal effects that cause a progressive decrease in LES pressure during pregnancy. A low LES pressure has been shown to occur in most pregnancies by week 36, but pressure returns to normal postpartum. With a decreased LES pressure, stomach acid easily refluxes into the esophagus, causing the symptoms associated with GERD. Heartburn that arises during pregnancy is most common in the first and second trimesters and may continue throughout the entire pregnancy, but it generally resolves upon delivery with no adverse effects on mother or fetus.[15]

Common factors that can trigger GERD during pregnancy are the same for the general population such as eating before bed, intake of fatty or spicy foods, caffeine, mints, chocolate, and side effects of medications. Simple lifestyle modifications can provide significant improvements for those who suffer from GERD. Such modifications are avoiding eating late at night, raising the head of bed to create an angle, and avoiding certain foods (fats, spices, carbonated and caffeinated beverages, chocolate) or medications that can cause heartburn symptoms.[15] In more severe cases in which lifestyle modifications do not result in symptomatic relief, drug therapy such as antacids may be warranted.

Gallstones

Pregnancy influences and alters many body organs, including the liver and the biliary tract. The liver plays an important part in digestion by storing fat-soluble vitamins and producing bile for digesting fats. Bile is carried through the biliary tract and stored in the gallbladder until eating signals its contraction and the subsequent release of bile into the duodenum. Thus, complications or injury to the biliary tract, including the formation of gallstones, can disrupt the normal, healthy digestive process. Pregnancy is associated with an increased risk in gallstone formation.

Bile consists of a mixture of cholesterol, bile salts, and bilirubin; when these components are imbalanced, gallstones may form. The cause or reason for such imbalances is not well understood, but the majority (80% in the United States) are stones consisting primarily of hardened cholesterol.[16] Gallstones are fairly common: 10–20% of Americans develop them at some time, with an incidence of gallstone formation during pregnancy of about 12%.[17] Gallstones in pregnancy are thought to be a result of hormonal changes that lead to decreased contractility of the gallbladder and changes in bile content characterized by increased cholesterol saturation. Although the majority of gallstones are asymptomatic and do not interfere with the gallbladder, liver, or pancreas, if a gallstone blocks the bile duct, pressure in the gallbladder is increased, which may initiate a painful gallbladder attack. These "attacks" usually occur after a large, high-fat meal and stop when the stone moves and is no longer blocking the duct. If the bile ducts remain blocked for an extended period of time, complications can be fatal.

Some risk factors for developing gallstones such as gender, genetics, and advancing age cannot be modified, but others, including diet, physical activity, obesity, and weight loss, may be addressed to prevent formation of gallstones. Women in general are more likely to develop gallstones because extra estrogen can increase cholesterol levels in bile and decrease gallbladder contractions, causing the formation of cholesterol stones. Pregnancy itself is therefore a risk factor because estrogen levels are increased at this time and can lead to the development of gallstones.[16] Other risk factors for developing gallstones include obesity because it increases the amount of cholesterol in bile; rapid weight loss, which causes the liver to secrete extra cholesterol into bile; and diet patterns—research suggests those who consume high-calorie, refined carbohydrates and low-fiber diets have an increased risk of developing gallstones. Therefore, to reduce risk of developing gallstones, it is recommended to maintain a healthy weight through proper diet and nutrition.

Treatment of gallstones during pregnancy is very conservative, especially in cases that are asymptomatic. In cases of persistent blockage with risk of more severe complications, cholecystectomy (or removal of the gallbladder) may be considered in the second trimester. Endoscopic retrograde cholangiopancreatography (ERCP), a nonsurgical method to remove stones, may also be used but has been associated with higher risk of preterm delivery and low birth weight when conducted in the first trimester of pregnancy.[18]

Inflammatory Bowel Disease: Ulcerative Colitis and Crohn's Disease

Inflammatory bowel disease (IBD) describes conditions with chronic or recurring immune response and inflammation of the GI tract. Crohn's disease (CD) and ulcerative colitis (UC) are the two most common forms in which inflammation can affect either the large intestine itself or the entire digestive tract. Both subtypes of IBD are characterized by periods of remission in which an individual is symptom free alternating with periods of active disease or flares. See **TABLE 5.1** for a comparison of the two subtypes.

Exacerbations of inflammatory bowel disease may occur during pregnancy and have been associated with

Table 5.1

Crohn's Disease Versus Ulcerative Colitis

	Crohn's Disease	Ulcerative Colitis
Location	Affects any part of GI tract from mouth to anus; common in the end of the small bowel (ileum) and beginning of large intestine (colon)	Limited to colon and rectum (large intestine)
Disease characteristics	May occur in patches that affect some areas leaving others untouched and healthy	Continuous inflammation occurring only in the innermost layer of intestinal lining
Symptoms	Frequent diarrhea	Frequent diarrhea
	Abdominal pain/cramping	Abdominal pain/discomfort
	Reduced appetite	Reduced appetite
	Weight loss	Weight loss
	Rectal bleeding	Blood or pus in stool
	Fever	Fever

increased risk of pregnancy complications such as low birth weight, small for gestational age (SGA), prematurity, and increased frequency of cesarean sections.[19]

It is estimated that about 1–1.6 million people suffer from IBD in the United States, with slightly higher incidence of UC versus CD.[20] With incidence rates of IBD most pronounced in persons between the ages of 20 and 35 years, potential for complications during pregnancy is a concern because the age of incidence coincides with likely childbearing years. The influence of pregnancy on IBD is related to whether disease activity is present at conception, meaning that if IBD is not active at the time of conception, it likely will remain inactive throughout the pregnancy, and if it is active at conception, it will continue throughout the course of pregnancy.[21]

For unclear reasons, women with UC are more likely to experience an exacerbation in their first trimester, whereas those suffering from CD are more likely to see flares in the third trimester.[21] Available data suggest that pregnancy does not seem to have any long-term detrimental effects on patients with IBD.[21] In fact, some studies suggest a beneficial effect of pregnancy on future IBD disease course and flares.[22]

Although the two identified subtypes of IBD differ in clinical presentation and their cause remains unclear, the etiology of both is thought to involve individual genetic susceptibility, alterations in the gut microbiome that stimulate the immune system, and environmental triggers. Both diseases can cause severe gastrointestinal symptoms such as persistent diarrhea, cramping and abdominal pain, fever, loss of appetite and weight loss, fatigue, and rectal bleeding.

IBD is not an easily preventable chronic disease, however, and management becomes important in both pregnant and nonpregnant individuals. Most drugs commonly used to treat IBD have not been associated with increased risk for adverse maternal or fetal outcomes and are therefore likely appropriate for use during pregnancy.[22]

Recap GI disorders are not uncommon among pregnant women. Changes in the GI tract as a result of pregnancy put the mother at risk for exacerbation of existing or development of new GI disorders. Understanding the risk factors and preventative measures, along with following recommendations for managing any GI conditions during pregnancy, are essential to avoid complications. GI conditions can be managed during pregnancy with successful outcomes.

1. How do morning sickness and hyperemesis gravidarum differ?
2. Make suggestions for decreasing the symptoms of GERD during pregnancy.
3. How do hormones affect the chance of getting gallstones during pregnancy?

Obesity and Malnutrition

Preview Healthy weight status and a healthy diet before and during pregnancy are crucial for mother and baby. Overweight status prior to and excessive weight gain during pregnancy are both associated with adverse maternal and fetal health outcomes, including reduced fertility.[23] This section explores how weight status before and during pregnancy, malnutrition, and nutrient deficiencies can affect mother and child during pregnancy.

Entering Pregnancy Overweight or Obese

For women who are overweight or obese prior to becoming pregnant, it is important to note that weight loss during pregnancy is never advised; however, overall weight gain goals will vary depending on the woman's pregravid BMI. Ideally, women who are overweight or obese should try to attain a healthy BMI prior to conception. Weight loss prior to pregnancy has been shown to improve menstrual functioning, ovulation, and fertility among obese women of childbearing age.[24] Women who are overweight or obese prior to pregnancy are more likely to exceed recommended weight gain and to maintain excess weight after delivery.[25] Studies have also shown that children of mothers who were obese prior to pregnancy and who do not breastfeed are six times more likely to be overweight when compared with children of normal-weight mothers who breastfeed for at least 4 months.[23]

Gaining more weight than recommended throughout gestation, regardless of pre-pregnancy weight classification, has also been correlated with both short- and long-term maternal health risks such as gestational diabetes and hypertension, preeclampsia, dyslipidemia, cardiovascular disease, and cesarean delivery. Postoperative complications of cesarean section, including wound infection, excess blood loss, deep vein thrombophlebitis, and postpartum endometritis, occur more often among obese and overweight mothers than among those of normal weight.[26] Recent research also shows that women who gain more weight than recommended in pregnancy are at substantially increased risk of excess weight retention 1 year later, and those who are unable to lose the weight within 6 months are at much higher risk of being obese 10 years later.[27] Evidence also suggests that maternal metabolic conditions, commonly found among overweight and obese individuals, may be associated with autism, developmental delays, and other neurodevelopmental problems in children.[28] Compared with children of normal-weight women, children of obese women are more likely to develop neural tube defects, oral clefts, heart anomalies, hydrocephaly, and abdominal wall abnormalities.[29]

Inadequate Weight Gain During Pregnancy and Entering Pregnancy Underweight

A BMI < 18.5 is considered underweight and suggests that weight gain during pregnancy should be at a higher rate than that for normal-weight (BMI 18.5–24.9) individuals.

An estimated 20% of pregnant women do not gain the recommended minimum amount of weight during pregnancy.[30] Some women make unhealthy nutrition and exercise decisions in an effort to prevent excess weight gain, with the hope that after delivery they can get back to their pre-pregnancy weight quickly. The consequences of too much weight gain during pregnancy are well understood, and maybe this is what leads some women to make unhealthy choices during pregnancy. For some women, seeing their body change and their weight increase week after week is a real struggle, particularly for those who are body image conscious before becoming pregnant. Over-exercising, cutting back on calories, avoiding nutrient-dense foods, and checking body weight daily are characteristics of this phenomenon sometimes referred to as "pregorexia" by the media.

Consequences of inadequate weight gain affect both the expecting mother and the developing fetus. During pregnancy, women are at an increased risk of bone and muscle loss, vitamin and mineral deficiencies, anemia, and fatigue. If an expecting mother is over-exercising or not eating enough calories, she is putting her baby at risk for intrauterine growth restriction (IUGR) and low birth weight.

LBW among infants in developing countries is primarily a result of IUGR, which is most often the result of maternal malnutrition. When compared with women of normal pregravid weight (BMI above 24) with normal gestational weight gain, women who are underweight prior to conception (BMI below 20) or who do not gain adequately throughout gestation experience a significantly greater incidence of IUGR births. Aside from underweight status or protein-calorie malnutrition, a lack of nutrients independent of weight status has also been implicated in poor maternal and fetal outcomes. Along with low birth weight comes a number of other health consequences such as infections or motor and social developmental delays.

During pregnancy (and otherwise), nutrition experts advise that instead of placing too much emphasis on calories, exercise, and body weight, women should eat a well-balanced diet of meals and snacks, listen to hunger and fullness cues, and engage in physical activity on a regular basis. Weight gain guidelines are in place to help expecting mothers have the best possible outcomes not only for their babies but also for their own bodies as well. An expecting mother's nutrition and lifestyle choices are key to the health of the next generation. TABLE 5.2 includes tips for expecting mothers who need to gain weight.

TABLE 5.3 and FIGURE 5.2 show weight gain recommendations for pregnancy based on pre-pregnancy weight, as suggested by the Institute of Medicine.

Iron

As a result of increased need for fetal and placental iron, as well as an increased volume of blood during pregnancy, iron deficiency is the most common cause of anemia among pregnant women. Women at increased risk for developing anemia in pregnancy include those who have had multiple pregnancies or two pregnancies close together, teenagers, and those with poor intake of iron-rich foods.

Table 5.2

Tips for Healthy Weight Gain During Pregnancy

- Do not skip meals. Aim for five to six small meals each day.
- Include snacks throughout the day. Try not to go longer than 3–4 hours without eating. Examples: nuts, cheese and crackers, peanut butter sandwich, yogurt, dried fruit and nuts.
- Add healthy oils, butter, cream cheese, sour cream, cheese, or gravy to your meals.
- Consume more healthy fats, including nuts, avocado, olive oil, and coldwater fish.

Table 5.3

Institute of Medicine Weight Gain Recommendations for Pregnancy

Pre-Pregnancy Weight Category	Underweight	Normal weight	Overweight	Obese (all classes)
Body Mass Index[a]	<18.5	18.5–24.9	25–29.9	≥30
Recommended Range of Total Weight (lb)	28–40	25–35	15–25	11–20
Recommended Rates of Weight Gain[b] in the Second and Third Trimesters (lb/wk)	1–1.3	0.8–1	0.5–0.7	0.4–0.6

[a] Body mass index is calculated as weight in kilograms divided by height in meters squared or as weight in pounds multiplied by 703 and divided by height in inches.

[b] Calculations assume a 1.1 to 4.4 lb weight gain in the first trimester.

Data from Institute of Medicine (US). Weight gain during pregnancy: reexamining the guidelines. Washington, DC: National Academies Press; 2009. ©2009 National Academy of Sciences.

Case Study

Rosa is now 20 weeks pregnant, and the episodes of nausea and vomiting have subsided. At this point, she has gained 6 pounds, which is 2 pounds under the suggested weight gain for her pre-pregnancy BMI. She describes her appetite as being okay, mostly low, with occasional times that she feels hungry throughout the day no matter what or how often she eats.

Questions

1. Provide suggestions on how Rosa can increase her kilocalorie intake throughout the day.
2. Which consequences of too little weight gain during pregnancy do you think are the most important for Rosa to understand and why?

The presence of iron-deficiency anemia in the first and second trimesters increases the risk for preterm labor, low-birth weight or small-for-gestational-age babies, maternal and infant mortality, and long-term fetal complications, including anemia during infancy, poor physical and mental growth, and impaired cognitive function. [31] Low iron stores in mothers may also increase their susceptibility to infection.

Symptoms of anemia are caused by lack of oxygen to the maternal tissues and include feeling tired, lethargy, pale skin, difficulty concentrating, rapid heartbeat, shortness of breath, and irritability.[32]

Iron-deficiency anemia can be prevented through a well-balanced diet. Because both maternal and fetal demand for iron are so high during pregnancy, absorption of iron increases and becomes more efficient; however, it is difficult for women to meet their increased

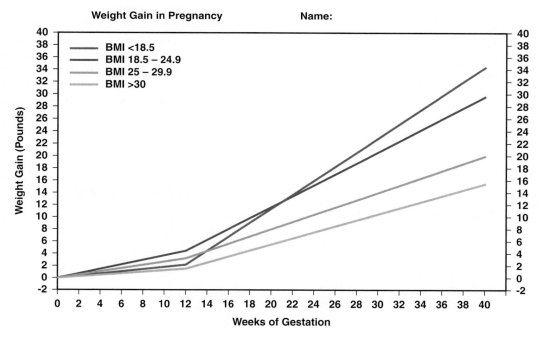

Figure 5.2
Suggested weight gain graph based on pre-pregnancy BMI.

Data from Institute of Medicine, May 2009

needs through diet alone. It is recommended that pregnant women be advised of dietary sources of iron and be encouraged to take a supplement containing iron. The U.S. Recommended Dietary Allowance (RDA) for iron is 27 mg/day for pregnant and lactating women.

It is important to note that iron intake does not necessarily equal iron absorption; the absorption capacity is greatest with meat sources of iron. Absorption of iron is enhanced by vitamin C, so pairing iron supplements or multivitamins with an orange, green peppers, broccoli, melon, strawberry, cabbage, or a small glass of orange or grapefruit juice may be beneficial. On the other hand, caffeine may inhibit the absorption of iron, so women should refrain from drinking coffee, tea, or colas for 1–3 hours before or after taking an iron supplement. Iron supplements have been known to cause some gastrointestinal discomfort and may best be taken with food or after a meal. Many foods are fortified with iron, such as cereals, breads, and pastas. Iron intake may be especially low in women who follow a vegetarian or vegan diet and those who consume limited meat. Iron supplements may be especially important among these groups. `TABLE 5.4` provides good sources of dietary iron.

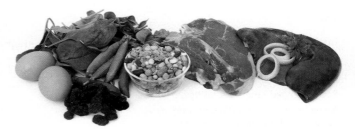

©Robyn Mackenzie/Shutterstock

Folic Acid

Folic acid is recognized as important both before and during pregnancy because it plays a crucial role in neural tube development, which occurs very early in gestation. Women of childbearing age and those who may become pregnant are advised to consume 400 mcg/day of folic acid from fortified foods and supplements in addition to consuming food sources of folate. Women are encouraged to take a prenatal multivitamin or folic acid supplement to ensure increased needs are met. Good dietary sources of folic acid are listed in `TABLE 5.5`.

Symptoms of folic acid and vitamin B_{12} deficiency may be similar, and it is therefore important to rule out a vitamin B_{12} deficiency, even though it is rare in pregnancy. Folic acid deficiency is characterized by low serum folate, whereas severe vitamin B_{12} deficiency shows a high serum folate.

Congenital Abnormalities

Congenital abnormalities, also known as birth defects, encompass all functional, morphologic, and biochemical/molecular defects presented at birth that developed at some point between conception and birth. `FIGURE 5.3` provides a time line of when congenital abnormalities occur. The most common congenital abnormalities caused by folate are neural tube defects (NTDs), which affect the central nervous system, including the brain and spinal cord. `FIGURE 5.4` shows spina bifida in an infant. NTDs are the easiest congenital abnormalities to prevent through

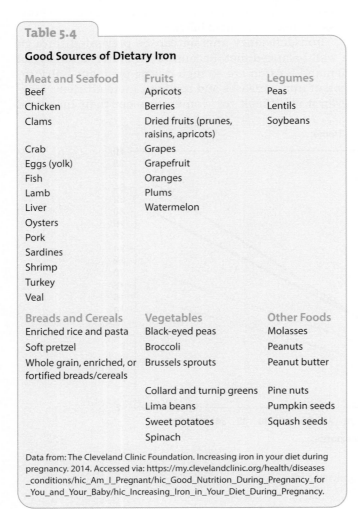

Table 5.4

Good Sources of Dietary Iron

Meat and Seafood	Fruits	Legumes
Beef	Apricots	Peas
Chicken	Berries	Lentils
Clams	Dried fruits (prunes, raisins, apricots)	Soybeans
Crab	Grapes	
Eggs (yolk)	Grapefruit	
Fish	Oranges	
Lamb	Plums	
Liver	Watermelon	
Oysters		
Pork		
Sardines		
Shrimp		
Turkey		
Veal		

Breads and Cereals	Vegetables	Other Foods
Enriched rice and pasta	Black-eyed peas	Molasses
Soft pretzel	Broccoli	Peanuts
Whole grain, enriched, or fortified breads/cereals	Brussels sprouts	Peanut butter
	Collard and turnip greens	Pine nuts
	Lima beans	Pumpkin seeds
	Sweet potatoes	Squash seeds
	Spinach	

Data from: The Cleveland Clinic Foundation. Increasing iron in your diet during pregnancy. 2014. Accessed via: https://my.clevelandclinic.org/health/diseases_conditions/hic_Am_I_Pregnant/hic_Good_Nutrition_During_Pregnancy_for_You_and_Your_Baby/hic_Increasing_Iron_in_Your_Diet_During_Pregnancy.

Table 5.5

Good Dietary Sources of Folic Acid

Fruits
   Citrus fruit and juice
Legumes
   Dried beans and peas
   Lentils
Vegetables
   Asparagus
   Broccoli
   Collard and turnip greens
   Okra
   Spinach

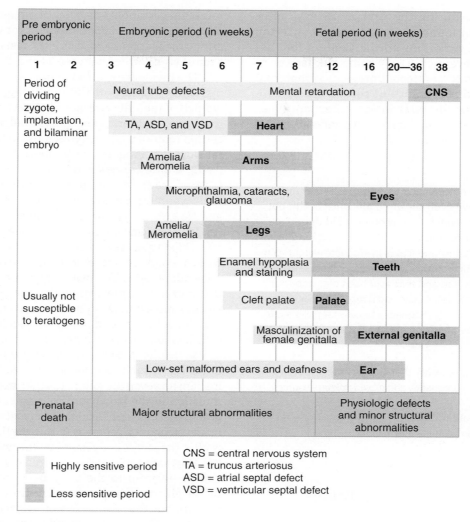

Pre embryonic period	Embryonic period (in weeks)						Fetal period (in weeks)				
1 2	3	4	5	6	7	8	12	16	20—36	38
Period of dividing zygote, implantation, and bilaminar embryo	Neural tube defects				Mental retardation					**CNS**
	TA, ASD, and VSD			**Heart**						
		Amelia/ Meromelia		**Arms**						
			Microphthalmia, cataracts, glaucoma			**Eyes**				
		Amelia/ Meromelia		**Legs**						
				Enamel hypoplasia and staining		**Teeth**				
Usually not susceptible to teratogens				Cleft palate	**Palate**					
					Masculinization of female genitalla	**External genitalla**				
		Low-set malformed ears and deafness			**Ear**					
Prenatal death	Major structural abnormalities						Physiologic defects and minor structural abnormalities			

☐ Highly sensitive period	CNS = central nervous system
▣ Less sensitive period	TA = truncus arteriosus
	ASD = atrial septal defect
	VSD = ventricular septal defect

Figure 5.3
Time line of when congenital abnormalities can occur.

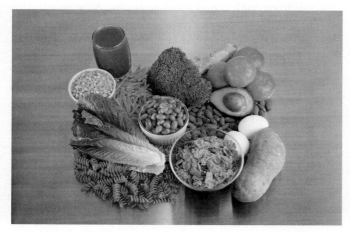

©Fertnig/iStock/Getty Images Plus/Getty

before a woman knows she is pregnant, folate recommendations are made for all women between the ages of 15 and 45 years.[33]

adequate folate supplementation before and during pregnancy. Because many pregnancies in the United States are unplanned and many congenital abnormalities occur within the first few weeks of pregnancy, maybe even

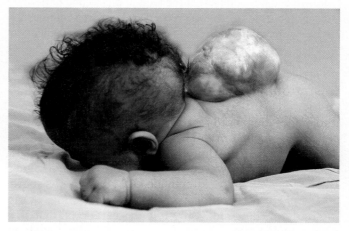

Figure 5.4
Spina bifida in an infant.

©Medicshots/Alamy Stock Photo

Adequate folate during the first 21–28 days after conception has been found to significantly reduce the likelihood of NTDs. According to the Centers for Disease Control and Prevention (CDC), some risk factors of NTDs are a previous NTD-affected pregnancy, maternal insulin-dependent diabetes, use of certain antiseizure medications, high temperatures in early pregnancy (i.e., prolonged fevers or hot tub use), certain race/ethnicity, and lower socioeconomic status.[33]

Recap Body weight, nutrition status, and overall diet quality during pregnancy have been shown to influence health outcomes. Gaining more weight than recommended throughout gestation has been correlated with both short- and long-term maternal health risks. Consequences of inadequate weight gain affect both the expecting mother and the developing fetus.

The micronutrients iron and folic acid both play important roles in development of a fetus. Folic acid is recognized as important both before and during pregnancy because it plays a crucial role in neural tube development, which occurs very early in gestation.

1. Name two micronutrients that women need more of before and during pregnancy and provide dietary sources for each.
2. Explain how folate fortification helps to decrease the prevalence of congenital abnormalities.

Endocrine and Metabolic Conditions

Preview The condition of pregnancy brings about rapid physiological changes in a woman's body and, hence, endocrine and metabolic conditions during pregnancy are common. Endocrine conditions such as gestational diabetes, thyroid disorder, and polycystic ovary syndrome (PCOS) have crucial effects on the growth and development of the fetus. If preexisting or newly diagnosed maternal endocrine conditions are well controlled, they may have little impact on maternal and fetal morbidity.

Gestational Diabetes

Gestational diabetes mellitus (GDM) is defined as glucose intolerance diagnosed for the first time in pregnancy, usually in the second or third trimester. GDM affects 1–14% of all pregnancies in the United States.[34] GDM usually resolves after child birth; however, women with GDM have higher risk for type 2 diabetes later in life. GDM has various short-term and long-term effects on the health outcomes of the mother and the child. Women with gestational diabetes have a higher risk for pregnancy complications such as cesarean section, macrosomia, and neonatal hypoglycemia that can occur during delivery. **FIGURE 5.5** outlines the

impact of gestational diabetes on pregnancy and fetal outcomes. Generally, risk assessment for GDM is carried out during the first prenatal visit. If the test for GDM is negative, a retest is performed between 24 and 28 weeks of gestation.

The incidence of GDM in pregnant women is increasing, likely because of the increasing rate of obesity in women of reproductive age. The prevalence of GDM tends to increase with increasing maternal age, increasing BMI, certain maternal ethnicity/race, use of Special Supplemental Nutrition Program for Women, Infants, and Children (WIC), and lower levels of education. The prevalence of GDM varies from state to state within the United States, with Wyoming having the lowest prevalence (2.2–5.6%) and New York City having the highest (5.4–11.7%).[35]

Physiological changes during pregnancy significantly affect blood glucose homeostasis in the expecting mother. A woman's body goes through extensive hormonal and endocrine adaptations because of the interactions between the placenta and the maternal endocrine system. The placenta, which supports the baby's growth, produces hormones that can block the action of the mother's insulin. This situation, called *insulin resistance*, makes it hard for the mother's body to use insulin. Most pregnant women's bodies can counteract this insulin resistance by increasing the secretion of insulin; however, the failure to do so results in glucose accumulation in the blood, and consequently the condition of gestational diabetes. Gestational diabetes affects the mother in late pregnancy, generally during the third trimester, which is after the baby's body has been formed.

Untreated or poorly controlled gestational diabetes can be harmful to the baby. Because of maternal high blood glucose levels, the expecting mother produces insulin, but the insulin is not utilized to help take glucose from the mother's blood into her cells. Insulin does not cross the placenta, but glucose and other nutrients do, and the extra glucose passed to the growing fetus give the baby high blood glucose levels. As a result, the baby's pancreas produces more insulin to rid the blood of glucose, which supplies the fetal cells with more energy than they need. This extra energy is stored as fat in the baby's body. In addition, because of the extra insulin the baby's pancreas produces, newborns may have very low blood glucose levels at birth. Babies born to mothers with poor control of their blood glucose levels during pregnancy tend to be large at birth, and they grow into children who are at risk for obesity and adults who are at risk for type 2 diabetes.[34]

More than 50% women who have GDM acquire type 2 diabetes within 20 years of delivery. Women who experience gestational diabetes are more likely to have this condition again in future pregnancies.

One of the key risk factors for development of GDM is advanced maternal age and increasing maternal weight. A first-degree relative with diabetes, family history of type 2 diabetes, history of GDM in a previous pregnancy, and history of PCOS are crucial non-modifiable risk factors for GDM. Women with GDM have a higher risk for

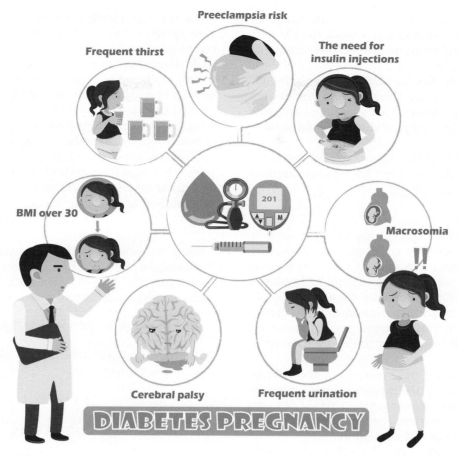

Figure 5.5
Impact of gestational diabetes on pregnancy and fetal outcomes.
©viyadaistock/Getty Images

obstetric complications and a sevenfold increase for developing type 2 diabetes 5–10 years from the delivery. Children born to mothers with GDM have a higher risk of developing metabolic complications and impaired glucose tolerance.[35] Studies suggest that maternal weight gain in previously normal-weight women at the rate of 1 to 5 pounds per year 5 years prior to pregnancy may increase the risk of GDM.[36] Low levels of physical activity and increased rates of obesity are also associated with increased risk for gestational diabetes.[36]

Risk factors for gestational diabetes include:

- Advanced maternal age
- Overweight/obesity
- Race/ethnicity
- First-degree relative with type 2 diabetes
- History of GDM or PCOS

Prevention strategies for GDM must involve dietary as well as exercise-related interventions. Systematic review and meta-analyses suggest that greater total physical activity pre-pregnancy and during pregnancy is associated with lower risk for GDM. Weight management strategies through nutritional interventions may help in reducing the risk of GDM.

The goal for treatment of GDM is to maintain normal blood glucose levels to minimize the risks associated with GDM. GDM must be first managed with lifestyle changes, which involve individualized medical nutrition therapy (MNT) as per the American Diabetes Association guidelines. Medications are added as and when needed. The glycated hemoglobin (HbA$_{1c}$) target in GDM women is <6% without running into the risk for hypoglycemia. Adequate calories and nutrients must be provided to meet the maternal nutrition goals as well as blood glucose goals set for the mother. Caloric intake of 25 kcal/kg/day with 35–40% of calories from carbohydrate has been associated with improved maternal and fetal outcomes in women with BMI >30. Unless contraindicated, moderate amounts of physical activity during pregnancy help to control blood glucose levels.

If medication is used, insulin is the preferred choice of treatment because the use of oral hypoglycemic drugs does not exhibit long-term safety during pregnancy. The glycemic targets are ≤95 mg/dL preprandial and ≤120 mg/dL 2 hours postprandial. Use of insulin therapy during pregnancy could be tricky and may require frequent monitoring and titration to meet the changing needs. Self-monitoring of blood glucose (SMBG) is mandatory for pregnant women with multiple-dose insulin. The pregnant woman must work closely with diabetes educators and evaluate the SMBG technique as well as results regularly.

Women with high risk for GDM must be screened when planning for pregnancy. These include women with BMI ≥30, high-risk ethnicities such as Asian, Latin, and African origins, family history of diabetes, and GDM in previous pregnancy.

The expected levels of blood glucose to minimize the maternal and fetal metabolic complications and improve outcomes are outlined in TABLE 5.6.

Thyroid Disorders

The physiological state of pregnancy brings a surge in the thyroid-binding globulins and thyroid hormones tri-iodothyronime (T_3) and thyroxine (T_4), elevating them to levels above the nonpregnant state. Thyroid-stimulating hormone (TSH) changes modestly as a result of an increase in human chorionic gonadotropin, which is structurally similar to TSH. Adverse pregnancy-related outcomes may result from uncontrolled thyrotoxicosis and hypothyroidism.[37]

Iodine is essential for the synthesis of thyroid hormones. During pregnancy, the mother's thyroid provides thyroid hormones to the developing fetus via the placenta until 18–20 weeks of gestation. The fetus uses these hormones for proper growth and development.

The most common etiology of hypothyroidism in the United States is the autoimmune disease Hashimoto's disease, which causes destruction of the thyroid gland.[38] Hypothyroidism is a leading cause of infertility; therefore, it is usually not undetected. However, undiagnosed hypothyroidism could be present in unplanned pregnancies. This poses a risk for maternal and fetal health and development. Uncontrolled hypothyroidism can lead to adverse pregnancy-related outcomes such as placental abruption, preterm deliveries, spontaneous abortion and fetal death, gestational hypertension and preeclampsia, developmental delays in the fetus, or mental retardation.[39]

It is recommended that pregnant women include a wide variety of food in their diet. It is important that they consume a healthy, balanced diet along with prenatal multivitamin and mineral supplements containing iodine to provide nutrients crucial for thyroid health. Physical activity and regular exercise further help in maintaining normal thyroid gland function and improve pregnancy-related outcomes. The fetus meets its iodine requirements through the mother's diet. It is important that the mother has adequate iodine intake; in the U.S. diet, this primarily comes from iodized salt used in food. Trimester-specific serum thyroid-stimulating hormone is an accurate method to check thyroid status during pregnancy.

Recap The endocrine and metabolic disorders gestational diabetes and thyroid disorder can complicate pregnancy. Successful management of these conditions during pregnancy results in little negative impact on baby and mother.

1. Discuss the strategies to prevent and treat gestational diabetes.
2. What measures can be taken to prevent thyroid insufficiency during pregnancy?

Cardiovascular Conditions

Preview Pregnancy brings about changes in cardiac output, blood pressure, and lipid levels in the maternal cardiovascular system to meet the metabolic demands of the mother and child. However, about 0.2–4% of pregnancies in Western countries are complicated by cardiovascular conditions that result in adverse pregnancy-related outcomes. The rates of cardiovascular events during pregnancy are increasing.[40] Obesity during pregnancy can lead to increased risk of cardiovascular conditions, hypertension, and diabetes in the mother as well as the offspring in later stages of life.[41]

Hypertension and Preeclampsia

Hypertension is defined as a systolic blood pressure of >140 mm Hg, a diastolic pressure of >90 mm Hg, or both. Hypertension in pregnancy can be classified into three common types: chronic hypertension, gestational hypertension, and preeclampsia. Hypertension affects the developing fetus because maternal hypertension prevents the placenta from getting enough blood, and therefore it delivers less oxygen and food to the fetus, which can result in low birth weight. If hypertension is severe, it can lead to preeclampsia.

Chronic hypertension occurs when women have hypertension before pregnancy, experience hypertension before the 20th week of gestation, or continue to have high blood

---

Table 5.6

Blood Glucose Targets During Pregnancy

Preprandial	≤95 mg/dL (5.3 mmol/L)
Fasting whole blood glucose	≤95 mg/dL (5.3 mmol/L)
Fasting plasma glucose	≤105 mg/dL (5.8 mmol/L)
1-h postprandial whole blood glucose	≤140 mg/dL (7.8 mmol/L)
1-h postprandial plasma glucose	≤155 mg/dL (8.6 mmol/L)
2-h postprandial whole blood glucose	≤120 mg/dL (6.7 mmol/L)
2-h postprandial plasma glucose	≤130 mg/dL (7.2 mmol/L)

Data from: Gestational Diabetes Mellitus. Diabetes Care. 2003;26(Supplement 1): S103-S105. doi:10.2337/diacare.26.2007.s103. Introduction. Diabetes Care. 2014;38 (Supplement_1):S1-S2. doi:10.2337/dc15-s001.

pressure after delivery. *Gestational hypertension* is when high blood pressure develops after 20 weeks of gestation and continues until after delivery. Risk factors for developing gestational hypertension include first pregnancy, a sister or mother who had pregnancy-induced hypertension, multiple births, age younger than 20 years or older than 40 years, and high blood pressure or kidney disease prior to pregnancy.[42]

Although there is no sure way to prevent hypertension during pregnancy, recommendations include following a low-salt diet, drinking plenty of water, decreasing the amount of fried foods and foods that are low in nutrient density, exercising regularly, elevating the feet several times during the day, and avoiding caffeinated beverages. Treatment for gestational hypertension includes rest, following a low-salt diet, and drinking at least 8 cups of water each day.

Preeclampsia is a syndrome that includes high blood pressure and protein in the urine that occurs after the 20th week of gestation. Preeclampsia occurs in up to 10% of first pregnancies and in 20–25% of women with history of chronic hypertension.[39] Untreated preeclampsia can lead to complications for both the mother and the baby. Women should be screened regularly throughout pregnancy for preeclampsia, and those at higher risk should be referred early for specialist care. Routine screening for preeclampsia includes measurement of blood pressure and urine analysis at each prenatal visit.

Hyperlipidemia

During a healthy pregnancy, there is a significant increase in the blood lipids. Concentrations of cholesterol, triglycerides, and lipoproteins increase significantly during the second trimester and reach maximum levels in the third trimester of pregnancy. Concentrations of both cholesterol and triglycerides decrease significantly after delivery. There is, however, a strikingly more rapid fall of plasma triglycerides and cholesterol in mothers who breastfeed their infants compared with women who never establish lactation.

The increase in triglyceride levels observed during the third trimester of pregnancy results from increased synthesis of triglyceride-rich lipoproteins and decreased clearance of triglycerides owing to hormonal suppression of lipoprotein lipase activity in the liver and adipose tissues.[43] Patients with triglyceride levels above 500 to 1,000 mg/dL have an increased risk of acute pancreatitis. Acute pancreatitis is the main consequence of hyperlipidemia, and gestational pancreatitis carries a significant risk of death for both mother (21%) and fetus (20%).

Patients with preexisting hyperlipidemia who become pregnant should continue a cholesterol-free or low-cholesterol diet with adequate amounts of vitamins, minerals, and calories to support the needs of pregnancy. Pharmacological agents are useful in reducing low-density lipoprotein (LDL) cholesterol in patients who cannot reach their treatment goal by diet alone.

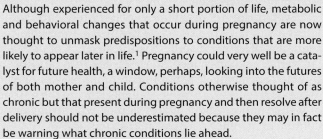

Let's Discuss

Although experienced for only a short portion of life, metabolic and behavioral changes that occur during pregnancy are now thought to unmask predispositions to conditions that are more likely to appear later in life.[1] Pregnancy could very well be a catalyst for future health, a window, perhaps, looking into the futures of both mother and child. Conditions otherwise thought of as chronic but that present during pregnancy and then resolve after delivery should not be underestimated because they may in fact be warning what chronic conditions lie ahead.

Preeclampsia, hypertension, and diabetes are examples of such conditions. A woman who experiences any of these conditions during pregnancy is at risk for developing various subsequent chronic issues. For example, women with preeclampsia during pregnancy have a higher incidence of cardiovascular disease, diabetes, and other disorders in the future.[2] Data suggest that women with hypertension during pregnancy are more likely to develop diabetes later in life.[3] Those who develop gestational diabetes have a greater risk of developing type 2 diabetes later.[4]

Perhaps an environmental factor plays a role as well. Is it possible that being pregnant can turn genes on and off, affecting how they "express" themselves? We understand that behavior and lifestyle choices such as diet, physical activity, stress, smoking, and sleep can modify the expression of our genes.

Just how much do you think we learn about the future health of expecting mothers and of their developing fetus during pregnancy? Just how much information can we learn by looking through the "window into future health" that is the condition of pregnancy?

References

1. Agrawal S, Fledderjohann J. Hypertensive disorders of pregnancy and risk of diabetes in Indian women: a cross-sectional study. *BMJ Open. August 5,* 2016;6:e011000.
2. Cheng SB, Sharma S. Preeclampsia and health risks later in life: an immunological link. *Semin Immunopathol.* [published online June 23, 2016].
3. Ehrlich S, Lambers D, Baccarelli A, Khoury J, Macaluso M, Ho SM. Endocrine disruptors: a potential risk factor for gestational diabetes mellitus. *Am J Perinatol.* [published online August 4, 2016].
4. Gilmore LA, Klempel-Donchenko M, Redman LM. Pregnancy as a window to future health: excessive gestational weight gain and obesity. *Semin Perinatol.* 2015;39(4):296–303.

Case Study

Rosa is now at 25 weeks gestation. Her appetite has improved over the past 5 weeks, and she does not have trouble tolerating foods. At her doctor visit today her blood pressure was elevated, with a reading of 150/100 mm Hg, her urine analysis revealed protein, and her ankles appear swollen (+1 pitting edema). She was diagnosed with preeclampsia. Rosa's diet history reveals that she has not been taking a prenatal multivitamin and mineral supplement consistently and that she eats meat protein three or four times a day; has bread, potatoes, rice, or corn with each meal; eats vegetables one to two times a week; eats one to two servings of fruit each day; and usually has ice cream or frozen yogurt in the evenings.

Questions

1. Although you currently do not have a family history for Rosa, what risk factors might she have that contribute to the condition of preeclampsia?
2. What diet recommendations would you give Rosa to help control her blood pressure at this time?

Recap Management of known cardiovascular disorders in women who intend to become pregnant should start before conception and continue throughout pregnancy. Unmanaged cardiovascular disease during pregnancy can have detrimental outcomes for both the expecting mother and the fetus.

1. List the dietary recommendations for pregnant women with preeclampsia that are thought to decrease the risk of eclampsia.
2. Describe how estrogen may affect lipid levels in pregnancy.
3. What are the dietary recommendations for pregnant women with preexisting hyperlipidemia?

Psychosocial Stressors

Preview It is important for practitioners to be alert to psychosocial stressors that may negatively affect the health of women who are of childbearing age, particularly those who plan to become or are pregnant. It is also important to screen for a history of eating disorders and explore feelings about weight gain and efforts to control weight.

Eating Disorders

During pregnancy, maternal body stores of carbohydrates, proteins, fats, vitamins, and minerals are utilized to nourish the fetus and support development. When nutrients are not restored sufficiently through a healthy diet, malnourishment, which can lead to depression, exhaustion, and other serious complications, may occur in the mother.

Although a concern for many pregnant women, those with a history of eating disorders may find the loss of control over their bodies during pregnancy to be terrifying, causing them to struggle to gain the recommended weight. Restrictive behaviors associated with disordered eating may therefore place them at higher risk for depleted stores and malnourishment, and both mother and baby are at risk for negative health outcomes. Studies show that women with past or active episodes of anorexia nervosa or bulimia nervosa have higher rates of maternal hypertension, miscarriages, breech deliveries, cesarean sections, premature births, low birth weights and lengths, smaller head circumference, microcephaly, fetal deaths, and postpartum depression.[44]

Though studies examining the effects of disordered eating patterns on neonatal outcomes offer conflicting results, eating disorders during pregnancy have been associated with dehydration, gestational diabetes, depression, preeclampsia, miscarriage, premature labor, increased risk of cesarean birth, complications during labor, stillbirth or fetal death, low birth weight, difficulty nursing and feeding, delayed fetal growth, and respiratory problems.[45]

Considering that eating disorders frequently occur during childbearing years, it is important for practitioners to recognize and address any potential restrictive behaviors prior to or early in pregnancy to prevent adverse outcomes. Three common eating disorders are anorexia nervosa, bulimia nervosa, and binge eating disorder. TABLE 5.7 provides characteristics of these disorders as defined by the fifth edition of the *Diagnostic and Statistical Manual of Mental Disorders* (DMS-V).

Even prior to pregnancy, disordered eating may affect a woman's reproductive health. One possible consequence of eating disorders is the absence of or irregular menstrual cycles, resulting in issues with fertility and trouble conceiving. It is not uncommon for women with anorexia to be amenorrheic, or experiencing the absence of menstruation. About 50% of women who struggle with bulimia experience irregular menstruation.[45]

During pregnancy, weight gain can be very unsettling for those who have body image issues, and though some are able to cope more easily, others may experience depression owing to their struggles with body image. Because disordered eating behavior tends to exist during childbearing years, any destructive behaviors associated with an eating disorder can have additional consequences. For example, women suffering from anorexia nervosa tend to be underweight and may not gain enough weight during pregnancy. Women with bulimia may suffer from dehydration that can result in chemical imbalances and resulting cardiac irregularities. Additionally, any laxatives or medications taken on a regular basis not only contribute to dehydration but also can negatively affect fetal development.[45] Laxative abuse can also lead to decreased

Table 5.7

Eating Disorders Defined

Disorder	Characteristics
Anorexia nervosa	• Distorted body image • A persistent lack of recognition of the seriousness of the current low body weight • A pathological fear of becoming fat, an intense fear of gaining weight, or a persistent behavior that interferes with weight gain Excessive dieting which can lead to severe weight loss
Bing Eating Disorder	• Recurrent episodes of binge eating - defined as: eating an amount of food that is definitely larger than most people would eat during a similar period of time and under similar circumstances accompanied by a sense of lack of control over eating during the episode • The binge eating episodes are associated with 3 or more of the following: 1) eating much more rapidly than normal; 2) eating until feeling uncomfortably full; 3) eating large amounts of food when not feeling physically hungry; 4) eating alone because of feeling embarrassed by how much one is eating; and 5) feeling disgusted with oneself, depressed or very guilty after binge eating • Recurring episodes of eating significantly more food in a short period of time than most people would eat under similar circumstances • May use eating as a coping mechanism for feelings of guilt, embarrassment, or disgust • Occurs on the average at least once per week over a period of 3 months • Generally associated with significant physical and psychological problems
Bulimia nervosa	• Recurrent episodes of binge eating followed by inappropriate behaviors such as self-induced vomiting to avoid weight gain. • Frequency of binge eating and compensatory behaviors occur at least 1 time a week for 3 months

Modified from: The Alliance for Eating Disorders Awareness. Eating disorders info. Retrieved from: http://www.allianceforeatingdisorders.com/. The American Psychiatric Association. Feeding and eating disorders. American Psychiatric Publishing; 2013. Retrieved from: http://www.dsm5.org/Documents/Eating%20Disorders%20Fact%20Sheet.pdf. Eating Disorders Victoria; November 25, 2015. Classifying eating disorders – DSM-5. Retrieved from: http://www.eatingdisorders.org.au/eating-disorders/what-is-an-eating-disorder/classifying-eating-disorders/dsm-5.

intestinal motility. Meanwhile, women who enter pregnancy overweight as a result of binging behaviors place themselves at a high risk for developing gestational diabetes and elevated blood pressure.[45] Complications of eating disorders may continue even after a healthy and successful birth; mothers suffering from anorexia and bulimia report more problems breastfeeding.[46]

Although exact causes of eating disorders remain unknown, genetics, emotional and psychological health, as well as pressures from society likely influence their development. Those at risk for developing an eating disorder include females in their teenage years and early 20s, those with a family member suffering from an eating disorder, anyone with other mental health disorders such as depression or anxiety disorder, people who lost significant weight and are consistently dieting, those suffering from stress, and athletes under pressure to maintain a certain weight or body image. Any woman with a history of disordered eating is at risk for the onset or continuation of such behaviors during pregnancy.

Even though some studies show a majority of pregnant women with eating disorders have normal pregnancies and healthy babies, pregnant women with past or current eating disorders should be viewed as being at high risk and monitored closely both during and after pregnancy to optimize maternal and fetal outcomes. Ideally, women with eating disorders should resolve related weight and behavioral problems prior to pregnancy. Women with eating disorders who become pregnant should continue to receive consistent and regular medical and psychological support throughout the duration of pregnancy.

Meal planning to include protein, complex carbohydrates, and fat at each meal or snack is essential and may help prevent episodes of binging or overeating. Consistent and regular monitoring of women's behavior and dietary intake should be conducted in an environment of trust and support. It is not uncommon for women with eating disorders to try to hide behaviors and tendencies, which can be challenging for practitioners. It is therefore recommended that psychologists, obstetricians, and dietitians collaborate in supporting any patient with an eating disorder prior to, throughout, and after her pregnancy to ensure optimal health for mother and baby. It is critical that healthcare providers screen for any irregular diet habits or negative body image perceptions associated with pregnancy to prevent the onset of such behaviors during pregnancy.

Depression

Many women suffer from depressive symptoms during pregnancy regardless of whether they have a history of clinical depression. However, it has been found that many do not receive adequate treatment. Numerous adverse outcomes of maternal depression, both occurring during pregnancy and postnatally (in the postpartum, within 12 months after pregnancy), have been well documented. It is also recognized that current prevalence records of depression occurring among women during and after pregnancy are conservative estimates given that depression is often underdiagnosed and underreported.[47] Therefore, it is important for practitioners to learn to identify signs of depression and encourage and ensure adequate treatment for women who demonstrate depressive symptoms.

In regard to the prevalence of depression among women of childbearing age, it is important to note that women are two to three times more likely than men to experience depression.[48] Although depression that occurs during pregnancy is much less studied than postpartum depression, reported data indicate that, conservatively speaking, antenatal depression may affect as many as 20% of women.[49] The prevalence of postpartum depression has been estimated to be around 12–16%.[49] Depression that occurs during pregnancy appears to peak in terms of prevalence during the first trimester, and among the postpartum group, depressive symptoms are most common at 12 weeks following delivery but can occur any time up to 1 year post delivery and last for months or even years following birth.

Several mechanisms have been proposed for the etiology of maternal depression. Although depression is likely a result of multiple factors, one commonality is nutrition. Specifically, associations with mood have been found with folate, vitamin B_6, vitamin B_{12}, vitamin D, calcium, iron, selenium, zinc, and polyunsaturated fatty acids (PUFAs). Though all of these nutrition correlations and associations are well researched, aside from the role of omega-3 fatty acids in perinatal depression, little is known about nutrient levels and maternal depression specifically because pregnant and lactating women are often excluded from investigational studies.

It is well understood that maternal depression can negatively influence both mother and child. For mothers, depression has been associated with poor maternal self-care and outcomes, including a decreased likelihood to seek medical attention during pregnancy and an increased likelihood to participate in risky behaviors such as alcohol or drug use. Additionally, depression during pregnancy has been linked to preeclampsia, birth difficulties including preterm delivery, increased risk for postpartum depression, and a reduced incidence of breastfeeding.[50]

For the newborn child, maternal depression has been associated with limitations in the child's cognitive,

The Big Picture

Schematic Overview of the Effects of Perinatal Depression on Maternal and Infant Outcomes

Maternal depression can cause negative fetal outcomes, but negative fetal outcomes may also affect postpartum depression.

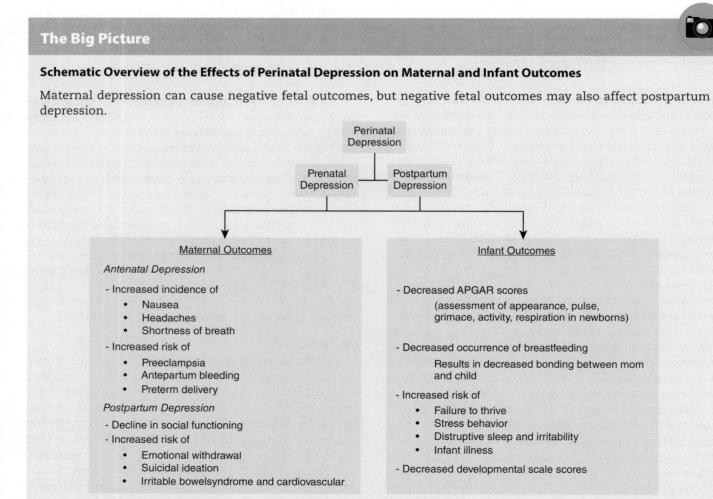

Modified from Leung BMY, Kaplan B. Perinatal depression: prevalence, risks, and the nutrition link – a review of the literature. *J Am Diet Assoc*. 2009; 109:1566-1575

Reference

1. Leung BMY, Kaplan B. Perinatal depression: prevalence, risks, and the nutrition link—a review of the literature. *J Am Diet Assoc.* 2009;109:1566–1575.

social, and developmental functioning as well as lower Apgar (American Pediatric Gross Assessment Record) scores, failure to thrive, malnutrition and poor growth, poor physical and emotional/behavioral development and overall developmental delays, increased risk of respiratory and diarrheal illnesses, behavioral problems including sleep disturbances and irritability, and an increased risk of depression later in life.

Regardless of the etiology, it is critical that, given the negative outcomes, maternal signs of depression be identified and addressed as early as possible.

Data show about 40–50% of the risk of depression is linked to genetics; however, research overall remains inconclusive on specific genes and susceptibility, and therefore it is likely that genetic predisposition in combination with environmental triggers may play a role in the onset of depression. Environmental factors include stress (physical, mental, and emotional), viral infections, hormonal disorders, chronic diseases, and some drugs and medications. Social, psychological, and biological factors may also contribute to the onset of depression such as lack of a partner; divorce or marital difficulties; financial insecurity or poverty; lack of social support or isolation; family violence or abuse; a history of depression, anxiety, or other psychiatric disorders; hormonal disturbances, disturbed neurotransmitter function; and nutrient deficiencies owing to malnutrition or poor diet quality. Although many of these factors cannot be prevented, any woman considering pregnancy should seek support in family, friends, or healthcare providers if currently affected by external stressors.

Several studies have found that among pregnant women intakes of energy, iron, zinc, calcium, magnesium, folate, n-3 essential fatty acids, and vitamins D and E were lower than recommended.[51] Given the link between certain nutrient deficiencies and depression, it is possible that ensuring a well-balanced diet that meets the minimum requirements could assist in the prevention of perinatal depression.

Signs of depression among pregnant women and new mothers are similar to those that occur in depression among the general population. They include depressed mood, loss of interest or pleasure, feelings of guilt or low self-worth, disturbed sleep or appetite, low energy, and poor concentration.

Although data suggest that some medications may be safely used in pregnancy and lactation, knowledge of the risks of prenatal exposure to such medications is not comprehensive, and the U.S. Food and Drug Administration (FDA) has yet to approve any psychotropic drug for use during pregnancy.[52] As a result, many women choose to discontinue their medications during pregnancy, but, given the maternal and fetal risks associated with untreated perinatal depression, it is important for women to discuss a treatment course with medical practitioners and that women suffering from depression be closely monitored throughout the duration of their pregnancy.

Pica

Food cravings and aversions are often reported during pregnancy; the most common cravings found in the United States among pregnant women include chocolate, citrus fruits, pickles, chips, and ice cream. Some of the most commonly reported aversions include coffee, tea, fried or fatty foods, highly spiced foods, meat, and eggs. Cravings for nonnutritive substances, including clay or dirt (**geophagia**), ice or freezer frost (**pagophagia**), cornstarch or laundry soap (**amylophagia**), soap, ashes, chalk, paint, burnt matches, and baking soda, may also occur. This condition is known as **pica**, and according to *DSM-5* criteria, an individual must meet the following criteria to be diagnosed:[53]

- Persistent eating of nonnutritive substances for a period of at least 1 month.
- The eating of nonnutritive substances is inappropriate to the developmental level of the individual.
- The eating behavior is not part of a culturally supported or socially normative practice.
- If occurring in the presence of another mental disorder (e.g., autistic spectrum disorder), or during a medical condition (e.g., pregnancy), it is severe enough to warrant independent clinical attention.

Pica has been occurring during pregnancy for thousands of years and was first mentioned by Hippocrates in 400 B.C.[54] Pica appears to occur more in areas of low economic status and is most common among women, especially pregnant women, although not exclusive to this population.

Pica is a common but often missed disorder with potential complications such as iron-deficiency anemia, lead poisoning, and other toxicities. Proper nutrition screening to evaluate for pica should include background information on a pregnant woman's socioeconomic status, regular questioning on the existence of specific cravings, as well as a complete medical history of psychiatric issues.

Like its prevalence, the etiology of pica is unknown, although it is likely a behavior pattern driven by multiple factors, with some evidence supporting pica as an obsessive-compulsive spectrum disorder. Pica may be multifactorial in origin, including medical explanations such as parasite infections, inappropriate levels of digestive enzymes or stomach acid, and iron deficiency. Other causes might be nutritional deficiencies other than iron, cultural factors, stress, learned behavior, or an underlying biochemical disorder.

Pica does not appear to increase the risk for complications during pregnancy; however, health complications can ensue depending on the nonfood substance consumed. Women who experience pica during pregnancy are more likely to have elevated blood lead levels and iron deficiency.[55] An association between pica and other micronutrient deficiencies has also been suggested.[56] Low hemoglobin, hematocrit, and plasma zinc have all been found to be associated with pica; however, the direction of the relationship between pica and these deficiencies is unclear.[56] Other conditions include complications of gestational diabetes especially with the continual consumption of starch, which can obstruct the intestines.[57]

Unfortunately, without more knowledge on risk factors and causes, it is impossible to predict and prevent pica. Because pica appears to be most common during pregnancy, pregnancy itself may be considered a risk factor. Nutrient deficiencies such as iron and zinc as well as potential gastrointestinal manifestations may be helpful in identifying occurrences of pica because ingestion of certain substances may be a driven by deficiency or result in mechanical bowel problems, constipation, ulcerations or perforations, and intestinal obstructions.[58]

Recap It is commonly accepted that pregnant women are especially susceptible to adverse outcomes associated with low nutrient intake because of their increased requirements during pregnancy and lactation needed to meet both maternal metabolic and fetal development needs. Given this increased susceptibility and the evidence of dietary inadequacy among pregnant women, a well-balanced diet rich in nutrients is recommended to help limit or control cognitive disorders such as eating disorders, pica, depression, and stress and anxiety.

1. Who is at risk for demonstrating disordered eating patterns during pregnancy? What are the most common behaviors and what are your concerns related to each?
2. Illustrate the impact of depression on maternal and fetal health.
3. Discuss pica and associated behaviors as well as potential complications and methods for addressing the condition.

Lifestyle Management

Preview Maternal lifestyle has a huge impact on the normal growth and development of the child. Physically active mothers have a reduced risk for gestational diabetes mellitus, preeclampsia, and excessive weight gain during pregnancy. Other lifestyle habits such as alcohol, tobacco, and substance use and abuse may have significant effects on the early stages of the child's development and long-term effects later in life.[59]

Exercise and Fitness

Regular physical activity and exercise during pregnancy and lactation have many benefits to both the mother and child. Strength-training exercises are associated with improved maternal fitness, appropriate weight gain for adequate growth of the fetus, faster postpartum recovery, and psychological health benefits.[60] In addition, regular

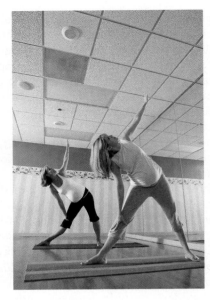

©Golden Pixels LLC/Alamy.

aerobic exercise may reduce a mother's risk of gestational diabetes and preeclampsia. Exercise should be accompanied by a well-balanced diet, proper hydration, and adequate rest to bestow its maximum benefits.

Most women who exercise regularly before pregnancy can continue the same exercise regime during pregnancy. Some women at high risk for miscarriage, preterm delivery, musculoskeletal injury, or poor fetal growth may be restricted from exercise during pregnancy.

Possible contraindications for exercise during pregnancy include the following:[60]

- Low placenta level
- Severe anemia
- Persistent second or third trimester bleeding
- Preeclampsia
- Multiple gestation at risk for preterm labor
- Previous history of miscarriage
- Premature labor during current pregnancy

Exercise recommendations for women with uncomplicated pregnancies include both moderate aerobic and strength-training exercises. Heavy weight lifting and similar strenuous activities are discouraged during pregnancy, especially in the second and third trimesters, and exercise in the supine and prone positions should be avoided after the first trimester. Unless medically contraindicated, every pregnant woman should aim for 20–30 minutes of moderate-intensity exercise on most or all days of the week.[60]

Exercises recommended during pregnancy include:

1. Swimming
2. Stationary bike
3. Walking
4. Jogging
5. Yoga
6. Low-impact aerobics

Exercises not recommended during pregnancy include:

1. Bike riding
2. Heavy weight lifting
3. High-impact aerobics/Zumba
4. Scuba diving/sky diving
5. Trekking to high altitudes
6. Hot yoga

Let's Discuss

Even if a woman has not followed a regular exercise routine prior to pregnancy, name some reasons she should start an exercise routine during pregnancy? Along with the benefits of exercising, discuss consequences of not exercising during pregnancy. Identify the contraindications to exercise during pregnancy.

Smoking

Smoking cigarettes during pregnancy is associated with increased risk of spontaneous abortion, prematurity, low birth weight, and congenital malformations.[61] Cigarette smoking during pregnancy exposes the fetus not only to the compound nicotine but also to more than 4,000 other compounds that can damage fetal tissues of the lungs and brain.[62] In addition, studies show that maternal smoking during pregnancy coupled with financial difficulty are related to poor quality of diet consumed during pregnancy.[63] Despite the fact that it is well known that smoking can lead to adverse pregnancy outcomes, 13–25% of pregnant women overall continue to smoke during this critical period.[64] For those who are not willing to give up smoking during pregnancy, it is important for health practitioners to counsel them on the benefits of prenatal multivitamin and mineral supplementation, because antioxidant supplementation during this time is significant.

Alcohol

Alcohol consumed by an expecting mother passes through the placenta into the circulatory system of the developing fetus, which has not yet developed the enzymes required to break it down. Toxic amounts of alcohol linger in the circulatory system, exposing the fetus to alcohol and interfering with proper growth and development. Prenatal alcohol exposure can be the cause of structural or functional defects of the heart, spine, brain, bones, kidneys, hearing, and vision. Alcohol exposure is associated with a higher incidence of attention-deficit/hyperactivity disorder and specific learning disabilities such as difficulties with mathematics and language, visual-spatial functioning, impulse control, information processing, memory skills, problem solving, abstract reasoning, and auditory comprehension.[65] Alcohol is especially harmful

during the first trimester when the brain and spinal cord of the fetus are developing quickly; consumption of alcohol during any point of the pregnancy can be harmful.

As a public health effort to reduce alcohol consumption during pregnancy, warning labels were added to alcoholic beverages in 1989 informing women of the risks of drinking during pregnancy. The American Academy of Pediatrics indicates that alcohol intake during pregnancy can cause thinking and behavioral problems that last a lifetime and that no amount of alcohol intake during pregnancy should be considered safe.[66]

Although there is no known safe level of alcohol intake during pregnancy, moderate (one to two drinks per week) and high intake (several drinks per day or binge drinking) contribute to the greatest risks. First-trimester drinking, compared to no drinking during that time, results in 12 times the odds of giving birth to a child with fetal alcohol syndrome disorder (FASD). First- and second-trimester drinking increases FASD odds 61 times, and women who drink during all trimesters increase the FASD odds by a factor of 65.[67]

Numerous risks are associated with alcohol intake during pregnancy. Fetal alcohol spectrum disorder (FASD) describes the various effects alcohol can have on a person exposed in utero. (See FIGURE 5.6 .) The most common

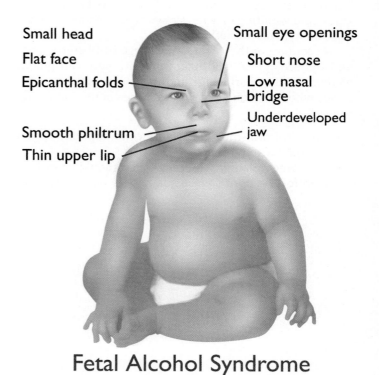

Small head
Flat face
Epicanthal folds
Smooth philtrum
Thin upper lip

Small eye openings
Short nose
Low nasal bridge
Underdeveloped jaw

Fetal Alcohol Syndrome

Figure 5.6
Effects alcohol can have on infants if they are exposed in utero.
Photo Researchers, Inc/Alamy Stock Photo

of these disorders is fetal alcohol syndrome (FAS), which affects 0.3 infants in every 1,000 live births in the United States.[68] FAS is characterized by abnormal facial features, growth deficiencies, central nervous system defects, behavioral and learning difficulties, poor social skills, and difficulties with vision and hearing. Other risks of alcohol intake during pregnancy include spontaneous abortion, birth defects, and mental retardation.[69]

Illegal Drug Use

Illicit drug use during pregnancy increases the risk of severe pregnancy complications for the mother and the fetus. Substances like cocaine, heroin, and methamphetamine pass from the mother's bloodstream through the placenta to the fetus and can result in a number of severe complications such as preterm delivery, miscarriage, high blood pressure, stillbirth, and sudden infant death syndrome (SIDS). Behavioral, learning, and cognitive difficulties, growth defects, and hyperactivity in the child can also result from use of illicit drugs during pregnancy.[70] The self-reported prevalence of marijuana use in pregnant women ranges from 2% to 5% in the United States, and use of marijuana for medicinal and recreational purposes is on the rise.[71]

Regular opioid drug (morphine, oxycodone, heroin, etc.) use in women during pregnancy can cause fetal dependency on the drug and can lead to withdrawal symptoms in the infant after birth. The extent of withdrawal symptoms depends on the particular drug and the length of use. Symptoms can vary from irritability, seizures, and vomiting to fever, slow weight gain, poor feeding, and hyperactive reflexes.[72]

According to the American College of Obstetricians and Gynecologists, healthcare practitioners can guide women of childbearing age and those considering pregnancy who have substance abuse issues in the following ways:[71]

- Abstain from smoking, alcohol consumption, use of marijuana and tobacco.
- All women planning for pregnancy should be evaluated for the use of these substances before, during, and after pregnancy for medical and nonmedical reasons.
- Women having a history of using addictive substances must be counseled about the potential adverse health and pregnancy-related outcomes for mother and child.
- Use of these substances during pregnancy must be discouraged.
- Use of multivitamin and mineral supplementation in these women needs to be evaluated.

TABLE 5.8 illustrates the prevalence of chemical use among pregnant and nonpregnant women. Mothers who smoke or consume alcohol should be counseled to abstain from smoking and drinking before, during, and after pregnancy.

Table 5.8

Comparison of Drug Use Among Women 15 to 44 Years of Age by Pregnancy Status (Data Collection 2012–2013)

	Pregnant Women,%	Nonpregnant Women,%
Illicit drug use	5.4	11.4
Alcohol use	9.4	55.4
Binge drinking	2.3	24.6
Cigarette use	15.4	24.0

Data from U.S. Department of Health and Human Services. Results from the 2013 National Survey on Drug Use and Health: Summary of National Findings. http://www.samhsa.gov/data/sites/default/files/NSDUHresultsPDFWHTML2013/Web/NSDUHresults2013.pdf

Recap Because of their influence on growth and development of the fetus, many nutrition and health-related behaviors must be considered during pregnancy. Women are encouraged to practice regular physical activity throughout their pregnancy as well as abstain from use of harmful chemicals such as alcohol, tobacco, and illicit drugs.

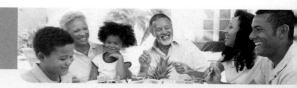

Learning Portfolio

Visual Chapter Summary

Gastrointestinal Conditions

- GI disorders are not uncommon among pregnant women.
- Changes in the GI tract as a result of pregnancy put the mother at risk for exacerbation of existing or development of new GI disorders.
- Understanding the risk factors and measures, along with following recommendations, for preventing and managing any GI conditions during pregnancy is essential to avoid complications. GI conditions can be managed during pregnancy with successful outcomes.

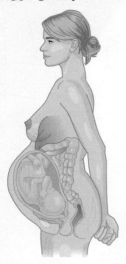

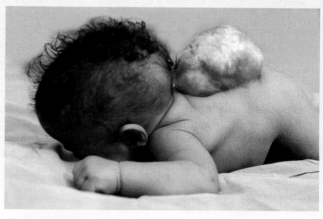

©Medicshots/Alamy Stock Photo

Consequences of inadequate weight gain affect both the expecting mother and the developing fetus.
- The micronutrients iron and folic acid both play important roles in development of a fetus. Folic acid is recognized as important both before and during pregnancy because it plays a crucial role in neural tube development, which occurs very early in gestation.

Endocrine and Metabolic Conditions

- The endocrine and metabolic disorders gestational diabetes, thyroid disorder, and polycystic ovary syndrome are all conditions that can complicate pregnancy. Successful management of these conditions during pregnancy results in little negative impact on the baby and mother.

Obesity and Malnutrition

- Body weight, nutrition status, and overall diet quality during pregnancy have been shown to affect health outcomes. Gaining more weight than recommended throughout gestation has been correlated with both short- and long-term maternal health risks.

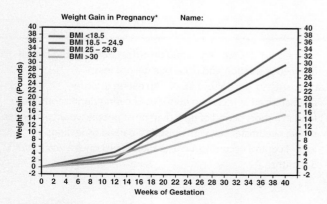

Weight Gain in Pregnancy*   Name:

Legend:
- BMI <18.5
- BMI 18.5 – 24.9
- BMI 25 – 29.9
- BMI >30

Y-axis: Weight Gain (Pounds)
X-axis: Weeks of Gestation

Data from Institute of Medicine, May 2009

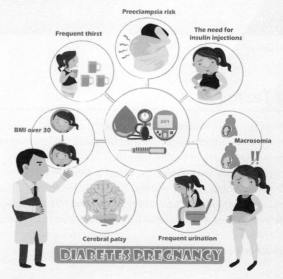

Preeclampsia risk
Frequent thirst
The need for insulin injections
BMI over 30
Macrosomia
Cerebral palsy
Frequent urination

DIABETES PREGNANCY

©viyadaistock/Getty Images

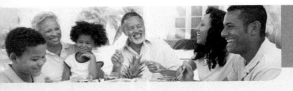

Learning Portfolio (continued)

Cardiovascular Conditions

■ Management of known cardiovascular disorders in women who intend to become pregnant should start before conception and continue throughout pregnancy. Consequences of unmanaged cardiovascular disease during pregnancy can have detrimental outcomes for both the expecting mother and the fetus.

■ It is commonly accepted that pregnant women are especially susceptible to adverse outcomes associated with low nutrient intake owing to their increased requirements during pregnancy and lactation to meet their own metabolic needs and the needs of the developing fetus.

Psychosocial Stressors

■ Given this increased susceptibility and the evidence of dietary inadequacy among pregnant women, a well-balanced diet rich in nutrients is recommended to help limit and control cognitive disorders such

as eating disorders, pica, depression, and stress and anxiety.

■ Because of their influence on growth and development of the fetus, many nutrition and health-related behaviors must be considered during pregnancy.

Lifestyle Management

■ Women are encouraged to include regular physical activity throughout their pregnancy as well as to abstain from using harmful chemicals such as alcohol, tobacco, and illicit drugs.

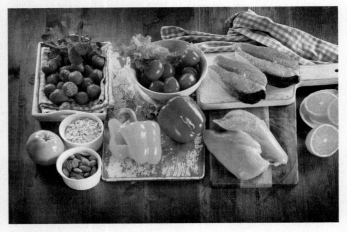

©Bitt24/Shutterstock

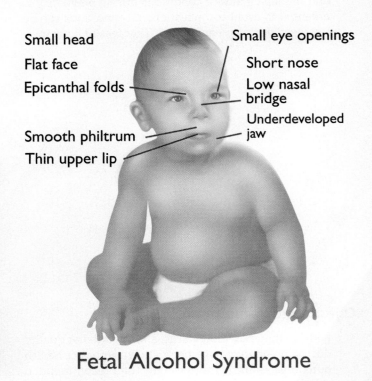

Small head
Flat face
Epicanthal folds
Smooth philtrum
Thin upper lip
Small eye openings
Short nose
Low nasal bridge
Underdeveloped jaw

Fetal Alcohol Syndrome

Photo Researchers, Inc/Alamy Stock Photo

Key Terms

amylophagia: A form of pica that is often observed in pregnant women. A condition involving the compulsive consumption of excessive amounts of purified starch.

anemia: A condition in which the blood is deficient in red blood cells, hemoglobin, or total volume. The World Health Organization, the United Nations Children's Fund, and United Nations University define anemia as a hemoglobin (Hb) concentration two standard deviations below the mean Hb concentration for a normal population of the same sex and age range.

anorexia nervosa: An eating disorder characterized by self-induced starvation and excessive weight loss.

binge eating disorder (BED): An eating disorder characterized as recurring episodes of eating significantly more food in a short period of time than most people would eat under similar circumstances, with episodes marked by feelings of lack of control occurring, on average, at least once a week over 3 months.

bulimia nervosa: An eating disorder characterized by binging (excessive or compulsive consumption of food) and purging (getting rid of food).

constipation: Development of hard, dry feces that results in difficulty emptying bowels or abnormally delayed or infrequent passage of hardened feces.

Crohn's disease: A subtype of inflammatory bowel disease; chronic ileitis that typically involves the distal portion of the ileum, often spreads to the colon, and is characterized by diarrhea, cramping, and loss of appetite and weight with local abscesses and scarring—also called regional enteritis, regional ileitis. It affects the entire digestive tract and all three intestinal mucosal layers.

diabetes mellitus: A disease of the pancreas that inhibits the production and utilization of the hormone insulin. Diabetes is a variable disorder of carbohydrate metabolism caused by a combination of hereditary and environmental factors and usually characterized by inadequate secretion or utilization of insulin, excessive urine production, excessive amounts of sugar in the blood and urine, and thirst, hunger, and loss of weight.

diarrhea: Abnormally frequent intestinal evacuations with more or less fluid stools.

dyslipidemia: A disorder of lipoprotein metabolism, including lipoprotein overproduction or deficiency, marked by abnormal concentrations of lipids or lipoproteins in the blood; dyslipidemias may manifest as elevation of total cholesterol, low-density lipoprotein (LDL) cholesterol, and triglyceride concentrations and a decrease in the high-density lipoprotein (HDL) cholesterol concentration in the blood.

eclampsia: Convulsions or coma late in pregnancy in an individual affected by preeclampsia.

gallstone: A calculus (as of cholesterol) formed in the gallbladder or biliary passages; also called biliary calculus or cholelith. Gallstones occur when the bile becomes concentrated in the gallbladder and becomes a stone-like material that can potentially block the flow of bile in the bile duct.

geophagia: Compulsive consumption of soil-like substances, including soil or clay.

gestational diabetes mellitus (GDM): Diabetes diagnosed during pregnancy and that cannot be categorized as overt diabetes.

hyperemesis gravidarum (HG): Severe persistent vomiting during pregnancy that results in weight loss and dehydration and that often requires hospitalization.

inflammatory bowel disease (IBD): A chronic condition with periodic immune responses combined with inflammation in the gastrointestinal tract. IBD encompasses two inflammatory diseases of the bowel: Crohn's disease or ulcerative colitis.

irritable bowel syndrome (IBS): A chronic functional disorder of the colon that is of unknown etiology. It is often associated with abnormal intestinal motility and increased sensitivity to visceral pain and characterized by diarrhea or constipation or diarrhea alternating with constipation, abdominal pain or discomfort, abdominal bloating, and passage of mucus in the stool; also called irritable colon, irritable colon syndrome, mucous colitis, and spastic colon.

macrosomia: "Fetal macrosomia" is used to describe a newborn who is significantly larger than average; a baby diagnosed with fetal macrosomia has a birth weight of more than 8 pounds, 13 ounces (4,000 g), regardless of his or her gestational age.

malnutrition: Inadequate intake of protein and/or energy over prolonged periods of time that results in loss of fat stores and/or muscle stores; includes starvation-related malnutrition, chronic disease or condition-related malnutrition, and acute disease or injury-related malnutrition.

nausea: A stomach distress that manifests as distaste for food and an urge to vomit.

neonatal hypoglycemia: The most common metabolic problem in newborns; defined as a plasma glucose level of less than 30 mg/dL (1.65 mmol/L) in the first 24 hours of life and less than 45 mg/dL (2.5 mmol/L) thereafter.

obesity: A condition characterized by excessive accumulation and storage of fat in the body. In an adult, obesity is typically indicated by a body mass index of 30 or higher. Although obesity may be subdivided into several categories: class 1: BMI ≥30; class 2: BMI of 35 to <40; and class 3: BMI of 40 or higher.

pagophagia: Compulsive consumption of ice or freezer frost.

perinatal depression: Major and minor depressive episodes during pregnancy (termed antenatal) or within the first 12 months after delivery (termed postpartum or postnatal).

pica: An eating disorder characterized by consuming nonnutritive substances such as clay, paper, starch, chalk, and soil.

postpartum (or postnatal) depression: Depression suffered by a mother following childbirth, typically arising from the combination of hormonal changes, psychological adjustment to motherhood, and fatigue.

preeclampsia: Hypertension with onset following 20 weeks of pregnancy that is characterized by a sudden rise in blood pressure, excessive weight gain, generalized edema, proteinuria, severe headache, and visual disturbances and that may result in eclampsia if untreated. It can lead to fetal growth restriction.

self-monitoring of blood glucose (SMBG): An empowering technique used by the patient and healthcare team to assess the effectiveness of a treatment plan in maintaining good glycemic control.

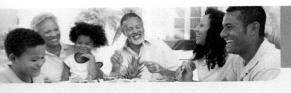

Learning Portfolio (continued)

ulcerative colitis (UC): A subtype of inflammatory bowel disease; a chronic inflammatory disease of the colon that is of unknown cause and that is characterized by diarrhea with discharge of mucus and blood, cramping abdominal pain,

and inflammation and edema of the mucous membrane with patches of ulceration.

vomiting: An act or instance of disgorging the contents of the stomach through the mouth; also called emesis.

Discussion Questions

1. Discuss why weight gain recommendations differ based on pre-pregnancy BMI category. Explain the complications that are associated with inadequate and excessive weight gain during pregnancy.

2. Explain the differences between hyperemesis gravidarum and morning sickness.

3. How is gestational diabetes tested during pregnancy? Summarize potential consequences of poorly controlled gestational diabetes.

Activities

1. With another student, practice nutrition-related counseling techniques. One person is the clinician, and the other is the pregnant patient who has a pre-pregnancy BMI of 25, is in her second trimester, and is already experiencing excessive weight gain. Remember to consider dietary intake, physical activity, edema, and other factors that may be influencing weight gain. Provide individualized nutrition recommendations.

2. When an expecting mother drinks alcohol during pregnancy, she is taking the risk of giving birth to a child who may suffer from mental and physical deficiencies for his or her entire life. Determine appropriate and effective ways of discussing the dangers of alcohol intake during pregnancy, and identify the signs and symptoms of an infant with fetal alcohol syndrome.

Study Questions

1. Which of the following dietary interventions is not used to manage mild nausea and vomiting during pregnancy?
   a. Drinking small amounts of water between and with meals
   b. Avoiding foods that are spicy
   c. Selecting foods that are tolerable and avoiding foods with strong odors
   d. Consuming high-fat foods

2. Oral hydration, correction of electrolyte imbalance, and having small, frequent meals that contain little fat, caffeine, and artificial sweeteners are diet recommendations to correct which of the following conditions?
   a. Heartburn
   b. Nausea and vomiting
   c. Diarrhea
   d. Constipation

3. Which of the following conditions is limited to affecting the colon and rectum and is characterized by continuous inflammation occurring only in the innermost layer of intestinal lining?
   a. Crohn's disease
   b. Ulcerative colitis
   c. Gallstones
   d. GERD

4. Low birth weight increases the risk for infant morbidity and mortality as compared with infants born at a healthy birth weight for which of the following reasons?
   a. Infants with low birth weight have a difficult time eating, fighting infection, and gaining weight.
   b. Infants with low birth weight are unable to absorb nutrients as readily.
   c. Infants with low birth weight produce hormones that increase the risk for infection and inflammation.
   d. Infants with low birth weight have been exposed to harmful substances in utero.

5. Which of the following statements about nutrient intake during pregnancy is not true?
   a. Increased iron is necessary to ensure the fetus receives adequate oxygen and to increase red blood cell count for production of fetal blood.
   b. Inadequate folate intake during the first 3 months of pregnancy can cause the neural tube to fail to close, resulting in neural tube defects.
   c. Iodine is vital during pregnancy for thyroid function, brain development of the fetus, and maternal energy production.
   d. Adequate vitamin D levels during pregnancy support bone health, immune function, and cell division and assist with the absorption and metabolism of calcium and phosphorus, which are vital for proper bone and tooth formation.

6. All of the following are characteristics of gestational diabetes *except* which one?
   a. Frequent thirst
   b. Frequent urination
   c. Risk for preeclampsia
   d. High blood pressure

7. Preeclampsia represents a syndrome characterized by all of the following *except* which one?
   a. Insulin resistance
   b. Oxidative stress
   c. High blood pressure
   d. Increased calcium and phosphorus excretion

8. Misdiagnosis of which condition can lead to potential complications, including iron-deficiency anemia, lead poisoning, and other toxicities?
   a. High blood pressure
   b. Pica
   c. Hypoglycemia
   d. Bulimia nervosa

9. Contraindications for exercise during pregnancy include all of the following *except* which one?
   a. Low placenta level
   b. Persistent second- or third-trimester bleeding
   c. Previous history of miscarriage
   d. First pregnancy with weight gain in the lower 10th percentile of recommendations

10. Which condition is characterized by abnormal facial features, growth deficiencies, central nervous system defects, behavioral and learning difficulties, poor social skills, and difficulties with vision and hearing?
    a. Fetal alcohol syndrome
    b. Gestational diabetes
    c. Attention-deficit disorder
    d. Intrauterine growth retardation

Weblinks

- **Academy of Nutrition and Dietetics**
  Pregnancy: http://www.eatright.org/resources/health/pregnancy
  Position of the American Dietetic Association and American Society for Nutrition: Obesity, Reproduction, and Pregnancy Outcomes: https://www.nutrition.org/media/news/fact-sheets-and-position-papers/ObesityReprodPreg.pdf

- **Centers for Disease Control and Prevention**
  Safe Medication Use During Pregnancy: http://www.cdc.gov/pregnancy/
  Breastfeeding: http://www.cdc.gov/breastfeeding/index.htm

- **Centers for Disease Control and Prevention Podcasts at CDC: "Don't Drink and Deliver"**
  http://www2c.cdc.gov/podcasts/player.asp?f=11983

- **Centers for Disease Control and Prevention Podcasts at CDC: "Folic Acid: Help Ensure a Healthy Pregnancy"**
  http://www2c.cdc.gov/podcasts/player.asp?f=7552

- **Fetal Alcohol Spectrum Disorders (video)**
  http://link.brightcove.com/services/player/bcpid3647051512001?bckey=AQ~~,AAABxqEDkXE~,hmZyzKR72h1kLXl6akqLG71Qb3dmzbsN&bctid=2034322528001

- **Hyperemesis Education and Research (HER Foundation)**
  http://www.helpher.org

- **MyPlate for Pregnancy and Breastfeeding**
  http://www.choosemyplate.gov/moms-pregnancy-breastfeeding

- **U.S. Department of Agriculture**
  Nutrition During Pregnancy: https://fnic.nal.usda.gov/lifecycle-nutrition/nutrition-during-pregnancy
  Nutrition During Lactation: https://fnic.nal.usda.gov/lifecycle-nutrition/nutrition-during-lactation

- **Visual Health Solutions Spina Bifida animation**
  http://www.visibleproductions.com/index.php?asset_id=vpl_0141_001&page=asset_detail

- **World Health Organization**
  Maternal, Newborn, Child and Adolescent Health: http://www.who.int/maternal_child_adolescent/en/

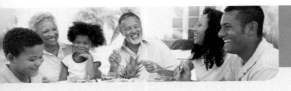

Learning Portfolio (continued)

References

1. Centers for Disease Control and Prevention; updated May 20, 2016. Birth defects. Retrieved from http://www.cdc.gov/ncbddd/birthdefects/index.html. Accessed September 20, 2016.

2. Martin JA, Hamilton BE, Osterman MJK, et al. Births: final data for 2013. *Nat Vital Stat Rep.* January 15, 2015;64(1). http://www.cdc.gov/nchs/data/nvsr/nvsr64/nvsr64_01.pdf. Accessed September 1, 2016.

3. Centers for Disease Control and Prevention; updated June 1, 2016. Births and natality. Retrieved from http://www.cdc.gov/nchs/fastats/births.htm. Accessed September 1, 2016.

4. Georgieff MK. Nutrition and the developing brain: nutrient priorities and measurement. *Am J Clin Nutr.* February 2007;85(2):614S–620S.

5. CORE Group. *Maternal Nutrition During Pregnancy and Lactation.* Washington, DC: LINKAGES; August 2014. Retrieved from: http://www.coregroup.org/storage/documents/Workingpapers/MaternalNutritionDietaryGuide_AED.pdf. Accessed September 1, 2016.

6. Saha S, Manlolo J, McGowan CE, et al. Gastroenterology consultations in pregnancy. *J Women Health.* November 3, 2011;20:359–363.

7. Christie JA, Rose S. Constipation, diarrhea, hemorrhoids and fecal incontinence. In *Pregnancy in Gastrointestinal Disorders.* Bethesda, MD: American College of Gastroenterology. http://gi.org/wp-content/uploads/2011/07/institute-PregnancyMonograph.pdf. Accessed September 1, 2016.

8. Strong TH Jr. Alternative therapies of morning sickness. *Clinc Obstet Gynecol.* 2001;44(4):653–660.

9. Ding MS, Leach M, Bradley H. The effectiveness and safety of ginger for pregnancy-induced nausea and vomiting: a systematic review. *Women Birth.* 2013;26(1):E26–E30.

10. Harvey-Banchik LP. Hyperemesis gravidarum and nutritional support. In *Pregnancy in Gastrointestinal Disorders.* Bethesda, MD: American College of Gastroenterology. http://gi.org/wp-content/uploads/2011/07/institute-PregnancyMonograph.pdf. Accessed September 1, 2016.

11. Family history linked to increased hyperemesis risk: adverse outcomes, such as low birth weight, are associated with hyperemesis. *Nursing Standard* 2010; 24(42):16.

12. Bonapace ES Jr, Fisher RS. Constipation and diarrhea in pregnancy. *Gastroenterol Clin North Am.* 1998;27(1):197–211.

13. Vazquez JC. Constipation, haemorrhoids, and heartburn in regnancy. *Clin Evid* (online). 2010;2010:1411. http://www.ncbi.nlm.nih.gov/pmc/articles/PMC3217736/.

14. Longo SA, Moore RC, Canzoneri BJ, et al. Gastrointestinal conditions during pregnancy. *Clin Colon Rectal Surg.* 2010; 23(2):80–89.

15. Richter JE. Heartburn, nausea, vomiting during pregnancy. In *Pregnancy in Gastrointestinal Disorders.* Bethesda, MD: American College of Gastroenterology. Retrieved from: http://gi.org/wp-content/uploads/2011/07/institute-Pregnancy-Monograph.pdf. Accessed September 1, 2016.

16. National Institute of Diabetes and Digestive and Kidney Diseases; updated November 27, 2013. Gallstones Retrieved from: http://www.niddk.nih.gov/health-information/health-topics/digestive-diseases/gallstones/Pages/facts.aspx. Updated November 27, 2013. Accessed September 1, 2016.

17. Almashhrawi AA, Ahmed KT, Rahman RN, et al. Liver disease in pregnancy: diseases not unique to pregnancy. *World J Gastroenerol.* November 21, 2013;19(43):7630–7638.

18. Tang SJ, Mayo MJ, Rodriguez-Frias E, et al. Safety and utility of ERCP during pregnancy. *Gastrointest Endosc.* 2009;69:453–461. doi:10.1016/j.gie.2008.05.024.

19. Boyd HA, Basit S, Harpsoe MC, et al. Inflammatory bowel disease and risk for adverse pregnancy outcomes. *PLoS ONE.* 2015;10(6): e0129567. doi:10.1371/journal.pone.0129567.

20. Centers for Disease Control and Prevention; updated September 4, 2014. Inflammatory bowel disease (IBD). Retrieved from: http://www.cdc.gov/ibd/. Accessed September 1, 2016.

21. Beaulieu DB, Kane S. Inflammatory bowel disease in pregnancy. *World J Gastroenterol.* June 14, 2011;17(22): 2696–2701.

22. Vermeire S, Carbonnel F, Coulie PG, et al. Management of inflammatory bowel disease in pregnancy. *J Crohn's Colitis.* 2012;6:811–823.

23. Kaiser LL, Campbell CG; Academy Positions Committee Workgroup. Practice paper of the Academy of Nutrition and Dietetics: nutrition and lifestyle for a healthy pregnancy outcome. *J Acad Nutr Diet.* 2014;114(7):1099–1103.

24. Sarwer DB, Allison KC, Gibbons LM, Markowitz JT, Nelson DB. Pregnancy and obesity: a review and agenda for future research. *J Womens Health* (Larchmt). 2006;15:720–733.

25. Jeric M, Roje D, Medic N, et al. Maternal pre-pregnancy underweight and fetal growth in relation to Institute of Medicine recommendations for gestational weight gain. *Early Hum Dev.* May 2013;89(5):277–281.

26. Vahratian A, Zhang J, Troendle JF, Savitz DA, Siega-Riz AM. Maternal prepregnancy overweight and obesity and the pattern of labor progression in term nulliparous women. *Obstet Gynecol.* 2004;104:943–951.

27. Office on Women's Health, U.S. Department of Health and Human Services; updated September 27, 2010. Pregnancy. WomensHealth.go. http://womenshealth.gov/pregnancy/you-are-pregnant/staying-healthy-safe.html. Accessed September 1, 2016.

28. Krawkowiak P, Walker CK, Bremer AA, et al. Maternal metabolic conditions and risk for autism and other neurodevelopmental disorders. *Pediatrics.* 2012;129(5):e1121–e1128.

29. Waller DK, Shaw GM, Rasmussen SA, et al. Prepregnancy obesity as a risk factor for structural birth defects. *Arch Pediatr Adolesc Med.* 2007;161:745–750.

30. Rasmussen KM, Kjolhede CL. Prepregnant overweight and obesity diminish the prolactin response to suckling in the first week postpartum. *Pediatrics.* 2004;113:465–471.

31. Goonewardene M, Shehata M, Hamad A. Anaemia in pregnancy. *Best Pract Res Clin Obstet Gynaecol.* 2012;26(1):3–24

32. Sridhar SB, Darbinian J, Ehrlich SF, et al. Maternal gestational weight gain and offspring risk for childhood overweight or obesity. *Am J Obstet Gynecol.* 2014;211(3):8.

33. Agopian AJ, Tinker SC, Lupo PJ, et al. Proportion of neural tube defects attributable to known risk factors. *Birth Defects Res A Clin Mol Teratol.* 2013;97(1):42–46.

34. Zhang C, Ning Y. Effect of dietary and lifestyle factors on the risk of gestational diabetes: review of epidemiologic

evidence. *Am J Clin Nutr.* 2011;94(6 suppl):1975S–1979S. doi:10.3945/ajcn.110.001032.

35. DeSisto CL, Kim SY, Sharma AJ. Prevalence estimates of gestational diabetes mellitus in the United States, Pregnancy Risk Assessment Monitoring System (PRAMS), 2007–2010. *Prev Chronic Dis.* June 19, 2014;11:130415. doi:10.5888/pcd11.130415.

36. Leddy MA, Power ML, Schulkin J. The impact of maternal obesity on maternal and fetal health. *Rev Obstet Gynecol.* 2008;1(4):170–178.

37. American Thyroid Association; 2015. Iodine deficiency. Retrieved from: http://www.thyroid.org/iodine-deficiency/. Accessed August 4, 2016.

38. Rebagliato M, Murcia M, Espada M, et al. Iodine intake and maternal thyroid function during pregnancy. *Epidemiology.* 2010;21(1):62–69.

39. Steegers EA, von Dadelszen P, Duvekot JJ, Pijnenborg R. Preeclampsia. *Lancet.* 2010;376(9741):631–644.

40. Regitz-Zagrosek V, Blomstrom Lundqvist C, Borghi C, et al. ESC guidelines on the management of cardiovascular diseases during pregnancy. *Eur Heart J.* 2011;32(24):3147–3197.

41. Li R, Jewell S, Grummer-Strawn L. Maternal obesity and breast-feeding practices. *Am J Clin Nutr.* 2003;77(4):931–936.

42. American Pregnancy Association; September 2015. Gestational hypertension: pregnancy induced hypertension (PIH). Retrieved from: http://americanpregnancy.org/pregnancy-complications/pregnancy-induced-hypertension/. Accessed September 1, 2016.

43. Hegele RA. Hyperlipidaemia in pregnancy. *CMAJ.* December 15, 1991;145(12):1596.

44. Lacey JH, Smith G. Bulimia nervosa: the impact on mother and baby. *Br J Psychiatry.* 1987;150:777–781.

45. American Pregnancy Association; July 2015. Pregnancy and eating disorders. Retrieved from: http://americanpregnancy.org/pregnancy-health/pregnancy-and-eating-disorders/. Accessed September 1, 2016.

46. Morgan JF, Lacey JH, Sedgwick PM. Impact of pregnancy on bulimia nervosa. *Br J Psychiatry.* 1999;174:135–140.

47. Leung BMY, Kaplan B. Perinatal depression: prevalence, risks, and the nutrition link—a review of the literature. *J Am Diet Assoc.* 2009;109:1566–1575.

48. Goldman LS, Nielsen NH, Champion HC. Awareness, diagnosis, and treatment of depression. *J Gen Intern Med.* 1999;14:569–580.

49. Flynn HA, Blow FC, Marcus SM. Rates and predictors of depression treatment among pregnant women in hospital-affiliated obstetrics practices. *Gen Hosp Psychiatry.* 2006;28(4):289–292.

50. Bowen A, Muhajarine N. Prevalence of antenatal depression in women enrolled in an outreach program in Canada. *J Obstet Gynecol Neonatal Nurs.* 2006;35:491–498.

51. Lee DT, Chung TK. Postnatal depression: an update. *Best Pract Res Clin Obstet Gynaecol.* 2007;21:183–191.

52. Massachusetts General Hospital Center for Women's Mental Health. Psychiatric disorders during pregnancy. Retrieved from: https://womensmentalhealth.org/specialty-clinics/psychiatric-disorders-during-pregnancy/?doing_wp_cron=1452160899.6538820266723632812500. Accessed September 1, 2016.

53. Ellis CR. Pica: Practice Essentials Medscape; updated April 1, 2016. Retrieved from: http://emedicine.medscape.com/article/914765-overview. Updated April 1, 2016. Accessed September 1, 2016.

54. Young SL. Pica in pregnancy: new ideas about an old condition. *Annu Rev Nutr.* August 21, 2010;30:403–422.

55. Thihalolipavan S, Candalla BM, Ehrlich J. Examining pica in NYC pregnant women with elevated blood lead levels. *Matern Child Health J.* 2013;17(1):49–55.

56. Miao D, Young S, Golden C. A meta-analysis of pica and micronutrient status. *Am J Hum Biol.* 2015;21(1):84–93.

57. López LB, Ortega Soler CR, de Portela ML. Pica during pregnancy: a frequently underestimated problem. *Arch Latinoam Nutr.* 2004;54(1):17–24.

58. Corbett RW, Ryan C, Weinrich SP. Pica in pregnancy: does it affect pregnancy outcomes? *MCN Am J Matern Child Nurs.* May–June 2003;28(3):183–189.

59. Gollenberg A, Pekow P, Markenson G, Tucker KL, Chasan-Taber L. Dietary behaviors, physical activity, and cigarette smoking among pregnant Puerto Rican women. *Am J Clin Nutr.* June 2008;87(6):1844–1851.

60. The American College of Obstetricians and Gynecologists Committee Opinion No. 650: Physical activity and exercise during pregnancy and the postpartum period. *Obstet Gynecol.* 2015;126(6):e135–142. http://www.acog.org/Resources-And-Publications/Committee-Opinions/Committee-on-Obstetric-Practice/Physical-Activity-and-Exercise-During-Pregnancy-and-the-Postpartum-Period. Accessed February 14, 2016.

61. Agrawal A, Scherrer JF, Grant JD, et al. The effects of maternal smoking during pregnancy on offspring outcomes. *Prev Med.* 2010;50(1–2):13–18.

62. U.S. Department of Health and Human Services. *A Report of the Surgeon General: How Tobacco Smoke Causes Disease: What It Means to You.* Washington, DC: U.S. Dept. of Health and Human Services, Centers for Disease Control and Prevention, National Center for Chronic Disease Prevention and Health Promotion, Office on Smoking and Health; 2010. Retrieved from: http://www.cdc.gov/tobacco/data_statistics/sgr/2010/consumer_booklet/pdfs/consumer.pdf. Accessed September 1, 2016.

63. Emmett PM, Jones LR, Golding J. Pregnancy diet and associated outcomes in the Avon Longitudinal Study of Parents and Children. *Nutr Rev.* 2015;73(suppl 3):154–174.

64. Bérard A, Zhao JP, Sheehy O. Success of smoking cessation interventions during pregnancy. July 8, 2016 *Am J Obstet Gynecol.* November, 2016;215(5):611.e1–611.e8 [published July 8, 2016 online ahead of print].

65. Kleiber ML, Laufer BI, Wright E, et al. Long-term alterations to the brain transcriptome in a maternal voluntary consumption model of fetal alcohol spectrum disorders. *Brain Res.* June 6, 2012;1458:18–33.

66. American Academy of Pediatrics. Fetal alcohol spectrum disorders: FAQs of parents and families. HealthyChildren.org; updated November 21, 2015 Retrieved from: https://www.healthychildren.org/English/health-issues/conditions/chronic/Pages/Fetal-Alcohol-Spectrum-Disorders-FAQs-of-Parents-and-Families.aspx. Accessed August 5, 2016.

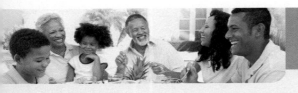

Learning Portfolio (continued)

67. American Academy of Pediatrics; October 19, 2015. AAP says no amount of alcohol should be considered safe during pregnancy. Retrieved from: https://www.aap.org/en-us/about-the-aap/aap-press-room/pages/AAP-Says-No-Amount-of-Alcohol-Should-be-Considered-Safe-During-Pregnancy.aspx. Accessed September 1, 2016.

68. Kobor MS, Weinberg J. Focus on: epigenetics and fetal alcohol spectrum disorders. *Alcohol Res Health*. 2010;34(1):29–37.

69. Ramsay M. Genetic and epigenetic insights into fetal alcohol spectrum disorders. *Genome Med*. 2010;2:8.

70. Behnke M, Smith VC, Committee on Substance Abuse; Committee on Fetus and Newborn. Prenatal substance abuse: short- and long-term effects on the exposed fetus. *Pediatrics*. 2013;131(3):e1009–e1024.

71. The American College of Obstetricians and Gynecologists Committee on Obstetric Practice. Committee Opinion No. 637: Marijuana use during pregnancy and lactation. *Obstet Gynecol*. 2015;126(1):234–238. doi:10.1097/01.AOG.0000467192.89321.a6. https://www.acog.org/-/media/Committee-Opinions/Committee-on-Obstetric-Practice/co637.pdf?dmc=1&ts=20160213T0655484056. Accessed February 14, 2016.

72. National Institute on Drug Abuse. Substance use in women: substance use while pregnant and breastfeeding. National Institutes of Health; updated July 2015. Retrieved from: https://www.drugabuse.gov/publications/research-reports/substance-use-in-women/substance-use-while-pregnant-breastfeeding. Accessed February 14, 2016.

CHAPTER 6

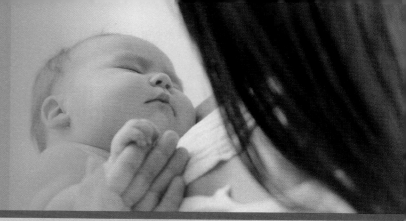

Infant Nutrition

April Litchford, MS, RD

Chapter Outline

Assessing Newborn Health

Infant Mortality

Infant Development

Infancy and Dietary Intake

Infant Feeding Skills Development

Nutritional Recommendations and Requirements During Infancy

Common Nutrition Considerations During Infancy

Promoting Healthy Lifestyles

Learning Objectives

1. Describe the normal stages of infant growth and development.

2. Summarize when and how solid foods should be introduced to infants.

3. List macronutrient and micronutrient needs of infants.

4. List common nutritional concerns encountered in infants.

5. List resources available to parents and caregivers of infants that promote a healthy lifestyle.

Case Study

©Nancy Brown/Photographer's Choice/Getty

Baby Clara is born at 36 weeks of gestation. Her mother's pregnancy was considered normal, however with low overall weight gain. Clara's mother gained a total of 15 pounds during her pregnancy. She followed a vegan type of diet throughout most of the pregnancy, with high intake of vegetable proteins, carbohydrates, fruits, and vegetables. During the pregnancy, Clara's mother walked between 1 and 3 miles each day.

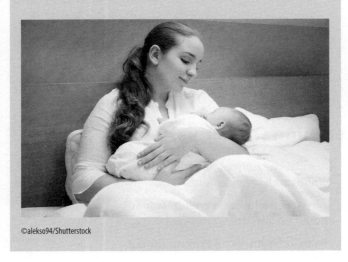

©alekso94/Shutterstock

An infant will experience an amazing rate of growth during the first year of life that requires a regular and adequate amount of nourishment. The birth of a child can evoke in parents a wide range of emotions, from excitement and joy to anxiety and worry. One of the first questions parents and caregivers explore after birth is feeding. Feedings become a major part of everyday routine during the first few days of life for an infant. Infants grow at an astounding rate, with gradual changes occurring each day. By the end of the first year, the baby barely resembles the newborn welcomed into the world.

Assessing Newborn Health

Preview The weight of an infant is an important measurement to help healthcare providers establish risk at birth and throughout infancy.

Infants experience a massive amount of growth in a relatively short amount of time. At 6 months of age, typical infants have doubled their birth weight, and they triple their birth weight by the end of their first year. The infant body is constantly growing and expanding its physical, cognitive, and social development. Infants rapidly learn how to move and use their tiny body to accomplish many

different tasks. A smile is usually the first sign of social interaction, and this occurs about 3 months from birth. At about this same time, a baby begins grabbing for objects within reach and cooing in attempts to communicate. (See **FIGURE 6.1**.)

Physical Growth Assessment

The most common criteria used to determine the health status of newborns are birth weight, length, and head circumference. During routine checkups throughout infancy, healthcare providers record these measurements on standard growth charts (see **FIGURE 6.2**).[1]

These charts reliably show growth of an individual child over time as well as allow comparison of one child's growth with that of children in the general population. Though it is normal to have a wide variety of measurements among children, some general trends in weight and length enable healthcare providers to diagnose an infant's potential for death, disease, or developmental delays. A few common designations include small for gestation age (SGA) and large for gestational age (LGA). A child that is SGA plots on the growth curve below the 10th percentile; an LGA infant plots above the 90th percentile. (See **FIGURE 6.3**.) An infant who falls into an average category for weight and length is termed appropriate for gestational age, or AGA.

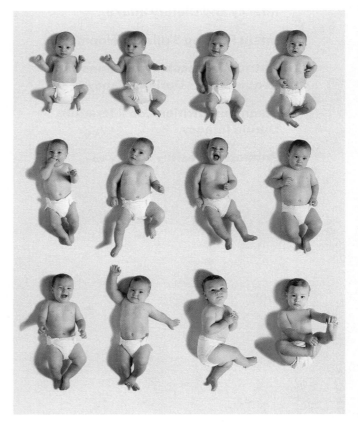

Figure 6.1
Growth rate of a child, month by month for the first year.
©Rob Goldman/The Image Bank/Getty

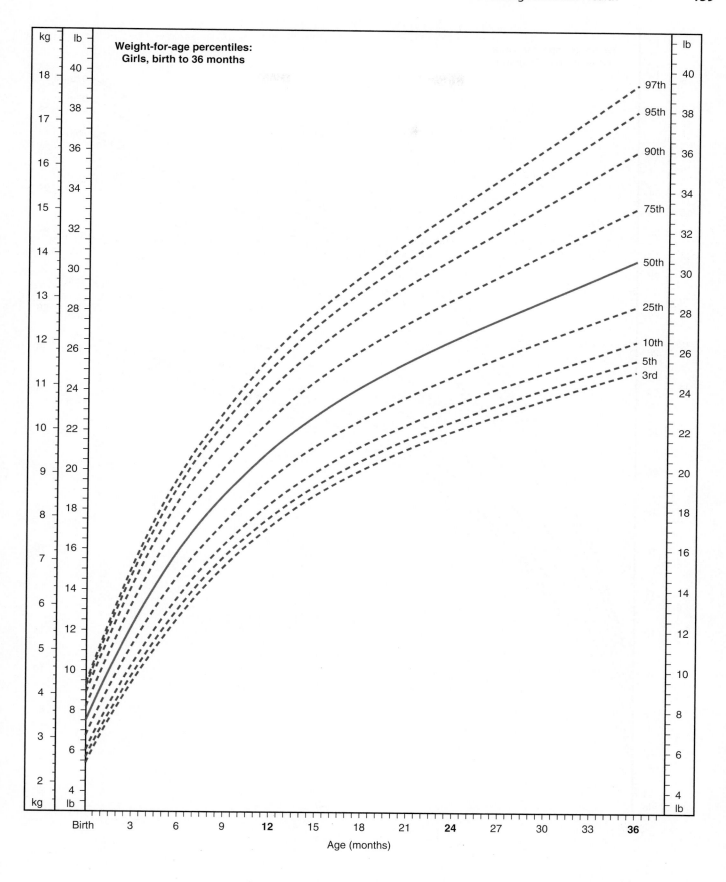

Weight-for-age percentiles:
Girls, birth to 36 months

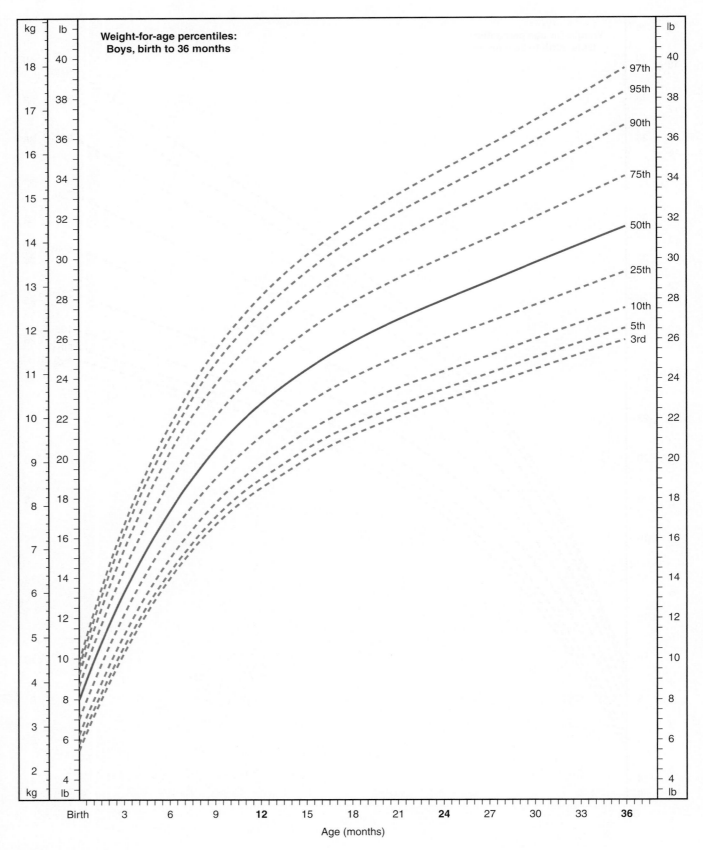

Figure 6.2

Center for Disease Control and Prevention growth charts for girls and boys.

Developed by the National Center for Health Statistics in collaboration with the National Center for Chronic Disease Prevention and Health Promotion (2000).

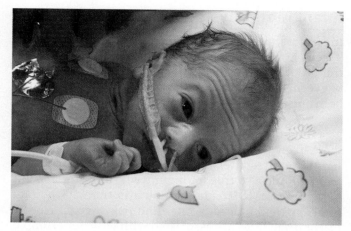

Figure 6.3
Infant born at a weight below the 10th percentile of weight for gestational age.
©Gert Vrey/Shutterstock

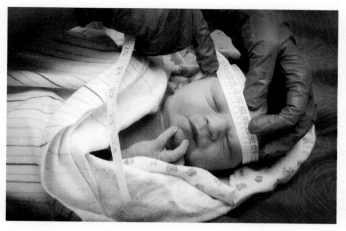

Figure 6.5
Measurement of an infant's head circumference.
©Alice Jeanette Brown/Shutterstock

To create data that are comparable among all infants, specific types of measurements are required. The length, or stature, of an infant is measured in a recumbent position (**recumbent length**) (see FIGURE 6.4). The child is stretched out on a measuring table with the head touching the top plate and the lower plate being adjusted to meet the bottom of the feet when the legs are stretched out straight. **Head circumference** is another common indicator. This is measured with a flexible measuring tape that is placed around the widest part the head, usually just above the ears (see FIGURE 6.5).

Tracking and Interpreting Data

Once proper measurements are taken, the data are then plotted on standardized growth charts. There are two different types of growth charts: the Growth Reference Charts, which are developed by the Centers for Disease Control and Prevention (CDC), and Growth Standard

Charts, which are developed by the World Health Organization (WHO).

Both the WHO and the CDC growth charts are used as standards for growth. The WHO international growth charts are established for children ages 0 to 5 years. Similar to the 2000 CDC growth charts, these charts describe weight for age, length for age, weight for length, and body mass index (BMI) for age. The differences between the two charts are that the WHO charts are growth standards based on data collected in the WHO Multicenter Growth Reference Study and they describe the growth of healthy children in optimal conditions, whereas the CDC charts are based on growth references that describe how certain children grew in a particular place and time.

In practice, clinicians use growth charts as standards rather than references. The CDC growth charts consist of a set of charts for infants birth to 36 months of age and a set of charts for children and adolescents from age 2 to 20 years. The charts for infants include sex-specific percentile curves for weight for age, recumbent length for age, head circumference for age, and weight for recumbent length. The CDC recommends that the WHO growth charts be used for children younger than 2 years of age, and the CDC charts for all children older than the age of 2. The WHO charts are based on information from a study engineered specifically for development of growth charts. These charts are standards that reflect how an infant should grow given optimal conditions. They also use breastfeeding as the standard method of feeding for optimal growth.[2]

To help establish an accurate assessment of how a child is growing, multiple measurements should be taken and plotted on a growth chart during the first 2 years of life. Ideally, measurements over time should be taken at regular intervals, such as every month or every 3 months. Regular plotted measurements can show drastic increases or decreases in growth, allowing for further investigation of why such a change occurred. Situations

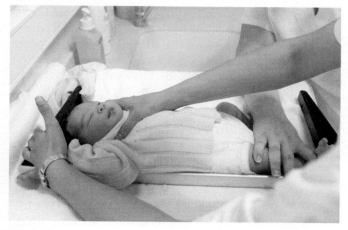

Figure 6.4
Measurement of an infant's length.
©CHASSENET/BSIP SA/Alamy Stock Photo

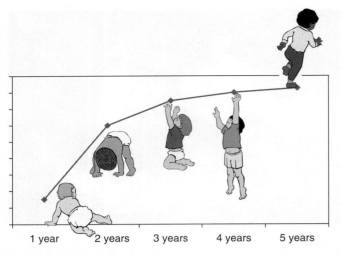

The WHO Child Growth Standards

Reprinted from WHO child growth standards : length/height-for-age, weight-for-age, weight-for-length, weight-forheight and body mass index-for-age : methods and development, Copyright 2006.

that warrant further investigation and possible interventions include: (1) if weight, length, or head circumference measurements do not increase for more than a 1-month period; (2) if weight and height do not increase over time; or (3) if there is a drop in weight that is not regained in a 3- to 4-week period.

Although an infant's measurements are essential in assessing overall health, gains in weight and length during infancy are not predictive of future patterns of growth. A child that is long and heavy during infancy does not predict a tall and heavy child or adult.

Case Study

Clara is now 6 months old.

1. Complete the following table to indicate her weight-for-age percentile and her length-for-age percentile.

Age	Weight	Weight-for-Age Percentile	Length	Length-for-Age Percentile
Birth	6 lb, 2 oz		18 inches	
2 weeks	6 lb, 4 oz		18¼ inches	
3 months	10 lb		20½ inches	
6 months	12 lb, 6 oz		24 inches	

2. At 3 months old, what does Clara's weight-for-age percentile and length-for-age percentile tell you about her size compared with other infants her age?

3. What is your assessment of Clara's weight, and should you be concerned?

4. Why is it important to have a series of growth measurements when tracking growth of an infant?

Infant Mortality

Infants are considered **full term** when they reach between 37 and 42 weeks of **gestation**. Most babies who are born full term weigh between 6 and 9 pounds and measure between 18.5 and 21.5 inches in length.[3] Infants can be born outside of the average guidelines and still be healthy.

Preterm infants are infants born before 37 weeks of gestation regardless of birth weight. Preterm infants are more likely to require intensive care and to have higher mortality rates after birth due to incomplete development. This is also true for infants who are born at a **low birth weight (LBW)**, defined as less than 5.5 pounds (2,500 g). High mortality rates and risk of cognitive and motor disabilities are associated with LBW; for example, research shows a potential link between LBW and development of autism spectrum disorder.[4] LBW is a major concern of healthcare providers worldwide, with the prevalence of LBW infants higher in developing countries, but it is still a major concern in the United States. The CDC reported a slight decrease (about 1%) in LBW infants from 2012 to 2013.[5]

The **infant mortality** rate is an estimate of the number of infant deaths, which occur within the first year of life, for every 1,000 live births. This rate is sometimes used as an indicator of the health and well-being of a nation because factors affecting the health of entire populations can also affect the mortality rate of infants. The statistics for infant mortality worldwide rank the United States well below other wealthy countries, a statistic especially concerning because the United States spends significantly more resources on health care than any other nation in the world.[6]

The CDC reported the top three causes of infant mortality in the United States as serious birth defects; LBW/preterm births; and sudden infant death syndrome (SIDS).[7] The rate of infant mortality reported in the United States was 5.96 per 1,000 live births in 2014.[8] This rate can be explained partially by reviewing the rates of LBW reported in infants for the same period. The national average rate of LBW reported in 2014 was 8%. This rate is generally steady for all ethnic groups except for children of non-Hispanic black origin. The current rate for this population was reported as 13.15%.[8] It is concerning that this ethnic group experiences such a large variation in the rate of infants born at LBW.

Reducing Incidence of Infant Mortality

Improvement of infant mortality rates (IMR) is a concern of healthcare professionals and government bodies in the United States. Every decade the government releases a set of goals and objectives designed to improve health outcomes in all individuals. The current goals are Healthy People 2020 and they include objectives related to infant health. **TABLE 6.1** lists some of the objectives that use public health tracking indicators to assess national progress toward the goals.

Table 6.1

Healthy People 2020 Objectives for Infants (birth to 1 year)

Relevant Goals for Infant Health	Baseline	Target
Reduce rate of fetal death of all fetal deaths within 1 year.	6.7 deaths per 1,000 live births	6.0 deaths per 1,000 live births
Reduce LBW.	8.6% of all live births	7.8% of all live births
Reduce total preterm births.	12.7% of all live births	11.4% of all live births
Increase the proportion of infants who are breastfed.	74% of all infants	81.9% of all infants

At the beginning of the 20th century, for every 1,000 live births in the United States, approximately 100 infants died before age 1 year. Over time this rate has declined significantly, with rate improvements from 7.0 deaths per 1,000 births in 2002 to a historically low rate of 5.96 deaths per 1,000 live births in 2013.[9] While the improvement is promising, the numbers are still too high. Factors contributing to infant mortality rate include the following:

- Birth defects
- Preterm birth (birth before 37 weeks of gestation) and low birth weight
- Maternal complications of pregnancy
- Sudden infant death syndrome
- Injuries

Currently, a large amount of government resources are in place to combat as many of the above factors as possible. They target at-risk populations in an effort to change birth outcomes. Some of the major programs capable of improving pregnancy and birth outcomes, such as Medicaid and the Child Health Initiatives Program (CHIP), focus on increasing individual access to medical care. Other programs focus on increasing nutrition quantity and quality and provide education and support to at-risk mothers: Special Supplemental Nutrition Program for Women, Infants, and Children (WIC), the Collaborative Improvement and Innovation Network (CoIIN), Healthy Start grants, Home Visiting program, and Title V block grants.

The role of nutrition in pregnancy and after birth is often underestimated by healthcare providers and the general public; however, inadequate nutrition for infants has been reported to be a key factor in infant mortality. Conclusive evidence links poor nutrition intake during pregnancy with birth defects, low birth weight, and poor maternal outcomes. Similar types of delays and poor outcomes are expected among newborns in the neonatal and postnatal stages when nutritional intake is inadequate.

Recap It is necessary to closely monitor infant growth to identify possible health problems. Growth can indicate the adequacy of a child's nutritional intake and ability to feed, and if an infant's growth slows, this may be an early sign of a disease or disorder. Standardized growth charts are used to monitor and evaluate an infant's growth patterns. Although it is normal to have a wide variety of birth weights and lengths, some general trends in weight and length allow healthcare providers to diagnose an infant's potential for death, disease, or developmental delays. Infants born before 37 weeks of gestation, regardless of birth weight, are considered preterm and are more likely to require intensive care and to have higher mortality rates after birth due to incomplete development. A large amount of government resources combat the factors that influence infant mortality.

1. Explain the difference between the WHO and the CDC growth charts.
2. Identify three warning signs that an infant may not be growing normally.
3. Describe how an infant's weight changes from birth to 6 months.
4. What does birth weight indicate about the mortality and morbidity risks associated with infants?
5. What U.S. regions have the highest mortality rates?
6. List factors that increase infant mortality.

Infant Development

Preview Stages of infant development are unique to each child, but a general expectation of when an infant should gain certain skills can aid in early detection of potential developmental delays.

A full understanding of the overall stages of infant development, starting with states of arousal, forms a basis for adequately monitoring the nutrition needs of infants. Infants demonstrate four general states of arousal, ranging from sleeping to fully alert. Recognizing these states of arousal can help increase feeding success because infants are more responsive to feeding during certain states of arousal. At the beginning of life, infants give subtle, inconsistent cues to suggest hunger or some other need. As infants grow, their ability to communicate develops and their messages become more consistent and direct.

An infant is born with certain protective **reflexes**. For example, the suck–swallow–breathe coordination is one of the first reflexes an infant demonstrates. This behavior is a vital part of the feeding process because it enables the infant to swallow milk while simultaneously sucking to draw out more. The behavior of suck–swallow can be seen during the 12th or 13th week of pregnancy when the fetus might suck its thumb, yawn, or make swallowing motions. By week 36 of gestation, the reflex is usually fully developed. If an infant is born before 36 weeks of gestation, the infant might need to rely on tube feedings for nourishment until the suck–swallow–breathe reflex develops.

Motor and Cognitive Development

One of the most rewarding experiences of which parents get to be a part is watching their child learn how to do new things. Clapping, waving, and crawling usually meet with excitement from those who love and care for infants. When an infant demonstrates a new skill the child has reached a **developmental milestone**. Each infant reaches developmental milestones at individual times, making it difficult to predict when an infant will learn which skill. However, knowing general ages when milestones usually occur can help parents and healthcare providers monitor infant growth and development over time. A delay in development can be a symptom of a larger problem. Early detection of certain problems can improve treatment outcomes. Common developmental milestones that occur in the first year are depicted in **FIGURE 6.6**.

The rapid advances in motor skills achieved in the first year of life can be astounding, and they generally occur in a predictable pattern. Infants first gain control of their head and neck. Once the head is under control, babies begin to develop their middle by attempting to roll over. After rolling over comes control over the legs as babies begin to push onto their knees and pull up onto their feet. Motor development also tends to move from center to peripheral. Infants can control their arms before they can grab toys or food with hands and fingers.

With motor control comes the ability to move more, which affects the amount of energy infants expend. Energy needs slowly increase as babies learn to control more and more of their body and move more. When infants have complete control of their head and neck and can sit without aid, they are usually ready to eat from a spoon. Infants who have not gained this control and who still have some early reflexes in place should not be spoon-fed because it increases their risk for **aspiration**, which occurs when infants breathe a foreign object, such as milk or juice, into their lungs.

Gaining motor skills is not the only development happening in the infant body. **Cognitive development**, learning or development that occurs in the mind, progresses rapidly during the first 2 years of life. Infants depend on interaction with the environment to learn and develop

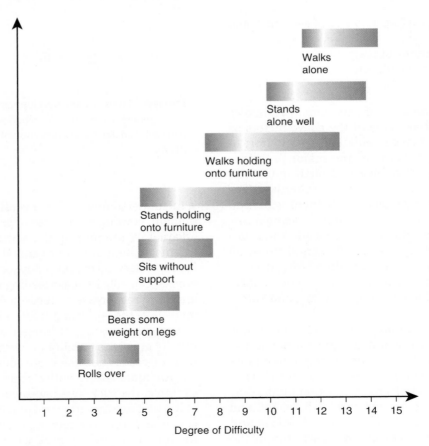

Figure 6.6
Usual infant motor development.

Table 6.2

Piaget's Stages of Cognitive Development

Stage	Age	Characteristics of Stage
Sensorimotor	0–2	The child: • Learns by doing: looking, touching, and viewing • Learns through physical interaction with the environment • Builds a set of concepts about reality and how it works • Has a primitive understanding of cause-and-effect relationships • Develops object permanence at about 9 months
Preoperational	2–7	The child: • Is not able to conceptualize abstractly and needs concrete physical situations • Uses language and symbols, including letters and numbers • Is egocentric • Conservation marks the end of the preoperational stage and the beginning of concrete operations
Concrete operations	7–11	The child: • Starts to conceptualize, creating logical structures that explain physical experiences • Demonstrates conservation, reversibility, serial ordering, and a mature understanding of cause-and-effect relationships • Begins abstract problem solving and continues with concrete thinking
Formal operations	12+	The child: • Begins to develop an abstract view of the world • Is able to apply reversibility and conservation to both real and imagined situations • Demonstrates abstract thinking, including logic, deductive reasoning, comparison, and classification • Has an increased understanding of the world and the idea of cause and effect; can develop theories about the world

Adapted from Piaget (1963).

---

ideas about the world. What they see, hear, touch, smell, and taste shapes their very earliest ideas about the world and how it works.

The **sensorimotor** stage of life allows infants to construct ideas as they experience different situations through their senses. Jean Piaget, the renowned psychologist, concluded that this first cognitive development stage encompasses six substages.[10] Feeding abilities change as infants meet the development goals of the various stages. For example, when infants gain the ability to coordinate single movements they will be able to pick up small pieces of food and develop the ability to self-feed (TABLE 6.2).[10] General motor skills, behavioral changes, and facial expressions also play important roles in the development of infants' eating habits and their ability to eat food and to drink.

For their brains to mature maximally, infants require not only adequate energy and protein but also social and emotional interactions. Genetics can also play a role in how and when the brain reaches certain stages.

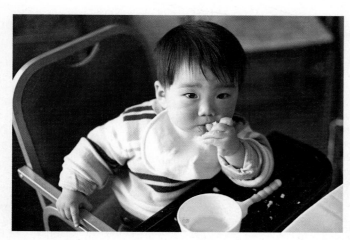
©Jack.Q/Shutterstock

Recap Understanding the overall stages of infant development is necessary to adequately monitor the nutrition needs of infants. The rapid advances in motor skills achieved in the first year of life can be astounding. Cognitive development progresses rapidly during the first 2 years of life. Research suggests that adequate nutrients and social and emotional interaction are necessary for successful development so that infants reach maximum brain maturity.

1. Give examples of reflexes that infants are born with that give them the ability to sustain life while their system continues to develop.
2. Using Piaget's model, describe what the sensorimotor stage of cognitive development is.

Infancy and Dietary Intake

Preview Infants are born with the ability to communicate their need for nourishment; however, interpretation of their messages can sometimes be difficult. It is helpful to understand the capacity of a newborn's stomach when assessing feeding intake.

The process of birth creates a dramatic shift in nutrient supply from the placenta to the infant gut. Until the first feeding, a newborn infant's gastrointestinal tract has not been exposed to anything different from amniotic fluid. To prepare the infant gut for food, particularly during the third trimester of pregnancy, infants swallow amniotic fluid, which stimulates the lining of the gastrointestinal (GI) tract to grow and mature. At birth, the infant digestive system is capable of breaking down fats, proteins, and simple sugars, and the intestinal lining is mature enough to absorb nutrients. At first, the rate of stomach emptying and peristalsis through the intestines is slow and generally inefficient, but it speeds up as the GI tract matures. By about 6 months, the infant GI tract is fully developed.

To stay alive, humans rely on **microbiomes**, the collective genomes of the microbes that live inside and on the human body. Overall, microbiomes protect humans against germs, and they break down food to release energy and produce vitamins. The gut microbiome begins to develop before birth and changes with the introduction of new foods. These microbes are essential for gut health and, as recent research is discovering,

determine the state of health an individual will enjoy over the lifetime.

Early development of healthy microbial colonies is a determinant of health in later years.[11] One factor that affects the diversity of the bacterial types found in an infant's gut is whether the infant is breastfed or formula-fed. Breastmilk contains **prebiotics** and **probiotics**, which, when introduced into an infant's gut, contribute to changing the state of the microflora and the development of intestinal mucosa. (See **FIGURE 6.7** .) Some infant formulas are fortified with prebiotics and probiotics.

The delicate balance of microflora can also be changed when infants develop diarrhea, vomit, or are given antibiotic medications. Several gut ailments are direct results of an immature gut, some which include colic, gastroesophageal reflux (GER), unexplained diarrhea, and constipation. Although the symptoms are unpleasant, these conditions do not usually hinder the growth of an infant.

Infant Feeding Patterns and Hunger Cues

Feeding a baby can become a consuming task for new parents, who are unsure how to feed the baby, when to feed the baby, and how much to feed the baby. Infants grow and develop at their own pace, requiring flexibility and adaptation with feedings. Infant feeding patterns should be based on hunger response.

The infant stomach is quite small but grows rapidly over the first 10 days of life. In the first few days of life, a newborn stomach can hold only 5–7 mL (about 1–1.5 teaspoons) of liquid per feeding. The infant will likely feed for 30 minutes to consume this volume owing to an immature feeding response, weak musculature, poor coordination of suck and swallow, and need for self-soothing through

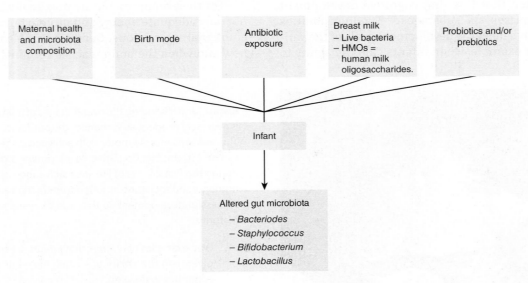

Figure 6.7
Factors that can modify the infant gut microbiome.

News You Can Use

The study of DNA sequences (genomics) has expanded into the area of the superorgans that live within our gut—our microbiome. In particular, research has focused on the microbiome of neonates. Studies have identified that the microbiome within the neonatal gut is influenced by the baby's mode of delivery (cesarean or vaginal delivery), whether the baby is breastfed or bottle-fed, and the gestational age of the infant.

Until recently, it was largely believed that the in utero environment was free of bacteria and that a fetus was not exposed to bacteria until the time of birth. Recent studies suggest, however, that the microbiome exists within the placenta, and because fetuses swallow large amounts of amniotic fluid during the last part of pregnancy, the fetal gut may in turn become colonized by these organisms.

How many organisms? An individual's microbiome is populated by approximately 100 trillion organisms. Gut bacteria are surmised to be a source of nutrients and vitamins for growing infants, and different gut bacteria carry out different roles within the human body. Understanding the role individual gut microbes play in metabolism, immunity, and even behavior is an active area of research. It cannot yet be determined whether any particular microbial profile is better than another, and indeed what is considered a healthy microbiome likely covers a wide spectrum.

It is important to include nutrients that enrich the microbiome environment as the infant diet progresses to solid foods. On the other hand, it is also essential to protect the microbiome. It is well known that altering the balance of bacteria in the digestive tract can weaken the immune system. Antibiotics, which are commonly prescribed, tend to disrupt the gut microbiome, and in infants this disruption may cause long-term consequences, including obesity, allergies, and autoimmune diseases.

---

sucking. By day 3, the stomach has expanded to accommodate 22–27 mL (less than 1 ounce) of fluid per feed. By day 10, and the onset of lactogenesis III, infant stomach capacity has grown to 60–81 mL (just under 3 ounces). The infant stomach continues to grow and the ability to take more volume per feeding continues to increase. At each increase in volume, the infant may decrease feed frequency. **FIGURE 6.8** represents the capacity of a baby's stomach during these first 10 days of life.

Shooter marble	=	Approximate stomach capacity of a newborn on day 1
Ping pong ball	=	Approximate stomach capacity on day 3
Extra-large chicken egg	=	Approximate stomach capacity on day 10

Shooter marble 5–7 mL

Ping pong ball 22–27 mL

Extra-large chicken egg 60–81 mL

Figure 6.8
The capacity of a baby's stomach during the first 10 days of life.

Recap An infant's GI tract is prepared for consumption of food well before the baby is born. A balanced gut microbiome is essential for gut health and may also determine the state of health an individual will enjoy over the lifetime. It is important to realize the capacity of a newborn's stomach to understand the amount and frequency of infant feedings.

1. Define gut microbiome and describe its role in health.
2. What is the difference in the stomach capacity of a 3-day-old infant compared with that of an adult?

Infant Feeding Skills Development

Preview Feeding skills develop gradually as an infant learns gross motor control and birth reflexes begin to disappear.

When and how quickly infants develop certain feeding skills depend on a variety of factors, ranging from their environment to parents' expectations. Infants are born with reflexes such as rooting, turning head, mouthing, gagging, and swallowing, all of which assist in the process of eating. Infants also are born with the ability to regulate appropriate amounts of food intake for their bodies at their specific stage of life. In the early stages of life, self-regulation is controlled by the sensation of pleasure associated with fullness. Hunger is regulated by this reflex until the infant is 4–6 weeks old; from this point, the infant develops the ability to purposely signal wants and needs for food.

It is difficult to outline an exact schedule of how often an infant should be eating, however; this should be dictated by the infant. Parents and caregivers should be aware of the unique hunger cues of their child and respond appropriately. In some phases, infants may eat more often than usual. This is referred to as cluster feeding and describes when a baby shifts from feeding every 2 or 3 hours to feeding every hour or feeding in spurts. Cluster feeding is most common during the evening hours and in young babies; however, older babies who are approaching a growth spurt or developmental changes may also cluster feed. Understanding a baby's stomach capacity, especially during the first 10 days of life, helps to explain why cluster feeds may occur.

Infant Feeding Position

Improper positioning of an infant for feedings from a bottle or a spoon is associated with choking, discomfort while eating, and ear infections. When infants are offered a bottle, they should be in a semiupright position as if they were sitting in a car seat or infant carrier. This allows infants to swallow all of their milk and prevents milk from sitting inside of the baby's mouth, or at the back of the ears, a situation called "pooling." When milk pools at the back of the ears, the risk of ear infections increases.[27] Unfortunately, some infants are fed in unsafe positions, such as when a baby is placed on a pillow or a bottle is propped with a blanket. This increases the risk of choking and aspiration.

The recommended position for infant sleeping is on the back without propping the head; this position is *not* recommended for feeding. Spoon-feeding is most successful when an infant is capable of controlling its head and mouth. Placing babies in a seated position with good support of their back and feet helps them control their mouth and head better. The person offering the food should sit directly in front of the infant, and the baby should not have to turn the head to receive the food. A high chair is the best support for infants when they are capable of sitting on their own. Ensure that the infant is sitting with legs and torso at a 90-degree angle. Lying back changes the position of the stomach and may contribute to spitting up.

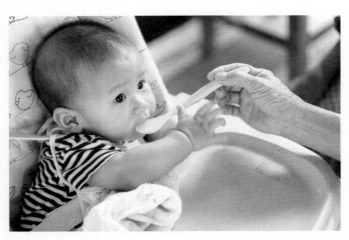

©BonNontawat/Shutterstock

Introducing Solid Foods

An infant's readiness for solid foods, around the age of 6 months, is judged with a model that looks for signs of readiness, such as moving the tongue from side to side, keeping the head upright, and sitting with little support. The solid food readiness milestone also depends on the strength of several inborn reflexes. The tongue thrust reflex is when an infant's tongue extends out of the mouth when the lips are touched. If this reflex is still strong, an infant will have a difficult time keeping food in the mouth. The gag reflex is strong in young infants to protect them from swallowing inappropriate foods or objects. If an object touches the back of the tongue, the object is propelled forward.

Once these reflexes have lessened and the baby has reached the other developmental milestones, the infant is ready for solid foods. Infants adapt quickly to different feeding practices and regiments. Recognizing an infant's specific cues of hunger, satiation, tiredness, and discomfort helps parents progress feedings appropriately. A few common infant cues include the following:

- Excitement when they see food might mean they are hungry.
- Tight fists or reaching for the spoon can indicate hunger.
- Crying or fussing when the pace of feeding is too slow or the feeder stops can indicate hunger.
- Slowed pace of eating can indicate satiation.
- Playing with food or the spoon as they start to get full.
- Refusing to open mouth or spitting food out indicates they are finished.

Solid foods should first be offered to an infant on a spoon. The amount of food eaten in this stage is minimal and is more for developing eating skills than for providing nourishment. Offering food from a spoon stimulates the muscles in the mouth and allows them to develop. Begin with 1–2 tablespoons of semisoft foods for each meal, one to two times a day. If the feedings become frustrating for caregiver or baby, feeding with a spoon can be stopped and reintroduced over time (2–5 days). Sometimes the infant has not mastered a necessary development stage. A bit more time may solve the problem and make solid food feeding more enjoyable.

Babies are sensitive to change, and new tastes and smells may be disturbing to them. Some techniques that can help improve an infant's first experience with solid foods are as follows:

- Feed babies when they are active and playful.
- Allow babies to signal when they will eat by waiting for them to open their mouth and extend the tongue forward.
- Place the bowl of the spoon on the tongue with a slight downward pressure toward the front of the mouth.
- Keep the spoon level; using the baby's gums to scrape food from spoon may increase the risk of choking.

- Infant should set the pace of feeding; food should not be offered to infants again until they have swallowed.
- First feedings should consist of 5–6 spoonfuls and last no longer than 10 minutes.

First Foods

One of the best foods to start with is infant rice cereal that has been thinned with breast milk or formula to a semiliquid consistency. Rice cereal is easy to prepare and has a very mild taste that is more familiar to the infant. It is also a safe food because it is hypoallergenic and easily digested. Fruits and vegetables are also common first foods, depending on culture and ethnicity. New foods should be offered one at a time and should be spaced over a day or two to determine whether any food allergies are present.

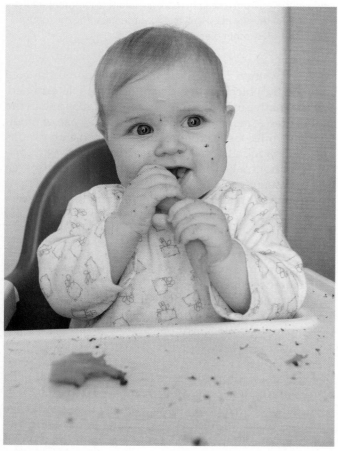

©rzucamokiem/Shutterstock

As infants progress to thicker, lumpier foods, they can eat many of the foods eaten by older children and adults. Some of these foods include applesauce, mashed potatoes, yogurt, soft green beans, and chopped cooked noodles. Although this is convenient, an infant's food intake should be based on need and not on what is available. Portion sizes should also be determined by the infant; when they are full they will stop eating. Caregivers should not force them to eat more than they need.

Care must be taken to avoid inappropriate foods that are unsafe for the baby. These include foods that increase the risk of choking. The following is a list of common foods associated with fatal choking incidences:

- Hot dog pieces
- Hard candy, jelly beans
- Nuts, including peanuts and chunky peanut butter
- Whole grapes
- Uncut tough meat, sausage
- Sticky foods like marshmallows, gum, and gummy candy
- Hard raw fruits and vegetables

These foods present a hazard because infant chewing ability is undeveloped. Pieces of underchewed foods can obstruct airways because an infant has not developed the ability to cough or clear the throat. Foods that break apart easily, such as potato chips, may also present choking hazards because such foods can crumble and be swallowed before they are chewed completely.

Drinking from a Cup

Transitioning from breastfeeding or bottle feeds to solid foods occurs toward the end of the first year and is usually complete by the time an infant becomes a toddler. Infants that are exclusively breastfed usually go from the breast to a cup, skipping the bottle completely. It is best to begin introducing a cup to breastfed infants around 6 months. Generally, infants begin to show interest in drinking from a cup at 6–8 months of age. They are usually not developmentally ready at this point and are incapable of elevating the tongue to control the liquid; however, by 10–12 months infants can control the cup and the movement of the tongue.

It is important to continue bottle- or breastfeeding while introducing new foods. Infants who stop taking bottle- or breastfeeding too early tend to have little or no change in weight following a period of active weight gain because they are not receiving an adequate amount of calories and fluid without the familiar technique of

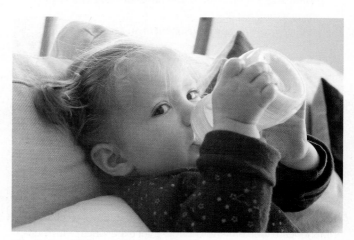

©PhotoAlto Agency RF Collections/Anne-Sophie Bost/Getty

bottle- or breastfeeding. The transition to solid foods is complete when the food and liquids that the infant takes in daily are equal in calories to the amount provided by bottle feeds or breast milk.

Food Preferences

Infants learn food preferences from their experiences with foods. Breastfed infants may be exposed to a wider variety of tastes through breastmilk. Studies have concluded that infants at the age of 4–7 months have a more rapid acceptance of new foods than those who are introduced to new foods after 12 months. A renowned pediatrician, Clara Davis, conducted many studies on infant self-selection of foods. Her studies demonstrate that older infants are capable of selecting a well-balanced diet. However, these results are susceptible to misinterpretation.

Food preferences are largely learned, but there is some evidence of genetic predisposition to sweet tastes and away from bitter tastes.[11] Also, parents and caregivers should be sensitive to the needs of their infants. An infant's refusal to eat may be a need for attention or a complaint against a discomfort rather than a message of dislike for that food.

Case Study

Clara is now 10 months old and weighs 16 pounds. She seems to have good body control, can stand, but cannot walk. She continues to feed from a bottle and eats about 8 ounces per feeding, five times per day. Occasionally, her parents offer her baby food, but they are hesitant to offer too much variety because they are concerned about various food allergies. Her formula is a regular cow's-milk-based formula. Clara struggles with fussiness and irritability.

Questions

1. Is the amount that Clara is eating adequate for her age?
2. What suggestions would you have for Clara's parents in progressing her diet?
3. Is Clara growing and developing at an acceptable rate?

Recap When and how quickly infants develop certain feeding skills depends on a variety of factors, ranging from their environment to their parents' expectations. Infants are born with the ability to regulate appropriate amounts of food intake for their bodies at their specific stage of life. They are also born with the ability to know their exact needs, so they should determine when and how much they eat. An infant's readiness for progressing to solid food is based on developmental changes. Infants learn food preferences from their experiences with foods,

and parents and caregivers need to be sensitive to the needs of their infants.

1. List three improper positions of an infant for feedings from a bottle or a spoon.
2. Identify signs of readiness for a 6-month-old infant to begin eating solid foods.
3. Why is it important to continue bottle- or breastfeeding while introducing new foods?

Nutritional Recommendations and Requirements During Infancy

Preview Nutritional recommendations are based on information gathered from research. There are infant recommendations in place for energy needs, all macronutrients, some micronutrients, and a few other diet components.

The composition of human milk is considered the gold standard by which infant nutrient needs are determined. The alternative to breastmilk is infant formula, and in the United States, most infant formulas have a base of modified cow's milk or soy protein, supplemented with various nutrients required to meet federal regulations.

Specific intake guidelines for infants are research based. Research enables various governmental and nongovernmental organizations to create comprehensive recommendations that provide for the overall health of most infants. These organizations include the following:

- The Academy of Pediatrics
- The National Academy of Medicine (develops Dietary Reference Intakes [DRIs])
- The Academy of Nutrition and Dietetics
- The European Society for Pediatric Gastroenterology, Hepatology, and Nutrition

Energy Needs

The typical infant needs more energy per pound of body weight during this stage of life compared with any other time. Relative to size, an infant's energy needs are twice those of an adult. Total energy intake is based on the weight of the infant in kilograms (kg), creating a broad range of energy requirements for infants; however, most newborns require about 100 kilocalories per kilogram of body weight.[12] **TABLE 6.3** provides equations for calculating infants' Estimated Energy Requirements (EERs).

As an infant grows and develops, allocation of energy changes. For example, infants 0–6 months of age require more calories for growth and fewer calories for physical activity compared with the same infant at 6–12 months old. Factors such as weight, growth rate, sleeping cycle, climate and temperature, physical activity, health status, and metabolic rate all determine infant kilocalorie needs.

Table 6.3

Estimated Energy Requirement Recommended Daily Allowance During Infancy

EER Equation	Age (months)
(89 × wt [kg] − 100) + 175 kcal/day	0–3
(89 × wt [kg]) + 56 kcal/day	4–6
(89 × wt [kg]) + 22 kcal/day	7–12

Modified from Institute of Medicine, Food and Nutrition Board. Dietary Reference Intakes for energy, carbohydrate, fiber, fat, fatty acids, cholesterol, protein, and amino acids (macronutrients). Washington, DC: National Academies Press; 2005.

The recommended distribution of calories in infancy is 40–50% from fat, 7–11% from protein, and the remainder from carbohydrates.[13] Because infants have high calorie needs but can consume only small amounts at a time, reliance on fat in the diet is essential. Fat is the most concentrated source of calories compared to carbohydrates and protein. A high-fat diet is also necessary for normal brain growth, which continues through 18 to 24 months of age.

Lipids

Triglycerides are the major energy source in human milk, providing about 50–55% of its total calories. Standard infant formulas match this composition. Infants should have at least 30 g of fat per day.[14]

Human milk provides essential fatty acids: the omega-6 fatty acid arachidonic acid (ARA) and two long-chain omega-3 fatty acids, eicosapentaenoic acid (EPA) and docosahexaenoic acid (DHA). Fatty acids such as DHA and ARA contribute to infant development in a variety of ways, most notably infant growth, brain and retinal development, immune function, and health.[15] DHA and ARA are naturally occurring in breastmilk and are commonly added to infant formula.

Protein

Protein needs are determined as grams per kilogram of body weight and change with infant growth and development. **TABLE 6.4** provides protein recommendations for infants 0 to 12 months of age.[16]

Human milk and infant formula provide protein that includes all of the essential amino acids needed for growth and development. Human milk protein is a more

Table 6.4

Protein Adequate Intake or Recommended Dietary Allowance for Infants

Age	
0–6 months	1.2 grams/kg
7–12 months	1.5 grams/kg or 11 grams/day

easily digested and absorbable source of protein than cow's milk.

Functions of protein for infants include the following:

- Build, maintain, and repair new tissues.
- Manufacture important hormones, enzymes, antibodies, and other components.
- Regulate specialized body functions.

The amount of protein needed to maintain a constant supply of essential amino acids for proper growth is high during the first year. For caregivers who are preparing infant formula, it is important that the formula be mixed according to package specifications. Mixing formula that is either too concentrated or too diluted affects the protein concentration, resulting in either excessive or inadequate protein intake.

Carbohydrates

Body metabolism is fueled by glucose, a major component of carbohydrates. Glucose is ready energy that infants use for growth, activity, and necessary bodily functions. When glucose is limited owing to infrequent feedings or other factors, a child's growth is limited by the amount of glucose the body is lacking. In a state of glucose depletion, the infant body uses amino acids as energy to maintain critical body processes. At the onset of need, the body first uses the amino acids circulating in the blood for glucose production; after this source is depleted, the body begins to break down protein in muscle to produce needed energy. Ongoing breakdown of protein may cause growth stunting because fats and proteins are being used for energy instead of as building blocks for new growth and development.

Vitamin D

Vitamin D is a fat-soluble vitamin that is required for bone mineralization and proper utilization of calcium and phosphorus in the blood. Evidence also suggests a role for vitamin D in maintaining innate immunity and preventing diseases such as cancer and diabetes.[17] Vitamin D is a unique substance that can be formed in the body but that requires ultraviolet (UV) rays from sunlight to activate it.

Breastmilk contains a small amount of vitamin D but that is not adequate for proper infant development; therefore, exclusively breastfed infants should receive a supplement of vitamin D shortly after birth.[17] The current American Academy of Pediatrics (AAP) recommendations for vitamin D intake is 400 IU per day for all infants, children, and adolescents, beginning the first few days after birth.[18]

Deficiency of vitamin D is known as rickets and can have severe and lasting effects on children as they grow. Inadequate intake of vitamin D also decreases intestinal absorption of calcium and phosphorus, causing improper mineralization of bones and teeth and resulting in swelled joints, bowed legs, and poor growth during childhood. (See **FIGURE 6.9**.)

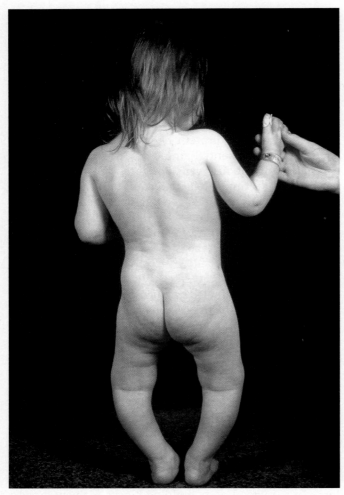

Figure 6.9
Infant with Rickets.

©Biophoto Associates/Science Source/Getty

Iron

A full-term infant is born with iron stores that reflect the mother's iron levels. If the mother consumes an iron-rich diet during pregnancy, the fetus builds iron stores to last the first 4–6 months of life. By 6 months, a breast-fed infant needs an additional iron source, at which time, iron-fortified infant cereals can meet this need. The AAP recommends iron-fortified formula for all formula-fed babies. Preterm infants have lower iron stores at birth that are depleted around 2–3 months of age.[19] Human milk is a source of iron, and compared with infant formula, a higher percentage of the iron in breastmilk is absorbed: 50% of the iron in breastmilk is absorbed, compared to about 4% of the iron in infant formula. The AAP makes the following recommendations concerning iron supplementation:[20]

- Full-term exclusively breastfed infants 4–6 months of age need 1 mg/kg/day of iron from a supplemental source, preferably from complementary foods. These foods include iron-fortified infant cereals and meats.

- Oral iron supplementation for breastfed infants unable to consume sufficient iron from complementary foods.
- Only iron-fortified formula should be used for infants younger than 1 year of age, including during weaning and when formula is a supplement to breast milk.

Iron-deficiency anemia is a direct result of low iron consumption. This condition can cause irreversible abnormalities in behavior and brain function.

Fluoride

Although fluoride is not considered an essential nutrient, it has beneficial effects on tooth formation. Fluoride is incorporated into the mineral structure of teeth, creating stronger teeth that are more resistant to decay. The current DRI for fluoride is 0.1 mg/day for infants younger than 6 months, and 0.5 mg/day for infants 7–12 months of age.[20] Care must be taken to avoid too much fluoride, which is possible if supplements are provided. Excessive fluoride can cause tooth discoloration later in life. Water fluoridation is common in many areas of the United States, and infants who live in areas with fluoridated water systems do not require supplementation. Supplementation is recommended in the following instances:

- Breastfed infants who live in areas with nonfluoridated water
- Formula-fed infants who live in areas with nonfluoridated water
- Infants who live in families that use bottled water as their regular water source for drinking and cooking. (If water is fortified with fluoride, it is adequate.)

Sodium

Sodium is an essential mineral needed for maintenance of fluid balance in the body. Infant requirements for sodium are 120 mg from birth to 5 months, and 200 mg for 6- to 12-month-old infants.[20] The amount of sodium found in breastmilk was used to set the adequate amount infants need daily. Aside from either formula or breastmilk, infants do not need added sodium to maintain adequate sodium levels.

Lead

Lead is not a nutrient, but an association is recognized between lead and calcium and iron stores. Elevated blood lead levels can be toxic to the human body. This toxicity can interrupt brain development, slow growth, and interfere with calcium and iron absorption. If an infant is exposed to lead, it is generally inadvertently. Lead contamination is sometimes found in water pipes of homes, particularly in homes built before 1950. Older homes may also contain lead-based paint, which can be toxic to infants. Also, lead is present in fuels and other chemicals to which adults may be exposed. They can unknowingly expose their infant to lead dust through infant contact with unwashed bodies or clothes. Lead dust can settle in laundry areas and can be transferred to baby clothes or bedding.

Fiber

An Adequate Intake (AI) for fiber in infants has been established. Breastmilk does not contain fiber, so typical infants do not consume dietary fiber until complementary foods are introduced. From 6 months to 12 months fiber-containing foods may be gradually introduced to infants until they consume 5 g of fiber per day.[20] Good sources of fiber for infants include whole-grain cereals, green vegetables, and legumes.

Water

Water is an essential nutrient required by infants for various functions, including regulation of body temperature, transport of nutrients and waste, metabolism in cells, and normal kidney function. An infant's water needs are typically met from consuming breastmilk, formula, and other foods. Supplemental water is not needed even in hot, dry climates. Excessive water intake may be detrimental to the health of an infant and can have severe consequences, including edema, irritability, hypothermia, reduced caloric intake, and seizures.[21]

Dehydration is a concern among infants because they have a limited ability to signal that they are thirsty. Common signs of dehydration include the following:

- Reduced amount of urine and urine that is dark in color
- Dry membranes in nose and mouth
- No tears when crying
- Sunken eyes
- Lethargy, restlessness, irritability

If an infant is noted to have any of these symptoms, medical attention is necessary.

Recap The typical infant needs more energy per pound of body weight during this stage of life compared with at any other time. Nutrient functions beginning in infancy stay consistent through the life span. Fat is used by infants to fuel the liver, brain, and muscles. An infant needs a constant source of high-quality protein to build, maintain, and repair new tissues; manufacture important hormones, enzymes, antibodies, and other components; and regulate specialized body functions. Carbohydrates are used for growth, activity, and necessary bodily functions. Vitamin D is required for bone mineralization and proper usage of calcium and phosphorus in the blood. Iron and fluoride are the most concerning, and inadequate intakes of these can alter infant growth and development. Sodium is an essential mineral needed for maintenance of fluid balance in the body. Lead is not a nutrient, but an association is recognized between lead and

calcium and iron stores. Water is an essential nutrient required by infants for various functions, including regulation of body temperature, transport of nutrients and waste, metabolism in cells, and normal kidney function. Adequate growth of infants is a good indicator that they are consuming all of the essential nutrients.

1. What are the intake recommendations for energy, lipids, carbohydrate, and protein for infants?
2. What is a consequence of excessive fluoride intake?

Common Nutrition Considerations During Infancy

Preview A few common nutritional concerns that affect infants are colic, lactose intolerance, constipation, and diarrhea. These conditions can have a large influence on the amount of food an infant eats. Cultural issues and breastfeeding mothers' vegetarian diet also introduce issues in regard to infant intake and possible supplement needs.

Colic

Colic is often defined by the "rule of three": crying for more than 3 hours per day, for more than 3 days per week, and for more than 3 weeks in an infant who is well fed and otherwise healthy.[22] Colic is a difficult condition to understand and usually has no specific determinable cause. Parents find this condition extremely frustrating and most often think the infant is experiencing abdominal pain. Because this condition is so ambiguous, opinions and ideas on how to cure colic proliferate.

Parents are usually bombarded with ideas on what works and what does not. One common practice includes changing formula if an infant is not breastfeeding, and many believe that what a breastfeeding mother eats may change the composition of the milk she produces, thus creating or eliminating symptoms of colic. Some studies suggest that the use of probiotics manages infantile colic.[23] For breastfeeding mothers, removing bananas from the diet and consuming protein-rich foods, grapes, lemons, and potatoes have been shown to act as protective mechanisms against colic.[24] A few simple actions may also help soothe the baby and reduce the severity or duration of colic episodes. These include rocking the infant, swaddling, bathing, burping, and other soothing actions.

Lactose Intolerance

Lactose intolerance is given as an excuse for many normal behaviors during infancy. True lactose intolerance should be based on a medical diagnosis that is confirmed by testing the gastrointestinal tract for specific bacteria. Symptoms of lactose intolerance include cramps, nausea, alternating diarrhea and constipation, or pain. These symptoms are similar to those of colic or those that occur with minor illnesses.

Lactose is the principal carbohydrate in dairy products and is found in all foods made from dairy. It is also present in cow's-milk-based formulas. Because the human body does not produce lactase, the enzyme needed to break down lactose, we depend on our gut bacteria to produce lactase. A change in the gastrointestinal tract resulting from illness or infection may temporarily change the infant's ability to digest lactose. Also, other infants may not have the correct strain of bacteria needed to produce lactase or enough of the bacteria to produce the correct volume of lactase. Lactose-free formulas replace the lactose with other sources of carbohydrates like sucrose or modified corn starch or the lactose has been broken into monosaccharides during the processing of the formula. Most infants who have been fed lactose-free formula will be able to eat dairy products as they get older and their gut flora become stronger.

Constipation and Diarrhea

Infant stool patterns can create concern among parents and caregivers. Constipation, or infrequent bowel movements, is usually not a concern of breastfed infants because their stool is generally soft and frequent. Formula-fed infants may deal with constipation at varying levels depending on the type of formula used. To avoid constipation, caregivers should ensure that the formula is mixed correctly so that the infant is getting enough water. Also, avoid use of medications unless they are prescribed for the infant. Some parents will use prune or other juices to encourage a bowel movement; this could potentially create a fluid imbalance and should be avoided. Excessive fruit juice intake is a common cause of diarrhea in this population. Increasing fiber intake among infants is also not recommended, the types of foods that are high in fiber are considered choking hazards.

Diarrhea can become a serious problem among infants. The cause of diarrhea is often not identifiable, but it is primarily caused by gastrointestinal infections, viral and bacterial, or other factors. It is recommended that infants be fed as usual during episodes of diarrhea because adequate fluid intake is usually enough to prevent dehydration during this time.[25]

Cross-Cultural Considerations

Culture can have a major impact on how an infant is fed and at what age solid foods are introduced. Breastfeeding may be expected in some cultures, whereas in others it is not generally accepted as normal and healthy. Also, the type of first foods given to an infant are unique to cultures and belief systems. Commercially prepared baby foods are considered normal and preferable in many American homes, but there is little ethnic variety in the baby foods for sale at the grocery store. Many ethnic foods can be a safe part of an infant's introduction to new foods;

however, parents should be educated on which foods are appropriate and which foods should be avoided. Education may be needed in some homes depending on the parents' level of understanding. Safe cultural practices should be encouraged and unsafe practices should be pointed out to parents with possible alternatives as part of the explanation. This respect for clients' and patients' ethnicity can promote open communication and increase willingness of families to participate in assistance programs such as WIC or early-intervention programs.

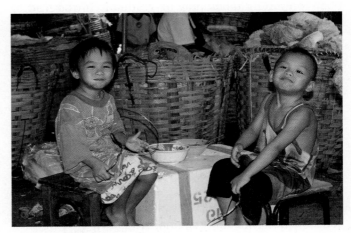
©Malcolm McDougall Photography/Alamy Stock Photo

Vegetarian Diets

Vegetarian diets can provide adequate nutrition for infants if they are carefully planned and executed. More restrictive diets such as vegan or macrobiotic diets can affect growth rates in infants. The degree to which vegetarian diets are considered adequate depends on the amount of restriction practiced in the diet. Mothers who practice vegan diets produce breastmilk with a different composition from breastmilk of mothers who eat a meat-based diet. When infants of vegan mothers are exclusively breastfed, mothers should pay particular attention to protein, omega-3 essential fatty acids, iron, calcium, and vitamin D and vitamin B_{12} intake.[26]

Case Study

Clara is now 12 months old. She can sit by herself with no support. She can stand but is not walking on her own. Over the past few months, she has transitioned to solid foods well and eats a wide variety of foods three times a day. She is still receiving formula three to five times a day and eats 6–8 ounces at each feeding. She has less fussiness and is sleeping 7–8 hours a night. She is still irritable at times, especially after a bottle feeding, and struggles with gassiness and regular bouts of diarrhea.

Upon examination at the doctor's office, Clara is diagnosed with an ear infection. In addition, Clara is diagnosed with an allergy to wheat.

Questions

1. Should Clara be experiencing the symptoms of colic at this age? What else could be causing her GI symptoms?
2. Explain what eating circumstances might contribute to Clara's ear infection.
3. Provide a list of foods that Clara should avoid because of her wheat allergy, and write a 2-day meal plan for her.

Recap Conditions of colic, lactose intolerance, constipation, and diarrhea should be addressed because they could be symptoms of a larger problem and can affect the amount of food infants eat. Cultural considerations and breastfeeding mothers who are vegetarian introduce unique feeding issues for infants.

1. How do colic, lactose intolerance, constipation, and diarrhea affect infant intake?
2. Vegan mothers who exclusively breastfeed their infants should pay particular attention to which nutrients?

Promoting Healthy Lifestyles

Preview Education, intervention programs, and newborn screenings can all contribute to better infant health as families adopt healthy lifestyles.

A common goal of many parents is to provide their babies with the type of care that encourages them to adopt healthy lifestyles, a task that can be hindered as a result of lack of education, resources, and monetary means. Many intervention programs such as WIC, Head Start, and the Bright Future in Practice initiative help parents reach the goal of raising healthy children from birth to adulthood. Following is a sample of topics covered in such education programs:

- Appropriate use of infant formula
- Baby food and sanitation
- Home-prepared baby foods
- Hunger and satiation cues
- Feeding position
- When to be concerned about spitting up, constipation, and diarrhea
- Keeping baby safe

Further education about how parents can create healthful home environments may be beneficial as well. Children exposed to smoking in the home have increased risk of disease. Also, the American Academy of Pediatrics recommends that infants should not be exposed to any screen time, including television, computers, or personal electronic devises. Early learning is often a draw for some parents to use these devices, but the exposure to this type of brain stimulation may be more detrimental than helpful.

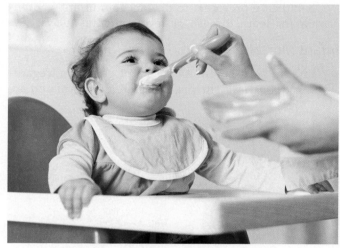

©Diego Cervo/Shutterstock

Some health conditions might be present at birth but not show symptoms until later in life. In many of these conditions, early diagnosis and nutrition intervention can prolong life and avoid disability. Newborn screening is conducted on all infants in the United States. Screenings include up to 60 different conditions. Phenylketonuria (PKU), and **galactosemia** are examples of conditions that, if detected, can be treated with a therapeutic diet to avoid detrimental side effects.

Recap Education, intervention programs, and newborn screenings all contribute to infant health. A common goal of parents is to provide their children with care that encourages them to adopt healthy lifestyles.

1. List three common subjects of nutrition education that are offered to new parents to help them adopt healthy lifestyles for their newborns.
2. Provide two examples of common newborn screenings conducted on all infants in the United States.

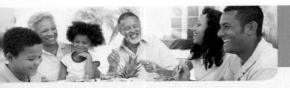

Learning Portfolio

Visual Chapter Summary

Assessing Newborn Health

■ Although it is normal for birth weights and lengths to vary, general trends in weight and length allow healthcare providers to diagnose an infant's potential for death, disease, or developmental delays.

Infant Mortality

■ Infants born before 37 weeks of gestation, regardless of birth weight, are considered preterm and are

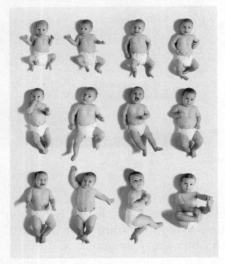

©Rob Goldman/The Image Bank/Getty

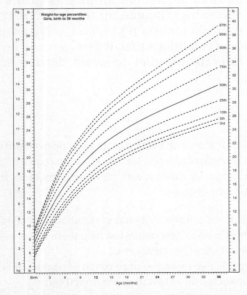

Developed by the National Center for Health Statistics in collaboration with the National Center for Chronic Disease Prevention and Health Promotion (2000).

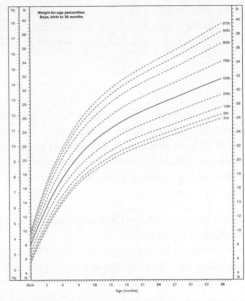

Developed by the National Center for Health Statistics in collaboration with the National Center for Chronic Disease Prevention and Health Promotion (2000).

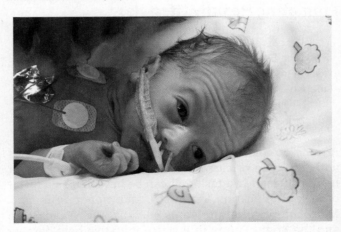

©Gert vrey/Shutterstock

more likely to require intensive care and to have higher mortality rates after birth because of incomplete development.

■ Large amounts of government resources are in place to support infant and maternal health before, during, and after pregnancy.

Infant Development

■ Understanding the overall stages of infant development is necessary to adequately monitor the nutrition needs of infants.

Table 6.2

Piaget's Stages of Cognitive Development

Stage	Age	Characteristics of Stage
Sensorimotor	0–2	The child: • Learns by doing: looking, touching, and viewing • Learns through physical interaction with the environment • Builds a set of concepts about reality and how it works • Has a primitive understanding of cause-and-effect relationships • Develops object permanence at about 9 months
Preoperational	2–7	The child: • Is not able to conceptualize abstractly and needs concrete physical situations • Uses language and symbols, including letters and numbers • Is egocentric • Conservation marks the end of the preoperational stage and the beginning of concrete operations
Concrete operations	7–11	The child: • Starts to conceptualize, creating logical structures that explain physical experiences • Demonstrates conservation, reversibility, serial ordering, and a mature understanding of cause-and-effect relationships • Begins abstract problem solving and continues with concrete thinking
Formal operations	12+	The child: • Begins to develop an abstract view of the world • Is able to apply reversibility and conservation to both real and imagined situations • Demonstrates abstract thinking, including logic, deductive reasoning, comparison, and classification • Has an increased understanding of the world and the idea of cause and effect; can develop theories about the world

Adapted from Piaget (1963).

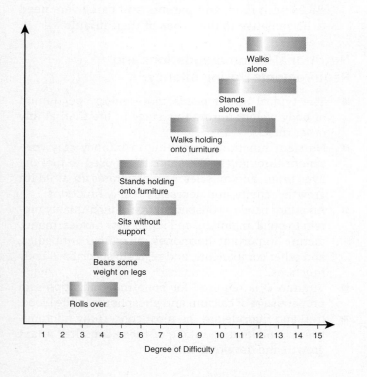

- The rapid advances in motor skills achieved in the first year of life can be astounding.
- Cognitive development progresses swiftly during the first 2 years of life.
- Research suggests that not only are adequate nutrients necessary for successful infant development but also social and emotional interaction is required for infants to reach maximum brain maturity.
- It is necessary to closely monitor infant growth to identify possible health problems.
- Growth can indicate the adequacy of a child's nutritional intake or ability to feed, and if an infant's growth slows, this may be an early sign of disease or disorder.
- Standardized growth charts are used to monitor and evaluate an infant's growth patterns.

Infancy and Dietary Intake

- An infant's GI tract is prepared for consumption of food well before the baby is born.

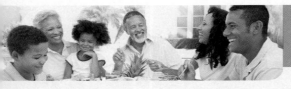

Learning Portfolio (continued)

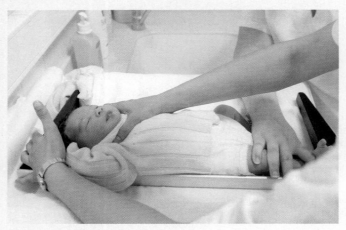

©CHASSENET/BSIP SA/Alamy Stock Photo

Shooter marble	=	Approximate stomach capacity of a newborn on day 1
Ping pong ball	=	Approximate stomach capacity on day 3
Extra-large chicken egg	=	Approximate stomach capacity on day 10

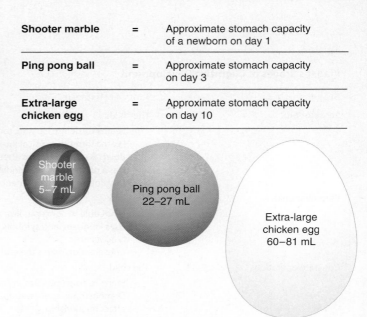

Shooter marble 5–7 mL

Ping pong ball 22–27 mL

Extra-large chicken egg 60–81 mL

- The gut's microbiome is essential for gut health and may also determine the state of health an individual will enjoy over the lifetime.
- It is important to know the capacity of a newborn's stomach to understand the amount and frequency of infant feedings.
- Infant feeding patterns are based on hunger response and, at times, are difficult for caregivers to assess.
- When and how quickly an infant develops certain feeding skills depends on a variety of factors, ranging from their environment to their parents' expectations.
- Infants are born with the ability to regulate food intake to an appropriate level for their body at their specific stage of life.

Infant Feeding Skills Development

- Infants are born with the ability to know their exact needs and should be the determinant of when and how much they eat.
- Assessing an infant's readiness for solid food is based on models that look for signs of readiness.
- Infants learn food preferences from their experiences with food, and parents and caregivers need to be sensitive to the needs of their infants.

Nutritional Recommendations and Requirements During Infancy

- The typical infant needs more energy per pound of body weight during this stage of life than at any other time.
- Nutrient functions beginning in infancy stay consistent through the life span. Fat is used to fuel the liver, brain, and muscles. Carbohydrates are used for growth, activity, and necessary bodily functions.
- An infant needs a constant source of high-quality protein to build, maintain, and repair new tissues; manufacture important hormones, enzymes, antibodies, and other components; and regulate specialized body functions.
- Vitamin D is required for bone mineralization and proper usage of calcium and phosphorus in the blood.
- Iron and fluoride are the most concerning micronutrients; inadequate intake of these can alter infant growth and development.

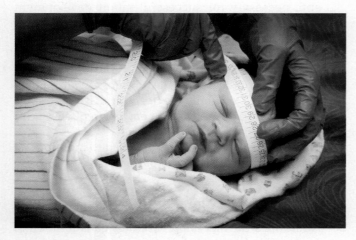

©Alice Jeanette Brown/Shutterstock

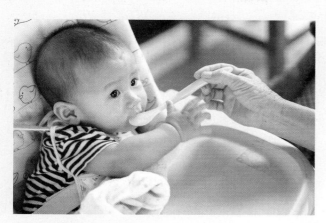

©BonNontawat/Shutterstock

Common Nutrition Considerations During Infancy

- Conditions of colic, lactose intolerance, constipation, and diarrhea should be addressed because they could be symptoms of a larger problem and can have a large impact on the amount of food an infant eats.
- Cultural considerations and breastfeeding mothers who are vegetarian introduce unique feeding issues for infants.
- Education, intervention programs, and newborn screenings all contribute to infant health.

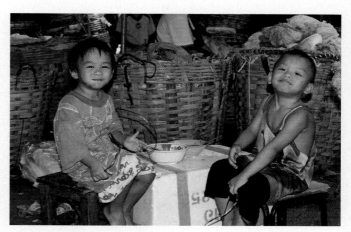

©Malcolm McDougall Photography/Alamy Stock Photo

Promoting Healthy Lifestyles

- A common goal of many parents is to provide their child with care that encourages them to adopt healthy lifestyles.

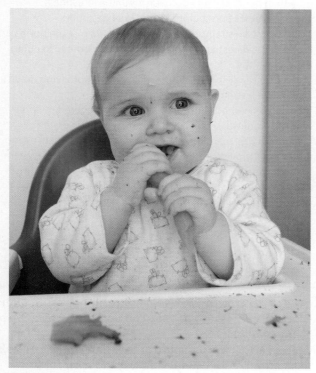

©rzucamokiem/Shutterstock

- Sodium is an essential mineral needed for maintenance of fluid balance in the body.
- Lead is not a nutrient, but an association is recognized between lead and calcium and iron stores.
- Water is an essential nutrient required by infants for various functions, including regulation of body temperature, transport of nutrients and waste, metabolism in cells, and normal kidney function.
- Adequate infant growth is a good indicator that infants are being provided with all of the essential nutrients.

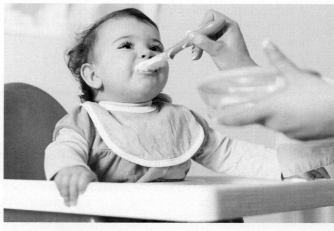

©Diego Cervo/Shutterstock

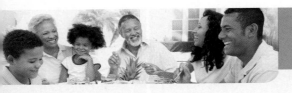

Learning Portfolio (continued)

Key Terms

appropriate for gestational age (AGA): Weight, head, and length within normal measurements for gestational age.

aspiration: Inhalation of food particles or water when the airway is not protected.

cluster feeding: When a baby shifts from feeding every 2 to 3 hours to feeding every hour or feeding in spurts.

cognitive development: Learning that occurs in the mind.

colic: Marked periods of irritability, fussiness, or crying in an infant between 2 weeks and 3 months who is generally healthy.

developmental milestone: Certain behaviors or physical skills infants gain as they grow and develop.

full term: Babies born between 37 and 42 weeks of gestation.

galactosemia: A genetic disorder that creates an inability to metabolize galactose, a common carbohydrate found in milk and a by-product of lactose metabolism. It results in an inability to use galactose to produce energy.

gestation: How long an infant is carried in the womb from conception to birth, usually measured in weeks.

growth stunting: A primary manifestation of malnutrition that results in reduced linear growth rate.

head circumference: A measurement of a child's head around its largest area. It measures the distance from above the eyebrows and ears and around the back of the head.

hypoallergenic: Foods that have a low risk of promoting food or other allergies.

infant mortality: Occurrence of death within the first 5 years of life.

large for gestational age (LGA): Weight, head, and length above the 90th percentile for gestational age.

low birth weight (LBW): Less than 2,500 g (5.5 pounds) at birth.

microbiomes: Collective colonies of different microbes that reside in the large intestine.

neonatal: Classification of infants directly after birth to 28 days.

postnatal: The period after childbirth.

prebiotics: A nondigestible food ingredient that promotes the growth of beneficial microorganisms in the intestine.

preterm: Babies born before 37 weeks of gestation.

probiotics: Live strains of bacteria and yeasts that are normally found in the digestive system and that contribute to keeping the gut healthy.

recumbent length: Measuring an infant's length lying down in a completely stretched out position.

reflexes: Unlearned, automatic responses triggered by some type of stimulus.

sensorimotor: Learning system where the infant's senses and motor skills provide information to the central nervous system to encourage further development.

small for gestational age (SGA): Weight below the 10th percentile for gestational age.

Discussion Questions

1. What are factors that contribute to infant mortality and which programs in the United States are in place to support infant health?
2. Explain the concept of developmental milestones and how it correlates with infant feeding.
3. How are growth charts useful for monitoring infant health over time, and how can points on the curve be interpreted?
4. What is the best indicator of adequate nutrition intake in infants? Discuss various ways to monitor this.

Activities

1. Find a new mother who is willing to talk with you about her child. Ask questions about the infant's birth, growth, and health concerns. Review growth charts and plot the rate of growth experienced by the infant.
2. During hot summer days, how much and what types of fluid should a caregiver provide to a 12-month-old infant to avoid dehydration?
3. If you were a parent following a vegetarian diet, what would be some of the questions you would have regarding nourishment of your infant?
4. Discuss reasons that parental attitude toward food might influence young children's attitude toward food. Consider food likes and dislikes, hunger/fullness cues, and so forth.

Study Questions

1. The most common criteria used to determine the health status of a newborn are weight, head circumference, and length.
   a. True
   b. False
2. What is it called when infant growth is disproportionately low in weight, length, or weight-for-length percentiles for gestational age?
   a. Small for gestational age
   b. Large for gestational age
   c. Intrauterine growth retardation
   d. Appropriate for gestational age
3. Infants are categorized as preterm infants if they are born before how many weeks of gestation?
   a. 37 weeks
   b. 38 weeks
   c. 39 weeks
   d. 40 weeks
4. In motor development, which part of the body do infants generally first gain control of?
   a. Arms
   b. Head and neck
   c. Abdomen
   d. Legs
5. Which of the following is *not* considered a stage in Piaget's model of cognitive development?
   a. Formal operational
   b. Preoperational
   c. Concrete operational
   d. Sensorimotor stage
   e. All of the above are considered stages in Piaget's model
6. Which type of growth chart is based on growth references that describe how certain children grew in a particular place and time?
   a. WHO growth charts
   b. WHO multicenter growth reference charts
   c. CDC growth charts
   d. National growth reference charts
7. The microbiome is defined as the collective genomes of the microbes that live inside and on the human body.
   a. True
   b. False

8. When introducing solid foods to an infant, which of the following is considered one of the best solid foods to start with?
   a. Cooked beans
   b. Canned peaches
   c. Dry cereal
   d. Rice cereal that has been thinned to a semiliquid consistency
9. Which nutrient is recommended to form a high percentage of overall kilocalorie intake because it is a concentrated source of energy that sustains infants through rapid growth and development?
   a. Carbohydrate
   b. Protein
   c. Amino acids
   d. Fat
10. Which nutrient is the body's first choice to fuel metabolism?
    a. Carbohydrate
    b. Protein
    c. Amino acids
    d. Fat
11. A 7-month-old infant weighting 16 pounds needs approximately how many kilocalories per day?
    a. 500
    b. 675
    c. 715
    d. 800
12. A deficiency of vitamin D is known to produce which condition?
    a. Scurvy
    b. Growth stunting
    c. Rickets
    d. Anemia
13. This toxicity can interrupt brain development, slow growth, and interfere with calcium and iron absorption.
    a. Sodium
    b. Fiber
    c. Fluoride
    d. Lead

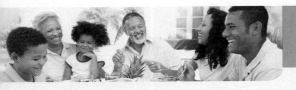

Learning Portfolio (continued)

14. Which of the following is *not* considered a common sign of dehydration in infants?
    a. Sunken eyes
    b. Reduced amount of urine that is dark in color
    c. Lethargy, restlessness, irritability
    d. Adequate skin elasticity

15. What is the recommended age for weaning an infant from the breast or bottle to a cup?
    a. 3 to 6 months
    b. 6 to 8 months
    c. 10 to 12 months
    d. 14 to 16 months

Weblinks

- **Nutrition.gov Life Stages**
  http://www.nutrition.gov/life-stages

- **USDA ChooseMyPlate.gov. Pregnancy and Breast-feeding Health and Nutrition Information**
  http://www.choosemyplate.gov/pregnancy-breast-feeding.html

- **USDA WIC Works Resource System**
  http://wicworks.nal.usda.gov/topics-z/myplate-resources

- **The WHO Child Growth Standards**
  http://www.who.int/childgrowth/en/

References

1. Blake JS, Munoz KD. *Nutrition from Science to You.* New York, NY: Pearson; 2010.
2. Kuczmarki RO. 2000 CDC growth charts for the United States: methods and development. *Vital Health Stat.* 2002;11(246).
3. American Pregnancy Association; updated August 2015. Monitoring your newborn's weight gain. Retrieved from: http://americanpregnancy.org/first-year-of-life/newborn-weight-gain/. Accessed September 6, 2016.
4. Pinto-Martin JA, Levy SE, Feldman JF, Lorenz JM, Paneth N, Whitaker AH. Prevalence of autism spectrum disorder in adolescents weighing <2000 grams. *Pediatrics.* November 11, 2009; 128(5) [published online before print October 17, 2011]. doi:10.1542/peds.2010-2846.
5. Hamilton, B., Martin J. Osterman M, Curtin, S. Births: preliminary data for 2013. *Nat Vital Stat Rep.* May 29, 2014; 63(2). http://www.cdc.gov/nchs/data/nvsr/nvsr63/nvsr63_02.pdf. Accessed September 6, 2016
6. Organization for Economic Co-Operation and Development; 2016. Infant mortality rates 2016. Retrieved from: https://data.oecd.org/healthstat/infant-mortality-rates.htm.
7. Mathews TJ, MacDorman MF, Thoma ME; Division of Vital Statistics. Infant mortality statistics from the 2013 period linked birth/infant death data set. *Nat Vital Stat Rep.* August 6, 2015;64(9). http://www.cdc.gov/nchs/data/nvsr/nvsr64/nvsr64_09.pdf. Accessed September 6, 2016.
8. Centers for Disease Control and Prevention; July 6, 2016. Infant health. Retrieved from: http://www.cdc.gov/nchs/fastats/infant-health.htm. Accessed September 6, 2016.
9. Centers for Disease Control and Prevention. CDC Grand Rounds: Public health approaches to reducing U.S. infant mortality MMWR. August 9, 2013; 62(31). Retrieved from: www.cdc.gov/mmwr/pdf/wk/mm6231.pdf. Accessed May 20, 2015.
10. Ormrod J. Piaget's sensorimotor stage. In Ormrod J, ed. *Human Learning.* New York, NY: Pearson; 2007:3.
11. Centers for Disease Control and Prevention; August 4, 2009. CDC growth charts: United States. Retrieved from: http://www.cdc.gov/growthcharts/background.htm. Accessed June 9, 2015.
12. Shin AC, Townsend RL, Patterson LM, Berthoud HR. "Liking" and "wanting" of sweet and oily food stimuli as affected by high-fat-diet induced obesity, weight loss, leptin, and genetic predisposition. *Am J Physiol Regul Integr Comp Physiol.* 2011;301(5):R1267–1280.
13. Voreades N, Kozil A, Weir TL. Diet and the development of the human intestinal microbiome. *Front Microbiol.* September v22, 2014;5:494.
14. Hadley KB, Ryan AS, Forsyth S, Gautier S, Salem N Jr. The essentiality of arachidonic acid in infant development. *Nutrients.* April 12, 2016;8(4):216.
15. Gartner LM, Morton J, Lawrence RA, et al. Breastfeeding and the use of human milk. *Pediatrics.* 2005;115(2):496–506.
16. Institute of Medicine. Dietary Reference Intakes. USDA National Agricultural Library. Retrieved from: http://fnic.nal.usda.gov/dietary-guidance/dietary-reference-intakes. Accessed July 1, 2015.
17. Centers for Disease Control and Prevention; June 17, 2015. Vitamin D supplementation. Retrieved from: https://www.cdc.gov/breastfeeding/recommendations/vitamin_d.htm. Accessed July 19, 2016.
18. Akkermans MD, Uijerschout L, Abbink M, et al. Predictive factors of iron depletion in late preterm infants at the postnatal age of 6 weeks. *Eur J Clin Nutr.* 2016;70(8):941–946 [published online ahead of print March 23, 2016].
19. Armstrong C. AAP reports on diagnosis and prevention of iron deficiency anemia. Practice guidelines. *Am Fam Phys.* March 1, 2011;83(5):624.

20. Food and Nutrition Board, Institute of Medicine, National Academies. Dietary Reference Intakes: elements. Retrieved from: http://www.nationalacademies.org/hmd/~/media/Files/Activity%20Files/Nutrition/DRIs/New%20Material/6_%20Elements%20Summary.pdf. Accessed September 6, 2016.

21. Milyamoto K, Ichikawa J, Okuya M, Tsuboi T, Hirao J, Arisaka O. Too little water or too much: hyponatremia due to excess fluid intake. *Acta Paediatr.* 2012;101(9):e390–391.

22. Vandenplas Y. Algorithms for common gastrointestinal disorders. *J Pediatr Gastroenterol Nutr.* 2016;63(suppl 1):S38–40.

23. Szajewska H, Dryl R. Probiotics for the management of infantile colic. *J Pediatr Gastroenterol Nutr.* 2016;63(suppl 1):S22–24.

24. Aksoy Okan M, Gunduz M, Okur M, Akgun C, Esin K. Does maternal diet affect infantile colic?. *J Matem Fetal Neonatal Med.* 2016;29(19):3139–3141 [published online ahead of print November 30, 2015].

25. Radlović N, Leković Z, Vuletić B, Radlović V, Simić D. Acute diarrhea in children. *Srp Arh Celok Lek.* November–December 2015;143(11–12):755–762.

26. Brzezinska M, Kucharska A, Sinska B. Vegetarian diets in the nutrition of pregnant and breastfeeding women. *Pol Merkur Lekarski.* 2016;40(238):264–268.

27. Samour PQ, King K. *Pediatric Nutrition.* Burlington, MA: Jones & Bartlett Learning. 2012; 87.

CHAPTER 7

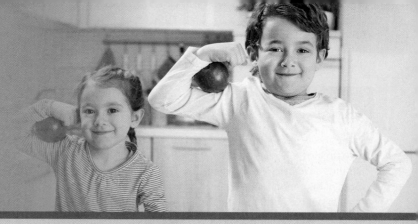

Early Childhood Nutrition

Kimberly Powell, PhD, MS, RD, **and Kimberley McMahon**, MDA, RD

Chapter Outline

Monitoring Growth in Early Childhood

Factors That Affect Dietary Intake

Nutrition Recommendations and Requirements

Common Nutrition Considerations During Preschool and Early Childhood

Promoting Healthy Lifestyles

Learning Objectives

1. Accurately make body size assessments, including weight and stature, and plot this information correctly on a growth chart.

2. Give examples of factors, such as food jags and food aversions, appetite and satiety, media influence, parental influence, the feeding relationship, and obesogenic environments, that affect dietary intake.

3. Create a meal plan for a toddler and preschool-age child using the Dietary Guidelines for Americans and Dietary Reference Intake values.

4. Provide practical ways to combat the common nutrition considerations of dental caries, constipation, and lead exposure during preschool and early childhood.

5. Describe suggested steps for preventing overweight and obesity as well as the physical activity recommendations for children.

Case Study

James is a 4-year-old boy who lives with his mother, father, and two siblings, a 2-year-old sister and a 7-year-old brother. James attends child care 3 days a week from 8 a.m. until 5 p.m. while both of his parents are at work.

James weighs 38 pounds and is 42 inches tall. James eats breakfast at home each day. On the days that he attends the child care center, he is offered a morning snack, lunch, and an afternoon snack. At home James does not eat at consistent times, and his mother allows him to eat foods that he chooses from the pantry throughout the day.

James is a generally happy boy who enjoys playing with his friends. He is active at home and at the child care center and seems to be interested in many different activities. James's mother describes his diet as being "limited" and that he does not like much variety and that his appetite does not seem to be consistent.

Toddlers and **preschoolers** make up the two age categories for early childhood. Children ages 2 and 3 years old are defined as toddlers, with this stage of development characterized by a rapid increase in gross and fine motor skills, an increase in independence, exploration of the environment, cognitive development, emotional development, social development, and language skills. Preschoolers are defined as children between the ages of 3 and 5 years, with improving fine motor skills, increased independence, expanded vocabulary, and improved control over their emotions.

Adequate energy and nutrient intake is essential for toddlers and preschool-age children to achieve their full growth potential. Eating habits established during these early years contribute to the development of subsequent eating habits; therefore, establishing good eating habits during this life stage is significant.[1] This chapter discusses normal growth and development, factors that affect dietary intake, nutrition recommendations, common nutrition considerations, and how to promote healthy lifestyles during preschool and early childhood.

Monitoring Growth in Early Childhood

Preview Although still significant, growth rate during the toddler and preschool years is slower than in infancy. As growth rate slows, independence increases, meal patterns change, and the importance of adequate nutrition and formation of food habits becomes significant.

Growth Rates

Growth rate varies considerably from child to child. However, during the second year of life, the average weight gain is about 3 to 5 pounds, and the average height or length gain is about 3 to 5 inches per year.[2] (See **FIGURE 7.1** .) For children 4 to 5 years of age, their weight gain average is about 4 to 6.5 pounds per year, with an average growth of about 3 inches per year. After the age of 2 years, body mass index (BMI) is used to assess appropriate weight for height.[3] (See **FIGURE 7.2** .)

Standards commonly used to interpret height and weight of children are the World Health Organization (WHO) growth charts and the Centers for Disease Control and Prevention (CDC) growth charts. WHO charts are based on growth data collected over time from children living in six different countries (including the United States) in environments believed to support optimal growth, which in this case includes being or having been breastfed. However, WHO growth charts are intended to be used on all children up to the age of 2 years, regardless of the type of feeding. CDC growth charts are based on data collected from children in the United States during the 1970s and 1990s. These national reference data are intended to be used for children ages 2 through 19 years, with the intent of tracking weight, stature, and BMI.

Accurate Measurement Techniques

Accuracy in both equipment and measurement technique is important because on the basis of these measurements medical and nutritional decisions will be made about the child.

Technique for weighing children and adolescents include (see **FIGURE 7.3**):[4]

- Children older than 36 months and who can stand on their own should be weighed on a beam-balance or digital scale; they should wear light undergarments or lightweight outer clothing.
- Weight should be measured to the nearest 0.1 kg.

Technique for measuring stature in children and adolescents include (see **FIGURE 7.4**):[4]

- Measuring stature requires a wall-mounted vertical board with an attached metric ruler and a horizontal headpiece that can be brought into contact with the superior part of the head.
- Stand the child against the ruler without shoes on, with heels together, legs straight, arms at sides, and shoulders relaxed.
- Ensure that the child is looking straight ahead.
- Bring the perpendicular headpiece down to touch the crown of the head.
- The measurer's eyes should be parallel with the headpiece.
- Measure to the nearest 0.1 cm.

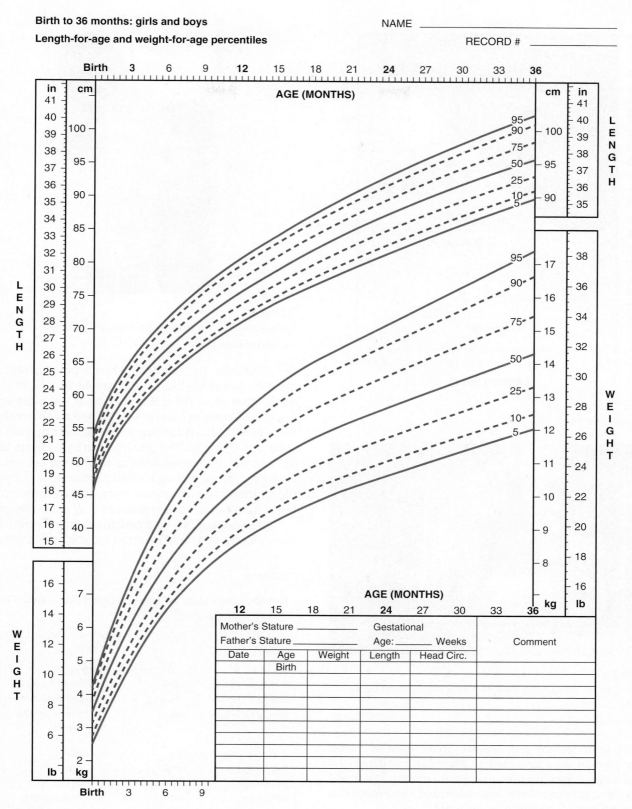

Figure 7.1

Centers for Disease Control and Prevention growth chart birth to 36 months old—girls and boys.

Developed by the National Center for Health Statistics in collaboration with the National Center for Chronic Disease Prevention and Health Promotion (2000)

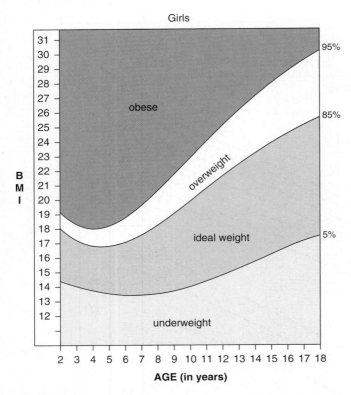

Figure 7.2
Body mass index.

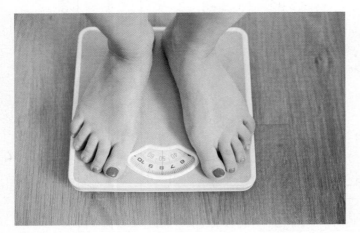

Figure 7.3
Technique for obtaining children and adolescent body weight.

©Rostislav_Sedlacek/Shutterstock

For both weight and stature, inaccurate or incorrectly plotted data can lead to errors in health status assessment. Choosing the appropriate growth chart and using standard procedures and calibrated equipment can ensure an overall accurate assessment.

Growth Chart Interpretation

Once measurements are taken and plotted on the corresponding chart, interpretations can be made. The curved lines on the growth charts indicate the percentiles and enable health practitioners to determine in which percentile

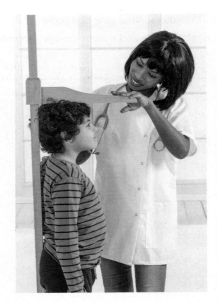

Figure 7.4
Technique for obtaining children and adolescent stature.

©Chassenet/BSIP SA/Alamy Stock Photo

the child falls. For example, when a point is plotted on the 95th percentile line on the weight-for-height chart, it means that 95 of 100 children (95%) of the same age and sex have a lower weight for age. Plotted measurements on these growth charts correspond to the nutrition indicators shown in TABLE 7.1 . The growth reference charts use the 5th and the 95th percentiles as the outermost percentile cutoff values indicating abnormal growth. If the percentile rank indicates a nutrition-related health concern, additional monitoring and assessment may be recommended.

Interpreting plots on a growth chart over time can create a picture of a child's overall growth status compared

Table 7.1

Nutrition Indicators as They Correspond to Growth Chart Measurements

Anthropometric Index	Percentile Cutoff Values	Nutritional Status Indicator
WHO Growth Charts 2nd and 98th percentiles		
Length for age	<2nd	Short stature
Weight for length	<2nd	Low weight for length
Weight for length	>98th	High weight for length
CDC Growth Charts 5th and 95th percentiles		
BMI for age	>95th	Obese
BMI for age	>85th and <95th	Overweight
BMI for age	<5th	Underweight
Stature for age	<5th	Short stature

National Center for Chronic Disease Prevention and Health Promotion, Division of Nutrition, Physical Activity, and Obesity. *Use and interpretation of the WHO and CDC growth charts for children from birth to 20 years in the United States.* Atlanta, GA: Centers for Disease Control and Prevention; May 2013. Retrieved from: http://www.cdc.gov/nccdphp/dnpao/growthcharts/resources/growthchart.pdf. Accessed September 9, 2016.

Case Study

Using the growth chart provided, plot James's weight of 38 pounds and his stature of 42 inches. According to the growth chart, in which percentile is James for weight and for height? Using Figure 7.2, plot his BMI and identify his BMI category.

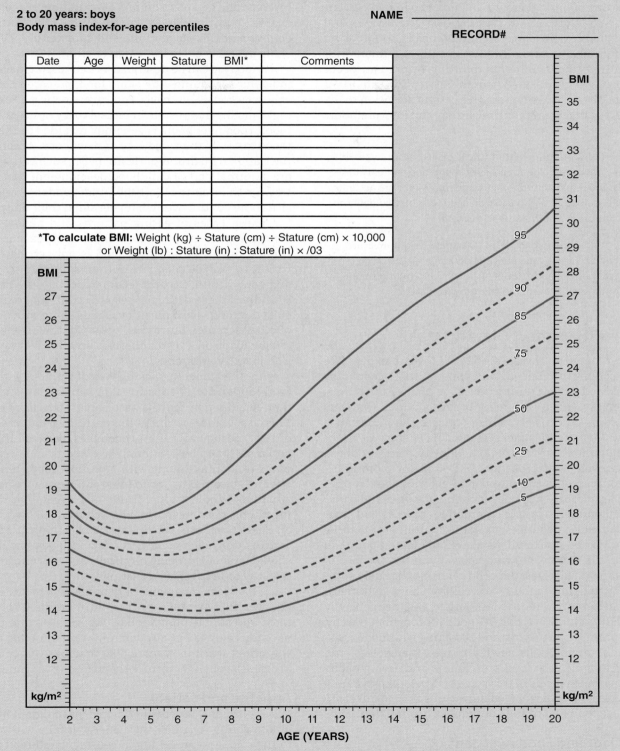

2 to 20 years: boys
Body mass index-for-age percentiles

NAME _____

RECORD# _____

Date	Age	Weight	Stature	BMI*	Comments

*To calculate BMI: Weight (kg) ÷ Stature (cm) ÷ Stature (cm) × 10,000
or Weight (lb) : Stature (in) : Stature (in) × /03

AGE (YEARS)

with that of other children in the same reference group and provides data on that child individually. It is interesting and informational to see how a child compares with others in the reference group; however, it is also important to evaluate the individual child's growth over time. Indications of normal growth include one to two percentile line changes, but, during the first 2 to 3 years and during puberty, crossing percentile lines is potentially a sign of growth disturbance.[4] As a result of human error or incorrect measurements, plotting errors can occur when growth charts are used; therefore, it is important that healthcare practitioners give careful attention to the processes of measurement, recording, and interpretation.

> **Recap** Monitoring a child's growth over time is a valuable method of assessing the adequacy of energy and nutrient intake. It is essential that anthropometric measurements are accurate and precise because inaccurate or incorrectly plotted data can lead to errors in health status assessment.
>
> 1. Consider the impact of an inaccurate height measurement, which is squared when determining BMI.
> 2. What is the main indicator of growth concern when monitoring a child over time on a growth chart?

Factors That Affect Dietary Intake

Children between the ages of 2 and 5 years experience decreased nutrition needs and appetite that accompany their slowed growth during this stage of life. At this time, children also have high activity levels and a relatively small stomach capacity, which stresses the importance of how meals and snacks should have high nutrient density rather than high caloric density. Nutrient dense foods provide a generous amount of one or more nutrients compared to the number of calories they supply. Examples of nutrient-dense food include eggs and fruit.

During this stage, it is common for parents and caregivers to notice changes in eating patterns and to be concerned about a toddler's seemingly low appetite. In general, if a child is growing normally in the absence of gastrointestinal issues, the child's nutrition is likely sufficient. By this time in their lives, children have identifiable eating patterns that tend to lack variety, and they generally eat small amounts of foods frequently throughout the day.

Learning about, trying, and accepting new foods, mastering the motor skills needed to feed themselves, and establishing healthy food preferences and eating habits are important aspects of this stage of development. Eating and health habits developed during this time are likely to influence food habits and subsequent health later in life.

Food Jags and Food Aversions

The need for independence, including self-feeding, becomes apparent during the toddler age. By preschool age, children are generally able to use utensils and drink from a cup, although not always without accidents. Adult supervision during eating episodes is still necessary, and care should be taken not to offer foods that can cause choking. Children at this age tend to be curious and want to be helpful, making this a good time for them to be involved in the selection and preparation of meals and snacks. Food jags, food aversion, and neophobia are also common at this stage of life and can identify a child as being a "picky" or "fussy" eater.

A food jag can be described as a condition in which an individual consumes the same food, prepared the same way, on a consistent basis. Food aversion is a strong feeling of dislike that results in refusal to try or to eat certain foods. Food neophobia is generally regarded as the reluctance to eat or the avoidance of new foods. According to the National Institutes of Health (NIH), such eating habits are a normal part of childhood development that offer a way for children to assert their independence and exercise some control over what goes on in their daily lives.

These types of eating patterns and behaviors are concerning to caregivers for a number of reasons. Often, caregivers worry that their child is not getting enough variety to provide adequate nutrients for optimal growth and good health. Experts recommend that the best way to address these eating issues is to continue to offer the child new or disliked nutritious foods along with a variety of other accepted nutritious foods. Continuous exposure to new foods on a regular basis is an effective way to get a child to try new foods.

Another concern of caregivers of children with these food tendencies is constipation. It has been suggested that constipation may be associated with picky eating.[5] This association is likely linked to low dietary intake of fiber, particularly from vegetables, because this food group seems to be commonly avoided by children. Adequate fluid intake along with high-fiber foods tend to be effective treatments for toddler and preschool-age constipation. Whole grains, fruits, and vegetables, including plums, peas, beans, and broccoli, are all high in fiber and help to relieve constipation. Foods that can increase constipation, such as fatty foods and foods low in fiber, should be avoided. Being physically active is also an effective way to help relieve constipation.

If food jags, aversions, or neophobia behavior continues over time, symptoms of malnutrition should be monitored and supplemental foods or beverages that provide not only calories but also vitamins and minerals may be warranted. It is important to note that these types of feeding issues generally resolve themselves over time.

Appetite and Satiety

It is a commonly accepted principle that children have the innate ability to adjust their energy intake with respect to their appetite, resulting in self-regulated food intake; therefore, a toddler or preschool-age child's food intake may fluctuate largely from meal to meal and from day to day. However, between the ages of 3 and 5 years, children become less responsive to internal cues of satiation and more responsive to external cues, which may result in eating in the absence of hunger, overeating, and potential weight gain.[6] Parents or caregivers who enforce strict feeding rules, such as "clean your plate before you can be excused from the meal," or who reward good behavior with food tend to interfere with the child's ability to self-regulate.

A child's personality traits tend to influence food intake as well; for example, studies indicate that impulsive children show normal sensitivity to internal hunger and satiety cues—meaning they could recognize and respond to internal cues for being hungry and for being full—but they tend to demonstrate an abnormal response to highly energy-dense foods—meaning that, when presented with foods such as candy or cookies, they tend to eat these even if they are not hungry and they avoid acknowledging the feeling of satiety, which leads to overeating.[7] It is important for parents to help children learn and practice self-regulating food intake by helping them recognize their hunger and fullness.

Media Influence

During the toddler and preschool-age years, children are forming their own food preferences and habits while observing and learning from others: their parents, caregivers, peers, and siblings, as well as what they see on TV and in other media. With regard to TV, U.S. children are frequently exposed to advertisements for high-fat, high-sugar foods, which is linked to greater demand for the consumption of those foods.[8] It is estimated that children see 12–16 TV advertisements per day for products generally high in saturated fat, sugar, or sodium. In addition, newer digital forms of unhealthy food and beverage marketing to youth are increasing; the Federal Trade Commission reported an inflation-adjusted 50.7% increase in new media marketing expenditures.

Children's exposure to unhealthy food marketing has long been recognized as a contributor to poor diets and weight gain. The link between television viewing and poor diet is strongest for children who watch the most commercial television and those who are exposed to advertisements embedded with programs.[9]

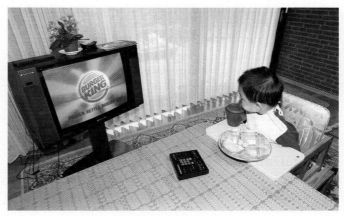

©Bernhard Classen/vario images GmbH &Co.KG/Alamy Stock Photo

was before CFBAI implementation. However, CFBAI company non-approved brands represent 65% of candy ads viewed by children, and 77% of these ads contained child-targeting techniques.

In 2016, the Council of Better Business Bureaus, in partnership with the National Confectioners Association, announced a new self-regulatory initiative that promotes responsible advertising to children. Under the Children's Confection Advertising Initiative, participating companies agree not to advertise directly to children younger than 12 years of age.

With continued focus on the negative correlation between advertisements for high-fat, high-sugar foods and the greater demand for those foods, the landscape of food advertising may change over time.

References

Harris JL, LoDoice M, Dembek C, Schwartz MB. Sweet promises: candy advertising to children and implications for industry self-regulation. *Appetite. 2015*;95:585–592.

Council of Better Business Bureaus. The National Partner Program: about the initiative. Retrieved from: https://www.bbb.org/council/the-national-partner-program/national-advertising-review-services/childrens-food-and-beverage-advertising-initiative/about-the-initiative/. Accessed April 28, 2016.

Council of Better Business Bureaus. New responsible advertising commitment by confectionery companies. Council of Better Business Bureaus; March 16, 2016. Retrieved from: http://www.bbb.org/council/news-events/news-releases/2016/03/new-responsible-advertising-commitment-by-confectionery-companies/. Accessed March 28, 2016.

Powell LM, Schembeck R, Chaloupka FJ. Nutritional content of food and beverage products in television advertisements seen on children's programming. *Child Obes.* 2013;9(6):524–531.

Food advertising may drive children's consumer behavior through four different modes. First, advertising creates expectations, which motivate individuals to want to purchase a particular food. Second, the purchase of advertised foods is accompanied by positive feelings. Third, the entertaining dimension of advertising generates a pleasant mood, which positively predisposes the evaluation of advertised foods. Fourth, children do not always possess the ability to recognize the persuasive nature of advertising.[10]

Parental Influence

Parental feeding practices have been linked to eating and weight status in young children.[11] Parents can influence a child's eating behaviors in a number of different ways, both direct and indirect. Choosing food for children can be a complex practice and many ideas and circumstances influence food choices that parents make for their children. The overall environment and individual circumstances combine to result in food choices influenced by beliefs, values, norms, and knowledge along with cost, quality, and availability of various foods.[12] Influences of time, social connections, and information sources are also apparent factors in parents' food choices for children.[12]

Modeling

Children follow the behavior modeled by those around them; therefore, they are likely to adopt the same eating habits as their parents or caregivers, which links parental influences to the eating and weight status of young children.[11] Learning through observation can increase consumption in two main ways: observation can change behavior directly or it can increase the possibility of consumption, therefore promoting a liking for a food through increased exposure.[13] Parents who eat a wide variety of foods, including seemingly less desirable foods, and parents who expose their children to a variety of healthy foods tend to have an overall healthy diet. Not only are parents the primary examples children observe but also they control the manner in which children are fed, both directly and indirectly influencing children's food preferences. Parents are the biggest influence in a child's life, which stresses the importance that they set good examples and maintain a positive attitude about food and the feeding environment. Parents' positive influences are vital for establishing healthy lifestyle behaviors in their children.[14]

Evidence suggests that the eating habits children develop during toddler and preschool age may in fact influence lifelong eating behaviors.[14] Once children begin school, most have already developed their food likes and

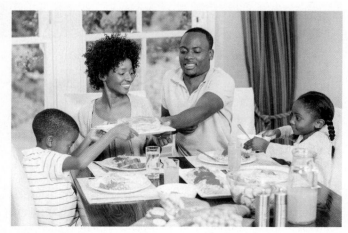

©wavebreakmedia/Shutterstock

dislikes, so achieving behavior change may be more difficult then.

Food Restrictions, Pressuring, and Serving Sizes

With the intent to create good eating habits in their children, well-meaning parents sometimes restrict certain foods—generally, low-nutrient-dense foods—or pressure a child to eat foods that are viewed as healthy choices. Both circumstances can have the opposite effect on a child's eating habits. Restricting certain foods from a child's diet generally increases the desire for those foods, whereas forcing a child to eat foods that he or she may not enjoy eating may create aversions to those foods. In addition, some studies have found that children with restrictive parents are more likely to be overweight later in life.[14] Many experts discourage pressuring because it can create a negative eating environment that decreases a child's ability to self-regulate hunger and satiety cues.

Evidence shows that 3- to 5-year-old children undergo important physical and behavioral changes that include being affected by the amount of food they are served, with larger portions of food served resulting in greater intake.[15] Generally, this finding is true even with adults: people eat more food when they are served larger portions and when the food is served in larger units (or bigger pieces). This association tends to be negative; for example, provide a whole bag of chocolate candy rather than one serving and a person is likely to overeat; offer a large bag of potato chips rather than a single serving and a person will eat more than one serving in one sitting.

Can this feeding situation of offering larger portions or larger units help a person eat more healthfully? One study examined whether these effects can be used for the good: to increase vegetable consumption among children. The study found that children's vegetable intake can be improved by serving larger portions in smaller-sized pieces.[15] Because parents of young children control the manner in which children are fed, educating parents regarding appropriate portion sizes is an important consideration. Teaching children appropriate serving sizes of all foods can affect their path of weight gain.[16]

Maternal Influences

Research demonstrates the significance of maternal feeding practices and children's eating behavior in the development of childhood obesity. People tend to eat as a result of either internal stimuli, such as the physical feeling of hunger, or external stimuli, such as it being a certain time of day or because a food that looks good is available. Studies demonstrate that a positive correlation exists between mothers who eat in response to outside stimuli, rather than as a result of internal hunger signals, and whether children are picky eaters as well as children's desire to eat.[17] Because mothers who often eat as a reaction to external stimuli also tend to have high control over what they offer or encourage their children to eat, or not to eat, they may be contributing to whether a child is a picky eater.

Mothers who eat for physical rather than emotional reasons and who have eating-related skills such as being mindful when eating and planning regular and nutritious eating opportunities for themselves were more likely to monitor their child's food intake and to divide feeding responsibilities with their child.[15] These findings suggest that parents who demonstrate intuitive eating—a nutrition philosophy based on the premise that becoming in tune with the body's natural hunger cues is a more effective way to attain a healthy weight rather than keeping track of calories—may create a more positive feeding environment for their young children.

The Feeding Relationship

As children develop eating habits, establishing a healthy feeding relationship between child and caregiver is an important step. This feeding relationship includes the division of responsibility in feeding young children with an emphasis on decreasing parental pressure on the child to eat. Internationally recognized authority on eating and feeding Ellyn Satter articulates this relationship well in what she calls "The Division of Responsibility for Feeding Toddlers Through Adolescents."[18] Satter describes the division of responsibility such that parents and caregivers allow the child to determine how much of the food that is presented to them will be eaten. In turn, the parent or caregiver takes responsibility of determining what food is offered to the child, when the food is offered, and where. For example, a child is offered a plate of cut-up fruit and cheese in the kitchen during the morning. The parent then gives the child the choice of whether to eat the food offered, and how much of it to eat, without forcing either of these issues. Additional responsibilities of the parent or caregiver include such things as providing regular meals and snacks, making mealtime an enjoyable experience, avoiding catering to child's likes and dislikes while being considerate of a child's lack of food experiences, not allowing eating between meals and snacks, and finally, letting the child grow and develop in the body that is right for her or him. In this model, the child's jobs include such things as learning to eat the food provided, and learning to behave well during mealtime.[19]

Obesogenic Environments

The current obesity epidemic across the United States has led to the recognition that the way we live, work, and play greatly affects our food intake and our activity level. Because children live in the environments that their parents or caregivers provide, they too share the consequences or the benefits of that living environment. Some factors that link lifestyle to body weight are controllable, such as how often people eat fast food and whether they choose to add physical activity to their day such as walking reasonable distances or taking the stairs instead of the elevator. Other factors may not be within a person's control, such as whether the neighborhood has safe walking paths or sidewalks or whether the grocery store carries fresh produce.

The term **obesogenic environment** is used to describe environments (within the home or workplace) that promote gaining weight and that are not conducive to weight loss.[20] In other words, an obesogenic environment contributes to obesity by encouraging people to eat unhealthy foods while discouraging physical activity. Common barriers to choosing healthful behaviors include lack of time; lack of neighborhood safety; limited knowledge of portion size, cooking methods, and ways to prepare healthy foods; the perceived cost of healthy options; and family members who are picky eaters.[21]

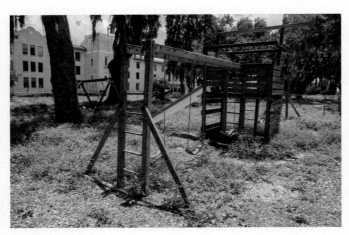

©David Mabe/Alamy Stock Photo

Consider, for example, a family with two young children and both parents who work full-time jobs. Lack of meal planning, busy schedules, and the convenience of ordering take-out or having fast food are all factors that can contribute to unhealthy eating. Fast-food hamburgers and french fries or pizza might be "easier" than spending the time required to prepare a more nutritious meal. Additionally, children who are allowed to spend a great amount of their time at home in front of a screen (TV, computer, or video game) and who are not encouraged to engage in physical activity are experiencing some of the negative factors of an obesogenic environment.

Suggestions to help avoid the consequence of unhealthy weight gain as a result of living in an obesogenic environment include planning meals and activities ahead of time, introducing new foods and behaviors often and in tandem with existing preferred foods and behaviors, and observing and learning healthy strategies from others.[21]

Recap A number of factors affect dietary intake of children, including food jags and food aversions, appetite and satiety, media influences, parental influences, the feeding relationship between child and caregiver, and obesogenic environments. Not only for their own health and wellness but also for that of their children, parents and caregivers should be aware that providing healthy foods while limiting unhealthy food choices and demonstrating healthy food habits are good building blocks for helping children develop healthy lifestyles.

1. Consider the different ways a potato can be cooked, such as baked or fried (as in french fries). Which of these options is considered more nutrient dense than others and why?
2. Describe a parent's or caregiver's role in the division of responsibility in feeding.

Nutrition Recommendations and Requirements

Preview Nutrition principles for toddlers and preschool-age children are the same as those for adults. Children need nutrients, such as carbohydrates, protein, fat, vitamins, and minerals; however, specific amounts are required at different ages. Following a healthy diet helps children grow and learn. Eating healthy foods during childhood also helps prevent obesity and weight-related diseases such as high cholesterol and diabetes later in life. Eating habits are formed during the preschool years, but at rates that vary from child to child, a situation that stresses the importance of establishing good eating attitudes, good eating habits, and adequate physical activity during this stage of life. An overview of the nutrients were discussed in Chapter 1. Here we will review the functions and food sources of these nutrients and focus on how each one plays a significant role in the diet of children.

Using the Dietary Guidelines for Americans to Estimate Calorie Needs and Establish Meal Patterns

The 2015–2020 *Dietary Guidelines for Americans* provides a table with estimated calorie ranges for children ages 2 to 5 years based on sex and activity level. (See **TABLE 7.2**.)

Creating a Meal Plan

The *Dietary Guidelines for Americans* also suggest daily meal plans based on particular calorie levels and provide daily food plan worksheets to help monitor daily intake. **TABLE 7.3** provides healthy eating patterns at recommended amounts of food for each food group at different calorie levels between 1,000 and 1,600 calories per day.

Table 7.2

Dietary Guidelines for Americans Estimated Calorie Ranges for Children

Age	Sex	Daily Physical Activity	Calorie Level of Food Plan
2 years	Boys and girls	Any level	1,000 calories
3 years	Boys	Less than 30 minutes	1,200 calories
		30–60 minutes	1,400 calories
		More than 60 minutes	
	Girls	Less than 30 minutes	1,000 calories
		30–60 minutes	1,200 calories
		More than 60 minutes	1,400 calories
4–5 years	Boys and girls	Less than 30 minutes	1,200 calories
		30–60 minutes	1,400 calories
	Boys	More than 60 minutes	1,600 calories
	Girls	More than 60 minutes	1,400 calories

Reproduced from: U.S. Department of Health and Human Services and U.S. Department of Agriculture. *2015–2020 Dietary Guidelines for Americans*. 8th ed. Washington, DC: U.S. Department of Health and Human Services and U.S. Department of Agriculture; December 2015. Retrieved from: http://health.gov/dietaryguidelines/2015/guidelines/. Accessed August 13, 2016; U.S. Department of Agriculture. MyPlate daily checklist for preschoolers. ChooseMyPlate.gov, updated July 22, 2016. Retrieved from: http://www.choosemyplate.gov/myplate-daily-checklist-preschoolers. Accessed September 6, 2016.

FIGURE 7.5 provides a suggested meal plan for 1,200 calories for 2- to 3-year-olds. **FIGURE 7.6** provides a suggested meal plan for 1,600 calories for 4- to 8-year-olds.

ChooseMyPlate **FIGURE 7.7** is the visual symbol used to summarize how the *Dietary Guidelines* can be used for each meal.[22] This tool is intended to help guide people of all ages on how much food from each food group they should include to make up meals. Once children can determine which foods fit into which food category (fruit,

Table 7.3

Healthy Eating Pattern Recommendations

Calorie Level of Pattern	1,000	1,200	1,400	1,600
Vegetables	1 c-eq	1½ c-eq	1½ c-eq	2 c-eq
Fruits	1 c-eq	1 c-eq	1½ c-eq	1½ c-eq
Grains	3 oz-eq	4 oz-eq	5 oz-eq	5 oz-eq
Dairy	2 c-eq	2½ c-eq	2½ c-eq	3 c-eq
Protein foods	2 oz-eq	3 oz-eq	4 oz-eq	5 oz-eq
Oils	15 g	17 g	17 g	22 g
Limit on calories for other uses	150	100	110	130

Food group amounts are shown in cup- (c-eq) or ounce-equivalents (oz-eq). Oils are shown in grams (g).

U.S. Department of Health and Human Services and U.S. Department of Agriculture. Appendix 3: USDA food patterns: healthy U.S.-style eating pattern. In *2015–2020 Dietary Guidelines for Americans*. 8th ed. Washington, DC: U.S. Department of Health and Human Services and U.S. Department of Agriculture; December 2015. Retrieved from: http://health.gov/dietaryguidelines/2015/guidelines/appendix-3/. Accessed September 6, 2016.

Food Group Amounts for 1,200 Calories a Day

Fruits
1 cup
Focus on whole fruits
Focus on whole fruits that are fresh, frozen, canned, or dried.

Vegetables
1 1/2 cups
Vary your veggies
Choose a variety of colorful fresh, frozen, and canned vegatables—make sure to include dark green, red, and orange choices.

Grains
4 ounces
Make half your grains whole grains
Find whole-grain foods by reading the Nutrition Facts lable and ingredients list.

Protein
3 ounces
Vary your protein routine
Mix up your protein foods to include seafood, beans and peas, unsalted nuts and seeds, soy products, eggs, and lean meats and poultry.

Dairy
2 1/2 cups
Move to low-fat or fat-free milk or yogurt
Choose fat-free milk, yogurt, and soy beverages (soy milk) to cut back on your saturated fat.

Limit
Drink and eat less sodium, saturated fat, and added sugars. Limit:
- Sodium to **1,500 milligrams** a day.
- Saturated fat to **13 grams** a day.
- Added sugars to **30 grams** a day.

Be active your way: Children 2 to 5 years old should play actively every day.

Figure 7.5
Suggested amount of food from each food group for 1,200 calories for 2- to 3-year-olds.

Reproduced from Choosemyplate.gov. Retrieved from: https://choosemyplate-prod.azureedge.net/sites/default/files/myplate/checklists/MyPlateDailyChecklist_1200cals_Age2-3.pdf

grain, protein, dairy, and vegetables), they can learn how much of each food should represent particular areas of their plate.

Carbohydrate, Protein, and Fat Needs
Carbohydrate
Carbohydrates are converted to glucose as a primary energy source for the body, making this a key component of any diet. Carbohydrates are found in a variety of foods, mainly bread, cereal, grains, fruits, and vegetables. Fiber is a key carbohydrate that provides many health benefits, and inadequate intakes can lead to health and digestion difficulties. Fiber intake in a child's diet plays an important role in reducing the child's risk for and lowering the incidence of numerous diseases.[23] Evidence has been found that dietary fiber from whole foods or supplements may reduce the risk of cardiovascular disease by improving serum lipids and reducing serum total and low-density lipoprotein (LDL) cholesterol concentrations in children.[24] Adequate fiber intake prevents constipation

Food Group Amounts for 1,600 Calories a Day

Fruits	Vegetables
1 1/2 cups	**2 cups**
Focus on whole fruits	**Vary your veggies**
Focus on whole fruits that are fresh, frozen, canned, or dried.	Choose a variety of colorful fresh, frozen, and canned vegatables—make sure to include dark green, red, and orange choices.

Grains	Protein
5 ounces	**5 ounces**
Make half your grains whole grains	**Vary your protein routine**
Find whole-grain foods by reading the Nutrition Facts lable and ingredients list.	Mix up your protein foods to include seafood, beans and peas, unsalted nuts and seeds, soy products, eggs, and lean meats and poultry.

Dairy	Limit
2 1/2 cups	
Move to low-fat or fat-free milk or yogurt	**Drink and eat less sodium, saturated fat, and added sugars. Limit:**
Choose fat-free milk, yogurt, and soy beverages (soy milk) to cut back on your saturated fat.	• Sodium to **1,900 milligrams** a day. • Saturated fat to **18 grams** a day. • Added sugars to **40 grams** a day.

Be active your way: Children 2 to 5 years old should play actively every day. Children 6 to 17 years old should move at least 60 minutes every day.

Figure 7.6
Suggested amount of food from each food group for 1,600 calories for 4- to 8-year-olds.

Reproduced from: Choosemyplate.gov. Retrieved from: https://choosemyplate-prod.azureedge.net/sites/default/files/myplate/checklists/MyPlateDailyChecklist_1600cals_Age4-8.pdf

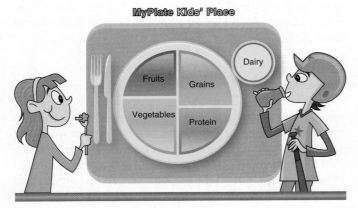

Figure 7.7
ChooseMyPlate for Kids.

Courtesy of ChooseMyPlate.gov

and has been linked to reducing the risk of certain types of cancer and decreasing the risk of obesity and diabetes in children.[25]

With regard to body weight, one study of children living in the United States showed that increasing levels of soluble fiber were associated with a small reduction of visceral body fat, whereas a decreased fiber intake was associated with a 10% increase in visceral body fat.[25]

Children benefit from a balance of fiber in their diet; however, in the United States children's fiber intake tends to be lower than recommended, especially in children from low-income and minority backgrounds. These studies reveal that children consume approximately one-half of the current Dietary Reference Intake (DRI) intake recommendations.[25] Good sources of dietary fiber include whole grains, nuts and seeds, fruits and vegetables.

The Recommended Dietary Allowance (RDA) for fiber for children ages 2 and 3 years is 19 g per day. The RDA for children ages 4 and 5 years old is 25 g per day. **TABLE 7.4** provides suggestions on how to incorporate fiber into children's diet.

The U.S. Department of Agriculture (USDA) recommends that between 45% and 65% of total daily calories come from carbohydrates. This equals about 19 g of carbohydrate per day for children ages 1 to 3 years and 24 g of carbohydrate for children ages 4 to 8 years. Important considerations of carbohydrate intake in children is that children consume adequate fiber and avoid excess added sugar. A balanced diet that provides variety by including whole grains, fruits, and vegetables should easily meet the carbohydrate needs of toddlers and preschool-age children.

Protein
Adequate protein intake is essential for maintaining the body's protein stores and keeping many bodily functions running smoothly. Because the body of a child between the ages of 2 and 5 years is growing and developing rapidly, consuming adequate protein is of particular importance during the toddler and preschool-age years.

Table 7.4	
Ways to Incorporate Fiber into Children's Diets	
Include oatmeal or other whole-grain cereal (which have 3 g or more fiber per serving) as a part of morning meals.	Top whole-grain pancakes with apples, berries, or raisins.
Offer whole-wheat bagels or English muffins instead of white bread.	Mix granola into low-fat yogurt.
Use whole-wheat bread instead of white bread.	Use whole-grain pasta instead of white pasta.
Add almonds, berries, chickpeas, artichoke hearts, or beans to salads.	Add lentils or whole-grain barley to soup.
Use whole-grain flour for baking.	Leave the skins on when serving fruits and vegetables.

Modified from: KidsHealth. Fiber and your child. The Nemours Foundation; reviewed September 2014. Retrieved from: http://kidshealth.org/en/parents/fiber.html#. Accessed September 8, 2016.

Protein is stored primarily in muscle and collagen, and the components of protein, which are amino acids, function as hormones, enzymes, and transporters of other nutrients. The RDA for protein for toddlers is 1.1 g/kg of body weight, and it decreases slightly to 0.95 g/kg of body weight for preschool-age children. (Divide weight in pounds by 2.2 to determine the weight in kilograms.) Protein needs per kg of body weight are higher in children than adults because of children's growth rates. Children grow significantly in both height and weight, and their brain, immune system, muscle, collagen, and hair are also developing.

Protein sources include foods made from animals—meat, poultry, seafood, and eggs—as well as plant based sources such as beans and peas, nuts, seeds, and soy. Protein from animal products is considered high-quality protein and offers a greater quantity of protein per calorie than vegetable or plant sources.

Protein has a unique role in in that it can be used as an energy source in the absence of adequate calorie intake; therefore, if a child is meeting recommended protein needs but not eating enough calories overall, protein's roles in muscle mass development and maintenance and hormone production will be compromised as the protein is used for energy instead.

Fat

Fats are nutrients used by the body in a variety of ways. Dietary fat builds nerve tissue and hormones; is essential for brain development; helps the body absorb the fat-soluble vitamins A, D, E, and K; insulates and protects systems and organs in the body; and contributes to the feeling of satiety after eating. As a food component, fat gives food flavor and texture, making many foods palatable and desirable.

Food sources of fat include foods made with butter or oils, such as cookies and cake, whole and 2% milk, and animal products such as beef, chicken, and pork. Fried food and processed foods also contain dietary fat. Getting enough fat from the diet is essential; however, getting too much has consequences, and therefore a child's fat intake should be monitored.

An adequate amount of fat is an important part of a child's diet; however, many children eat more than the recommended amounts, particularly of trans and saturated fats. Excessive fat intake generally leads to excessive calorie intake, which is associated with weight gain and obesity. Increased fat intake is also associated with greater risk for heart disease, high blood pressure, and diabetes. For children ages 1 to 3 years, the recommendation of fat intake is 30% to 35% of calories, and for children ages 4 and older, the recommendation is 25% to 35% of total calories. See TABLE 7.5 for tips on how to follow a low-fat diet.

Vitamins and Minerals
Calcium and Vitamin D

During childhood, the body uses calcium to build bones. Vitamin D aids in calcium absorption and is an important component in the process of bone formation. Children

---

Table 7.5

Tips for Following a Low-Fat Diet

Ideas for keeping fat intake within the recommended ranges

- Offer low-fat foods such as fruit, vegetables, low-fat dairy, and lean meat and cheese as snacks.
- Use unsaturated fats in cooking and baking.
- Avoid fried foods.
- Make low-fat choices when eating out.
- Avoid high-fat sauces and salad dressings.

---

who do not get enough calcium and vitamin D are at risk for **rickets**, a bone-softening disease that causes severe bowing of the legs, poor growth, and sometimes muscle pain and weakness. Calcium also plays a role in proper function of muscles and nerves and in the release of hormones and enzymes. (See TABLE 7.6 .)

Food sources of calcium include milk and other dairy products. Milk is fortified with vitamin D, making it good source of both minerals. Beans, almonds, broccoli, and dark-green leafy vegetables are also good sources of calcium. Some foods, such as orange juice, breads, and soy products, are fortified with calcium, making them good sources as well. For children who are lactose intolerant, allergic to milk, or vegetarian, calcium and vitamin D supplements may be warranted.

Vitamin D is a fat-soluble vitamin found naturally in only a few sources. Small amounts of vitamin D are found in cheese and egg yolks. Fortified foods provide most of the vitamin D in the American diet. With the help of skin exposed to sunlight, the human body can convert an inactive form of vitamin D to the vitamin's active form, contributing to vitamin D stores in the body. Roles of vitamin D include promoting calcium absorption in the gut and maintaining adequate serum calcium and phosphate concentrations to assist with bone mineralization and bone growth. In addition, vitamin D assists with cell growth and immune function and reduces inflammation.[26]

Table 7.6

RDAs for Calcium and Vitamin D

Age	Calcium	Vitamin D
2 to 3 years old	700 mg/day	600 IU/day
4 to 5 years old	1,000 mg/day	600 IU/day

IU, international unit.

Data from: Institute of Medicine Committee to Review Dietary Reference Intakes for Vitamin D and Calcium; Ross AC, Taylor CL, Yaktine AL, Del Valle HB, eds. *Dietary Reference Intakes for Calcium and Vitamin D.* Washington, DC: National Academies Press; 2011. Retrieved from: https://www.nationalacademies.org/hmd/~/media/Files/Report%20Files/2010/Dietary-Reference-Intakes-for-Calcium-and-Vitamin-D/Vitamin%20D%20and%20Calcium%202010%20Report%20Brief.pdf. Accessed September 8, 2016.

Iron

The mineral iron has many roles in the human body. Iron is an essential component of hemoglobin, which transfers oxygen from the lungs to the tissues, and is a component of myoglobin, which provides oxygen to muscles. Iron supports metabolism, and is necessary for growth, development, normal cell functioning, and synthesis of some hormones and connective tissue.[27]

Toddlers need 7 mg of iron each day. Kids ages 4 and 5 years old need 10 mg of iron each day. Tolerable Upper Intake Levels (ULs) for children ages 2 to 5 years old is 40 mg per day. Iron is stored in the body as ferritin; therefore, the serum ferritin level is a good indicator of iron status in children.[28]

Dietary iron has two main forms: heme and nonheme. Heme sources of iron include meat and poultry; nonheme sources include fruits, vegetables, fortified bread, and grain products such as cereal. **TABLE 7.7** lists good sources of iron.

The amount of iron absorbed depends on the iron status of the individual as well as the form of iron (heme or nonheme) consumed. Heme iron sources are more easily absorbed than the iron from plants, dairy products, fortified foods, and supplements. The absorption of nonheme iron is strongly influenced by enhancers and inhibitors eaten at the same meal.[29] Vitamin C enhances iron absorption; therefore, eating foods such as orange juice, tomatoes, broccoli, and strawberries with foods that contain iron maximizes iron absorption. Inhibitors of iron absorption include polyphenols found in some fruits, some vegetables, coffee, tea, and spices; phytic acid, which is found in almonds, walnuts, sesame seeds, dried beans, lentils, and peas; calcium; and eggs. Drinking milk at the same meal as eating red meat decreases iron absorption from the meat. In addition, nonheme iron absorption is lower for those consuming vegetarian diets than for those eating nonvegetarian diets. For this reason, it has been suggested that the iron requirement for those consuming a vegetarian diet is approximately twofold greater than that of those consuming a nonvegetarian diet.[27]

Table 7.7
Good Sources of iron
Red meat
Poultry (dark meat)
Tuna fish
Salmon
Eggs
Tofu
Enriched grains
Dried beans and peas
Dried fruits
Leafy-green vegetables
Ironfortified breakfast cereal

Recap Using the *Dietary Guidelines for Americans* as a basis for helping toddlers and preschool-age children develop healthy attitudes about food and good eating habits can help prevent consequences of poor food choices not only in this life stage but across the life span.

1. Describe why fiber is an important component of a child's diet.
2. Explain the role of calcium in the diet of a child.
3. Identify enhancers and inhibitors of iron absorption.

Common Nutrition Considerations During Preschool and Early Childhood

Preview A number of considerations for toddlers and preschool-age children are of particular interest. Dental caries, constipation, and lead exposure are a few that have nutrition implications. Being aware of these conditions and knowing how to combat them with nutrition interventions helps to minimize the negative effects that can result.

Dental Caries

Tooth decay is one of the most common chronic conditions among children.[30] CDC statistics indicate an increase in the number of preschoolers with dental caries, and this trend appears across income levels, with a typical incidence rate of 6–10 caries per individual.[31]

Our mouths are home to different bacteria, some good, some harmful. The bacterium *Streptococcus mutans* is one such harmful species. *S. mutans* in the mouth excretes acid that helps cause tooth decay. This type of bacteria feeds off of carbohydrates; therefore, the more often and longer teeth are exposed to carbohydrates, the longer the environment in the mouth is conducive to the development of tooth decay.[32]

All throughout the day, a tug of war wages inside the mouth. On one side are dental plaque, a sticky, colorless film of bacteria, and residues of foods and drinks such as milk, bread, candy, and juice that contain sugar and starch. The bacteria and sugar mix, which creates an acid that begins to act on the teeth's outer surface, the enamel. On the other side of this tug of war are the minerals in saliva such as calcium and phosphate plus fluoride from toothpaste, water, and other sources. This side helps tooth enamel repair itself by replacing minerals lost when the teeth are exposed to the acidic bacterial mixture.

This tug of war occurs as a result of the natural and continuous process of the teeth losing minerals and regaining minerals.[33] Repeated or prolonged exposure of the teeth to the acidic bacterial mixture causes the enamel to lose minerals, which can cause white spots to appear on the surface of the teeth. White spots indicate decay; however, at this point tooth decay can be stopped or reversed. Enamel can repair itself using minerals from saliva and fluoride from toothpaste and other sources. But if the process of tooth decay continues, more minerals are lost, and over time, the enamel is weakened, destroyed, and the permanent damage of a cavity results.[34] Some issues that make toddlers and preschool-aged children at risk for dental caries include frequent eating, juice intake, naps, and challenges in proper teeth brushing. While children need to eat frequently due to their small stomach size, care should be taken to limit high sugary foods and juices that can coat the teeth with substrate preferred by the bacteria. During sleep there is low saliva so it is important to brush teeth before nap and bed time. Teeth cleaning should begin as soon as the first tooth erupts by wiping with cloth and water. Around 18 months, children can use special fluoride-free toothpaste and move to fluoride-containing children's toothpaste when they can spit. Setting up good teeth brushing habits of at least twice a day can reduce the risk for dental caries. Tooth decay can cause pain and infection and can lead to problems with eating, speaking, and learning.[30]

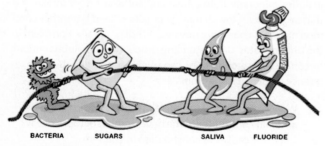

BACTERIA   SUGARS   SALIVA   FLUORIDE

Courtesy of the National Institutes of Health

Fluoride is a mineral that can prevent tooth decay from progressing. It can even reverse, or stop, early tooth decay. Fluoride works to protect teeth in two ways: (1) fluoride prevents mineral loss in tooth enamel and replaces lost minerals; and (2) fluoride reduces the ability of bacteria to make acid. Sources of fluoride include fluoridated water and toothpaste that contains fluoride.

The National Institutes of Health (NIH) recommends the following tooth-friendly tips:[35]

- Limit between-meal snacks. This reduces the number of acid attacks on teeth and gives teeth a chance to repair themselves.
- Save candy, cookies, soda, and other sugary drinks for special occasions.

Let's Discuss

The human mouth is filled with bacteria—more than 600 species of bacteria. Most of these are harmless; however, when it comes to tooth decay, the bacterium *Streptococcus mutans* is a major culprit. *S. mutans* converts sugar from the foods we eat into tooth-dissolving acids. Reducing this species of bacteria in the mouth is associated with fewer cavities.

Some healthy bacteria, also called probiotics, contribute to decreasing the numbers of *S. mutans* inside the mouth. With the help of food science, probiotics can be added to common foods we eat, such as yogurt and other dairy products. Studies show that short-term daily ingestion of probiotics in the diet shows marked salivary pH elevation and reduction of salivary *S. mutans* counts, two factors that are key in preventing dental caries.

It can be suggested that supplements containing such probiotics, either in pill or food form, may indeed help prevent enamel demineralization. Do you think that candy or chewing gum filled with probiotics could become a recommendation for preventing tooth decay in the future?

Reference

Data from Shivangi Srivastava, Sabyasachi Saha, Minti Kumari, et al. Effect of Probiotic Curd on Salivary pH and *Streptococcus mutans*: A Double Blind Parallel Randomized Controlled Trial. *J Clin Diagn Res*. 2016 Feb;10(2):ZC13-ZC16.

- Limit fruit juice.
- Make sure children do not eat or drink anything with sugar in it after brushing their teeth before they go to bed. Saliva flow decreases during sleep. Without enough saliva, teeth are less able to repair themselves after an acid attack.
- Children should brush their teeth two times per day.
- Children should see a dentist for regular checkups.

In addition, the American Academy of Pediatric Dentistry offers the following tips for toddlers and young children:[36]

- Encourage children to drink from a cup by their first birthday; a training cup is only meant to serve as a transitional tool from helping kids adjust from the bottle to a cup.
- Only put water in training cups—except during mealtime. Filling a cup with juice or even milk and allowing a child to drink from it throughout the day bathes the child's teeth in cavity-causing bacteria.
- Parents should dispense a "pea-size" amount of toothpaste and perform or assist with their child's tooth brushing.

- Supervise children brushing their teeth and teach them to spit out, not swallow, the toothpaste.
- Help children develop good eating habits early and choose sensible, nutritious snacks.

Constipation

Constipation is a condition in which a child has fewer than two bowel movements a week or has hard, dry, and small bowel movements that are painful or difficult to pass. Studies indicate that 10% of children in the United States suffer from chronic constipation.[37] Likely causes of constipation in children include the following: ignoring the urge to have a bowel movement; diets low in fiber; certain medicines; health problems involving the gastrointestinal (GI) tract; or functional GI disorders.

Strong evidence supports an association between low intakes of fiber and the high prevalence of childhood constipation as well as a positive effect of dietary fiber intake in the treatment of constipation in children.[37] Fiber helps stool stay soft, which allows it to move smoothly through a child's colon. Adequate fluid intake in the form of water or fruit juices is also important in helping fiber do its job of moving stool through the GI tract.

Adequate fluid intake, sufficient fiber intake, and avoiding foods low in fiber, such as cheese, potato chips, fast food, ice cream, and processed foods, are generally effective treatments for children with constipation; however, medical management may also be necessary.[38] Fecal impaction, anal fissures, and rectal prolapse are all possible treatment methods used by doctors if necessary.

Lead Exposure

Lead is a naturally occurring toxic metal found in the earth's crust. Young children are particularly vulnerable to the toxic effects of lead, which involve the developing brain and nervous system. Lead can adversely affect children's brain development, resulting in reduced intelligence quotient (IQ), behavioral changes such as shortening of attention span and increased antisocial behavior, and reduced educational attainment. The neurological and behavioral effects of lead are believed to be irreversible.[39]

People can be exposed to lead through occupational and environmental sources, resulting mainly in inhalation of lead particles generated by burning materials containing lead or from lead-contaminated dust, water, or food. Young children are especially at risk because they absorb four to five times as much ingested lead as adults do from a given source. Furthermore, children's innate curiosity and their age-appropriate hand-to-mouth behavior result in their putting potentially lead-contaminating or lead-coated objects in their mouth.

Once lead enters the body, it is distributed to organs such as the brain, kidneys, liver, and bones. The body stores lead in the teeth and bones, where it accumulates over time. Lead stored in bone may be remobilized into the blood during pregnancy, thus exposing the fetus. Undernourished children are more susceptible to lead because their bodies absorb more lead if other nutrients such as calcium are lacking.[39]

Recap Tooth decay and constipation are both common conditions experienced during childhood, and both can be prevented or at least minimalized with certain nutrition considerations. Constipation in children can be treated by following a diet that includes adequate fluid intake and sufficient fiber intake and that avoids foods low in fiber. Exposure to lead is another common nutrition condition; however, is not generally a problem in the United States. Understanding proper nutrition interventions to combat these conditions can minimize the negative consequences that can result from each.

1. What is the name of the bacteria that resides in the mouth and that contributes to the development of tooth decay?
2. List likely causes of constipation in children.
3. What effects can lead exposure have on children?

News You Can Use

The human gut contains a microbial community composed of tens of trillions of organisms that is formed prior to birth and normally assembled during the first 2–3 years of life. Much is being studied and learned about the microorganisms that make up our gut ecosystem, which differ significantly from person to person.

Studies suggest that the gut microbiome is involved in the control of body weight and energy metabolism. It affects the two main causes of obesity: energy acquisition and storage, and insulin resistance and the inflammatory state, both of which characterize obesity.[a] Many factors affect gut microorganisms, including food choices and the environment.

One area of research is the link between antibiotic use and microbial imbalance within the digestive tract. Antibiotic-induced gut microbiota imbalance has been associated with obesity.[b] Because early development of obesity increases the risk of obesity later in life, antibiotics should be used with caution and concern in childhood, and measures should be taken to determine what, if anything, can reverse the damaging effects of microbial imbalance in the gut.

Not all of the mechanisms that explain how antibiotics destroy some of the beneficial bacteria, which help us maintain a healthy body weight, have been defined. However, it is believed that the inclusion of prebiotics and probiotics in the diet can help prevent obesity.[c] The take-home message:

Children should use antibiotics when medically necessary and when effective alternatives are not available. In addition, the incorporation of foods that contain prebiotics and probiotics (such as yogurt) can be helpful to the gut microbiota in children.

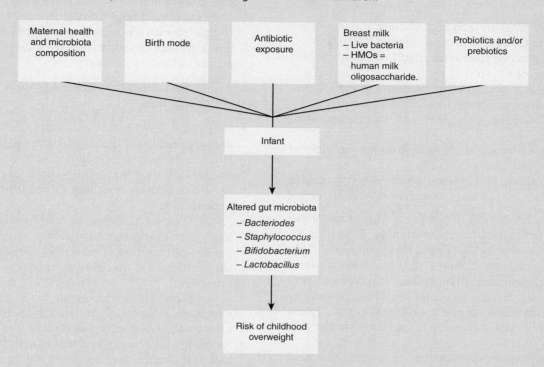

References

a. Isolauri E, Salminen S. The impact of early gut microbiota modulation on the risk of child disease: alert to accuracy in probiotic studies. *Benef Microbes*. 2015;6(2):167–171.
b. Principi N, Esposito S. Antibiotic administration and the development of obesity in children. *Int J Antimicrob Agents*. 2016;47(3):171–177.
c. Koleva PT, Bridgman SL, Kozyrskyj AL. The infant gut microbiome: evidence for obesity risk and dietary intervention. *Nutrients*. March 31, 2015;7(4):2237–2260.

Promoting Healthy Lifestyles

Preview Preventing overweight and obesity during the toddler and preschool years goes a long way in warding off overweight and obesity later in life. Following guidelines for a healthy lifestyle, including eating and exercise, are key components in helping to curb the obesity epidemic among children.

Preventing Overweight and Obesity

The most common measurement used to determine childhood overweight and obesity is body mass index (BMI). Overweight is defined as a BMI at or above the 85th percentile and below the 95th percentile for children and teens of the same age and sex; obesity is defined as a BMI at or above the 95th percentile. According to the CDC, the prevalence of obesity among children ages 2 to 5 years was 8.4% during the years 2011–2012, with highest rates among children in families with a household income that is at or below the poverty threshhold.[40]

Regardless of age, behavior and genetics are both strong causes of overweight and obesity. Behavior factors include dietary patterns, level of physical activity, medication use, education and skills, the environment, and food marketing and promotion. Genetic changes in humans occur slowly; therefore, it is unlikely that genetics alone can be the cause of excess weight. However, the different ways in which people respond to the same environment suggests that genes do play a role in the development of obesity.[41]

Obesity during childhood can have a harmful effect on the body in a variety of ways. Children who are obese have a greater risk of the following:[42]

- High blood pressure and high cholesterol, which are risk factors for cardiovascular disease (CVD)
- Impaired glucose tolerance, insulin resistance, and type 2 diabetes
- Breathing problems, such as sleep apnea and asthma
- Joint problems and musculoskeletal discomfort
- Fatty liver disease, gallstones, and gastroesophageal reflux
- Psychological stress such as depression, behavioral problems, and issues in school
- Low self-esteem and low self-reported quality of life
- Impaired social, physical, and emotional functioning

Children who are obese are likely to become obese adults. Significant health consequences of childhood overweight and obesity that occur in adulthood include cardiovascular disease, diabetes, musculoskeletal disorders (especially osteoarthritis), and certain types of cancer (endometrial, breast, and colon).[42] Having a healthy diet pattern and engaging in regular physical activity are both important in the prevention of excessive weight gain in children.

The obesogenic environment plays a significant role in the development of childhood overweight and obesity. In the home, child care center, school, or community, children are exposed to a number of factors that contribute to a lifestyle that promotes increased consumption of unhealthy food while discouraging physical activity. Some factors include the following:[43]

- *No safe and desirable place to play or be active:* Many communities are built in ways that make it difficult or unsafe for community members to be physical active. For example, getting to a park or recreation center may be difficult. For many children, safe routes for walking or riding a bike to school may not exist. Safe areas to play outside may not be available.
- *Limited access to healthy affordable foods:* Some people have limited access to stores and supermarkets that sell healthy, affordable food such as fruits and vegetables, especially in rural, minority, and lower-income neighborhoods. Choosing healthy food is also difficult for people who live in an area where most of the food retailers, such as convenience stores and fast-food restaurants, sell less-healthy food.
- *Greater availability of high-energy-dense foods and sugar-sweetened beverages:* Sugar-sweetened beverages are the largest source of added sugar and an important contributor of calorie to the diets of U.S. children. High consumption of sugar-sweetened beverages, which have few if any nutrients, has been associated with obesity. On a typical day, 80% of youth drink sugar-sweetened beverages.
- *Increased portion sizes:* Portion sizes of less-healthy foods and beverages have increased in restaurants and grocery stores. Research shows that when children are served larger portions, they eat more food compared with when they are offered a standard portion size. This can mean that they are overeating at a number of eating occasions.

Additional factors that contribute to childhood overweight include these:[44]

- *Food choices:* Diets higher in calories and lower in fruits and vegetables are linked with overweight.
- *Physical activity vs. sedentary activity:* Less physical activity and more time spent participating in activities such as watching TV result in less energy expenditure.
- *Parental obesity:* Children of obese parents are more likely to be overweight themselves. An inherited component of childhood overweight makes it easier for some children to become overweight compared with others.
- *Eating patterns:* Skipping meals or failure to maintain a regular eating schedule tends to contribute to overeating at the next eating occasion.
- *Parenting style:* Some researchers believe that excess parental control over children's eating might lead to poor self-regulation of children's energy intake.
- *Diabetes during pregnancy:* Overweight and type 2 diabetes occur with greater frequency in the offspring of diabetic mothers.
- *Excessive weight gain during pregnancy:* Studies have shown that excessive maternal weight gain during pregnancy is associated with increased birth weight and overweight later in life.
- *Formula feeding vs. breastfeeding:* Although the exact mechanism is not known, studies suggest that breastfeeding may prevent excess weight gain as children grow.
- *Parental eating and physical activity habits:* Parents with poor nutritional habits and who lead sedentary lifestyles role model these behaviors for their children, thereby creating an obesogenic home environment.
- *Demographic factors:* Certain demographic factors are associated with an increased risk of being overweight in childhood. For example, there is evidence that black and Hispanic children 6 to 11 years old are more likely to be overweight than are non-Hispanic white children of the same age. Asian and Pacific Islander children of the same age were slightly less likely to be overweight.

There are multiple causes of childhood overweight and obesity, some considered preventable. The World

Health Organization (WHO) recognizes that prevention is the most feasible option for decreasing childhood obesity and calls to attention that current treatment practices largely aim at bringing the problem under control rather than effecting a cure. The WHO goal in fighting the childhood obesity epidemic is to achieve an energy balance that can be maintained throughout the individual's life span. General recommendations include the following:[45]

- Increase consumption of fruit and vegetables as well as legumes, whole grains, and nuts.
- Limit energy intake from total fats and shift fat consumption away from saturated fats to unsaturated fats.
- Limit the intake of sugars.
- Be physically active—accumulate at least 60 minutes of developmentally appropriate, regular, moderate- to vigorous-intensity activity each day.

The Obesity Society provides these tips on ways to establish healthy eating patterns with kids:[43]

- Parents should choose highly nutrient-dense foods for children and let the child determine how much to eat.
- Fruits and vegetables, as compared with high-calorie snacks, should be readily available in the home.
- Use small portions—child portions are usually very small, particularly compared with adult portions.
- Bake, broil, roast, or grill meats instead of frying them.
- Limit use of high-calorie, high-fat, and high-sugar sauces and spreads.
- Use low-fat or nonfat and lower calorie dairy products for milk, yogurt, and ice cream.
- Support participation in play, sports, and other physical activity at school, church, or community leagues.
- Be active as a family—go on walks, bike ride, swim, and hike together.
- Limit screen time.
- Avoid eating while watching TV.
- Replace high-sugared drinks, especially sodas, with water or low-fat milk.
- Limit fruit juice intake to two servings or less per day.
- Encourage free play in young children and provide environments that allow children to play indoors and outdoors.
- Role model through healthy dietary practices, nutritional snacks, and lifestyle activities. Avoid badgering children, restrictive feeding, labeling foods as "good" or "bad," and using food as a reward.

Physical Activity Recommendations

It has been determined that inactive children are likely to become inactive adults.[46] According to the American Heart Association, physical inactivity is a major risk factor for developing coronary artery disease; it increases the risk of stroke and other cardiovascular risk factors such as obesity, high blood pressure, low HDL (high-density lipoprotein) cholesterol, and diabetes. On the other hand, regular physical activity is important for bone health. Weight-bearing exercises such as jumping rope, running, and walking can also help develop and maintain strong bones. Children who engage in physical activity tend to be leaner and less likely to become overweight. Parents and caregivers of children are in a position to role model an active lifestyle and provide children with opportunities for physical activity. Physical activity should be enjoyable, be age-appropriate, and offer variety.

Movement and physical activity throughout the day is an important comment of the development of toddlers and preschool-aged children. Specific duration and intensity recommendations have been set for children over 6 years of age. For younger children, physical activity is thought of less as specific sports or activities; rather it is a constant presence throughout the day and as a component of play. Young children need opportunities to develop gross motor skills and have active play both inside and outside. The Institute of Medicine recommends that toddlers and preschool-age children in child care have "light, moderate, and vigorous physical activity for at least 15 minutes per hour while children are in care" including outdoor time, developmental appropriate structured and unstructured physical activity, and integration of physical activity in cognitive and social development.[47]

Children who exercise on a regular basis experience many of the same benefits that adults do. For example, they feel less stress; feel better about themselves; feel more ready to learn in school; keep a healthy weight; keep bones, muscles, and joints healthy; and sleep better at night.

Case Study

Four-year-old James is described as an active child at the preschool he attends. During free time, he likes to be active on the playground, running, jumping, and climbing on the apparatus. James plays on a recreation league soccer team and practices 1 day a week, with games on the weekends.

Questions

1. Within a typical week, do you think that James is meeting the suggested criteria for physical activity? Suggest how he can meet the activity guidelines throughout the year.
2. Describe benefits associated with young children being engaged in regular physical activity.

Recap BMI is a good guideline to use to determine the weight status of toddlers and preschool-age children. Behavior and genetics are both strong causes of overweight and obesity, and the obesogenic environment plays a significant role in the development of childhood overweight and obesity. Exercise is an important component in warding off obesity; children who exercise on a regular basis experience many benefits to their health and well-being.

1. List three risk factors of childhood obesity.
2. Describe the American Heart Association physical guidelines for children.

At least 60 minutes of moderate to vigorous intensity aerobic activity is recommended everyday for kids.

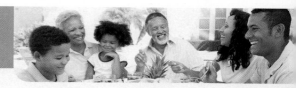

Learning Portfolio

Visual Chapter Summary

Monitoring Growth in Early Childhood

- Monitoring a child's growth over time is a valuable tool in assessing the adequacy of energy and nutrient intake.

- It is essential that measurements used as assessment tools are accurate and precise because inaccurate or incorrectly plotted data can lead to errors in health status assessment.

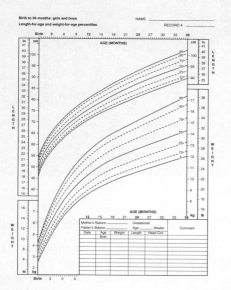

Developed by the National Center for Health Statistics in collaboration with the National Center for Chronic Disease Prevention and Health Promotion (2000)

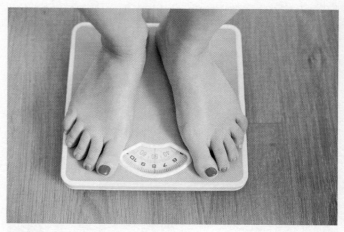

©Rostislav_Sedlacek/Shutterstock

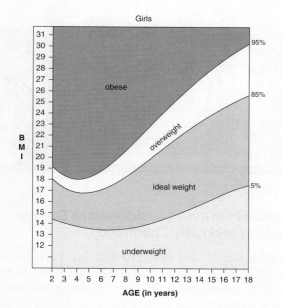

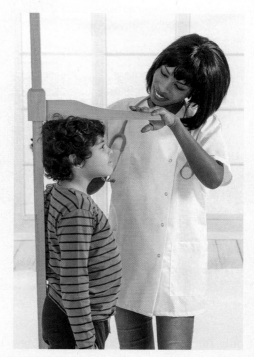

©Chassenet/BSIP SA/Alamy Stock Photo

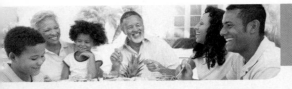

Learning Portfolio (continued)

Factors that Affect Dietary Intake

- Toddlers and preschool-aged children show a decreased appetite and a much slower rate of growth compared with infants. A number of factors affect dietary intake of children, including food jags and food aversions, appetite and satiety, media influences, parental influences, the feeding relationship between child and caregiver, and the obesogenic environment.

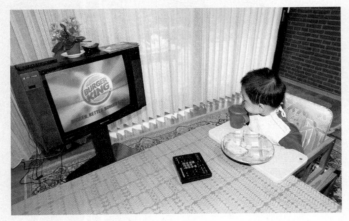

©Bernhard Classen/vario images GmbH &Co.KG/Alamy Stock Photo

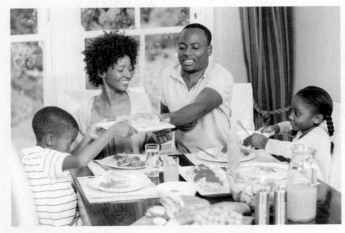

©David Mabe/Alamy Stock Photo

- Not only for their own health and wellness but for that of their children, parents and caregivers should be aware that providing healthy foods while limiting

unhealthy food choices and demonstrating healthy food habits are good building blocks for helping children develop healthy lifestyles.

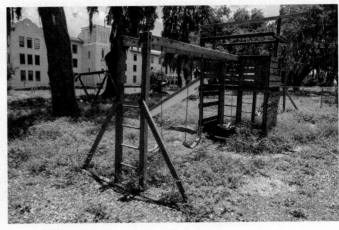

©wavebreakmedia/Shutterstock

Nutrition Recommendations and Requirements

- Using the *Dietary Guidelines for Americans* as a basis for helping toddlers and preschool-age children develop healthy attitudes about food and good eating habits can help prevent consequences of poor food choices not only in this life stage but across the life span.

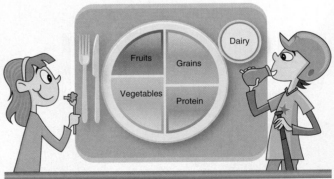

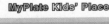

Courtesy of ChooseMyPlate.gov

Common Nutrition Considerations During Preschool and Early Childhood

- Tooth decay and constipation are both common conditions experienced during childhood, and both can be prevented or at least minimalized with certain nutrition considerations.

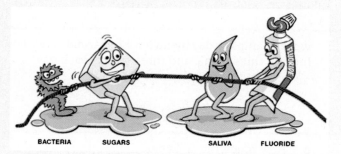

BACTERIA   SUGARS   SALIVA   FLUORIDE

Courtesy of the National Institutes of Health

Promoting Healthy Lifestyles

- BMI is a good guideline to use to determine the weight status of toddlers and preschool-age children.
- Behavior and genetics are both strong causes of overweight and obesity, and the obesogenic environment plays a significant role in the development of childhood overweight and obesity.
- Exercise is an important component in warding off obesity, and children who exercise on a regular basis experience many benefits to their health and well-being.

- Constipation in children can be treated by following a diet that includes adequate fluid intake and sufficient fiber intake and that avoids foods that are low in fiber.
- Exposure to lead is another common nutrition condition; however, it is not generally a problem in the United States. Understanding proper nutrition interventions to combat these conditions can minimize the negative consequences that can result.

At least 60 minutes of moderate to vigorous intensity aerobic activity is recommended everyday for kids.

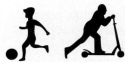

Key Terms

food aversion: A strong feeling of dislike that results in refusal to try or to eat certain foods.

food jags: When an individual consumes the same food, prepared the same way, on a consistent basis.

intuitive eating: A nutrition philosophy based on the idea that becoming more in tune with the body's natural hunger signals is a more effective way to attain a healthy weight than keeping track of the amounts of kcalories and macronutrients eaten.

neophobia: Generally regarded as the reluctance to eat or the avoidance of new foods.

nutrient density: A characteristic of foods that provide a generous amount of one or more nutrients compared to the number of calories they supply.

obesogenic environment: An environment that promotes gaining weight and that is not conducive to weight loss within the home or workplace.

preschoolers: Children between the ages of 3 and 5 years.

rickets: A bone-softening disease the results from vitamin D deficiency and that causes severe bowing of the legs, poor growth, and sometimes muscle pain and weakness.

toddlers: Children 2 to 3 years of age.

Discussion Questions

1. What is the difference between a child demonstrating a food jag and neophobia toward food? Give examples of when these two stages of eating might occur together. What advice would you give a caregiver in an effort to ease a food jag or neophobia toward food?

2. As discussed in this chapter, studies show that a child's personality traits tend to influence food intake. Think of your eating habits as a child, or think of children you have observed. Have you seen a link between a child's impulses and their ability to self-regulate food intake based on hunger? Discuss ways you could advise caregivers or teach children to recognize their hunger and fullness cues.

3. Think about the environments in which you live, work, and play. Do these environments contribute to a healthy or an unhealthy lifestyle? Why or why not?

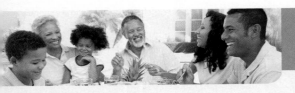

Learning Portfolio (continued)

Activities

1. Using the *Dietary Guidelines for Americans* eating pattern recommendations (Table 7.4 and Figure 7.5), write a sample 2-day menu for a 3-year-old active boy. Include three meals and three snacks each day.

Study Questions

1. Using the BMI chart (Figure 7.2), identify the weight category of a 4-year-old with a BMI of 16.6.
   a. About 25th percentile
   b. About 30th percentile
   c. About 50th percentile
   d. About 60th percentile
2. Which of the following is the most likely reason for the observed decrease in nutrition and appetite of children ages 2 to 5 years of age?
   a. Children this age tend to want to eat low-nutrient-dense foods and therefore do not seem to be hungry as often throughout the day.
   b. At this age, children generally grow more slowly and it requires less energy production.
   c. At this age, children tend to have a rapid growth rate but small stomach capacity, requiring less energy intake each day.
   d. Children at this age are not in tune with their hunger and fullness cues, and they tend to "forget" about eating.
3. Examples of foods that are high in nutrient density include which of the following?
   a. Candy bar and soda
   b. Watermelon
   c. Eggs
   d. Cucumbers
4. According to the author Ellyn Satter's division of responsibility for feeding toddlers and adolescents, the parent or caregiver is responsible for which of the following?
   a. How much the child eats
   b. Whether the child eats
   c. What, when, and where the child eats
   d. Answers a and b are both correct
5. Which of the following is the best description of how the bacteria *Streptococcus mutans* acts inside the human mouth?
   a. Produces acid-fighting saliva to prevent tooth decay.
   b. Fights against sugar in preventing tooth decay.
   c. Extracts other bacteria that increase saliva production and accelerate tooth decay.
   d. Excretes acid that causes tooth decay.
6. Which of the following recommendations would likely cause constipation in children?
   a. Eating a diet high in fruit and high in complex carbohydrates
   b. Limiting fluids and eating foods low in fiber
   c. Eating a high-fiber diet
   d. Having adequate fluid intake and increased consumption of dairy products
7. Childhood obesity is associated with a higher risk of each of the following *except* which one?
   a. Breathing problems such as sleep apnea
   b. Fatty liver disease, gallstones, and gastroesophageal reflux
   c. High blood pressure and high cholesterol
   d. Impaired social, physical, and emotional functioning
   e. All of the above

Weblinks

■ **CDC Growth Charts: United States**
   http://www.cdc.gov/growthcharts/clinical_charts.htm

■ **Ellyn Satter Institute:**
   http://ellynsatterinstitute.org

References

1. Nicklaus S. The role of food experiences during early childhood in food pleasure learning. *Appetite*. September 1, 2016;104:3–9 [published online ahead of print August 20, 2015].

2. National Center for Health Statistics, National Center for Chronic Disease Prevention and Health Promotion. Clinical growth charts: birth to 36 months: girls. Centers for Disease Control and Prevention; May 30, 2000. Retrieved from: http://www.cdc.gov/growthcharts/data/set1clinical/cj41l018.pdf. Accessed April 21, 2016.

3. National Heart, Lung, and Blood Institute. Calculate your body mass index. Retrieved from: http://www.nhlbi.nih.gov/health/educational/lose_wt/BMI/bmicalc.htm. Accessed April 21, 2016.

4. The health professional's guide to using growth charts. *Paediatr Child Health*. March 2004;9(3):174–176. Copyright © 2004, Pulsus Group Inc.

5. Taylor CM, Northstone K, Wernimont SM, Emmett PM. Picky eating in preschool children: associations with dietary fibre intakes and stool hardness. *Appetite*. May 1, 2016; 100:263–271.

6. Remy E, Issanchou S, Chabanet C, et al. Impact of adiposity, age, sex and maternal feeding practices on eating in the absence of hunger and caloric compensation in preschool children. *Int J Obes* (London). 2015;39(6):925–930.

7. Nederkoorn C, Dassen FC, Franken L, et al. Impulsivity and overeating in children in the absence and presence of hunger. *Appetite*. 2015;93:57–61.

8. Tripicchio G, Heo M, Diewald L, et al. Restricting advertisements for high-fat, high-sugar foods during children's television programs: attitudes in a US population-based sample. *Child Obes*. 2016;12(2):113–118.

9. Kelly B, Freeman B, King L, et al. Television advertising, not viewing, is associated with negative dietary patterns in children. *Pediatr Obes*. 2016;11(2):158–160.

10. Lioutas ED, Tzimitra-Kalogianni I. I saw Santa drinking soda! Advertising and children's food preferences. *Child Care Health Dev*. 2015;41(3):424–433.

11. Damiano SR, Hart LM, Paxton SJ. Correlates of parental feeding practices with pre-schoolers: parental body image and eating knowledge, attitudes, and behaviours. *Appetite*. March 4, 2016;101:192–198.

12. Boak R, Virgo-Milton M, Hoare A. Choosing foods for infants: a qualitative study of the factors that influence mothers *Child Care Health Dev*. May 2016;42(3):359–369 [published online ahead of print March 3, 2016].

13. Wardle J, Coole L. Genetic and environmental determinants of children's food preferences. *Br J Nutr*. 2008;99: S15–S21.

14. Gibson EL, Kreichauf S, Wildgruber A, et al. (2012). A narrative review of psychological and educational strategies applied to young children's eating behaviours aimed at reducing obesity risk. *Obes Rev*. 2012;13(1):85–95.

15. Small L, Lane H, Vaughan L, Melnyk B, McBurnett D. A systematic review of the evidence: the effects of portion size manipulation with children and portion education/training interventions on dietary intake with adults. *Worldviews Evid Based Nurs*. 2013;10(2):69–81.

16. van Kleef E, Bruggers I, de Vet E. Encouraging vegetable intake as a snack among children: the influence of protein and unit size. *Public Health Nutr*. 2015;18(15):2736–2741.

17. Micali N, Rask CU, Olsen EM, Skovgaard AM. Early predictors of childhood restrictive eating: a population-based study. *J Dev Behav Pediatr*. May 2016;37(4):314–321 [published online ahead of print February 17, 2016].

18. Satter E. *How to Get Your Kid to Eat … But Not Too Much*. Palo Alto, CA: Bull Publishing; 2012.

19. Agras WS, Hammer LD, Huffman LC, Mascola A, Bryson SW, Danaher C. Improving healthy eating in families with a toddler at risk for overweight: a cluster randomized controlled trial. *J Dev Behav Pediatr*. Sept. 2012;33(7):529–534.

20. Swinburn B, Eggar G, Raza F. Dissecting obesogenic environments; the development and application of a framework for identifying and prioritizing environmental interventions for obesity. *Prevent Med*. 1999;29(6):563–570.

21. Martin-Biggers J, Spaccarotella K, Hongu N, et al. Translating it into real life: a qualitative study of the cognitions, barriers and sports for key obesogenic behaviors of parents of preschoolers. *BMC Public Health*. February 26, 2015;15:189.

22. U.S. Department of Health and Human Services and U.S. Department of Agriculture. *2015–2020 Dietary Guidelines for Americans*. 8th ed. Washington, DC: U.S. Department of Health and Human Services and U.S. Department of Agriculture; December 2015. Retrieved from: http://health.gov/dietaryguidelines/2015/guidelines/. Accessed August 13, 2016.

23. Mackowiak K, Torlinska-Walkowiak N, Torlinska B. Dietary fibre as an important constituent of the diet. *Postepy Hig Med Dosw* (online). February 25, 2016;70:104–109.

24. Kranz S, Brauchia M, Slavin JL, et al. What do we know about dietary fiber intake in children and health? The effects of fiber intake on constipation, obesity, and diabetes in children. *Adv Nutr*. January 2012;3:47–53.

25. Davis JN, Alexander KE, Ventura EE, Toledo-Corral CM, Goran MI. Inverse relation between dietary fiber intake and visceral adiposity in overweight Latino youth. *Am J Clin Nutr*. 2009;90:1160–1166.

26. Institute of Medicine Committee to Review Dietary Reference Intakes for Vitamin D and Calcium; Ross AC, Taylor CL, Yaktine AL, Del Valle HB, eds. *Dietary Reference Intakes for Calcium and Vitamin D*. Washington, DC: National Academies Press; 2011.

27. National Institutes of Health; February 11, 2016. Health information: iron [dietary supplement fact sheet]. Retrieved from: https://ods.od.nih.gov/factsheets/Iron-HealthProfessional/. Accessed September 9, 2016.

28. Owens A, Cloud HH. Special topics in toddler and preschool nutrition: vitamins and minerals in childhood and children with disabilities. In: Edelstein S, Sharlin J, eds. *Life Cycle Nutrition: An Evidence-Based Approach*. Sudbury, MA: Jones & Bartlett Publishers; 2009:183–225.

29. Amah SM, Carriquiry AL, Reddy MB. Total iron bioavailability from the US diet is lower than the current estimate. *J Nutr*. 2015;145(11):2617–2621.

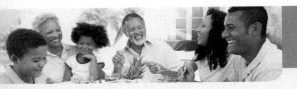

Learning Portfolio (continued)

30. Griffin S, Barker L, Wei L, et al. Use of dental care and effective preventive services in preventing tooth decay among U.S. children and adolescents—Medical Expenditure Panel Survey, United States, 2003–2009 and National Health and Nutrition Examination Survey, United States, 2005–2010. *MMWR Suppl.* September 12, 2014;63(2):54–60.

31. Centers for Disease Control and Prevention; December 16, 2014. Hygiene-related diseases: dental caries (tooth decay). Retrieved from: http://www.cdc.gov/healthywater/hygiene/disease/dental_caries.html. Accessed September 9, 2016.

32. Srivastava S, Saha S, Kumari M, Mohd S. Effect of probiotic curd on salivary pH and *Streptococcus mutans*: a double blind parallel randomized control trial. *J Clin Diagn Res.* February 2016;10(2):ZC13–16.

33. Deyhle H, White SN, Bunk O, et al. Nanostructure of carious tooth enamel lesion. *Acta Biomater.* 2014;10(1):355–364.

34. Kayes PH, Rams TE. Dental calculus arrest of dental caries. *J Oral Biol* (Northborough). February 2016;3(1):pii: 4.

35. National Institute of Dental and Craniofacial Research; May 2013. The tooth decay process: how to reverse it and avoid a cavity. Retrieved from: http://www.nidcr.nih.gov/oralhealth/OralHealth-Information/ChildrensOralHealth/ToothDecay-Process.htm. Accessed September 9, 2016.

36. American Academy of Pediatric Dentistry. Early childhood caries (ECC). Chicago, IL: American Academy of Pediatric Dentistry. Retrieved from: http://www.mychildrensteeth.org/assets/2/7/ECCstats.pdf. Accessed September 9, 2016.

37. Walia R, Mahajan L, Steffen R. Recent advances in chronic constipation. *Curr Opin Pediatr.* 2009;21:661–666.

38. National Institute of Diabetes and Digestive and Kidney Disease; November 13, 2014. Eating, diet, and nutrition for constipation in children. Retrieved from: http://www.niddk.nih.gov/health-information/health-topics/digestive-diseases/constipation-in-children/Pages/eating-diet-nutrition.aspx. Accessed September 9, 2016.

39. World Health Organization; August 2016. Lead poisoning and health [fact sheet]. Retrieved from: http://www.who.int/mediacentre/factsheets/fs379/en/. Accessed September 9, 2016.

40. Centers for Disease Control and Prevention; updated June 19, 2015. Childhood obesity facts: prevalence of childhood obesity in the United States, 2011–2012. Retrieved from: http://www.cdc.gov/obesity/data/childhood.html. Accessed September 9, 2016.

41. Centers for Disease Control and Prevention; last reviewed May 10, 2013. Behavior, environment, and genetic factors all have a role in causing people to be overweight and obese. Retrieved from: http://www.cdc.gov/genomics/resources/diseases/obesity/. Accessed September 9, 2016.

42. World Health Organization. Global Strategy on Diet, Physical Activity and Health: why does childhood overweight and obesity matter? Retrieved from: http://www.who.int/dietphysicalactivity/childhood_consequences/en/. Accessed September 9, 2016.

43. Wardle J, Carnell S, Haworth CMA, Plomin R. Evidence for a strong genetic influence on childhood adiposity despite the force of the obesogenic environment. *Am J Clin Nutr.* 2008;87:398–404.

44. Obesity Society; last updated May 2014. Childhood overweight. Retrieved from: http://www.obesity.org/obesity/resources/facts-about-obesity/childhood-overweight. Accessed September 9, 2016.

45. World Health Organization. Global Strategy on Diet, Physical Activity and Health: what can be done to fight the childhood obesity epidemic? Retrieved from: http://www.who.int/dietphysicalactivity/childhood_what_can_be_done/en/. Accessed September 9, 2016.

46. Non AL, Roman JC, Gross CL, et al. Early childhood social disadvantage is associated with poor health behaviours in adulthood. *Ann Hum Biol.* 2016;43(2):144–153.

47. Institute of Medicine; June 2011. Early childhood obesity prevention policies: goals, recommendations, and potential actions. Retrieved from: http://www.nationalacademies.org/hmd/~/media/Files/Report%20Files/2011/Early-Childhood-Obesity-Prevention-Policies/Young%20Child%20Obesity%202011%20Recommendations.pdf. Accessed September 18, 2016.

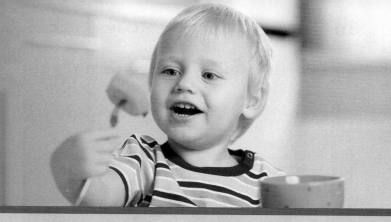

CHAPTER 8

Nutrition for Health and Disease in Infancy Through Early Childhood

Kathryn L. Hunt, RDN, CD, CSO; **Kim Nowak-Cooperman**, MS, RDN, CD;
Mary Verbovski, MS, RDN, CD, CSO; **Nila Williamson**, MPH, RDN, CNSC;
Susan Casey, RDN, CD; **Melissa Edwards**, MS, RDN, CD; **Camille L. Lanier**, RDN, CD;
Barb York, MS, RDN, CD, **and Regina Nagy-Steinert**, RDN, CD

Chapter Outline

Gastrointestinal Conditions

Food Allergies and Sensitivities

Malnutrition

Failure to Thrive

Cancer

Iron Deficiency

Newborn Screening and Genetics

Selected Pediatric Conditions

Learning Objectives

1. List the various dietary recommendations for children with diarrhea, constipation, reflux, and celiac disease.

2. Discuss how the different food allergy tests assess an individual for food allergy.

3. Describe the difference between malnutrition and failure to thrive.

4. Describe nutrition strategies that support growth needs of the child with cancer.

5. Explain genetic conditions and newborn screening.

6. Describe the nutritional implications and recommendations for infants and children with these pediatric conditions.

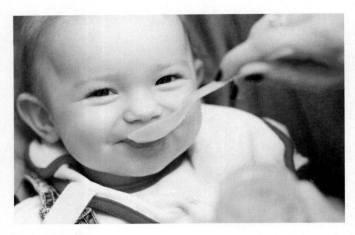

©Olena Zaskochenko/Shutterstock

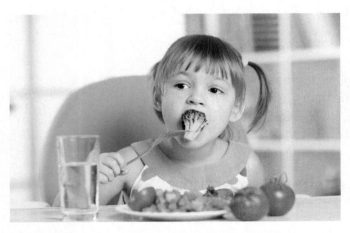

©Oksana Kuzmina/Shutterstock

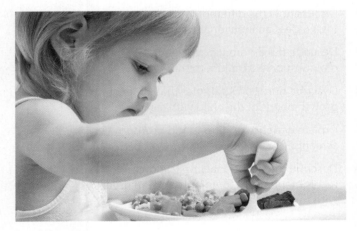

©Maryna Pleshkun/Shutterstock

Infancy and early childhood are stages of life characterized by rapid growth and development. Adequate nutrition during this time is essential for a child's overall physical, social, emotional, and cognitive development. Although most children learn to eat and consume adequate nutrients with ease, some experience feeding difficulties that place them at risk for faltered growth and impaired development.

This chapter summarizes details for special health-care conditions of children from infancy to 5 years of age with special healthcare and nutrition needs, including gastrointestinal disease, food allergies, cancer, failure to thrive, malnutrition, genetic conditions such as Down syndrome and cystic fibrosis, children born with cleft palate, and autism spectrum disorders.

Gastrointestinal Conditions

Preview This section reviews nutritional needs of infants and children with gastrointestinal conditions, including diarrhea, constipation, reflux, and celiac disease.

Diarrhea

Diarrhea refers to an increase in frequency and looseness of stools. Although stool frequency and consistency vary among individuals, diarrhea is generally defined as having three or more loose or liquid stools per day in older children, and an increase in stool frequency to twice the usual number per day in infants. Diarrhea lasting fewer than 7 days and no longer than 14 days is considered acute diarrhea, whereas diarrhea lasting for more than 4 weeks is considered chronic diarrhea.[1]

Particularly in infants and young children, diarrhea can be serious because it can quickly result in dehydration. According to the World Health Organization (WHO), there are 1.6 billion cases of diarrheal illnesses each year around the world.[2] Diarrhea is the second leading cause of death in children younger than 5 years old, killing approximately 760,000 children each year, and is the leading cause of malnutrition in this age group.[3] Among adults and children, it is estimated that almost 100 million cases of acute diarrhea occur annually in the United States, many as the result of foodborne illness.[4]

Diarrhea is a symptom of a variety of conditions and diseases. Most frequently, an individual experiences

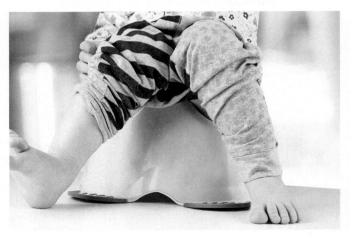

©Saklakova/Shutterstock

diarrhea as a symptom of a gastrointestinal (GI) tract infection caused by bacteria, a virus, or a parasite. Rotavirus is the primary cause of severe infectious diarrhea in Western countries, whereas parasites are the main cause in developing nations. In addition to infectious causes, diarrhea can also be a side effect of a medication, such as an antibiotic, or a symptom of a variety of chronic GI conditions and diseases such as Crohn's disease, celiac disease, and lactose intolerance.

Individuals with an impaired immune system are the most at risk for developing diarrhea. Each episode of diarrhea in an infant or child puts that individual at greater risk for developing undernutrition, and undernourished children are then more susceptible to further episodes of diarrhea.[5]

Prevention of infectious diarrhea for all children requires access to safe drinking water and proper sanitation, which is particularly needed in developing countries. According to the WHO, the most effective strategies that individuals can use to prevent the spread of infection are proper handwashing and safe food preparation. The probiotic *Lactobacillus rhamnosus* GG has been shown to be effective prevention for antibiotic-associated diarrhea in children and adults.[6]

Dehydration is the main complication of diarrhea. Mild and moderate dehydration are typically treated at home with oral rehydration. **Hypotonic fluids** that contain salt, potassium, and bicarbonate in combination with sugar are recommended for rehydration to replace nutrients lost in diarrhea, urine, sweat, and vomiting. Once rehydrated, it is important that the child's usual diet be offered and resumed. Enterocytes, the cells that line the small intestine, obtain needed nutrients from the GI tract to stay healthy. During periods of fasting, these needed nutrients are unavailable, which may further prolong recovery. For this reason, dietary restrictions should be avoided, and feedings should be maintained as much as possible during times of illness.

In instances of severe dehydration when infants or children are not able to replace fluids by mouth, using a feeding tube is necessary. A feeding tube is placed through the nose into the stomach or a part of the intestine. **Enteral Tube feedings** provide nutrition to individuals who cannot obtain nutrition by mouth or who are unable to swallow safely. **Total parenteral nutrition (TPN)** is a method of feeding that bypasses the stomach and gastrointestinal tract. Fluids are administered into a vein and provide nutrients that the body needs.

Lack of appetite often temporarily occurs during diarrheal illness; however, food should be offered in small portions and be available as requested by the child. Higher energy intake during episodes of diarrheal illness is associated with shorter duration of illness and less subsequent malnutrition.[7] A temporary lactose and fructose intolerance can sometimes accompany diarrhea, particularly in the malnourished. This is because the enzymes that digest these disaccharides are produced by the brush border cells of the GI tract, which can atrophy during diarrhea, reducing enzyme production. In these instances, it would be recommended that children temporarily avoid lactose-containing dairy products and fructose-containing fruit juices until diarrhea resolves.[8]

In situations of chronic diarrhea, determining the underlying cause guides nutrition interventions. Examples include possible lactose or gluten intolerance.

Constipation

Constipation, a condition in which there is difficulty emptying the bowels, usually associated with hardened feces, is a common pediatric problem. Although constipation can be associated with underlying medical conditions such as prematurity, developmental delay, or hypotonia (poor muscle tone) and is common in children with special healthcare needs, it can just as easily affect healthy children. Most cases of constipation are considered functional, meaning there is no underlying anatomic or physiological cause. Irritability, abdominal pain, and decreased appetite/early satiety are symptoms that often accompany the criteria for a diagnosis of constipation, and they may or may not resolve with passage of a bowel movement.[9]

For some children, constipation may be related to their diet and lifestyle. Diet should be evaluated for adequate fiber intake with the inclusion of whole grains, fruits, vegetables, nuts, and legumes. Also important are adequate fluid intake and meal structure/routine. Individuals who skip meals and follow an inconsistent eating pattern are at increased risk for inconsistent stooling patterns. Daily physical activity is an important lifestyle strategy for children to prevent constipation.[10] See **TABLE 8.1** and **TABLE 8.2** for current fiber and fluid recommendations for children.

Treatment of constipation includes optimizing dietary and lifestyle habits in combination with use of **laxatives**, which stimulate and facilitate stooling, as necessary. Normal fiber and fluid intake is recommended as

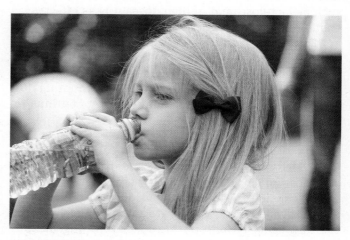

©Andrey Arkusha/Shutterstock

Table 8.1

Daily Fiber Recommendations: Dietary Reference Intake Standards (DRIs)

Children 1–3 years of age	19 g/day
Children 4–6 years of age	25 g/day
Boys 9–13 years	31 g/day
Girls 9–13 years	26 g/day

Data from Agricultural Research Services. Retrieved from: https://www.ars.usda.gov/ARSUserFiles/80400530/pdf/DBrief/12_fiber_intake_0910.pdf

Table 8.2

Estimated Fluid Requirements

Weight	Amount of Fluid
<10 kg	100 mL/kg
11–20 kg	1,000 mL + 50 mL/kg over 10 kg
≥21 kg	1,500 mL + 25 mL/kg over 20 kg
Adolescents	40–60 mL/kg

Data from U.S. Department of Agriculture. Nutrition and Your Health: Dietary Guidelines for Americans. Part D: Science Base, Section 7: fluid and electrolytes. Retrieved from: https://health.gov/dietaryguidelines/dga2005/report/HTML/D7_Fluid.htm.

well as normal physical activity levels and a routine toileting schedule. If a child's diet is not meeting fiber recommendations, it is important that fiber and fluid intake be increased together and gradually. Increasing fiber without fluid can worsen constipation and symptoms of pain, gas, and bloating. The use of fiber supplements or a high-fiber diet with intake greater than the DRI has not been found to be effective and is not recommended.[11]

Stool softeners and laxatives are prescribed frequently in treating functional constipation with several options safe for use in children. Polyethylene glycol is a laxative that works to draw water into the intestine, softening stool for easier defecation. In children, it has been found to be more effective than other common laxatives such as lactulose, and in high doses it is as effective as enemas for treating fecal impaction.[12]

Fortunately, treatment for constipation is effective. Fifty percent of children referred to a pediatric gastroenterologist for their constipation recover and no longer require laxatives after 6–12 months, with another 10% remaining asymptomatic as long as they continue on laxatives.[13]

Reflux

Gastroesophageal reflux (GER) is defined as the passage of stomach contents into the esophagus, or throat. GER is considered a normal physiological process that affects all ages and is not always accompanied by symptoms of regurgitation, spitting up, or vomiting. Spitting up occurs daily in at least half of infants younger than

4 months of age, but despite being considered a normal process it results in approximately 20% of U.S. caregivers seeking medical attention for their infant.[14] Frequency of daily episodes varies among individuals, but fortunately the majority of infant reflux typically resolves by 12–14 months of age. There is no difference in frequency of episodes between breastfed and formula-fed infants.[15]

Gastroesophageal reflux disease (GERD) occurs when GER is accompanied with the symptoms and complications of: weight loss or poor weight gain, wheezing/cough, reoccurring pneumonia, irritability, refusal of feedings, inflammation of the esophagus, and, in severe cases, apnea. **Apnea** is when breathing temporarily stops, and it occurs more frequently in sleep. GERD affects nutritional status when the regurgitation or vomiting is associated with feedings and is so significant that it results in inadequate energy intake to support growth and hydration.[16]

Children with special healthcare needs, such as neurologic impairment, decreased muscle tone, esophageal atresia, chronic lung disease, and some genetic syndromes, and infants with a history of premature birth are at higher risk for GERD than the normal population.[17]

Unfortunately, there is no way to prevent GER or GERD in infancy and early childhood. Treatment consists of nutrition and feeding modifications as well as positional modifications to elevate the head while feeding and sleeping. Medications to reduce acid secretion and protect the lining of the GI tract from damage from stomach acid are routinely employed but may not alter the underlying cause of the reflux. In severe cases of children experiencing life-threatening complications of GERD, aggressive therapies may be needed.

The goal of nutrition management of GER and GERD in infants and children is to decrease symptoms while promoting expected growth and development. For healthy infants who are growing and eating well but experiencing symptoms of reflux, parents can be reassured that GER is common and their child should outgrow it. Small, frequent feedings and avoiding overfeeding are strategies used to reduce frequency of GER. If reducing the volume of feedings is needed to improve reflux, increasing the energy density of feedings with formula may be needed in some cases to meet energy needs for appropriate growth. In older children who eat more variety in their diet, there is no evidence that routine eliminations of certain foods treats reflux; but caffeine, chocolate, and spicy foods are known irritants in the diet that could worsen symptoms.[18] Keep in mind that most irritants are individualized, and parents should use trial and error, as well as food/symptom diaries, to identify foods that worsen symptoms for their children. Foods should not be eliminated unnecessarily because this could narrow the diet and put the child at risk for inadequate intake and growth concerns.

For infants, thickening feedings with rice cereal is a common strategy to reduce GER, and infant formulas that contain rice starch that thickens once it contacts gastric acid are now commercially available. A systematic review of the research on this topic concluded that thickened feedings are only moderately effective in treating the reflux of otherwise healthy infants.[19] Potential safety concerns of this strategy can include the unknown allergenicity of additives to an infant's diet, that adding cereal to breastmilk/formula substantially increases the energy density of the liquid and might result in rapid weight gain, and that thickened liquids often require an enlarged hole in the bottle nipple to allow adequate flow, and this can result in increased feeding difficulties.

In infants experiencing regurgitation and vomiting, allergy may be the cause. In these cases, dietary change, such as eliminating dairy from the diet of a breast-feeding mother or changing infant formula, should significantly reduce frequency of vomiting within approximately 2 weeks. It is rare that reflux symptoms of allergy are so severe that breastfeeding needs to be discontinued.[20]

Celiac Disease

Celiac disease is an immune-mediated disease of the small intestine that can develop in genetically susceptible individuals when they consume **gluten**. Epidemiological studies in the United States and Europe estimate the prevalence of celiac disease as 1 in every 130 to 300 people.[21] The prevalence is slightly higher in children; it is estimated as affecting 1 out of every 80 to 300 children younger than age 15 years.[22] With this disease, the ingestion of gluten triggers an inflammatory response within the body, which results in destruction of the epithelium, or lining of the GI tract. The intestinal villi that protrude from the epithelial layer of the GI tract become flattened, with reduced surface area, resulting in decreased absorption of nutrients from the intestinal contents (FIGURE 8.1).

Gluten, the trigger of this damage, is a protein found in the grain products wheat, barley, and rye. Treatment

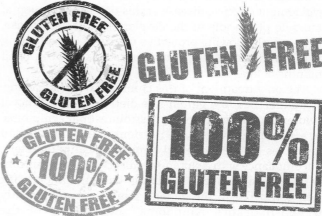

©ducu59us/Shutterstock

consists of removing gluten completely from the diet, because once gluten is no longer consumed, the damage to the small intestine stops and the GI tract can heal.

Celiac disease can develop and be diagnosed at any age; however, presenting symptoms may vary with age (TABLE 8.3). Children diagnosed younger than 3 years of age typically present with classic symptoms of the disease following introduction of gluten into the diet, with malnutrition and insufficient weight gain or inappropriate weight loss occurring if diagnosis is delayed. Onset at a later age could be triggered by stress or viral infections, with the possibility of other triggers not yet identified. Symptoms can be highly variable and atypical. When symptoms suggest celiac disease, serologic tests are used to screen for it. If serologic tests are elevated, an intestinal mucosal biopsy is used to confirm whether the disease is present. This biopsy remains the gold standard for diagnosis but can only be obtained with an upper GI endoscopy.[23]

Celiac disease requires that an individual carry one of two genes, *HLA DQ2* or *DQ8*; however, with 40% of the general population carrying these genes, they are not a reliable indicator of those at risk.[24] An increased risk for celiac disease is associated with the following conditions: type 1 diabetes, various syndromes (Down, Turner,

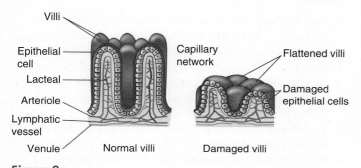

Labels: Villi, Epithelial cell, Lacteal, Arteriole, Lymphatic vessel, Venule, Capillary network, Flattened villi, Damaged epithelial cells, Normal villi, Damaged villi

Figure 8.1
Damaged villi as occurs in celiac disease.

Table 8.3

Classic and Atypical Symptoms of Celiac Disease

Classic	Atypical (Less Common)
Weight loss	Iron-deficiency anemia
Vomiting	Dermatitis herpetiformis
Diarrhea/constipation	Dental enamel defects
Abdominal pain	Bone disease
Gas/bloating	Pubertal delay
Irritability	Short stature
Failure to thrive	

and Williams), autoimmune thyroiditis, immunoglobulin A (IgA) deficiency, and a first-degree relative with celiac disease. Individuals in these groups benefit from routine screening.[25] Unfortunately, there is no strategy to prevent development of celiac disease at this time. Environmental factors do play a role in the development of the disease, with research showing protective effects of breastfeeding and of introducing gluten-containing solids between 4 and 7 months of age.[26]

The only treatment of this chronic disease is lifelong, strict adherence to a gluten-free diet. Complete removal of gluten in the diet resolves gastrointestinal symptoms, corrects any growth and nutrient deficiencies, and normalizes biochemical and hematological parameters. Noncompliance with a gluten-free diet can have significant health consequences, doubling overall cancer risk when compared to the general population, particularly for non-Hodgkin's lymphoma and cancers of the gastrointestinal tract and system.[27] Fortunately, however, when celiac disease is diagnosed in childhood and the gluten-free diet adopted early, there appears to be no increased cancer risk.[28]

Because of the importance of adherence to the gluten-free diet, a team approach when educating newly diagnosed individuals is ideal. According to the National Institutes of Health (NIH), six elements are essential for management of celiac disease, and they can be remembered using the acronym CELIAC:[29]

C: Consultation with skilled dietitian
E: Education about celiac disease
L: Lifelong adherence to a gluten-free diet
I: Identification/treatment of nutritional deficiencies
A: Access to advocacy group
C: Continuous long-term follow-up

Because even small amounts of gluten can be harmful, education on removal of wheat, barley, and rye from the diet must also include instruction on avoiding cross-contamination and hidden sources of gluten that could be found in anything ingested, including medications and supplements. Fortunately for those with celiac disease, in 2014 the U.S. Food and Drug Administration (FDA) issued a final rule on gluten-free labeling that makes identification of gluten-free foods easier and safer. Food manufacturers can now use the gluten-free label on inherently gluten-free foods and foods with gluten content less than 20 parts per million (ppm). The FDA has the authority to enforce compliance by food manufacturers with this rule using inspections, testing, and other tools.[30]

Recap Episodes of constipation, diarrhea, and reflux are common for infants and young children. A balanced diet plays a role in minimizing symptoms for these conditions while providing the nourishment needed for optimal growth and development. For those with celiac disease, a gluten-free diet is the only treatment available, and proper adherence leads to resolution of gastrointestinal symptoms as well as recovery from any growth or nutrient deficiencies.

1. What are fluid and fiber recommendations for a child experiencing constipation?
2. How effective is the treatment of celiac disease with a gluten-free diet?

News You Can Use

Not just individuals with celiac disease are following a gluten-free diet these days. The media has popularized the gluten-free diet, and a growing number of people feel eating gluten free is healthier and fashionable. Households purchasing gluten-free products increased from 5% to 11% between 2010 and 2014, and the sale of gluten-free products is a multimillion-dollar industry.

Many people eating a gluten-free diet do not have celiac disease but do report feeling better when they avoid intake of gluten. This condition was coined nonceliac gluten sensitivity (NCGS) in 2012 by celiac researchers in an effort to differentiate it from celiac disease. NCGS is different from celiac disease in that ingestion of gluten does not lead to inflammation and damage to the lining of the GI tract. One of the first studies to show gluten could induce symptoms in nonceliac patients was published in 2011.[a] This same group of researchers published a follow-up study in 2013 but found that gluten alone may not be responsible for causing symptoms.[b] When a broader group of fermentable carbohydrates, including gluten, were removed from the diet, study participants had more significant improvements in their symptoms compared with when only gluten was removed. Research in this area is ongoing and will hopefully shed light on this knowledge gap and help guide clear evidence-based recommendations for future patients.[c]

References

a. New York Times Article: Stephanie Strom. A Big Bet on Gluten Free. Mar 1, 2016. http://www.nytimes.com/2014/02/18/business/food-industry-wagers-big-on-gluten-free.html.

b. Biesiekierski JR, et al. Gluten causes gastrointestinal symptoms in subjects without celiac disease: a double-blind randomized placebo controlled trial J Am Gastroenterol. 2011;106:508-14.

c. Biesiekierski JR, et al. No effects of gluten in patients with self-reported non-celiac gluten sensitivity after dietary reduction of fermentable, poorly absorbed, short-chain carbohydrates Gastroenterol. 2013;145:320-8.

Food Allergies and Sensitivities

Preview This section discusses some of the most common food allergies, how they are identified, and appropriate nutritional management.

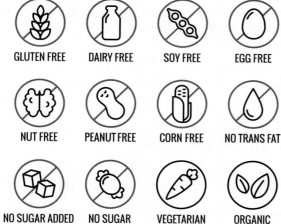

GLUTEN FREE DAIRY FREE SOY FREE EGG FREE

NUT FREE PEANUT FREE CORN FREE NO TRANS FAT

NO SUGAR ADDED NO SUGAR VEGETARIAN ORGANIC

©Sudowoodo/Shutterstock

A **food allergy** is any adverse reaction to a food or ingredient in a food that involves the body's immune system. Food allergies occur in 2–8% of children.[31] The major "players" in a food allergy are mast cells, their circulating counterparts, basophils, and antibodies called immunoglobulin E (IgE). An allergic reaction occurs when the immune system treats a generally harmless substance (antigen) as if it were trying to attack the body. The immune system overreacts by producing B cells, which produce IgE antibodies and travel to cells in various parts of the body, causing symptoms of allergic reactions. These symptoms usually occur in the nose, lungs, throat, sinuses, ears, lining of the stomach, or on the skin. It is not fully understood why some substances trigger allergies and others do not, or why some people have allergies and others do not. A family history of allergies is one of the factors that puts a person at risk for particular allergies.

It is not uncommon for individuals to have some sort of reaction to a variety of foods. Sometimes it is difficult to tell whether the symptoms are a result of a food allergy or something else. Food intolerances and food sensitivities can share some of the same symptoms as food allergies, such as nausea, stomach pain, diarrhea, or

The Big Picture

1. The antigen (allergen) enters the body.

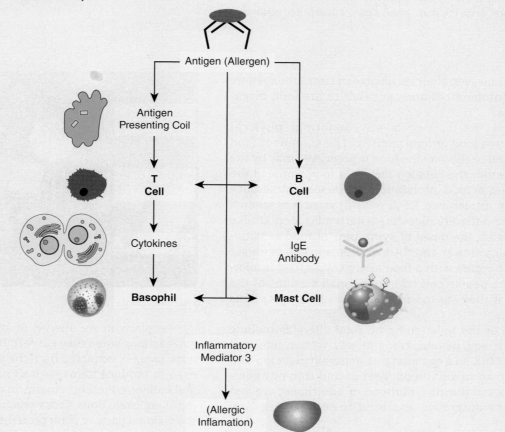

2. Body reacts by producing B cells that produce IgE antibodies to the antigen (allergen). IgE is one of five different antibodies that the immune system makes.

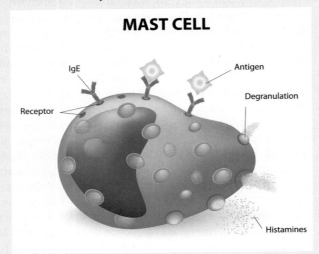

MAST CELL

©Designua/Shutterstock

3. Mast cells reside in tissues in the body, and basophils are in the bloodstream. These cells have thousands of receptors specific for the IgE antibody. When the allergen enters the immune system, the antigen binds to these IgE receptors on the surface of cells.

4. These antibodies travel to cells in various parts of the body (generally in the nose, lungs, throat, sinuses, ears, lining of the stomach, or on the skin). When a person is exposed again to

the same allergen that initiated the response, the IgE is able to bind to that allergen. When IgE antibodies next to each other bind to the antigen, this interaction causes the mast cell or basophil to release chemicals that result in the allergic reaction.

5. Each mast cell or basophil contains hundreds of granules that contain different allergy-causing chemicals. One of the better understood of these chemicals is histamine. When histamine is released in the skin, itching results. When histamine is released in the lungs, wheezing results.

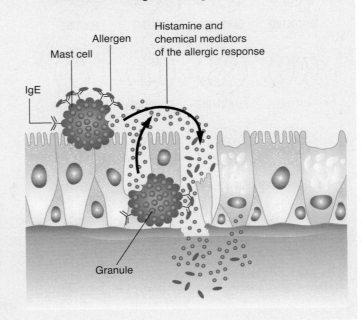

vomiting; however, allergies involve the immune system, whereas intolerances and sensitivities are food digestion issues.

A **food intolerance** is any abnormal physical response to a food or food additive. The amount of food that is eaten or the way the food is processed may be the key to whether the person reacts to a food. Some of the more common food intolerances are lactose intolerance and gluten intolerance. **Food sensitivity** occurs when a person has difficulty digesting a particular food. Unlike food allergies, the onset of symptoms of food sensitivity is usually slower and the symptoms may last longer than what occurs with a food allergy. With food intolerance, some people can tolerate a small amount of the food, but if they eat too much or too often, symptoms may result.

Some of the most common food allergies include cow's milk, egg, peanut, tree nut, soy, wheat, fish, and shellfish. Milk and egg allergies generally develop and are outgrown in childhood. Peanut and tree nut allergies can occur during childhood or adulthood, are less likely to be outgrown, and tend to cause more fatal reactions.[32]

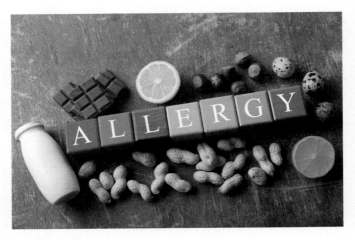

©Africa Studio/Shutterstock

People who are allergic to latex may express allergic reactions when they eat certain fruits, vegetables, and nuts. Latex is extracted from the sap of a gum tree and is used to produce items such as rubber gloves, catheters, and balloons. Protein remains in the latex product, causing allergic reactions. Cross-reactions may occur between the residual parts of plant proteins in the latex rubber and proteins in foods, just like cross-reactions in foods, such as banana, avocado, kiwi, and chestnut.[33] About 30–80% of people with latex allergy experience symptoms when they eat one or more of these foods.[33]

News You Can Use

In June 2015, the American Academy of Pediatrics issued a policy by the name of "Consensus Communication on Early Introduction and the Prevention of Peanut Allergy in High-Risk Infants". The policy provides guidance regarding early peanut introduction based on data generated in a study conducted in the United Kingdom which looked at 640 high-risk infants between the ages of 4 and 11 months, all of whom had severe eczema, egg allergy, or both.

The policy indicates that there is no scientific evidence supporting the idea that health care providers should recommend introducing peanut-containing products into the diets of infants between the ages of 4 and 11 months of age who are at "high risk" of these allergies in countries where peanut allergy is prevalent, because delaying the introduction of peanuts can be associated with increased risk of developing peanut allergy.[a]

Further recommendations suggest that infants with early-onset atopic disease, such as severe eczema or egg allergy in the first 4 to 6 months of life, might benefit from evaluation by an allergist or physician trained in the management of allergic disease in this age groups. Such specialists can possibly diagnose any food allergy and assist in implementing suggestions regarding when it is appropriate to introduce peanuts into the diet of an infant.[a]

Additionally, it is expected that more specific guidelines regarding early-life, complementary feeding practices, and the risk of allergy development will be provided in the future from the National Institute of Allergy and Infectious Disease-sponsored Working Group, as well as the European Academy of Allergy and Clinical Immunology.[b]

References

a. Fleischer DM, Scott S, Greenhawt M, et al. Consensus Communication on Early Peanut Introduction and the Prevention of Peanut Allergy in High-Risk Infants. Pediatrics 2015; 136(3)600-604.

b. DuToit G, Roberts G, Sayre PH, et al. Randomized Trial of Peanut Consumption in Infants at Risk for Peanut Allergy. NEJM 2015; 372(9)803-813.

If a food allergy is suspected, it is important to seek the advice of a physician or board-certified allergist. Self-diagnosis of food allergies can lead to unnecessary dietary restrictions and even inadequate nutrition. Proven diagnostic methods for testing food allergies include skin prick test, radioallergosorbent test (RAST) blood test, and oral food challenge with trial elimination diet.

A *skin prick test* is performed by putting a droplet of an extract of a suspected food on the surface of the skin. The surface is then pricked. At the end of a specific time, the size of the reaction, or wheal, is measured and graded from 0 to 5, with 0 being no reaction and 5 being a significant reaction. *RAST* is a small blood sample sent to a lab that tests the amount of IgE measured with a specific food. Radioallergosorbent measures the amount of IgE to a specific food. "High" levels indicate an allergy to the specific food.

An *oral food challenge* consists of a double-blind placebo-controlled food challenge. A suspected food is eliminated from a child's diet and, when the allergy symptom or symptoms are no longer apparent, if the symptoms reappear when the suspected food is given to the child, it is considered diagnostic. A healthy respect for anaphylaxis should provide an abundance of caution, and a true food challenge should be conducted only with the proper medical equipment.

Nutrition Management

If the test used to diagnosis the food allergy is legitimate, removal of the offending food or foods from the child's diet is the first step. Detailed education, such as patient education material, should be given to the family and carefully reviewed in any nutrition counseling sessions.

The Food Allergy Labeling and Consumer Protection Act (FALCPA) requires food companies to indicate whether a food product has any of these potentially allergenic foods as ingredients: milk, wheat, eggs, peanuts, tree nuts, fish, shellfish, and soy.

To help ensure that children with food allergies are safe both inside and outside of their homes, it is important for healthcare providers to be advocates for the child in day care, preschool, and school by helping to supply appropriate education and printed material.

Recap Food allergies occur when an adverse reaction results from ingestion of a food or ingredient in a food. These are different from food intolerances and food sensitivities. The correct method of diagnosis, appropriate nutritional assessment, and guidance on foods to avoid, foods to allow, and advocacy and education in community settings for nonfamily caregivers are crucial for safe management of food allergies in the pediatric population.

1. Name three tests recommended for diagnosing food allergies.
2. List common cross-reactive foods associated with latex allergy.

Malnutrition

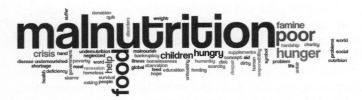

©ibreakstock/Shutterstock

Preview Pediatric malnutrition (also referred to as undernutrition) is defined as an imbalance between nutrient requirements and intake that results in cumulative deficits of energy, protein, or micronutrients that may negatively affect normal growth and development.

Prevalence

Pediatric malnutrition is an underdiagnosed problem among chronically ill and hospitalized patients. In the developed world, malnutrition is predominantly related to disease, chronic conditions, trauma, burns, and surgery.[34] The Academy of Nutrition and Dietetics (AND), along with the American Society for Parenteral and Enteral Nutrition (ASPEN), developed a standardized approach for treating malnutrition.[35] **Wasting** refers to when a child is too thin for his or her height as a result of sudden or acute malnutrition. In these situations, the child is not getting enough calories to support energy needs and faces an immediate risk of death. **Stunting** refers to when a child is too short for his or her age and is defined as the failure to grow both physically and cognitively as a result of chronic or recurrent malnutrition.[36] **FIGURE 8.2** shows how the three conditions of wasted, stunted, and underweight might appear in a child. Effects of stunting often last throughout a person's life. The primary contributors to malnutrition are poverty, famine, and war, all of which limit food distribution and access.[36]

In 2014, approximately 1 out of every 13 children in the world was malnourished.[36] Malnutrition most often occurs in developing countries that also struggle with acute or chronic infectious diseases because these are separate and devastating factors that affect malnutrition. In developed countries, malnutrition generally occurs in the setting of acute or chronic illness or in children with special healthcare needs. Often, the diagnosis occurs in the hospital setting.

The prevalence of malnutrition varies depending on the underlying medical conditions. Some common conditions that contribute to malnutrition include neurologic disease, infectious disease, cystic fibrosis, cardiovascular disease, oncology treatment, and GI diseases.[37] According to the World Health Organization, the prevalence of malnutrition worldwide has declined over time. Although parameters indicate less malnutrition in children overall, there is still room for continued efforts to reduce prevalence worldwide.

Wasted	No	Yes	No
Stunted	No	No	Yes
Underweight	No	Yes	Yes

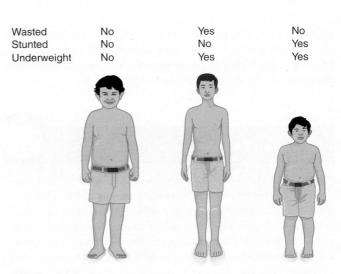

Figure 8.2
Visual differences between body size of a child who is wasted, stunted, and underweight.

Etiology

The etiology of malnutrition has become increasingly complex over recent decades. Historically, malnutrition was thought to be caused most often by food insecurity or starvation. Presently, the etiology suggests multiple factors that can contribute to its development. The Academy of Nutrition and Dietetics defines five domains categorizing malnutrition: anthropometric parameters, growth, chronicity of malnutrition, etiology/pathogenesis, and developmental/functional status. Based on its etiology, malnutrition is characterized as illness related (secondary to disease, condition, surgery, or injury) or non-illness related (secondary to environmental factors) or potentially both.[34] The role of the registered dietitian nutritionist (RDN) is to assess and define the type and degree of malnutrition and develop a care plan to ultimately improve or even reverse the process and bring the child to a well-nourished state. Suggested data collection during patient assessment to determine presence, type, and degree of malnutrition includes the following:

- Intake/diet history
- Mid-upper arm circumference (MUAC)
- Triceps skin fold (TSF)
- Arm muscle area (AMA)
- Z-score and reference charts (CDC or WHO)
- Growth history
- Weight gain velocity
- Functional assessment, for example: handgrip strength, get up and go, muscle testing

Table 8.4		
Diagnosis Criteria for Malnutrition		
Identification of at least 2 of the following criteria can indicate a diagnosis of malnutrition		
Criteria	Does the criteria exist	
	Yes	*No*
Insufficient energy intake		
Weight loss		
Loss of muscle mass		
Localized or generalized fluid accumulation that may sometimes mask weight loss		
Diminished functional status as measured by hand grip strength		

Modified from: Cederholm T, Bosaeus I, Barazzoni R, et al. Diagnostic criteria for malnutrition – An ESPN Consensus Statement. Clin Nutr. 2015 Jun;34(3):335-40.

- Presence of disease, for example: cancer, autoimmune disorder, cystic fibrosis
- Metabolic stressors, for example: burn, injury, surgery
- Utilization of nutrients in the body (malabsorption)

Prevention

The purpose of nutrition screening and assessment is to identify patients who are at risk for malnutrition or who are already malnourished.[36] Early intervention that provides an individualized nutrition management plan is effective in preserving the health, well-being, and growth potential of the child. In addition, routine follow-up with a healthcare provider is essential to catch signs or see trends that are concerning.

Treatment/Pathogenesis

For effective treatment, it is important to understand the specific pathway initially leading to malnutrition. These pathways may include one or more of the following: (1) decreased nutrient intake (starvation), (2) increased requirement for nutrients, (3) increased nutrient losses, and (4) altered nutrient utilization.[34] Once determined, the appropriate treatment supported by a multidisciplinary healthcare team can follow.

A myriad of outcomes result from malnutrition left untreated, for example, loss of lean body mass, delayed wound healing, developmental delay, muscle weakness, infections, immune dysfunction, and prolonged hospital stay. Specific nutrition intervention includes raising awareness of malnutrition of the patient and to the family, providing nutrition education, and determining what food, formula, or nutrients are needed to meet energy needs and thereby supporting the child and family with ways to meet those needs for catch-up growth and weight gain.

Certain foods or food groups may need to be augmented or restricted to optimize nutrient utilization and encourage expected growth and development. A step-by-step approach developed in collaboration with the patient and family with routine follow-up to collect accurate data is essential to supporting the child in achieving an optimally nourished state. TABLE 8.4 provides diagnosis criteria for three levels of malnutrition.

Recap Approximately 1 out of every 13 children in the world is malnourished. This includes conditions of wasting and stunting. The pathway to malnutrition may include one or more of the following: decreased nutrient intake, increased requirements for nutrients, increased nutrient losses, and altered nutrient utilization. Once the cause of malnutrition is determined, the appropriate treatment can be followed.

1. List examples of data to collect when assessing a child for malnutrition.
2. Define the five domains categorizing the etiology of malnutrition.

Failure to Thrive

Preview Malnutrition and Failure to Thrive are caused by inadequate intakes of nutrients. These conditions can be detrimental to infants.

Failure to thrive (FTT) is a complex clinical syndrome that describes infants and children who require nutrition intervention because of unexplained deficits in growth.[38] Failure to thrive is caused by malnutrition but differs from it: FTT is due to inadequate intake rather than shortage of food or starvation.[39] FTT can be further described as **growth faltering**, which occurs when weight crosses three percentiles on standard growth charts over 3 months in infancy and over 6 months in the second and third years of life.[40]

Table 8.5	
Failure to Thrive Characteristics	
BMI	< 5th percentile for age
Weight for length	< 3rd percentile on a CDC growth chart, or < 2nd percentile on WHO growth chart
Weight gain history	Poor or no weight gain over a period of time • 3-6 months an interval of one to two weeks with poor or no weight gain • 6 months and older an interval of at least one month of poor or no weight gain
Weight percentiles	Significant downward trend

Modified from Leon C, Goday P. Failure to thrive. Pediatric Nutrition Practice Group Building Block for Life. Spring 2012;35(2).

Table 8.6
Summary of Risk Factors Associated with Failure to Thrive
Prematurity
Transition to solids
Inexperienced parents
Lack of nutrition knowledge
Poor eating habits and lack of adequate opportunities for eating
Lack of financial resources
Disturbed parent–child interaction/attachment
Child temperament
Difficulty sucking, chewing and swallowing, and moving the tongue
Difficulty with food textures
Child refusal to eat
Aversion to eating because of allergic reactions, gastroesophageal reflux, negative experiences with tube feedings
Child anxiety
Parental worry, anxiety, and tension
Behavioral, interactional, and environmental issues between the child and caregiver

Etiology

FTT can result from a number of factors, some brought on when the child is not presented with adequate nutrition, and other cases caused by the child's inability to take in adequate amounts of nutrients. **TABLE 8.5** When FTT develops as a result of caregiver treatment, a mild problem of weight faltering might occur as a result of feeding problems, parental anxiety, or lack of experience in child rearing. FTT can also stem from a more difficult problem of inadequate parenting, distorted perceptions, neglect, and abuse.[41]

FTT can also result from subtle neuromotor problems such as difficulty sucking, chewing and swallowing, and moving the tongue. Some children have difficulties with food textures and refuse foods, leading to being "force fed" by a caregiver, which creates an aversive eating relationship and damages the parent–child feeding relationship. Other children may develop aversion to eating because of allergic reactions, gastroesophageal reflux, or negative experiences with gavage or nasogastric tube feeding in infancy.

Some children have significant psychiatric disorders such as anxiety that manifests as rumination or eating refusal.[41] Parental reactions to growth and feeding concerns such as worry, anxiety, and tension have been shown to exacerbate these problems. Behavioral, interactional, and environmental issues between the child and caregivers can contribute. **TABLE 8.6** summarizes risk factors that are associated with FTT.

Assessment

Because children with FTT may have issues related to medical, oral-motor, and psychosocial conditions, assessment and interventions are more effective with an interdisciplinary approach. It is paramount to involve all caregivers when developing treatment plans and goals, and it is important to address any unrealistic expectations and to be sensitive to caregivers' interpretations of the diagnosis.

When evaluating for FTT, normal variations in growth should be taken into account. Children may have short stature as a result of genetics, so it is useful to calculate midparental height to predict a child's stature potential. It is also important to determine the growth history of parents and whether they were malnourished as children because that would negate the accuracy of determining the child's growth potential.[39] Leanness may be genetic as well, with characteristics of frame size and muscle mass or tone contributing.

Treatment

Treatment should target the suspected cause or causes, address feeding difficulties, and provide treatment or therapy. Behavioral issues need to be evaluated and caregivers given useful strategies to reinforce desired behaviors while avoiding power struggles. The temperament of the child, such as distractibility, hypersensitivity, passivity, or impulsivity, often contributes to feeding problems. Environmental issues such as lack of resources, lack of education, inadequate parenting, neglect, and abuse need to be overcome. Effective nutrition intervention should focus on increased calorie and nutritional intake to support improved weight gain and growth.

Recap Malnutrition and failure to thrive (FTT) are serious conditions that affect infants and toddlers. Both are caused by deficits of energy, protein, and macro- and micronutrients. Malnutrition can occur at any age as a result of food shortages and starvation as well as acute or chronic illnesses that interfere with adequate intake. FTT, though caused by malnutrition, is due to inadequate intake in the setting of an adequate food supply.

1. List three infant/child characteristics that can contribute to FTT.

Cancer

Preview This section covers common cancers in infants and toddlers and defines strategies to monitor nutritional status throughout cancer treatment. Improvements in cancer detection and treatment have improved survival rate for childhood cancer patients. Research shows that childhood cancer may be explained by the interaction of multiple factors. The primary treatments for childhood cancer are chemotherapy, surgery, radiation therapy, and bone marrow transplant. Nutritional assessment requires an understanding of the type of cancer and the potentially negative side effects of treatment to formulate an appropriate nutritional care plan.

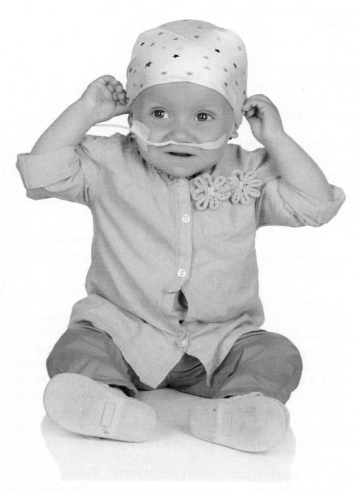

©Gelpi/Shutterstock

Oncology

Prevalence

Despite recent advances in research and treatment, childhood cancer continues to be a significant national health problem. Approximately 2,300 children and adolescents in the United States die of some form of pediatric cancer each year, which makes cancer the most common disease-related cause of death for children 1–19 years of age.[42] Current data show that approximately 12,400 children and adolescents younger than 20 years are diagnosed with cancer every year in the United States.[42]

Leukemia is a cancer of the white blood cells (WBCs). The bone marrow produces and accumulates abnormal, cancerous WBCs, which both reduces and compromises the function of the body's normal blood cells. The largest form of leukemia, acute lymphoblastic leukemia (ALL), comprises about 33% of pediatric cancer cases and was incurable in the 1950s. However, since the mid-1970s, improvements in leukemia treatment and gains in our understanding of both the biology and treatment of other childhood cancers have increased the 5-year survival rate of ALL to almost 90%.[44] This increased survival rate is principally attributed to advances in intensified therapy, including the addition of chemotherapy agents high-dose methotrexate, vincristine, asparaginase, and dexamethasone.[43]

The increase survival rates of ALL and other childhood cancers has also improved through patient participation in well-designed, randomized, cooperative group clinical trials and through advances in **nutrition support**, which is the provision of enteral or parenteral nutrients to treat or prevent malnutrition.[45]

Common Cancers in This Age Group

Unlike adult cancers, which are usually tabulated by primary site, childhood cancers are grouped by histologic type and primary site based on the International Classification of Childhood Cancer (ICCC). The **Surveillance, Epidemiology, and End Results (SEER)** program of the National Cancer Institute provides information on cancer statistics in an effort to reduce the burden of cancer among the U.S. population. The ICCC identifies the most common types of cancer from birth to 5 years of age in **TABLE 8.7**.

Why Do Children Develop Cancer?

No single factor determines whether a child from birth to 5 years of age will develop cancer. Although exposure to environmental conditions may explain the occurrence of a specific cancer, research shows that childhood cancer may be explained by the interaction of multiple factors. These factors include but are not necessarily limited to the genetic composition of the child, hormonal reactions, immune deficiencies, diet, and viral infections.[42]

Cancer Treatment and Nutritional Side Effects

Children younger than age 5 years who have cancer are often treated with a combination of therapies, depending on the type and location of the cancer and the stage of its malignancy. The four primary treatments are chemotherapy, surgery, radiation therapy, and hematopoietic cell transplant (bone marrow transplant). Each primary treatment causes nutrition-related issues, either mild and transient or that lead to severe and permanent problems.[46]

Table 8.7			

Age-Adjusted and Age-Specific SEER Cancer Incidence Rates, 2009–2013
By International Classification of Childhood Cancer (ICCC) Group and Subgroup and Age at Diagnosis (1–4 yrs), All Races and Sexes

Cancer Group	Incidence per 1,000,000 children in 1–4 yrs age group	Cancer Subgroup	Incidence per 1,000,000 children in 1-4 yrs age group
Leukemias	94.8	Acute lymphoid	78.6
		Acute myeloid	11.6
		All other leukemias	4.7
CNS and miscellaneous intracranial (brain tumors) and intraspinal neoplasms	49.2	Astrocytoma	19.9
		Ependymomas and choroid plexus tumors	6.8
		All other brain and CNS tumors	22.5
Sympathetic nervous system tumors	21.8	Neuroblastoma	21.6
		Other sympathetic nervous system tumors	0.2
Renal tumors	19.1		
Retinoblastoma (eye tumor)	8.7		
Soft tissue sarcomas	10.8	Rhabdomyosarcoma	7.4
		Other soft tissue sarcomas	3.4
Hepatic tumors	6.7	Hepatoblastoma	6.4
		Other hepatic tumors	0.3

CNS=central nervous system.

Dorota Iwaniec. Children Who Fail to Thrive A Practical Guide. Institute of Child Care Research, Queen's University of Belfast, Northern Ireland. John Wiley & Sons, Ltd. 2004

National Cancer Institute, SEER Pediatric Monograph, 3. Retrieved from: http://seer.cancer.gov/csr/1975_2013/browse_csr.php?sectionSEL=29&pageSEL=sect_29_table.01. html. Accessed September 16, 2016; Steliarova-Foucher E, Stiller C, Lacour B, Kaatsch P. International Classification of Childhood Cancer, Third Edition. Cancer. April 1, 2005;103(7):1457–1467.

Chemotherapy

Chemotherapies work by inhibiting DNA synthesis of both normal tissues and malignant cells. Most of the adverse nutritional side effects associated with chemotherapy stem from damage to rapidly proliferating cells, including the epithelial cells of the gastrointestinal (GI) tract.[46] The degree of the GI alterations depends on the specific medication administered, the dosage given and duration of use, the rate of the child's metabolism, and the child's tolerance to the drug.[47] Potential side effects of chemotherapy include these:

- Nausea and vomiting
- Alterations in taste and smell
- Mucositis and esophagitis
- Diarrhea
- Constipation
- Anorexia
- Early satiety
- Steroid-induced hyperglycemia
- Pancreatitis
- Typhlitis (inflammation of the cecum)
- Pneumatosis (gas in the bowel wall)
- Electrolyte and mineral wasting (magnesium, phosphorus, and potassium)
- Interruption in oral feeding skills

Managing the side effects of cancer treatment can be complex. **TABLE 8.8** offers suggestions for treating some common side effects.

Surgery

Surgery is a required therapy for the removal of solid tumors at certain stages of treatment. For example, Wilms' tumor (a type of kidney tumor) and most brain tumors are surgically removed before administering chemotherapy and, if applicable, radiation. Some brain tumors are unresectable because of their location and will be treated by radiation and chemotherapy. Other solid tumors, such as neuroblastoma, receive several courses of chemotherapy to shrink the tumor mass before they can be surgically removed.

Neuroblastoma is an embryonal tumor of the autonomic nervous system that develops from neural-crest tissues of the sympathetic nervous system. It can occur in many areas of the body, including abdomen, adrenal glands, neck, skull, pelvis, spinal column, and bone marrow. Neuroblastoma generally occurs in very young children; the median age at diagnosis is 17 months. Surgical removal of a tumor may lead to insufficient oral intake of nutrition for several days during a period of increased nutritional requirement.[46] Depending on the surgical site, nutrient intake and absorption issues may be significant.

Table 8.8

Managing Common Cancer Treatment Side Effects

Oral and esophageal mucositis (inflammation of the oral and esophageal mucosa)
- Try soft or pureed foods.
- Avoid rough-textured or hard foods, such as dry toast, chips, crackers, and raw vegetables.
- Avoid acidic or spicy foods and overly hot or cold foods.
- Offer milk, ice cream, homemade shakes or smoothies, and bland moist foods such as mashed potatoes and cream soups.
- Try high-calorie/protein liquid nutrition supplements.
- Use a straw when drinking to bypass mouth sores.
- Encourage frequent mouth rinsing to remove food and bacteria (1 tsp baking soda + 1 tsp salt mixed in 1 quart of water).

Alterations in taste and smell
- Offer cold, nonodorous foods.
- Try adding herbs, spices, marinades, and teriyaki to foods to enhance flavor.
- Offer beverages in a container with a lid and with a straw.

Nausea and vomiting
- Sip water, juice, sports drinks throughout the day. Popsicles and gelatin are also good ways to get in fluid.
- When vomiting has decreased, try easy-to-digest foods, such as crackers, plain toast, dry cereal, and rice.
- Encourage small, frequent meals, five to six times per day.
- Avoid greasy, fried, and overly sweet foods.
- Avoid feeding in a room that is overly warm or that has strong cooking odors that may trigger nausea.
- Encourage rest periods after meals.
- Avoid offering favorite foods when nauseated to prevent permanent dislike of the food.

Loss of appetite
- Offer nutrient-dense foods, such as nut butters, cheese, and avocados. Add half-and-half or heavy cream to appropriate foods to boost calories.
- Try high-calorie liquid nutrition supplements.
- Provide smaller, more frequent meals and snacks (five to six times per day).
- Use smaller plates and arrange food creatively.
- Avoid nagging or arguing around mealtimes.

Constipation
- Encourage plenty of fluids throughout the day.
- Offer high-fiber foods (whole grains, washed fresh fruits and vegetables, nuts, legumes).
- Increase physical activity as able.

Diarrhea
- Avoid high-fiber and high-fat foods (greasy or fried foods).
- Avoid caffeine and apple juice.
- Limit lactose-containing foods, such as regular milk and cheese. Try low-lactose milk, yogurt, and buttermilk.
- Encourage adequate fluids to prevent dehydration.
- Increase soluble fiber foods such as applesauce, bananas, white rice, and oatmeal.

Data from Medical Nutrition Therapy Services, Seattle Cancer Care Alliance, Seattle, WA; American Cancer Society. Caring for the patient with cancer at home. Last revised June 8, 2015. Retrieved from: http://www.cancer.org/treatment/treatmentsandsideeffects/physicalsideeffects/dealingwithsymptomsathome/caring-for-the-patient-with-cancer-at-home-poor-appetite. Accessed September 22, 2016.

Surgery involving the head or neck areas, such as brain tumors, or in the GI tract may result in acute nutritional implications, including problems chewing and swallowing, occurrence of diarrhea, malabsorption of nutrients, and imbalances of fluids and electrolytes.[46]

Radiation Therapy

Radiation therapy is the initial treatment modality for brain tumors that are unresectable, and in such cases it is applied locally and often used in combination with chemotherapy. Radiation is also used locally following surgical removal of resectable brain tumors and to treat other cancers, including high-risk neuroblastoma and certain stages of Wilms' tumor. One radiation modality, total body irradiation (TBI), is administered to leukemia patients who do not respond to conventional chemotherapy and who require radiation throughout their bodies to prepare them for bone marrow transplantation. The nutritional implications of radiation therapy depend on many factors, including the following:

- The region and field size of the body receiving the radiation
- The dose of radiation administered
- Fractionation
- The duration of treatment
- The extent of concurrent use of other antitumor therapy such as surgery or chemotherapy
- The child's current nutritional status

Table 8.9

Nutritional Implications of Radiation Therapy

Site of Radiation Therapy	Potential Side Effects
Central nervous system	Anorexia
	Nausea and vomiting
Head and neck	Nausea and vomiting
	Mucositis
	Esophagitis
	Altered taste and smell
	Tooth decay
	Altered salivation (saliva becomes thick and viscous)
	Dysphagia
	Fatigue
Gastrointestinal tract	Nausea and vomiting
	Diarrhea
	Steatorrhea and malabsorption
	Fluid and electrolyte imbalances
Total body	Nausea, vomiting, diarrhea
	Mucositis, esophagitis
	Altered taste acuity and salivation
	Anorexia
	Delayed growth and development

Like chemotherapy, radiation destroys both malignant cancer cells and rapidly replicating normal tissues and cells, including in the GI tract. Nutritional side effects associated with radiation therapy are listed in **TABLE 8.9** .[47]

Nutrition Assessment

Understanding the specific type and stage of the cancer, the treatment protocol, and the potential side effects of therapy is necessary to effectively formulate an appropriate nutrition care plan for the child. Three basic elements of a nutrition assessment should begin at diagnosis and be repeated periodically throughout treatment: nutrition history, physical assessment, and estimation of nutritional needs.[45]

Nutrition History

Food and nutrient intake are the primary elements of nutritional status. The nutrition assessment of the child includes taking a comprehensive feeding and diet history to identify the child's use of infant formulas or breastfeeding and to determine the stage of eating development. This includes whether the child is able to self-feed, requires pureed food, or has advanced to eating table food, and whether the child is fed by bottle, cup, or a combination of the two.

The history should also include the use of special diets, presence of food allergies, food aversions or intolerances, and use of vitamin, mineral, and herbal supplements.[46] A paramount concern for infants and toddlers is their ability to meet their nutrient needs for proper growth, weight gain, and development, given their current clinical situation and treatment protocol.

After the initial history, the child should frequently be monitored for changes in oral and gastrointestinal symptoms, such as chewing or swallowing difficulties, mucositis, esophagitis, taste alterations, xerostomia (dry mouth), heartburn, nausea and vomiting, early satiety, changes in appetite, and altered bowel habits (diarrhea or constipation).[46]

Physical Assessment

Careful clinical observation is valuable to detect the presence of obesity, undernutrition, dehydration, or edema. The child's age and baseline anthropometric measurements help determine his or her nutritional status. Accurate weight, length, and height measurements are critical to calculate body surface area, which is used to determine dosages of chemotherapy and other medications during treatment.

The initial assessment includes the child's age and measurements for height (or recumbent length in children younger than 2 years of age), weight, and, in children younger than 2 years, head circumference. Any measurement below the 10th percentile should be investigated as a sign of growth impairment due to inadequate nutrition.[46] Growth measurements for children younger than 36 months should include the child's weight-for-length percentile. However, once the child turns 2 years old, his or her proportionality should be measured using the body mass index (BMI), which over the years has become the most reliable anthropometric indicator of nutrition status in children with cancer. Current literature supports also taking measurements of the child's mid-upper arm circumference (MUAC) and triceps skin fold (TSF) to obtain an even more accurate assessment of nutritional status and body composition. Because changes in hydration, fluid shifts (edema or ascites), and tumor mass can influence BMI measurements, MUAC and TSF tests are more reliable and accurate assessments of changes in the child's muscle mass and fat stores.[48]

Estimation of Nutrient Needs

It is critical to evaluate and monitor the ongoing energy needs and intake of each child, especially those identified with a risk of malnutrition. Energy needs are determined by many methods and are satisfied by sufficient caloric intake.[49] All methods determine energy needs at least in part by measuring the child's age, weight, gender, therapy, and growth requirements.[50] The 2005 Dietary Reference

Intakes (DRIs) set forth specific equations for calculating energy and protein needs, but the equations were determined solely from children with normal growth, body composition, and activity.[49] Therefore, this method of measurement may underestimate energy needs in the pediatric oncology population, especially patients younger than 5 years old.

The 1989 Recommended Dietary Allowance (RDA) calculations for infants and children and the WHO equation, which uses the basal metabolic rate with additions for growth, infection, and stress, are also commonly used to estimate energy needs. By multiplying the basal metabolic rate by a stress factor of 1.6 to 1.8 for very young or malnourished children, the WHO equation estimates the caloric intake to allow for growth, stress, and light activity. Other factors affecting energy needs include humoral (primarily cytokines) and tumor-secreting factors from the tumor itself, cancer treatment, bacterial sepsis, and fever secondary to neutropenia.[46] These factors can all drive up the metabolic needs of young cancer patients.

Measuring energy and protein needs properly for the child oncology patient is described in the following subsections.

Calculating Energy Needs

- *Infants 0–12 months:* Use the RDA for age for appropriate-weight infants. The RDA accurately predicts energy needs in the infant cancer patient who often has higher energy requirements. Use a catch-up growth calculation if the child is underweight.

> [RDA for weight age = (kcal/kg) × ideal body weight for height] ÷ actual weight [kg]

- *Children older than 12 months:* Use the WHO basal metabolic rate (BMR) table multiplied by stress factors:

Calculations using BMR and Stress Factors for Estimating Energy Needs

> If normal weight: Age 2 years and older: BMR × 1.6
> If underweight: Age 2 years and older: BMR × 1.8–2.0
> If obese: BMR for adjusted ideal body weight (AIBW) × 1.3
> AIBW: Use adjusted ideal body weight calculation for obese patients:
> IBW + 0.25 (Actual weight – Ideal weight)

Estimating Protein Needs

Protein needs are elevated during cancer treatment because of the rapid turnover of tissue and cells, muscle wasting, and skin breakdown, which are side effects of steroids used to treat leukemia, and the child's ongoing growth requirements. Most children need 2 g/kg protein

©Billion Photos/Shutterstock

Case Study

Kevin is a 12-month-old boy with high-risk neuroblastoma admitted to the hospital with vomiting and failure to thrive. His current weight is 17 pounds, or 7.7 kg (2nd percentile channel). His length is 79.4 cm (95th percentile channel). Weight for length is <2nd percentile channel. Ideal body weight for length is 10.4 kg.

Questions

1. Using the WHO equation for age and sex, calculate the estimated nutrient requirements for this patient.
   Equation: (60.9 × weight [kg]) – 54.
   This provides only estimated needs in a resting state without factors for activity or stress.
2. Now calculate the estimated caloric intake for this same child to account for his malnourished state.
3. Using the RDA formula below to calculate catch-up needs for weight gain/growth if underweight, calculate Kevin's calorie needs using this method for infants 0–12 months. Note: Average energy allowance for children 1–3 years is 102 kcal/kg/day.
4. Which method would you be more likely to use to assess energy needs in this patient?

per day. Infants up to 6 months old require 2.5–3.0 g/kg/day. Protein may need to be restricted in the following situations:

- Renal failure due to tumor lysis syndrome
- Rising blood urea nitrogen (BUN)/creatinine blood levels due to nephrotoxic drugs

Estimating Fluid Needs

The fluid needs of the child with cancer are based on the child's weight and are usually similar to the needs of the healthy population. The standard methodology for calculating fluid requirements in children who weigh less than 40 kg is outlined in Table 8.2.

As with any pediatric disease or condition, ongoing monitoring of the oncology patient's weight, growth, and nutritional status enables the nutrition plan of care to be adjusted as needed. The care provider should always ask these questions:

- Is the child growing and gaining at an appropriate rate based on his or her growth pattern prior to diagnosis?
- Is the child's growth faltering because of undernutrition?
- Is the child's rate of weight gain exceeding expectation for age?
- Is the child able to take in adequate fluid, food, and nutrients on his or her own to sustain growth during treatment?

Supporting the Child Undergoing Cancer Treatment

The incidence of malnutrition in children with newly diagnosed cancers is highly variable and dependent upon such factors as advanced or metastatic disease, the degree of tumor burden, histology, and treatment protocols.[51] Children with cancer tolerate anticancer treatments better if they receive proper nutrition throughout treatment and do not become malnourished.[52] Infants and young toddlers with leukemia, hepatoblastoma, and brain tumors, and whose development of self-feeding skills is often interrupted, are highly vulnerable to malnutrition and chemotherapy-related toxicities. They often suffer pain, mucositis, and vomiting and are, therefore, unable to accept breastmilk, infant formula, or solid foods at sufficient energy and protein levels to sustain growth and weight gain.[46]

Strategies to Keep the Child Nourished
Oral Diet

The optimal goal for infants and children undergoing cancer treatment is to meet their nutritional needs for growing and gaining weight in the least invasive way possible. Suboptimal oral intake of short duration during treatment can be acceptable if the child is initially well nourished and can return to a normal eating pattern when feeling well.

Children may benefit from calorically dense foods that increase energy. Suggestions for boosting the nutrient density of foods consumed are shown in TABLE 8.10. Although breastfeeding and breastmilk have clinical benefits that support an infant's growth and immune system and are the primary nutrition sources for most infants, without calorie and protein fortification the protein content is often inadequate to support normal growth during treatment.[53] Although many commercial liquid medical

Table 8.10

Increasing Nutrient Density of Food

Dairy Products

• Milk	• Use whole milk for drinking and in recipes because it has more calories than lower-fat milks. • Use in milk-based drinks and in cooking to replace water. • Use in preparing hot cereals, soups, cocoa, and pudding.
• Powdered milk	• Mix 1 cup dry milk powder in 4 cups of liquid milk. Use this milk for recipes in cooking and baking. • Add milk powder directly to hot or cold cereals, scrambled eggs, soups, gravies, casserole dishes, mashed potatoes, and desserts.
• Cream and half-and-half	• Use in soups, sauces, egg dishes, batters, puddings, and custards. • Use on cold and hot cereals. • Mix with pasta, mashed potatoes, and rice. • Make cocoa with half-and-half or cream and add marshmallows.
• Cheese	• Add grated cheese or chunks of cheese to sauces, vegetables, soups, salads, casseroles, and refried beans.
• Sour cream	• Add to soups, baked potatoes, vegetables, sauces, salad dressings, gelatin desserts, bread and muffin batter. • Use as dip for raw fruits and vegetables.

Fats

• Butter, margarine, and oils	• Add to soup, mashed and baked potatoes, hot cereal, grits, rice, noodles, and cooked vegetables. • Stir into sauces and gravies.
• Avocados	• Add to sandwiches, salads, and as a topping on eggs and main course dishes. • Prepare guacamole and use as a dip.

Eggs

	• Add eggs to soups and casseroles. • Cook eggs in sauces and cook in stir fry dishes served over rice or noodles. Add cooked sliced eggs to buttered toast, or hot biscuits. • Prepare egg salad with mayonnaise and use on sandwiches and salads, or eat on crackers.

Nut Butters

Peanut, cashew, almond butters	• Add nut butters to make sauces (such as peanut sauce), use on crackers, waffles, pancakes, celery sticks, or apples. • Spread peanut butter on hot buttered bread, tortilla shells.

Granola

	• Use in cookie, muffin, and bread batters. • Sprinkle on yogurt, ice cream, pudding, custard, and fruit. • Mix with dried fruits and nuts for a snack.

Dried Fruit and Nuts

	• Add to muffins, cookies, breads, cakes, rice and grain dishes, cereals and puddings, and stuffing. • Bake in pies and turnovers. • Combine with cooked vegetables such as carrots, sweet potatoes, and acorn and butternut squash.

Pasteurized Honey (use in children older than 1 year)

	• Add to cereal, milk drinks, fruit desserts, smoothies, and yogurt. • Use as a glaze for meats such as chicken or ham.

Modified from Medical Nutrition Therapy Service. Seattle Cancer Care Alliance.

nutritional supplements designed for pediatric patients are available, the child may not like the taste, which will ultimately limit their effectiveness. Children usually better tolerate shakes and smoothies made with familiar ingredients, such as yogurt, fruit, and other less noticeable modular components such as protein powders or fats. Supplements are often acceptable if offered for short durations and as a part of the regular meal or snack pattern. Lactose-free or soy-based products can be useful for a child who is lactose intolerant.

Oral and esophageal lesions may limit tolerance for oral supplements, and hyperosmolar or lactose-containing products may aggravate diarrhea. Encouragement from the healthcare providers along with parent education on the benefit of nutrition supplements can help improve acceptance during treatment. Feeding a child during intense therapy may be a slow process because appetite and tolerance for food fluctuate widely. Individualizing the child's diet, offering small and frequent servings of nutrient-dense foods and fluids that he or she enjoys, and encouraging parents to be involved in the process support enhance the child's oral intake.

Young children with preexisting delays in feeding development should receive intervention from an interprofessional feeding team, which may include an occupational therapist, speech pathologist, and dietitian trained in feeding therapy. Daily food intake records must be thoroughly evaluated to provide a basis for decisions regarding the need for supplemental feedings from alternative interventions, such as tube feeding or parenteral nutrition (PN) support. Patients and family members may assist with record keeping and provide valuable intake information.

Tube Feeding

Enteral tube feeding (ETF) is used for patients who cannot meet nutrition needs through oral intake. A complete formula which contains protein, carbohydrate, fiber, fat, water, minerals, and vitamins is administered through a medically placed tube from the nose to the stomach or intestine. Enteral tube feeding is recognized as a primary nutrition intervention strategy for infants and children undergoing cancer treatment and is the preferred method of providing the patient with safe, beneficial, and physiologic nutrition support.[54] Tube feeding is a type of nutrition support that maintains the function and integrity of the GI tract, therefore reducing risk for infection. For children who have difficulty taking oral medications, tube feeding provides a safe route for administration.

Parenteral Nutrition

During cancer therapy, if a child's GI tract is not tolerating an oral diet or enteral tube feedings, total parenteral nutrition (TPN) may be provided. In this case, an intravenous (IV) administration of nutrients, which include carbohydrate, protein, lipids, electrolytes, vitamins, and minerals, is provided. TPN may be necessary because of complications associated with cancer treatment such as recovery from surgical resection of the tumor (ileus), nausea and vomiting, being unresponsive to antiemetic therapy, secretory-type diarrhea, colitis, pancreatitis, intestinal graph versus host disease (GVHD), radiation enteritis, or esophagitis. Children can also develop conditions in the bowel known as **pneumatosis**, which is s gas cyst in the bowel wall, or **typhlitis**, which is inflammation of the cecum. Both of these conditions indicate use of TPN because resting the GI tract is required.[45]

Other Considerations

Children undergoing cancer treatment are typically not on special diets but often follow an immunosuppressed or low-microbial diet to minimize the risks of foodborne illness. The goal of the diet for the immunosuppressed child is to maximize healthy food options while minimizing GI exposure to pathogenic organisms.[55] Although this diet does not prevent the incidence of infection in children with neutropenia, most facilities impose dietary restrictions, which include avoidance or strict washing of raw, fresh fruits or vegetables; no sprouts (alfalfa, bean, etc.); no raw or undercooked meats, eggs, or fish; and total avoidance of moldy cheeses. Pasteurization of dairy products and juice is also recommended.[56]

Vitamins and Minerals

Specific vitamin and mineral requirements for children with cancer are undefined. Current guidelines are to give vitamins and minerals per DRI guidelines for age and gender if oral intake is suboptimal. Iron-containing vitamins are to be avoided during cancer treatment because of blood transfusions that are frequently needed to support the patient. Supplements containing folic acid should be avoided during administration of oral high-dose methotrexate and IV methotrexate.

The American Academy of Pediatrics (AAP) recommends that infants who receive cancer treatment and who are exclusively breastfeeding or receiving human milk via bottle or tube feeding be supplemented on a daily basis with 400 IUs of vitamin D. Vitamin D supplementation

Case Study

Kevin is now 4 years and 2 months old and has recurrent leukemia. He has just received a course of chemotherapy. His weight is stable, but Kevin is now developing sores in his mouth from the chemotherapy and is starting to refuse to eat food. Kevin has an enteral feeding tube in place that is used to deliver medications.

Question

1. Identify strategies you would recommend to support Kevin's nutritional status and prevent weight loss while the sores in his mouth heal.

should begin in the first few days of life and continue until the infant is weaned to at least 1 L/day or 1 quart/day of vitamin D–fortified formula or whole milk.

Recap Infants and children from birth to 5 years who develop cancer pose unique challenges to their medical providers. The cancer and its treatment can interfere with the child's physical and cognitive development, especially if nutritional intake is compromised. Children with cancer may experience various nutrition-related side effects from both the cancer and treatment that may interfere with growth and development. Understanding how to support children in this age group get back to health through diet or specialized nutrition support is essential and requires the expertise and intervention of a team of qualified healthcare professionals.

1. What are the components of a nutrition assessment for the cancer patient in this age group?
2. List three ways to add additional calories and protein to foods to increase caloric density and improve protein content of meals and snacks.
3. Name three potential side effects related to chemotherapy.

Iron Deficiency

Preview Iron is a necessary nutrient for neuronal energy metabolism, the metabolism of neurotransmitters, myelination, and memory function. Iron deficiency in children presents unique medical challenges.

Iron deficiency (ID) and **iron-deficiency anemia (IDA)** in young children are worldwide health concerns. Iron is a vital nutrient for biologic function, including respiration, energy production, DNA synthesis, and cell proliferation.[57,58]

Elements of blood include white blood cells, platelets, and red blood cells (**FIGURE 8.3**). Blood transports oxygen and nutrients to body tissues and removes waste and carbon dioxide. Anemia develops when the body does not have enough healthy red blood cells to carry oxygen to body tissues. Iron helps to make red blood cells, so a lack of iron in the body may lead to the condition of anemia.

ID is the most common single-nutrient deficiency among children in the developing world. In industrialized nations, despite a decline in prevalence, ID remains a common cause of anemia in young children, especially those between 18 months and 3 years.[59] A rising concern for this age group is recent research that shows a possible adverse effect of ID/IDA on a child's long-term neurodevelopment and behavior; some cognitive effects may

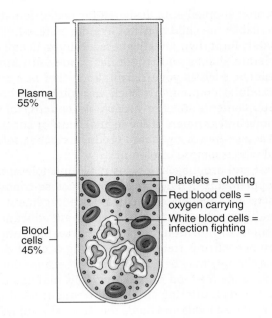

Figure 8.3
Components of blood.

be irreversible.[59] Further study is needed to fully understand the relationship of ID/IDA and cognitive deficits in children. The challenge for the medical community is to develop more effective universal screening systems to identify infants and toddlers who are at risk of ID.[60]

Prevalence
Statistics in the United States currently do not exist on the prevalence of ID or IDA in infants younger than 12 months.[59] Data from 1999–2002 derived from the National Health and Nutrition Examination Survey show that ID and IDA occur in 6.6% to 15.2% of toddlers (1–3 years of age), depending upon ethnicity and socioeconomic status.[61] Without dietary fortification or enrichment of iron in cereals, noodles, and other foods, the reported prevalence of ID increases to approximately 40% in toddlers, which shows the increased physiological demand for dietary iron during this specific life stage.[58]

Risk Factors or Causes
The body obtains iron from food sources, and it reuses iron from old red blood cells. A diet without adequate iron intake is the most common cause of iron deficiency, and in developing countries, ID and IDA typically result from insufficient dietary intake as a result of poverty, malnutrition, or intestinal loss of blood.[58] A common cause of ID and IDA in developed countries is diet by choice. For example, strict vegan (no animal products) or vegetarian diets (no beef, pork, fowl, or seafood) may contribute to ID. More likely in the toddler age group, a limited food palette of low-iron-containing foods, particularly diets where most calories are provided by cow's milk, other dairy products, and low-iron foods such as rice and bread,

increase the risk of ID leading to IDA. Other causes of iron deficiency are nonabsorption of iron even if the child is eating adequate iron, infections, and blood loss from gastrointestinal conditions such as allergy, celiac disease, or inflammatory bowel disease.[58]

Symptoms

The most common symptoms of anemia appear when cells cannot get enough oxygen and are likely to present as a child seeming more tired, weak, and with lower energy than normal or being more irritable. Other signs and symptoms might be as follows:

- Pale skin, lips, or nail beds compared with the normal color
- Dizziness or lightheadedness
- Headaches
- Cold hands and feet
- Rapid heartbeat or irregular heartbeat

Diagnosis

Diagnosing ID and IDA is challenging and complex, requiring the medical and nutrition history of the patient together with laboratory analysis. This complexity requires multiple measures of iron status to determine iron sufficiency or deficiency; no single measurement is currently available that can reliably characterize the iron status of a child. Once an iron deficiency is suspected, the least invasive way to identify ID or IDA is by obtaining and assessing the following laboratory data (see also TABLE 8.11):

- Hemoglobin (Hb) concentration
- Hematocrit (HCT)
- Mean corpuscular volume (MCV)
- Reticulocyte Hb concentration (CHr)
- Total iron-binding capacity

- Transferrin saturation
- Serum ferritin (SF)
- A simultaneous measurement of C-reactive protein (CRP) is required to rule out inflammation.

Hemoglobin concentration is mandatory because it determines the adequacy of the circulating red cell mass and whether anemia is present. A hemoglobin concentration of less than 11 mg/dL starting at 12 months of age is in indicator of IDA. Serum ferritin is a sensitive measurement of iron stores in healthy subjects; however, it is also an acute-phase reactant and may be elevated in the presence of inflammation, both acute and chronic, infection, malignancy, or liver disease.

Prevention

Breastfed Infants

Infants born at term usually have sufficient iron stores until 4 to 6 months of age. Exclusive breastfeeding after 6 months without iron supplementation places infants at increased risk of developing IDA at around 9 months of age. Studies demonstrate that exclusively breastfed infants given iron supplements between 1 and 6 months of age had higher Hb concentration and higher MCV than did their unsupplemented peers.[62] Supplementation also resulted in better visual acuity and higher Bayley Psychomotor Development Indices at 13 months. These findings support that exclusively breastfed term infants should be supplemented with 1 mg/kg/day of iron starting no later than at 4 months of age and continuing until age-appropriate iron-containing foods, such as iron-fortified cereals, are successfully introduced in the diet.

Formula-Fed Infants

For the past 25 years, the standard infant formula for term babies born in the United States has contained 12 mg of

---

Table 8.11

Spectrum of Iron Status

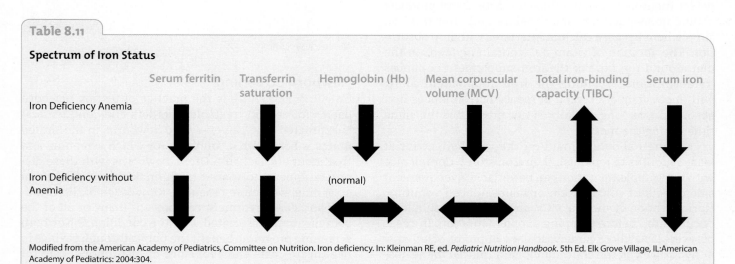

	Serum ferritin	Transferrin saturation	Hemoglobin (Hb)	Mean corpuscular volume (MCV)	Total iron-binding capacity (TIBC)	Serum iron
Iron Deficiency Anemia	↓	↓	↓	↓	↑	↓
Iron Deficiency without Anemia	↓	↓	↔ (normal)	↔	↑	↓

Modified from the American Academy of Pediatrics, Committee on Nutrition. Iron deficiency. In: Kleinman RE, ed. *Pediatric Nutrition Handbook*. 5th Ed. Elk Grove Village, IL:American Academy of Pediatrics: 2004:304.

iron per liter. The recommended level was determined by calculating the total iron needs of the child from 0–12 months, assuming average birth weight and average weight gain during the first year of life. Iron needs for the first 12 months of life can be met by standard infant formula and the introduction of iron-containing solid foods. Because cow's milk is not fortified with iron, this should not take the place of an iron-fortified formula before 12 months of age.[59,60]

Toddlers (1–3 Years of Age)

The iron requirement for toddlers is 7 mg/day. Ideally, the toddler should consume adequate amounts of iron contained in iron-rich foods, such as heme iron sources found in red meat and nonheme sources found in legumes, iron-fortified cereals, raisins, nut butters, and enriched pastas. Although fortification of cereals and other foods has decreased the incidence of IDA, toddlers in the United States often gravitate to foods low in dietary iron, such as milk and other dairy products, or they do not eat enough foods fortified with iron or that are higher in iron content, such as meat. Some toddlers may fill up on milk, which can displace other iron-rich foods in the child's diet. Because of such diet preferences, iron intake may need to be supplemented with oral iron sulfate drops, chewable iron tablets, or a pediatric multivitamin. Liquid supplements are safer for babies 12 to 36 months, and chewable multivitamins should be reserved for children 3 years and older.

Treatment for ID and IDA

Children diagnosed with ID or IDA should receive oral iron supplementation, the most common of which is iron sulfate. The recommended daily dose of a liquid preparation is 3 to 6 mg/kg of body weight. The supplement should be given alone, in divided doses via syringe, and never mixed into food or liquid because the child will detect the iron and may refuse its taste. Dairy products should be avoided for 1 hour before and after the iron supplement because calcium interferes with iron absorption. The addition of vitamin C–containing foods in the diet around the time of the iron supplement enhances its absorption. Providing the iron supplement along with meat, fish, or chicken at meals also enhances iron absorption, as long as dairy is not present at the same time during the meal.

Children should remain on the supplement for at least 3 months to replenish their iron stores. Compliance with iron supplementation can be variable given frequent side effects of constipation or taste-induced vomiting. Normalization of anemia, MCV, and iron stores should be documented before stopping supplementation. In cases of severe IDA, where cardiovascular symptoms of lethargy or hypoxia exist, the child should be admitted to the hospital under the care of physicians trained to treat severe anemia; in such cases, red blood cell transfusion may be indicated.

Recap Infants and children from birth to 5 years with iron deficiency pose unique challenges to their medical providers. ID can interfere with the child's physical and cognitive development, especially if nutritional intake is compromised.[59] Iron is a vital nutrient for biologic and cognitive function, especially for children in this age group. Iron deficiency refers to the depletion of iron stores, which can eventually progress to full-onset iron-deficiency anemia. Once identified, both ID and IDA are largely preventable and curable through dietary intervention.

1. List four important functions in the body of the nutrient iron in infants and children between 1 and 5 years of age.
2. Discuss strategies for preventing ID and IDA in this age group.

Newborn Screening and Genetics

Preview The practice of screening newborns for different disorders and conditions is important because a number of complications associated with certain disorders can be prevented with early diagnosis and treatment.

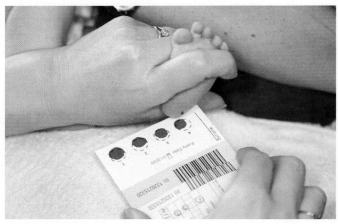

©David Gee/Alamy Stock Photo

Newborn Screening

Newborn screening is the practice of testing newborn babies for certain treatable disorders and conditions. It is estimated that 1 in every 800 newborns in the United States is born with a condition for which screening and treatment are available. Often, newborns with these disorders appear normal at birth, making the process of screening even more essential. Knowledge of the condition and early treatment can prevent many or all of the complications associated with the condition.[63] Newborn screening programs benefit the public through savings in healthcare costs and avoidance of institutional care for affected individuals; thus, newborn screening is nationally recognized as an essential program, and it is a model for other public health-based interventions.[64]

Newborn screening began when Robert Guthrie developed a test that allowed for presymptomatic screening of patients with phenylketonuria (PKU).[65] The test that Guthrie developed was specifically for PKU; however, the simple methodology of collecting blood from a newborn through heel prick, which is then spotted onto filter paper, remains the foundation of newborn screening today.[65] (See **FIGURE 8.4**.)

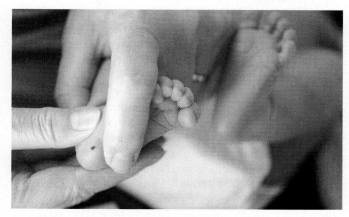

Figure 8.4
Newborn screening through heel prick to have blood draw.

©crozstudios/Alamy Stock Photo

Although newborn screening is now much expanded, it is a screening program only, and follow-up testing is required to confirm or rule out a diagnosis.

Recent publications for newborn screening recommendations by the American College of Medical Genetics have made unifying recommendations across the nation for newborn screening programs.[66] According to the American College of Medical Genetics, a successful newborn screening system consists of the following steps: (1) education of professionals and parents, (2) screening (specimen collection, submission, and testing), (3) follow-up of abnormal and unsatisfactory test results, (4) confirmatory testing and diagnosis, (5) medical management and periodic outcome evaluation, and (6) system quality assurance, including program evaluation, validity of testing systems, efficiency of follow-up and intervention, and assessment of long-term benefits to individuals, families, and society.[66]

Many of the newborn screening conditions are considered to be inborn errors of metabolism that require nutrition interventions as part of their treatment. Examples of such conditions include amino acid metabolism disorders, organic acid metabolism disorders, fatty acid oxidation disorders, carbohydrate metabolism disorders, and various endocrine disorders.

The Big Picture

The following diagram represents the careful coordination of doctors involved with the birth of a child and primary and secondary care services in an effort to prevent undiagnosed severe disabilities.

Reference

Washington State Department of Health State Board of Health. Newborn screening. Policy number 246-650 WAC.

NEWBORN SCREENING

CORE FUNCTION: PREVENTION of severe physical disability or death

METHOD: PREVENTION BASED SCREENING of all newborns carefully coordinated with providers of birthing, primary, and specialty care service

FOCUS: PREVENTION DISEASE that would go undetected without this screening and result in catastophic outcomes

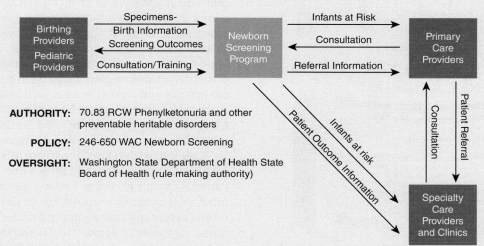

AUTHORITY: 70.83 RCW Phenylketonuria and other preventable heritable disorders

POLICY: 246-650 WAC Newborn Screening

OVERSIGHT: Washington State Department of Health State Board of Health (rule making authority)

Amino Acid Metabolism Disorders

Amino acid metabolism disorders are characterized by the body's inability to correctly metabolize specific amino acids, which often results in accumulation of specific amino acids that are neurologically toxic. Examples include phenylketonuria (PKU), maple syrup urine disease (MSUD), and tyrosinemia type 1 (TYR1).

One example of an amino acid metabolism disorder is maple syrup urine disease, which is caused by a defect in the branched-chain α-ketoacid dehydrogenase complex and which results in the inability to metabolize the branched-chain amino acids (BCAAs) leucine, isoleucine, and valine. MSUD is an autosomal recessive genetic condition. The incidence of patients with MSUD varies between populations, with worldwide incidence for MSUD estimated at 1 in 185,000 individuals.[67] The treatment for MSUD involves restriction of BCAAs to amounts that allow individuals to achieve target plasma BCAA levels while providing all other nutrients (carbohydrates, amino acids, fats, and vitamins and minerals) that support normal growth and development.[68] This is primarily achieved by use of special metabolic formulas that have special protein sources with no leucine, isoleucine, or valine. The amino acid levels in patients with MSUD are monitored closely, and intakes are adjusted frequently depending on labs, growth, illness, and other factors.

Organic Acid Metabolism Disorders

Organic acid metabolism disorders are characterized by errors in metabolism of certain amino acids that result in the accumulation of nonamino organic acids and buildup of toxic intermediates, which can cause metabolic crises and increases in blood acids and ammonia.[69] Examples of organic acid metabolism disorders that are a part of the newborn screening panel are isovaleric acidemia (IVA), glutaric acidemia type 1 (GA1), methylmalonic acidemia (MMA), and propionic acidemia (PA).[66]

Fatty Acid Oxidation Disorders

Fatty acid oxidation disorders are characterized by the body's inability to use stored fat for energy. During times of increased energy needs, such as illnesses or prolonged fasting, infants with fatty acid oxidation disorders can suffer from dangerously low blood glucose levels that can result in serious damage to many organs and possibly cause death. Many historic sudden infant death syndrome (SIDS) cases are thought to be a result of undiagnosed fatty acid oxidation disorders.[70] Examples of fatty acid oxidation disorders that are part of newborn screening panels include medium-chain acyl-CoA dehydrogenase deficiency (MCAD), long-chain 3-hydroxyacyl-CoA dehydrogenase deficiency (LCHAD), and very long chain acyl-CoA dehydrogenase deficiency (VLCAD).

Carbohydrate Metabolism Disorders

Carbohydrate metabolism disorders are characterized by errors in metabolism of certain carbohydrates (sugars). An example of a carbohydrate disorder that is part of newborn screening panels is galactosemia.[71] Galactosemia is a disorder of galactose metabolism, which is treated with a galactose-restricted diet.[72]

Other disorders screened for as part of newborn screening programs include various endocrine disorders such as congenital adrenal hyperplasia, congenital hypothyroidism, various hemoglobinopathies, and cystic fibrosis (CF).

Cystic Fibrosis

Cystic fibrosis (CF) is an autosomal recessive genetic disorder and is the result of a defective cystic fibrosis transmembrane conductance regulator (CFTR). CFTR is a protein that allows chloride to cross all cell membranes. With a defect in CFTR, secretions become sticky and thick and affect some or all of the following systems and organs: gastrointestinal tract, lungs, pancreas, liver, sinuses, and reproductive system. From a nutritional aspect, the result of this defect is often poor weight gain and growth throughout infancy and toddlerhood as well as throughout the life span. Both parents have to be carriers of a CF gene to have a child affected by cystic fibrosis. CF affects 1 in 2,500 Caucasian live births, and to a lesser degree all races.[73]

Children with cystic fibrosis are followed by a primary care provider for well-child issues and are followed concurrently by an accredited cystic fibrosis center a minimum of four times a year. A cystic fibrosis center offers multidisciplinary management and includes a physician, nurse, registered dietitian, social worker, and respiratory therapist. Many centers also have a child life therapist and clinical psychologist on staff.

Courtesy of Abbott Laboratories

Nutritional management in CF includes nutritional assessment; increasing caloric, protein, and fat intake (including by supplements and tube feedings); management of pancreatic insufficiency and pancreatic enzyme replacement; and fat-soluble vitamin replacement.

Distal Intestinal Obstruction Syndrome

Distal intestinal obstruction syndrome (DIOS) is a complete or partial intestinal blockage by fecal material in the ileum and cecum and is a complication of cystic fibrosis. Symptoms include abdominal distention, abdominal pain, and, with a complete blockage, vomiting. DIOS is described as more acute than standard constipation, which can be long-standing with fecal material throughout the colon.[74] Poorly controlled fat malabsorption can be a factor in some cases of DIOS. Treatment for incomplete blockage includes oral rehydration and stool softeners or an enema. If blockage is complete, oral or nasogastric administration of an electrolyte osmotic solution may be administered. Rare cases require surgical intervention.[74] The importance of nutrition in DIOS includes guidance, both at the time of occurrence and at each cystic fibrosis clinic visit, on adequate fluid intake.

Pancreatic Insufficiency

Pancreatic insufficiency is a common GI complication of cystic fibrosis. It is caused by the inability of lipase, protease, and amylase to transit from the pancreas to the small intestine resulting from the blockage of the duct from the pancreas to the small intestine. This leads to fat, carbohydrate, and protein malabsorption and steatorrhea and, left untreated, mild, moderate, or severe malnutrition. In addition, malabsorption of fat-soluble vitamins (A, D, E, K) may also occur. Treatment for pancreatic insufficiency is pancreatic enzyme and fat-soluble vitamin replacement.

Pancreatic Enzyme Replacement Therapy

An adequately functioning pancreas is necessary for proper digestion of food. In situations in which the pancreas does not make enough enzymes to digest food properly (for example, in individuals with cystic fibrosis), medication can be used to help improve digestion of fats, proteins, and sugars from food. Fecal elastase is a medical test that measures how well the pancreas is functioning and can be used to diagnose pancreatic insufficiency (PI). PI can be detected at birth, or up to several months later, with a normal fecal elastase test, and it usually declines gradually over the first year of life.

Pancreatic enzymes used in pancreatic enzyme replacement therapy (PERT) to treat this condition are capsules typically taken orally. They have an acid-resistant coating meant to help them bypass the stomach and dissolve in the alkaline pH of the duodenum.

Because newborns and infants are not able to swallow capsules, the capsules are opened and the microspheres are fed with the infant food followed by whatever liquid (breast or bottle) the infant is expected to drink. When Children are able to safely swallow capsules whole, this is the preferred form of enzyme administration. Enzymes are administered prior to each feeding.[73]

Enzyme therapy adjustment is based on clinical response, such as appropriate weight gain and growth, plus review of symptoms of PI such as increase in stools. If appropriate and necessary, the dose can be increased.

Fat-Soluble Vitamins

Patients with CF should be monitored for evidence of vitamin deficiency and may require supplemental nutrients.[74] Supplementation of fat-soluble vitamins A, D, E, and K are a priority because pancreatic enzyme insufficiency often results in malabsorption of these nutrients.

Tube Feeding in CF Patients

Based on guidelines from the CF Foundation, children are prescribed many different types of nutrition supplements.[75] Initially, high-calorie formula or breastmilk by mouth is recommended for infants who struggle with maintaining adequate weight and weight/length percentiles equal to or greater than the 50th percentile. Likewise, an escalation to high-calorie foods or commercial liquid supplements is often prescribed in older infants and children. Tube feeding may be recommended in infants and children who, despite aggressive oral intervention, are unable to gain and grow adequately.

CF Nutrition Assessment and Recommendations

Nutrition management for infants and children with CF is a carefully coordinated effort to combine normal age-related nutrition and feeding while treating pancreatic insufficiency, low serum vitamin levels, and gastrointestinal-related illness, and preventing malnutrition.[73]

Infants are followed in a CF center immediately after diagnosis. The focus of nutrition management is determining how sufficiently the pancreas is working based on the fecal elastase results and determining the status of fat-soluble vitamins. Initiation of a multivitamin that includes what is needed to correct any fat-soluble vitamin deficiencies generally occurs at this time.[75] Anticipatory guidance on calorie, enzyme, vitamin, and salt requirements is given as is information on feeding methods and the possibility of nutrition support.[73] Although increased caloric density of nutrition sources is essential, both breastfeeding and bottle feeding can be successful feeding methods for infants with cystic fibrosis.[73] At each CF clinic visit, nutrition assessment is completed, including measurements of weight, length, and head circumference, which are plotted on the WHO growth grids. The infant's goal or "ideal" weight is calculated at a point between the 50th and 75th percentile. Requirements for infants with CF or pancreatic insufficiency are approximately 130% of the RDA for calories at the ideal body weight and up to 200% of the RDA for protein. Fat is expected to contribute 40% of daily calories. The nutrition assessment continues with stool history and history of reflux and aspiration episodes.[76]

Table 8.12

Nutrition for the Toddler with Cystic Fibrosis

Noodles with Alfredo sauce (with butter, cream, and cheese)	Grated whole-milk cheese	Crackers with cheese or peanut butter
Blueberry muffins	Pancakes or waffles	Sliced avocado
Soft-cooked vegetables with butter and cheese	Scrambled eggs with cream and cheese	Tuna or egg salad sandwich with mayonnaise
Breaded fish or fish sticks	Ice cream	Cooked cereal with cream, butter, and brown sugar
Whole-milk cottage cheese or yogurt	Pudding made with whole milk and cream	Refried beans

Cystic Fibrosis Foundation Education Committee; 2006. Nutrition for your toddler with cystic fibrosis (one to three years). Retrieved from: https://www.cff.org/PDF-Archive/Nutrition-for-Your-Toddler-(1-to-3-Years)/. Accessed September 9, 2016.

Nutrition assessment and recommendations for toddlers ages 1 to 3 years with CF are similar to those for infants in regard to calorie and protein needs. Additional calories and protein can be added to liquids and solid foods, and full-fat foods such as dairy, proteins, salad dressings, and snack foods are encouraged as a way to meet the higher calorie needs.

Additional considerations for preschoolers with CF include the importance of educating caregivers on enzyme administration, adequate calories in the foods provided during meals, adequate access to a restroom, and the ability to offer snacks, particularly if a child's physical activity during the day is increased. See TABLE 8.12 for suggestions on high-calorie foods for children with CF.

Down Syndrome

Down syndrome, also called trisomy 21, is a chromosomal abnormality characterized by an extra chromosome 21. The parents of an affected child are typically genetically normal; the extra chromosome occurs by chance. No known behavior or environmental factors change the risk; however, an association exists between the age of the mother and the risk of her baby having Down syndrome. As a woman gets older, her risk of having a child with Down syndrome steadily increases.[77] Prenatal screening can identify Down syndrome as can a blood test performed after birth to confirm the diagnosis. One in every 700 newborns is affected.[78] Down syndrome is characterized by hypotonia (low muscle tone), developmental delay, short stature, and mild to moderate intellectual disability. Children with Down syndrome have an increased incidence of congenital heart disease, hypothyroidism, type 1 diabetes, celiac disease, gastrointestinal atresia, autism, seizure disorders, leukemia, and hearing or vision problems.[78]

The American Academy of Pediatrics (AAP) recently published health supervision guidelines for children with Down syndrome from birth through 21 years. Infants with

Down syndrome may have feeding problems, such as slow feeding or increased sleeping that requires them to be woken for routine feedings. Like all other infants, feeding progression should proceed on the basis of developmental readiness; however, in children with Down syndrome, this progression may be delayed. If infants choke with feeding or have recurrent respiratory problems such as pneumonia, they should be referred for a feeding evaluation and radiographic swallowing assessment.[79]

Children with Down syndrome are at increased risk for becoming overweight and obese because they have reduced calorie requirements resulting from the lower energy requirements associated with low muscle tone. Basal metabolic rate has been reported to be 10–15% lower in children with Down syndrome than in children without Down symdrome.[80,81] Excessive weight may also be a result of hypothyroidism. Nutritional education should focus on creating healthy eating habits and incorporating physical activities.

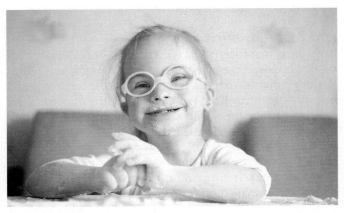

©Eleonora_os/Shutterstock

Numerous products claim to improve the nutrition of those with Down syndrome; however, no scientifically rigorous evidence supports the benefit of any specific vitamin/mineral or alternative therapies other than the use of a general multivitamin to help boost the immunity of people with Down syndrome.[79]

Recap Many different genetic conditions require specialized nutrition management in infants and children. Newborn screening can identify most of these conditions early, which supports improved nutritional outcomes.

1. Infants with Down syndrome are at risk for what type of feeding problems?
2. What is the recommendation for calories, protein, and fat for infants and children with cystic fibrosis?
3. Describe the nutritional management for genetic conditions affecting carbohydrate, fat and protein metabolism.

Selected Pediatric Conditions

Preview Pediatric conditions such as spina bifida, cerebral palsy, cleft lip and palate, and autism spectrum disorder all require specific nutrition recommendations and, in some cases, particular modes of feeding. Addressing these issues is essential for optimal growth and development.

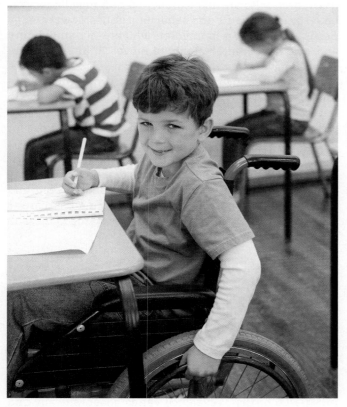

©wavebreakmedia/Shutterstock

Spina Bifida (Myelomeningocele)

Spina bifida is a neural tube defect characterized by abnormal development of the spinal canal during the first trimester of pregnancy. *Spina bifida* means "split spine."[82] The result is a sac on the spine that contains meninges and spinal nerves. The location of the lesion determines the severity of weakness or paralysis, with higher lesions having the greatest severity.[83] Conditions often found with spina bifida include the following:[84]

- *Hydrocephalus:* A condition that develops as the result of excess fluid in the ventricles in the brain that affects 85% of children born with spina bifida.
- *Arnold-Chiari malformation type II:* A brain stem malformation that results in weaknesses in the neck and arm muscles, leading to dysphagia or swallowing difficulties.
- *Neurogenic bowel and bladder:* Lack of control of urination and defecation caused by nerve damage.
- *Intellectual disability*
- *Epilepsy (seizure disorders)*

Spina bifida is associated with the folate status of the mother. Incidence is 0.5–1.0 per 1,000 live births and 20–40 per 1,000 live births of a mother who previously had a pregnancy affected by neural tube defect. It is more common in women with poor economic status; poor maternal diet; exposure to chemicals, anticonvulsants, or amphetamines; maternal febrile illness; and maternal diabetes. It is recommended that all women who may become pregnant take 400 mcg of folate daily. This dose is increased to 4 mg for women who have had a previous pregnancy affected by neural tube defect. The U.S. Food and Drug Administration (FDA) released regulations in 1996 requiring the addition of folic acid to fortify and enrich grain products such as breads, cereals, pastas, and flour as a way to reduce the risk of neural tube defects.[85] In 1998, these regulations were made mandatory.[86]

Neonates with spina bifida typically have their lesions repaired immediately after birth. This increases energy and protein as well as vitamin/mineral requirements in an effort to promote optimal wound healing. Children with spina bifida are at risk for the development of wounds because of lack of feeling in their lower body, below their lesion.[87]

Energy needs are similar in infancy to those of healthy infants but are decreased by as much as 50% by 1 year of age. This is directly related to decreased activity due to paralysis. Children with lower lesions, such as a sacral lesion, may be ambulatory and have typical energy needs. Children with spina bifida are shorter in stature than typically developing children. Linear growth usually slows around 2 years of age. Lean body mass is decreased as well, depending on the severity of paralysis, and is an issue that can lead to increased incidence of overweight and obesity.

Feeding difficulties may be present in children with spina bifida as a result of complications in the part of the brain that controls balance (a condition called Arnold-Chiari malformation type II), reducing the ability to suck and swallow. This may lead to the need for adjustments in feeding technique, equipment, food and liquid texture or consistency, and caloric density, or ultimately the need for gastrostomy tube placement.

Children with spina bifida also experience bladder and bowel dysfunction associated with constipation and increased risk of urinary tract infections. Children typically have a bowel and bladder "program" that includes bowel medications as well as typical constipation management strategies such as increased fiber, fluids, and exercise. Bladder programs involve routine catheterizations to release urine from the bladder. Adequate fluid intake as well as clean catheterization procedures are needed to decrease the risk of infection.

The risk of developing a latex allergy is high for children with spina bifida because of repeated exposures to latex during procedures in the hospital and at home (such as bladder catheterization with latex catheters).[82] The risk is decreased by using latex-free products. Children who develop latex allergy may also be allergic to certain foods that "cross-react" with latex, including banana, avocado, chestnut, kiwi, apple, carrot, celery, papaya, tomato, and melon. These foods should not be avoided unless there is a reaction to them.[82]

Cerebral Palsy

Cerebral palsy is a condition caused by brain injury or abnormal brain development that results in difficulties with motor control and muscle tone. Cerebral palsy can occur during the prenatal, perinatal, or postnatal period, caused by brain structure malformation or events such as abnormalities of blood flow, asphyxia, brain hemorrhage, or traumatic brain injury or infection.[88] It is a nonprogressive disorder that can affect an infant and young child in a variety of ways. Children with cerebral palsy are at increased risk for cognitive impairment, learning difficulties, and intellectual disabilities. Vision and hearing can be affected, and seizure disorders can affect up to 30% of individuals.[88]

Typically, cerebral palsy is difficult to diagnose prior to the age of 2 years and cannot be considered until infants reach the age when they would typically roll or sit.[89] Cerebral palsy is classified by severity of functional movement problems and level of self-sufficiency in activities of daily living (ADLs). There are five categories of gross motor function, with category 1 being the least affected and category 5 the most affected.[89] Children who fall into the fourth and fifth categories are more likely to have feeding problems and to have a gastrostomy tube for some or all of their nutritional needs.

Common nutrition-related problems include feeding problems related to **dysphagia**, which is difficulty or discomfort in swallowing, difficulty gaining weight, which leads to growth retardation, gastrointestinal problems such as gastroesophageal reflux and constipation, and drug–nutrient interactions. Oral motor function is affected by decreased jaw, tongue, and lip control that reduces the ability to chew, swallow, and eat efficiently. This lack of control may also increase the risk of aspirating food and can affect dental health. Children with feeding difficulties benefit from a formal feeding evaluation by a feeding therapist such as an occupational or speech therapist. These professionals are trained to evaluate anatomy and swallowing function and can educate families in using proper positioning, using therapeutic feeding techniques, and providing proper food textures.

Nutrition Assessment

Nutrition assessment of individuals with cerebral palsy includes assessment of: (1) dysphagia/aspiration risk; (2) proper positioning; (3) proper food texture; (4) need for therapeutic feeding techniques; (5) appropriate duration of meals; (6) appropriate amounts of food and fluids; and (7) need for tube feeding for part of or all nutritional needs.

Goals for nutrition include meals that last no longer than 30 minutes because children become fatigued coordinating the work of eating with breathing and swallowing. Oral eating efficiency decreases over time with this fatigue, and the risk of aspiration increases. High-calorie and nutrient-dense foods and fluids are recommended. If the child is unable to meet nutritional needs orally, a gastrostomy tube is placed to provide for these needs.

Some children with cerebral palsy have increased energy needs resulting from **athetosis**, which is excessive movement. Other factors that contribute to increased energy needs are wearing braces that are heavy, frequent illness, and frequent infection. Underweight is common in children who are 100% orally fed and may be exacerbated by low appetite and behavioral issues. Lower energy needs are common in children who are nonambulatory and who have limited ability to move. Children who are tube fed have lower muscle mass as a result of **hypotonia**, which is also known as "floppy baby syndrome." Hypotonia results in a low amount of tension or resistance to stretch in a muscle and often involves reduced muscle strength, causing weight goals to be lower than those for typical children the same age.

Infants and children with cerebral palsy are best managed by interdisciplinary teams that include primary care; developmental medicine; occupational, speech, and physical therapy; nutrition; and specialty medical care as needed such as orthopedics, rehabilitation medicine, and gastroenterology.

Cleft Lip and Palate

Cleft lip and palate (CLP) are congenital anomalies that result in incomplete closure of the skin, muscle, and bone of the upper lip and gum line (cleft lip) and incomplete closure of the tissues that form the roof of the mouth (cleft palate). CLP are also known as orofacial clefts.

Prevalence/Etiology

CLP are common birth defects, with an incidence of 1 in 500–700 births. Prevalence varies geographically and by ethnicity, with lowest incidence in infants of African descent (1:2,500 births) and highest incidence among Native American infants and Asian infants (1:500 births). Incidence in infants of European descent is 1:1,000.[90]

CLP can be described by the anatomy they affect. **Bilateral cleft lip and palate** involve the lip having two clefts, dividing the lip into three segments, and may be present in varying degrees: unilateral or bilateral cleft lip without involvement of the **palate**; unilateral or bilateral cleft lip with involvement of the hard or soft palate; isolated cleft palate; **submucous cleft palate**; midline cleft of the palate; or **bifid uvula**. (See **FIGURE 8.5**, **FIGURE 8.6**, **FIGURE 8.7**, and **FIGURE 8.8**.)

CLP can also be described as syndromic and nonsyndromic. Twenty percent of all clefts and 40% of isolated cleft palates are syndromic, meaning they are associated with additional physical or cognitive abnormalities.[91] **TABLE 8.13** describes orofacial clefts and the associated nutrition implications.

The etiology of CLP can be genetic, environmental, or idiopathic, with syndromic clefts most likely to have a genetic etiology. The developmental changes that cause clefting occur between 5 and 12 weeks of gestation.

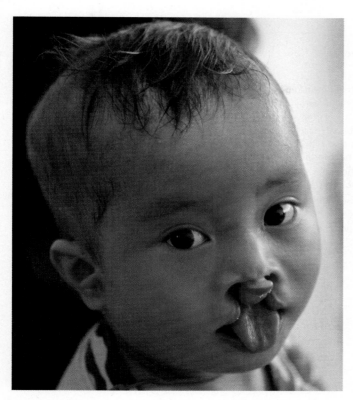

Figure 8.5
Bilateral cleft lip and palate.

©Nguyen Huy Kham/Reuters

Risk Factors

Risk of having a child with CLP increases slightly if the family already has one affected child or the parent has an orofacial cleft. Risk is increased further with two affected children or other family members. Certain teratogens, which are substances in the environment of an embryo that can cause birth defects, such as alcohol, smoking, or **antiepileptic medications**, can increase risk.[92,93]

Risk factors associated with orofacial clefts include feeding difficulties with subsequent poor growth; increased energy requirement; Eustachian tube dysfunction resulting in increased incidence of **otitis media** (ear

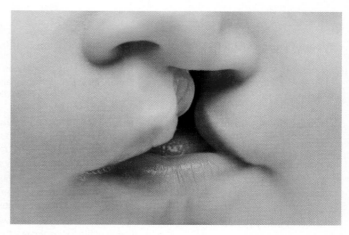

Figure 8.7
Unilateral cleft lip and palate.

©Malgorzata Ostrowska/Alamy Stock Photo

infections) and conductive hearing loss; dental, orthodontic, and/or speech problems; gastroesophageal reflux; breathing difficulty (Pierre Robin sequence); and endocrine dysfunction (midline clefting).

Prevention

To increase understanding, parents who have had a previous child with a cleft can consider genetic counseling to help determine the risk of having more children with the same condition. Taking prenatal vitamins prior to pregnancy as well as avoiding known teratogens during pregnancy may help decrease the risk of cleft.

Treatment

CLP are surgically repaired in a series of age/development-determined surgeries.[94] Nonsurgical treatment primarily addresses how to feed infants until their clefts are repaired. Infants with cleft lip and a normal palate may

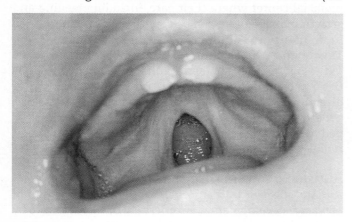

Figure 8.6
Isolated cleft palate.

©BIOPHOTO ASSOCIATES/Science Source/Getty

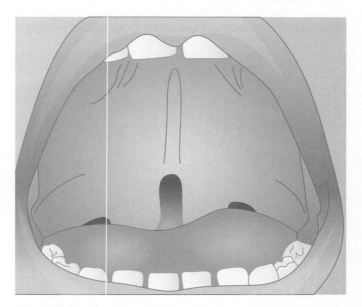

Figure 8.8
Submucous cleft palate.

Table 8.13	
Types of Orofacial Clefts with descriptions and nutrition implications[a]	
Syndrome	**Description and Nutrition Implications**
Velocardiofacial syndrome or DiGeorge syndrome	Genetic disorder with anomalies that can include any combination of the following: cleft palate, cardiac abnormalities, facial differences, learning disabilities, and speech difficulties. Feeding difficulties associated with cleft palate.
Pierre Robin sequence (RS)	Birth defect characterized by abnormal small lower jaw and tendency for the tongue to fall backward toward the throat. Is usually associated with cleft palate and Gastroesophageal reflux is common. Increased energy needs and may need fortified breastmilk or kcal fortified formula.
Treacher Collins syndrome	Genetic condition which affects the bones, jaw, skin, and muscles of the face; anomalies include cleft palate, small oral cavity, airway problems, and feeding problems. Feeding difficulties similar to RS
Stickler syndrome	Genetic disorder of connective tissue affecting the eye and joints. Anomalies include cleft palate, high risk of retinal detachment, deafness, and arthritis. Feeding difficulties similar to RS
Van der Woude syndrome	Genetic disorder associated with pits or mounds of tissue in the lower lip, cleft lip, cleft palate, or both. Feeding difficulties similar to cleft lip and palate

[a] This table does not present all syndromes associated with orofacial clefting.

be able to breastfeed or use a standard bottle effectively. Infants with cleft lip and palate and those with isolated cleft palate cannot close their mouth and shape their palate adequately and therefore do not have the intraoral pressure needed for sucking and successful breastfeeding or (standard) bottle feeding. To overcome this difficulty, specialty bottles that do not require sucking are used.

An individualized assessment of feeding by a craniofacial nurse with experience in feeding infants with clefts determines the best specialty bottle to use and best position for feeding (**FIGURE 8.9**). A feeding therapist evaluates more difficult feeding issues. An upright feeding position helps prevent milk flowing into the nasopharynx, which is the space above the soft palate at the back of the nose that connects the mouth with the nose. An upright feeding position helps in infants with glossoptosis, or a downward displacement of the tongue; an elevated, side-lying position helps the tongue stay forward for better milk flow management. Frequent burping is recommended because infants with cleft tend to swallow more air during feedings.

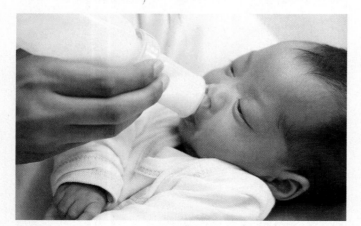

Figure 8.9
Specialty bottles used for infants with CLP and corresponding descriptions of how they work.

©PeopleImages/iStock/Getty Images Plus/Getty

During the first 6 months of life, the preferred nutrition for an infant with CLP is breastmilk. However, because adequate breastfeeding is not possible, this would require that the mother extract breastmilk by using a breast pump. When breastmilk is not available, standard infant formula is an acceptable substitute.

The introduction of complementary foods and the cup is typical at 6 months of age or when the baby is showing readiness. At this time, nasal regurgitation of food is common and does not harm the baby. Weaning from breastmilk or formula to whole milk is typical at age 1 year but may be delayed per family preference or for increased nutrition until after the palate repair. Normal feeding and nutrition continue, with temporary alteration in food textures (soft, no-chew) after surgical repairs as needed. Timing of surgeries, feeding modalities, and nutrition interventions may vary between craniofacial centers. **TABLE 8.14** describes typical surgical, feeding, and nutrition management of cleft lip and palate.

Recommendations

Infants with orofacial clefts should be referred to a craniofacial center where their care, including feeding and growth management, can be coordinated and monitored from infancy to adulthood by an interdisciplinary team. This team includes a minimal core of speech-language pathology, surgery (plastic and oral), and orthodontics specialists and access to professionals in other disciplines, including psychology, social work, audiology, genetics, general and pediatric dentistry, otolaryngology, pediatrics/primary care, neurosurgery, ophthalmology, radiology, and nutrition.[94]

Autism Spectrum Disorders

Autism spectrum disorders (ASD) represent a group of pervasive developmental disorders (PDD) characterized by complex developmental disabilities with severe impairments in social interaction and communication accompanied by behavioral inflexibility, repetitive behaviors, and/or

Table 8.14

Surgical, Feeding, and Nutrition Management of Cleft Lip and Palate

Age	Surgical Management	Feeding Modality	Nutrition Management
3–6 months	Lip repair	Cleft lip only: breastfeeding or bottle feeding with wide-based nipple. Cleft palate: Specialty bottle. Upright position helps keep milk out of nasopharynx. Side-lying position if tongue-based obstruction (Pierre Robin). Burp often secondary to increased air swallowing. After lip repair: Resume typical feeding modality soon after lip repair.	Breastmilk or standard infant formula. 400 IU vitamin D for babies receiving breastmilk. Introduction of complementary foods at 6 months or when baby is showing readiness. Progression of textures typical for age. After lip repair: Resume breastmilk or formula.
9–15 months	Palate repair (syndromic clefts at late end) Ear tubes for otitis media	See above. Introduction of cup typical for age. Cup must not contain valve. Wean from bottle to cup typical for age (~age 1) or after palate repair. After palate repair: For 2–4 weeks, bottle feed with specialty bottle and/or use open cup or unvalved cup without a hard or long spout; nothing hard (no utensils or straws or fingers/hands) in the mouth.	Wean to whole milk typical for age (age 1), but may wait until after palate is repaired. Toddler diet typical for age. Ensure meeting calcium and vitamin D requirements. After palate repair: For 2–4 weeks, soft, no-chew diet.
2–5 years	Velopharyngeal insufficiency (VPI) surgery ("speech surgery") Nose and lip revision considered	After VPI surgery: Nothing hard (no utensils or straws) in mouth for 4–6 weeks.	Preschool diet typical for age. After VPI surgery: Soft, no-chew diet for 4–6 weeks.

Case Study

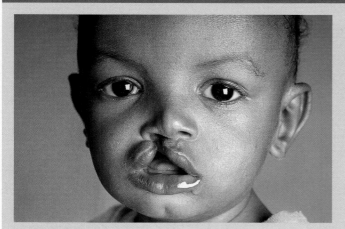

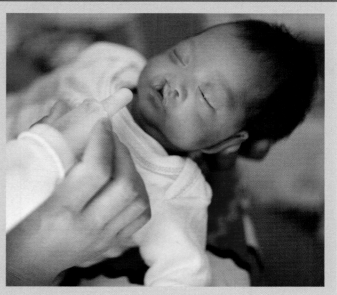

Ben is a full-term 2-month-3-week-old boy with a right **unilateral cleft lip and palate**. He was born in another state and moved to his current residence after 1 month of life. His parents were unaware of cleft palate during pregnancy. The parents report that at birth they were given a Haberman bottle and then were sent home without instructions or support. Mom read the instructions included in the packaging of the Haberman bottle. Ben took 1 hour to feed and demonstrated signs of fatigue near the end of the feedings. He was provided Enfamil formula made to a standard 20 kcal/oz.

At age 2 months, Ben was seen by a pediatrician near the family's new residence. His anthropometric measurements were charted as shown below. Growth parameters were <2nd percentile for weight, 16th percentile for length, <2nd percentile weight-to-length ratio, and 2nd percentile occipitofrontal circumference (OFC). The pediatrician changed the concentration of the formula to

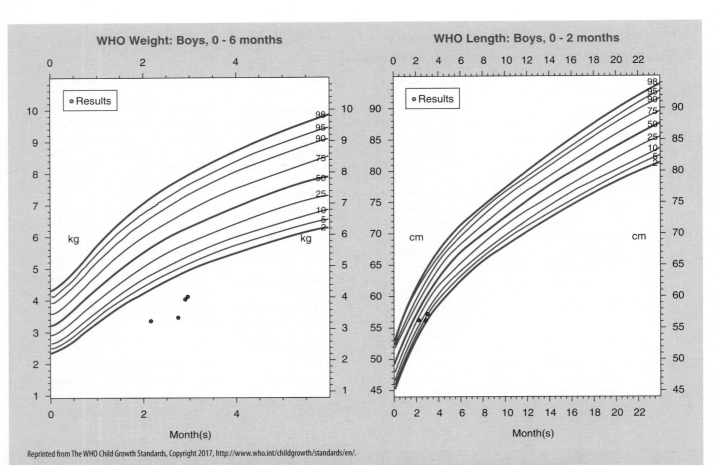

24 kcal/oz. Ben was referred to the craniofacial team for poor weight gain and growth and for management of his cleft lip and palate.

A craniofacial registered nurse observed Ben feeding with a Haberman bottle and tried a Dr. Brown bottle with a cleft valve. This new bottle and valve proved to be more efficient for the infant. Diet history showed that the parents were offering Ben 3 ounces every 3–4 hours and 1 feeding at night: estimated 6 feedings per day = 18 ounces of intake = 122 kcal/kg.

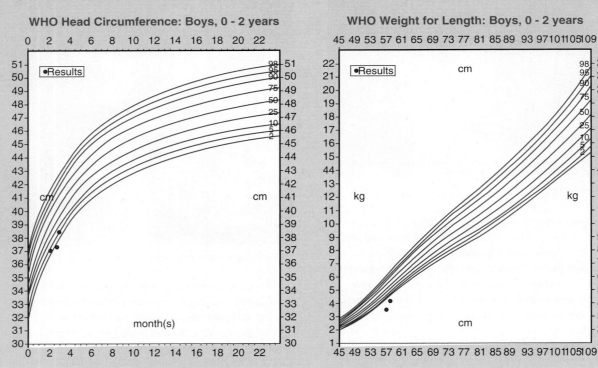

The new plan was for the parents to offer more formula volume in the bottle, 4–6 ounces per feeding, 7 or more feedings per day, and have 1 week follow-up with craniofacial. Recipes for 24 kcal/oz in 4-ounce and 6-ounce total volumes were provided to the parents.

At the follow-up visit, the parents report significant improvement in energy and increased volume intake of 4–5 ounces per feeding. Ben has 6–7 feedings daily but has started to spit up occasionally. Current growth parameters are <2nd percentile weight, 5th percentile length, <2nd percentile weight to length,

and 4th percentile OFC, as shown in the growth charts provided. Ben demonstrated catch-up weight gain and is growing in length appropriately.

Questions

1. What factors contributed to Ben's slowed weight gain?
2. What interventions helped achieve improvement in growth parameters?

restricted interests.[95] Generally speaking, autism spectrum disorder refers to the three most common PDDs: autism, Asperger syndrome, and pervasive development disorder—not otherwise specified.

Prevalence/Etiology

Recent reports from the Centers for Disease Control and Prevention indicate the prevalence of ASD in U.S. children to be 1 in 68.[96] This number is four to five times higher for U.S. males compared with females.[97] The etiology of ASD is unknown. A number of epidemiologic studies also show a 2–8% higher rate of ASD among siblings and a 60–90% higher rate of ASD for identical twins.[96] The risk of a child having ASD is also greater in families with a first-degree relative with ASD and in families with a first-degree relative who exhibits similar deficits in communication, social skills, transitional inflexibility, and stereotypical behaviors. All point to the likelihood of a strong genetic component.

Risk Factors

An estimated 50% to 90% of children with ASD have feeding problems that negatively affect their social interactions at home and at school.[98] Feeding problems common to children with ASD are categorized as behavioral feeding disorders, including avoidant eating behaviors (food refusal, turning away, throwing food, pushing food away, packing food in their mouth, swallowing whole foods without chewing, crying, choking, gagging, or vomiting without a medical basis), and sensory-based feeding difficulties (food selectivity by type, texture, sight, smell, and/or presentation, touch avoidance, and lack of self-feeding). Other difficult feeding behaviors common to children with ASD include behavioral rigidity around food, often manifesting as repetitive rituals in the sequence or manner with which food is eaten, or patterns of food choice relative to certain environments or daily activities.

There is a greater prevalence of reported GI symptoms, including constipation, diarrhea, and general abdominal pain, in children with autism than in those without.[99] On the other hand, research that looks at objective markers of GI dysfunction, including GI inflammation, digestive enzyme deficiencies, and intestinal permeability, shows little statistical difference in either pathology or frequency of abnormal GI inflammation, intestinal permeability,

and digestive enzyme activity in children with and without autism.[100] These results support the observance that common GI problems occur in children with autism and suggest that additional GI evaluations may be beneficial for children with autism, particularly those who exhibit stereotypical or self-injurious behaviors.[100]

The emergence of feeding problems in children with ASD most commonly occurs without an identifiable organic cause such as GI, respiratory, or oral motor delays.[101] These findings suggest that feeding difficulties manifest instead from deficits in social compliance, communication, a heightened concentration on detail, fear of novelty, perseveration, impulsivity, and sensory impairments. This, in turn, is consistent with both research and anecdotal reports by parents and clinicians suggesting that the occurrence of GI problems may be a secondary component of restricted eating patterns, which also appear to be compounded by sensory sensitivities that intensify the GI-associated pain and discomfort. Language delays common to children with ASD may exacerbate or mask all aforementioned feeding difficulties and GI disturbances as a result of a child's limited ability to communicate pain and other problems, including fear.[102]

Additional risk factors resulting from such inherent feeding problems in children with ASD include underdeveloped oral motor muscles and chewing dysfunction, which in many cases can compromise a child's ability to efficiently and effectively prepare food into a bolus and propel it. Immature oral motor skills also appear to exacerbate avoidant eating of certain textures or may give way to swallowing difficulties and risk of aspiration.[103]

Children with ASD demonstrate an overall narrower range and quantity of accepted foods compared with children without ASD but with feeding problems.[98] And, by the same comparison, children with ASD also display higher rates of disruptive behavior (gagging, vomiting, temper tantrums) when presented with nonpreferred foods.[103] Interestingly, in spite of having significant feeding problems, the majority of toddlers and school-age children do not typically have faltered growth patterns.[104]

The emergence of feeding problems during the toddler years can be significantly challenging with regard to day-to-day family activities. A parent's subsequent anxiety and stress can lead to maladaptive home-based feeding practices such as lack of structure and the modeling of inappropriate eating habits, both of which can inadvertently shape and strengthen problematic feeding behaviors. As a result, children learn additional avoidant or disruptive feeding behaviors as a means to escape negative feeding experiences or gain attention from a parent or caregiver.[105]

Children with ASD have a greater risk for the numerous comorbidities associated with chronic feeding problems, including faltered growth, particularly after 8 years of age, malnutrition, the need for tube feedings, and limitations in social, emotional, and educational functioning.[104] More recent studies have also demonstrated a higher incidence of bone fractures among children with ASD than among children without ASD.[106]

Higher rates of nutritional deficits or toxicity in children with ASD may also stem from a generally higher rate of caregiver experimentation with complementary and alternative therapies, including elimination diets and megadosing of vitamins and minerals.[102] Commonly used elimination diets include the gluten-free casein-free (GFCF) diet and the specific carbohydrate diet (SCD). Although research supporting the use of such diets to date is inconclusive, many parents report a reduction in ASD symptoms, including disruptive behavior and poor GI function, when following elimination diets. Such diets are recognized to pose some nutritional risks. For example, the GFCF diet eliminates dairy proteins, which may place a child at risk for deficits in calcium and protein.[106] Elimination diets also tend to target starches and snack foods that, in many cases, function as a child's primary source of calories. Eliminating a child's preferred food increases the risk of poor growth and, for some, may heighten food-seeking behaviors and emotional outbursts related to food.[107] Parents of children with ASD also tend to use supplements at higher rates than parents of children without ASD.[98]

Prevention
Prevention efforts include genetic counseling for parents with one or more first-degree family members with ASD or ASD traits. Prevention measures that specifically target feeding problems include screening for early identification and treatment for feeding difficulties with or without growth concerns.[103]

Treatment
The most effective intervention for individuals with ASD is achieved with use of behavioral assessment and treatment in an interdisciplinary team setting consisting of feeding experts in applied behavioral analysis, child psychology, medicine, occupational therapy, speech therapy, and nutrition.[105] The primary goals of such behavioral intervention are to achieve the closest approximation of age-appropriate mealtime behavior. For example, goals may include decreasing reliance on supplemental feedings by bottle or tube, increasing food variety, increasing acceptance of textured foods, and decreasing rigid mealtime routines. Nonbehavioral goals include improvements in language and speech, oral motor abilities, GI functioning, and other medically related concerns as well as nutritional intake.

Concurrent nonbehavioral intervention with medical providers, occupational therapists, and speech therapists addresses cumulative health-related issues such as constipation, vomiting, and food sensitivities, underdeveloped oral muscles and coordination, and speech delays.[98] Concurrent nutrition intervention involves nutrition education to help parents select, prepare, and present foods in a way and at a frequency that optimizes balanced nutrient intake and structured eating patterns. Dietitians can provide counseling for safe use of supplements and elimination diets and can coordinate care for intensive intervention to address nutrition-related GI issues and adjust supplemental oral or tube feedings to enhance hunger recognition and subsequent interest and engagement in behavioral feeding therapy.

Recommendations
Primary care providers are encouraged to screen for, identify, and help parents of children with ASD access appropriate intervention at an early age.[102]

Current research supports early access to a comprehensive, behaviorally focused interdisciplinary assessment that can better direct treatment to match the individual needs of a child, parent, and the overall functioning level of the family system. The benefits of such treatment not only provide appropriate treatment without the risk of reinforcing maladaptive behaviors, but can help generalize skill acquisition to different social settings such as home and school, and identify short and long-term risks to guide appropriate monitoring and adjustments in treatment intensity to meet the changing needs for the child and parent with eminent change in developmental drives and family functioning.[108]

> **Recap** Infants and children with pediatric conditions often have unique feeding and nutrition issues. These issues include how the child receives nutrition (e.g., as oral intake with adaptations of feeding modality, food texture, fluid viscosity, positioning while feeding/eating, or as enteral intake) and what the child's nutrition requirements are (i.e., increased or decreased energy requirement). Addressing these issues is essential for optimal growth and development.
>
> 1. Name two pediatric conditions that might have increased energy requirements. Explain why.
> 2. Describe feeding modifications (how the child receives nutrition) for three pediatric conditions and explain why they are needed.
> 3. Describe a condition that puts an infant or child at risk for nutrition deficiencies. Explain why there is increased risk, and how you would address this.

Learning Portfolio

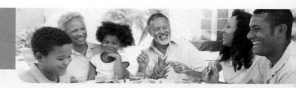

Visual Chapter Summary

Gastrointestinal Conditions

- Episodes of constipation, diarrhea, and reflux are common for infants and young children. A balanced diet plays a role in minimizing symptoms for these conditions while providing the nourishment needed for optimal growth and development.

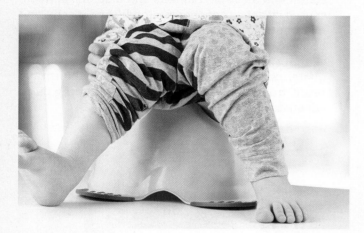

©Saklakova/Shutterstock

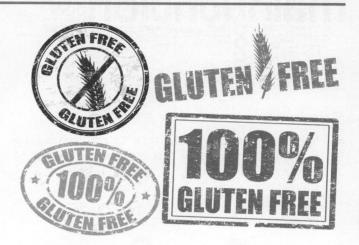

©ducu59us/Shutterstock

Food Allergies and Sensitivities

- Food allergies occur when an adverse reaction results from ingestion of a food or ingredient in a food. These are different from food intolerances and food sensitivities.

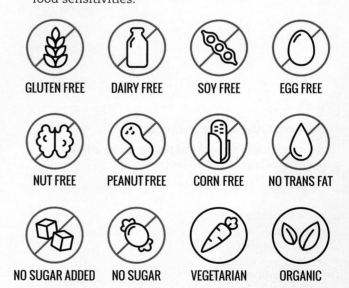

GLUTEN FREE   DAIRY FREE   SOY FREE   EGG FREE

NUT FREE   PEANUT FREE   CORN FREE   NO TRANS FAT

NO SUGAR ADDED   NO SUGAR   VEGETARIAN   ORGANIC

©Sudowoodo/Shutterstock

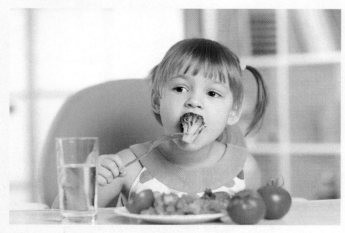

©Oksana Kuzmina/Shutterstock

- For those with celiac disease, a gluten-free diet is the only treatment available, and proper adherence leads to resolution of gastrointestinal symptoms as well as recovery from any growth or nutrient deficiencies.

- Correct method of diagnosis, appropriate nutritional assessment, guidance in foods to avoid and foods to allow, and advocacy and education in community settings for nonfamily caregivers are all crucial for safe management of food allergies in the pediatric population.

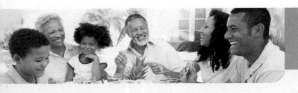

Learning Portfolio (continued)

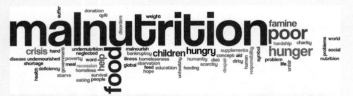

©ibreakstock/Shutterstock

Malnutrition

- Approximately 1 out of every 13 children in the world is malnourished. This includes conditions of wasting and stunting.

Wasted	No	Yes	No
Stunted	No	No	Yes
Underweight	No	Yes	Yes

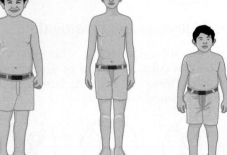

Table 8.4

Diagnosis Criteria for Malnutrition

Identification of at least 2 of the following criteria can indicate a diagnosis of malnutrition

Criteria	Does the criteria exist	
	Yes	*no*
Insufficient energy intake		
Weight loss		
Loss of muscle mass		
Localized or generalized fluid accumulation that may sometimes mask weight loss		
Diminished functional status as measured by hand grip strength		

Modified from Cederholm T, Bosaeus I, Barazzoni R, et al. Diagnostic criteria for malnutrition – An ESPN Consensus Statement. Clin Nutr. 2015 Jun;34(3):335-40.

- The pathway to malnutrition may include one or more of the following: decreased nutrient intake, increased requirements for nutrients, increased nutrient losses, and altered nutrient utilization. Once the cause of malnutrition is determined, the appropriate treatment can be followed.

Failure to Thrive

- Malnutrition and failure to thrive (FTT) are serious conditions that affect infants and toddlers. Both are caused by deficits of energy, protein, and macro- and micronutrients. Malnutrition can occur at any age because of food shortages and starvation as well as acute or chronic illnesses that interfere with adequate intake. FTT, though caused by malnutrition, result from inadequate intake in the setting of an adequate food supply.

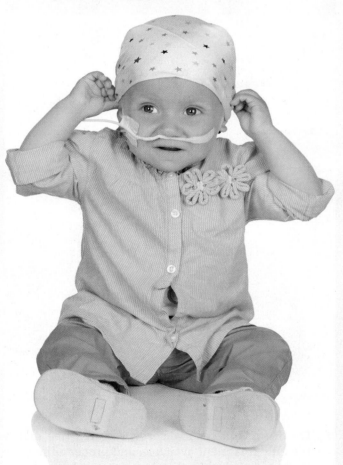

©Gelpi/Shutterstock

Cancer

- Children from birth to 5 years who develop cancer pose unique challenges to their medical providers. The cancer and its treatment can interfere with the child's physical and cognitive development, especially if nutritional intake is compromised.
- Children with cancer may experience various nutrition-related side effects from both the cancer and the treatment that may interfere with growth and development.
- Understanding how to support the child with cancer in this age group back to health through diet or specialized nutrition is essential and requires the expertise and intervention of a team of qualified healthcare professionals.

Iron Deficiency

- Elements of blood include white blood cells, platelets, and red blood cells, which transport oxygen and nutrients to body tissues and remove waste and carbon dioxide.

Plasma 55%

Blood cells 45%

Platelets = clotting
Red blood cells = oxygen carrying
White blood cells = infection fighting

- Children from birth to 5 years with iron deficiency pose unique challenges to their medical providers. The deficiency can interfere with the child's physical and cognitive development, especially if nutritional intake is compromised.

- Iron is a vital nutrient for biologic and cognitive function, especially for children in this age group.
- Iron deficiency refers to the depletion of iron stores, which can eventually progress to full-onset iron-deficiency anemia. Once identified, both ID and IDA are largely preventable and curable through dietary intervention.

Newborn Screening and Genetics

- Many different genetic conditions require specialized nutrition management in infants and children. Newborn screening can identify many of these conditions early, which supports improved nutritional outcomes.

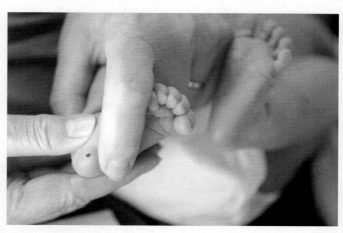

©crozstudios/Alamy Stock Photo

Selected Pediatric Conditions

- Infants and children with pediatric conditions often have unique feeding and nutrition issues. These issues include how the child receives nutrition (e.g., as oral intake with adaptations of feeding modality, food texture, fluid viscosity, positioning while feeding/eating, or as enteral intake) and what the child's nutrition requirements are (i.e. increased or decreased energy requirement). Addressing these issues is essential for optimal growth and development. Spinal bifida, cerebral palsy, cleft lip and palate, autism spectrum disorder, and mental retardation and developmental disabilities are examples of such conditions.

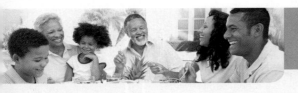

Learning Portfolio (continued)

Key Terms

antiepileptic medication: Medication used to treat seizures.

apnea: When breathing temporarily stops; it usually occurs more frequently in sleep.

athetosis: A condition in which abnormal muscle contractions cause excessive, involuntary movements.

autism spectrum disorder (ASD): A diagnosis given to children and adults with pervasive developmental disorders characterized by complex developmental disabilities with severe impairments in social interaction and communication accompanied by behavioral inflexibility, repetitive behaviors, and/or restricted interests.

bifid uvula: A split or cleft uvula that results from incomplete fusion of the palate.

bilateral cleft lip and palate: Split on two sides.

cleft lip and palate (CLP): Congenital split of the lip and palate that varies from a notching to a complete division of the lip or a cleft that may extend through the uvula and soft palate and into the hard palate.

constipation: Development of hard, dry feces that results in difficulty emptying bowels or abnormally delayed or infrequent passage of hardened feces.

diarrhea: Abnormally frequent intestinal evacuations with more or less fluid stools.

dysphagia: The inability to swallow properly. Swallowing is a complex cascade of reactions. Dysphagia occurs more frequently in older adults and can result in inhaling food and a lung infection or choking. Dysphagia may result from a neurologic disorder that impairs esophageal motility or a mechanical obstruction of the esophagus.

enteral tube feeding (ETF): The delivery of a nutritionally complete feeding, which contains protein or amino acids, carbohydrate, fiber, fat, water, minerals and vitamins, directly into the gut via a tube.

failure to thrive (FTT): Unexplained deficits in growth in infants and children that require nutrition intervention.

food allergy: An immune system reaction that occurs soon after eating a certain food.

food intolerance: Any abnormal physical response to a food or food additive.

food sensitivity: A condition which occurs when a person has difficulty digesting a particular food.

gastroesophageal reflux (GER): The passage of stomach contents into the esophagus, or throat.

glossoptosis: Downward displacement (retraction) of the tongue.

gluten: A protein found in the cereal grains wheat, barley, and rye that causes illness when ingested by those with celiac disease. Gluten, which is a is mixture of two proteins, is responsible for the elastic texture of dough.

growth faltering: When weight measurements cross three percentiles over 3 months in infancy and over 6 months in the second and third years of life.

hypotonia: Also known as "floppy baby syndrome"; a low amount of tension or resistance to stretch in a muscle and often involving reduced muscle strength that causes weight goals to be generally lower than that for a typical child of the same age.

Hypotonic fluids: a solution that contains fewer dissolved particles, such as salt, and potassium, then is found in normal cells and blood.

iron deficiency (ID): A state in which there is insufficient iron to maintain normal physiologic functions.

iron-deficiency anemia (IDA): A condition characterized by low hemoglobin levels, paleness, exhaustion, and rapid heart rate. Signs of iron deficiency are also present and include short attention span, poor appetite, irritability, and susceptibility to infection.

laxative: Medication that stimulate sand facilitates stooling.

leukemia: A cancer of the white blood cells (WBCs) where the bone marrow produces abnormal WBCs. This leads to an increased accumulation of cancerous cells in the blood, with a variable reduction in normal blood cells, affecting the normal function of blood cells.

nasopharynx: The space above the soft palate at the back of the nose that connects the mouth with the nose.

neuroblastoma: An embryonal tumor of the autonomic nervous system that develops from neural crest tissues of the sympathetic nervous system. It can occur in many areas of the body, including the abdomen, adrenal glands, neck, skull, pelvis, spinal column, and bone marrow. Neuroblastoma generally occurs in very young children; the median age at diagnosis is 17 months.

newborn screening: The practice of testing newborn babies for certain treatable disorders and conditions.

nutrition support: The provision of enteral or parenteral nutrients to treat or prevent malnutrition. Nutrition support therapy is part of nutrition therapy, which is a component of medical treatment that can include oral, enteral, and parenteral nutrition to maintain or restore optimal nutrition status and health.

otitis media: Ear infection.

palate: The top (roof) of the mouth, including the hard palate (front portion, includes bone) and soft palate (back portion, includes muscle).

parenteral nutrition (PN): The intravenous administration of nutrients, which include carbohydrate, protein, lipids, electrolytes, vitamins, and minerals.

pneumatosis: Gas cyst in the bowel wall.

stunting: Failure to grow both physically and cognitively; when a child is too short for his or her age. Stunting is the result of chronic or recurrent malnutrition.

submucous cleft palate: A split of the muscle layer of the soft palate with an intact layer of mucosa lying over the defect.

Surveillance, Epidemiology, and End Results (SEER): Program of the National Cancer Institute to provide information on cancer statistics in an effort to reduce the burden of cancer among the U.S. population.

total parenteral nutrition (TPN): A method of feeding that bypasses the stomach and gastrointestinal tract. Fluids are administered into a vein to provide nutrients that the body needs.

tube feeding: When a medical device is used to provide nutrition to individuals who cannot obtain nutrition by mouth or who are unable to swallow safely.

typhlitis: Inflammation of the cecum.

unilateral cleft lip and palate: A cleft defect that affects one side of the mouth and that may be present in varying degrees.

wasting: The result of sudden or acute malnutrition, when a child is not getting enough calories and faces an immediate risk of death. A child who is too thin for his or her height is undergoing wasting.

Discussion Questions

1. Celiac disease is a chronic disease that requires life-long adherence to a gluten-free diet. Compare and contrast potential challenges and advantages that you might foresee with following a gluten-free diet for an individual diagnosed at 2 years of age and someone diagnosed as an adult.

2. Explain the challenges that parents of young children with food allergies face in ensuring 100% avoidance of allergens. Consider potential caregivers in the child's life as well as the child's developmental transition toward independence.

3. Failure to thrive is a complex condition that requires an interdisciplinary approach. Discuss the limitations of nutritional counseling.

4. Childhood cancer treatment can have both short-term and long-term nutrition-related consequences. Discuss potential effects children in this age group may experience in regard to growth and feeding. Also, identify secondary disease conditions that may occur.

5. Briefly describe the purpose of newborn screening and features of a successful newborn screening program.

6. Describe the various interdisciplinary approaches to evaluating and treating the following pediatric conditions: spina bifida, cerebral palsy, cleft lip and palate, and autism spectrum disorders.

Activities

1. Analyze nutrition deficits and make recommendations for supplemental vitamin and minerals for a 14-year-old male with ASD whose daily intake is consists of 1 quesadilla, 3 cups of Goldfish crackers, and 2 gallons of 1% milk.

2. Plan 3 days of menus (three meals per day and three snacks per day) for a 10-year-old boy with cystic fibrosis. His weight is 45 kgs.

Study Questions

1. Which evidence-based dietary intervention is recommended for the treatment of infant reflux?
   a. A 2-week trial of feedings with hydrolyzed formula for a breastfed infant not responding to reflux medications
   b. Thickening breastmilk or formula with cereal or a commercial thickening product
   c. Small, frequent feedings and evaluation of intake for overfeeding
   d. Dietary elimination of all citrus foods, dairy products, and high-fat foods consumed by the mother of breastfed infants

2. Adherence to a gluten-free diet includes all of the following *except* which one?
   a. Selecting only foods labeled as gluten free or those without gluten-containing ingredients
   b. Using only gluten-free cosmetics and toiletries

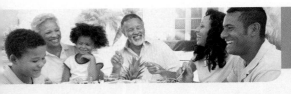

Learning Portfolio (continued)

c. Avoiding cross-contamination when eating out at restaurants

d. Using only gluten-free supplements and medication

3. Which of the following is a recommendation for the treatment of acute diarrhea?
   a. Fasting, intravenous rehydration, reintroduction of food once symptoms are gone
   b. Fasting, oral rehydration, resume lactose-free and sugar-free diet
   c. Oral rehydration, maintain adequate food intake, use medications sparingly
   d. Intravenous rehydration, maintain adequate food intake, use medications sparingly

4. Which three foods are the most common causes of food allergy?
   a. Cow's milk, eggs, fin fish
   b. Sugar, oatmeal, cow's milk
   c. Chicken, beef, eggs
   d. Cow's milk, chocolate, and gluten

5. Which of the following is one specific pathway leading to malnutrition?
   a. Increased nutrient intake
   b. Decreased requirement of nutrients
   c. Decreased nutrient losses
   d. Normal nutrient utilization

6. According to the World Health Organization, what is the prevalence of malnutrition worldwide doing?
   a. Decreasing
   b. Increasing

7. What child characteristics are important to evaluate in FTT? (Choose all that apply.)
   a. Medical
   b. Oral motor
   c. Psychosocial
   d. Gastrointestinal
   e. Metabolic
   f. Genetic

8. Strategies to keep the child with cancer nourished during treatment include all of the following except for which one?
   a. Add half-and-half to mashed potatoes, hot cereal, and other appropriate foods.
   b. Initiate a tube feeding.
   c. Wait to feed the child because it is only a matter of time before the child's appetite returns to normal.
   d. Try a commercially prepared oral supplement.

9. Common side effects of chemotherapy include all of the following except for which one?
   a. Diarrhea or constipation
   b. Early satiety

c. Nausea and vomiting

d. Thick, viscous saliva

10. Treatment for iron-deficiency anemia includes all of the following except which one?
    a. Add the iron supplement to foods or liquids to guarantee the child or infant will receive the medication.
    b. Provide a therapeutic iron supplement for at least 3 months to replenish iron stores.
    c. Incorporate foods high in iron into the diet such as red meat, chicken, legumes.
    d. Offer orange juice or orange slices after giving the iron supplement.

11. Maple syrup urine disease is which type of disorder?
    a. Amino acid metabolism disorder
    b. Organic acid metabolism disorder
    c. Fatty acid metabolism disorder
    d. Carbohydrate metabolism disorder

12. Children with Down syndrome are at increased risk for which conditions? (Choose all that apply.)
    a. Celiac disease
    b. Renal insufficiency
    c. Hypothyroidism
    d. Seizure disorders

13. Cerebral palsy is classified by what characteristic?
    a. Cognitive status
    b. Motor function
    c. Ability to walk (ambulatory status)
    d. Brain malformation

14. What is the recommendation for folate supplementation for women who have had a previous pregnancy affected by a neural tube defect?
    a. 400 mcg/day
    b. 4,000 mcg/day
    c. 4 mg/day
    d. 40 mg/day

15. Infants with cleft palates are rarely able to breastfeed. What kind of bottle do they need?
    a. Standard bottle works fine
    b. Haberman or squeeze bottle
    c. Pigeon or Dr. Brown bottle with a special valve
    d. Answers B and C

16. Feeding problems in children with autism spectrum disorders are categorized as behavioral feeding disorders and include which of the following?
    a. Turning away from food
    b. Packing mouth with food
    c. Swallowing food whole without chewing
    d. Gagging and vomiting without medical cause
    e. All the above

17. Research suggests that the majority of feeding problems in children with autism spectrum disorders manifest from which source?
    a. Deficits in social and language skills
    b. A heightened concentration on detail
    c. Fear of novelty
    d. Sensory impairments
    e. All the above

Weblinks

- **FARE (Food Allergy Research and Education)**
  http://www.foodallergy.org
  FARE is the world's largest private source of funding for food allergy research. FARE invests in basic and clinical research to develop new therapies to prevent life-threatening food allergy reactions, to discover the cause of food allergies, and to understand the economic and psychosocial impact of this disease.

- **GIKids**
  http://www.gikids.org

Resources for parents and kids on pediatric digestive disorders. Includes information on conditions, symptoms, and treatment options.

- **Washington State Department of Health**
  http://www.doh.wa.gov/YouandYourFamily/InfantsChildrenandTeens/NewbornScreening
  Each state has a website with information on which disorders its newborn screening program screens for, and reports of annual results, as do many other state programs.

References

1. Guarino A, Ashkenazi S, Gendrel D, et al. European Society for Pediatric Gastroenterology, Hepatology, and Nutrition/European Society for Pediatric Infectious Diseases evidence-based guidelines for the management of acute gastroenteritis in children in Europe: update 2014. *JPGN*. 2014;59:132–152.
2. World Health Organization; April 2013. Diarrhoeal disease [Fact Sheet no. 330]. Retrieved from: http://www.who.int/mediacentre/factsheets/fs330/en/. Accessed October 2, 2015.
3. Brandt KG, de Castro Antunes MM, da Silva GAP. Acute diarrhea: evidence-based management. *J Pediatr (Rio J)*. 2015;91(6 suppl 1):S36–S43. http://dx.doi.org/10.1016/j.jped.2015.06.002.
4. Nahikian-Nelms MN, Sucher K, Long S. Diseases of the lower gastrointestinal tract. In: Nelms M, Sucher KP, Lacey K, Long Roth S, eds. *Nutrition Therapy and Pathophysiology*. Belmont, CA: Wadsworth/Thomson Learning; 2007.
5. World Health Organization. *The Treatment of Diarrhea—A Manual for Physicians and Other Senior Health Works*. 4th ed. Geneva, Switzerland: WHO; 2005.
6. Szajweska H, Kolodziej M. Systematic review with meta-analysis: *Lactobacillus rhamnosis* GG in the prevention of antibiotic-associated diarrhea in children and adults. *Aliment Pharmacol Ther*. 2015;42(10):1149–1157.
7. Islam M, Roy SK, Begum M, Chisti MJ. Dietary intake and clinical response of hospitalized patients with acute diarrhea. *Food Nutr Bull*. 2008;29:25–31.
8. Gaffey MF, Wazny K, Bassani DG, Bhutta ZA. Dietary management of childhood diarrhea in low- and middle-income countries: a systematic review. *Am J Public Health*. 2013;13:S17.
9. Liem O, Harman J, Benninga M, et al. Health utilization and cost impact of childhood constipation in the United States. *J Pediatr*. 2009;154:258–262.
10. Rasquin A, Di Lorenzo C, Forbes D, et al. Childhood functional gastrointestinal disorders: child/adolescent. *Gastroenterology*. 2006;130:1527–1537.
11. National Institute for Health and Care Excellence (NICE). Constipation in children and young people: diagnosis and management. NICE Guidelines CG99; May 2010. Retrieved from: http://www.nice.org.uk/guidance/CG99. Accessed September 9, 2016.
12. Tabbers MM, DiLorenzo C, Berger MY, et al. Evaluation and treatment of functional constipation in infants and children: evidence-based recommendations from ESPGHAN and NASPGHAN. *JPGN*. 2014;58(2):258–274.
13. Banaszkiewicz A, Bibik A, Szajewska H. Functional constipation in children: a follow-up study. *Pediatr Wspol*. 2006;8:21–23.
14. Nelson SP, Chen EH, Syniar GM, et al. Prevalence of symptoms of gastroesophageal reflux during infancy. A pediatric practice-based survey. Pediatric Practice Research Group. *Arch Pediatr Adolesc Med*. 1997;151:569–572.
15. Campanozzi A, Boccia G, Pensabene L, et al. Prevalence and natural history of gastroesophageal reflux: pediatric perspective survey. *Pediatrics*. 2009;123:779–783.
16. Vandenplas Y, Rudolph CD, Di Lorenzo C, et al. Pediatric gastroesophageal reflux clinic practice guidelines: joint recommendations of the North American Society for Pediatric Gastroenterology, Hepatology, and Nutrition (NASPGHAN) and the European Society of Paediatric Gastroenterology, Hepatology, and Nutrition (ESPGHAN). *J Pediatr Gastroenterol Nutr*. 2009;49:498–547.
17. Khoshoo V, Ross G, Brown S, Edell D. Smaller volume, thickened formulas in the management of gastroesophageal reflux in thriving infants. *J Pediatr Gastroenterol Nutr*. 2000;31:554–556.
18. Tsou MV, Bishop PR. Gastroesophageal reflux in children. *Otolaryngol Clin North Am*. 1998;31:419–434.

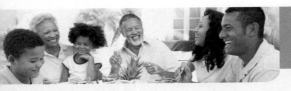

Learning Portfolio (continued)

19. Hovarth A, Dziechciarz P, Szajewska H. The effect of thickened-feed interventions on gastroesophageal reflux in infants: systematic review and meta-analysis of randomized, controlled trials. *Pediatrics*. 2008;122(6):e1268–1277.

20. Cavataio F, Carroccio A, Iacono G. Milk-induced reflux in infants less than one year of age. *J Pediatr Gastroenterol Nutr*. 2000:30(suppl):S36–44.

21. Fasano A, Berti I, Gerarduzzi T, et al. Prevalence of celiac disease in at-risk and not-at-risk groups in the United States: a large multicenter study. *Arch Intern Med*. 2003;163: 286–292.

22. Hill ID, Dirks MH, Liptak GS, et al. Guideline for the diagnosis and treatment of celiac disease in children: recommendations of the North American Society for Pediatric Gastroenterology, Hepatology and Nutrition. *J Pediatr Gastoenterol Nutr*. 2005;40(1):1–19.

23. Niewinski MM. Advances in celiac disease and gluten-free diet. *J Am Diet Assoc*. 2008;108(4):661–672.

24. Fasano A, Catassi C. Current approaches to diagnosis and treatment of celiac disease: an evolving spectrum. *Gastroenterology*. 2001;120:636–651.

25. Askling J, Linet M, Gridley G, et al. Cancer incidence in a population-based cohort of individuals hospitalized with celiac disease or dermatitis herpetiformis. *Gastroenterology*. 2002;123:1428–1435.

26. Corrao G, Corazza GR, Bagnardi V, et al; Club del Tenue Study Group. Mortality in patients with coeliac disease and their relatives: a cohort study. *Lancet*. 2001;358:356–361.

27. Ivarsson A, Hernell O, Stenlund H, Peterson LA. Breastfeeding protects against celiac disease. *Am J Clin Nutr*. 2002;75:914–921.

28. Norris JM, Barriga K, Hoffenberg EJ, et al. Risk of celiac disease autoimmunity and timing of gluten introduction in the diet of infants at increased risk of disease. *JAMA*. 2005;293:2343–2351.

29. National Institutes of Health. NIH Consensus Development Conference on Celiac Disease, June 28–30, 2004. *Gastroenterology*. 2005;128(suppl.1):S1–9.

30. U.S. Food and Drug Administration; last updated May 2, 2016. Gluten-free labeling of foods. Retrieved from: http:// www. fda.gov/gluten-freelabeling. Accessed October 7, 2015.

31. Valenta R, Hochwallne H, Linhart B, Pahr S. Food allergies: the basics. *Gastroenterology*. 2015;148(6):1120–1131.

32. Patel BY, Viocheck GW. Food allergy: common causes, diagnosis, and treatment. *Mayo Clin Proc*. 2015;90(10):1411–1419.

33. American College of Allergy, Asthma, & Immunology. Food allergy: a practice parameter. *Ann Allergy Asthma Immunol*. 2006;96(3 suppl 2):S1–68.

34. Mehta N, Corkins MR, Lyman B, et al. Defining pediatric malnutrition: a paradigm shift toward etiology-related definitions. *J Parenter Enteral Nutr*. 2013;37(4):460–481.

35. Beer S, Juarez M, Vega M, Canada N. Pediatric malnutrition: putting the new definition and standards into practice. *Nutr Clin Pract*. October 2015;30(5):609–624.

36. United Nations Children's Fund, World Health Organization, The World Bank. *UNICEF-WHO-The World Bank Joint Child Malnutrition Estimates*. New York, NY: UNICEF; Geneva, Switzerland: WHO; Washington, DC: The World Bank; 2012. Retrieved from: http://www.who.int/nutgrowthdb/jme_unicef_who_wb.pdf. Accessed September 9, 2016.

37. de Onis M, Blössner M, Borghi E, Frongillo EA, Morris R. Estimates of global prevalence of childhood underweight in 1990 and 2015. *JAMA*. 2004;291(21):2600–2606. doi:10.1001/jama.291.21.2600.

38. Kessler DB. Failure to thrive and pediatric undernutrition historical and theoretical context. In Kessler DB, Dawson P, eds. *Failure to Thrive and Pediatric Undernutrition: A Transdisciplinary Approach*. Baltimore, MD: Paul H. Brooks Publishing Co.; 1999:3–15.

39. Berhane R, Dietz WH. Clinical assessment of growth. In Kessler DB, Dawson P, eds. *Failure to Thrive and Pediatric Undernutrition: A Transdisciplinary Approach*. Baltimore, MD: Paul H. Brooks Publishing Co.; 1999:195–214.

40. Iwaniec D. Failure to thrive: definition, prevalence, manifestation and effect. In Iwaniec D, ed. *Failure to Thrive: A Practice Guide*. New York, NY: Wiley; 2004:28–44.

41. Kleinman RE, ed. Failure to thrive. In *Pediatric Nutrition Handbook*. 6th ed. Elk Grove Village, IL: American Academy of Pediatrics; 2009:601–636.

42. Ries LAG, Smith MA, Gurney JG, et al, eds. *Cancer Incidence and Survival Among Children and Adolescents: United States SEER Program 1975–1995, National Cancer Institute, SEER Program*. NIH Pub. No. 99-4649. Bethesda, MD: National Cancer Institute Surveillance, Epidemiology, and End Results Program; 1999:1–15.

43. Smith MA, Altekruse, SF, Adamson, PC, Reaman, GH, Seibel NL. Declining childhood and adolescent cancer mortality. *Cancer*. August 15, 2014:2497–2506.

44. Orgel E, Sposto R, Malvar J, et al. Impact on survival and toxicity by duration of weight extremes during treatment for pediatric acute lymphoblastic leukemia: a report from the Children's Oncology Group. *J Clin Oncol*. 2014;32:1331–1337.

45. Ladas EJ, Sacks N, Meachum L, et al. A multidisciplinary review of nutrition considerations in the pediatric oncology population: a perspective from the Children's Oncology Group. *Nutr Clin Pract*. 2005;20:377–393.

46. Charuhas PM, Hunt K. Hematology and oncology. In Queen PS, King K, eds. *Pediatric Nutrition*. 4th ed. Burlington, MA: Jones & Bartlett Learning; 2012:364–383.

47. Barale KV, Charuhas PM. Oncology and hematopoietic cell transplantation. In: Queen PS, King K, eds. *Handbook of Pediatric Nutrition*. 3rd ed. Sudbury, MA: Jones & Bartlett Publishers; 2005:459–481.

48. Rogers PC. Nutritional status as a prognostic indicator for pediatric malignancies [editorial]. *J Clin Oncol*. 2014;32:1–2.

49. Becker PJ, Carney LN, Corkins MR, et al. Consensus statement of the Academy of Nutrition and Dietetics/American Society for Parenteral and Enteral Nutrition: indicators recommended for the identification and documentation of pediatric malnutrition (undernutrition). *J Acad Nutr Diet*. 2014;114(12):1988–2000.

50. Charuhas PM. Pediatric hematopoietic stem cell transplantation. In Hasse JM, Blue LS, eds. *Comprehensive Guide to Transplant Nutrition*. Chicago, IL: American Dietetic Association; 2002:226–247.

51. Mauer AM, Burgess JB, Donaldson SS, et al. Special nutritional needs of children with malignancies: a review. *J Parenter Enteral Nutr*. 1990;14:315–324.

52. Mosby TT, Barr RB, Pencharz PB. Nutritional assessment of children with cancer. *J Pediatr Oncol Nurs*. 2009;26(4):186–197.

53. Denne SC. Neonatal nutrition. *Pediatr Clin N Am.* 2015;62:427–438.

54. Sacks N, Hwang WT, Lange BJ, et al. Proactive enteral tube feeding in pediatric patients undergoing chemotherapy. *Pediatr Blood Cancer.* 2014;61(2):281–285.

55. Moody K, Finlay J, Mancuso C, Charlson M. Feasibility and safety of a pilot randomized trial of infection rate: neutropenic diet versus standard food safety guidelines. *J Pediatr Hematol Oncol.* 2006;28(3):126–133.

56. French MR, Levy-Milne R, Zibrik D. A survey of the use of low microbial diets in pediatric bone marrow transplant programs. *J Am Diet Assoc.* 2001;101:1194–1198.

57. Denne SC. Neonatal nutrition. *Pediatr Clin N Am.* 2015; 62:427–438.

58. Camaschella C. Iron-deficiency anemia. *N Engl J Med.* 2015; 372(19):1832–1843.

59. Barker RD, Greer FR; Committee on Nutrition. Clinical report—diagnosis and prevention of iron deficiency anemia in infants and young children (0–3 years of age). *Pediatrics.* 2010;126(5):1040–1050.

60. Friel JK, Aziz K, Andrews WL, Harding SV, Courage ML, Adams RJ. A double-masked, randomized control trial of iron supplementation in early infancy in healthy term breast-fed infants. *J Pediatr.* 2003;143(5):582–586.

61. Centers for Disease Control and Prevention; last updated February 24, 2106. National Health and Nutrition Examination Survey. Retrieved from: http://www.cdc.gov/nchs/nhanes.htm. Accessed September 9, 2016.

62. Seattle Children's Hospital. Iron-deficiency anemia: symptoms and diagnosis. Retrieved from: http://www.seattlechildrens.org/medical-conditions/heart-blood-conditions/iron-deficiency-anemia-symptoms/. Accessed August 23, 2016.

63. La Marca G. Mass spectrometry in clinical chemistry: the case of newborn screening. *J Pharm Biomed Anal.* 2014;101: 174–172.

64. Mak CM, Lee HC, Chan AY, Lam CW. Inborn errors of metabolism and expanded newborn screening: review and update. *Crit Rev Clin Lab Sci.* 2013;50(6):142–162.

65. Frazier DM, Allgeier C, Homer C, et al. Nutrition management guidelines for maple syrup urine disease: an evidence- and consensus-based approach. *Mol Genet Metab.* 2014;112(3): 210–217.

66. American College of Medical Genetics [press release]. *American College of Medical Genetics Affirms Importance of Newborn Screening (NBS) Dried Blood Spots in New Position Statement: National Public Health Officials and NBS Experts Also Show Support of Position.* Bethesda, MD: American College of Medical Genetics. https://www.acmg.net/StaticContent/NewsReleases/Blood_Spot_News_Release2009.pdf. Accessed January 27, 2016.

67. Marriage B. Nutrition management of patients with inherited disorders of branched-chain amino acid metabolism. In Acosta P, ed. *Nutrition Management of Patients with Inherited Metabolic Disorders.* Sudbury, MA: Jones & Bartlett Publishers; 2010:175–236.

68. Frazier D. Newborn screening by mass spectrometry. In Acosta P, ed. *Nutrition Management of Patients with Inherited Metabolic Disorders.* Sudbury, MA: Jones & Bartlett Publishers; 2010:21–65.

69. Yanicelli S. Nutrition management of patients with inherited disorders or organic acid metabolism. In Acosta P, ed. *Nutrition Management of Patients with Inherited Metabolic Disorders.* Sudbury, MA: Jones & Bartlett Publishers; 2010:283–341.

70. Saudubray JM, Martin D, de Lonlay P, et al. Recognition and management of fatty acid oxidation defects: a series of 107 patients. *J Inherit Metab Dis.* 1999;22(4):488–502.

71. Berry GT. Galactosemia: when is it a newborn screening emergency? *Mol Genet Metab.* 2012;106:7–11.

72. VanCalcar SC, Bernstein LE, Rohr FJ, Scaman CH, Yannicelli S, Berry GT. A re-evaluation of life-long severe galactose restriction for the nutrition management of classic galactosemia. *Mol Genet Metab.* 2014;112(3):191–197.

73. Casey S. Medical nutrition therapy in cystic fibrosis. *Support Line, PPG Building Block For Life.* Pediatric Nutrition Practice Group. April 2015; 37(2).

74. Colombo C, Ellemunter H, Howen R, Munck A, Taylor C, Wilschanski M. Guidelines for the diagnosis and management of distal intestinal obstruction syndrome in cystic fibrosis patients. *J Cyst Fibrosis.* 2001;10(suppl 1): 524–528.

75. Cystic Fibrosis Foundation, Borowitz D, Robinson KA, Rosenfeld M, et al. Cystic Fibrosis Foundation evidence-based practice guidelines for management of infants with cystic fibrosis. *J Pediatr.* 2009;155(6 suppl):S73–93.

76. Michel S, Magbool A, Hanna M, Mascaarenhas M. Nutrition management of pediatric patients who have cystic fibrosis. *Pediatr Clin North Am.* 2009;58:1123–1141.

77. Eunice Kennedy Shriver National Institute of Child Health and Human Development; reviewed January 17, 2014. What are common treatments for Down syndrome? Retrieved from: https://www.nichd.nih.gov/health/topics/down/conditioninfo/Pages/treatments.aspx. Accessed January 26, 2016.

78. Bull MJ. Health supervision for children with Down syndrome. *Pediatrics.* 2011;128:393–406.

79. Capone G, Muller D, Ekvall S. Down syndrome. In *Pediatric Nutrition in Chronic Diseases and Developmental Disorders.* 2nd ed. New York, NY: Oxford University Press; 2005:126.

80. Medlen JEG. *The Down Syndrome Nutrition Handbook.* Bethesda, MD: Woodbine House Publishing; 2002:212.

81. Centers for Disease Control and Prevention; last updated January 7, 2016. Growth charts for children with Down syndrome. Retrieved from: http://www.cdc.gov/ncbddd/birthdefects/downsyndrome/growth-charts.html. Accessed September 9, 2016.

82. Spina Bifida Association. What is spina bifida? Retrieved from: http://spinabifidaassociation.org/what-is-sb/. Accessed October 15, 2015.

83. Kreutzer C, Wittenbrook W. Nutrition issues in children with myelomeningocele (spina bifida). *Nutr. Focus.* September 1, 2013;28(5). http://depts.washington.edu/nutrfoc/webapps/?p=840. Accessed September 9, 2016.

84. National Institute of Neurological Disorders and Stroke; June 2013. Spina bifida fact sheet. Retrieved from: http://www.ninds.nih.gov/disorders/spina_bifida/detail_spina_bifida.htm. Accessed August 28, 2016.

85. Daly S, Mills JL, Molloy AM, et al. Minimum effective dose of folic acid for food fortification to prevent neural tube defects. *Lancet.* 1997;350(9092):1666–1669.

86. Centers for Disease Control and Prevention. Spina bifida and anencephaly before and after folic acid mandate—United States, 1995–1996 and 1999–2000. *MMWR Morb Mortal Wkly Rep.* 2004;53(17):362–365.

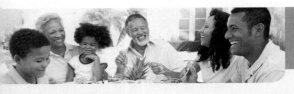

Learning Portfolio (continued)

87. Wittenbrook W. Best practices in nutrition for children with myelomeningocele. *ICAN.* 2012;2(4):237–245.

88. Krick J, Miller P. Nutritional implications in children with cerebral palsy. *Nutr Focus.* May/June 2003; 18(3).

89. Palisano R, Rosenbaum P, Bartlett D, Livingston M. *GMFCS-E&R. Gross Motor Function Classification System Expanded and Revised.* Hamilton, ON, Canada: Canada Child Centre for Childhood Disability Research, Institute for Applied Health Sciences, McMaster University; 2007. Retrieved from: https://www.cpqcc.org/sites/default/files/documents/HRIF_QCI_Docs/GMFCS-ER.pdf. Accessed September 9, 2016.

90. Mossey P, ed. *Addressing the Global Challenges of Craniofacial Anomalies: Report of a WHO Meeting on International Collaborative Research on Craniofacial Anomalies.* Geneva, Switzerland: World Health Organization; 2005:1–135. Retrieved from: http://www.who.int/genomics/publications/CFA%20Completed%20text.pdf. Accessed September 9, 2016.

91. Leslie EJ, Marazita ML. Genetics of cleft lip and cleft palate. *Am J Med Genet C Semin Med Genat.* 2013;163C:246–248.

92. Little J, Cardy A, Munger RG. Tobacco smoking and oral clefts: a meta-analysis. *Bull World Heath Organ.* 2004;82:213–218.

93. Margulis AV, Mitchell AA, Gilboa SM, Werler MM, Glynn RJ, Hernandez-Diaz S. National Birth Defects Prevention Study. Use of topiramate in pregnancy and risk of oral clefts. *Am J Obstet Gynecol.* 2012;207:405.e1–e7.

94. American Cleft Palate-Craniofacial Association. *Parameters for Evaluation and Treatment of Patients with Cleft Lip/Palate or Other Craniofacial Anomalies.* Rev. ed. Chapel Hill, NC: American Cleft Palate-Craniofacial Association; November 2009. Retrieved from: http://www.acpa-cpf.org/uploads/site/Parameters_Rev_2009.pdf. Accessed September 9, 2016.

95. American Psychiatric Association. *Diagnostic and Statistical Manual of Mental Disorders.* 4th ed. text revision. Washington DC: American Psychiatric Association; 2000.

96. Centers for Disease Control and Prevention. Prevalence of autism spectrum disorders among children aged 8 years—Autism and Developmental Disabilities Monitoring Network, United States, 2010. *MMWR Surveillance Summary.* 2014;63(SS02):1–21.

97. Kim YS, Leventhal BL, Koh YJ, et al. Prevalence of autism spectrum disorders in a total population sample. *Am J Psychiatry,* 2011;168(9):904–912.

98. Centers for Disease Control and Prevention. Prevalence of autism spectrum disorders—Autism and Developmental Disabilities Monitoring Network, 14 sites, United States, 2008. *MMWR Surveillance Summaries.* March 30, 2012;61(SS03):1–19. https://www.cdc.gov/mmwr/preview/mmwrhtml/ss6103a1.htm. Accessed September 9, 2016.

99. McElhanon BO, McCracken C, Karpen S, Sharp WS. Gastrointestinal symptoms in autism spectrum disorder: a meta-analysis. *Pediatrics.* 2014;133:872–883.

100. Kushak RI, Buie TM, Murray KF, et al. Evaluation of intestinal function in children with autism and gastrointestinal symptoms. *J Pediatr Gastroenterol Nutri.* 2016;62(5):687–691.

101. Sharp WG, Jaquess DL, Morton JF, Herzinger CV. Pediatric feeding disorders: a quantitative synthesis of treatment outcomes. *Clin Child Fam Psychol Rev.* 2010;13:348–365.

102. Kerwin MLE. Empirically supported treatments in pediatric psychology: severe feeding problems. *J Pediatr Psychol.* 1999;24(3):193–214.

103. Kerwin MLE, Eicher PS, Gelsinger J. Parental report of eating problems and gastrointestinal symptoms in children with pervasive developmental disorders. *Child Health Care.* 2005;34(3):221–234.

104. Ledford JR, Gast DL. Feeding problems in children with autism spectrum disorders: a review. *Focus Autism Other Develop Dis.* 2006;21(3):153–166.

105. Sharp WG, Berry RC, McCracken C, et al. Feeding problems and nutrient intake in children with autism spectrum disorders: a meta-analysis and comprehensive review of the literature. *J Autism Dev Disord.* 2013;43:2159–2173.

106. Schwartz SM. Feeding disorders in children with developmental disabilities. *Infants Young Child.* 2003;16:317–330.

107. Neumeyer AM, O'Rourke JA, Massa A, et al. Brief report: bone fractures in children and adults with autism spectrum disorders. *J Autism Dev Disord.* 2015;45(3):881–887.

108. Sharp, W.G., et.al., (2010) Pediatric feeding disorders: a quantitative synthesis of treatment outcomes. *Clin Child Fam Psychol Rev.* 13: 348–365

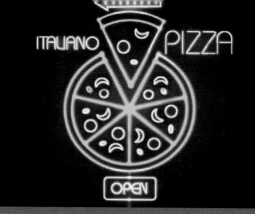

CHAPTER 9

Childhood and Preadolescent Nutrition

Christina Stella, MS, RDN, CDN, CDE **and Stephanie Lakinger**, MS, RD

Chapter Outline

Normal Growth and Development of Children and Preadolescents

Factors Affecting Dietary Intake During Childhood and Preadolescence

Nutritional Recommendations During Childhood and Preadolescence

Food and Nutrition Programs and Physical Activity

Common Nutritional Considerations During Childhood and Preadolescence

Learning Objectives

1. Discuss the factors that affect growth and development in childhood and preadolescence.

2. Describe anthropometric measurements that assess pediatric growth.

3. Describe the utility of pediatric height, weight, body mass index, and growth charts to evaluate childhood growth and development.

4. Explain factors that influence food choice of children and preadolescents.

5. List suggestions for children and preadolescents to guide nutrition and exercise habits to support healthy growth and development.

6. Identify health concerns and nutrition-related problems that affect children and preadolescents.

7. List suggestions to prevent dental caries.

8. Explain why oral health is important during the childhood and preadolescent stage.

9. Describe the role of calcium in bone health.

To optimize health, proper nutrition should be supported throughout childhood and preadolescence. Nutrient needs vary at different stages of life. During childhood and preadolescence, approximately defined as children ages 6 to 9 years old, the focus of nutrition should be to support the physiological process of growth and development, including maintenance of age-appropriate body weight, achievement of optimal cognitive development, and prevention of early onset of adult-related chronic disease.

This time period offers a child an opportunity to independently explore new foods and establish taste preferences, which can also be influenced by genetics and environment. Several programs assist health professionals in promoting healthy eating and lifestyles. This chapter discusses the nutritional health of preadolescents, focusing on the role of nutrition in growth and development, the development of eating habits and factors that shape these behaviors, the specific nutrient needs of children 6 to 9 years old, common preadolescent health conditions managed through nutrition, and programs available to health professionals to promote healthy living and eating right.

©All_about_people/Shutterstock

Case Study

Peter is an 8-year-old boy who lives in an urban setting described as an obesogenic environment. He lives with his mother, who is a homemaker, father, who works nights and sleeps during the day, and twin younger brothers. Peter's hobbies include going to basketball once a week for 1 hour and playing video games. Peter says he doesn't like to go outside and play because the parks have a lot of litter and limited playground equipment, so he plays video games instead. There is a family history of cardiovascular disease on his father's side.

Peter skips breakfast, receives school lunches with a rotating schedule but with pizza always available, and eats fast food for dinner on nights he has basketball, mostly from McDonald's. The rest of the week for dinner Peter has home-cooked meals. Mom likes to cook white rice and beans with meals because she is Mexican, and she serves canned vegetables on occasion because there is no good fresh produce in close proximity to their home. He thinks his diet is more healthy than unhealthy because he eats fruits with school lunches. Peter says his favorite food is pizza and soda.

Height: 124 cm (48.8 inches)

Weight: 28 kg (61.6 pounds)

BMI: 18.3

Medications/supplements: Chewable multivitamin

Normal Growth and Development of Children and Preadolescents

Preview Growth and development are human stages of life that have specific characteristics and are affected by nutrition. Although differences in these processes exist depending on age, gender, and ethnicity, childhood and preadolescent growth needs to be supported by adequate nutrition. The proper understanding and evaluation of the growth process helps health practitioners better assess overall health and risk for disease development.

Growth and Development

Growth, a fundamental trait of all natural organisms, is an anabolic process that occurs at different rates for all children and adolescents. It is defined as increase in size of various body parts and organs by multiplication of cells and intercellular components.[1] The manifestations of growth become visible with changes in height, weight, and head circumference. Children also develop, which refers to the increase of their functional capacity.[1] Although they are not identical processes, growth and development occur simultaneously and are interdependent as children progress through different life stages.

Different definitions of growth and development after the postnatal period exist. Three phases have been used to classify human physical growth and development in this period: infancy, childhood, and adolescence, with childhood separated into early and middle childhood.[1] When human and ape development were compared, the comparison suggested that major life stages can be described as infancy, juvenile period, short adolescent phase, and adult stage (see **FIGURE 9.1**).[2] However, modern humans have inserted an additional stage, early

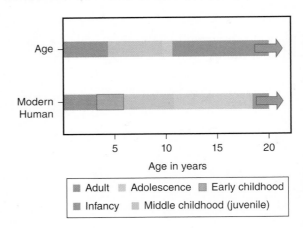

Figure 9.1
Acquisition of height of modern humans compared with ape ancestors.

Data from Rogol A, Clark P, Roemmich J. Growth and pubertal development in children and adolescents: effects of diet and physical activity. J Clin Nutr. 2000;72:521S–528S.

childhood, which comes before the juvenile period, and humans have a greatly elongated adolescent stage.[3] The whole growth period is extended, taking almost twice as long as that of apes.[3] Common to both definitions of growth and development is the presence of **permanent teeth**, less dependency on parents, assertion of independence, further brain development, and better understanding of the world around a child.

Genetics and Hormones Influence Growth

Growth and development processes are the result of the combined actions of genetics, hormones, and nutrition. Genetic information, specifically, genes, inherited from parents determine height and body size.[1] Hormones are regulatory substances produced by the endocrine system, and they represent the biochemical aspect of growth. The endocrine system, hypothalamus, and pituitary gland secrete and stimulate hormones during periods of growth, and hormones regulate growth and development using the instructions they receive from genes.[1,4] Numerous hormones are involved in growth and development. **Growth hormone**, for example, although it has an indirect effect on growth, is the most important hormone involved in the growth process. The pituitary secretes growth hormone in response to the hypothalamus releasing growth-hormone-releasing hormone and the stomach releasing ghrelin.[1,5] Growth hormone affects growth by stimulating insulin-like growth factors, which activate cell growth, with the end result being bone and muscle growth (**FIGURE 9.2**).[5] Other key hormones involved in growth include glucocorticoids, thyroid hormones, and sex steroids.[6] Much that is known about the hormonal regulation of childhood growth is derived from studies of children with various deficiencies or other endocrine dysfunctions.[4]

For children between the ages of 6 and 9 years, the growth of anatomy slows in comparison with the growth that took place during the toddler stage and the growth surge that is yet to come in adolescence secondary to puberty (which is measured by the **Tanner Scale**). Despite

slower skeletal growth, in general consistent annual growth in height and weight can be expected; around 6 to 7 years of age a mild growth spurt associated with **adiposity rebound** occurs.

Measuring height and weight in this population is essential to a nutrition assessment. There are several ways to measure growth, including height, weight, and body composition. Length is measured in children too young to stand; height is measured once the child can stand.[7] Height growth in children older than 2 years of age is measured with the child standing.[8] Children should be measured without shoes while standing against the vertical plane to which the measuring tape is attached.[8] The child's heels, buttocks, shoulders, and back of head should be touching the wall.[8] Health practitioners can use the general rule of thumb that a child's height will increase by 5–6 cm (2–2.4 inches) each year until puberty while keeping in mind that after 12 months height is mostly genetically driven.[8] Because extremities grow faster than the trunk it is common for children of this age group to have an awkward appearance. **FIGURE 9.3** demonstrates proper technique for measuring height in the preadolescent population.

In addition to measuring height, it is important to analyze growth or height velocity, which is defined as the rate of change in height over a set period of time. Height velocity is a more sensitive measure of growth than are time-specific height measurements. A prepubertal child whose height velocity is less than 5 cm (2 inches) per year should be monitored closely.[9] Height velocity can be derived as often as height measurements are taken; however, it is suggested that yearly growth velocities be measured because children have growth spurts.[8] Some children have a small increase in **growth**

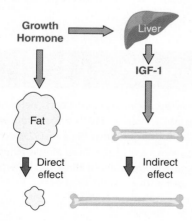

Figure 9.2
Role of growth hormone.

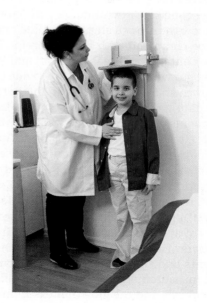

Figure 9.3
Measuring height in the preadolescent population.
©Levent Konuk/Shutterstock

velocity between the ages of 4 and 8 years, known as the midgrowth spurt. The midgrowth spurt was defined and has been researched as far back as 1915; it occurs well before the onset of puberty, can occur for up to 2 years, and is observed in some but not all children.[10] The Fels Longitudinal Study found that the midgrowth spurt occurred in up to 79% of boys studied and in 36% of girls.[10] Differences in height measurements exist between sexes, and differences in height velocity exist between seasons.

Careful measurement of weight is an essential component of the physical and nutrition assessment because it is another technique for measuring growth. It is recommended that children remove shoes, bulky clothing, and pocket contents. Children older than 2 should sit or stand on a calibrated scale. Children gain 2 kg (4.4 pounds) per year between 2 years and puberty.[9] Knowing height and weight, practitioners can calculate body mass index (BMI), which is a nondiagnostic measurement of weight to height; in children and teens BMI is age and gender specific.[11] For this population, BMI can be considered an alternative technique to measure body fatness.[11] Body mass index is expressed on an age- and gender-specific growth chart, which is a major difference between calculating BMI for adults and for children. Although the same calculation is used, BMI levels among children and teens must be expressed relative to other children of the same sex and age because of the growth process.[11]

In 1978, the American Academy of Pediatrics and the Maternal and Child Health Program of the Bureau of Community Health Services included growth charts as part of the evaluation of pediatric growth. The National Center for Health Statistics developed growth charts for the United States when nationally representative cross-sectional survey data became available for most of the pediatric age range.[12] Growth curves are growth references and allow the growth status of a child or a group of children to be compared with that of a reference population.[13] The Centers for Disease Control and Prevention (CDC) revised growth charts in 2000 to provide better estimates of growth and physical size, and this version is the most up to date tool that clinicians should be using in their assessments of growth. The new features of the 2000 growth charts, which were created using nationally representative data, include the following: new sex-specific BMI for age charts, extended age range, added percentile ranking and corresponding percentiles, and Z-scores.[13]

The CDC recommends using the World Health Organization (WHO) growth standards for children younger than 2 years of age and using the CDC growth charts for children 2 years of age and older. After obtaining accurate measurements and selecting appropriate charts, practitioners plot measurements by finding the child's age on the horizontal axis and the growth measurement on the vertical axis, and plotting the point where the child's age and growth measurement intersect. This point identifies where the child ranks relative to other children of the same sex and a similar age.[14] For example, when a plotted weight is on the 90th percentile for weight-for-age, it means that only 10 of 100 children (10%) of the same age and sex in the reference population have a higher weight-for-age.[14] Specifically, by plotting on BMI growth charts, practitioners can help determine whether children can be described as underweight, normal weight, overweight, or obese (**TABLE 9.1**). It is normal in the first few years of life to see children jump percentiles, but crossing percentile lines is potentially a sign of growth disturbance.[14] Special

---

Table 9.1

Nutritional Indicators Determined by Measuring Body Mass Index on Age-/Gender-Specific Growth Charts

Growth Measurement	Percentile Measurements	Nutritional Indicator
BMI for age/gender	<5th percentile	Underweight
BMI for age/gender	≥5th percentile and <85th percentile	Normal nutrition
BMI for age/gender	≥85th percentile and <95th percentile	Overweight
BMI for age/gender	≥95th percentile	Obesity

Let's Discuss

Children diagnosed with certain diseases, especially chromosomal disorders, demonstrate growth and development patterns that do not follow a normal trajectory; therefore, measuring height and weight in these populations as part of a nutrition assessment is more difficult. Disease-specific growth charts have been developed.

Questions

1. What are the strengths and limitations of using disease-specific growth charts?
2. Should these growth charts be updated more frequently or less frequently than standard growth charts?

Let's Discuss

On age- and sex-appropriate growth charts, determine the percentiles for height, weight, and BMI using the following anthropometrics: 12-year-old girl who is 134.2 cm (52.8 inches), 41.2 kg (90.6 pounds), with a BMI of 22.8. After plotting these measurements what do you know about this child in terms of being classified as normal, overweight, or obese?

Questions

1. What guidance would you offer about how this child is growing?

growth curves have been developed for Turner syndrome, Down syndrome, Williams syndrome, achondroplasia, and prematurity.[9] Growth and development are dynamic processes that provide valuable clinical information about children's overall health, and practitioners should not overlook assessment of these parameters.

Cognitive Development

In addition to physical changes, growth and development also include cognitive changes. It is a stage of life biologists label as when individuals who are not yet reproductively capable are responsible for feeding themselves but are still under the social influence of their parents.[15] The transition to this phase of development is closely related to the timing of brain development.[15] Anthropologist Benjamin Campbell says about this life stage, "In middle childhood, kids start to make sense."[15] Understanding emotions and making emotional adjustments along with social independence are other characteristics of early childhood development. Transition from infancy to early childhood and from puberty to adulthood always earn more attention because the somatic changes of growth become more visible. In 1975, a landmark study to estimate the age at which cultures assigned children a more mature social, sexual, and cultural role determined that in 16 of the categories studied, children ages 6 and 7 years were assigned new cultural roles and responsibilities.[16]

Nutrition

Nutritionally, growth is supported through a sufficient intake of **macronutrients** and **micronutrients**. An adequate supply of calories serves as the fuel to ensure the above functions continue to happen under the normal physiological state. Nutritional needs vary with each phase of development but likely parallel the rate of growth with the greatest nutrient demands occurring during the peak velocity of growth.[1,6] The dynamic nature of growth and development is highly individualized, but overall it is a well-defined age period influenced by genetics, hormones, and nutrition.

Recap Growth and development are human processes that occur as children age and that are affected by age, gender, and adequate nutrition. Preadolescence is defined by a midgrowth spurt, continued need for tracking of anthropometrics on age- and gender-appropriate growth charts, and expansion of functional capacity, which ultimately leads to increased development. These processes do not take place when children are not fed or cannot feed themselves adequate nutrition.

1. Discuss the factors that affect growth and development.
2. Explain the development of growth charts and importance of tracking anthropometrics.
3. Demonstrate how to measure anthropometrics.
4. Identify anthropometrics that indicate over- and underweight status, and describe development of preadolescence.

Case Study

At his last well-child visit, Peter's pediatrician informed his mom that his growth velocity was slower than that of other children his age.

Question

1. Discuss what the doctor meant with this assessment and what should be considered next steps for Peter at this point in time.

News You Can Use

The CDC's First New Growth Charts in Years!

In October 2015, for the first time since 1988, a new set of growth charts was developed for children with Down syndrome. The results of the Down Syndrome Growing Up Study (DSGS) funded by the CDC led to the creation of these new graphs.

Question

1. How are the 2015 Down syndrome growth charts different from charts that were previously developed?

Reference

a. Children's Hospital of Philadelphia. New growth charts developed for U.S. children with Down syndrome. PR Newswire; October 27, 2015. Retrieved from: http://www.prnewswire.com/news-releases/new-growth-charts-developed-for-us-children-with-down-syndrome-300167191.html. Accessed September 13, 2016.

Factors Affecting Dietary Intake During Childhood and Preadolescence

Preview Food choice is a complex human behavior that begins in early childhood when children exert independence in selecting what to eat and what not to eat. Dietary intake is driven mainly by the feelings of being hungry and full, but many factors influence food choice. It is important for all parameters that affect dietary intake to promote healthy eating because dietary intake during this development period can influence health later in life. Family, peers, schools, culture, and food marketing play roles and build the environment that shapes dietary intake during preadolescence.

Establishing Food Behaviors

The foundation of food behaviors is laid early in life and continues to form during preadolescence. These practices affect a child's overall health status. Many factors shape children's decisions about what to eat. Though parents and peers likely remain role models for proper nutrition, preadolescents exert more personal choice over their eating habits. This is an age when children either continue to avoid or be reluctant to try new foods or begin to experiment with new foods and flavors because of increased independence in selection. Healthy eating habits and personal preferences are further influenced by culture and religion. Schools are important determinants of eating habits because schools not only offer meals and snacks but also sometimes teach nutrition education, and schools are the environment in which children spend most of their time. When they are exposed to food marketing through increased media, children may develop stronger opinions about what they want to eat. Factors affecting dietary intake during adolescence are influenced by an assortment of variables, all of which impact overall health.

Because of an inability to vocalize hunger, satiety, and preferences, the nutrient needs of babies and young children are met according to what parents find acceptable and adequate. As children become older, they learn about food through personal experiences, which continue to be influenced by parents but are not determined by parents. This age group is historically defined as consuming a diet of adult foods influenced by their parents. In children as young as 2 years old, research has shown that food preferences were associated with their mothers' foods preferences.[17] One of the most likely reasons children eat like their parents is because parents keep foods they like in the home, increasing the number of exposures a child has to parents' favorite foods. Sometimes the reason children will not eat a certain food is because it is unfamiliar to them. Children like what they know, and they eat what they like.[18] If a child becomes more familiar with a food through parents' actions and responses to the food, the acceptance of new foods can increase. The threat of parental monitoring and actual parental presence decrease children's intake of nonnutritious foods.[19]

Parents should not only encourage their children to try new foods but also model eating the foods they want their children to eat. Children are more likely to sample unfamiliar foods after they have seen an adult eating the food, and they are more likely to eat when they see their mother eating rather than a stranger.[20] It is of utmost importance to therefore also keep in mind that modeling can expose children to unhealthy habits and restrictive dieting patterns that more often characterize an adult's eating pattern. For example, dieting mothers were more likely to have dieting daughters.[21] Health professionals know modeling improves a child's food choices and eating habits; however, simply listening to parents speak about what are good and bad foods and monitoring facial expressions can also affect food choices. Food selection is most often a joint decision, especially between children and parents and influenced by culture and environment; therefore, children have the opportunity to mimic how those in their surroundings choose, cook, eat, and react to different foods.[22]

Food Rewards

Another way parents influence preadolescent food selection is when they use food as reward or punishment. When food is used as a reward or a punishment, it makes food a privilege rather than fuel for healthy living. Usually, foods high in calories, fat, and sugar are used as rewards. When using these foods as a reward, parents make an association between unhealthy foods and good behaviors or achievements. A mother might say, for example, "I will give you your favorite cookie if you clean your room." A child might then think that every time he cleans, he'll receive a cookie, which would not only increase consumption of calories, fat, and sugar but also cause a child to eat when he might not be hungry.

The common ways in which parents can use control over food are as follows: pressuring children to eat only healthy foods like fruits and vegetables, restricting access to sweets and snacks, and using food as a reward.[23] Although the intentions of these controlling behaviors might be good, these practices are associated with negative outcomes; restriction is strongly correlated with children's disinhibited eating behaviors.[23] In addition, when food is used as a punishment—restricting dessert because a child failed to eat all the vegetables on the plate, for example—children can develop further distaste for vegetables or continue not to eat these foods out of defiance. Using food as punishment also undermines the emerging independence children have over their eating habits by telling children they cannot have something. According to the American Academy of Pediatrics, in the long run food as a reward or bribe usually creates more problems than it solves.[24] To prevent poor eating habits, health professionals should encourage parents not to use food as a privilege.

Cultural Food Preferences

Parents and community bring culture to life for children, and cultural traditions related to food can influence a child's eating habits. Culture is defined as knowledge, beliefs, customs, and habits a group of people share that is learned, not inherited. Each culture has different core foods and preparation methods, and children may learn to accept culturally specific foods or meals over others for a number of reasons. Cultural influences apply to eating patterns of adults as well as what and how adults feed their children and how the children are socialized to choose foods for themselves.[25] A child of Latin American descent, for example, would not be expected to choose sushi, pasta, or curried meats over rice and beans. Because rice and beans is specific to Latin American cultural cuisine, we would anticipate a child would have positive associations with these specific foods, the family would model it as a healthy food choice, and likely the child would have numerous exposures to these foods on any given day. Although the most common foods of cultures might differ, usually all cultures share the belief that food is used as the foundation for health and human interactions.

Peer Influence

During preadolescence, peer influence over children's food choices might not be as strong as it will become during adolescence. Reasons peer influence is more limited in preadolescence are that social networks are still forming and peer acceptance is not as strong a motivator for younger children. Peer influence, however, should still be considered a factor affecting dietary habits. In 3- to 7-year-olds, children are more likely to eat a novel food if they see a peer positively modeling consumption.[26] Acceptance of novel foods was also noted to be stronger if the peer was older and there were repeat exposures.[26] Peers also have the ability to change a child's opinions about foods. When a preschooler with a strong dislike for a vegetable, for example, was seated with peers who had a strong preference for the same vegetable, the preschooler was significantly likely to alter food preferences over time and eventually select the initially disliked vegetable.[27] Although children may have more freedom to make their own meal choices as they age, who children eat with is important in determining what they are eating.

Food Likes and Dislikes

Another factor that affects a child's nutritional status during childhood is whether the child is considered a picky eater or has demonstrated food neophobia, defined as reluctance to try new foods or avoidance of certain foods and food groups. There is no formal definition of picky eating habits, and it is not a diagnosis, as is Avoidant/Restrictive Food Intake disorder, which was added to the fifth edition of the *Diagnostic and Statistical Manual of Mental Disorders*. More recent research suggests that for some children and parents, picky eating habits continue to be a problem for many years, with 47% having duration longer than 2 years.[28] Picky eating habits usually develop between the ages of 2 and 6 years old, but it is quite common for preadolescent children to continue to demonstrate food neophobia.[29] TABLE 9.2 lists some typical food-related habits of picky eaters. It is important for preadolescents to accept new foods because their requirements for certain nutrients will increase during puberty and adolescence. A registered dietitian, nutritionist may be helpful is suggesting techniques and foods to improve food acceptance.

Advertising and Marketing

Preadolescents are an age group that is vulnerable to the suggestive powers of food companies and their marketing and advertising campaigns. Nearly one-third of American children and adolescents are affected by overweight or obesity.[30] The rapid increase in obesity rates led health professionals to regard food marketing of nutritionally poor foods as a potential factor contributing to obesity. The Institute of Medicine (IOM) has called on food, beverage, restaurant, and entertainment industries to work closely with government, scientific, and public health associations to establish and enforce the highest standards for the marketing of foods, beverages, and meals to children and youth.[31] To achieve the standards recommended by the IOM, two key aspects of food marketing to children must be addressed: (1) the identification of food marketing practices and venues aimed at children, and (2) nutrition criteria for foods and beverages appropriate to market to children.[31] Since the release of these recommendations, the Council of Better Business Bureaus' Children's Food and Beverage Advertising Initiative (CFBAI) established a uniform set of voluntary category-specific nutrition standards that took effect in 2014. Dairy products are shown as an example in TABLE 9.3.[32] The full table is available from the Better Business Bureau.

Food and beverage companies spend more than $1.6 billion per year on advertising targeted toward young consumers.[33] Advertising efforts include using catchy slogans, intimation, and cartoons as a few tactics to capture the attention of young consumers and influence their dietary choices. A recent systematic review concluded that companies use characters on products to build an emotional relationship between children and products.[34]

In 2007, SpongeBob SquarePants and Dora the Explorer, for example, began to appear on fruits and vegetables, and Shrek became a spokesman for various U.S. Department of Health and Human Services campaigns and had his image appear on products from Kellogg's, McDonald's, Mars (M&Ms), Frito Lay (Cheetos), and Keebler.

Table 9.2

Typical Food Habits of Picky Eaters

Refuses specific foods or food groups, especially fruits and vegetables.

Unwilling to try and refuses new foods.

Accepts limited types of food (usually less than 10).

Limits quantity of food eaten and/or eats only preferred foods.

Prefers drinks over foods.

Has strong food preferences.

Mealtime exceeds 30 minutes.

Eats food camouflaged in others or liquids.

Uses distractions to limit food intake.

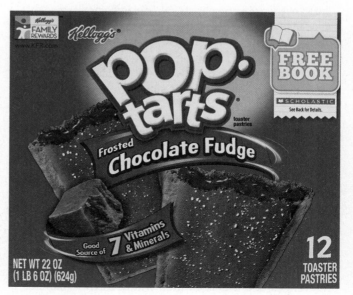

©Sheila Fitzgerald/Shutterstock

Table 9.3

Children's Food and Beverage Advertising Initiative Standards for Promoting Dairy Products to Children

Product Category	Unit	Nutrients to Limit (NTL)				Example
		Calories	Saturated Fat	Sodium	Total Sugars	
Dairy products						
Milks and milk substitutes	8 fl oz	≤150	≤2 g	≤200 mg	≤24 g	1 glass of almond milk
Yogurts and yogurt-type products	6 oz	≤170	≤2 g	≤140 mg	≤23 g	2 children's yogurt sticks
Dairy-based desserts	½ c	≤120	≤2 g	≤110 mg	≤20 g	1 small ice cream sandwich
Cheese and cheese products	LSS	≤80	≤3 g	≤290 mg	≤2 g	1 cheese stick

LSS = labeled serving size.

Data from Children's Food & beverage Advertising Initiative. CFBAI's Category-Specific Uniform Nutrition Criteria. Available at: http://www.bbb.org/storage/16/documents/cfbai/CFBAI%20Uniform%20Nutrition%20Criteria%20Fact%20Sheet%20-FINAL.pdf. Accessed August 6th, 2016.

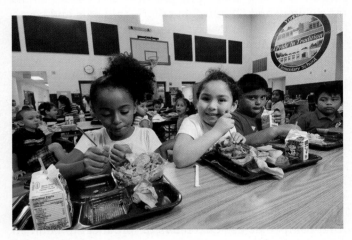

Courtesy of U.S. Department of Agriculture

Let's Discuss

Research has correlated food marketing and the rise in childhood overweight and obesity. Do you agree or disagree that food marketing is a contributing factor to weight problems in this population?

Current standards regulate food marketing of food products to consumers up the age of 14 years. Should marketing regulations expand to older age groups?

More than advocating for the use of licensed characters for healthy foods, research points to the need to regulate and curtail the use of this marketing approach on high-energy, low-nutrient foods.[35] Because food companies most often attempt to establish an emotional connection between the child and the food product, efforts to change food marketing should focus on reduction of that emotional connection so a child is less influenced. We are limited, however, in understanding the specific mechanisms by which cartoon characters influence children's preferences and this is an area where further research is needed.[34] Companies market food products to children on television, radio, toys, clothing, posters, and billboards, on the Internet, and in magazines and video games. Food marketing can be detrimental to children's health not only because of the unhealthy foods frequently being promoted but also because it accesses children easily through almost all outlets associated with pediatric leisure activities.

Schools

The foods that surround children most often on a daily basis will likely become part of their normal repertoire of food choices regardless of nutritional value; therefore schools and the learning environment are factors affecting dietary choice. Schools influence children's food choices through the foods they serve at school meals and snack times, through the sale of foods in vending machines and school stores, as well as foods available in less structured settings such as bake sales, fundraisers, and parties, and formally by offering nutrition education as part of a curriculum. The Institute of Medicine's action plan for the prevention of childhood obesity observes that schools are in a unique position to influence the diets and **physical activity** of U.S. children.[30] No other institution has as much continuous and intensive contact with children; most U.S. children attend school for 6 or more hours per day, 180 days per year, from ages 5 through 17 years.[30] Public and private schools have access to federally funded school breakfast and lunch programs, which make low-cost, nutritious food available to children for selection on a daily basis. These programs are discussed in detail later in this chapter.

Vending Machines

School vending machines traditionally offer opportunities for children to make poor food choices because vending machines are usually stocked with foods known to exceed recommendations for calories, fat, and sugar per serving. A long-term study of high school students provided evidence that availability of foods in schools affects choices, and less healthy snack and drink offerings in vending machines and school stores may even have undesirable effects on body weight.[36] Regular access to foods that are high in energy and sugar and of low nutritional quality, however, remains a significant issue at schools.[37] To get children to choose more healthy foods in schools, it is important nutritious foods be made available to them and to educate children about why these foods are their best options. By integrating nutrition education in cafeterias and classrooms, the nutritional status of preadolescents can be positively affected.

Food Availability

Access to food can be a persuasive factor in children's food selection choices. We cannot expect preadolescents, for example, to select fruits and vegetables when their local markets, schools, and homes do not offer these foods. In the ongoing study of the causes of pediatric obesity, the built environment has been targeted as one determinant of pediatric obesity. The term *obesogenic environment* refers to "an environment that promotes gaining weight and one that is not conducive to weight loss" within the home or workplace.[38] An obesogenic environment includes factors that influence eating outside of education and behaviors. Usually, in obesogenic environments inhabitants have closer proximity to fast-food establishments than to supermarkets. Studies link the obesogenic environment to adverse health consequences such as obesity and diabetes. Both child and adult obesity are lowest in neighborhoods with environments that are most favorable to healthy eating, defined by supermarket proximity and/or lower fast-food restaurant density, and physical activity, defined as having a built environment that is more conducive to walking and access to higher-quality parks.[39] Fast food has become routine for some children because of the concentration of these restaurants in neighborhoods where they live. Families can improve a child's eating habits by not allowing fast-food meal consumption to be the norm.

Recap A child's dietary intake is shaped over time and influenced by a variety of factors. It is important to foster healthy eating during this developmental age so that children understand the importance of good nutrition and that disease prevention begins at an early stage. Family, friends, schools, culture, environment, and innate human behaviors all play a role in the development of diet.

1. Name the factors affecting a child's dietary intake during preadolescence.
2. Discuss how exposure to television and food marketing affect children's health status.
3. Explain the role of environment as a factor influencing nutritional choices of young children.
4. Support the role of culture as a factor shaping food choices.
5. Describe governmental efforts within schools to improve the nutritional status of children and assist in developing healthy eating habits.

Case Study

Peter's pediatrician suggested that Peter and his family meet with a dietitian, but mom is reluctant because she feels the reason Peter doesn't have a good diet is because of the meals he gets in school.

Questions

1. How can the pediatrician and dietitian address mom's concerns?
2. Discuss how Peter's environment could be contributing to his poor diet.

News You Can Use

Cartoon Characters Can Influence Children to Make Better Nutrition Choices

Cartoon characters can influence children to choose junk food in promotions, but new research suggests that cartoon characters can also be used to influence children to eat healthier foods! A study from the University of Bari Aldo Moro in Italy used stickers with a cartoon character on fruits and vegetables to promote the foods. Children's perceptions were changed when the characters were used.

Questions

1. Can marketing healthy foods to children improve the diets of children in the United States?
2. How can the food industry change to improve the health of children?

Reference

a. MedicalXpress; December 15, 2015. Cartoon characters can influence children to make better nutrition choices. Retrieved from: http://medicalxpress.com/news/2015-12-cartoon-characters-children-nutrition-choices.html. Accessed September 13, 2016.

Nutritional Recommendations During Childhood and Preadolescence

Preview The principles of nutrition during early childhood are based on the principles for adults; however, the amounts of specific nutrients differ because of children's needs for well-being, growth, and development, all of which depend on age and gender. Dietary guidelines provide information on the specific amounts of nutrients needed and appropriate daily servings for all food groups.

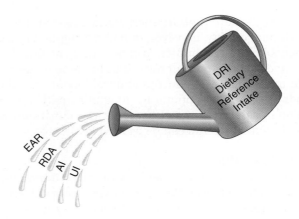

Table 9.4

Dietary Reference Intakes

Estimated Average Requirement (EAR)	The intake value that meets the estimated nutrient needs of 50% of individuals in a specific lifestage and gender group.
Recommended Dietary Allowances (RDAs)	The nutrient intake levels that meet nutrient needs of almost all (97% to 98%) individuals in a lifestage and gender group.
Adequate Intake (AI)	The nutrient intake that appears to sustain a defined nutritional state or some other indicator of health (e.g., growth rate or normal circulating nutrient values) in a specific population or subgroup. AI is used when there is insufficient scientific evidence to establish an EAR.
Tolerable Upper Intake Level (UL)	The maximum level of daily nutrient intake that is unlikely to pose health risks to almost all the individuals in the group for whom the UL is designed.
Estimated Energy Requirement (EER)	Dietary energy intake that is predicted to maintain energy balance in a healthy adult of a defined age, gender, weight, height, and level of physical activity consistent with good health.
Acceptable Macronutrient Distribution Ranges (AMDR)	Range of intakes for a particular energy source that is associated with reduced risk of chronic disease while providing adequate intake of essential nutrients.

Nutrient Recommendations

Though all individuals need the same macro- and micronutrients to ensure the body functions appropriately, people have different needs during infancy, adolescence, and adulthood. Young children, for example have increased nutrient requirements because their bodies demand more nutrition to keep up with bodily functions, especially growth. National organizations have been able to quantify and subsequently develop standards for most nutrients. Developed by the Food and Nutrition Board of the Institute of Medicine, the Dietary Reference Intakes (DRIs) are used to plan and assess the nutrients needed by healthy individuals; they include Recommended Dietary Allowances (RDAs), Adequate Intakes (AIs), and Tolerable Upper Intake Levels (ULs).[40] **TABLE 9.4** defines the DRIs. DRIs expand on the periodic reports called Recommended Dietary Allowances, which have been published since 1941.[40] DRIs are based on age, life stage, and gender; even with statistical measurements, DRIs remain an overall estimate of general needs. It is important for health professionals to educate parents on how they can meet the DRIs for their children to ensure proper growth and development and prevent chronic disease.

Recommendations on energy, macronutrient, and micronutrient needs for this age come from the Dietary Guidelines for Americans. Macronutrients are nutrients needed by the human body in relatively large quantities; carbohydrates, fats, and protein are the three

macronutrients. Micronutrients are chemical elements needed in trace amounts for normal growth of living organisms. Every 5 years the government updates the *Dietary Guidelines for Americans* intended for healthy Americans ages 2 and up. The most recent set of *Dietary Guidelines*, published in 2015, recommends Americans eat a diet of healthy foods and beverages to maintain an appropriate calorie level and that each eating pattern be adapted to the individual.[41] An eating pattern is defined as what people routinely consume. The *Dietary Guidelines for Americans* make childhood nutrition an important focus because studies support optimizing nutrition at a young age continuing throughout the life span, and because too many children are consuming diets with excess calories and sugar and spend limited time engaged in physical activity. The key concepts of the 2015 *Dietary Guidelines* are shown in **FIGURE 9.4** and **FIGURE 9.5**.

Let's Discuss

Access the *Dietary Guidelines for Americans 2015–2020* at https://health.gov/dietaryguidelines/. Find Appendix 2 and look at the Estimated Calorie Needs per Day for Children and Preadolescents. What are the needs of a 7-year-old girl?

Next, find one recommendation you can use to improve the health of a child/preadolescent. What is one way you can implement this recommendation at a school?

Last, find how boys ages 4–8 are doing in the category of dairy intake compared with the recommendations. Are boys in this age group consuming the recommended amount of this important food group?

Although the number of calories a person needs on a daily basis is influenced by a number of factors, children need more calories per kilogram of body weight compared with adults 19 years and older. Depending on age, weight status, and activity level, the daily calorie guidelines for girls and boys ages 6 to 9 are 1,400–2,000.[41]

The Guidelines

1. **Follow a healthy eating pattern across the lifespan**. All food and beverage choices matter. Choose a healthy eating pattern at an appropriate calorie level to help achieve and maintain a healthy body weight, support nutrient adequacy, and reduce the risk of chronic disease.

2. **Focus on variety, nutrient density, and amount**. To meet nutrient needs within calorie limits, choose a variety of nutrient-dense foods across and within all food groups in recommended amounts.

3. **Limit calories from added sugars and saturated fats and reduce sodium intake**. Consume an eating pattern low in added sugars, saturated fats. and sodium. Cut back on foods and beverages higher in these components to amounts that fit within healthy eating patterns.

4. **Shift to healthier food and beverage choices**. Choose nutrient-dense foods and beverages across and within all food groups in place of less healthy choices. Consider cultural and personal preferences to make these shifts easier to accomplish and maintain.

Figure 9.4
The *Dietary Guidelines for Americans 2015–2020*.

Data from The National Academies of Sciences, Engineering, Medicine; updated May 31, 2016. Dietary Reference Intakes tables and application. Retrieved from: http://www.nationalacademies.org/hmd/Activities/Nutrition/SummaryDRIs/DRI-Tables.aspx. Accessed September 13, 2016.

Key Recommendations

Consume a healthy eating pattern that accounts for all foods and beverages within an appropriate calorie level.

A healthy eating pattern includes:[2]

- A variety of vegetabkes from all if the subgroups—dark green, red and orange, legumes (beans and peas), Starchy, and other

- Fruits, especially whole fruits

- Grains, at least half of which are whole grains

- Fat-free or low-fat dairy, including milk, yogurt, cheese, and/or fortified soy beverages

- A variety of protein foods, including seafood, lean meats and poultry, eggs, legumes (beans and peas), and nuts, seeds, and soy products

- Oils

Figure 9.5
2015–2020 Dietary Guidelines for Americans: Key Recommendations.

U.S. Department of Health and Human Services and U.S. Department of Agriculture. 2â€"2. 8th ed. Washington, DC: U.S. Department of Health and Human Services and U.S. Department of Agriculture; December 2015. Retrieved from: https://health.gov/dietaryguidelines/2015/guidelines/chapter-1/key-recommendations/. Accessed September 14, 2016.

The National Academy of Science Health and Medicine Division has established ranges for the percentage of calories in the diet that should come from macronutrients; these ranges take into account both chronic disease risk reduction and intake of essential nutrients (see TABLE 9.5).[42] In addition, the Recommended Daily Allowances for grams of carbohydrates and protein have been set. Total dietary fat intake remains an acceptable percentage range of total calories[42] (see TABLE 9.6).

The U.S. Department of Agriculture (USDA) is responsible for developing not only the DRIs but also a food guidance system for all Americans. The Center for Nutrition Policy and Promotion is the group with the USDA responsible for these programs, which include MyPlate

Table 9.5

Acceptable Macronutrient Distribution Range for Children 4–18 Years

Fat	25–35%
Carbohydrate	45–65%
Protein	10–30%

Data from The National Academies of Sciences, Engineering, Medicine; updated May 31, 2016. Dietary Reference Intakes tables and application. Retrieved from: http://www.nationalacademies.org/hmd/Activities/Nutrition/SummaryDRIs/DRI-Tables.aspx. Accessed September 13, 2016.

My Daily Food Plan

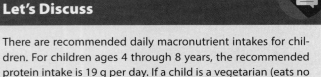

Based on the information you provided, this is your daily recommended amount for each food group.

GRAINS 5 ounces	VEGETABLES 2 cups	FRUITS 1 1/2 cups	DAIRY 3 cups	PROTEIN FOODS 5 ounces
Make half your grains whole Aim for at least **3 ounces** of whole grains a day	**Vary your veggies** Aim for these amounts each week: **Dark green veggies** = 1 1/2 cups **Red & orange veggies** = 4 cups **Beans & peas** = 1 cup **Starchy veggies** = 4 cups **Other veggies** = 3 1/2 cups	**Focus on fruits** Eat a variety of fruit Choose whole or cut-up fruits more often than fruit juice	**Get your calcium-rich foods** Drink fat-free or low-fat (1%) milk, for the same amount of calcium and other nutrients as whole milk, but less fat and Calories Select fat-free or low-fat yogurt and cheese, or try calcium-fortified soy products	**Go lean with protein** Twice a week, make seafood the protein on your plate Vary your protein routine—choose beans, peas, nuts, and seeds more often Keep meat and poultry portions small and lean

Courtesy of U.S. Department of Agriculture

method, MyPyramid, Food Guide Pyramid, Healthy Eating Index, U.S. Food Plans, Nutrient Content of the U.S. Food Supply, and Expenditures on Children by Families. The MyPlate method is one of the newest programs targeting the nutritional health of all Americans, and it encourages Americans to think about what goes on their plate or in their cup or bowl before they eat.[43] Along with the MyPlate method, daily food group plans have been created that show the food groups and how much of each food group to consume based on age and calorie requirements.

Let's Discuss

There are recommended daily macronutrient intakes for children. For children ages 4 through 8 years, the recommended protein intake is 19 g per day. If a child is a vegetarian (eats no meat or fish), which foods would you recommend to meet his or her protein needs?

Trends in children's diets are important to study to understand potential causes for development and progression of chronic diseases, especially obesity. There have been changes in overall food intake and nutrient intake among children. From 1989 to 2004, there was a significant increase in per capita total daily energy intake for U.S. children aged 2 to 18 years.[44] Starting in 1989, the total mean energy intake among children and

adolescents ages 6 to 11 years increased until 2005, when it began to decrease to 1,863 mean calories in 2010.[44] Seven specific food and beverage categories remained the highest contributors to calorie intake across all six groups of years studied. These food groups were sugar-sweetened beverages, pizza, full-fat milk, grain-based desserts, breads, pasta dishes, and savory snacks.[44] These findings are similar to other studies examining the sources of intake among U.S. children and adolescents. These foods represent top dietary sources of excessive energy, solid fats, and added sugar.[45] The 2015 *Dietary Guidelines* makes quantitative recommendations for nutrients that are of particular concern for all Americans, such as added sugars, saturated fat, and sodium. Because the most common foods in this age group's diet are high in these nutrients, these recommendations are especially important for preadolescents. **FIGURE 9.6** lists the recommendations.

Let's Discuss

The *Dietary Guidelines for Americans* include foods that are part of a healthy eating pattern. They also contain foods that should be limited and in what quantities.

How can practitioners and parents teach children how to implement these dietary limitations? Be specific. Hint: Think of replacing unhealthy foods with healthy ones, healthy role models, and limiting unhealthy foods.

Table 9.6

Acceptable Macronutrient Distribution Range for Children 4–18 Years

	Protein	Carbohydrate	Fiber	Fat (Total)	α-Linolenic Acid (n-3)	Linoleic Acid (n-6)
Children 4–8 years	19 g	130 g	25 g	25–35%	0.9 g	10 g
Boys 9–13 years	34 g	130 g	31 g	25–35%	1.2 g	12 g
Girls 9–13 years	34 g	130 g	26 g	25–35%	1.0 g	10 g

Data from The National Academies of Sciences, Engineering, Medicine; updated May 31, 2016. Dietary Reference Intakes tables and application. Retrieved from: http://www.nationalacademies.org/hmd/Activities/Nutrition/SummaryDRIs/DRI-Tables.aspx. Accessed September 13, 2016.

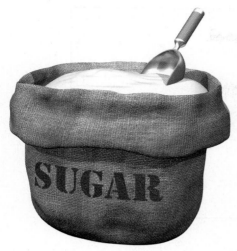

Consume less than 10% of calories per day from added sugars.

©Paul Fleet/Shutterstock

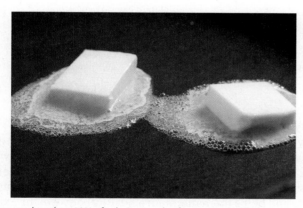

Consume less than 10% of calories per day from saturated fats.

©Kulinarni studio Bauermedia/Profimedia.CZ a.s./Alamy Stock Photo

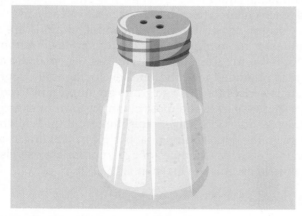

Consume less than 2,300 mg per day of sodium.

©Vasilyevalara/iStock / Getty Images Plus/Getty

Figure 9.6

Key Recommendations for Diet Components that Should Be Limited in Children and Adolescents.

U.S. Department of Health and Human Services and U.S. Department of Agriculture. *2015–2020 Dietary Guidelines for Americans*. 8th ed. Washington, DC: U.S. Department of Health and Human Services and U.S. Department of Agriculture; December 2015. Retrieved from: http://health.gov/dietaryguidelines/2015/guidelines/. Accessed August 13, 2016.

Recap Children and preadolescents need the same nutrients during this stage of life as all other life stages, just in different amounts. Caloric intake should not exceed what is needed to support normal growth and development. To meet their nutritional needs, children should eat a variety of foods to reach the RDAs for each nutrient while staying within the recommended AMDRs for their age group. The *Dietary Guidelines for Americans* and MyPlate are helpful in guiding healthy food choices.

1. Define the four dietary reference intakes values.
2. Explain different methods for calculating energy needs.

Food and Nutrition Programs and Physical Activity

Preview In addition to food choices in childhood and preadolescence, physical activity plays an important role in shaping healthy habits into adulthood. Schools have a large influence on children's health habits. Programs such as Let's Move!, school breakfast and lunch programs, and physical education are designed to teach children healthy habits.

Federal Nutrition Assistance Programs

The **National School Lunch Program (NSLP)** and **National School Breakfast Program (NBLP)** are federal food assistance programs that support school meals for children in high school or younger. These are only two of many programs funded by the Food and Nutrition Services division of the USDA. The NSLP started providing school lunches under the National School Lunch Act in 1946, and the NSBP started providing school breakfast meals in 1975 in schools and child care institutions. Another benefit of the programs is that they provide snacks and summer meals, which are served after school during educational and enrichment programs and in the summer when school is not in session.[46]

In 2012, NSLP served 31 million lunches, and the NSBP serviced 12.9 million children. Total school lunch participation increased from 28.9 million students on an average day in the 2003–2004 school year to an all-time high of 31.8 million in 2010–2011, and then dropped to 30.3 million in 2013–2014 (FIGURE 9.7).[47]

For a student to receive the benefits, families can qualify for free or reduced meals based on household income (TABLE 9.7).[46] Schools receive cash reimbursement for USDA foods for the meals they serve in the program.[46] (See TABLE 9.8 .) Schools need the support of federally funded programs because increasing food costs limit their ability to provide nutritious food without help. Lunches served by schools participating in the NSLP and NSBP must meet minimum nutritional requirements on

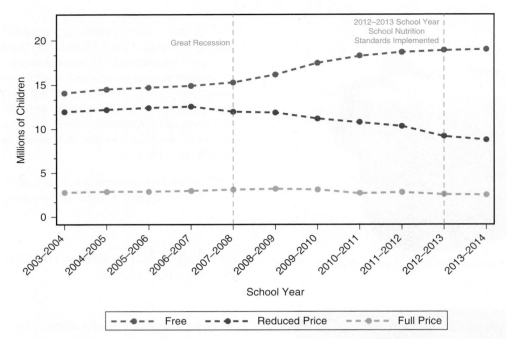

Figure 9.7
Average daily participation in the National School Lunch Program (NSLP).

U.S. Department of Agriculture Food and Nutrition Service.

<table>
<tr><td colspan="2">

Table 9.7

</td></tr>
</table>

Annual Household Income to Qualify for Free and Reduced Meals in the National School Lunch and National School Breakfast Programs

Program	Qualified Income Level
Free Lunch/Breakfast	<130% poverty level
Reduced Lunch/Breakfast	130–185% poverty level

Reproduced from U.S. Department of Agriculture; September 2013. National School Lunch Program [fact sheet]. Retrieved from: http://www.fns.usda.gov/sites/default/files/NSLPFactSheet.pdf. Accessed December 2015.

the basis of tested nutritional research. The meal requirements are shown in **TABLE 9.9** .[48]

Another program created by the USDA as part of the Healthy, Hunger-Free Act of 2010 is the Smart Snacks in Schools. This program restricts the types of food and drinks schools can serve to children at school. The act requires that foods be **nutrient-dense** snacks and drinks. Elementary schools can serve 8-ounce portions of milk and juice. Drinks they can serve are plain water, unflavored low-fat milk, unflavored or flavored fat-free milk, 100% fruit or vegetable juice, and 100% fruit or vegetable juice diluted with water and no added sweeteners. Snacks must be whole grains, fruits, vegetables, dairy products, proteins, a combination food that contains ¼ cup of fruit or vegetable or that contains 10% the Daily Value (DV) of calcium, potassium, vitamin D, or dietary fiber. Additional restrictions for snacks and entrees of calories, sodium, total fat, saturated fat, trans fat, and sugar must be met.[49]

Physical Activity

Physical activity is an important part of maintaining a healthy body in preadolescents. Physical activity improves the health of children's emotional state, musculoskeletal system, cardiovascular system, and neuromuscular awareness and helps them maintain a healthy body weight. Exercise also prevents diseases such as cancer, diabetes, and heart disease.[50] In reality, physical activity decreases from childhood to adulthood; therefore, it is crucial to promote and teach children to maintain active at an early age.[51]

Current physical activity recommendations are 60 minutes or more of physical activity per day.[52] Aerobic, **strength training**, and **bone-strengthening exercises** are all recommended for children. Developmentally appropriate exercises for this age group are important to consider. Active play is the most common form of exercise in the preadolescent stage![52] It is important that children are given the opportunity for active play, including a safe place for activity. Examples of age-appropriate exercises for preadolescents are listed in **TABLE 9.10** .

Let's Move

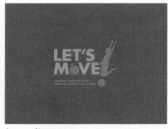

Courtesy of Letsmove.gov

Table 9.8

Reimbursement to Schools

School Programs Meal, Snack, and Milk Payments to States and School Food Authorities (expressed in dollars or fractions thereof; effective from July 1, 2016–June 30, 2017)

National School Lunch Program[1]		Less Than 60%	Less Than 60% + 6 Cents[2]	60% or More	60% or More + 6 Cents[2]	Maximum Rate	Maximum Rate + 6 Cents[2]
Contiguous states	Paid	0.30	0.36	0.32	0.38	0.38	0.44
	Reduced price	2.76	2.82	2.78	2.84	2.93	2.99
	Free	3.16	3.22	3.18	3.24	3.33	3.39
Alaska	Paid	0.49	0.55	0.51	0.57	0.60	0.66
	Reduced price	4.72	4.78	4.74	4.80	4.98	5.02
	Free	5.12	5.18	5.14	5.20	5.38	5.44
Hawaii	Paid	0.35	0.41	0.37	0.43	0.44	0.50
	Reduced price	3.29	3.35	3.31	3.37	3.49	3.55
	Free	3.69	3.75	3.71	3.77	3.89	3.95
Puerto Rico[3]	Paid	0.35	0.41	0.37	0.43	0.44	0.50
	Reduced price	3.29	3.35	3.31	3.37	3.49	3.55
	Free	3.69	3.75	3.71	3.77	3.89	3.95

School Breakfast Program		Nonsevere Need	Severe Need
Contiguous states	Paid	0.29	0.29
	Reduced price	1.41	1.74
	Free	1.71	2.04
Alaska	Paid	0.44	0.44
	Reduced price	2.43	2.98
	Free	2.73	3.27
Hawaii	Paid	0.33	0.33
	Reduced price	1.69	2.08
	Free	1.99	2.38
Puerto Rico[3]	Paid	0.33	0.33
	Reduced price	1.69	2.08
	Free	1.99	2.38

Special Milk Program	All Milk	Paid Milk	Free Milk
Pricing programs without free option	0.1975	N/A	N/A
Pricing programs with free option	N/A	0.1975	Average cost per ½ pint of milk
Nonpricing programs	0.1975	N/A	N/A

After-School Snacks Served in After-School Care Programs		
Contiguous states	Paid	0.07
	Reduced price	0.43
	Free	0.86
Alaska	Paid	0.12
	Reduced price	0.70
	Free	1.40
Hawaii	Paid	0.09
	Reduced price	0.50
	Free	1.01
Puerto Rico[3]	Paid	0.09
	Reduced price	0.50
	Free	1.01

[1] Payment listed for Free and Reduced Price Lunches include both section 4 and section 11 funds.

[2] Performance-based cash reimbursement (adjusted annually for inflation).

[3] Beginning July 1, 2016, FNS approved Puerto Rico to receive a 17% increase in school meal reimbursement rates.

Reproduced from USDA Food and Nutrition Service. National School Programs: meal, snack and milk payments to states and school food authorities (July 1, 2016 – June 30, 2017). Retrieved from: http://www.fns.usda.gov/sites/default/files/cn/SY2015-16table.pdf. Accessed September 20, 2016.

Table 9.9

Required Meal Patterns for the National School Lunch Program and National School Breakfast Program

Meal Pattern	Breakfast Meal Pattern			Lunch Meal Pattern		
	Grades K–5[a]	Grades 6–8[a]	Grades 9–12[a]	Grades K–5	Grades 6–8	Grades 9–12
	Amount of food[b] per week (minimum per day)					
Fruits (cups)[c,d]	5 (1)[e]	5 (1)[e]	5 (1)[e]	2½ (½)	2½ (½)	5 (1)
Vegetables (cups)[c,d]	0	0	0	3¾ (¾)	3¾ (¾)	5 (1)
Dark green[f]	0	0	0	½	½	½
Red/orange[f]	0	0	0	¾	¾	1¼
Beans/peas (legumes)[f]	0	0	0	½	½	½
Starchy[f]	0	0	0	½	½	½
Other[g]	0	0	0	½	½	¾
Additional veg to reach total[h]	0	0	0	1	1	1½
Grains (oz eq)[i]	7–10 (1)[j]	8–10[l] (1)[j]	9–10[l] (1)[j]	8–9 (1)	8–9 (1)	10–12 (2)
Meats/meat alternates (oz eq)	0[k]	0[k]	0[k]	8–10 (1)	9–10 (1)	10–12 (2)
Fluid milk (cups)[l]	5 (1)	5 (1)	5 (1)	5 (1)	5 (1)	5 (1)
Other Specifications: Daily Amount Based on the Average for a 5-Day Week						
Min-max calories (kcal)[m,n,o]	350–500	400–550	450–600	550–650	600–700	750–850
Saturated fat (% of total calories)[n,o]	<10	<10	<10	<10	<10	<10
Sodium (mg)[n,p]	≤430	≤470	≤500	≤640	≤710	≤740
Trans fat[n,o]	Nutrition label or manufacturer specifications must indicate 0 g of trans fat per serving.					

[a] In the SBP, the above age–grade groups are required beginning July 1, 2013 (SY 2103–14). In SY 2012–2013 only, schools may continue to use the meal patterns for grades K–12 (see §220.23).

[b] Food items included in each food group and subgroup and amount equivalents. Minimum creditable serving is 1/8 cup.

[c] One quarter-cup of dried fruit counts as 1/2 cup of fruit; 1 cup of leafy greens counts as 1/2 cup of vegetables. No more than half of the fruit or vegetable offerings may be in the form of juice. All juice must be 100% full strength.

[d] For breakfast, vegetables may be substituted for fruits, but the first 2 cups per week of any such substitution must be from the dark green, red/orange, beans and peas (legumes), or "Other vegetables" subgroups as defined in § 210.10(c)(2)(iii).

[e] The fruit quantity requirement for the SBP (5 cups/week and a minimum of 1 cup/day) is effective July 1, 2014 (SY 2014–2015).

[f] Larger amounts of these vegetables may be served.

[g] This category consists of "Other vegetables" as defined in § 210.10(c)(2)(iii)(E). For the purposes of the NSLP, "Other vegetables" requirement may be met with any additional amounts from the dark green, red/orange, and beans/peas (legumes) vegetable subgroups as defined in § 210.10(c)(2)(iii).

[h] Any vegetable subgroup may be offered to meet the total weekly vegetable requirement.

[i] At least half of the grains offered must be whole grain-rich in the NSLP beginning July 1, 2012 (SY 2012–2013), and in the SBP beginning July 1, 2013 (SY 2013–2014). All grains must be whole grain-rich in both the NSLP and the SBP beginning July 1, 2014 (SY 2014–15).

[j] In the SBP, the grain ranges must be offered beginning July 1, 2013 (SY 2013–2014).

[k] There is no separate meat/meat alternate component in the SBP. Beginning July 1, 2013 (SY 2013–2014), schools may substitute 1 oz. eq. of meat/meat alternate for 1 oz. eq. of grains after the minimum daily grains requirement is met.

[l] Fluid milk must be low-fat (1 percent milk fat or less, unflavored) or fat-free (unflavored or flavored).

[m] The average daily amount of calories for a 5-day school week must be within the range (at least the minimum and no more than the maximum values).

[n] Discretionary sources of calories (solid fats and added sugars) may be added to the meal pattern if within the specifications for calories, saturated fat, trans fat, and sodium. Foods of minimal nutritional value and fluid milk with fat content greater than 1% milk fat are not allowed.

[o] In the SBP, calories and trans fat specifications take effect beginning July 1, 2013 (SY 2013–2014).

[p] Final sodium specifications are to be reached by SY 2022–2023 or July 1, 2022. Intermediate sodium specifications are established for SY 2014–2015 and 2017–2018. See required intermediate specifications in § 210.10(f)(3) for lunches and § 220.8(f)(3) for breakfasts.

Reproduced from U.S. Department of Agriculture Food and Nutrition Service. Nutrition standards in the National School Lunch and School Breakfast Programs. *Federal Register.* January 26, 2012;77(17):4102. Retrieved from: https://www.gpo.gov/fdsys/pkg/FR-2012-01-26/pdf/2012-1010.pdf. Accessed September 21, 2016.

Let's Discuss

The recommendation for physical activity is 60 minutes per day. Do you think U.S. children and preadolescents are meeting the daily physical activity recommendation? Why or why not?

Let's Move! is a federal program focusing on reducing and preventing childhood obesity. The goal of the program is to "Solve the problem of childhood obesity within a generation." The program focuses on a multiperson approach and on five pillars recommended by the Let's Move Initiative, as shown in **FIGURE 9.8** .[53]

Getting children a healthy start on life

- With good prenatal care for their parents; support for breastfeeding; adherence to limits on "screen time"; and quality child care settings with nutritious food and ample opportunity for young children to be physically active.

Empowering parents and caregivers

- With simpler, more actionable messages about nutritional choices based on the latest *Dietary Guidelines for Americans*; improved labels on food and menus that provide clear information to help make healthy choices for children; reduced marketing of unhealthy products to children; and improved health care services, including BMI measurement for all children.

Providing healthy food in schools

- Through improvements in federally-supported school lunches and breakfasts; upgrading the nutritional quality of other foods sold in schools; and improving nutrition education and the overall school environment.

Improving access to healthy, affordable foods

- By eliminating "food deserts" in urban and rural America; lowering the relative prices of healthier foods; developing or reformulating food products to be healthier; and reducing the incidence of hunger, which has been likened to obesity.

Getting children more physically active

- Through quality physical education, recess, and other opportunities in and after school; addressing aspects of the "built environment" that make it difficult for children to walk or bike safely in their communities; and improving access to safe parks, playgrounds, and indoor and outdoor recreational facilities.

Figure 9.8
Five-pillar approach to the Let's Move! initiative.

Modified from White House Task Force on Childhood Obesity. Letsmove.gov. America's Move to Raise A Healthier Generation of Kids | Let's Move!. 2015. Retrieved from: http://www.letsmove.gov/about. Accessed December 18, 2015.

Table 9.10

Types of Physical Activity, Recommendations, and Examples of Exercises for Children

Aerobic Activity	Strength Activity	Bone Strengthening
Most of physical activity each day	At least 3 days per week	At least 3 days per week
Moderate activity: brisk walking, dancing, skateboarding, martial arts, etc.	Play on jungle gyms, climb trees, gymnastics, etc.	Running, jump rope, hop scotch, skipping, etc.
Vigorous activity: running, bicycle riding, games, jumping rope, swimming, soccer, etc.		

Modified from Centers for Disease Control and Prevention; updated June 4, 2015. How much physical activity do children need? Retrieved from: http://www.cdc.gov/physicalactivity/basics/children/. Accessed September 14, 2016.

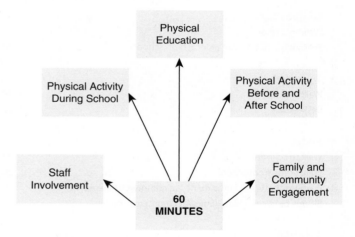

Figure 9.9
Comprehensive school physical activity program.

Reproduced from Centers for Disease Control and Prevention; updated September 25, 2015. Healthy schools: Comprehensive School Physical Activity Program (CSPAP). Retrieved from: http://www.cdc.gov/healthyschools/physicalactivity/cspap.htm. Accessed December 2015.

Physical Education

Physical education (PE) is required in most states. The frequency and duration varies by state, school, and grade level. Health-related PE provides educational opportunities for students to learn about health and wellness. Schools can make time to promote these healthy practices (**FIGURE 9.9**).[54]

Recess, intramurals, well-designed playgrounds and other school programs can provide opportunities to meet the 60-minutes-per-day recommendation for physical activity. The majority of elementary schools provide recess, which is an excellent time for students to be physically active. However, not all schools provide an environment that allows for this activity.[54]

Let's Discuss

Children and preadolescents require 60 minutes of physical activity per day. One way to incorporate more daily physical activity is with after-school programs. Brainstorm ideas for more opportunities for after-school physical activities. Remember to keep it age appropriate and fun!

Case Study

How can Peter meet his physical activity goals?

Below is an example of how Peter can meet 60 minutes of activity per day, including bone-strengthening and strength training exercises 3 days per week. To start, Peter can walk to and from school some days of the week. This adds a moderate activity of brisk walking. He has been going to basketball 1 day per week, but his mom can sign him up to go twice per week. This adds a whole extra hour of vigorous physical activity per week. In addition, the local high school is offering open swim. He attends open swim after school with his siblings on Wednesdays. Outside of scheduled after-school activities, Peter can incorporate some strength training exercises during video games or commercial breaks. Adding fun activities that are active such as playing outside with friends and siblings is the last change Peter can make to meet his physical activity goals as well as have fun!

Activity	Amount of Time	Type of Activity
Monday		
Basketball	60 minutes	Aerobic
Walk to school	20 minutes	Aerobic
	Total = 80 minutes	
Tuesday		
Walk to school	20 minutes	Aerobic
Walk home from school	20 minutes	Aerobic
Jumping jacks between video games/at commercial breaks	20 minutes	Aerobic and bone strengthening
	Total = 60 minutes	
Wednesday		
Walk to school	20 minutes	Aerobic
Swimming: open swim at local high school	40 minutes	Aerobic
	Total = 60 minutes	
Thursday		
Walk to school	20 minutes	Aerobic
Basketball	60 minutes	Aerobic
	Total = 80 minutes	
Friday		
Walk to school	20 minutes	Aerobic
Walk home from school	20 minutes	Aerobic
Push-ups between video games/at commercial breaks	10 minutes	Strength
Sit-ups between video games/at commercial breaks	10 minutes	Strength
	Total = 60 minutes	
Saturday		
Jump rope at home	20 minutes	Aerobic and bone strengthening
Skateboard or rollerblade outside with friends	40 minutes	Aerobic
	Total = 60 minutes	
Sunday		
Bike ride with siblings or friends	45 minutes	Aerobic
Push-ups between video games/at commercial breaks	15 minutes	Strength
	Total = 60 minutes	

MyPlate

The current food guidance visual, **MyPlate**, separates foods into five groups: fruit, vegetables, grains, protein, and dairy, and places them on a "plate." The simple visual represents the proportion of the food groups that make up a healthy meal. The diagram has been modified to visually appeal to kids and is part of the many child-specific tools and resources the USDA offers (FIGURE 9.10). The website offers games, videos, songs, and activities for kids older than preschool age.[43] Key messages of MyPlate Kids' Place are shown in TABLE 9.11 .

MyPlate Kids' Place

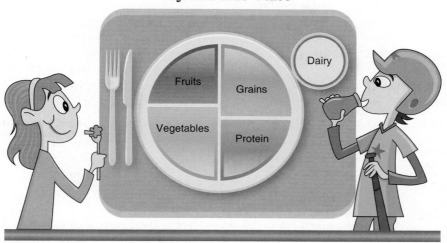

Figure 9.10
MyPlate Kids' Place.

Reproduced from U.S. Department of Agriculture. Choose MyPlate. Retrieved from: http://www.choosemyplate.gov/MyPlate. Accessed January 5, 2016.

Case Study

Today in school Peter learned about MyPlate and the *Dietary Guidelines for Americans*. He went home and asked his mom to help him set some goals for himself. Peter and his mom want to figure out the following using the MyPlate My Daily Food Plan (**FIGURE 9.11**):

1. How many servings of fruits and vegetables does Peter need to try to eat per day?
2. How many servings of dairy does Peter need to eat per day?
3. Peter eats only two vegetables. What can you do to help him vary his vegetable intake?

My Daily Food Plan

Based on the information you provided, this is your daily recommended amount for each food group.

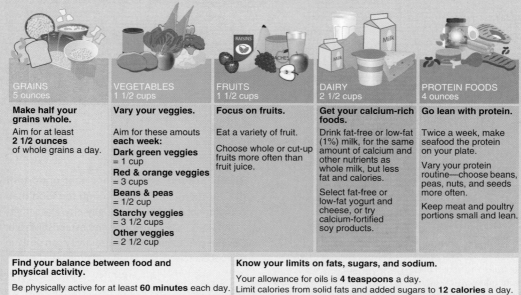

GRAINS 5 ounces	VEGETABLES 1 1/2 cups	FRUITS 1 1/2 cups	DAIRY 2 1/2 cups	PROTEIN FOODS 4 ounces
Make half your grains whole. Aim for at least **2 1/2 ounces** of whole grains a day.	**Vary your veggies.** Aim for these amouts **each week:** **Dark green veggies** = 1 cup **Red & orange veggies** = 3 cups **Beans & peas** = 1/2 cup **Starchy veggies** = 3 1/2 cups **Other veggies** = 2 1/2 cup	**Focus on fruits.** Eat a variety of fruit. Choose whole or cut-up fruits more often than fruit juice.	**Get your calcium-rich foods.** Drink fat-free or low-fat (1%) milk, for the same amount of calcium and other nutrients as whole milk, but less fat and calories. Select fat-free or low-fat yogurt and cheese, or try calcium-fortified soy products.	**Go lean with protein.** Twice a week, make seafood the protein on your plate. Vary your protein routine—choose beans, peas, nuts, and seeds more often. Keep meat and poultry portions small and lean.

Find your balance between food and physical activity.

Be physically active for at least **60 minutes** each day.

Know your limits on fats, sugars, and sodium.

Your allowance for oils is **4 teaspoons** a day.
Limit calories from solid fats and added sugars to **12 calories** a day.
Reduce sodium intake to less than **2300 mg** a day.

Your results are based on a 1400 calorie pattern.   Name:_____

This calorie level is only an estimate of your needs, Monitor your body weight to see if you need to adjust your calorie intake.

Figure 9.11
MyPlate Food Plan for Peter.

Reproduced from U.S. Department of Agriculture. Choose MyPlate. Retrieved from: http://www.choosemyplate.gov/MyPlate. Accessed January 5, 2016.

4. How many minutes of physical activity per day does Peter need?

5. Peter does not meet his physical activity goal currently. Name some ideas to help him achieve this goal.

Peter can use the following worksheet (**FIGURE 9.12**) to track whether he is meeting his goals for food and physical activity. In addition, Peter can track how he is feeling each day and set goals for the next. Why not make it a family affair? Peter's mom and sister now also want to create their own customized My Daily Food Plan!

My Daily Food Plan Worksheet

Check how you did today and set a goal to aim for tomorrow.

Write In Your Food Choices for Today	Food Group	Tip	Based on a 1400 Calorie Pattern. Your Goals Are:	Match Your Food Choices with Each Food Group	Estimate Your Total
_____ _____ _____	GRAINS	Make at least half your grains whole grains.	**5 ounce equivalents** (1 ounce equivalent is about 1 slice bread; 1 ounce ready-to-eat cereal; or ½ cup cooked rice, pasta, or cereal.)	_____ _____ _____	ounce equivalents
_____ _____ _____	VEGETABLES	Aim for variety every day; pick vegetables form several subgroups: dark green, red & orange, beans & peas, starchy, and other veggies.	**1 ½ cups** (1 cup is 1 cup raw or cooked vegetables, 2 cups leafy salad greens, or 1 cup 100% vegetable juice.)	_____ _____ _____	cups
_____ _____ _____	FRUITS	Select fresh, frozen, canned, and dried fruit more often than juice.	**1 ½ cups** (1 cup is 1 cup raw or cooked fruit, ½ cup dried fruit, or 1 cup 100% fruit juice.)	_____ _____ _____	cups
_____ _____ _____	DAIRY	Include fat-free and low-fat dairy foods every day.	**2 ½ cups** (1 cup is 1 cup milk, yogurt, or fortified soy beverage; 1 ½ ounces natural cheese; or 2 ounces processed cheese.)	_____ _____ _____	cups
_____ _____ _____	PROTEIN FOODS	Aim for variety—choose seafood, lean meat & poultry, beans, peas, nuts, and seeds each week.	**4 ounce equivalents** (1 ounce equivalent is 1 ounce lean meat, poultry, or seafood; 1 egg; 1 Tbsp peanut butter; ¼ cup cooked beans or peas; or ½ ounce nuts or seeds.)	_____ _____ _____	ounce equivalents
_____ _____ _____	PHYSICAL ACTIVITY	Be active every day. Choose activities that you like and fit into your life.	Be physically active for at least **60 minutes** each day.	Some foods and drinks, such as sodas, cakes, cookies, donuts, ice cream, and candy, are high in fats and sugars. Limit your intake of these.	minutes

How did you do today? ☐ Great   ☐ So-So   ☐ Not So Great

My food goal for tomorrow is: _____

My activity goal for tomorrow is: _____

Figure 9.12
MyPlate Daily Food Plan worksheet.

Reproduced from U.S. Department of Agriculture. Choose MyPlate. Retrieved from: http://www.choosemyplate.gov/MyPlate. Accessed January 5, 2016.

Table 9.11

MyPlate Key Messages

Balancing Calories

- Enjoy your food, but eat less.
- Avoid oversized portions.

Foods to Increase

- Make half your plate fruits and vegetables.
- Make at least half your grains whole grains.
- Switch to fat-free or low-fat (1%) milk.

Foods to Reduce

- Compare sodium in foods like soup, bread, and frozen meals and choose foods with lower numbers.
- Drink water instead of sugary drinks.

Reproduced from U.S. Department of Agriculture. Choose MyPlate. Retrieved from: http://www.choosemyplate.gov/MyPlate. Accessed January 5, 2016.

Recap Schools offer an important opportunity to improve the nutrition of children through the food that is offered and educational opportunities. Daily physical activity is essential to maintaining a healthy body and establishing a healthy lifestyle. Developmentally appropriate activity can be a fun and engaging form of exercise for children and preadolescents. Food plans such as MyPlate Kids' Place are a helpful resource to aid children and adolescents in food choices and meal planning.

1. Explain why physical activity is important to preadolescents.
2. Discuss the importance of regular physical activity.
3. List the benefits of school nutrition programs.
4. Summarize the key features of the Let's Move! campaign.
5. Describe the unique recommendations for children ages 6–9 of the MyPlate program.

Let's Move! Turns 5 … Is It Working?

The Let's Move campaign to tackle childhood obesity turned 5 years old in 2015. The White House Task Force on Childhood Obesity came about as part of the Let's Move campaign, and its goal is to reduce obesity within a generation. Recently, the task force put together 170 recommendations to reach that goal.

Question

1. Do the White House and the Let's Move campaign have the power to create the change we need to improve pediatric obesity rates?

References

a. Barnes, M. Take a look at our action plan to solve the problem of childhood obesity. White House blog; May 11, 2010. Retrieved from: https://www.whitehouse.gov/blog/2010/05/10/take-a-look-our-action-plan-solve-problem-childhood-obesity. Accessed September 13, 2016.

b. White House Task Force on Childhood Obesity report to the president, last updated February 2011. Let's Move! Retrieved from: http://www.letsmove.gov/white-house-task-force-childhood-obesity-report-president. Accessed September 13, 2016.

Common Nutritional Considerations During Childhood and Preadolescence

Preview Many nutrition considerations for the preadolescent stage are unique to this age group. These habits will set the stage for a healthy body through adulthood. Dental caries is a preventable disease that can be avoided with proper oral health. Proper oral health includes avoiding sugar-sweetened beverages, which are detrimental not only to teeth but also to the whole body of a child. Proper vitamin D and calcium intake builds a strong bone structure through adulthood.

Oral Health

Primary teeth fall out and are replaced by permanent teeth generally between the ages of 7 and 13 years. It is important for long-term health that primary teeth are kept healthy during the childhood stage and that permanent teeth are kept healthy during the preadolescent stage (FIGURE 9.13 and FIGURE 9.14). Proper oral care and nutrition can keep children's teeth healthy (TABLE 9.12). Many factors affect tooth decay (TABLE 9.13), including a balanced, healthy diet. The type, form, and frequency of foods and beverages consumed have a direct effect on oral health. Fermentable carbohydrates are metabolized in the mouth by bacteria, in turn decaying teeth.[55] The

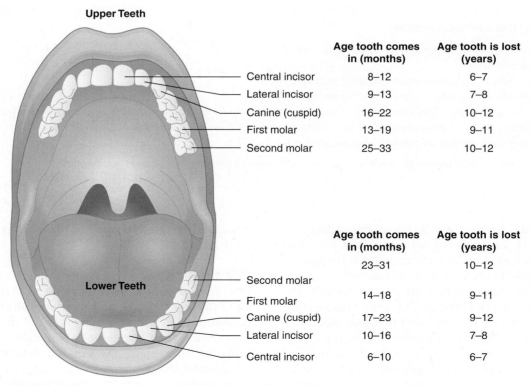

Upper Teeth

	Age tooth comes in (months)	Age tooth is lost (years)
Central incisor	8–12	6–7
Lateral incisor	9–13	7–8
Canine (cuspid)	16–22	10–12
First molar	13–19	9–11
Second molar	25–33	10–12

Lower Teeth

	Age tooth comes in (months)	Age tooth is lost (years)
Second molar	23–31	10–12
First molar	14–18	9–11
Canine (cuspid)	17–23	9–12
Lateral incisor	10–16	7–8
Central incisor	6–10	6–7

Figure 9.13
Primary teeth eruption chart.

Data from Mouth Healthy. Eruption charts. Retrieved from: http://www.mouthhealthy.org/en/az-topics/e/eruption-charts. Accessed September 14, 2016.

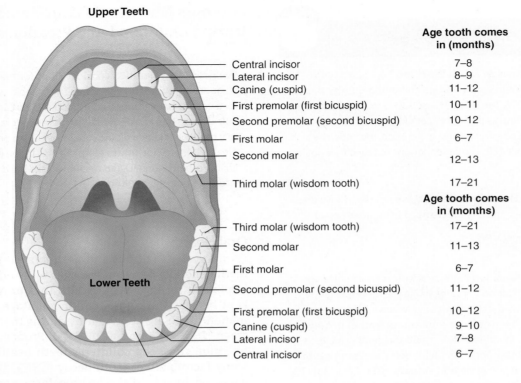

	Age tooth comes in (months)
Upper Teeth	
Central incisor	7–8
Lateral incisor	8–9
Canine (cuspid)	11–12
First premolar (first bicuspid)	10–11
Second premolar (second bicuspid)	10–12
First molar	6–7
Second molar	12–13
Third molar (wisdom tooth)	17–21

	Age tooth comes in (months)
Third molar (wisdom tooth)	17–21
Second molar	11–13
First molar	6–7
Second premolar (second bicuspid)	11–12
First premolar (first bicuspid)	10–12
Canine (cuspid)	9–10
Lateral incisor	7–8
Central incisor	6–7
Lower Teeth	

Figure 9.14
Permanent teeth eruption chart.

Data from Mouth Healthy. Eruption charts. Retrieved from: http://www.mouthhealthy.org/en/az-topics/e/eruption-charts. Accessed September 14, 2016.

Table 9.12

Tips for Keeping Preteens' Teeth Healthy

Always brush your teeth twice a day with fluoride toothpaste for 2 minutes.

Floss between your teeth daily.

Avoid sugary and starchy snacks such as soda, potato chips, and candy.

Wear a mouthguard when you're playing sports or other recreational activities.

Stay away from tobacco. Cigarettes, cigars, and chewing tobacco all increase your risk for tobacco-related health problems. They also give you bad breath!

Don't pierce your lips or any part of your mouth because you could crack a tooth or worse if part of the jewelry breaks off in your mouth.

See your dentist. Regular dental visits will help set you up to be Mouth Healthy for Life.

Modified from Mouth Healthy Kids. For preteens. Retrieved from: http://www.mouthhealthykids.org/en/preteens/. Accessed December 2015.

American Dental Association (ADA) recommends that children should limit sugary beverages and snacking between meals and should brush their teeth frequently, at least twice per day to prevent tooth decay.[56]

Nutrient deficiencies can affect oral health (see **TABLE 9.14**). Fluoride, calcium, and vitamin D are essential vitamins and minerals for tooth mineralization and enamel formation. Nutrition intake affects the development, maintenance, and repair of the teeth and oral tissues, which is imperative to general health in childhood and preadolescence. Dental caries are preventable; therefore, it is important to promote and educate preadolescents on good oral care at a young age. An

example of age-appropriate promotion of good oral health is in **FIGURE 9.15** .

Bone Health

Muscle and bone growth is rapid in this stage of life. Optimal bone growth and development are important to maintain health and movement of the human body over the life span. The essential functions of bones in the body are for support, movement, protection, blood cell production, calcium storage, and endocrine regulation.[57] Keeping bones, including teeth, healthy in the childhood and adolescent stages sets the stage for healthy adulthood.

Table 9.13

Dietary Factors and Eating Patterns Associated with Dental Caries Risk

Dietary factors that increase risk of dental caries

- Sugar-sweetened beverages, such as soda, fruit drinks, sports drinks, and sweetened teas and coffees
- Sticky foods, such as dried fruit
- Sticky and slowly dissolving candies, such as chewing gum, taffy, and lollipops
- Sugary starchy snacks and desserts, such as cookies, cakes, etc.
- Simple sugars added to foods such as white sugar, brown sugar, and honey

Dietary factors that lower risk of dental caries

- Sugar-free candy and chewing gum
- Fresh fruits and vegetables
- Unprocessed foods with high-quality protein, such as meat, fish, poultry, eggs, milk, cheese, beans, and legumes
- Whole grains such as wild rice, quinoa, kamut, farro, and wheatberries
- Whole-grain breads, grains, and cereals made with minimal sugar
- Beverages that contain no sugar such as unflavored water

Eating patterns that increase risk of dental caries

- Frequently eating foods rich in simple sugars
- Eating sticky foods alone and those that stay in the mouth a prolonged time
- Prolonged sipping of sugar-sweetened beverages

Eating patterns that lower risk of dental caries

- Food and beverage consumption is spaced out with least 2 hours between eating/drinking events
- Choosing fresh, whole, unprocessed/minimally processed foods to stimulate salivary output
- Brushing teeth or chewing sugarless gum immediately after a meal or snack
- Being well hydrated and drinking fluoridated water

Modified from Touger-Decker R, Mobley C; Academy of Nutrition and Dietetics. Position of the Academy of Nutrition and Dietetics: oral health and nutrition. *J Acad Nutr Diet.* 2013;113(5):693–701. http://www.eatrightpro.org/~/media/eatrightpro%20files/practice/position%20and%20practice%20papers/position%20papers/oral-health-and-nutrition-final-paper.ashx. Accessed September 13, 2016.

Bones go through a remodeling process in which they continually lose calcium that needs to be replaced. If the body does not supply enough calcium to replace what is lost, bones become weakened.[57] The body can build up calcium stores in the bones at an early age to prevent future calcium deficiency, in turn creating healthier and stronger bones. Maintaining healthy bones is essential for health at older ages. The DRI for calcium for ages 4–8 years is 1000 mg per day.[41] According to a study in 2010 based on National Health and Nutrition Examination Survey (NHANES) data, children in this age group met their calcium needs through diet and supplements.[58]

Vitamin D

Optimal bone growth and development not only depend on calcium but also require adequate intake of vitamin D. Vitamin D is a fat-soluble vitamin that is naturally present in very few foods, added to others, available as a dietary supplement, and synthesized as sunlight strikes the skin.[59] Vitamin D is a nutrient of particular concern

Table 9.14

Nutrient Deficiencies that Affect Dental Caries

Nutrient	Effect on Tissue	Effect on Caries
Protein-calorie malnutrition	Delayed tooth eruption, decreased tooth size and enamel solubility, salivary gland deficiency	Yes
Calcium, vitamin D and phosphorus	Hypomineralization, compromised tooth integrity, delayed eruption patterns	Yes
Vitamin A deficiency	Decreased epithelial tissue development, tooth morphogenesis dysfunction, decreased odontoblast differentiation, increased enamel hypoplasia, hypomineralization, compromised tooth integrity	Yes
Vitamin C deficiency	Dental pulpal alterations, odontoblastic degeneration, aberrant dentition	No
Iodine deficiency	Delayed tooth eruption, altered growth patterns, malocclusions	No
Iron deficiency	Slow growth, salivary gland dysfunction	Yes
Fluoride presence	Increased stability of enamel crystal, inhibition of demineralization, stimulation of remineralization, mottled enamel (excess)	Yes

Data from Touger-Decker R, Ragassio Radler D, Depaola DP. Nutrition and Dental Medicine. In Ross AC, Caballero B, Cousins R. et al. eds. *Modern Nutrition in Health and Disease.* 11th ed. Baltimore MD: Lippincott Williams & Wilkins; 2014:Table 73.2.

The Big Picture

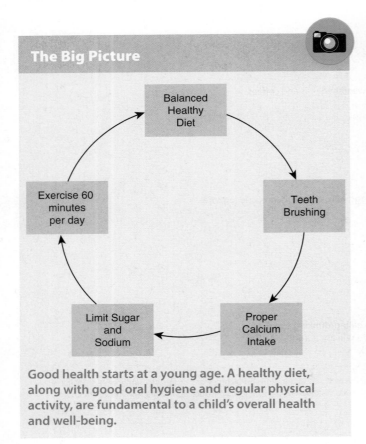

Good health starts at a young age. A healthy diet, along with good oral hygiene and regular physical activity, are fundamental to a child's overall health and well-being.

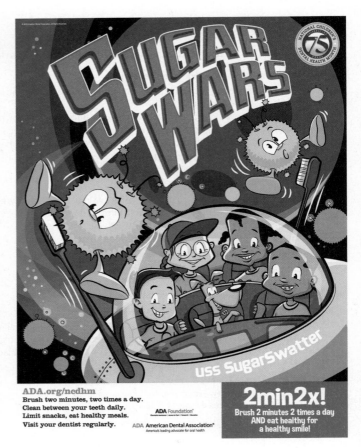

ADA.org/ncdhm
Brush two minutes, two times a day.
Clean between your teeth daily.
Limit snacks, eat healthy meals.
Visit your dentist regularly.

2min2x!
Brush 2 minutes 2 times a day
AND eat healthy for
a healthy smile!

Figure 9.15
Age-appropriate oral health promotion.

for preadolescents because deficiency is common and can compromise adequate bone health. The vital role of vitamin D in bone health became evident as researchers studied the prevention of rickets. Previously, the National Academy of Science and Institute of Medicine established the RDA for vitamin D as from sun, diet, or supplements, to reliably prevent rickets in almost any child.[60] More recently, the RDA for vitamin D represents a daily intake that is sufficient to maintain bone health and normal calcium metabolism in healthy people.[59] **TABLE 9.15** lists the Recommended Dietary Allowances for vitamin D for infants through preadolescents.

Vitamin D promotes calcium absorption in the gut and maintains adequate serum calcium and phosphate concentrations to enable normal mineralization of bone. Without sufficient vitamin D, bones can become thin, brittle, or misshapen. In addition to bone health, because

vitamin D can act as a hormone as well, it is involved in other aspects of health. Vitamin D has a role in cell growth, neuromuscular and immune function, and reduction of inflammation.[59]

Preadolescents can meet their vitamin D requirements through diet, sunlight, and supplements. Vitamin D is not common in the food supply, and because of this more foods have begun to be fortified. The flesh of fatty fish, fish liver oils, beef, liver, cheese, and eggs yolks all contain varying amounts of natural vitamin D. Almost all of the U.S. milk supply is voluntarily fortified with 100 IU per 1 cup. Ready-to-eat breakfast cereals often contain added vitamin D as do some brands of orange juice, yogurt, and margarine. Time spent in the sun can also provide some of the needed amounts of vitamin D for preadolescents. Research suggests approximately 5–30 minutes of sun exposure to the face, arms, legs, or back without sunscreen between 10 a.m. and 3 p.m. at least twice a week usually leads to sufficient vitamin D synthesis.[59] Currently, the American Academy of Pediatrics recommends supplementation only for exclusively breastfed infants, but it is suggested that preadolescents who do not consume 400 IU of vitamin D daily and/or maintain exposure to

Table 9.15

Vitamin D Recommendations Ages 1–13 Years

Age	Male	Female
1–13 years	600 IU	600 IU

National Institutes of Health, Office of Dietary Supplements; updated February 11, 2016. Vitamin D: fact sheet for health professionals. Retrieved from: https://ods.od.nih.gov/factsheets/VitaminD-HealthProfessional/. Accessed January 17, 2016.

Table 9.16

CDC Strategies for Reducing Consumption of Sugar-Sweetened Beverages

- Ensure ready access to potable drinking water.
- Limit access to sugar-sweetened beverages.
- Promote access to and consumption of more healthful alternatives to sugar-sweetened beverages.
- Limit marketing of sugar-sweetened beverages and minimize marketing's impact on children.
- Decrease the relative cost of more healthful beverage alternatives through pricing of sugar-sweetened beverages.
- Include screening and counseling about sugar-sweetened beverage consumption as part of routine medical care.
- Expand the knowledge and skills of medical care providers to conduct nutrition screening and counseling regarding sugar-sweetened beverage consumption.

Centers for Disease Control and Prevention. *The CDC Guide to Strategies for Reducing the Consumption of Sugar-Sweetened Beverages.* Atlanta, GA: Centers for Disease Control and Prevention; March 2010. Retrieved from: http://www.cdph.ca.gov/sitecollectiondocuments/stratstoreduce_sugar_sweetened_bevs.pdf. Accessed September 22, 2016.

Recap Childhood and preadolescence is a critical time to lay the foundations for a healthy life. Good oral health, the prevention of dental caries, and a healthy skeleton are dependent on balanced nutrition during these formative years. Foods that contain added sugar and sugar-sweetened beverages should be limited to reduce the risk of developing overweight and obesity as well as other chronic degenerative diseases.

1. Explain the difference between primary and permanent teeth.
2. List strategies to maintain healthy teeth.
3. Describe the role of calcium and vitamin D in bone development.
4. State the prevalence of consumption of sugar-sweetened beverages in preadolescents.
5. Explain why sugar-sweetened beverages are unhealthy for preadolescents and children.
6. Suggest strategies to decrease consumption of sugar-sweetened beverages.

sunlight should receive a vitamin D supplement.[59] This recommendation did not change when recommendations were increased from 400 IU to 600 IU; recommendations for supplementation can and should change as requirements for vitamin D evolve.

Sugar

Sugar is found in many foods such as sweets, desserts, and juice. Drinks that contain sugar are a large portion of sugar-containing foods that children consume. Sugar-sweetened beverages include regular soda pop, soft drinks, fruit juice and fruit drinks, sports drinks, energy drinks, tea and coffee drinks, and flavored milk. Although the consumption of sugar-sweetened beverages decreased between 1999–2000 and 2007–2008 (76% to 66%), the incidence still remains high.[61] In 2010, a staggering 80% of youth still consumed sweetened beverages.[62]

Sugar is associated with many health risks, including overweight and obesity, diabetes, elevated triglycerides, cardiovascular disease, nonalcoholic fatty liver disease, elevated uric acid levels, gout, and dental caries.[63–71] It adds nutritionally empty calories that may cause a decrease in consumption of nutrient-dense foods, leading to imbalances in the diet. The additional calories consumed by eating large amounts of sugary foods can increase body weight and add body fat. Decreasing the consumption of sugar-sweetened beverages, for example can help children and preadolescents decrease body weight and improve body composition.

The CDC recommends a number of strategies to reduce the consumption of sugar-sweetened beverages (**TABLE 9.16**). All settings where sugar-sweetened beverages might be found need to be addressed, such as schools, homes, worksites, and communities.[62]

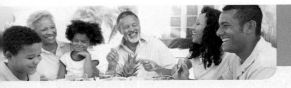

Learning Portfolio

Visual Chapter Summary

Normal Growth and Development of Children and Preadolescents

- During this stage in life, there is rapid physical growth and development, although they are less rapid than in other life stages such as for toddler and adolescents.
- Growth can be evaluated using techniques such as growth charts.

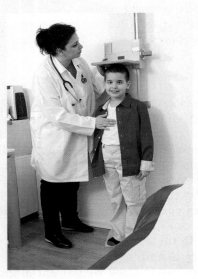

©Levent Konuk/Shutterstock

Factors Affecting Dietary Intake During Childhood and Preadolescence

- Children's eating habits at this age are influenced by peers, schools, culture, religion, media, and family.
- Children are starting to make personal choices of what to eat. Some children are picky eaters and some are adventurous eaters. Either way, the eating habits formed in this stage shape eating habits in the future.

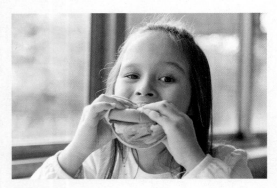

©Images By Kenny/Shutterstock

Nutritional Recommendations During Childhood and Preadolescence

- Good nutrition is needed for well-being, growth, and development.
- Minimizing added sugars, saturated fats, and sodium promotes health and well-being.

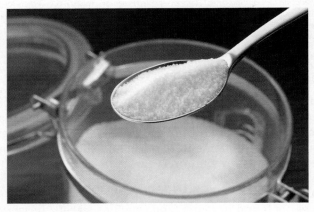

©sumire8/Shutterstock

Food and Nutrition Programs and Physical Activity

- Healthy eating and physical activity habits form in childhood when children learn how to live a healthy life.
- Childhood is an important time to shape kids' habits with schools, education, and government programs.

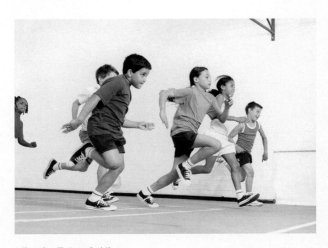

©Alistair Berg/The Image Bank/Getty

Common Nutritional Considerations During Childhood and Preadolescence

■ Preventing dental caries with good oral health habits and building strong bones by consuming adequate calcium are especially crucial between the ages of 6 and 9 years.

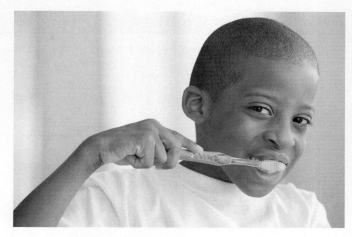

©Jose Luis Pelaez Inc/Blend Images/Getty

Key Terms

adiposity rebound: A second rise in body mass index that occurs in children between the ages of 3 and 7 years.

bone-strengthening exercise: Exercises that strengthen the bone structure of the human body.

core foods: Foods consumed by particular demographics over many generations.

culture: Beliefs and customs that shape the behaviors of a particular group of people.

food neophobia: Reluctance to try new foods and/or avoidance of certain foods or food groups.

growth: Anabolic biological function where size of body parts and organs increases.

growth chart: Measurement tool that tracks height, length, weight, head circumference, and body mass index changes over time.

growth hormone: A hormone released by the brain that causes the growth process.

growth velocity: Changes in growth measurements that occur over a set period of time.

macronutrient: Nutrient the human body needs in relatively large quantities to promote growth.

micronutrient: Chemical element or substance required in small amounts for normal growth and development of all living organisms.

midgrowth spurt: Small increase in the velocity of growth that precedes puberty development.

MyPlate: Federal government's newest health education model that illustrates a healthy diet, including food groups and place setting.

National School Breakfast Program (NSBP): A federal program that provides cash assistance to states to operate nonprofit breakfast programs in schools and residential child care facilities.

National School Lunch Program (NSLP): A federally assisted meal program for federal and nonprofit private schools where on a daily basis children receive nutritionally balanced meals either for free or for low cost.

novel food: Food that does not have a significant history of consumption or that is produced by a method that has not previously been used for food.

nutrient dense: Relatively large amount of nutrients in a small serving of calories.

oral health: The health and well-being of a person's mouth.

permanent teeth: Second set of teeth in humans, also known as the adult teeth.

physical activity: Any bodily movement produced by skeletal muscles that requires energy expenditure.

primary teeth: The first set of teeth in humans; also known as the baby teeth.

strength training: Exercises that strengthen the muscles of the body.

sugar-sweetened beverage: Beverage that contains caloric sweeteners such as sugar, honey, and high-fructose corn syrup.

Tanner scale: A scale that measures the variability in puberty development.

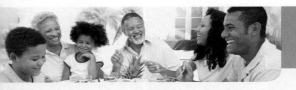

Learning Portfolio (continued)

Discussion Questions

1. Brainstorm ideas to create more after-school program physical activities.

2. With obesity on the rise, what strategies can schools use to prevent and reduce overweight and obesity in children? How about parents?

Activities

1. Create a 1-day meal plan that meets the dietary guidelines for a 10-year-old boy with a normal BMI. Hint: Use the MyPlate method as a guide.

2. Create a 1-week exercise program that meets all physical activity guidelines for the same 10-year-old boy with normal BMI. Hint: Make sure to include all three types of exercises and make them age appropriate.

Study Questions

1. Which form of physical activity is most common during preadolescence?
   a. Participation in structured sports team
   b. School-based physical education classes
   c. Active play in safe environments
   d. Exercise-based video and computer games

2. Children can be classified as overweight when their body mass index plots on which percentiles?
   a. Greater than 95th percentile BMI for age and gender
   b. Greater than 85th percentile BMI for age and gender
   c. Greater than or equal to 80th percentile but less than 85th percentile BMI for age and gender
   d. Greater than or equal to 85th percentile but less than 95th percentile BMI for age and gender

3. What does an obesogenic environment refer to?
   a. Environmental surroundings that promote weight gain and ultimately obesity
   b. A neighborhood that limits access to fast-food establishments
   c. Living spaces that have a significant number of supermarkets per square mile
   d. Neighborhood environments where schools are not permitted to participate in federally assisted meal programs

4. The goal of the Let's Move! campaign is what?
   a. Prevent development of childhood obesity.
   b. Prevent type 1 juvenile diabetes.
   c. Prevent childhood hunger.
   d. Promote school lunch programs.

5. Children are eligible for the National School Lunch Program based on which criterion?
   a. Their current academic grade
   b. Parents' incomes

   c. Parents' financial contribution to school
   d. Child's health status

6. What does food neophobia refer to?
   a. Parents' fear of serving certain foods to children
   b. Peer pressure to avoid certain foods
   c. Child's own personal reluctance to try new foods and/or food groups
   d. Fear of certain foods that developed because of cultural influences

7. Dietary guidelines are updated every ___ years.
   a. 10
   b. 4
   c. 2
   d. 5

8. Calorie needs for preadolescents depend on the all the following *except* which one?
   a. Disease status
   b. Age
   c. Weight
   d. Physical activity

9. Which is the most recent USDA program aimed at illustrating the building blocks of a healthy diet?
   a. MyPlate
   b. MyPyramid
   c. Healthy Food Index
   d. *Dietary Guidelines for Americans*

10. All of the following are micronutrients needed for tooth mineralization and enamel formation *except* for which one?
    a. Fluoride
    b. Iron
    c. Calcium
    d. Vitamin D

11. The general rule of thumb is that preadolescents will grow how many centimeters per year until puberty?
    a. 3–4 cm
    b. 1–2 cm
    c. 5–6 cm
    d. More than 6 cm

12. If a child plots at the 70th percentile weight for age, what does this mean?
    a. 30% of children the same age and sex have a higher weight than the child.
    b. 70% of children the same age and sex have a higher weight than the child.
    c. 30% of children the same age and sex have a lower weight than the child.
    d. 70% of children the same age and sex have a lower weight than the child.

13. The greatest demand for nutrients occurs during which phase?
    a. Times of catabolic illness
    b. Every year until 19 years of age
    c. From birth to 2 years of age
    d. Peak velocity of growth

14. Current research tells us what about preadolescent behaviors and vending machine choices?
    a. Selection from vending machines is associated with higher BMI in preadolescents, but not in adolescent children.
    b. Selection from vending machines is associated with lower BMI in preadolescents than in adolescents.
    c. Selection from vending machines is associated with higher BMI in preadolescents and adolescents.
    d. Selection from vending machines does not influence health of preadolescents or adolescents.

15. Length is measured in children _____, and height is measured in children _____.
    a. 12–24 months of life; for all other ages
    b. who are sick; who are well
    c. who can stand; once a child can stand
    d. up until the midpoint growth spurt; who are in puberty

Weblinks

- **PediTools**
  http://peditools.org/ Interactive tools for nutritional assessment of pediatric growth and development.

- **MyPlate Kids' Place**
  https://www.choosemyplate.gov/kids

- **Let's Move! Kids Take Action**
  http://www.letsmove.gov/kids

References

1. Bose K. Concept of human physical growth and development. Human Resource Development Group, Council of Scientific & Industrial Research, India; 2007. Retrieved from: http://nsdl.niscair.res.in/jspui/bitstream/123456789/243/1/PDF%205.5CHAPTER%20ON%20HUMAN%20GROWTH%20FOR%20CSIR.pdf. Accessed December 2015.

2. Thompson J, Nelson A. Middle childhood and modern human origins. *Hum Nat.* 2001;22:249–280.

3. Bogin B. *Patterns of Human Growth.* Cambridge, England: Cambridge University Press; 1999.

4. Ulijaszek S Johnston F Preece M. Hormonal regulation of growth in childhood and puberty. In: *The Cambridge Encyclopedia of Human Growth and Development.* Cambridge, England: Cambridge University Press; 1998:225–229.

5. Bowden R; last updated December 24, 2006. Growth hormone (somatotropin). Retrieved from: http://arbl.cvmbs.colostate.edu/hbooks/pathphys/endocrine/hypopit/gh.html. Accessed October 2015.

6. Marcovecchio M, Chiarelli F. Obesity and growth during childhood and puberty. *World Rev Nutr Diet.* 2013;106:135–141.

7. Doyle DA. Physical growth of infants and children. Merck Manual Professional Version. Retrieved from: http://www.merckmanuals.com/professional/pediatrics/growth-and-development/physical-growth-of-infants-and-children. Accessed October 2015.

8. Rogol A, Clark P, Roemmich J. Growth and pubertal development in children and adolescents: effects of diet and physical activity. *J Clin Nutr.* 2000;72:521S–528S.

9. Nichols J. Normal growth patterns in infants and prepubertal children. UpToDate; May 26, 2016. Retrieved from: http://www.uptodate.com/contents/normal-growth-patterns-in-infants-and-prepubertal-children. Accessed September 2016.

10. Towne B, Williams K, Blangero J. Presentation, heritability, and genome-wide linkage analysis of the midchildhood

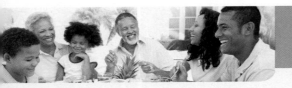

Learning Portfolio (continued)

growth spurt in healthy children from the Fels Longitudinal Study. *Human Biol*. 2008;6:623–636.

11. Centers for Disease Control and Prevention; updated May 15, 2015. Healthy weight: about child and teen BMI. Retrieved from: http://www.cdc.gov/healthyweight/assessing/bmi/childrens_bmi/about_childrens_bmi.html. Accessed October 2015.

12. Hamill P, Drizd T, Johnson C, Reed RB, Roche AF. NCHS growth curves for children birth–18 years. United States. *Vital Health Stat 11*. 1977;(165):i–iv, 1–74.

13. Kuczmarski RJ, Ogen CL, Gio SS. 2000 CDC growth charts for the United States. methods and development. *Vital Health Stat*. 2002;11:246.

14. Dietitians of Canada and Canadian Paediatric Society. A health professional's guide to using growth charts. *Paediatr Child Health*. 2004;9(3):174–176.

15. Campbell B. An introduction to the special issue on middle childhood. *Human Natr*. 2001;22:247–248.

16. Rogoff B, Sellers M, Pirrotta S. Age assignment of roles and responsibilities to children: a cross cultural survey. *Hum Develop*. 1975;22:247–248.

17. Patrick H, Nicklas T. A review of family and social determinants of children's eating patterns and diet quality. *J Am Coll Nutr*. 2005;24(2):83–92.

18. Cooke L. The importance of exposure for healthy eating in childhood: a review. *J Hum Nutr Diet*. 2007;20(4):294–301.

19. Salvy SJ, de la Haye K, Bowker J. Influences of peers and friends on children's and adolescent's eating. *Physiol Behav*. 2012;106(3):369–378.

20. Harper LV, Sanders KM. The effects of adults' eating on young children's acceptance of unfamiliar foods. *J Exp Child Psychol*. 1975;20:206–214.

21. Pike KM, Rodin J. Mothers, daughters, and disordered eating. *J Abnorm Psychol*. 1991;100:198–204.

22. Shuttsm K, Kinzler K, DeJesus J. Understanding infants' and children's social learning about foods: previous research and new prospects. *Develop Psychol*. 2013;49(3):419–425.

23. Scaglioni S, Arrizza C, Vecchi F, Tedeschi S. Determinants of children's eating behavior. *Am J Clin Nutr*. 2011;94(6):2006S–2011S.

24. American Academy of Pediatrics; 2011, updated November 21, 2015. Tips for preventing food hassles. Retrieved from: http://www.healthychildren.org/English/Healthy-living/nutrition/Pages/Tips-for-Preventing-Food-Hassles.aspx. Accessed December 12, 2015.

25. Kumanyika S. Environmental influences on childhood obesity: ethnic and cultural influences in context. *Physiol Behav*. 2008;94:61–70.

26. Greenlagh J, Horne P, Lowe C, Whitaker C, Griffiths J. Positive and negative peer modeling effects on the young children's consumption of novel blue foods. *Appetite*. 2009;52(3):646–653.

27. Birch LL. Effects of peer models' food choices and eating behaviors on preschoolers' food preference. *Child Develop*. 1980;51:489–496.

28. Mascola A, Bryson S, Agras W. Picky eating during childhood: a longitudinal study to age 11 years. *Eat Behav*. 2010;11(4):253–257.

29. Lafraire J, Rioux C, Giboreau A, Picard D. Food rejection in children: cognitive and social/environmental factors involved in food neophobia and picky/fussy eating behavior. *Appetite*. 2016;1(96):347–357.

30. Ogden CL, Carroll MD, Kit BK, Flegal KM. Prevalence of childhood and adult obesity in the United States, 2011–2012. *JAMA*. 2014;311(8):806–814.

31. Institute of Medicine. *Food Marketing to Children: Threat or Opportunity?* Washington, DC: National Academies Press; 2006.

32. Children's Food and Beverage Advertising Initiative; June 2013. CFBAI's Category-Specific Uniform Nutrition Criteria. Retrieved from: http://www.bbb.org/storage/16/documents/cfbai/CFBAI%20Uniform%20Nutrition%20Criteria%20Fact%20Sheet%20–FINAL.pdf. Accessed August 6, 2016.

33. Linn S, Novosat C. Calories for sale: food marketing to children in the twenty-first century. *Ann Am Acad Pol Soc Sci*. 2008;615:133–155.

34. Kraak V, Story M. Influence of food companies brand mascots and entertainment companies cartoon media characters on children's diet and health: a systematic review and research needs. *Obesity*. 2015;16:107–126.

35. Roberto C, Baik J, Harris J, Brownell K. Influence of licensed characters on children's taste and snack preferences. *Pediatrics*. 2010;126(88):88–93.

36. Nanney MS, MacLehose RF, Kubik MY, et al. School obesity prevention Policies and practices in minnesota and student outcomes: a longitudinal cohort study. *Am J Prev Med*. November 2016;51(5):656–663. doi: 10.1016/j.amepre.2016.05.008 [Epub ahead of print June 16, 2016].

37. Council on School Health; Committee on Nutrition. Snacks, sweetened beverages, added sugars, and schools. *Pediatrics*. March 2015;135(3):575–83. doi: 10.1542/peds.2014–3902.

38. Swinburn B, Eggar G, Raza F. Dissecting obesogenic environments: the development and application of a framework for identifying and prioritizing environmental interventions for obesity. *Prevent Med*. 1999;29(6):563–570.

39. Saelens B, Sallis J, Frank L, Couch S, Zhou C, Colhour T. Obesogenic neighborhood environment, child and parent obesity; the Neighborhood Impact Kids Study. *Am J Prev Med*. 2012;42(5):57–64.

40. Food and Nutrition Board, Institute of Medicine. *Dietary Reference Intakes: A Risk Assessment Model for Establishing Upper Intake Levels for Nutrients*. Washington, DC: National Academies Press; 1998.

41. U.S. Department of Health and Human Services and U.S. Department of Agriculture. *2015–2020 Dietary Guidelines for Americans*. 8th ed. Washington, DC: U.S. Department of Health and Human Services and U.S. Department of Agriculture; December 2015. Retrieved from: http://health.gov/dietaryguidelines/2015/guidelines/. Accessed August 13, 2016.

42. The National Academies of Sciences, Engineering, Medicine; updated May 31, 2016. Dietary Reference Intakes tables and application. Retrieved from: http://www.nationalacademies.org/hmd/Activities/Nutrition/SummaryDRIs/DRI-Tables.aspx. Accessed September 13, 2016.

43. U.S. Department of Agriculture. Choose MyPlate. Retrieved from: http://www.choosemyplate.gov/MyPlate. Accessed January 5, 2016.

44. Slining M, Popkin B, Mathias K. Trends in food and beverage sources among US children and adolescents: 1989–2010. *J Acad Nutr Diet*. 2013;113:1683–1694.

45. Reedy J, Krebs-Smith S. Dietary sources of energy, solid fats, and added sugars among children and adolescents in the United States. *J Am Diet Assoc.* 2010;110(10):1477–1484.

46. U.S. Department of Agriculture Food and Nutrition Service; September 2013. The School Breakfast Program [fact sheet]. Retrieved from: http://www.fns.usda.gov/sites/default/files/sbpfactsheet.pdf. Accessed September 13, 2016.

47. Food Research and Action Center. National School Lunch Program: Trends And Factors Affecting Student Participation. Washington, DC: Food Research and Action Center; 2015. http://frac.org/pdf/national_school_lunch_report_2015.pdf. Accessed January 12, 2016.

48. Gunderson GW. National School Lunch Act. USDA Food and Nutrition Service; August 26, 2015. Retrieved from: http://www.fns.usda.gov/nslp/history_5. Accessed October 2015.

49. U.S. Department of Agriculture Food and Nutrition Service; July 10, 2014. Healthier School Day. Retrieved from: Available at http://www.fns.usda.gov/healthierschoolday. Accessed August 7, 2016.

50. World Health Organization. Global strategy on diet, physical activity and health: physical activity and young people. Retrieve from: http://www.who.int/dietphysicalactivity/factsheet_young_people/en/. Accessed December 12, 2015.

51. National Center for Chronic Disease Prevention and Health Promotion, Centers for Disease Control and Prevention. Guidelines for school and community programs to promote lifelong physical activity among young people. *J Sch Health.* 1997;67(6):202–219.

52. Centers for Disease Control and Prevention; updated June 4, 2015. How much physical activity do children need? Retrieved from: http://www.cdc.gov/physicalactivity/basics/children/. Accessed December 18, 2015.

53. White House Task Force on Childhood Obesity. About Let's move! Retrieved from: http://www.letsmove.gov/about. Accessed December 18, 2015.

54. Pate R. Promoting physical activity in children and youth: a leadership role for schools: a scientific statement from the American Heart Association Council on Nutrition, Physical Activity, and Metabolism (Physical Activity Committee) in collaboration with the Councils on Cardiovascular Disease in the Young and Cardiovascular Nursing. *Circulation.* 2006;114(11):1214–1224. doi: 10.1161/circulationaha.106.177052.

55. Touger-Decker R, Mobley C; Academy of Nutrition and Dietetics. Position of the Academy of Nutrition and Dietetics: oral health and nutrition. *J Acad Nutr Diet.* 2013;113(5):693–701.

56. American Dental Association. Nutrition. Mouth Healthy. Retrieved from: http://www.mouthhealthy.org/en/Teens/nutrition. Accessed December 18, 2015.

57. Eunice Kennedy Shriver National Institute of Child Health and Human Development. What is calcium and how does it build strong bones? Retrieved from: https://www.nichd.nih.gov/health/topics/bonehealth/conditioninfo/pages/calcium.aspx. Reviewed May 6, 2014. Accessed December 18, 2015.

58. Bailey RL, Dodd KW, Goldman JA, et al. Estimation of total usual calcium and vitamin D intakes in the United States. *J Nutr.* 2010;140(4):817–822.

59. National Institutes of Health, Office of Dietary Supplements; updated February 11, 2016. Vitamin D: Fact sheet for health professionals. Retrieved from: https://ods.od.nih.gov/factsheets/VitaminD-HealthProfessional/. Accessed January 17, 2016.

60. Holick MF. Resurrection of vitamin D deficiency and rickets. *J Clin Invest.* 2006;116:2062–2072.

61. Han E, Powell LM. Consumption patterns of sugar sweetened beverages in the United States. *J Acad Nutr Diet.* 2013;113(1):43–53.

62. Centers for Disease Control and Prevention. *The CDC Guide to Strategies for Reducing the Consumption of Sugar-Sweetened Beverages.* Atlanta, GA: Centers for Disease Control and Prevention; March 2010. http://www.cdph.ca.gov/sitecollection documents/stratstoreduce_sugar_sweetened_bevs.pdf. Accessed August 18, 2016.

63. Apovian CM. Sugar-sweetened soft drinks, obesity, and type 2 diabetes. *JAMA.* 2004;292(8):978–979.

64. Montonen J, Järvinen R, Knekt P, Heliövaara M, Reunanen A. Consumption of sweetened beverages and intakes of fructose and glucose predict type 2 diabetes occurrence. *J Nutr.* 2007;137(6):1447–1454.

65. Dhingra R, Sullivan L, Jacques PF. Soft drink consumption and risk of developing cardiometabolic risk factors and the metabolic syndrome in middle-aged adults in the community. *Circulation.* 2007;116(5):480–488.

66. Stanhope KL, Griffen SC, Bair BR, Swarbrick MM, Keim NL, Havel PJ. Twenty-four-hour endocrine and metabolic profiles following consumption of high-fructose corn syrup-, sucrose-,fructose-, and glucose-sweetened beverages with meals. *Am J Clin Nutr.* 2008;87(5):1194–1203.

67. Fung TT, Malik V, Rexrode KM, Manson JE, Willett WC, Hu FB. Sweetened beverage consumption and risk of coronary heart disease in women. *Am J Clin Nutr.* 2009;89(4):1037–1042.

68. Ouyang X, Cirillo P, Sautin Y, et al. Fructose consumption as a risk factor for non-alcoholic fatty liver disease. *J Hepatol.* 2008;48(6):993–999.

69. Choi JW, Ford ES, Gao X, Choi HK. Sugar-sweetened soft drinks, diet soft drinks, and serum uric acid level: the Third National Health and Nutrition Examination Survey. *Arthritis Rheum.* 2008;59(1):109–116.

70. Choi HK, Curhan G. Soft drinks, fructose consumption, and the risk of gout in men: prospective cohort study. *BMJ.* 2008;336(7639):309–312.

71. Sohn W, Burt BA, Sowers MR. Carbonated soft drinks and dental caries in the primary dentition. *J Dent Res.* 2006;85(3):262–266.

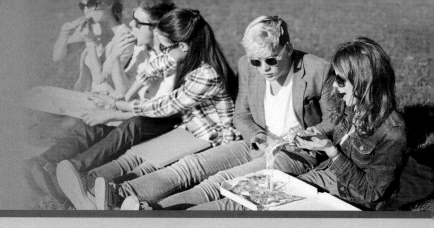

CHAPTER 10

Adolescent Nutrition

Katarina Berry, MS, RD, LDN, **and Julie Cooper,** MS, RD, LDN

Chapter Outline

Growth and Development During Adolescence

Factors Affecting Dietary Intake During Adolescence

Nutritional Recommendations and Requirements During Adolescence

Common Nutrition Considerations During Adolescence

Promoting Healthy Lifestyles

Learning Objectives

1. Describe normal physical and psychological growth and development during adolescence.

2. List the influential factors present during adolescence and how they affect dietary intake.

3. Summarize the nutrients of importance during adolescence.

4. Describe assessment of growth and nutritional status of adolescents, indications for intervention, and concepts for counseling toward behavior change.

5. Use the theoretical model presented to create an effective intervention program that appeals to adolescents.

©KateStone/Shutterstock

Case Study

Carla is a 14-year-old girl who lives with her mom and 17-year-old brother. She has had annual preventive health care from birth and has grown along average height and weight trends. Her medical history includes only seasonal allergies. Carla's parents divorced when she was very young, and she does not see her dad. Her mom has a full-time job and is comfortably able to provide food for the family. Carla is a strong student at her public middle school and has enjoyed participating in team sports for the past several years.

Adolescence is a period of great physical, psychological, and emotional development that spans ages 10 to 19 years.[1] Perhaps the simplest way to define its endpoints is the entrance of a child and emergence of a young adult. Changes over this near decade of life are constant, with internal influences such as hormonal shifts and external factors such as family, school, media, and daily social interactions. Adequate nutrition is necessary for adolescents to achieve their growth potential, and with this period of development comes increased and unique nutrient needs. The American Academy of Pediatrics (AAP) recommends discussion of nutrition and physical activity with during annual preventive care appointments.[2] The role for registered dietitian nutritionists and other healthcare providers in supporting healthy adolescent development is increasingly vital.

Growth and Development During Adolescence

Preview Physical and psychological developments occur side by side during adolescence, though each can progress at different paces. This section discusses these two formative processes.

Normal Physical Growth and Development
Although adolescence encompasses the entirety of this period of transformation from childhood to young adulthood, the process of puberty includes only the physical changes that occur as a child attains reproductive capacity.[3] The most familiar changes of puberty are likely the development of visible secondary sexual characteristics, such as appearance of pubic hair and breast growth. Progress through puberty is defined by sexual maturity ratings (SMRs) 1 through 5, also called Tanner stages. Developed by Marshall and Tanner in the 1960s, this scale

is a well-accepted method of evaluation in adolescent health care.[4,5] A child with an SMR of stage 1 has no visual signs of change, which indicates prepuberty, whereas SMR stage 5 is reached once adult characteristics have developed. Secondary sexual characteristics at each stage are outlined in TABLE 10.1. [4,5]

Gonadarche is the first visual sign of puberty and heralds the child's transition from stage 1 to stage 2. Boys generally reach this milestone about 2 years behind girls. Gonardarche in girls is marked by breast budding, also called thelarche, and usually occurs between 9 and 13 years of age.[6] In boys, gonadarche is marked by an increase in testicular size. On average for boys, this occurs at 11.5 to 12 years of age,[7] with the vast majority of boys beginning pubertal genital development by age 13.[3]

During normal development of both boys and girls, changes associated with progression through SMR stages appear in a specific sequence and do not vary. This sequence is shown in TABLE 10.2. [8] The pace, or tempo, at which an adolescent moves through these stages is unique to each person. On average, it takes 4 years for a girl to progress from breast budding (SMR stage 2) to adult breast development (SMR stage 5). Boys, on average, take 3 years to move from SMR stage 2 to stage 5.[6] Total time of puberty, however, can range from these averages and can take as little as 1.5 years to as long as 8 years in girls, and from 2 to 5 years in boys.[9] Varied tempo of puberty is important to keep in mind because nutritional needs change during progression through SMR stages, and age itself is therefore not a good determinant of dietary requirements.[6]

Contrary to common thinking, menarche, or first menstruation, is not a sign of the start of puberty. This milestone actually occurs during SMR stage 3 or 4, when, in fact, girls will have already experienced a breast budding and a height growth spurt about 1 year after thelarche and before their first period.[3] Similarly, boys generally will not experience spermarche, or first evidence of ejaculation of sperm, until SMR stage 3 and will not attain fertility until SMR stage 4.[9]

Average age of menarche is a topic of focused discussion because much research shows a gradual decline over several generations. Records from the 18th century report menarche at 17 or 18 years old, with a clear decline to present day in industrialized nations.[10] Theories propose that this trend is due to improved nutrition and health care over this same period.[11] From the 1960s to 1990s, there was a decline in menarcheal age of approximately 2.5 months from an average of 12.75 to 12.54 years. A correlation between higher body mass index (BMI) and earlier menarche has been observed, as have differences between ethnicities. black girls, for example, reach menarche before non-Hispanic white girls, and Hispanic American girls fall in the middle. Other groups have not been individually studied closely enough to

Table 10.1			
SMR and Tanner Stages			
Sexual Maturity Rating/Tanner Stage	Males (Genitalia)	Females (Breasts)	Pubic Hair (Males and Females)
1	• Preadolescent • Testes, scrotum, and penis about the same size and proportion as early childhood	• Preadolescent • Elevation of papilla only	• Preadolescent • No pubic hair
2	• Scrotum and testes enlarged • Change in texture of scrotal skin • Some reddening of scrotal skin	• Breast buds; elevation of breast and papilla as small mound • Enlargement of areola diameter	• Sparse growth of long, slightly pigmented, downy hair • Straight or slightly curled hair • Appears mainly at base of penis (males) or along the labia (females)
3	• Growth of penis, length and then breadth • Further growth of testes and scrotum	• Further enlargement of breast and areola • No separation of breast and areola contours	• Darker, coarser, and more curled hair • Hair spreads sparsely over junction of pubes
4	• Penis further enlarged, length and breadth • Development of glans • Further growth of testes and scrotum • Further darkening of scrotal skin	• Projection of areola and papilla to form secondary mound above the level of the breast	• Adult-type hair • Smaller area covered with hair compared to most adults • No spread to medial surface of thighs
5	• Genitalia are adult size and shape. No further enlargement after stage 5	• Mature stage • Projection of papilla only	• Adult hair in quantity and type • Distributed as inverse triangle • Spread to medial surface of thighs

Modified from Marshall WA, Tanner JM. Variations in pattern of pubertal changes in girls. *Arch Dis Child*. 1969;44:291–303; Marshall WA, Tanner JM. Variations in pattern of pubertal changes in boys. *Arch Dis Child*. 1970;45:13–23.

place them in this time line, and researchers found that the effects of race and weight on menarcheal age are mutually independent.[12] Based on data from the National Health Examination Survey and the Third National Health and Nutrition Examination Survey, the observed decline in overall menarcheal age was concurrent with racial population changes and increased mean BMI in adolescent girls.[13] Of note, the amount that menarcheal age has declined within individual races has been considerably smaller than the average decline in the overall population. This could mean that, rather than a true population-wide shift, changes in racial proportions could have influenced the average menarcheal age. This is important to keep in mind when evaluating the trend of earlier menarche.[12,13]

Height

Linear growth is significant during adolescence, when adolescents gain about 20% of their adult stature.[14] In adolescence, both boys and girls go through growth spurts during which the rate of height growth, or height velocity, reaches its peak. Though boys' **peak height velocity** is more rapid, males hit their growth spurt about 2 years behind girls. Girls reach peak velocity at about 11.5 years and SMR stages 2 to 3, as compared with boys, who peak at approximately 13.5 years and SMR stages 3 or 4.[9] Boys can then continue to grow taller

for a longer period of time than girls. These variations between genders in pace and duration of linear growth can be seen in adult men, who on average are taller than women. Interestingly, girls generally will not grow more than 2 to 3 inches after menarche, which can be a good rule of thumb when reviewing growth curves and projecting height potential.

Bone Mass

Bone mass approximately doubles over the course of puberty, with 90% of peak skeletal mass reached by age 18 in healthy adolescents. Bone mineral content is similar between sexes before puberty. Both sexes experience an increased rate of bone mass accumulation during puberty, with peak accrual occurring after peak height velocity. Accrual tends to slow in girls around age 15 and in boys at approximately age 17.[15] Peak bone mass in boys tends to be greater than in girls, owing in great part to the fact that boys generally have 2 more years of prepubertal growth than girls and a longer duration of their pubertal growth spurt.[16] It is very important to guide adolescents in establishing healthy behaviors for bone health given these limited "windows of opportunity" of rapid rate of bone turnover and accrual during puberty.[17] This includes adequate micronutrient intake, namely, calcium and vitamin D, to be discussed in more detail later in this chapter.

Table 10.2

Tanner Stages of Development

(A) Pubertal sequence: girls

Stage	Age Range (Years)	Breast Growth	Pubic Hair Growth	Other Changes
I	0–15	Preadolescent	None	Preadolescent.
II	8–15	Breast budding (thelarche); areolar hyperplasia with small amount of breast tissue	Long downy pubic hair near the labia, often appearing with breast budding or several weeks or months later	Peak growth velocity often occurs soon after stage II.
III	10–15	Further enlargement of breast tissue and areola, with no separation of their contours	Increase in amount and pigmentation of hair	Menarche occurs in 2% of girls late in stage III.
IV	10–17	Separation of contours; areola and nipple form secondary mound above breasts tissue	Adult in type but not in distribution	Menarche occurs in most girls in stage IV, 1–3 years after thelarche.
V	12.5–18	Large breast with single contour	Adult in distribution	Menarche occurs in 10% of girls in stage V.

(B) Pubertal sequence: boys

Stage	Age Range (Years)	Testes Growth	Penis Growth	Pubic Hair Growth	Other Changes
I	0–15	Preadolescent testes (≤ 2.5 cm)	Preadolescent	None	Preadolescent.
II	10–15	Enlargement of testes; pigmentation of scrotal sac	Minimal or no enlargement	Long downy hair, often appearing several months after testicular growth; variable pattern noted with pubarche	Not applicable.
III	1½–16.5	Further enlargement	Significant enlargement, especially in diameter	Increase in amount; curling	Not applicable.
IV	Variable: 12–17	Further enlargement	Further enlargement, especially in diameter	Adult in type but not in distribution	Development of axillary hair and some facial hair.
V	13–18	Adult in size	Adult in size	Adult in distribution (medial aspects of thighs; linea alba)	Body hair continues to grow and muscles continue to increase in size for several months to years; 20% of boys reach peak growth velocity during this period.

Reprinted from WHO. (2010). Antiretroviral Therapy for HIV Infection in Infants and Children: Towards Universal Access: Recommendations for a Public Health Approach: 2010 Revision. Annex H: *Sexual MaturityRating (Tanner Staging) in Adolescents*, pp. 162–163, Copyright 2010.

Theories that carbonated beverage consumption could have an adverse effect on bone density in adolescents have circulated for many years. The most commonly suggested mechanism for this relationship is the displacement of calcium-rich milk in the diet[18] by the regular consumption of beverages containing phosphorus (in colas),[19] fructose,[20] and high acid content.[21] Caffeine has also been suggested, though doubt of its impact on bone mineral density in young women has been raised.[22,23] Much of the research has found associations between carbonated beverage intake and bone health in girls. In a nationally representative sample of adolescents in Ireland, for example, researchers found an association between lower bone mineral density and consumption of carbonated soft drinks in girls, but they did not find the same in boys.[24] An association between carbonated beverage intake, especially cola, and bone fractures in a sample of active high school girls has also been seen in the United States.[25] Similarly, in Canada, consumption of low-nutrient-dense beverages was associated with lower bone mineral accrual and lower total bone mineral content in adolescent girls, and the authors of this study concluded that higher intake of low-nutrient-dense beverages was inversely associated with milk consumption in both boys and girls.[18]

Weight and Body Composition

In addition to height growth, adolescents gain approximately 50% of their adult weight around puberty.[7] Girls will experience peak weight gain before their growth spurt, spurring sayings such as "An adolescent girl first has to grow out to grow up." This type of phrasing might ring true but should be used with caution in the presence of an adolescent girl and her parents because it can be interpreted negatively. Such messages can spark ideas about the need for dieting and weight loss, which are not appropriate at this age. Alternatively, this fact should not be viewed as a green light for excessive weight gains that could lead to chronic overweight and obesity. Boys, in contrast, experience the majority of their weight gain concurrent with their growth spurt.

In the setting of weight gain and height growth, body composition during puberty shifts and contributes heavily to developing adult characteristics of sexual dimorphism, or the differences in appearance between men and women. These shifts are driven by gonadal steroid hormones and growth hormone. Differences in appearance are greatly due to variations in total body fat, percentage of body fat, and fat distribution.

Before puberty, boys and girls have similar total fat mass, with girls having slightly more percent body fat than boys (19% in girls compared with 15% in boys).[6] Around the age of 12, fat-free body mass gain in girls begins to slow, whereas boys' rate of gaining fat-free mass accelerates under the influence of testosterone.[15] During puberty, females, influenced by estrogen and progesterone, also gain more fat mass than males. Males' total fat mass does not change significantly during puberty, but their percent fat mass decreases as a result of increases in fat-free mass.[15] By adulthood, women on average have 25% body fat compared with 13% in men;[15] men have 150% of the lean body mass of women.[7] Sexual dimorphism is usually apparent by adulthood, with females generally having a gynoid body shape, or fat deposition around hips and thighs. Males develop an android shape, with body fat concentrated near the abdomen.[7,15] See `FIGURE 10.1`.

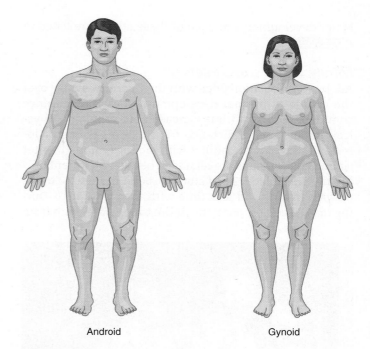

Android   Gynoid

Figure 10.1
Fat deposition in gynoid and android body shapes.

Normal Psychosocial Development

Popular thought about adolescence views it as a time of emotional turmoil and "normative disturbance," though recent scholarly thought disputes this theory and posits that the majority of teenagers handle this developmental process fairly well and without significant, lasting difficulty.[26,27] In contrast to puberty, during which physical stages occur in a set sequence in normal development, psychosocial development of adolescents does not necessarily follow a linear path. Timing of emotional and social growth can vary among individuals and does not always align with physical changes. A young teen girl might appear physically developed, for instance, but might not yet be able to make informed decisions about sex.

Cognitive development during adolescence is characterized by development of reasoning skills and the ability to think abstractly and hypothetically, allowing an adolescent to develop decision-making abilities. Adolescents might daydream more and can imagine situations they have not yet experienced. This is demonstrated in newfound ability to think philosophically or spiritually about a topic and to develop a deeper capacity to love. Adolescents also begin to think about their own feelings and how others perceive them.[27,28]

Adolescent psychosocial development can be divided into three different stages, on the basis of age, though individual development might not correlate exactly with this breakdown:

- Early adolescence (10–13 years)
- Middle adolescence (14–17 years)
- Late adolescence (17–21 years)

Case Study

Carla reached menarche just before her 13th birthday after experiencing a height growth spurt. She is finding that she is now taller than a lot of the boys in her class.

Questions

1. How does Carla's height growth and age at menarche compare to other girls her age? Review the sequence of physical changes in girls' puberty. Was it normal to grow taller before reaching menarche?
2. Should Carla expect to always be taller than many of her male peers?

Major developments at each of these stages are listed in FIGURE 10.2 [27]

Family, Friends, and Peers

Adolescents' relationships with their parents evolve over the course of normal development. Early adolescence commonly brings with it increased bickering and physical and emotional distance from parents.[26] Early adolescents have most conflict with siblings, though better sibling relationships are related to better adjustment during this life stage.[29] They start to spend more time alone or with friends and less time with their parents.[30] During middle adolescence, the desire to separate more from

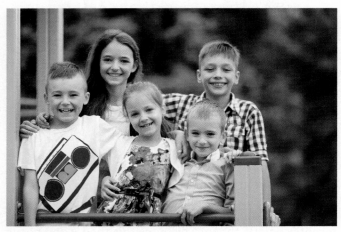

©Olesia Bilkei/Shutterstock

family and spend time with school activities, friends, or an after-school job are of great importance to a teen.[31] Over time, however, the parent–child relationship again improves and becomes more equal and less explosive.[26] By late adolescence, young adults have developed a separate identity from parents; however, at this stage they might return to seek parental advice, something they likely initially shunned in earlier stages.[27,28]

In early adolescence, peer contact is mainly with the same gender, though there may be the beginning of contact with the opposite gender in group settings. By middle adolescence, assimilation with peer groups of both genders and involvement in group activities such as sports, clubs, or gangs become strong motivators. Boys and girls who do not feel a connection with a specific peer group might struggle more psychologically, though a study of children near early adolescence showed that the support and feeling of protection from even a single friend can help to offset such challenges.[32] In late adolescence, developing closeness in one-on-one relationships is valued.[27]

Development of romantic relationships is a significant and normative part of adolescence. These relationships not only occupy a great amount of adolescent thought but also can provide significant individual support that affects current and future development. By the end of high school, almost three-quarters of U.S. teens report involvement in a romantic relationship in the prior 18 months. Timing for initiation of dating can vary by culture, ethnicity, gender, and influences of friend groups; however, earlier dating has been associated with earlier

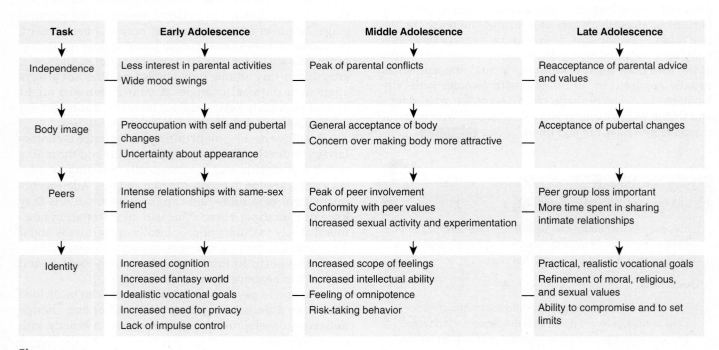

Task	Early Adolescence	Middle Adolescence	Late Adolescence
Independence	Less interest in parental activities Wide mood swings	Peak of parental conflicts	Reacceptance of parental advice and values
Body image	Preoccupation with self and pubertal changes Uncertainty about appearance	General acceptance of body Concern over making body more attractive	Acceptance of pubertal changes
Peers	Intense relationships with same-sex friend	Peak of peer involvement Conformity with peer values Increased sexual activity and experimentation	Peer group loss important More time spent in sharing intimate relationships
Identity	Increased cognition Increased fantasy world Idealistic vocational goals Increased need for privacy Lack of impulse control	Increased scope of feelings Increased intellectual ability Feeling of omnipotence Risk-taking behavior	Practical, realistic vocational goals Refinement of moral, religious, and sexual values Ability to compromise and to set limits

Figure 10.2
Psychosocial Development of Adolescents

Data from Radzik M, Sherer S, Neinstein LS. Psychosocial development in normal adolescents. In Neinstein LS, ed. *Adolescent Health Care: A Practical Guide.* 5th ed. Philadelphia, PA: Wolters Kluwer Heath/Lippincott Williams & Wilkins; 2007:52–57.

sexual activity, lower self-esteem, increased alcohol and substance abuse, and inferior academic performance.[29] Research on the role of romantic relationships in adolescents is limited, and further investigation is warranted to help elucidate the impact of these interactions on body image and dietary habits.

Self-Esteem and Body Image

In early adolescence, there is often self-focus on body changes and uncertainty about appearance. At this age, kids commonly compare themselves physically to peers. Teenage girls, in general, report lower self-esteem and more negative body image than boys. Differences may exist between girls of different ethnicities. In a multicultural study of adolescents, for example, Hispanic girls self-reported more negative body image and depressive feelings, and black girls reported the most positive body image, perhaps because of differing cultural ideals.[33]

There also may be gender differences in self-esteem related to body changes and development. Interestingly, girls who perceive that they are developing early report lower self-esteem, whereas boys who feel they are maturing earlier than peers report higher self-esteem. Early-maturing boys are often seen as leaders or more popular, whereas early-maturing girls are at increased risk for poor body image, depression, and behavioral problems.[28]

By the time middle adolescence occurs, teens spend significant time on their appearance in an effort to look more attractive. In addition, they might be more comfortable than earlier in adolescence with the physical changes that accompany puberty.[27] Body image is usually not of critical concern to emerging adults in late adolescence, though they will certainly contend with continued media messaging into adulthood about sometimes unattainable body ideals.

Identity and Psychological Development

Establishing a sense of self and individual identity is a process that occurs over the course of adolescence. In earlier adolescence, this is evidenced by distancing from family and involvement in activities outside of the household. It is not until later adolescence that a true sense of identity seems to form. "The process of discovering *that* one has a separate identity (the process of individuation) precedes the process of discovering *what* that identity is (the process of identity development)."[34]

The mind-set of an adolescent can be egocentric, especially in early development. A child or young teen might feel that adults around him or her should share the same priorities and values. A young teen, for example, might not understand why his school work has to get in the way of an important game over a weekend. Another might feel as if "the world will end" if she cannot attend a dance. Adolescents may experience an "imaginary audience," where they tend to feel that others around them are especially focused on them. If a dietitian notices that a teen is not getting adequate nutrition, for example, and asks that he or she eat a larger, more balanced lunch meal at school, fear of peer judgment at the lunch table might race through a teen's mind. In late adolescence, a young adult has a stronger sense of identity, and self-image is less defined by peers.[31]

Risk Taking

Adolescents are presented with many new situations in which they have to make decisions about participating in potentially risky behavior, such as sexual relations, driving, drugs, and alcohol. Earlier theory proposed that teens often make poor decisions to take risks because of limited decision-making capacity and cognitive skills.[35] More recently, research has shown that adolescents make such decisions fully aware of risks, but that they are greatly influenced by impulsive emotions in the moment and social influences.[36] Studies have also demonstrated that adolescents might feel greater emotional satisfaction in risk taking, which can influence their decision to participate in such behavior despite potential dangers.[28] In boys, there is a potential association between age of onset of puberty, either earlier or later than the norm, and increased likelihood of risk-taking behaviors.[37] Healthcare practitioners, including dietitians, need to be aware that these behaviors are potentially a part of an adolescent client's life. It is important to create an environment in which a teen feels comfortable addressing such concerns and to identify opportunities to discuss the potential risks of such behavior.[28]

Role of Technology

The role of technology in adolescent development is no longer an up-and-coming influence; it has become a standard. By 2010, kids 11 to 18 years of age spent an average of over 11 hours per day exposed to electronic media.[38] Social networking sites play a major role in day-to-day interaction, and adolescents check these sites at the start, throughout, and at the conclusion of their days. Their solitary activities and face-to-face interactions with friends are now interrupted by social media messaging. Use of social media feeds seamlessly into adolescents' increased desire to participate in group activities and compare themselves to others.[39] Students in both high school and college report that most of their social media connections, or "friends," are made up of their "offline" or face-to-face friends.[39,40]

Social media unfortunately increases the possibility of experiencing negative feedback or disheartening self-comparison to peers.[39] With increased reliance on social media, the topic of "cyber-bullying" has become a focus of concern. Cyber-bullying is defined as "any behavior performed through electronic or digital media by individuals or groups that repeatedly communicates hostile or aggressive messages intended to inflict harm or discomfort on others."[41] On average 20–40% of youths have been victims of cyber-bullying and rarely do victims inform parents or adults of their experience.[41] The existing research on associations between age, gender, demographics, and prevalence of cyber-bullying is inconsistent, though it seems adolescents are most susceptible at 12 to 14 years of age.[41]

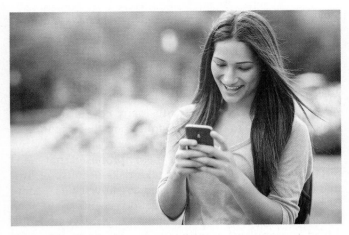

©arek_malang/Shutterstock

Recap The physical developments of adolescence, or puberty, progress through a specific sequence of changes as boys and girls develop reproductive capacity and become young adults. During this time, physical differences between sexes become more apparent. Psychosocial development also takes place three stages of early, middle, and late adolescence, during which a child's identity and relationships with family and peers evolve.

1. What is a sexual maturity rating (SMR)? What does it mean if an adolescent has an SMR of stage 1? Of stage 5?
2. What is the difference between sequence and tempo of puberty?
3. How does the timing of weight gain differ between girls and boys during puberty?
4. Why is menarche (the start of a girl's period) not a good marker of the start of puberty?
5. How does concern about body image usually change over the course of adolescent development?

Case Study

Carla always used to be happy to sit and talk with her mom and brother at the dinner table on school nights. Lately, Carla has been moody and quieter, distracted by her cellular phone for most of the meal. She looks at images of peers on social media and sends text messages to her friends from her lunch table at school. Some of her friends have recently been skipping lunch period to go smoke cigarettes.

Questions

1. In which stage of adolescent development is Carla at 14 years of age?
2. Is her behavior at the dinner meal typical of normal adolescent psychosocial development?

Factors Affecting Dietary Intake During Adolescence

Preview The adolescent years draw many parallels to the toddler years. Much like toddlers, adolescents are exposed to a wide array of new life experiences and are continuously seeking their own freedom and independence. With this desire for independence, all aspects of their life undergo change, especially dietary intake and nutrition. This section reviews factors that may affect an adolescent's life and their potential impact on dietary intake.

Family

Adolescents' home environment is one of the greatest influences on all aspects of their life, which is why it is no surprise that family is a large factor affecting dietary intake. Quality of nutritional intake has been linked to family meals. The frequency of family meals has been found to be positively associated with fruit, vegetable, grain, and calcium-rich food intake and negatively associated with soft drink intake.[42] In addition, the frequency of family dinners is positively associated with increased intake of fiber, calcium, folate, iron, vitamins B_6, B_{12}, C, and E,[42,43] as well as a lower intake of saturated fat, soda, and fried food among those who ate meals more often with their families.[44]

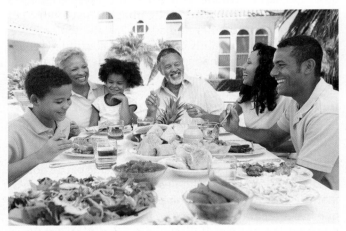

©Monkey Business Images/Getty Images

Family mealtimes are constantly changing during this life stage, especially as adolescents make the transition from middle school to high school. During the high school years, adolescents separate themselves more from their families as they get their driver's license, become more involved in after-school activities, and hold jobs outside of the home. The number of family meals tends to drop off with the transition from middle school to high school.[45,46] This of course is not surprising, given the increased independence that occurs during this stage of life.

Although families may want to have mealtimes together, meals are often missed because of the high demands of everyone's busy schedules. And though 74% of adolescents from one survey enjoyed having meals with their families, 53% reported different schedules inhibited frequent/consistent family meals.[47] Adolescents tend to take on more extracurricular activities and academic demands increase, both of which can contribute to decreased time at home with family. Despite their busy schedules, a study that looked at frequency of family meals found that although adolescents report eating meals with "all or most" of the members in their household 4.5 times a week, 14% of adolescents reported no family meals.[42] In light of the positive outcomes observed linking family meals and nutritional intake, adolescents and their families should be encouraged to find time to incorporate family meals several times per week.

Peers

As children move from childhood to adolescence, they have an increased need for acceptance by their peers. General opinion is that peer groups have influence on dietary intake; however, studies have not consistently demonstrated a strong association between friends and food choices.[48–50] Peers have minimal influence on the adolescent's fruit and vegetable intake, but they do appear to influence consumption of whole grain foods, dairy products, and breakfast.[51] This finding is of importance because these foods are often lacking in the adolescent's diet. Not surprising, an individual's snack and soft drink consumption was greater when the adolescent's peers had high consumption of these items as well as when snack food and soft drinks were easily accessible within schools and vending machines.[52] Adolescents and their friends exhibit some similarities in eating patterns, making friend groups a good target population for future nutrition interventions.

Time and Convenience

Because adolescents are always on the go, they tend to prefer foods that meet their busy lifestyle needs. Fast food appeals to teenagers because it is quickly satisfying, relatively inexpensive, tasteful, socially acceptable, and easy to access. Fast-food restaurants are also common employers of adolescents, making them widely accepted by this group.[53] Common menu items of fast-food establishments are energy dense and high in sodium.[53] Fast-food companies have made great strides in attempting to improve items on their menu by offering salads and lower-fat food options. However, just because these items are offered on the menu does not necessarily mean they are chosen more often, especially by this population.

Time constraints have been perceived as a significant and pervasive barrier to consuming a healthful diet in this population. Adolescent focus groups have noted commonalities that adversely affect dietary intake, including preferring to sleep in in the mornings over preparing breakfast, selecting foods at home that had short preparation times, and choosing to eat at fast-food restaurants because the serve time is short.[49,50] It is clear that adolescents feel their schedules do not allow time for worrying about consuming healthy foods.

Difficulty managing busy schedules makes meal skipping a common practice among adolescents. The most commonly skipped meal among teenagers is breakfast.[48] Skipping meals can cause disturbances to appetite regulation and can lead to overeating during subsequent mealtimes but can also lead to undereating.[54–57] Indeed, adolescents who consume fewer than three meals per day have diets that are of poorer quality compared with those who eat more frequently.[53] Adolescents have also reported skipping meals as a method to lose weight. The 2013 U.S. High School Youth Risk Behavior Survey found that 13% of individuals did not eat for 24 hours or more in order to lose weight or to keep from gaining weight in the 30 days preceding the survey.[58] Adolescents should be closely monitored, and concerning behaviors (such as skipping meals) should be further investigated.

Media

As technology has continued to advance, media has gained a greater reach into our lives. Adolescents are constantly connected to various social media outlets at nearly all hours of the day. Media is no longer restricted to television and print but is on cell phones, tablets, computers, and even watches. Young adults spend more time on various media outlets than in school, and it is the leading activity for children and teenagers besides sleeping.[38,59,60] Seventy-one percent of children and teenagers have reported having a television in their bedroom, which is especially concerning because evidence shows that having a television in the bedroom increases risk of obesity.[38,59,61,62]

Food items that are typically advertised to young consumers are sweetened cereals, fast food, snack foods, and candy—items typically high in sugar, fat, and sodium.[53] With advertisement of this type of food, it is no surprise that empty calories from solid fat and added sugar comprise 40% of total daily calories consumed by children and adolescents.[63]

Compounding the challenges are media advertisements that set very unrealistic body image expectations to which adolescents compare themselves. In addition, as the number of social media outlets continues to grow, offering innumerable images of models, actors/actresses, and athletes, the exposure to unrealistic body images is relentless. During the adolescent years, boys and girls are hyperaware of their body as they undergo a multitude of physical changes. Body image issues apply to both girls and boys, with boys reporting that their predominant fear is they are not muscular or big enough and girls generally reporting fear of not being thin enough.[64] It is important to help the adolescent understand that advertisements are airbrushed, photoshopped, and touched up to create a "perfect" photo. With media messages and images having a potentially harmful effect, pediatricians are encouraged to take a media history during all well-child visits to assess amount of daily screen time, social media exposure, and risks.[59]

School

Adolescents spend the majority of their day in school, and a large proportion of students has at least one meal per day at school. Two programs that play an important role in providing nutrition and ensuring students' nutritional needs are met are the School Breakfast Program and National School Lunch Program. Both are administered by the U.S. Department of Agriculture (USDA), and guidelines regarding food groups and portion sizes are established at the federal level. Federal guidelines require that a school lunch provide one-third of the Recommended Dietary Allowance (RDA) or Adequate Intake (AI) for participating students.[65] Although meal requirements are set at the federal level, local school food authorities decide which foods to serve.

Common criticisms of the School Lunch Program include poor acceptance of menu items by students, food waste, and the amount of fat, sugar, and sodium in the foods served.[53] These criticisms have been addressed by the USDA in the following ways: encouraging school lunch participants to aid in menu planning, limiting saturated fat to less than 10% of the weighted average based on what is offered over the week, and allowing individuals to refuse or substitute items for something that is nutritionally comparable.[65] In the 2014–2015 school year, the USDA responded to criticism that meals were not healthy enough by requiring that all grains served be whole grain.[65]

Schools are in a powerful position to significantly affect students' dietary choices. One critical area in which schools can influence student meals and snacking is through vending machines. Schools have been criticized over the availability and content of on-campus vending machines because the content of the vending machines can influence student eating behavior. A study administered by the U.S. Health Behavior in School-Aged Children Survey to sixth- through tenth-graders found that 83.1% of the schools had vending machines; in particular, schools with higher grades were more likely to have vending machines.[66] Students who attend schools offering fruits and vegetables in vending machines consumed more fruits and vegetables as compared with students from schools where these items are not available. On the other hand, students from schools that sell sweets in vending machines consumed more sweets than those students whose schools did not sell these items.[66] Unfortunately, reports indicate that the most common items sold in school vending machines are soft drinks, chips, and sweets.[66–69] Schools have now begun to replace available

snacks with the Smart Snacks in School program. The program, rolled out in the 2014–2015 school year, affects over 100,000 schools participating in the National School Lunch Program.[70] Smart Snacks in School applies to foods sold at schools including vending machines, at the school store, and à la carte and limits the amount of calories, fat, sugar, and sodium permitted in foods made available at schools.[70] Smart Snacks encourages children to make healthier snack choices that give them the nutrition they need to grow and learn. Given the influential position of schools to make a positive impact on children's dietary choices, more nutritionally mindful options should be available to students, and the Smart Snacks in Schools program is a great leap in the right direction.

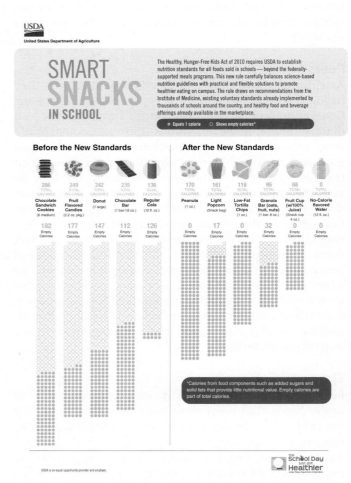

Reproduced from: http://www.fns.usda.gov/healthierschoolday/tools-schools-focusing-smart-snacks

Food Availability

Parents may have minimal influence on items their adolescents consume outside of the home, but inside the home parents should make healthy, nutrient-dense options readily available. Availability simply means something that is easy to get to or access. Teenagers tend to prefer foods that are readily available, hence the popularity of fast-food establishments in this population. At home, when possible the approach of "out of sight, out of mind" should be taken with energy-dense, nutrient-poor items. Fresh fruits and vegetables should be made easily accessible, such as a fruit bowl on the table, to promote intake of these nutritious foods on a more regular basis. Findings from the project EAT (Eating Among Teens) suggest positive associations between availability of healthy foods at home and vegetable and fruit food patterns and inverse associations with the fast-food pattern.[71]

Food Security

The majority of U.S. households have reliable access to adequate amounts of food to support a healthful lifestyle. A minority of U.S. households, however, undergo periods of food insecurity throughout the year, meaning they do not have access to enough food owing to inadequate resources during those times. In 2014, 9.4% of households with children were food insecure at some point in the year.[72] Of the food-insecure households, 61% reported participating in at least one of the three major federal food and nutrition assistance programs (Special Supplemental Nutrition Program [SNAP], Women, Infants, and Children [WIC], and National School Lunch Program) during the preceding month.[72] Food insecurity is more common in large cities and rural areas than in suburban areas and exurban areas surrounding large cities.[72] It is extremely important to know about an adolescent's home life and to work with both the individual and his or her family to ensure nutritional needs are being sufficiently met with available resources.

Recap Adolescents are a population highly susceptible to exterior and interior influences. When working with adolescents, it is important to understand the many influences in their lives and their part in affecting nutritional intake.

1. List factors affecting dietary intake during adolescence and provide an example of how each affects the adolescent's intake.

Let's Discuss

Today's adolescent population has grown up nearly from birth with the Internet, mobile phones, and social media. Give some thought to how these technologies influence daily interactions with peers as well as health and diet. How could an adolescent today use these media in a positive way to make and promote safe and healthy choices?

News You Can Use

How accurate are activity trackers?

Electronic wristbands are gaining in popularity among exercise enthusiasts. The wearable gadgets come with a multitude of features, including counting steps, monitoring heart rate, and estimating energy expenditure. The gadgets continue to gain popularity among individuals of all age groups and activity levels. However, the question that often surfaces with these wildly popular wristbands is how accurate are they? Recent research at Iowa State University tested the accuracy of four popular consumer fitness trackers and two research monitors. Researchers monitored participant's involvements in common exercise activities as well as daily living activities and examined where the errors occurred.[a] The results found that the research monitors and consumer fitness trackers provided reasonably accurate energy expenditure estimates with the error rate ranging from 15.3% to 18.2% for the devices studied, except for one, which had a much greater error rate of 30.4%.[a] Larger margins of error were seen when resistance training was looked at individually, with the error rate ranging from 20% to 52.6% for the devices studied.[a] Although fitness trackers do have some limitations, more research is needed to further examine these monitors and understand the activities most compatible with these tracking systems. In the meantime, consumers should not shy away from these fitness sidekicks, especially if one keeps them motivated and accountable to taking steps toward a healthy lifestyle.

Reference

a. Bai Y, Welk G, Nam YH, et al. Comparison of consumer and research monitors under semistructured settings. *Med Sci Sport Exer*. 2015;48:151–158.

Case Study

Carla's mom recently got a new job that requires her to be out of the home during dinnertime several nights per week. There is always adequate food in the house, but Mom is finding herself too busy to pack a lunch for Carla every day. On the days when she is unable to pack lunch, she gives Carla money to purchase food at school.

Questions

1. What are some factors that might influence Carla's food choices on days when she buys lunch at school?
2. When Mom is unable to be home for dinner, what resources can be utilized to ensure Carla eats an adequate dinner?

Nutritional Recommendations and Requirements During Adolescence

Preview During the adolescent years, growth is more rapid than at any other time in life with the exception of infancy. Puberty is a staple of adolescence, and this is the first time nutrient needs are distinguished between boys and girls as they enter this stage of monumental change. Given the many physical changes that occur during this time, nutrient needs greatly increase. Adequate nutrient intake is therefore crucial to adequately support the biological changes taking place. As adolescents take hold of their independence, they begin making more food choices for themselves. Often, these choices are not healthy or nutritionally sound. This section highlights key nutrients that are of importance in this population as well as areas to focus on for improvement.

Table 10.3

Children and Adolescents 3–18 Years

Estimated Energy Requirement (kcal/day) = Total Energy Expenditure + Energy Deposition

Boys

3–8 yrs	EER = 88.5 − (61.9 × age [y]) + PA^b × [(26.7 × weight [kg]) + (903 × height [m])] + 20
9–18 yrs	EER = 88.5 − (61.9 × age [y]) + PA × [(26.7 × weight [kg]) + (903 × height [m])] + 25

Girls

3–8 yrs	EER = 135.3 − (30.8 × age [y]) + PA × [(10.0 × weight [kg]) + (934 × height [m])] + 20
9–18 yrs	EER = 135.3 − (30.8 × age [y]) + PA × [(10.0 × weight [kg]) + (934 × height [m])] + 25

Note: These equations provide an estimate of energy requirement. Relative body weight (i.e., loss, stable, gain) is the preferred indicator of energy adequacy.

^{a}EER = Estimated Energy Requirement.

^{b}PA = Physical Activity Coefficient.

Data from Otten JJ, Hellwig JP, Meyers LD. *DRIs: The Essential Guide to Nutrient Requirements*. Washington, DC: Institute of Medicine, The National Academies Press; 2006.

Macronutrients

Energy

Guidelines for daily energy needs are defined by the Dietary Reference Intakes (DRIs) as the Estimated Energy Requirement (EER). EER is determined by an individual's basal metabolic rate, age, sex, weight, height, and physical activity (see **TABLE 10.3** and **TABLE 10.4**).[73] The energy needs as determined by the EER are based on children with normal metabolic rate, activity, growth, and body composition.

Table 10.4

Physical Activity Coefficients (PA Values) for Use in EER Equations

	Boys 3–18 y	Girls 3–18 y
Sedentary (PAL* 1.0–1.39) Typical daily living activities (e.g., household tasks, walking to the bus)	1.00	1.00
Low Active (PAL 1.4–1.59) Typical daily living activities PLUS 30–60 minutes of daily moderate activity (e.g., walking at 5–7 km/h)	1.13	1.16
Active (PAL 1.6–1.89) Typical daily living activities PLUS at least 60 minutes of daily moderate activity	1.26	1.31
Very Active (PAL 1.9–2.5) Typical daily living activities PLUS at least 60 minutes of daily moderate activity PLUS an additional 60 minutes of vigorous activity or 120 minutes of moderate activity	1.42	1.56

*PAL = physical activity level.

Data from Otten JJ, Hellwig JP, Meyers LD. *DRIs: The Essential Guide to Nutrient Requirements*. Washington, DC: Institute of Medicine, The National Academies Press; 2006.

Carbohydrates, protein, and fat should be consumed in appropriate proportions to meet energy needs, and no food group should be omitted from the diet. The Acceptable Macronutrient Distribution Range (AMDR) is defined as an intake range that is related to a decreased risk of chronic disease while meeting essential nutrient needs.[53] Intakes above the AMDR reference range may increase the risk of chronic diseases and may lead to inadequate intake of essential nutrients. Adolescents should try to maintain the following macronutrient distribution of their total caloric intake: carbohydrates 45–65%, fat 25–35%, and protein 10–30%.

Protein

Protein is a fundamental building block of the human body and is found in all cells and tissues, ranging from muscles and bones to skin and hair. In the United States, most individuals exceed the Recommended Dietary Allowance (RDA) for protein, and the incidence of protein malnutrition is rare.

Rapid growth and development are staples of the adolescent years, making adequate consumption of high-quality protein important. Protein requirements are greatest during times when height velocity peaks. Protein needs steadily decline following the rapid growth phase during infancy and then increase again during puberty. Protein RDAs for adolescence can be found in **TABLE 10.5**.

When obtaining a diet history, it is good practice to assess not only the quantity but also the quality of the protein that is consumed. Vegetable protein sources may be considered inferior to animal protein because they are not complete proteins, meaning they lack essential amino acids. This is crucial to remember when working with adolescents who follow a vegetarian diet.

Fluid

In general, healthy adolescents are typically able to self-regulate their fluid intake without risking dehydration or overhydration. With this in mind, adolescent hydration becomes more of a question of quality than quantity. Adolescents generally have high intake of sweetened beverages such as soda. Although these beverages meet hydration needs, they provide minimal nutritional value and the "empty calories" can contribute to undesired weight gain. Adolescents should be encouraged to drink water, nutrient-rich beverages such as skim or low-fat milk, or 100% fruit juice to meet fluid needs. Fruit juice should be limited to 8–12 ounces per day in 7- to 18-year olds per recommendations from the American Academy of Pediatrics.

Hydration status can most easily be assessed by urine color and urination frequency. When individuals are adequately hydrated, their urine appears "straw like" in color. Underhydration can lead to dark-colored urine and should be a sign to increase fluid intake. The Holliday–Segar equation is the most commonly used method in calculating maintenance fluid needs in children and adolescents. This equation equates the estimated number of kilocalories expended to fluid needs.[74] **TABLE 10.6** shows for the Holliday–Segar equation in calculating maintenance fluid needs in children.

Fiber

Americans generally meet their requirements for daily total carbohydrates; however, most consume added sugar and refined grains in excess and do not eat enough fiber.[75] Foods rich in fiber include fruits, vegetables, and whole grains, all of which are usually lacking in the typical adolescent diet. According to the findings of a large national dietary survey, less than 1% of adolescents meet daily recommendations for both fruits and vegetables.[76] Furthermore, a 2010 report noted that 28.5% of high school students consumed less than one fruit per day and 33.2% of high school students consumed less than one vegetable per day.[77] Adolescents should be encouraged to increase fiber intake and to make at least half of their grain choices whole grains to meet daily recommendations outlined in **TABLE 10.7**.

Table 10.5

Dietary Reference Intakes for Protein.

	Source of goal[a]	Female 9-13	Male 9-13	Female 14-18	Male 14-18
Calorie level(s) assessed		1,600	1,800	1,800	2,200, 2,800, 3,200
Protein, g	RDA	34	34	46	52
Protein,% kcal	AMDR	10-30	10-30	10-30	10-30

Data from U.S. Department of Health and Human Services and U.S. Department of Agriculture. *2015-2020 Dietary Guidelines for Americans.* 8th ed. Washington, DC: U.S. Department of Health and Human Services and U.S. Department of Agriculture; December 2015. Retrieved from: https://health.gov/dietaryguidelines/2015/guidelines/appendix-7/. Accessed September 13, 2016.

Table 10.6

Holliday–Segar Equation for Maintenance Fluid

Weight (kg)	Fluid Requirement
1–10 kg	100 cc/kg
10–20 kg	1,000 cc + 50 cc for each kg >10 kg
> 20 kg	1,500 cc + 20 cc for each kg over 20 kg

Modified from Holliday MA, Segar WE. The maintenance need for water in parenteral fluid therapy. *Pediatrics*.1957; 19:823–832.

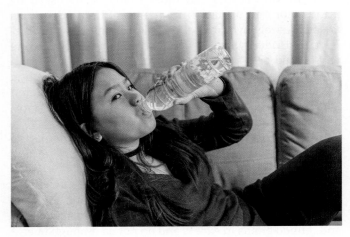

©9george/Shutterstock

Vitamins and Minerals

Vitamin and mineral needs increase during adolescence because of the rapid physical changes that occur during this stage of life. Vitamin and mineral deficiencies are rare in the United States. **TABLE 10.8** and **TABLE 10.9** list the DRIs for vitamins and minerals. It is important to remember

Table 10.7

Fiber requirements

Age (in years)	Total Fiber Intake (g/day)
1–3	19
4–8	25
Boys	
9–13	31
14–18	38
Girls	
9–13	26
14–18	26

Fiber recommendations are based on data for adults, 14 grams fiber/1000 kcal, using median energy intake from United States, Continuing Survey of Food Intakes by Individuals (CSFII), 1994–1996, 1998.

Information compiled from http://www.nal.usda.gov/fnic/DRI//DRI_ Energy/339-421.pdf.

that the DRIs are recommendations for a healthy population. With various disease states, vitamin and mineral needs may change.

The DRIs provide guidelines for recommended intake; however, the nutrients most commonly lacking in the diets of children and adolescents are calcium, iron, vitamin A, folic acid, zinc, vitamin E, and vitamin B_6.[53] Interestingly, a study investigating the association between the frequency of family meals and dietary intake found positive associations between frequency of family meals and intake of calcium, iron, folate, fiber, and vitamins A, C, E, and B_6.[42] Increasing the frequency of family meals positively affects adolescents' dietary intake and should be encouraged.

Fruits and vegetables are rich sources of vitamins and minerals, and adolescents are commonly poor consumers of these foods. A large cohort study analyzed 2 days of 24-hour recalls reported by adolescents and found that fruit intake was primarily composed of 100% orange juice and the main contributors of total vegetable intake were fried and nonfried potatoes.[76] When fried potatoes were not included as vegetable intake, the median vegetable intake decreased by over half.[76] These findings highlight the need for education and programs to increase adolescent exposure to a greater variety of fruits and vegetables. Encouraging a more varied intake will hopefully bridge the gap between actual and recommended intake.

Although adequacy and variety of all essential micronutrients is important, the following are of specific significance for the adolescent population.

Calcium

Calcium plays a vital role in bone health and is needed for bone mineralization. The adolescent years are prime time for calcium retention so adolescents achieve peak bone mass, especially in girls because they are at greater risk of osteoporosis later in life.[53] Unfortunately, calcium intake decreases during the adolescent years and soda intake increases. Adolescent males drink an average of 22 ounces and females average 14 ounces of regular soda per day, respectively. In comparison, average milk consumption is much less at 10 ounces and 6 ounces per day for males and females, respectively.[78] **TABLE 10.10** lists the calcium content of common calcium-rich food sources.

Vitamin D

Vitamin D is also crucial for optimal bone health development, with the primary function of facilitating calcium absorption. Adequate intake of vitamin D can be difficult to obtain via food alone and this vitamin is best absorbed from sunlight exposure. Adolescents with minimal sunlight exposure may need supplementation. Checking serum 25-hydroxy vitamin D is an excellent method for

Table 10.8

Dietary Reference Intakes for Vitamins and Minerals.

	Ages 9–13		Aes 14–18	
	Female	Male	Female	Male
Minerals				
Calcium, mg	1300	1300	1300	1300
Iron, mg	8	8	15	11
Magnesium, mg	240	240	360	410
Phosphorous, mg	1250	1250	1250	1250
Potassium, mg	4500	4500	4700	4700
Sodium, mg	2200	2200	2300	2300
Zinc, mg	8	8	9	11
Copper, mcg	700	700	890	890
Manganese, mg	1.6	1.9	1.6	2.2
Selenium, mcg	40	40	55	55
Vitamins				
Vitamin A, mg RAE	600	600	700	900
Vitamin E, mg AT	11	11	15	15
Vitamin D, IU	600	600	600	600
Vitamin C, mg	45	45	65	75
Thiamin, mg	0.9	0.9	1	1.2
Riboflavin, mg	0.9	0.9	1	1.3
Niacin, mg	12	12	14	16
Vitamin B6, mg	1	1	1.2	1.3
Vitamin B12, mcg	1.8	1.8	2.4	2.4
Choline, mg	375	375	400	550
Vitakin K, mcg	60	60	75	75
Folate, mcg DFE	300	300	400	400

Data from the 2015-2020 Dietary Guidelines. Retireved from: https://health.gov/dietaryguidelines/2015/guidelines/appendix-7/.

Table 10.9

Tolerable Upper Levels for Vitamins and Minerals.

	UL 9–13	UL 14–18
Minerals		
Calcium, g/d	2.5	2.5
Iron, mg/d	40	45
Magnesium, mg/d	350	350
Phosphorous, g/d	4	4
Sodium, g/d	2.2	2.3
Zinc, mg/d	23	34
Copper, mg/d	5,000	8,000
Manganese mg/d	6	9
Selenium	280	400
Vitamins		
Vitamin A	1700	2800
Vitamin E	600	800
Vitamin D	50	50
Vitamin C, mg/d	1200	1800
Niacin, mg/d	20	30
Vitamin B6, mg/d	60	80
Choline, g/d	2	3
Folate	600	800

Data from the DRI report; http://www.nap.edu; Dietary Guidelines 2015.

Table 10.10

Calcium rich food sources and their respective calcium equivalents.

1 cup milk* = approx. 300 mg calcium	1 cup (8 oz) yogurt†
	1 cup calcium-fortified orange juice
	1 cup calcium-fortified soy milk‡
	1 cup calcium-fortified rice milk or almond milk‡,§
3/4 cup milk =	1 oz cheddar, jack, or Swiss cheese
2/3 cup milk =	1 oz mozzarella or American cheese
	2 oz canned sardines (with bones)
1/2 cup milk =	2 oz canned salmon (with bones)
	1/2 cup custard or milk pudding
	1/2 cup cooked greens (mustard, collards, kale)
1/4 cup milk =	1/2 cup cottage cheese
	1/2 cup ice cream
	3/4 cup dried beans, cooked or canned

*Some low-fat or skim milks and some low-fat yogurts have additional nonfat dry milk (NFDM) solids added. Some labels will read "fortified." Such products will contain more calcium than indicated here.

†Most commercially prepared yogurt does not contain vitamin D.

‡The amount of calcium varies; not all milks are fortified with calcium and/or vitamin D.

§Rice and almond milks (and other nut milks) have significantly less protein than cow's milk and soy milk.

assessing vitamin D status. Serum 25(OH)-D levels of ≤ 37.5 nmol/L (15 ng/mL) are considered deficiency, and greater than 50 nmol/L (20 ng/mL) is classified as vitamin D sufficiency.[79] The most common treatment strategy for vitamin D deficiency in adolescents is administration of a high-dose vitamin D supplement of up to 50,000 International Units (IU) and rechecking the 25(OH)-D level in 6 to 8 weeks to reevaluate vitamin D status.[79]

Iron

It is estimated that up to 6.5 million teenage girls and women are iron deficient.[80] Iron needs significantly increase during adolescence largely because of increases in blood volume and muscle mass. Ensuring adequate iron intake is especially important for adolescent females because menses increases their risk of iron deficiency. Iron deficiency can cause fatigue and weakness and may lead to deregulation of homeostasis and impair immune function.[80] Although iron deficiency can also lead to anemia, isolated iron deficiency is more common than iron-deficiency anemia in the United States. Iron-rich foods should be encouraged as well as iron-fortified foods. Animal sources of iron (i.e., heme iron) are more bioavailable, and thus more readily absorbed, as compared with plant sources (i.e., nonheme iron). To maximize iron absorption, nonheme iron should be consumed concurrently with a vitamin C–rich food source.

Folate

Folate is needed for protein synthesis, and daily needs of folate are heightened during the adolescent years. Intake studies have shown that adolescents do not consume an adequate amount of folate daily.[53] Good sources of folate that should be encouraged are dark leafy-green vegetables (asparagus, spinach, and broccoli), legumes (lentils and dried beans), and folate-fortified foods (breakfast cereal and bread).

Sexually active adolescent females should be especially mindful to consume sufficient folate. Inadequate folate intake has been shown to greatly increase risk of neural tube defects in fetuses. Thus, adolescents and women of childbearing age should consume 600 mcg of folate daily.

Recap The adolescent years are a time of rapid physical change, and adequate nutritional intake is needed to support the changes taking place. Adolescents' diets have been shown to have several shortcomings and close attention should be paid to ensure they are meeting nutritional needs for continued growth and development.

1. Which micronutrients are most commonly lacking in the adolescent's diet?

2. Which micronutrients are important for bone health development?

3. You have a 25-kg female client and are asked to calculate her maintenance fluid needs. What equation would you use and how much fluid in milliliters does she need per day?

Case Study

Carla has recently complained to her mother of heavy menstrual flow and fatigue. Her mom took her to the doctor for medical assessment, and her lab values indicated iron deficiency.

Question

1. Carla's medical doctor will address concerns related to her menstrual cycle but asks you for dietary guidance related to her iron deficiency. What strategies could you provide to Mom and Carla?

Common Nutrition Considerations During Adolescence

Preview A multitude of physical, psychological, and environmental factors can affect an adolescent's nutritional status and growth. It is important, therefore, that a healthcare practitioner complete a thorough assessment that includes each of these areas. Support of a multidisciplinary healthcare team in establishing healthy behaviors is critically important in adolescence because positive well-being during teenage years can influence adult patterns.[81]

Nutrition Screening and Assessment

The American Academy of Pediatrics' *Bright Futures Nutrition* is a national health promotion and disease prevention initiative for infants, children, adolescents, and families that aims to promote positive attitudes towards nutrition and offer suggestions for choosing healthy foods.[82] *Bright Futures Nutrition* outlines important categories for adolescent nutrition screening, including eating behaviors, food choices, food resources, weight and body image, physical activity, and lifestyle.[82] Numerous questionnaires have been developed to screen for food-related issues and assist in providing dietary guidance. A sample questionnaire to screen for nutritional well-being from the California Department of Public Health is shown in TABLE 10.11. This questionnaire can provide basic information about

Table 10-11

Food Habits

Client name _____

For each question, **circle** the answer which best describes the client's usual behavior.

1. How many days each week do you skip breakfast, lunch, or dinner?

   None   1–2 days   3–5 days   6–7 days

2. Do you limit or avoid any food or food groups (such as meat or dairy)?

   Yes   No   If yes, explain: _____

3. How often do you eat any of these foods?

   - Candy, chocolate, chips, cookies
   - Donuts, muffins, biscuits, cake, sweet bread
   - Ice cream, frozen yogurt
   - Sour cream, mayonnaise

   Never   Rarely   A few times per week   Daily

4. Yesterday, did you drink any sweetened beverages or energy drinks (e.g. regular soda, fruit drinks, sweetened tea/coffee drinks, Kool-Aid® punch, or sports drinks)?

   Yes   No   If yes, which: _____

   If yes, how much did you drink? _____

5. How often do you eat or take out a meal from a fast-food restaurant?

   Never   Rarely   A few times per week   Daily

6. How often do you take a multivitamin or folic acid supplement in a week?

   Never   1–2 days   3–5 days   6–7 days

7. Do you take any other vitamin or mineral supplements, such as iron and calcium?

   Yes   No

   If so, what brand or type?

   _____

8. Do you use home remedies or herbal supplements, such as chamomile or ginseng?

   Daily   Weekly   Rarely   Never

   If so, what brand or type?

   _____

9. Do you use any pills or teas to lose weight?

   Yes   No

10. Do you eat, drink, or take anything to build muscle or increase your weight?

    Daily   Weekly   Rarely   Never

    If so, what brand or type?

    _____

11. Are you a vegetarian?

    Yes   No

12. Are you on a special diet?

    Yes   No   If yes, explain: _____

13. Has your doctor ever told you that you have anemia or another nutrition-related health issue?

    Yes   No   If yes, explain: _____

14.   **Ask if pregnant:**

   A.   Do you ever eat any of the following?

   - Raw or undercooked eggs, meat, shellfish, fish, including sushi
   - Deli meat or hot dogs without heating or steaming
   - Unpasteurized milk, cheese, or juice, including soft cheeses such as feta, blue cheese, queso de crema, asadero, queso fresco, panela, or homemade
   - Alfalfa/mung bean sprouts
   - Shark, swordfish, king mackerel, or tilefish
   - Albacore tuna >6 ounces/week

   B.   Do you eat fish or shellfish more than 2x/week?

   Yes   No   If yes, explain: _____

   C.   Do you eat fish caught locally by self, friends, or family more than 1x/week?

   Yes   No   If yes, explain: _____

   D.   Have you fasted during this pregnancy, or do you plan to fast?

   Yes   No   If yes, explain: _____

Interpreting Responses:

The responses in gray indicate the client may be at high risk nutritionally and may need a referral.

Skipped Meals: Frequently missed meals can result in the inadequate intake of calories and nutrients or can lead to overeating at other meals and snacks. Explore the client's reasons for skipped meals with them. See the *Weight Management* section for healthy snack ideas and tips for healthy eating.[a]

Unhealthy Beverages: Sugar-sweetened beverages, such as soda, sports drinks, juice, and energy drinks can contribute to weight gain due to the extra calories and sugar. Note that the American Academy of Pediatrics recommends that energy drinks never be consumed by children and adolescents due to the high caffeine content.[b] Sweetened or non-nutritive beverages also displace healthier beverages such as lowfat milk or water.

Convenience/Fast Food: Convenience and fast foods are popular and easily available. Frequent consumption increases fat, calorie, and salt intake and reduces intake of fiber and some vitamins and minerals. Use the handout below to discuss options for healthier food choices at fast-food restaurants: www.ces.ncsu.edu/EFNEP/fesmm_handouts/makingSmartChoicesEatingFastFood.pdf.

Vegetarian Diets: Because the term "vegetarian" is often used loosely, refer to the *Vegetarian Teens* section for additional screening questions for clients who say they are vegetarian.[a]

Vitamin and mineral supplements, although helpful in some instances, such as in the case of folic acid, cannot take the place of a healthy diet. If the client insists on taking supplements, emphasize the need to avoid high doses that can be toxic. This can be done by encouraging or helping a teen to choose a multivitamin that meets all her or his needs, rather than taking multiple pills. Encourage her or him to talk to her/his healthcare provider, registered dietitian, or a pharmacist if she or he has any questions about what quantity is safe for her or him to take. Herbal supplements are not regulated by the U.S. Food and Drug Administration (FDA) and have not been satisfactorily researched to determine their safe use for adolescents.

Protein Powders and Creatine: Protein recommendations even for athletes can generally be met through diet alone, without the use of protein or amino acid supplements.

The effect of creatine on the growing adolescent body is unknown. Like herbal supplements, creatine is not regulated by the FDA. There is no monitoring of the purity or strength of the supplement.

If an adolescent is using supplements, refer to a registered dietitian.

Special Diets: Clients on special diets for medical reasons, such as diabetes, should be instructed by a registered dietitian and should receive ongoing monitoring of their medical condition by their healthcare provider.

Food Safety: Pregnant women and infants are at greater risk from food poisoning because their immune systems are weaker than healthy adults and children. The foods listed in Question 14 may contain harmful bacteria or toxic chemicals.

Fasting: Fasting is not recommended during pregnancy. Most religions and cultures give exceptions to fasting practices during pregnancy.

Resource(s):

[a] The *Weight Management, Vegetarian Teens* and *Folic Acid and Folate* sections can be found in the California Department of Public Health

Adolescent Nutrition Guidelines found at www.cdph.ca.gov/HealthInfo/healthyliving/nutrition/Pages/TeenGuidelines.aspx .

Steps to Take nutrition, physical activity, and breastfeeding handouts in English and Spanish can be found at www.cdph.ca.gov/programs/ NutiritionandPhysicalActivity/Pages/NutritionPhysicalActivityandBreastfeeding.aspx .

WIC educational materials for women in English and Spanish can be found at www.cdph.ca.gov/programs/wicworks/Pages/ WICEducationMaterialsWomen.aspx.

Food Security

Client name _____

For each question, **circle** the answer which best describes the client's usual behavior or situation.

1. In the past month, were you worried whether your food would run out before you or your family had money to buy more?

   Yes   No

2. In the past month, were there times when the food that you or your family bought just did not last and you did not have money to get more?

   Yes   No

3. Do you use any of the following food resources?
   - CalFresh (food stamps)   Yes   No
   - WIC   Yes   No
   - Free food, such as from food banks, pantries, or soup kitchen   Yes   No
   - Free or reduced-price school meals   Yes   No

Interpreting Responses:

The responses in gray indicate the client may be at high risk nutritionally and may need a referral.

Encourage the client to use available resources. Refer to food assistance and nutrition programs, such as WIC, if the client is eligible.

Resource(s):

Steps to Take nutrition, physical activity and breastfeeding handouts in English and Spanish can be found at www.cdph.ca.gov/programs/NutiritionandPhysicalActivity/Pages/NutritionPhysicalActivityandBreastfeeding.aspx.

WIC educational materials for women in English and Spanish can be found at www.cdph.ca.gov/programs/wicworks/Pages/WICEducationMaterialsWomen.aspx.

Choosemyplate.gov has useful information and tips for meeting food and physical activity recommendations.

Food Shopping and Preparation

Client name _____

For each question, **circle** the answer which best describes the client's usual behavior or facilities.

1. Who buys the food that you and your family eat?

   I do   My parent(s)   My spouse or partner   Other: _____

   If not you, is the person who does open to suggestions and education?   Yes   No

2. Is a shopping list used?

   Yes   No   Sometimes

3. Who plans and prepares the meals that you eat?

   I do   My parent(s)   My spouse or partner   Other: _____

   If not you, is the person who does open to suggestions and education?   Yes   No

4. Where you live, do you have …
   - Enough space for food preparation?   Yes   No
   - Electricity?   Yes   No
   - Clean running water?   Yes   No
   - A working stove?   Yes   No
   - A working oven?   Yes   No
   - A working microwave?   Yes   No
   - A working hot plate?   Yes   No
   - A working refrigerator?   Yes   No

Interpreting Responses:

The responses in gray indicate the client may be at high risk nutritionally and may need a referral.

Resource(s):

If appropriate, share healthy recipes with the client or other person responsible for the family's meals. This resource can be found at www.cdph.ca.gov/programs/NutiritionandPhysicalActivity/Pages/EasyMealsandSnacks.aspx.

Steps to Take nutrition, physical activity and breastfeeding handouts in English and Spanish can be found at www.cdph.ca.gov/programs/NutiritionandPhysicalActivity/Pages/NutritionPhysicalActivityandBreastfeeding.aspx.

WIC educational materials for women in English and Spanish can be found at www.cdph.ca.gov/programs/wicworks/Pages/WICEducationMaterialsWomen.aspx.

Choosemyplate.gov has useful information and tips for meeting food and physical activity recommendations.

Modified from California Department of Public Health. California Nutrition and Physical Activity Guidelines for Adolescents. Retrieved from: http://www.cdph.ca.gov/HealthInfo/healthyliving/childfamily/Documents/MO-NUPA-02NutritionalRiskScreening.pdf. Accessed September 13, 2016.

an adolescent's food intake and food security but cannot replace a complete nutrition assessment and dietary recall. Asking adolescents about their sleep patterns can also be useful because it can provide background information about meal timing and because inadequate sleep may negatively influence dietary quality.[83]

A comprehensive and accurate dietary recall of both food and drink is critical for appropriate nutrition assessment and can be obtained via several methods. A 24-hour recall is common, in which the adolescent reports intake from the day prior to the assessment. Starting with the most recent eating occasion has been found to sometimes aid memory.[84] A general food recall, which asks an adolescent to describe a typical school day of eating, can also provide an estimate of intake. Rather than prompting a teenager with "What do you normally eat for breakfast?" it can be better to ask, "When is the first time you eat on a typical day?" and progressing to ask about the next eating occasion, and so on. Asking in this manner does not assume that breakfast or any other meal is part of a daily eating pattern, which is often the case for teens. If an adolescent will be returning for follow-up visits in an outpatient setting, a 3-day food record (usually 2 weekdays and 1 weekend day) can provide more detail about typical eating patterns. A drawback to using a 3-day food record is that an adolescent might alter his or her food choices during these 72 hours, knowing that someone will be evaluating what is recorded.[84] Depending on the age of the adolescent, parental assistance with completing a food record might be necessary. A food frequency questionnaire yields the same limited information as in Table 10.11 and does not provide specifics about portion sizes. It can, however, be useful as an initial screening tool.[85]

Objective data from an adolescent's health record are also of critical importance to piecing together a full picture of nutritional status. These data include a general medical and growth curve history that likely includes sexual maturity rating, family medical history, current anthropometrics (i.e., weight, height, BMI), vital signs (e.g., blood pressure, pulse), and laboratory test results.[86] Elements of an initial nutrition assessment are illustrated in **TABLE 10.12**. Close coordination and sharing of exam data with a physician or nurse practitioner, likely the primary care provider (PCP), helps elucidate what a dietitian cannot evaluate. The PCP will also likely be the best resource for obtaining growth curve history. If prior growth curves are unavailable, any known anthropometrics should be plotted on age-appropriate growth curves to aid with nutritional assessment.

It is important to establish a trusting relationship with an adolescent during the nutrition visits. For successful adolescent care, a practitioner must genuinely like clients in this age group and be interested in their development.[87] If the context of the nutrition visit allows, it can be very beneficial to interview the patient both in the presence of the parent/caregiver and alone to provide the adolescent freedom to speak and to build rapport and trust with the dietitian. In some situations it is also helpful to interview parents/caregivers individually. It can help to ask permission of a teen to do this so that the dietitian is not perceived to be breaking trust. Often, a comprehensive picture can be gained by gathering information from both child and parental sides.

Also important to keep in mind is that data provided by adolescents are not always accurate. Reliance solely on self-reported height and weight, for instance, has led to missed cases of adolescents who, when accurately measured, fall within overweight or obese BMI ranges as a result of underreporting of weight.[88,89] Height and weight measurements should ideally be physically obtained during a nutrition assessment, especially if recent medical records are unavailable. With regard to dietary recall, early adolescents younger than the age of 12 might struggle with providing accurate food and portion size recall without the assistance of parents. As adolescents get older, general underreporting of energy intake has been observed. Accuracy of food recalls in adolescents can also be made difficult by changing factors in their lives, such as unstructured eating patterns, eating out of the home, and concerns with self-image.[90]

Nutrition Intervention

Information gleaned from a thorough nutrition assessment can inform a dietitian or other healthcare practitioner about the potential need for further evaluation or counseling. Adolescents who are greater than or equal to the 95th percentile for BMI for age and gender are considered to be obese. Those who are greater than or equal to the 85th percentile BMI, but less than the 95th percentile, are considered overweight.[91] Of note, from the age of 20 onward, BMI can no longer be plotted on a standard growth curve. Obesity after this point is measured by the adult BMI value of greater than or equal to 30 kg/m^2. This is important to remember because older adolescents (but younger than the age of 20) who plot at greater than or equal to the 95th percentile on a growth curve might indeed have a BMI of greater than or equal to 30 kg/m^2. Therefore, the recommended definition of obesity in this subset of adolescents is 95th percentile BMI or BMI greater than or equal to 30 kg/m^2, whichever is lower.[91]

Guidelines recommend that medical practitioners provide interventional counseling for adolescents categorized as obese. For adolescents who fall into overweight BMI percentiles, practitioners are encouraged to further evaluate the health risk posed by a teen's BMI score. Risk can be influenced by an adolescent's medical history, family medical history, BMI trend, diet, activity, and relevant laboratory values.[91] Coincidentally, a thorough initial nutrition assessment will have already covered these areas of concern and can therefore inform a dietitian or physician about the need for medical attention. Once this

Table 10.12

Elements of an Initial Nutrition Assessment for Adolescents

General	• Age (including date of birth to help correctly plot on growth curves) • Grade or level of schooling
Diet and physical activity	• Food allergies and/or intolerances • General intake of food and beverage (via 24-hour diet recall, 3-day food record, or other) • Meals eating inside vs. outside the home • Vitamin/mineral/supplement intake • Cultural or religious dietary needs • Adherence to a diet (e.g., vegetarianism, veganism, calorie counting) • Physical activity and competitive sports
Anthropometrics	• Height • Weight • BMI • Growth curve history of the above • Biological parents' heights to calculate midparental height

Medical history	• Disease(s) that might affect intake, growth, or mobility
	• Surgery or injury that could affect intake or mobility
	• Psychological conditions
	• Sexual maturity rating
	• Menstrual history (girls)
	  • Age at menarche
	  • Regularity
	  • Biological mother's age at menarche

Pertinent family history	• History of underweight, overweight, or obesity • History of nutrition-related disease states (e.g., cardiac, diabetes) • Menstrual difficulties (women)
Nutrition-focused physical findings	• Constipation • Diarrhea • Nausea • Vomiting • Dizziness or blurry vision upon standing • Feeling cold more often (associated with underweight)
Laboratory values and vital signs	• Cholesterol panel • Iron studies • Vitamin levels if suspicion for deficiency (e.g., vitamin D) • Electrolytes (especially with report of diarrhea or suspicion of disordered eating) • Blood pressure • Biopsy results (e.g., celiac disease)
Social history (if appropriate)	• Members of household • Food insecurity • Extracurricular activities • Alcohol intake

background information is reviewed, a practitioner might determine that a teen who falls in the overweight category is not at increased risk of health concerns related to his or her weight. In this case, preventive health care that includes messaging about healthy diet and activity should be provided, as with any normal-weight teenager.[91]

Historically, adolescents who have a BMI of less than the 5th percentile have been considered underweight, and accepted guidelines have directed them for referral to a doctor.[86] In 2014, updated guidelines for evaluating pediatric malnutrition (up to 18 years of age) were published by the Academy of Nutrition and Dietetics and the American Society for Parenteral and Enteral Nutrition (ASPEN).[92]

The purpose of these guidelines was to identify standardized parameters for diagnosis and documentation of malnutrition. Rather than focus on BMI percentiles, these new parameters are based on **Z-scores** of anthropometric measurements. Under these guidelines, malnutrition, if present, can be categorized as mild, moderate, or severe. Mild malnutrition is generally related to short-term or acute events such as illness, whereas moderate and severe malnutrition are related to longer-term undernutrition. A diagnosis of any level of malnutrition indicates a need for further medical evaluation and potential nutrition intervention. The published parameters are shown in TABLE 10.13,[92] and indicators that are applicable to the adolescent population are highlighted.

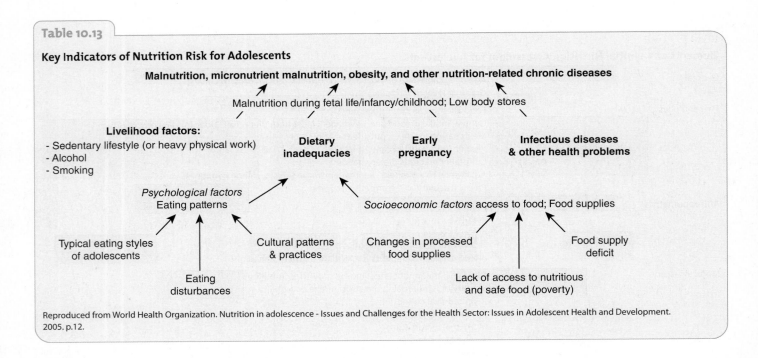

Table 10.13

Key Indicators of Nutrition Risk for Adolescents

Reproduced from World Health Organization. Nutrition in adolescence - Issues and Challenges for the Health Sector: Issues in Adolescent Health and Development. 2005. p.12.

Delayed puberty can have significant influence on whether a child attains his or her height potential and therefore should be watched closely.[9] When assessing an adolescent's growth curves, it is valuable to remember that weight is a shorter-term indicator of nutrition, and height is a longer-term indicator of nutritional status. It is important to investigate, therefore, percentile changes over time and, more importantly, changes in Z-score values. A useful practice when evaluating adolescent girls' growth curves is to mark age at menarche on the height curve. Because girls generally do not grow more than 2–3 inches after menarche, seeing a plateau begin within a couple of years of menarche is to be expected. If an adolescent girl has not yet reached menarche, asking about her biological mother's age of menarche can be a useful because menarcheal age is in part influenced by heredity.[93] If an otherwise normally developing girl is premenarchal and plotting below her anticipated midparental height, she likely still has time for catch-up growth, and additional medical and nutrition evaluation is warranted. A similar approach can be taken in an otherwise normal adolescent male if he seems to be plotting below his projected midparental height and has not yet completed puberty. See FIGURE 10.3 for an example of a normal female height curve compared with a height trend for which intervention is indicated.

Counseling for Adolescent Behavior Change

Initially, developing adolescents lack the ability to project or plan into the future or evaluate long-term consequences of their actions. Discussion of healthy behavior change should therefore focus on short-term goals. A child at this age might not respond to advice such as, "Eating breakfast will help you focus in class so you can get into college," but he or she might respond more to "Breakfast will give you energy so you can outrun your competitors in sports practice this week." As they transition into young adulthood, adolescents develop the ability to be forward thinking, which will aid them in planning for higher education, career, and/or adult responsibilities. These can then become motivating topics for behavior change. For example, if an older adolescent is making poor food choices or partaking in risky behavior, discussion might focus on how healthier choices can improve energy or focus for an impending college course or job responsibilities. Strategies to promote healthy eating and physical activity in adolescents are listed in TABLE 10.14.

Recap A thorough assessment of adolescent growth and nutritional status includes medical history, growth records, and self-report of behaviors related to eating and activity. Intervention can be indicated when an adolescent's growth varies significantly from expectations, lab results or vital signs are abnormal, or a teen reports unhealthy patterns of behavior. Counseling for behavior change must be age appropriate and relate to an adolescent's stage of physical and psychosocial development.

1. In addition to a dietary recall, what types of objective data can be useful during an initial nutrition assessment?
2. What are potential drawbacks of relying on an adolescent's self-report for anthropometric measurements and dietary recall?
3. How do guidelines suggest a medical practitioner intervene for an adolescent categorized as obese? As overweight?

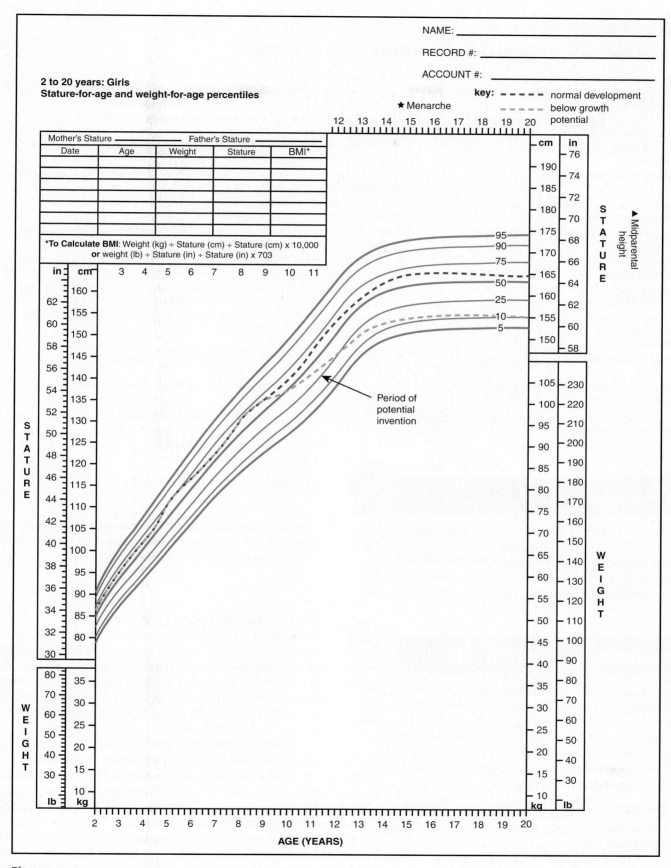

2 to 20 years: Girls
Stature-for-age and weight-for-age percentiles

★ Menarche

key: normal development

below growth potential

Mother's Stature _____ Father's Stature _____

Date	Age	Weight	Stature	BMI*

***To Calculate BMI**: Weight (kg) ÷ Stature (cm) ÷ Stature (cm) x 10,000
or weight (lb) ÷ Stature (in) ÷ Stature (in) x 703

▲ Midparental height

Period of potential invention

Figure 10.3
Stature for age and weight for age percentiles.

Table 10.14	
General Strategies to Promote Healthy Eating and Physical Activity to Adolescents	
Strategies	Applications/Questions
Ask the adolescent about changes in eating and physical activity behaviors at every visit.	"How are you doing in changing your eating and physical activity behaviors?"
Emphasize to the adolescent the consumption of foods rather than nutrients.	For example, say, "Drink more milk and eat cheese or yogurt," rather than "Increase your calcium intake."
Build on positive aspects of the adolescent's eating behaviors.	It's great that you're eating breakfast. Would you be willing to try cereal, fruit, and toast instead of bacon and doughnuts 4 days out of the week?"
Provide "how to" information.	Share behaviorally-oriented information (e.g., what, how much, and when to eat and how to prepare food) rather than focusing on why the information is important.
Provide counseling that integrates realistic behavior change into the adolescent's lifestyle.	"I understand that your friends eat lunch at fast-food restaurants. Would it help you to learn how to make healthier food choices at these restaurants?"
Discuss how to make healthy choices in a variety of settings.	Talk about how to choose foods in various settings such as fast-food and other restaurants, convenience stores, vending machines, and friends' homes.
Provide the adolescent with learning experiences and skills practiced.	Practice problem solving and role playing (e.g., having the adolescent ask the food server to hold the mayonnaise).
Introduce the concept of achieving balance and enjoying all foods in moderation.	"Your food diary indicates that after having pepperoni pizza for lunch yesterday, you ate a healthier dinner. That's a good way to balance your food intake throughout the day."
Make record-keeping easy, and tell the adolescent that you do not expect spelling, handwriting, and behaviors to be perfect.	"Be as accurate and honest as you can as you record your food intake. This food diary is a tool to help you reflect on your behaviors."
Make sure the adolescent hears what you are saying.	"What eating and physical activity behaviors are you planning to work on before your next appointment?"
Make sure that you and the adolescent define terms the same way to avoid confusion.	Discuss the definition of words that may cause confusion, such as "fat," "calories," "meal," and "snack."

Reproduced from California Nutrition and Physical Activity Guidelines for Adolescents, http://www.cdph.ca.gov/HealthInfo/healthyliving/childfamily/Documents/MO-NUPA-02NutritionalRiskScreening.pdf

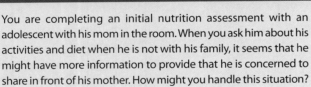

Let's Discuss

You are completing an initial nutrition assessment with an adolescent with his mom in the room. When you ask him about his activities and diet when he is not with his family, it seems that he might have more information to provide that he is concerned to share in front of his mother. How might you handle this situation?

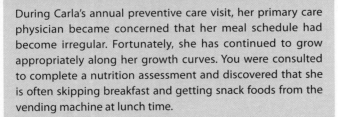

Case Study

During Carla's annual preventive care visit, her primary care physician became concerned that her meal schedule had become irregular. Fortunately, she has continued to grow appropriately along her growth curves. You were consulted to complete a nutrition assessment and discovered that she is often skipping breakfast and getting snack foods from the vending machine at lunch time.

Questions

1. What methods might you have used to obtain this dietary recall from Carla?
2. When counseling Carla about behavior change, what might you discuss as motivators for her to make changes to her dietary habits?

Promoting Healthy Lifestyles

Preview Keeping adolescents motivated and engaged is no easy task. This section discusses theoretical models to building an effective health promoting intervention.

Models for Nutrition Intervention

Adolescents have a difficult time envisioning themselves as susceptible to disease, and this can make implementation of and compliance with nutrition interventions challenging. Still, there are methods that should be used to motivate adolescents. Nutrition interventions that have been found to be most effective in this population fall into three categories: behavioral, theoretical, and environmental.

Interventions that are behaviorally focused are effective in yielding and maintaining the desired dietary change in adolescents.[94–96] Nutrition-related behaviors have been shown to start at an early age and typically follow individuals over time as they progress from one life stage to the next. Therefore, it has been suggested that intervening at an earlier age may be cost effective by influencing future chronic disease development.[96] Behavior-based interventions can be incorporated into school programs, and when additional behaviors, such as physical activity, are targeted, programs have demonstrated greater success.[96] The aim of behaviorally focused programs is to promote health by reducing risk factors.[96]

For adolescent programs the prevailing framework used is social cognitive theory (SCT) for promoting nutritional interventions.[71,96] The SCT framework allows for behavioral, personal, and environmental factors to continually interact. Adolescents may intend to drink more water and less soda, for example, but if the school vending machines only offer soda and few water fountains are available, the school environment may be limiting their ability to follow their intentions. As discussed in previous sections, adolescents are a highly influenced population and tend to conform to their peers and their environment. Therefore, nutrition interventions may be most effective in group settings that incorporate not only the individual but also peers. Schools are an opportune location to reach many teens.

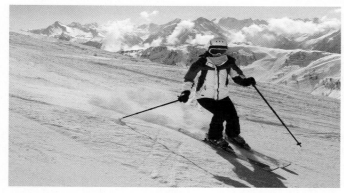

©Hisom Silviu/Shutterstock

Physical Activity

With the prevalence of childhood obesity on the rise, a proactive approach with physical activity promotion is critical. According to the U.S. High School Youth Risk Behavior Survey of 2013, 52.7% of students reported they were not physically active for at least 60 minutes per day on 5 or more days.[58] In addition, 15.2% of students reported they did not participate in at least 60 minutes of physical activity on at least 1 day in the 7 days preceding the survey.[58] Given the large number of students reporting inadequate physical activity, adequate attention should be given to promoting physical activity in this population.

Programs promoting physical activity interventions among adolescents that utilize an "education only" approach have little effect on increasing participation in physical activity.[97] Instead multicomponent interventions that take place in school environments, and employ the ecological approach have been used in the past to elicit behavior change.[97] The ecological model accounts for the fact that adolescents are a group influenced by a multitude of variables such as the individual, social, physical, and societal environment.[50,53] It is not surprising that the most effective interventions promoting physical activity among

adolescents utilized school-based interventions with community or family involvement.[97] Additionally, environmental elements, such as policy changes affecting physical education in schools can significantly influence physical activity promotion. A multicomponent approach that includes policy, schools, families, and community should be taken to promote physical activity because studies have shown this to be highly effective among adolescents.[97]

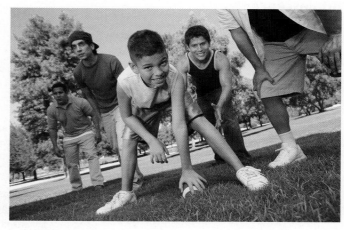

©bikeriderlondon/Shutterstock

Recap Adolescents have a difficult time envisioning themselves as susceptible to disease and can be a difficult population to keep motivated. When planning interventions targeted toward adolescents, it is best to take an interactive approach and to incorporate the adolescent's surroundings such as their friends or family.

1. What is the aim of a behaviorally focused nutrition intervention program?
2. What variables does the ecological model take into account?

Case Study

Soccer season has just started for Carla, and she has practice for 1 hour 3 days per week and is active during a soccer game for about an hour each weekend. On other days of the week, she watches television or plays video games on the couch.

Questions

1. According to the U.S. Department of Health and Human Services, children and adolescents should be physically active for 60 minutes per day. Is Carla meeting these recommendations with her current schedule?
2. In what setting might intervention to encourage Carla to be more active be most effective?

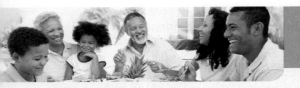

Learning Portfolio

Visual Chapter Summary

Growth and Development During Adolescence

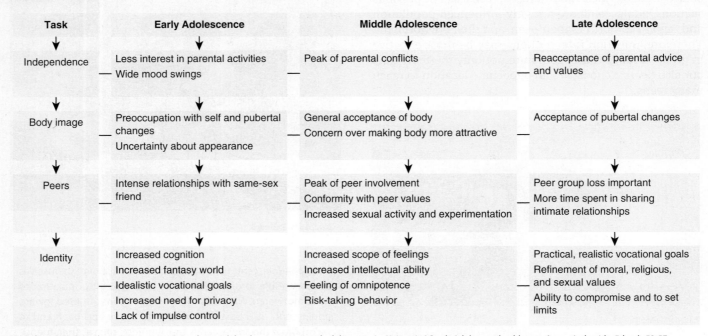

Task	Early Adolescence	Middle Adolescence	Late Adolescence
Independence	Less interest in parental activities Wide mood swings	Peak of parental conflicts	Reacceptance of parental advice and values
Body image	Preoccupation with self and pubertal changes Uncertainty about appearance	General acceptance of body Concern over making body more attractive	Acceptance of pubertal changes
Peers	Intense relationships with same-sex friend	Peak of peer involvement Conformity with peer values Increased sexual activity and experimentation	Peer group loss important More time spent in sharing intimate relationships
Identity	Increased cognition Increased fantasy world Idealistic vocational goals Increased need for privacy Lack of impulse control	Increased scope of feelings Increased intellectual ability Feeling of omnipotence Risk-taking behavior	Practical, realistic vocational goals Refinement of moral, religious, and sexual values Ability to compromise and to set limits

Data from Radzik M, Sherer S, Neinstein LS. Psychosocial development in normal adolescents. In: Neinstein LS, ed. Adolescent health care: A practical guide. 5th ed. 52-57. Philadelphia, PA: Wolters Kluwer Heath/Lippincott Williams & Wilkins; 2007:52-5

- Pubertal progress is defined by sexual maturity ratings (SMR) 1 through 5, also called Tanner stages. An SMR of stage 1 has no visual signs of change (prepuberty); SMR stage 5 is reached once adult characteristics have developed. SMR stages occur in a specific sequence and do not vary. The pace, or tempo, at which an adolescent moves through these stages is unique to each person.

- Gonadarche is the first visual sign of puberty. Boys generally reach this milestone about 2 years behind girls. Gonardarche in girls is marked by breast budding, also called thelarche. In boys, gonadarche is marked by an increase in testicular size. Menarche, or first menstruation, is not a sign of the start of puberty in girls. It usually occurs during SMR stage 3 or 4. Research shows a gradual decline in average age at menarche over several recent generations.

- About 20% of adult stature is gained during adolescence. Boys and girls go through growth spurts during which the rate of height growth, or height velocity, reaches its peak during adolescence. Variations between genders in pace and duration of linear growth results in adult men, on average, being taller than women. Girls generally will not grow more than 2 to 3 inches after menarche.

- Bone mass approximately doubles over the course of puberty, with 90% of peak skeletal mass reached by age 18 in healthy adolescents. Peak bone mass in boys tends to be greater than in girls. It is important to guide adolescents in establishing healthy behaviors for bone health.

- Adolescents gain approximately 50% of their adult weight during puberty. Girls experience peak weight gain before their growth spurt, and boys gain the majority of weight concurrent with their growth spurt.

- Body composition during puberty shifts and contributes to adult characteristics of sexual dimorphism, or the differences in appearance between men and women. Females generally having a gynoid body shape, or fat deposition around hips and thighs. Males develop android shape, with body fat concentrated near the abdomen.

- Psychosocial development can be divided into three stages based on age: early, middle and late

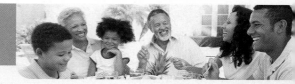

adolescence. Timing of emotional and social growth can vary between adolescents and does not always align with physical changes.

- Distancing from parents is typical of early adolescence, a focus on activities outside of the home in middle adolescence, and a transition into more balanced family relationships in late adolescence.
- Self-consciousness about body changes often occurs in early adolescence, and much time is devoted to an adolescent's own attractiveness by middle adolescence. Body image is usually less of a concern by late adolescence.
- Adolescents are often confronted with decisions about risk-taking behaviors such as driving, smoking, drinking alcohol, and sex. Technology and social media are also part of the fabric of adolescent life, and with this comes the potential for cyber-bullying.

Factors Affecting Dietary Intake During Adolescence

- The frequency of family meals has been found to be positively associated with fruit, vegetable, grain, and calcium-rich food intake and negatively associated with soft drink intake.[42]
- Snack and soft drink consumption is greater when the adolescent's peers have high consumption of these items as well as when snack food and soft drinks are easily accessible within schools and vending machines.[52]

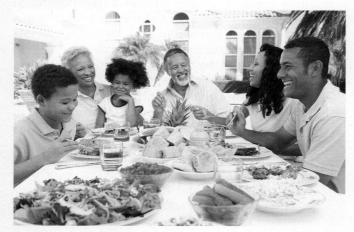

©Monkey Business Images/Getty Images

- Time constraints have been perceived as a significant and pervasive barrier to consuming a healthful diet.

- Common adverse influences on dietary intake, include preferring to sleep in the mornings over preparing breakfast, selecting foods at home that have short preparation times, and choosing to eat at fast-food restaurants because the serve time is short.[49,50]
- Difficulty managing busy schedules makes meal skipping a common practice among adolescents. The most commonly skipped meal among teenagers is breakfast.[48]
- Food items that are commonly advertised to young consumers are sweetened cereals, fast food, snack foods, and candy—all items that are typically high in sugar, fat, and sodium.[53] Empty calories from solid fat and added sugar comprise 40% of total daily calories consumed by children and adolescents.[63]
- Two programs that play an important role in providing and ensuring students' nutritional needs are met are the School Breakfast Program and National School Lunch Program.
- Of the food insecure households, 61% reported participating in at least one of the three major federal food and nutrition assistance programs (SNAP, WIC, and the National School Lunch Program) during the preceding month.[72]
- Adolescents are susceptible to a multitude of influences, including, but not limited to, family, peers, time, convenience, media, school, food, availability, and food security.

Nutritional Recommendation and Requirements During Adolescence

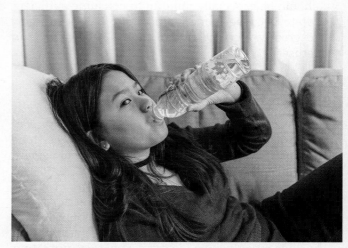

©9george/Shutterstock

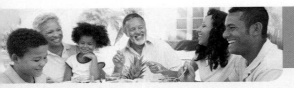

Learning Portfolio (continued)

- During the adolescent years, growth is more rapid than at any other time in life with the exception of infancy.
- Guidelines for daily energy needs are defined by the Dietary Reference Intakes (DRIs) as the Estimated Energy Requirement (EER). EER is determined by an individual's basal metabolic rate, age, gender, weight, height, and physical activity.[73]
- Protein requirements are greatest during times when height velocity peaks. Protein needs steadily decline following the rapid growth phase during infancy and then increase again during puberty.
- The Holliday–Segar equation is the most commonly used method in calculating maintenance fluid needs in children and adolescents. This equation equates the estimated number of kilocalories expended to fluid needs.[74]
- The nutrients most commonly lacking in the diets of children and adolescents are calcium, iron, vitamin A, folic acid, zinc, vitamin E, and vitamin B_6.[53]
- The adolescent years are essential for calcium retention in order to achieve peak bone mass, and this is especially true for girls because they are at greater risk of osteoporosis later in life.[53]
- Vitamin D is crucial for optimal bone health development, with its primary function being facilitating calcium absorption.
- Iron needs significantly increase during adolescence largely because of increases in blood volume and muscle mass.
- Folate is needed for protein synthesis, and daily needs of folate are heightened during the adolescent years. Sexually active adolescent females should be especially mindful to consume sufficient folate because inadequate intake has been show to greatly increase risk of neural tube defects in fetuses.

Common Nutrition Considerations During Adolescence

- Important categories for adolescent nutrition screening include eating behaviors, food choices, food resources, weight and body image, physical activity, and lifestyle. A dietary assessment can be completed using a 24-hour recall, 3-day food record, or a food frequency questionnaire. Each tool has strengths and weaknesses for gathering information.
- Objective data for an initial nutrition assessment include growth curve history, sexual maturity rating,

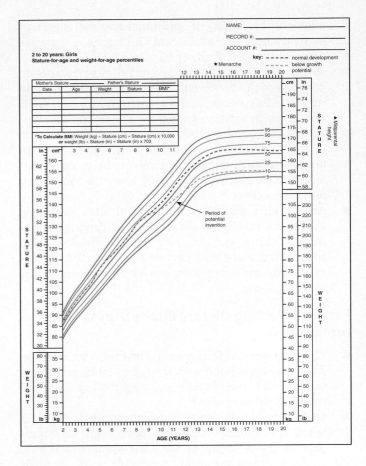

family medical history, current anthropometrics, vital signs, and laboratory test results.[86] Some of this information will come from other healthcare providers; close team coordination is critical.

- Establishment of trust between healthcare providers and adolescents is important. Even with trust, some adolescents can have difficulty providing accurate dietary and anthropometric recalls. Parents can aid with these shortcomings.
- Nutrition intervention should occur when an adolescent demonstrates factors of being at nutritional risk. Intervention should always occur with obese or malnourished adolescents. Further evaluation of overweight adolescents is important to determine whether their health is at risk. Healthy adolescents should receive appropriate preventive counseling.
- Motivators for behavior change should be age specific. Adolescents are often focused on short-term goals.

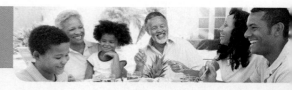

Promoting Healthy Lifestyles

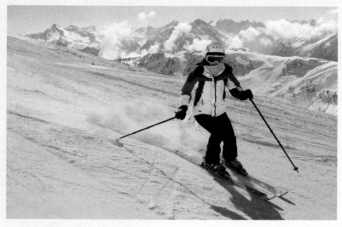

©Hisom Silviu/Shutterstock

- Nutrition interventions that have been found to be most effective among adolescents fall into three categories: behavioral, theoretical, and environmental.
- Interventions that are behaviorally focused are effective in yielding and maintaining the desired dietary change in adolescents.[94–96] Nutrition-related behaviors have been shown to start at an early age and typically follow individuals over time as they progress from one life stage to the next.
- Adolescent programs use the social cognitive theory (SCT) model for promoting nutritional interventions.[71,96] The SCT framework allows for behavioral, personal, and environmental factors to continually interact.
- A multicomponent approach that includes policy, schools, families, and community should be taken to promote physical activity among adolescents.[97]

Key Terms

android: Possessing characteristics of the male form; relating to fat deposition around abdomen.

gonadarche: First visual sign of puberty. Seen as breast budding in girls and as testicular enlargement in boys.

gynoid: Also called gynecoid. Possessing characteristics of the female form; relating to fat deposition around the hips and thighs.

menarche: Onset of menses, or the female period.

midparental height: A height calculated using an equation based on parents' height and adjusted for the child's sex; provides an indication of a child's linear growth potential.

peak height velocity: The time period of fastest rate of linear (height) growth.

puberty: Physical changes that occur as a child attains reproductive capacity.

sequence: In relation to puberty, the order in which physical changes occur during development. This order does not vary among individuals.

sexual maturity ratings (SMRs): Also called Tanner stages. Stages 1 through 5 of physical developments of puberty, visually assessed by gonadal and pubic hair changes.

sexual dimorphism: Variation of physical characteristics and body composition between the sexes.

spermarche: The first ejaculation of seminal fluid.

tempo: In relation to puberty, the pace at which physical changes occur during development. This can vary among individuals.

thelarche: Breast budding, a sign of pubertal onset in girls.

Z-scores: Measurements of how far a point is from the mean or average. A Z-score can be a positive or negative number.

Discussion Questions

1. What are three psychosocial factors for a developing adolescent that could influence decision making? Describe how each could potentially affect nutritional status.

2. Discuss at least three factors that affect an adolescent's dietary intake and how each factor can act as a potential barrier and facilitator to nutritional intake.

3. Discuss three shortcomings in the adolescent's diet and what you would recommend to help the individual better meet nutritional needs.

4. Discuss how guidelines for intervention of underweight children and adolescents have changed. How is malnutrition now categorized and when should intervention occur?

5. Suggest an nutritional intervention to help adolescents increase their daily physical activity. Use the social cognitive theory model as the framework for your intervention.

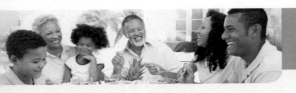

Learning Portfolio (continued)

Activities

1. Create a 1-day menu (include three meals and two snacks) for a 14-year-old healthy adolescent athletic male who is 5 feet 9 inches tall and who weighs 170 pounds. Figure out how many calories and how much protein and fluid he would need based on the information provided, and create a menu that appropriately meets these needs.

2. In partners or small groups, each participant should pretend to be an adolescent girl, 15 years of age.

Create a history for yourself, including typical food intake, activity level, height, weight, food beliefs, and social background (family and friends). Take turns completing a mock assessment with your partner or group members, asking about these issues. Then, together, discuss points where intervention might be warranted.

Study Questions

1. Which of the following does the process of puberty include?
   a. Physical changes
   b. Psychological changes
   c. Emotional changes
   d. All of the above
2. In comparison to girls, when do boys reach the first visible stages of puberty?
   a. 2 years earlier
   b. At nearly the same time
   c. 1 year later
   d. 2 years later
3. Which of the following are potential factors to assess in normal adolescent psychosocial development?
   a. Risk-taking behaviors
   b. Romantic relationships
   c. Use of social media and technology
   d. All of the above
4. How much do girls generally grow after menarche?
   a. They stop growing taller after menarche.
   b. 0.5–1 inch.
   c. 2–3 inches.
   d. They often grow 3+ inches.
5. Which government programs can influence dietary intake during the adolescent years?
   a. National School Lunch Program
   b. School Breakfast Program
   c. Supplemental Nutrition Program
   d. All of the above
6. Which is the most commonly skipped meal among this group?
   a. Dinner
   b. Lunch
   c. Breakfast

7. Which food items are most commonly advertised to young consumers?
   a. Rich in calcium
   b. Nutrient dense
   c. High in sugar, fat, and sodium
   d. High in cholesterol
8. Sexually active adolescent females should be mindful of consuming adequate amounts of what micronutrient?
   a. Calcium
   b. Iron
   c. Riboflavin
   d. Folate
9. Which of the following food sources would be considered a heme source of iron?
   a. Beef
   b. Iron-fortified cereal
   c. Spinach
   d. Both B and C
10. When assessing a patient for a vitamin D deficiency, which lab value would you ask for?
    a. DEXA scan
    b. 25(OH)-D
    c. 1, 25(OH)-D
    d. B and C
11. When assessing an adolescent, how can the best information be gathered?
    a. Interviewing the teen alone
    b. Interviewing the parent or caregiver alone
    c. Interviewing the teen at the same time as the parent or caregiver
    d. All of the above

12. When should interventional counseling be immediately provided?
    a. When an adolescent plots as obese
    b. When an adolescent plots as overweight
    c. When an adolescent plots at median BMI
    d. Both A and B
13. Which elements make up the social cognitive theory (SCT)?
    a. Behavioral
    b. Environmental
    c. Theoretical
    d. All of the above

14. When creating a physical activity intervention program for adolescents, what kind of approach would you use?
    a. Education only
    b. Ecological model
    c. Behavioral
15. What is an ideal environment to implement an effective physical activity program using the social cognitive theory?
    a. Group setting including an individual's peers
    b. Individualized setting
    c. School program
    d. Both A and C

Weblinks

- **American Academy of Pediatrics Bright Futures**
  https://brightfutures.aap.org/Pages/default.aspx
  From the American Academy of Pediatrics, this site provides tools for well-child care from birth to age 21. Contains age-specific tools and guidelines, including nutrition-focused tools for adolescents.

- **World Health Organization Adolescent Health**
  http://www.who.int/topics/adolescent_health/en/
  Age-specific data and healthcare recommendations for adolescent populations.
- **Centers for Disease Control and Prevention Adolescent and School Health**
  http://www.cdc.gov/healthyyouth/.

References

1. World Health Organization; 2015. Health topics: adolescent health. Retrieved from: http://www.who.int/topics/adolescent_health/en/. Accessed October 1, 2015.
2. Hagan JF, Shaw JS, Duncan P, eds. *Bright Futures: Guidelines for Health Supervision of Infants, Children, and Adolescents.* 3rd ed. Elk Grove Village, IL: American Academy of Pediatrics; 2008.
3. Craig KR, Biro FM. Normal pubertal physical growth and development. In: Fisher MM, ed. *Textbook of Adolescent Health Care.* 1st ed. Elk Grove Village, IL: American Academy of Pediatrics; 2011:23–31.
4. Marshall WA, Tanner JM. Variations in pattern of pubertal changes in girls. *Arch Dis Child.* 1969;44:291–303.
5. Marshall WA, Tanner JM. Variations in pattern of pubertal changes in boys. *Arch Dis Child.* 1970; 45: 13–23.
6. Spear, BA. Adolescent growth and development. *J Am Diet Assoc.* 2002;102(3):S23–S29.
7. Rogol AD, Roemmich JN, Clark PA. Growth at puberty. *J Adolesc Health.* 2002;31:192–200.
8. Root AW. Endocrinology of puberty. *J Pediatr.* 1973;83(1):1–19.
9. Carswell JM, Stafford DEJ. Normal physical growth and development. In Neinstein LS, ed. *Handbook of Adolescent Health Care.* Philadelphia, PA: Lippincott Williams & Wilkins; 2009:1–13.
10. Lee Y, Styne D. Influences on the onset and tempo of puberty in human beings and implications for adolescent psychological development. *Horm Behav.* 2013;64:250–261.
11. Gluckman PD, Hanson MA. Evolution, development and timing of puberty. *Trends Endocrin Met.* 2006;17(10):7–12.
12. Anderson SE, Dallal GE, Must A. Relative weight and race influence average age at menarche: results from two nationally representative surveys of US girls studied 25 years apart. *Pediatrics.* 2002;111(4):844–850.
13. Anderson SE, Must A. Interpreting the continued decline in the average age at menarche: results from two nationally representative surveys of girls studied 10 years apart. *J Pediatr.* December 2005;147(6):753–760.
14. Chulani VL, Gordon LP. Adolescent growth and development. *Prim Care.* 2014;41:465–487.
15. Loomba-Albrecht LA, Styne DM. Effect of puberty on body composition. *Curr Opin Endocrinol Diabet Obes.* 2009; 16:10–15.
16. Saggese G, Baroncelli GI, Bertelloni S. Puberty and bone development. *Best Pract Res Cl En.* 2002;16(1):53–64.
17. Weaver CM. Adolescence: the period of dramatic bone growth. *Endocrine.* 2002;17(1):43–48.
18. Whiting SJ, Healey A, Psiuk S, Mirwald R, Kowalski K, Bailey DA. Relationship between carbonated and other low nutrient dense beverages and bone mineral content of adolescents. *Nutr Res.* 2001;21:1107–1115.
19. Wyshak G, Frisch RE. Carbonated beverages, dietary calcium, the dietary calcium/phosphorus ratio, and bone fractures in girls and boys. *J Adolesc Health.* 1994;15:210–215.
20. Milne DB, Nielsen FH. The interaction between dietary fructose and magnesium adversely affects macromineral homeostasis in men. *J Am Coll Nutr.* 1999;19(1):31–37.

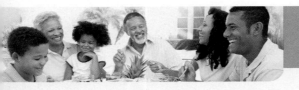

Learning Portfolio (continued)

21. Barzel US. The skeleton as an ion-exchange system: implications for the role of acid–base imbalance in the genesis of osteoporosis. *J Bone Miner Res.* 1995;10(10):1431–1436.

22. Massey LK, Whiting SJ. Caffeine, urinary calcium, calcium metabolism and bone. *J Nutr.* 1993;123:1611–1614.

23. Conlisk AJ, Galuska DA. Is caffeine associated with bone mineral density in young adult women? *Prev Med.* 2000;31:562–568.

24. McGartland C, Robson PJ, Murray L, et al. Carbonated soft drink consumption and bone mineral density in adolescence: the Northern Ireland Young Hearts Project. *J Bone Miner Res.* 2003;18:1563–1569.

25. Wyshak G. Teenaged girls, carbonated beverage consumption, and bone fractures. *Arch Pediat Adolesc Med.* 2000;154:610–613.

26. Steinberg L, Morris AS. Adolescent development. *Annu Rev Psychol.* 2001;52:83–110.

27. Radzik M, Sherer S, Neinstein LS. Psychosocial development in normal adolescents. In Neinstein LS, ed. *Adolescent Health Care: A Practical Guide.* 5th ed. Philadelphia, PA: Wolters Kluwer Heath/Lippincott Williams & Wilkins; 2007:52–57.

28. Sanders RA. Adolescent psychosocial, social, and cognitive development. *Pediatr Rev.* 2013;34(8):354–359.

29. Smetana JG, Campione-Barr N, Metzger A. Adolescent development in interpersonal and societal contexts. *Annu Rev Psychol.* 2006;57:255–284.

30. Larson R, Richards MH. Daily companionship in late childhood and early adolescence: changing developmental contexts. *Child Dev.* 1991;62(2):284–300.

31. Hornberger LL. Adolescent psychosocial growth and development. *J Pediatr Adolesc Gynec.* 2006;19:243–246.

32. Hodges EVE, Boivin M, Vitaro F, Bukowski WM. The power of friendship: protection against an escalating cycle of peer victimization. *Dev Psychol.* 1999;35(1):94–101.

33. Siegel JM, Yancey AK, Aneshensel CS, Schuler R. Body image, perceived pubertal timing, and adolescent mental health. *J Adolesc Health.* 1999;25(2):155–165.

34. Steinberg L, Collins WA. Adolescent psychosocial development and behavior. In Fisher MM, ed. *Textbook of Adolescent Health Care.* 1st ed. Elk Grove Village, IL: American Academy of Pediatrics; 2011:39–44.

35. Elkind D. Egocentrism in adolescence. *Child Dev.* 1967;38(4):1025–1034.

36. Steinberg L. Cognitive and affective development in adolescence. *Trends Cogn Sci.* 2005;9(2):69–74.

37. Williams JM, Dunlop LC. Pubertal timing and self-reported delinquency among male adolescents. *J Adolescence.* 1999;22:157–171.

38. Ridout VJ, Foehr UG, Roberts DF. Generation M2: media in the lives of 8- to 18-year olds. Kaiser Family Foundation; January 20, 2010. Retrieved from: http://kff.org/other/event/generation-m2-media-in-the-lives-of/. Accessed October 1, 2015.

39. Shapiro LAS, Margolin G. Growing up wired: social networking sites and adolescent psychosocial development. *Clin Child Fam Psych.* 2014;17(1):1–18.

40. Reich SM, Subrahmanyam K, Espinoza G. Friending, IMing and hanging out face-to-face: overlap in adolescents' online and offline social networks. *Dev Psychol.* 2012;48(2):356–368.

41. Tokunaga RS. Following you home from school: a critical review and synthesis of research on cyberbullying victimization. *Comput Hum Behav.* 2010;26(3):277–287.

42. Neumark-Sztainer D, Hannan PJ, Story M, Croll J, Perry C. Family meal patterns: associations with sociodemographic characteristics and improved dietary intake among adolescents. *J Am Diet Assoc.* 2003;103(3):317–322.

43. Munoz KA, Krebs-Smith SM, Ballard-Barbash R, Cleveland LE. Food intakes of US children and adolescents compared with recommendations. *Pediatrics.* 1997;100(3):323–329.

44. Kann L, Warren CW, Harris WA, et al. Youth Risk Behavior Surveillance: United States, 1995. *J Sch Health.* 1996;66:365–377.

45. Gillman MW, Rifas-Shiman SL, Frazier AL, et al. Family dinner and diet quality among older children and adolescents. *Arch Fam Med.* 2000;32:235–240.

46. Boutelle KN, Lytle LA, Murray DM, Birnbaum AS, Story M. Perceptions of the family mealtime environment and adolescent mealtime behavior. Do adults and adolescents agree? *J Nutr Educ.* 2001;33:128–133.

47. Neumark-Sztainer D, Story M, Ackard D, Moe J, Perry C. Family meals among adolescents: findings from a pilot study. *J Nutr Educ.* 2000;32:335–340.

48. Lin BH, Guthrie J Blaylock J. *The Diets of America's Children: Influences of Dining Out, Household Characteristics, and Nutrition Knowledge.* Washington, DC: U.S. Department of Agriculture; 1996. Economic Report no. 46 (AER-746).

49. Neumark-Sztainer D, Story M, Perry C, Casey M. Factors influencing food choices of adolescents: findings from focus groups discussion with adolescents. *J Am Diet Assoc.* 1999;99:929–937.

50. Story M, Neumark-Sztainer D, French S. Individual and environmental influences on adolescent eating behaviors. *J Am Diet Assoc.* 2002;102(3):S40–S51.

51. Bruening M, Eisenberg M, MacLehose R, Nanney MS, Story M, Neumark-Sztainer D. Relationship between adolescents' and their friends' eating behaviors: breakfast, fruit, vegetables, whole-grain, and dairy intake. *J Acad Nutr Diet.* 2012;112(10):1608–1613.

52. Wouters EV, Larsen JK, Kremers SP, Dagnelie PC, Greenen R. Peer influence on snacking behavior in adolescence. *Appetite.* 2010;55:11–17.

53. Lucas B Ogata B, Feucht S. Normal nutrition from infancy through adolescence. In Queen Samour P, King K, eds. *Pediatric Nutrition.* 4th ed. Burlington, MA: Jones & Bartlett Learning; 2012:103–126.

54. Neumark-Sztainer D, Hannan PJ, Story M, Perry CL. Weight-control behaviors among adolescent girls and boys: implications for dietary intake. *J Am Diet Assoc.* 2004;104(6):913–920.

55. Neumark-Sztainer D, Wall M, Story M, Standish AR. Dieting and unhealthy weight control behaviors during adolescence: associations with 10-year changes in body mass index. *J Adolesc Health.* 2012;50(1):80–86.

56. Savige G, MacFarlane A, Ball K, Worsley A, Crawford D. Snacking behaviours of adolescents and their association with skipping meals. *Int J Behav Nutr Phys Act.* September 17, 2007;3:36.

57. Castle J, Jacobsen M. Fearless feeding for your teenager (thirteen to eighteen years). In *Fearless Feeding.* San Francisco, CA: Jossey-Bass; 2013:189–246.

58. Kann L, Kinchen S, Shanklin SL, et al. Youth Risk Behavior Surveillance—United States, 2013. *MMWR Suppl.* 2014;63(4):1–168.

59. Council on Communications and Media. Children, adolescents, and the media. *Pediatrics.* 2013;132:958–961.

60. Strasburger VC, Jordan AB, Donnerstein E. Health effects of media on children and adolescents. *Pediatrics.* 2010;125(4):756–767.

61. Staiano AE, Harrington DM, Broyles ST, Gupta AK, Katzmaryzk PT. Television, adiposity, and cardiometabolic risk in children and adolescents. *Am J Prev Med.* 2013;44(1):40–47.

62. Gruber EL, Want PH, Christensen JS, Grube JW, Fisher DA. Private television viewing, parental supervision, and sexual and substance use risk behaviors in adolescents [abstract]. *J Adolesc Health.* 2005;36(2):107.

63. Reedy J, Krebs-Smith SM. Dietary sources of energy, solid fats, and added sugars among children and adolescents in the United States. *J Am Diet Assoc.* 2010;110(10):1477–1484.

64. Klawitter B. Nutrition counseling. In Queen Samour P, King K, eds. *Handbook of Pediatric Nutrition.* 3rd ed. Sudbury, MA: Jones & Bartlett Publishers; 2005:131–141.

65. Nutrition Standards in the National School Lunch and School Breakfast Programs. *Federal Register.* 2012;77(17):4088–4164. Retrieved from: http://www.fns.usda.gov. Accessed October 2015.

66. Rovner AJ, Nansel TR, Wang J, Iannotti RJ. Foods sold in school vending machines are associated with overall student dietary intake. *J Adolesc Health.* 2011;48(1):13–19.

67. Committee on Nutrition Standards for Foods in Schools. *Nutrition Standards for Foods in Schools: Leading the Way Toward Healthier Youth.* Washington, DC: Institute of Medicine; 2007.

68. Fox MK, Gordon A, Nogales R, Wilson A. Availability and consumption of competitive foods in US public schools. *J Am Diet Assoc.* 2009;109(2):S57–S66.

69. O'Toole TP, Anderson S, Miller C, Guthrie J. Nutrition services and foods and beverages available at school: results from the School Health Policies and Programs Study 2006. *J Sch Health.* 2007;77(8):500–521.

70. U.S. Department of Agriculture, Food and Nutrition Services; August 17, 2016. Healthier school day: tools for schools: focusing on smart snacks. Retrieved from: http://www.fns.usda.gov/healthierschoolday/tools-schools-focusing-smart-snacks. Accessed December 28, 2015.

71. Cutler GJ, Flood A, Hannan P, Neumark-Sztainer D. Multiple sociodemographic and socioenvironmental characteristics are correlated with major patterns of dietary intake in adolescents. *J Am Diet Assoc.* 2011;111(2):230–240.

72. Coleman-Jensen A Rabbitt MP Gregory C Singh A. *Household Food Security in the United States in 2014.* Washington, DC: U.S. Department of Agriculture, Economic Research Service; 2015. Economic Research Report no. 104.

73. Kohn MR. Nutrition. In Neinstein LS, ed. *Handbook of Adolescent Health Care.* Philadelphia, PA: Lippincott Williams & Wilkins; 2009:66–73.

74. Holliday MA, Segar WE. The maintenance need for water in parenteral fluid therapy. *Pediatrics.* 1957;19:823–832.

75. U.S. Department of Agriculture and U.S. Department of Health and Human Services. *Dietary Guidelines for Americans, 2010.* 7th ed. Washington, DC: U.S. Government Printing Office; December 2010.

76. Kimmons J, Gillespie C, Seymour J, Serdula M, Blanck HM. Fruit and vegetable intake among adolescents and adults in the United States: percentage meeting individualized recommendations. *Medscape J Med.* 2009;11(1):26.

77. Kim SA, Grimm KA, Harria DM, Scanion KS. Fruit and vegetable consumption among high school students—United States. MMWR. 2011;60:1583–1586.

78. Forshee RA, Anderson PA, Storey ML. Changes in calcium intake and association with beverage consumption and demographics: comparing data from CSFII 1994–1996, 1998 and NHANES 1999–2002. *J Am Coll Nutr.* 2006;25:108–116.

79. Misra M, Pacaud D, Petryk A, Collett-Solberg PF, Kappy M. Vitamin D deficiency in children and its management: review of current knowledge and recommendations. *Pediatrics.* 2008;122:398–417.

80. Deegan H, Bates HM, McCargar LJ. Assessment of iron status in adolescents: dietary, biochemical and lifestyle determinants. *J Adolesc Health.* 2005;37(1):75.

81. Hoyt LT, Chase-Lansdale PL, McDade TW, Adam EK. Positive youth, healthy adults: does positive well-being in adolescence predict better perceived health and fewer risky health behaviors in young adulthood? *J Adolesc Health.* 2012;50:66–73.

82. American Academy of Pediatrics. *Bright Futures: Nutrition.* 3rd ed. Elk Grove Village, IL: American Academy of Pediatrics. Retrieved from: https://brightfutures.aap.org/materials-and-tools/nutrition-and-pocket-guide/Pages/default.aspx. Accessed October 1, 2015.

83. Bel S, Michels N, De Vriendt, T, et al. Association between self-reported sleep duration and dietary quality in European adolescents. *Brit J Nutr.* 2013;110:949–959.

84. Academy of Nutrition and Dietetics. *Normal nutrition, adolescents, nutrition assessment. Pediatric Nutrition Care Manual.* Retrieved from: https://www.nutritioncaremanual.org/topic.cfm?ncm_category_id=12&lv1=144613&lv2=145229&ncm_toc_id=145229&ncm_heading=&. Accessed September 3, 2015.

85. Stang J. Assessment of nutritional status and motivation to make behavior changes among adolescents. *J Am Diet Assoc.* 2002;102(3):S13–S22.

86. Stang J, Story M. Nutrition screening, assessment, and intervention. In Stang J, Story M, eds. *Guidelines for Adolescent Nutrition Services.* Minneapolis, MN: University of Minnesota; 2005:35–54.

87. Woods ER Neinstein LS. Office visit, interview techniques, and recommendations to parents. In Neinstein LS, ed. *Adolescent Health Care: A Practical Guide.* 5th ed. Philadelphia, PA: Wolters Kluwer Heath/Lippincott Williams & Wilkins; 2007:52–57.

88. Elgar FJ, Roberts C, Tudor-Smith C, Moore L. Validity of self-reported height and weight and predictors of bias in adolescents. *J Adolesc Health.* 2005;37:371–375.

89. Tokmakidis SP, Christodoulos AD, Mantzouranis NI. Validity of self-reported anthropometric values used to assess body mass index and estimate obesity in Greek school children. *J Adolesc Health.* 2007;40(4):305–310.

90. Livingstone MBW, Robson PJ, Wallace JMW. Issues in dietary intake assessment of children and adolescents. *Brit J Nutr.* 2004;92(suppl 2):S213–S222.

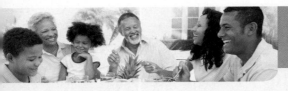

Learning Portfolio (continued)

91. Barlow SE. Expert committee recommendations regarding the prevention, assessment, and treatment of child and adolescent overweight and obesity: summary report. *Pediatrics.* 2007;120:S164–S192.

92. Becker P, Carney LN, Corkins MR, et al. Consensus statement of the Academy of Nutrition and Dietetics/American Society for Parenteral and Enteral Nutrition: indicators recommended for the identification and documentation of pediatric malnutrition (undernutrition). *Nutr Clin Pract.* 2014;114(12):1988–2000.

93. Graber JA, Brooks-Gunn J, Warren MP. The antecedents of menarcheal age: heredity, family environment, and stressful life events. *Child Dev.* 1995;66(2):346–359.

94. Nader PR, Stone EJ, Lytle LA, et al. Three-year maintenance of improved diet and physical activity. *Arch Pediatr Adolesc Med.* 1999;153:695–704.

95. Lytle LA. Nutrition education for school aged children. *J Nutr Educ.* 1995;27:298–311.

96. Hoelscher DM, Evans A, Parcel GS, Kelder SH. Designing effective nutrition interventions for adolescents. *J Am Diet Assoc.* 2002;102(3):S52–S63.

97. van Slujia EMF, McMinn AM, Griffin SJ. Effectiveness of interventions to promote physical activity in children and adolescents: systematic review of controlled trials. *BMJ.* October 6, 2007;335(7622):703. doi:113/bmj.39320.84394.BE.

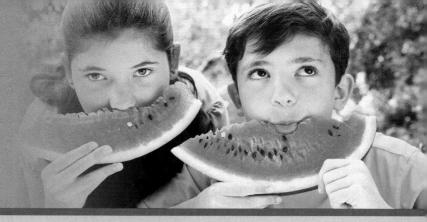

CHAPTER 11

Nutrition for Health and Disease in Childhood and Adolescence

Shelly Ben Harush Negari, MD **and Sigalit Cohen Zabar**, RD, **with contributions from Rachel Fine**, MS, RD, CSSD, CDN

Chapter Outline

Celiac Disease in Children and Adolescents

Pediatric Overweight and Obesity

Adolescent Eating Disorders

Pediatric Diabetes

Nutrition for Young Athletes

Adolescent Alcohol and Substance Abuse

Vegetarian Children and Adolescents

Learning Objectives

1. Describe the presentation and management of celiac disease.

2. Suggest three different strategies to address adolescent obesity.

3. Discuss three nutritional recommendations in the treatment of eating disorders.

4. Describe the differences between type 1 and type 2 diabetes in youth.

5. Explain the unique nutritional needs of young athletes.

6. Identify risk factors for adolescent substance abuse.

Case Study

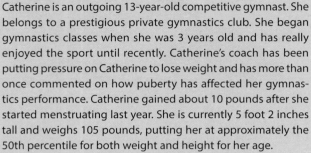

Catherine is an outgoing 13-year-old competitive gymnast. She belongs to a prestigious private gymnastics club. She began gymnastics classes when she was 3 years old and has really enjoyed the sport until recently. Catherine's coach has been putting pressure on Catherine to lose weight and has more than once commented on how puberty has affected her gymnastics performance. Catherine gained about 10 pounds after she started menstruating last year. She is currently 5 foot 2 inches tall and weighs 105 pounds, putting her at approximately the 50th percentile for both weight and height for her age.

In school, Catherine's grades begin to suffer and her friends have noticed she's quiet and withdrawn—not her usual bubbly self. Over the lunch period, Catherine can be seen walking the halls at a vigorous pace in an effort to burn calories. She skips eating lunch with her friends altogether. At home, Catherine's family is becoming concerned because she often skips dinner, saying she does not feel well. They also notice Catherine has been losing weight at a rapid pace. Catherine's coach, on the other hand, is pleased with Catherine's recent weight loss and praises her physique and commitment.

Childhood into adolescence is a unique time in the life span marked by profound physical, emotional, and mental development, increasing independence, significant social pressures, and maturation to adulthood. The developmental importance of this life stage is significant because it lays the foundation for future health and well-being. The dramatic physical growth during childhood and adolescence can be challenged by various health conditions, compounding the traditional nutrition-compromising behaviors such as meal skipping, convenience food and beverage consumption, and fad dieting. Diseases and conditions that have unique nutritional features during childhood and adolescence are discussed in this chapter.

Celiac Disease in Children and Adolescents

Preview Gastrointestinal conditions can have a profound effect on normal nutrient digestion and absorption and can challenge normal growth and development. Diseases of the gastrointestinal tract, such as celiac disease, that interfere with adequate nutrition also can increase risk of chronic conditions later in life.

Diseases and conditions that limit nutrient digestion and absorption can have a profound effect on growth and development. Many factors can disrupt the normal functioning of the gastrointestinal tract, including diet, disease, injury, infection, medication use, bacterial overgrowth and parasites, and environmental contamination. Gastrointestinal disease can occur along the length of the gastrointestinal tract; symptoms can range from mild to severe and can occur locally in the gut or present in other areas of the body. Common pediatric gastrointestinal disorders are listed in **TABLE 11.1**.

Prevalence and Etiology

Celiac disease is a chronic, systemic, autoimmune disorder.[1] Gluten proteins and related prolamins, especially gliadin, found in grains such as wheat, barley, and rye trigger an autoimmune response in the gut that damages intestinal villi. With continued exposure to the offending proteins, eventual **villous atrophy** results in malabsorption of macronutrients and micronutrients.

According to serological screening studies, celiac disease occurs in 1% of the population of Europe and the United States. The prevalence is higher in some countries (Finland) and lower in others (Germany).[2] Females are diagnosed twice more frequently than males.

HLA-DQ is a cell surface receptor protein found on antigen-presenting cells. Specific genetic haplotypes are at risk for developing celiac disease: 90–95% of the patients with celiac are found to have HLA-DQ2, and 5–10% have HLA-DQ8.[3] Several syndromes are known to have higher rates of celiac: trisomy 21, Turner syndrome, and Williams syndrome. There is an increased risk for celiac disease in first-degree relatives of patients with celiac and in patients with other autoimmune diseases such as diabetes mellitus type 1, autoimmune hepatitis, autoimmune thyroiditis, and rheumatoid arthritis.[4]

Celiac manifests with gastrointestinal as well as systemic symptoms. Gastrointestinal symptoms include abdominal distention, chronic diarrhea, and poor weight gain. Adolescents are more likely have with atypical gastrointestinal complaints such as constipation and vomiting.[2] Systemic manifestations include iron deficiency, short stature, chronic fatigue, **aphthous stomatitis**, and reduced bone mineral density. Some patients are asymptomatic and are diagnosed by screening of at-risk groups.

Diagnosis and Treatment

Celiac is diagnosed by clinical symptoms and serological testing such as for antibodies to tissue transglutaminase (anti-tTG) and endomysial antibodies, but a small-bowel biopsy is considered the gold standard for confirming the diagnosis.[4]

Celiac disease is a lifelong disorder requiring consistent dietary management with a gluten-free diet (GFD).[1] The GFD should be continued for life even when symptoms resolve. The gluten threshold, which is the amount

Table 11.1

Common Pediatric Gastrointestinal Disorders

Presenting Symptom	Differential Diagnosis	Treatment
Stomach and Esophagus		
Vomiting/regurgitation	Congenital anomaly of the gastrointestinal tract	Surgery
	Gastroesophageal reflux	Infants: positioning, medications such as antacids, H2 blockers, and proton pump inhibitors (PPIs). If preceding fails, consider surgical treatment.
		All ages: medications, antacids, H2 blockers, PPIs, avoid caffeine-containing foods and other personal triggers
	Eosinophilic esophagitis	Elimination diet, swallowed steroids
	Eosinophilic gastritis	Steroids, immunosuppressive medication
	Peptic disease	Medications such as antacids, H2 blockers, and PPIs; avoid caffeine-containing foods and other personal triggers
	H. pylori	Antibiotics, PPIs
	Gastroparesis	Prokinetics, diet changes such as multiple small low-fat meals per day, or postpyloric feeds
Dysphagia (choking after eating), odynophagia (pain with swallowing)	Congenital anomalies, strictures, webs	Surgery
	Eosinophilic esophagitis	Elimination diet, swallowed steroids
	Esophageal spasms/dysmotility	Calcium channel blockers and nitrates; avoid extreme temperatures in foods
	Peptic strictures	Medications such as antacids, H2 blockers, and PPIs; dilation
Liver and Pancreas		
Jaundice	Extrahepatic biliary tract obstruction, such as biliary atresia	Surgical correction; diet/formula with medium chain triglycerides (MCT), fat-soluble vitamin supplementation, choleretic agents such as ursodeoxycholate
	Autoimmune hepatitis	Steroids, evaluation for fat malabsorption, fat-soluble vitamin supplementation, protein restriction only if encephalopathic
Jaundice with recurrent abdominal pain	Gallstones	Surgery
	Choledochal cyst	Surgery
Nausea, vomiting, abdominal pain	Pancreatitis	No food by mouth (NPO) if severe or prolonged course expected then postplyoric tube feeds or parenteral nutrition; pain control, H2 blockers; when clinically able, resume low-fat oral diet
	Pancreatic pseudocyst	Monitor cyst size; if cyst increases with enteral nutrition, may require parenteral nutrition
Chronic diarrhea, failure to thrive	Pancreatic insufficiency, such as cystic fibrosis	Enzyme replacement therapy, fat-soluble vitamin supplementation, high-calorie balanced diet
	Cholestatic disease	Diet/formula with MCT, fat-soluble vitamin supplementation
Small Bowel and Colon		
Anemia, gastrointestinal bleeding	Congenital malformations, such as Meckel's diverticulum, duplication cysts	Surgery
Vomiting	Food allergies	Hydrolysate formula, elimination diet
	Infectious enteropathies	Oral rehydration solutions, followed by lactose and/or sucrose restrictions

Presenting Symptom	Differential Diagnosis	Treatment
Diarrhea in neonatal period	Congenital disorders of carbohydrate absorption and transport	Restriction of the problematic carbohydrate, balanced nutrition, vitamin/mineral supplementation, enzyme replacement
Diarrhea, perioral and perianal rash	Zinc deficiency	Zinc supplementation
Diarrhea	Food allergies	Elemental formula and/or elimination diet
	Infectious enteropathies	Intravenous fluids, oral rehydration solutions, followed by lactose and/or sucrose restrictions if clinically indicated
	Crohn's disease	Enteral feeds for therapy and/or malnutrition, replete iron, fat-soluble vitamins, and zinc as necessary; monitor vitamin B_{12} if severe ileal disease or resection
	Ulcerative colitis	Enteral feeds for weight gain, replete iron as necessary, low-residue diet if strictures
	Celiac disease	Gluten-free diet
	Short bowel syndrome	Parenteral nutrition progressing to enteral nutrition to oral feeds; vitamin and mineral supplements specific to patient's condition
	Fructose intolerance	Dietary restrictions of fructose-containing foods
	Lactose intolerance	Dietary restrictions of lactose-containing foods
Diarrhea, normal growth pattern	Irritable bowel syndrome, chronic nonspecific diarrhea, toddler's diarrhea	Normal diet for age, increased soluble fiber intake, decreased intake of sorbitol-containing beverages (apple and pear juice) and other personal triggers
Abdominal distention/pain	Celiac disease	Gluten-free diet
	Short bowel syndrome	Total parenteral nutrition progressing to MCT-predominate hydrolysate formula; vitamin and mineral supplements
	Functional constipation	Complete bowel clean-out using saline enemas, mineral oil, Miralax; high-fiber diet and adequate fluids; bowel habit training
	Congenital disorders of carbohydrate absorption and transport	Restriction of the problematic carbohydrate, balanced nutrition, vitamin/mineral supplementation, enzyme replacement
	Fructose intolerance	Dietary restrictions of fructose-containing foods
	Lactose intolerance	Dietary restrictions of lactose-containing foods
Constipation	Hirschsprung's disease; post-necrotising enterocolitis (NEC) strictures	Surgery
	Functional constipation	Complete bowel clean-out using saline enemas, mineral oil, Miralax; high-fiber diet and adequate fluids; bowel habit training

of daily gluten consumed that can harm the intestinal mucosa, is 10–50 mg/day. The Codex regulations of the World Health Organization limit gluten contamination to 20 ppm in gluten-free products.[5]

Adhering to a strict gluten-free diet is difficult for patients. Common sources of gluten are wheat, barley, and rye. Oatmeal consumption is controversial because, although oats do not contain gliadin, they do contain avenin, which has lower toxic effect. However, occasionally patients are also oat sensitive. Often, oats are contaminated by wheat, and this has led to recommendations for celiac patients to avoid oats. It is suggested that celiac patients add oats to their diet only when they are

established on a conventional gluten-free diet and they can stop eating oats if they develop any symptoms.[6] Gluten is found in many food products, and therefore careful attention to food labels is necessary. **TABLE 11.2** summarizes common sources of gluten.

It is necessary for celiac patients to maintain a balanced and age-appropriate nutritional plan that includes all required vitamins and minerals. Folic acid, iron, zinc, and calcium deficiencies are common and therefore should be screened for and supplemented accordingly. It is critical that those diagnosed have a support team. This may include nannies, school nurses, teachers, and school kitchen staff who are educated about the GFD.

Table 11.2

Sources of Gluten

Sources of Gluten	Potential Sources of Gluten or Food Contaminated with Gluten	Gluten-Free Foods
Wheat (and food products made from wheat):	Starch, dextrin	Rice
Wheat berries, durum, emmer, semolina, spelt, farina, farro, graham flour, Khorasan wheat, einkorn wheat		
Rye	Soy sauce	Corn
Barley	Malt, brewer's yeast, beer	Potatoes
Triticale	Meat substitute made with seitan	Tapioca
	Emulsifiers	Quinoa
	Preservatives	
	Oats that are not gluten free	
	Medications	
	Nuts	

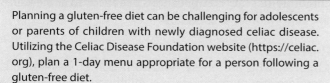

Let's Discuss

Planning a gluten-free diet can be challenging for adolescents or parents of children with newly diagnosed celiac disease. Utilizing the Celiac Disease Foundation website (https://celiac.org), plan a 1-day menu appropriate for a person following a gluten-free diet.

Education should include information about the specific functions of the small intestine because this will help patients understand potential symptoms and risks associated with celiac disease and a GFD.[1] Visual aids of normal and abnormal mucosa help to depict the damaging effects that continued exposure to gluten has in patients with celiac disease. Furthermore, the use of visual aids can help raise awareness to the potential of mucosal healing, which encourages patients to adhere to the GFD. Support should also addresses the psychological and social implications of maintaining a gluten-free diet through adolescence.

Clinical symptoms and antibodies resolve gradually after a gluten-free diet is started. Patients should be followed annually for growth assessment and evaluation of complications. Poor adherence to a gluten-free diet may result in complications such as neurologic disorders, osteoporosis, impaired splenic function, infertility, ulcerative jejunoileitis, and cancer.[5]

Recap Adequate nutrition management is essential for the treatment and prevention of diseases of the gastrointestinal tract such as celiac disease. Grains such as wheat, barley, and rye trigger an autoimmune response in the gut, which leads to damage of the intestinal villi. With continued exposures to the offending proteins, eventual villous atrophy results in malabsorption of various macronutrients and micronutrients. Educational support should be considered in addition to the psychological and social implications of maintaining a gluten-free diet through adolescence.

1. Define celiac disease.
2. Describe the nutritional challenges for children and adolescents with celiac disease.
3. List dietary recommendations and specific food choices for children with celiac disease.

Pediatric Overweight and Obesity

Preview Pediatric overweight and obesity are significant public health nutrition problems that affect a large number of children and adolescents. Overweight and obese children have increased risk for a number of chronic health conditions and for becoming overweight and obese as adults.

Obesity is the most prevalent pediatric nutritional disorder, affecting approximately 17% of children and adolescents.[7] Overweight and obesity during this early life stage predispose children and adolescents to a host of health conditions as they age, including insulin resistance, type 2 diabetes, hypertension, unfavorable blood lipids, and heart disease and dramatically increase their risk of adult obesity. Pediatric obesity is a complex and significant public health concern. Prevention is challenging because the majority of cases are multifactorial and idiopathic in origin, and treatments have been largely unsuccessful.

Prevalence and Etiology

The prevalence of obesity (body mass index [BMI] ≥ 95th sex-specific CDC percentile for age) among U.S. children ages 6 to 11 years is 17.5% and is 20.5% among adolescents ages 12 to 19 years.[7] The prevalence of extreme obesity (BMI ≥ 120% of 95th sex-specific CDC percentile for age) is 4.3% and 9% at the ages 6–11 years and 12–19 years, respectively. The prevalence of obesity in adolescents tripled in the last three decades in all socioeconomic status levels (**FIGURE 11.1** and **FIGURE 11.2**).

There are racial disparities in obesity. Rates are higher for Mexican and non-Hispanic black American adolescents than for non-Hispanic whites. Contributing factors to the rise in obesity prevalence in the last decades are increased consumption of total energy, soft drinks, and snacks; frequent fast food consumption; and inadequate amount of fruits and vegetables in the daily menu. The world's population has access to low-cost, highly

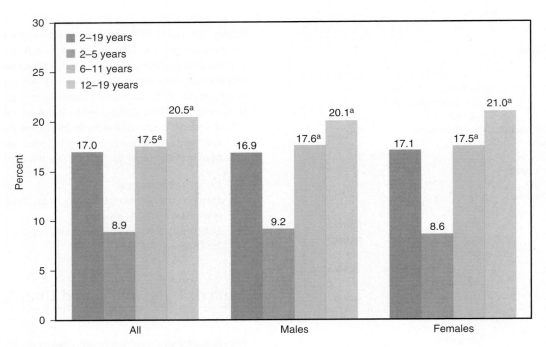

a Significantly different from those aged 2–5 years.

Figure 11.1

Prevalence of obesity among American youth, 2011-2014.

Reproduced from Centers for Disease Control and Prevention/National Center for Health Statistics. National Health and Nutrition Examination Survey, 2011-2014. Hyattsville, MD: National Center for Health Statistics; 2015.

processed, energy-dense, and nutrient-poor food products.[8] Food portion size has also increased significantly in the past decades.[9]

The level of daily physical activity is decreased in modern life. Environmental research suggests that geographic areas of low socioeconomic status have lower availability of physical activity facilities and decreased availability of fresh, nonprocessed food. This disparity contributes to the increased rates of obesity in population that live in these areas.[10] Childhood adiposity is associated with poor health outcomes in adulthood.[11] The comorbidities and complications of obesity in adolescents are summarized in TABLE 11.3 .

Prevention

Children who are obese tend to become obese adults; therefore, interventions during childhood are essential to establish healthier eating habits and to prevent adolescent

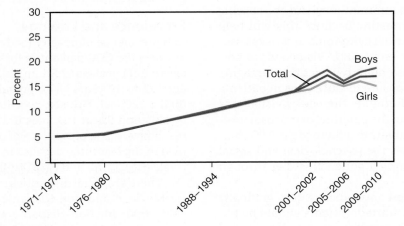

Figure 11.2

Obesity trends among children and adolescents aged 2–19 years, by sex: the United States 1971–1974 through 2009–2010.

Reproduced from Centers for Disease Control and Prevention/National Center for Health Statistics. National Health and Nutrition Examination Survey. s (NHANES) I–III; and NHANES 1999–2000, 2001–2002, 2003–2004, 2005–2006, 2007–2008, and 2009–2010. Hyattsville, MD: National Center for Health Statistics.

Table 11.3

Comorbidities of Obesity in Adolescents

Body System	Complication
Endocrine	Impaired glucose tolerance
	Type 2 diabetes
	Metabolic syndrome
	Hyperandrogenism
Cardiovascular	Hypertension
	Dyslipidemia
	Major cardiovascular events during adulthood
Gastrointestinal	Nonalcoholic fatty liver disease
	Cholelithiasis
Renal	Proteinuria
	Focal segmental glomerulosclerosis
Pulmonary	Obstructive sleep apnea
Orthopedic	Slipped capital femoral epiphysis
	Musculoskeletal pain (back, knee, foot)
	Impaired mobility
	Blount disease
Psychosocial	Poor self-esteem
	Distorted body image
	Anxiety and depression
	Distorted peer relationships
Neurological	Pseudotumor cerebri

Table 11.4

Approaches to Target Weight-Related Behaviors

- Computer-based weight control plans.
- In-person clinician visits to discuss the adolescent's physical activity, nutrition, and sedentary behaviors. Of note, in-person group education sessions have been shown to be effective.[a]
- Adolescent and parent sessions to learn about self-monitoring of physical activity and food intake.
- Adolescent phone coaching sessions.
- Informational materials provided to the adolescent and parent.
- Telehealth.

[a] Stark LJ, Spear S, Boles R, et al. A pilot randomized controlled trial of a clinic and home-based behavioral intervention to decrease obesity in preschoolers. *Obesity* (Silver Spring). 2011;19(1):134–141. doi:10.1038/oby.2010.87.

Treatment and Recommendations

Intensive lifestyle modification remains the primary treatment for pediatric overweight and obesity.[17] Behavioral changes are hard to achieve, but are possible. Discussion of specific weight targets with the patient and family is often not helpful and can cause adolescents to withdraw from weight control efforts. It is better to emphasize behavior goals for specific dietary habits than discussing weight loss goals. Target weight should be evaluated by the pediatrician to ensure the patient's weight goal is safe and appropriate.

For children and adolescents who are overweight (BMI > 85th percentile) or mildly obese, the goal of maintaining the current body weight is appropriate because height growth will lead to a final decrease in BMI. With higher degrees of obesity (BMI ≥ 99th percentile) gradual weight loss is recommended. It is safe for adolescents with obesity and comorbidities to lose up to 2 pounds per week, but a weight loss of 1–2 pounds per month is more realistic.[18–20]

Effective interventions focus directly on weight management and regular monitoring of weight and weight-related behaviors such as dietary intake and physical activity.[11] It is important to assess the patient's readiness for change and to adjust the treatment accordingly. Treatment strategies include environmental control (reducing the availability of food and increasing cues to be active); behavioral monitoring; setting goals that are specific, explicit, and subject to self-monitoring; rewarding successful behavioral change; identifying barriers and solving problems; and teaching parenting skills.[21]

Treatment plans should incorporate self-monitoring activities, such as weekly weighing and food diaries. Additionally, encouraging and monitoring daily or weekly physical activity patterns to meet individualized goals are crucial.[22] Previous studies have placed less emphasis on weight and calorie tracking when working with adolescent females.[15] However, weight measurements should still be included at each intervention session, with additional self-monitoring and guidelines related to food intake, physical activity, and sedentary behaviors (screen time). Elementary-school-aged children benefit from

obesity and medical complications during adult life. Pediatric primary care providers play a significant role in the prevention and treatment of pediatric obesity.[12] It is critical that those working with obese children and adolescents educate parents about the potential risks associated with childhood obesity so that preventative measures are established. Healthcare providers should keep any potential barriers in mind, finding ways to overcome such obstacles. Common barriers to prevention and treatment include the following:

- Time constraints in the clinical setting, which make education difficult[13]
- High cost of primary care providers' services and suboptimal reimbursement for provider activities[14]
- Lack of parental motivation to make weight-related behavioral modifications for themselves and their family
- Low parent concern about child's weight[11]

Although effective interventions may successfully target adolescents, interventions that demonstrate true impacts on obesity-related outcomes (including BMI and weight-for-height percentile) include parent-targeted interventions.[15,16] Healthcare providers should consider multiple approaches to target weight-related behaviors, as listed in TABLE 11.4. At a population level, regulation of energy density and portion size and reformulation of food products to support weight control are useful for obesity prevention.[8]

parent inclusion and parent modeling of healthy behaviors and physical activity, including targeted parental weight loss.[11]

Parents are known to sometimes inaccurately perceive their child's weight status and risk for obesity.[23] This false perception makes it challenging for a clinician to motivate parents to engage in behavior change. Using behavioral counseling techniques, such as motivational interviewing, healthcare providers can encourage parents to address sensitive topics, such as their child's weight. Another strategy that may help increase overall parental awareness of childhood obesity is for healthcare providers to discuss BMI in relation to the individual child's weight status and obesity risk. Use of growth charts can specifically help depict trends in weight, making it easier for parents to understand and see the importance of weight monitoring over time.

Interventions in the treatment of childhood obesity remain a large burden in the primary care setting in relation to provider time, staff time, cost of services, and participation time.[24] It is critical that healthcare providers create ways to render burdensome interventions into more sustainable practices. For example, utilizing social media platforms (apps) and smartphone technology may help to link interventions with families at little or no cost. Community-based programs and resources for families with children at risk should be encouraged.

Nutritional recommendations for the treatment of obesity include increased consumption of dietary fibers. Children and adolescents should be encouraged to consume five to eight servings of fruits and vegetables per day for sufficient minerals, micronutrients, fiber, and vitamins. Fiber can also be found in whole grains. It is recommended that children avoid saturated and trans fats and choose instead unsaturated fats, such as those found in olive oil, avocado, nuts, and almonds). Nutritional consultation should include guidance to decrease salt and simple carbohydrates in the diet and avoid any sugary drinks. Research has shown that consuming a Mediterranean diet (that consists of nuts, vegetables, and olive oil and no restriction on fat intake) can aid in the prevention of obesity and type 2 diabetes and can help in weight management.[25,26] Recent data suggest that noncaloric artificial sweetener consumption increases the risk of glucose intolerance and metabolic abnormalities and, therefore, paradoxically, has the potential to cause harm.[27]

According to the stepped care approach, the level and intensity of treatment should be adapted to the level of obesity and comorbidities.[28,29] The U.S. Food and Drug Administration (FDA) has approved the use of lipase inhibitor Orlistat in obese adolescents age 12 years and older with comorbidities. This drug serves as a pharmacologic adjunct to behavioral interventions for severely obese adolescents. Potential adverse effects include gastrointestinal symptoms. The risks of medication use should be weighed against the lack of evidence of persistent weight reduction after active treatment ends.[30]

Bariatric surgery is not generally recommended for children. It may be considered for adolescents with severe obesity (BMI > 40 or BMI > 35 with comorbidities) if they have achieved or nearly achieved physiological maturity. Roux-en-Y gastric bypass surgery makes the stomach smaller and allows food to bypass part of the small intestine. This procedure results in early satiety and lower absorption in the intestine. Sleeve gastrectomy is a procedure in which a large portion of the stomach is removed surgically and the open edges are staples together to form a sleeve. Bariatric surgeries result in significant improvement in weight, cardiometabolic health (remission of type 2 diabetes, prediabetes, and dyslipidemia), and weight-related quality of life. The risks associated with bariatric surgeries include micronutrient deficiencies (specifically, iron, vitamin B_{12}, and vitamin A deficiency) and the need for additional abdominal procedures.[31] There are not enough data regarding long-term effects of bariatric surgeries in adolescents.

News You Can Use

Advertisements and Children's Diet Choices

One in six American children is now considered obese.[a] Unhealthy behaviors, including poor diet, play a key role in the development of childhood overweight and obesity. In a recent systematic review of evidence based on 29 randomized trials, it was found that kids exposed to the marketing of unhealthy foods and beverages via product packaging, TV, and/or the Internet increased their short-term caloric intake.[b] The marketing also increased their preference for junk food. This is particularly concerning because children are exposed to an average of five food ads per hour, with unhealthy foods accounting for more than 80% of all televised food advertisements in Canada, the United States, and Germany.[c]

References

a. Centers for Disease Control and Prevention; updated November 9, 2015. Childhood overweight and obesity. Retrieved from: http://www.cdc.gov/obesity/childhood/index.html. Accessed September 25, 2016.

b. Sadeghirad B, Duhaney T, Motaghipisheh S, Campbell NR, Johnston BC. Influence of unhealthy food and beverage marketing on children's dietary intake and preference: a systematic review and meta-analysis of randomized trials [published online ahead of print July 18, 2016]. *Obes Rev.* October 2016;17(10):945–59. doi:10.1111/obr.12445.

c. Wilson T. Children make poor dietary choices shortly after advertisements of unhealthy foods and beverages: study. McMaster University; July 5, 2016. Retrieved from: http://fhs.mcmaster.ca/main/news/news_2016/poor_diet_choices_after_advertisements.html. Accessed July 29, 2016.

Recap Pediatric obesity is a complex and significant public health concern that predisposes children and adolescents to a host of health conditions. Rising rates can be attributed to a combination of increased access to low-cost, highly processed, energy-dense, and nutrient-poor food products and decreased levels of daily physical activity. Interventions should include combined efforts of self-monitoring and parent modeling of healthy behaviors, physical activity, and calorie goals.

1. Describe the long-term health consequences of pediatric overweight and obesity.
2. List strategies for the prevention and treatment of pediatric overweight and obesity.

Adolescent Eating Disorders

Preview Anorexia nervosa and bulimia nervosa are lethal psychiatric disorders characterized by disturbances in eating that impair health and psychosocial functioning. Anorexia nervosa is characterized by restriction of energy and nutrient intake to a level that is incompatible with healthy and normal body function. Bulimia nervosa involves high caloric intake in a limited period of time followed by compensating purging. Purging behavior may include vomiting, excessive physical activity, diet medication, or laxative abuse.

Following obesity and asthma, eating disorders are the third most common chronic illness in adolescents. And though much public health attention is focused on the nutritional implications of overweight and obesity, many adolescents become obsessively preoccupied with their physical appearance in effort to remain thin.

Prevalence and Etiology

Eating disorders are characterized by persistent disturbance of eating that impairs health and psychosocial functioning. The *Diagnostic and Statistical Manual of Mental Disorders* (DSM), published by the American Psychiatric Association (APA), defines diagnosis criteria for the various eating disorders. **TABLE 11.5** and **TABLE 11.6** provide diagnostic criteria for anorexia nervosa and bulimia nervosa, respectively. Anorexia nervosa has a lifetime prevalence of 0.3–0.9%, and bulimia nervosa has a lifetime prevalence of 0.9–1.5%.[32] The *DSM-5* criteria broaden the diagnosis of anorexia nervosa, and epidemiologic studies based on the new criteria report higher lifetime prevalence of anorexia nervosa of up to 4.2%.[33] Females are diagnosed more often than males. The male-to-female ratio is 1:4 before the age of 14 years and 1:10 after the age of 14. There is a peak incidence of eating disorders during adolescence. Many adolescents with eating disorders (20%) do not seek treatment owing to shame, denial, or lack of recognition by the medical system.[34]

Eating disorders have a complex biopsychosocial etiology. Twin studies demonstrate that anorexia nervosa and bulimia nervosa run in families and a portion of this familiarity is due to genetic factors.[35,36] Genetic factors become more prominent after puberty.[37] Several personality traits put people at risk for anorexia nervosa. Years before developing anorexia nervosa, children may display perfectionism, anxiety, depression, people-pleasing behaviors, harm avoidance, and obsessiveness.[32] Neurobiologic changes in the brains of eating disorder patients interfere with reward processing, hedonic motivation, and response to hunger and appetite. It is believed that the networking center of the brain, which is involved in processing of information from the various systems of the brain, developing awareness of physiological processes, and initiating a response, malfunctions.[38]

Environmental factors, such as early life stress and parental behavior, play a role in remodeling gene expression and contribute to the susceptibility of developing an eating disorder. Observations of overcontrolling family members or dysfunctional families as contributors to the development of eating disorders should be evaluated.

Table 11.5

DSM-5 Diagnostic Criteria for Anorexia Nervosa

A. **Restriction of energy intake**. Avoidance of food leading to significantly low body weight compromising physical health.

B. **Intense fear of weight gain or becoming fat or persistent behavior that interferes with weight gain, even though at a significantly low weight**. Purposeful behavior to avoid weight gain. Steadfast pursuance and maintenance of low body weight.

C. **Disturbance in the way in which one's body weight or shape is experienced**, undue influence of body weight or shape on self-evaluation, or persistent lack of recognition of the seriousness of the current low body weight.

Restricting type vs. binge eating/purging type

Modified from American Psychiatric Association. *Diagnostic and Statistical Manual of Mental Disorders*. 5th ed. (DSM-5) Arlington, VA: American Psychiatric Association; 2013.

Table 11.6

DSM-5 Diagnostic Criteria for Bulimia Nervosa

A. **Recurrent episodes of binge eating** that includes eating large amount of food in a distinct period of time (usually 2 hours), an inability to stop eating, and feeling of lack of control of what and how much is being eaten

B. **Recurrent purging behavior** to compensate for binge in attempt to prevent weight gain such as self-induced vomiting, misuse of laxatives and diuretics, prolonged fasting, and excessive exercise

C. Binge and purge behaviors that both occur at least once per week for 3 months

D. Self-evaluation that is excessively influenced by body shape and weight

E. Excessive concern about body weight or shape not exclusive to anorexia nervosa episodes

Modified from American Psychiatric Association. *Diagnostic and Statistical Manual of Mental Disorders*. 5th ed. (DSM-5) Arlington, VA: American Psychiatric Association; 2013.

Starvation by itself results in psychological changes similar to those seen in anorexia nervosa. In 1950, Ancel Keys published landmark research demonstrating that starvation of healthy young men can result in depression, irritability, intense preoccupation with thoughts of food, decreased self-initiated activity, loss of sexual drive, and social introversion.[39]

Anorexia nervosa is characterized by restriction of energy and nutrient intake to a level that is incompatible with healthy and normal body function. FIGURE 11.3 lists the medical complications of anorexia nervosa according to body system. Bulimia nervosa involves high caloric intake in a limited period of time followed by purging. Purging is a compensating behavior such as vomiting, excessive physical activity, use of diet medication, or laxative abuse.

Bulimia nervosa results in medical complications that include electrolyte abnormalities, impaired satiety, gastrointestinal bleeding, abdominal pain, constipation, malabsorption, acute pancreatitis, cardiac arrhythmia, depression, anxiety, and guilt.[40] The severity of malnutrition in adults is diagnosed according to the BMI. In adolescents the severity is staged according to growth percentiles. Factors contributing to favorable outcomes are short duration of symptoms prior to treatment and good parent–child relationship. Factors contributing to unfavorable outcomes are vomiting, bulimia nervosa, chronicity of anorexia nervosa, and obsessive-compulsive features.

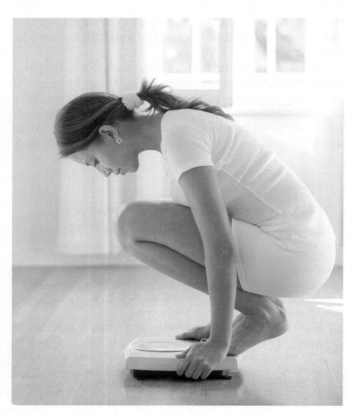

Figure 11.3
Complications of anorexia nervosa.

©Mark Scott/The Image Bank/Getty

Case Study

Catherine continues to skip lunch in order to exercise and also often skips dinner with her family. She avoids going out to eat with friends and is fearful of gaining back the weight she lost through exercise and restricting her calorie intake. Her gymnastics coach continues to be pleased with her weight loss, and she doesn't want to let him down. Catherine recently stopped menstruating and has noticed her hair has become brittle and is falling out in the shower. She continues to feel down and her personality has changed drastically. Her friends are very concerned.

Questions

1. Based on what you've learned so far, do you think Catherine might be suffering from an eating disorder?
2. What details helped you to come to this conclusion?

Prevention and Treatment

Recognizing the risk factors for eating disorders, such as a history of sexual abuse, female gender, peer teasing about weight, and dieting behavior, helps focus the prevention resources. Prevention programs have been suggested in different levels, as described in TABLE 11.7.

The treatment of eating disorders includes medical stabilization, treatment of complications, refeeding, and psychosocial rehabilitation. After a long starvation and catabolic state, refeeding and a load of carbohydrate intake carry the risk of electrolyte abnormalities secondary to insulin secretion and anabolic state. Refeeding syndrome is characterized by hypokalemia, hypophosphatemia, hypomagnesemia, and thiamin deficiency. Refeeding should be done cautiously and while monitoring for complications. Traditionally, feeding was started at a low caloric level and increased gradually. Recent data demonstrate that higher-calorie diets increase rate of weight gain and shorten the hospital stay in hospitalized adolescents with anorexia nervosa. Therefore, it is feasible to start at a higher caloric level (1,400 kcal/day) and advance energy intake while monitoring for electrolyte abnormalities and providing needed supplementation of minerals.[41] Hemodynamic instability such as bradycardia, orthostatic hypotension, postural tachycardia, hypothermia, or severe malnutrition might require hospital admission for medical stabilization.

It is important to adjust nutrition recommendations to enable growth and development. In anorexia nervosa, nutrition therapy and correction of malnutrition can reverse most of the medical complications, improve cognitive function, and enable the adolescent to participate in psychotherapy. Goal weight should be set according to growth measures prior to the illness. A weekly weight gain goal of 0.5–2 pounds can be achieved. Activity should be limited until energy intake is sufficient to support continued weight gain. Daily multivitamin should be added and fat-free and sugar-free dietetic food products should be avoided.

Table 11.7

Levels in Eating Disorder Prevention Programs

Family	More frequent family meals are considered a protective factor and associated with: • Better dietary intake • Higher levels of psychosocial well-being, academic success • Lower levels of substance abuse[a] Recommendations for families are to: • Talk less about weight. • Facilitate healthy eating and physical activity.
Schools	School-based programs that work at: • Improving student self-esteem • Providing positive web-based prevention programs • Interventions at ballet and gymnastic schools • Programs to educate about teasing-free environment at schools
Teachers	Teacher programs that teach educators: how to treat their own bodies and how to discuss dieting, **body dissatisfaction**, eating, and physical activity. Teachers should avoid discussing their own dieting behaviors with students.
Health care	Healthcare providers should discourage dieting, support physical activity, and promote positive body image, helping teenagers feel better about their bodies so that they will nurture themselves through healthy eating.
Society	Legislative efforts that help change societal norms by requiring advertisers improve the messages in the media about size, weight, and beauty.

Neumark-Sztainer D, Larson NI, Fulkerson JA, Eisenberg ME, Story M. Family meals and adolescents: what have we learned from Project EAT (Eating Among Teens)? *Public Health Nutr.* 2010;13(7):1113–1121. doi:10.1017/S1368980010000169.

Bulimia nervosa treatment aims at cessation of binging and purging activity and normalization of weight gain. The cycle of food restriction followed by binge eating and purging results in a hypometabolic state. Regular intake of frequent small meals improves metabolic efficiency, enables normal hunger and satiety cues, and reduces the binging and purging behavior, hence minimizing weight gain. Balanced exercise can improve mood, decrease stress, and improve metabolic efficiency, but excessive exercise should be avoided. Patients with anorexia nervosa and bulimia nervosa should be encouraged not to measure their weight.

There are several psychotherapy strategies to treat eating disorders in adolescents. Family-based therapy (FBT) is an evidence-based method that empowers families to take part in the treatment of their sick child. FBT takes an agnostic view of the cause of illness: neither the patient nor the parents are to blame. It is a pragmatic method that focuses initially on the symptoms and nutrition, and only when goal weight is achieved is the responsibility gradually returned to the patient and comorbidities addressed. In cases with unsupportive family members, older patients, or bulimia nervosa, cognitive behavioral therapy, dynamic therapy, or other methods may be used.[32,34]

Depression and anxiety, which may accompany eating disorders, often improve with nutritional rehabilitation and psychotherapy. Medications may be useful in dual diagnoses, when the depression or anxiety preceded the eating disorder or when it persists after weight has been restored. Selective serotonin reuptake inhibitors (SSRIs) are not effective on malnourished brains; therefore, their use in anorexia should be considered only after the nutritional state has been restored. In bulimia nervosa, SSRIs reduce binge–purge frequency.[42] Several studies report the use of antipsychotic medications to augment treatment for eating-related obsessions and compulsions.

Anorexia nervosa is the most lethal psychiatric disorder, with a mortality rate of 6%. More than 50% of the deaths result from physical complications such as cardiac arrhythmia. Suicide mortality rates are 1.3%. Full recovery is found in less than 50% of anorexia nervosa survivors, and 20% develop chronicity.[32]

Let's Discuss

Do you have or have you ever known someone with an eating disorder? What behaviors and symptoms did you recognize first? *Treatment can be life-saving!* Familiarize yourself with the eating disorder treatment centers in your area. What types of services and treatments do they offer? Who provides these services and treatments?

Recap Adolescent eating disorders encompass a broad range of complex biopsychosocial issues that affect physical well-being and that lead to a future of detrimental health impacts. Depending on disease severity, the treatment of eating disorders may include medical stabilization, treatment of complications, refeeding, and long-term psychosocial rehabilitation. Regular intake of frequent small meals improves metabolic efficiency and enables normal hunger and satiety cues.

1. Describe the key features of anorexia nervosa.
2. Describe the key features of bulimia nervosa.
3. Summarize eating disorder treatment strategies.

Pediatric Diabetes

Preview Diabetes can be classified into several categories. Type 1 diabetes results from beta cell destruction and usually leads to absolute insulin deficiency. In type 2 diabetes, there is a progressive loss of insulin secretion against a background of insulin resistance. Type 2 diabetes is appearing with increasing frequency in younger age groups. Challenges faced by youth with diabetes include minimizing current and future disease burden and lowering risk of associated medical conditions, while also providing adequate nutrition for growth and development and taking into consideration the emotional and social well-being of the child.

Pediatric Type 1 Diabetes: Prevalence and Etiology

Three-quarters of all cases of type 1 diabetes (T1DM) are diagnosed in individuals younger than 18 years of age.[43] Children with T1DM typically present with the hallmark symptoms of increased thirst and frequency of urination (polyuria and polydipsia) and weight loss, and about one-third present with diabetic ketoacidosis (DKA), an emergency situation when blood glucose levels are high, but because of a lack of insulin, glucose is not inserted into cells and the body uses alternative pathways to supply energy needs at the cost of acid production.

The pathophysiology in T1DM is autoimmune destruction of pancreatic islet cells. Patients with T1DM are at increased risk for other autoimmune diseases (thyroid abnormalities, celiac disease, etc.); therefore, patients should be screened for these conditions at the initial assessment and routinely in follow-up.

Pediatric Type 1 Diabetes: Treatment

The treatment of T1DM includes supplementation of the missing insulin. Insulin is provided through injections or insulin pump in accordance with the patient's food supply and level of activity. To reach glycemic control, glucose levels should be monitored either by taking measurements several times a day before and after meals or by sensor.

Medical nutrition therapy (MNT) plays an essential part in diabetes management and requires patient education and personalized adjustment of the menus to the patient's needs. The goal of nutrition therapy in diabetes is to promote healthful eating patterns. Patients should learn to be mindful of their eating and adjust the insulin therapy to their eating but, on the other hand, not be afraid of eating or avoid insulin treatment. It is recommended that patients with diabetes have frequent follow-ups with a dietitian to improve eating habits. The dietitian can educate about carbohydrate counting or estimation to determine mealtime insulin dosing and improve glycemic control.

There is no single ideal dietary distribution of calories among carbohydrates, fats, and proteins for people with diabetes. The macronutrient distribution should be individualized. Carbohydrate intake from whole grains, vegetables, fruits, legumes, dairy products, and food higher in fiber and lower in glycemic load is recommended. Sugar-sweetened beverages should be avoided.

Pediatric Type 2 Diabetes: Prevalence and Etiology

Insulin is an anabolic hormone produced by pancreatic beta cells. It regulates the metabolism of carbohydrates, proteins, and fats. Type 1 diabetes results from beta cell destruction and is characterized by insulin deficiency. Type 2 diabetes (T2DM) is characterized by insulin resistance: the demand for insulin rises, yet there is inadequate insulin secretion and relative insulin deficiency, and the cells are unable to use the insulin effectively. In T2DM, the insulin resistance results from genetic, metabolic, and environmental causes and, unlike in type 1 diabetes, there is no identified autoimmune process.[44] Insulin resistance is also associated with other metabolic abnormalities such as dyslipidemia, fatty liver disease, polycystic ovary syndrome, and hypertension. T2DM was previously considered an adult illness, but in the past three decades, it has increased in prevalence among children and adolescents.[45] **FIGURE 11.4** summarizes the four methods used to diagnose diabetes.[43,46]

Youth-onset type 2 diabetes rarely occurs prior to puberty. It usually occurs during the second decade of life and the median age of onset is 1 year later in boys than in girls.[46] Risk factors for developing type 2 diabetes are listed in **TABLE 11.8**.

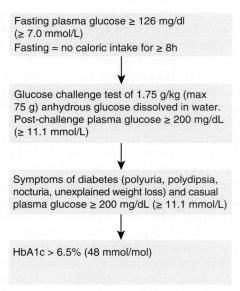

Figure 11.4
Methods to diagnose diabetes.

The Big Picture

Race: Blacks, Hispanics, Native Americans, Asian Americans and Pacific Islanders are at higher risk for type 2 diabetes.

Weight: Being overweight is a primary risk factor. Weight is impacted by both diet and activity levels in children and adolescents.

Inactivity: The less active a child is, the greater risk of type 2 diabetes.

Family History: The risk of type 2 diabeties significancy increases if a parent/sibling has type 2 diabetes; may be related to lifestyle, genetics, or both.

Data from: Mayo Clinic. Type 2 Diabetes in Children. http://www.mayoclinic.org/diseases-conditions/type-2-diabetes-in-children/basics/definition/con-20030124. Published May 3, 2014. Accessed July 29, 2016.

Table 11.8

Risk Factors for Type 2 Diabetes

- Being a first- or second-degree relative of family members with type 2 diabetes increases the risk of developing type 2 diabetes.
- Males who are born to mothers who had gestational diabetes and who were born large for gestational age have a higher risk of developing type 2 diabetes than females.[a]
- Youth-onset type 2 diabetes occurs in all races but with higher prevalence among nonwhite adolescents not of European descent (for example, blacks, Native Americans, Hispanics, Asians, and South Asians).
- In the United States and Europe, youth-onset type 2 diabetes is related to obesity, but in Asia type 2 diabetes is often seen in normal-weight adolescents.
- Sex ratio (male:female) of youth-onset type 2 diabetes varies from 1:4 to 1:6 in native North Americans and to 1:1 in Asians.
- In the United States and Europe, youth-onset type 2 diabetes disproportionately affects populations with low socioeconomic and low education levels, whereas in developing countries youth-onset type 2 diabetes is seen in children from higher socioeconomic levels.[a]

[a] Copeland KC, Zeitler P, Geffner M, et al. Characteristics of adolescents and youth with recent-onset type 2 diabetes: the TODAY cohort at baseline. *J Clin Endocrinol Metab.* 2011;96(1):159–167. doi:10.1210/jc.2010-1642.

Pediatric Type 2 Diabetes: Prevention and Treatment

Screening for type 2 diabetes in asymptomatic patients is currently considered not cost effective owing to the low prevalence of type 2 diabetes. Hypertension, dyslipidemia, and microalbuminuria can exist during a prediabetic state, but they can also occur with obesity alone; therefore, it is recommended healthcare providers screen for these comorbidities and promote weight loss, increased physical activity, and nutritional changes, even when dysglycemia is absent.

The ideal care for patients with type 2 diabetes is provided by a team that includes a pediatric endocrinologist, diabetes nurse educator, registered dietitian nutritionist, and behavioral specialist.[45] Behavioral changes should promote healthy lifestyle and weight reduction. The behavioral changes should be achieved gradually and be individualized. The care team and the patient should set achievable goals together.

A registered dietitian nutritionist should guide the patient to achieve the following objectives: eliminate sugar-containing beverages, increase consumption of vegetables and fruits, reduce consumption of simple carbohydrates and refined grains, decrease consumption of processed food, incorporate more whole grains, and control food portion sizes. It is recommended that the family establish family mealtime, avoid other activities while eating, limit the availability of high-caloric, high-fat food products, and promote parental modeling of healthy eating habits. Youth with type 2 diabetes should be encouraged to engage in moderate to vigorous physical activity 1 hour per day. Sedentary time (computer-related activity, TV) should be limited to less than 2 hours per day. House routines that increase sleep duration and limit screen time are recommended.

Comorbidities of type 1 diabetes are often seen many years after initial diagnosis. In type 2 diabetes, on the other hand, comorbidities often exist at the time of the initial diagnosis. These include other insulin resistance–related abnormalities, cardiovascular disease, hypertension, polycystic ovary syndrome (PCOS), nonalcoholic fatty liver disease, kidney damage, and obstructive sleep apnea. These comorbidities should be screened for early after the diagnosis of type 2 diabetes. Because type 2 diabetes comorbidities include cardiovascular disease, it is recommended that youth with type 2 diabetes be counseled about the additive harmful effect of tobacco.

Recommendations for Pediatric Diabetes Management

Asymptomatic metabolically stable (HbA$_{1c}$ < 9) T2DM patients should be treated with metformin. If HbA$_{1c}$ levels are greater than 9, insulin is used to improve glycemic control. Treatment should aim for HbA$_{1c}$ levels of less than 6.5. Microalbuminuria (the secretion of protein in the urine) should be checked and if present in three repeated tests should be treated medically. Blood

pressure (BP) should be measured; if BP is higher than the 95th percentile for age and sex, hypertension should be treated by weight reduction, dietary salt limitation, and increased physical activity. Medications should be used if no improvement is seen within 6 months. Lipid profile should be evaluated every 6 months and treated with lifestyle and nutritional changes; statins or fibrates should be used if no improvement is seen within 6 months. Screening for retinopathy and nonalcoholic fatty liver disease should be conducted annually. Type 2 diabetes patients should be asked about menstrual history and assessed for PCOS. Youth with type 2 diabetes are at increased risk for major depression; therefore, an evaluation of their mental status should be incorporated into the treatment.

Recap The pathophysiology in T1DM is autoimmune destruction of pancreatic islet cells that then requires lifelong medical and dietary intervention to maintain normal blood glucose levels. Type 2 diabetes is characterized by insulin resistance, which can lead to other metabolic abnormalities if left uncontrolled. Care for pediatric patients with diabetes is provided through an interdisciplinary approach with a team that includes a pediatric endocrinologist, diabetes nurse educator, nutritionist, and behavioral specialist. Nutritional management is critical and should work to achieve consistent normal blood glucose levels and healthy body weight and support normal growth and development.

1. Discuss the differences in etiology, symptoms, management and treatment of type 1 vs type 2 diabetes.
2. List the risk factors for development of type 2 diabetes in children and adolescents.
3. Describe the short- and long-term health consequences of pediatric type 2 diabetes.
4. Provide two to four nutrition recommendations for children and adolescents with type 2 diabetes.

Nutrition for Young Athletes

Preview Optimal nutrition directly affects both physical and mental performance. Involvement in physical activity at an early age is beneficial for growth and development, overall health, social and emotional well-being, as well as chronic disease prevention. The nutritional plan for young athletes needs to consider the type of sport activity; the age, weight, and body composition of the athlete; the amount of training; and seasonal variability.

Adolescents often have insufficient, imbalanced, and disorganized nutrition. This behavior may lead to nutritional deficits that can cause early as well as long-term complications. The nutrition challenges an adolescent athlete faces are more difficult than those of an adult athlete **TABLE 11.9** .

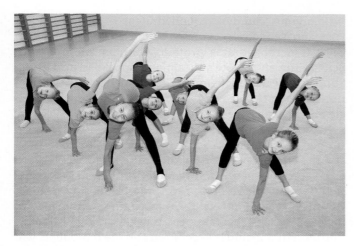

©alexkatkov/Shutterstock

Child and Adolescent Athletes

One of the goals of sport activity is achieving and constantly improving the body's performance. Physical activity involves mental and physical exertion even when sport is for pleasure purposes only. Optimal nutrition directly affects performance physiologically by supplying energy for muscle activity; preventing injury, fatigue, and weakness; and shortening the postexercise recovery period and mentally in the form of mental relaxation following the focused physical exertion.[47] To reach maximum

athletic potential, every training program should include a nutrition plan.[48,49]

Sedentary lifestyle and lack of physical activity during childhood and adolescence are strongly related to obesity in Western society.[50–52] Physical activity at an early age has beneficial effects on growth and development as well as morbidity and mortality prevention,[52] specifically the prevention of obesity, diabetes, cardiac illnesses,[50] and insulin resistance (Table 11.9). Physical activity improves bone mass, posture, self-esteem, and mood. In men more than in women, physical activity in childhood significantly improves their chances of being physically active in adulthood.[53,54]

Adolescence is characterized by accelerated growth, weight gain, increased height, and the development of the adult body structure. Adequate nutrition during this period is crucial.[47] Eating habits are important for sport activity. Balanced and varied nutrition usually satisfies the body's needs without requiring external dietary supplements. Prolonged exertion and strain and increased sweating may require supplementation of specific minerals according to professional recommendations.[49]

Sports nutrition is defined as the consumption of appropriate amounts of nutrients at the right time to achieve the body's best performance during exertion while maintaining health. Personal needs vary among individuals. Balanced nutrition does not automatically increase physical strength, athletic ability, or endurance and does

---

Table 11.9

Complications of Inadequate Nutrition in Children and Adolescent Athletes

- **Growth delay:** Lack of sufficient energy during a growth spurt may damage growth irreversibly.
- **Fertility:** Delayed menarche and amenorrhea can result even when there is no concern about body image and not enough diagnostic criteria present to diagnose an eating disorder. The combination of low energy availability, functional hypothalamic amenorrhea, and osteoporosis is called female athlete triad.
- **Bone mineral density:** Osteoporosis and osteopenia can be seen as part of the female athlete triad.
- **Eating disorders:** The prevalence of eating disorders is higher among athletes compared with controls.[a,b] Eating disorders are more common among female athletes than among male athletes. Disordered eating is more frequent in sports that emphasize leanness, have a high power-to-weight ratio, and use weight categories.[c]
- **Nutritional deficit:** Young athletes are at risk for negative energy balance and nutritional deficit of protein, vitamins, and minerals.[d]
- **Dehydration:** Inadequate hydration can decrease athletic performance and put athletes at risk for heat stroke.[e]
- **Water intoxication:** Long-distance runners, bike riders, and triathlon participants are at risk for exercise-induced hyponatremia. The condition results from the loss of sodium in the sweat or excessive water intake. Water intoxication may lead to diluted blood minerals, hyponatremia, renal failure, and even death.[f–h]
- **Sport injury:** Inadequate nutrition decreases athletic performance and may increase the risk of injury. Negative energy balance results in the use of fat and lean tissue for energy. Loss of lean tissue mass results in the loss of strength and endurance and poor musculoskeletal function.

[a] Martinsen M, Sundgot-Borgen J. Higher prevalence of eating disorders among adolescent elite athletes than controls. *Med Sci Sports Exerc*. 2013;45(6):1188–1197. doi:10.1249/MSS.0b013e318281a939.

[b] Sundgot-Borgen J, Torstveit MK. Aspects of disordered eating continuum in elite high-intensity sports. *Scand J Med Sci Sports*. 2010;20(suppl 2):112–121. doi:10.1111/j.1600-0838.2010.01190.x.

[c] Maïano C, Morin AJ, Lanfranchi MC, Therme P. Body-related sport and exercise motives and disturbed eating attitudes and behaviours in adolescents. *Eur Eat Disord Rev*. 2015;23(4):277–286. doi:10.1002/erv.2361.

[d] Petrie HJ, Stover EA, Horswill CA. Nutritional concerns for the child and adolescent competitor. *Nutrition*. 2004; 20(7–8):620–631. doi:10.1016/j.nut.2004.04.002.

[e] Purcell LK, Section EM. Sport nutrition for young athletes. *Paediatr Child Health*. 2013;18(4):200.

[f] Hew TD, Chorley JN, Cianca JC, Divine JG. The incidence, risk factors, and clinical manifestations of hyponatremia in marathon runners. *Clin J Sport Med*. 2003;13(1):41–47.

[g] Hew-Butler T, EAH Consensus Panel 2015. Inadequate hydration or normal body fluid homeostasis? *Am J Public Health*. 2015;105(10):e5–6. doi:10.2105/AJPH.2015.302825.

[h] Peters EM. Nutritional aspects in ultra-endurance exercise. *Curr Opin Clin Nutr Metab Care*. 2003;6(4):427–434. doi:10.1097/01.mco.0000078986.18774.90.

Table 11.10

Beneficial Effect of Sport Activity in Children and Adolescents

Obesity prevention
Improved body image
Improved self-esteem
Improved mood
Decreased anxiety and depression
Improved bone mass
Improved posture
Improved cognitive function
Improved quality of life
Disease prevention: diabetes, stroke, osteoporosis, cardiovascular disease

not transform an average athlete into an elite athlete. But insufficient and unbalanced nutrition does affect athletic performance physiologically (increased injuries, fatigue, and athletic ability) and mentally (reduced attention, learning ability, alertness).[49] Inadequate nutrition in athletic children and adolescents may cause several complications (TABLE 11.10).

Nutritional Challenges for Young Athletes

Child and adolescent athletes face nutritional challenges. During growth and development, requirements for energy, fluid, and nutrients need to be maintained. Puberty causes an increase in metabolic needs. Nutritional plans for adolescents must consider the type of sport activity; the age, weight, and body composition of the athlete; the amount of training; and seasonal variability, for example, lower energy requirements off-season, higher energy needs during training camp.

Fluids

Physical activity results in excessive sweating and hyperventilation that lead to the loss of fluids and minerals. Warm and humid climates increase fluid and mineral losses. Dehydration of as little as 2% of the body weight impairs exercise performance, increases the risk for muscle damage and cramps, and harms the athlete's attention and alertness.[55,56] Thirst decreases during physical activity; therefore, it is crucial athletes drink before, during, and after exercise to maintain optimal fluid balance and prevent dehydration.[47] In intense sport activities, athletes must drink isotonic beverages that include carbohydrates and minerals in similar concentrations to those in the human body and not just water.

Macronutrients

Adequate carbohydrates are needed to maintain blood glucose levels during exercise and replace muscle glycogen. Glucose is the preferred energy source for muscle activity. As muscular glycogen storage increases, muscle performance improves and the exhaustion threshold is delayed. Carbohydrates are essential for extended strain.

Whole-grain, complex carbohydrates are recommended. Postexercise recovery requires balanced nutrition, rich in calories, carbohydrates, protein, vitamins, and minerals. Scheduling an athlete's meals and snacks is important. Supplying the correct energy requirements at the correct time accelerates recovery and replenishes liver and muscle glycogen storage.

Adolescent athletes require higher protein intake than the general population. Protein needs depend on the age, sex, the type of sport and its intensity. Protein can be used as a source of energy during prolonged physical activity; therefore supplementation of protein may be needed. Optimal protein intake at the right timing combined with physical activity increases the muscle mass.[49] Balanced nutrition that includes vegetarian and meat products will usually provide the necessary protein needs without the need for dietary supplements.[49] Overconsumption of protein may cause an increase in the fat tissue, dehydration, and kidney burden.

Consumption of fat in the diet is necessary for essential fatty acids and the absorption of fat-soluble vitamins.[47] It is recommended young athletes consume unsaturated fat such as olive oil and almonds and avoid saturated fat and fast food. Fat is a valuable source of energy during prolonged activities of moderate intensity.

Micronutrients

During physical activity, there is an increase in the need for minerals and vitamins.[57] It is essential to maintain sufficient levels of calcium, vitamin D, magnesium, and iron.[47,49]

Iron is an essential mineral that is part of the hemoglobin that serves as an oxygen carrier to the cells. Iron deficiency is common among athletes and adolescents. Physical activity increases the need for iron. Females, runners, and vegetarians are at increased risk for iron deficiency. Meat, poultry, lentils, and other iron-containing foods eaten with high vitamin C foods helps to enhance the absorption of dietary iron. Iron supplements should be used only in the case of iron-deficiency anemia that is not sufficiently treated with nutrition.[49]

Nutritional Schedule

Food composition and meal schedule affect the body's performance both during training and during competitions. Research shows that spreading energy intake over five meals a day (breakfast, lunch, dinner, and two snacks) prevents gastrointestinal overload, provides for energy needs, and improves physical performance. An individual's menu and meal schedule should be adjusted to the training schedule to provide the needed energy, enable recovery postphysical strain, and avoid gastrointestinal discomfort during effort.[47,49]

The pretraining meal should be a full meal, low in fat, and eaten at least 3 hours prior to training.[47] A low-fat granola bar or a low-fat sandwich can be eaten an hour or two before the training, and a fruit an hour before the training. Endurance training that lasts longer than an hour requires the addition of carbohydrates such as an isotonic drink[47] or a piece of fruit.[49] In endurance training that lasts longer than 90 minutes, it is recommended the athlete schedule a protein and carbohydrate meal post-training. A training that lasts less than an hour requires posttraining drinking.[49]

Recommendations for Young Athletes

Athletes' menus should be planned according to their individual needs relative to age, weight, body composition, sports type, training schedule and intensity,[49] training goals, medical condition, and any other relevant information. Nutritional plans should include detailed instructions about what should and should not be eaten and include substitutions if it is necessary to deviate from the plan. It is recommended that parents of adolescent athletes be made aware of the importance of nutrition. In a period of accelerated growth, weight gain, and height growth, it is important to adjust the adolescent's and specifically the athlete's nutritional habits to ensure optimal mental and physical growth and development. The nutritional plan of the young athlete should be incorporated into the training plan to improve performance, achieve the training goals, and ensure posttraining recovery.

Athletes should be assessed prior to sport participation for female athlete triad (**FIGURE 11.5**). Trainers and coaches should be educated to discourage unhealthy diets and weight loss practices.

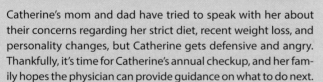

Case Study

Catherine's mom and dad have tried to speak with her about their concerns regarding her strict diet, recent weight loss, and personality changes, but Catherine gets defensive and angry. Thankfully, it's time for Catherine's annual checkup, and her family hopes the physician can provide guidance on what to do next.

During the appointment, Catherine's family discusses Catherine's physical and social history, including her participation in competitive gymnastics, her recent diet changes, weight loss, cessation of menstruation, and personality changes.

Catherine's physical examination shows the following:
Height: 5 feet 2 inches
Weight: 89 pounds
Muscle loss noted in the extremities, thinning hair, and lanugo (fine hair) noted on the body.

Catherine's physician discusses his concerns that Catherine is suffering from anorexia nervosa and likely the female athlete triad.

Questions

1. What other symptoms will Catherine need to exhibit to be diagnosed with the female athlete triad?
2. What treatment might be necessary to help Catherine regain her health?

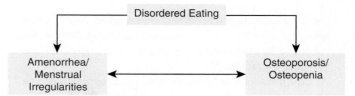

Disordered Eating

Amenorrhea/ Menstrual Irregularities ↔ **Osteoporosis/ Osteopenia**

Disordered Eating

The athlete develops one or more harmful eating behaviors in an attempt to lose weight. The result is an energy deficit.

Amenorrhea

Insufficient energy availability, which leads to a decrease in estrogen production, eventually results in menstrual irregularities and amenorrhea.

Osteoporosis/Osteopenia

The lack of estrogen decreases calcium absorption and retention. Dietary deficiency of calcium also is common. Left untreated, this lack of calcium leads to bone loss, stress fractures, and osteoporosis.

Figure 11.5
The female athlete triad.

Recap Nutrition directly affects both physiologic and mental performance. An optimal nutritional plan is critical for adolescent athletes and must take into consideration the type of sport activity; the age, weight, and body composition of the athlete; the amount of training; and seasonal variability, for example, lower energy requirements off-season, higher energy needs during training camp. Appropriate amounts of fluids, macronutrients, and micronutrients at the right times enables the body to achieve optimal performance during exertion.

1. Describe the unique nutritional needs of young athletes.
2. List the benefits of participation in sports for children and adolescents.

Adolescent Alcohol and Substance Abuse

Preview Substance abuse during adolescence can result in physical, psychiatric, and social complications and is associated with increased rates of comorbid mental health disorders and neurocognitive deficits, use of other illicit drugs in the future, and higher likelihood of abuse or dependence in adulthood. Several treatments have been developed to reduce youth alcohol consumption including behavioral interventions, cognitive therapies and motivational interviewing provided as interventions directly to the adolescent or as part of family therapy in attempt to reduce risk factors.

The midadolescent period is often characterized by danger-seeking behavior. Adolescents are exposed to substances with addictive potential and their use can lead to abuse. Substance abuse during adolescence can result in physical, psychiatric, and social complications. Alcohol misuse during adolescence places youth at increased risk for subsequent adult alcohol abuse.[58]

Prevalence and Etiology of Adolescent Substance Abuse

Since early history, people have used alcohol to socialize, celebrate, and relax. About 10 minutes after alcohol consumption blood alcohol concentration (BAC) rises. Higher BAC increases alcohol's effects and can cause reduced inhibition, motor impairment, confusion, and impaired memory and attention. Adolescence is an important developmental period. Alcohol and marijuana use during this crucial time when the brain is still developing is associated with increased rates of comorbid mental health disorders and neurocognitive deficits, use of other illicit drugs in the future, and higher likelihood of abuse or dependence in adulthood.[59] Youth dependent on alcohol demonstrate reduced motivation for academic success. Marijuana use is associated with greater academic unpreparedness, lower academic performance, and greater delinquency.[60]

Alcohol is the substance most frequently used by teens (alcoholism). In a 2014 report, 2.7% of teens ages 12–17 years reported alcohol use disorder, and 13.8% of teens ages 12–20 years reported binge drinking.[61] In another study, 1 in 10 adolescents ages 13–14 years reported regular alcohol use, and this number increased to 47.1% at the ages of 17–18 years. The median age of onset was 13 years for first alcohol use and 14 years for regular use or abuse (with and without dependence).[62]

White and Hispanic youth have higher rates of alcohol and other drug use initially and increase their use more rapidly over time than nonwhite youth; however, racial differences lessen as nonwhite youth reach their 20s and 30s.[60] The highest rates of substance use disorders are seen at the ages of 18–25 years.[63] Most cases of drug abuse in the United States had their initial onset during adolescence:[62] 36.6% of adolescents who used illicit drugs developed abuse.

The prevalence of marijuana use has increased, prevalence of cigarette smoking has decreased, but hookah and electronic cigarettes have emerged as a method of nicotine use. Cannabis is the most frequently used substance of all illicit drugs used during adolescence.

Risk Factors for Adolescent Substance Abuse

The initiation of alcohol use is strongly influenced by genetics and modeling within the family environment.[64]

There are variations in alcohol use according to the place of birth and cultural norms. Adolescents with African or Asian backgrounds were much less likely to consume alcohol than Australian-born adolescents. However, regardless of adolescents' country of birth, high levels of parental disapproval of alcohol use and parental monitoring strongly inhibited recent alcohol use.[65]

Males have higher rates of illicit drug use than females, with the exception that female adolescents have higher rates of nonmedical use of amphetamines, sedatives, and tranquilizers. Childhood poverty and socioeconomic stress increase the risk for adulthood substance use and abuse.[66]

Psychotropic effects of a substance may affect adolescents differently from how they affect adults because of biological, social, or cognitive reasons. Initiation of marijuana use during adolescence prior to 18 years of age is associated with increased risk of developing dependence on the substance and addiction. This risk is increased specifically with daily use.[59]

Substance Use Disorder

The fifth edition of the *Diagnostic and Statistical Manual of Mental Disorders* (DSM-5) combined the terms *substance abuse* and *substance dependence* into a single disorder measured on a continuum from mild to severe. Each specific substance is addressed as a separate use disorder. There are 11 criteria, and meeting 2–3 criteria is diagnosed as mild. Moderate disorder is diagnosed with the presence of 4–5 criteria, and the presence of 6 or more criteria defines a severe degree of substance use disorder (**TABLE 11.11**).

Withdrawal Syndrome

Cessation or reduction in substance use that has been heavy and prolonged may lead to withdrawal syndrome, which is characterized by typical signs and symptoms. The symptoms cause significant discomfort and impairment in social, occupational, and other important areas of functioning. Alcohol withdrawal can present with autonomic hyperactivity (sweating, tachycardia), hand tremor, insomnia, nausea and vomiting, transient visual tactile or auditory hallucinations or illusions, psychomotor agitation, anxiety, or seizures.

Treatment of Adolescent Substance Abuse

Several treatments have been developed to reduce youths' alcohol consumption. The interventions are provided either directly to the adolescent or in the context of the family. Individual treatments include behavioral interventions that identify triggers for alcohol use and teach refusal skills, relaxation techniques, and behavioral management; cognitive therapies (that focus on distorted thoughts and maladaptive perceptions that lead to addictive behaviors), and motivational interviewing, which helps the patient build internal motivation toward behavioral change. Family therapies attempt to

Table 11.11

DSM-5 Criteria for Alcohol Use Disorder

1. Alcohol is often taken in a large amounts or over a longer period than was intended.
2. Persistent desire or unsuccessful efforts to cut down alcohol use.
3. A great deal of time is spent in activities necessary to obtain alcohol, use alcohol, or recover from its effects.
4. Strong desire or urge to use alcohol.
5. Recurrent alcohol use resulting in a failure to fulfill major obligations at work, school, or home.
6. Continued alcohol use despite having recurrent social or interpersonal problems caused by the effect of alcohol.
7. Important social, occupational, or recreational activities are given up or reduced because of alcohol use.
8. Recurrent alcohol use in situations in which it is physically hazardous.
9. Alcohol use is continued despite knowledge of having persistent or recurrent physical or psychological problems that are likely to have been caused or exacerbated by alcohol.
10. Tolerance, as defined by either of the following:
    a. A need for markedly increased amounts of alcohol to achieve intoxication or desired effect.
    b. A markedly diminished effect with continued use of the same amount of alcohol.
11. Withdrawal, as manifested by either of the following:
    a. The characteristic withdrawal syndrome for alcohol.
    b. Alcohol or closely related substance is taken to relieve or avoid withdrawal symptoms.

Data from American Psychiatric Association. *Diagnostic and Statistical Manual of Mental Disorders*. 5th ed. Arlington, VA: American Psychiatric Association; 2013.

reduce risk factors for substance use that present in the youth's social environment and family. Some interventions are brief and others have long follow-up. An analysis that compared individual versus family intervention to reduce alcohol use among adolescents showed that individual counseling had a larger influence on the reduction of alcohol use for adolescents with alcohol use disorders than family-based intervention.[58]

Brief interventions to treat drug-abusing adolescents were found to be useful when they worked with the adolescent alone or involved a parent. The efficacy was higher when parents were involved in the treatment.[67] Motivational interviewing is an essential part of treatment. Factors that influence the ability to change include peer drug use, parenting practices, and coexisting mental disorders. In severe cases of drug use disorders, an admission to a rehabilitation facility might be required.

Recommendations for Adolescent Substance Abuse

Parents should be encouraged to be involved in their adolescent's daily life. Parental monitoring for alcohol and drug abuse is recommended. Teachers, dietitians, physicians, and any care providers should be encouraged to use the routine meetings with the adolescent to screen for drug use or abuse. If drug use is noted, an assessment should be made about the level of use, the triggers for use, and the motivation for change. Schools can serve as a venue to screen for alcohol and drug use, and brief interventions can be planned. Discussing with teens their plans regarding alcohol and drug use is important, and raising awareness of the harm caused by these substances is essential because early use has long-term effects.

Recap Substance abuse during adolescence places youth at increased risk for multiple health and behavioral consequences and a higher likelihood of abuse or dependence in adulthood. Interventions can be designed to identify triggers for alcohol use and behavioral management, address distorted thoughts that lead to addictive behaviors, build internal motivation toward behavioral change, and reduce risk factors for substance use in the social environment and family. Parents should be encouraged to be involved in their adolescent's daily life preventing and monitoring for alcohol and drug abuse.

1. Describe two short- and two long-term harmful effects of alcohol or marijuana use.
2. Define the way to diagnose substance use disorder.

Vegetarian Children and Adolescents

Preview A balanced diet is critical for children and adolescents. Food restrictions can inhibit them from receiving the adequate nutrients needed for proper growth and development. It is possible to achieve a balanced diet following vegetarian and vegan patterns; however, risk of various micronutrient deficiencies persists. Individual nutrition planning must incorporate education about acceptable foods that can help the child or adolescent obtain any nutrients that may be missing.

Vegetarianism is a dietary lifestyle that avoids intake of any meat, poultry, or fish. Vegetarian diets are defined by the foods that they include.[68] Common subclassifications include lacto-ovo vegetarians (avoidance of meat but inclusion of dairy and eggs) and pesco-vegetarians (avoidance of meat but inclusion of fish). Similar to vegetarianism, veganism is the avoidance of all animal products and any food products derived from animals or that may include animal by-products. The reasons children and adolescents follow vegetarian dietary patterns may range from religious beliefs to cultural influences and family or personal preferences.

Health Advantages of a Vegetarian Diet

It is well accepted that a well-planned vegetarian or vegan diet can supply all nutrients needed to maintain adequate nutrition status.[68] Scientific evidence suggests there are multiple health benefits for those who choose to follow a vegetarian lifestyle. Though total energy intake does not differ significantly among vegetarians, vegans, and omnivores, the total fat (specifically saturated fat) intake is lowest in vegans and highest in omnivores.[69] Furthermore, vegans eat the most amounts of polyunsaturated fatty acids when compared to both vegetarians and omnivores.[69] When compared with nonvegetarians, self-reported prevalence of diabetes mellitus in semivegetarians, lacto-ovo-vegetarians, and vegans is approximately half.[68] Although research remains inconclusive, limited evidence suggests that the risk for cancer at all sites combined is slightly lower in vegetarians than in nonvegetarians.[68] More specifically, those who eat fish, but not meat, may have a lower risk of colorectal cancer.[68]

Health Risks for Pediatric Vegetarians

Although a balanced diet is possible with vegetarian and vegan diets, the risk of various micronutrient deficiencies persists.[69] Subsequently, these micronutrient deficiencies may coincide with more serious adverse health effects. Low intakes of vitamin B_{12}, vitamin D, calcium, and omega-3 fatty acids are potential risks with the avoidance of dairy products and meat. Despite high intakes, lower iron status in vegetarians and vegans may be a result of lower iron bioavailability from plant foods when compared to animal foods.[69] Nonheme iron, the form found in plants, is absorbed less efficiently when compared to heme iron, the form found in meat. Additionally, natural inhibitors of iron absorption such as polyphenols and phytic acid reduce the bioavailability of iron even further.[69] Similar to iron, zinc-rich plant foods such as legumes, whole grains, nuts, and seeds also contain high amounts of phytic acid, inhibiting overall absorption of zinc.

Relatively low vitamin B_{12} levels commonly observed in vegetarians and especially in vegans may be associated with relatively high plasma homocysteine, a precursor to impaired heart health and stroke.[68] It has been suggested that above-average levels of plasma homocysteine, which may be caused either by genetic defects in the enzymes involved in homocysteine metabolism or by nutritional deficiencies in B-group vitamin cofactors, may be associated with cardiovascular risk and impaired bone health.[70,71] Research also suggests that vegetarians and especially vegans who avoid calcium-rich dairy products may be at greater risk of low bone mineral density and fracture than nonvegetarians.[68-70] Nutritional recommendations for children and adolescents following a vegetarian diet are listed in **TABLE 11.12**.

> **Recap** A vegetarian or vegan diet can supply all necessary nutrients to maintain adequate nutrition status for adolescents. Careful planning ensures adequate needs are met at this critical age. Vegetarian and vegan adolescents may be at risk for deficiencies of vitamin B_{12}, vitamin D, calcium, and omega-3 fatty acids.
>
> 1. List at least three nutrient deficiencies that vegetarian and vegan adolescents may be at risk for.
> 2. Formulate a plan of food substitutes that may benefit a vegetarian and vegan adolescent.

Table 11.12

Recommendations for Pediatric Vegetarians

1. When combined with adequate caloric intake, a variety of foods can offer many healthy advantages in a well-planned vegetarian diet.
2. Educational efforts should be provided to ensure adequate intake of various supplemental and fortified products:

   Vitamin B_{12}: Consider vitamin supplements, vitamin-enriched cereals, and fortified soy products.

   Vitamin D: Fatty fish (salmon, tuna, halibut), fortified milk products, and milk substitutes (requires appropriate education on label reading).

   Zinc: Whole grains, soy products, legumes, nuts, chia seeds, flax seeds, and wheat germ.

   Omega-3 fatty acids: Many vegetarian diets that do not include fish and eggs are generally low in active forms of omega-3 fats. Because conversion of the plant-based omega-3 to the types used by humans is inefficient, consider fortified products or supplements as needed. Intake of avocados, nuts, nut butters, flaxseeds, chia seeds, and olive oil should be encouraged.

   Calcium: Calcium-enriched and fortified products, including milk substitutes (such as almond milk), fortified cereals, leafy-green vegetables, and tofu.

3. Supplemental calcium, vitamin D, and vitamin B_{12} are often required if not consumed via fortified foods.

Data from Appleby PN, Key TJ. The long-term health of vegetarians and vegans. *Proc Nutr Soc.* 2016;75(3):287–293; Schüpbach R, Wegmüller R, Berguerand C, Bui M, Herter-Aeberli I. Micronutrient status and intake in omnivores, vegetarians and vegans in Switzerland [published online October 26, 2015]. *Eur J Nutr.*; Krivosıkova Z, Krajcovicova M, Spustová V, et al. The association between high plasma homocysteine levels and lower bone mineral density in Slovak women: the impact of vegetarian diet. *Eur J Nutr.* 2010;49:147–153.

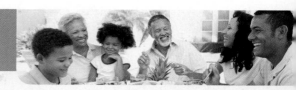

Learning Portfolio

Visual Chapter Summary

Celiac Disease in Children and Adolescents

- Celiac disease is a chronic, systemic, autoimmune disorder.
- Gluten proteins and related prolamins found in grains such as wheat, barley, and rye trigger an autoimmune response in the gut that damages intestinal villi.
- Villous atrophy results in malabsorption of various macronutrients and micronutrients.
- Celiac disease occurs in 1% of the population in Europe and the United States.
- Females are diagnosed twice more frequently than males.
- Specific genetic haplotypes are at risk for developing celiac disease.
- First-degree relatives of patients with celiac and patients with other autoimmune disorders are at increased risk for celiac disease.
- Gastrointestinal presentations include abdominal distention, chronic diarrhea, and poor weight gain.
- Celiac disease is diagnosed by clinical symptoms, serological testing, and small-bowel biopsy, which is the gold standard for confirmation of diagnosis.
- Celiac disease is a lifelong disorder that requires consistent dietary management with a gluten-free diet.
- Poor adherence to a gluten-free diet may result in complications such as neurologic disorders, osteoporosis, impaired splenic function, infertility, ulcerative jejunoileitis, and cancer.

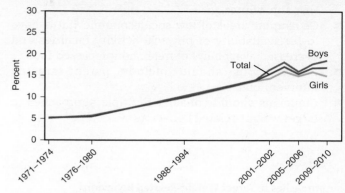

Reproduced from Centers for Disease Control and Prevention/National Center for Health Statistics. National Health and Nutrition Examination Survey. s (NHANES) I–III; and NHANES 1999–2000, 2001–2002, 2003–2004, 2005–2006, 2007–2008, and 2009–2010. Hyattsville, MD: National Center for Health Statistics.

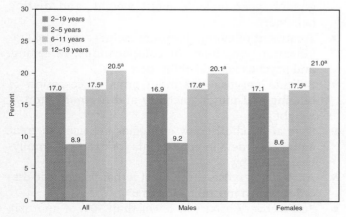

a Significantly different from those aged 2–5 years.

Reproduced from Centers for Disease Control and Prevention/National Center for Health Statistics. National Health and Nutrition Examination Survey, 2011-2014. Hyattsville, MD: National Center for Health Statistics; 2015.

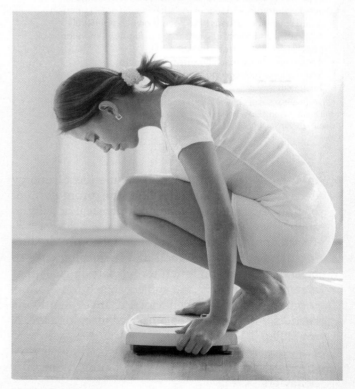

©Mark Scott/The Image Bank/Getty.

Pediatric Overweight and Obesity

- The prevalence of obesity in adolescents tripled in the last three decades in all socioeconomic status levels.
- Causes of pediatric overweight and obesity include increased consumption of total energy, soft drinks, and snacks; frequent fast-food consumption; inadequate amount of fruits and vegetables in the diet; and decreased levels of daily physical activity.

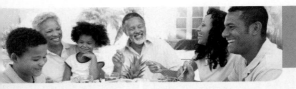

Learning Portfolio (continued)

- Rates of obesity are higher for Mexican and non-Hispanic black American adolescents than for non-Hispanic whites.
- Geographic areas of low socioeconomic status have lower availability of physical activity facilities and decreased availability of fresh, nonprocessed food.
- Interventions should include parent-targeted interventions.
- Clinicians should consider multiple approaches to target weight-related behaviors

Table 11.4

Approaches to Target Weight-Related Behaviors

- Computer-based weight control plans.
- In-person clinician visits to discuss the adolescent's physical activity, nutrition, and sedentary behaviors. Of note, in-person group education sessions have been shown to be effective.[a]
- Adolescent and parent sessions to learn about self-monitoring of physical activity and food intake.
- Adolescent phone coaching sessions.
- Informational materials provided to the adolescent and parent.
- Telehealth.

[a] Stark LJ, Spear S, Boles R, et al. A pilot randomized controlled trial of a clinic and home-based behavioral intervention to decrease obesity in preschoolers. *Obesity* (Silver Spring). 2011;19(1):134–141. doi:10.1038/oby.2010.87.

- Interventions should include regulation of energy density and portion size and the promotion of healthy food choices along with physical activity to support weight control.
- Treatment strategies: environmental control (reducing the availability of food and increasing cues to be active); behavioral monitoring; setting goals that are specific, explicit, and subject to self-monitoring; rewarding successful behavioral change; identifying barriers and solving problems; and teaching parenting skills.
- Effective interventions for preschool-aged children should include parent modeling of healthy behaviors.
- Elementary-school-aged children also benefit from parent inclusion, including target parent weight loss.

Adolescent Eating Disorders

- Eating disorders are the third most common chronic illness in adolescents.

Table 11.5

DSM-5 Diagnostic Criteria for Anorexia Nervosa

A. **Restriction of energy intake**. Avoidance of food leading to significantly low body weight compromising physical health.

B. **Intense fear of weight gain or becoming fat or persistent behavior that interferes with weight gain, even though at a significantly low weight**. Purposeful behavior to avoid weight gain. Steadfast pursuance and maintenance of low body weight.

C. **Disturbance in the way in which one's body weight or shape is experienced**, undue influence of body weight or shape on self-evaluation, or persistent lack of recognition of the seriousness of the current low body weight.

Restricting type vs. binge eating/purging type

Modified from American Psychiatric Association. *Diagnostic and Statistical Manual of Mental Disorders*. 5th ed. (DSM-5) Arlington, VA: American Psychiatric Association; 2013.

Modified from: American Psychiatric Association. Diagnostic and Statistical Manual of Mental Disorders. 5th ed. (DSM-5) Arlington, VA: American Psychiatric Association; 2013.

- Eating disorders are characterized by persistent disturbance of eating that impairs health and psychosocial functioning.
- Females are diagnosed with anorexia nervosa more often than males.
- There is a peak incidence of eating disorders during adolescence.
- Twenty percent of adolescents with eating disorders do not seek treatment because of shame, denial, or lack of recognition by the medical system.
- Genetic and environmental factors play roles in the development of eating disorders.
- Prevention of eating disorders focuses on addressing risk factors (history of sexual abuse, female gender, peer teasing about weight, and dieting behavior).
- Treatment of eating disorders includes medical stabilization, treatment of complications, refeeding, and psychosocial rehabilitation.
- Bulimia nervosa treatment aims at cessation of binging and purging activity and normalization of weight gain.
- Several psychotherapy strategies are used to treat eating disorders in adolescents for example: family-based therapy.
- Anorexia nervosa is the most lethal psychiatric disorder, with a mortality rate of 6%.
- Full recovery occurs in fewer than 50% of anorexia nervosa survivors, and 20% develop chronicity.

Table 11.7

Levels in Eating Disorder Prevention Programs

Family	More frequent family meals are considered a protective factor and associated with:
	• Better dietary intake
	• Higher levels of psychosocial well-being, academic success
	• Lower levels of substance abuse[a]
	Recommendations for families are to:
	• Talk less about weight.
	• Facilitate healthy eating and physical activity.
Schools	School-based programs that work at:
	• Improving student self-esteem
	• Providing positive web-based prevention programs
	• Interventions at ballet and gymnastic schools
	• Programs to educate about teasing-free environment at schools
Teachers	Teacher programs that teach educators: how to treat their own bodies and how to discuss dieting, body dissatisfaction, eating, and physical activity.
	Teachers should avoid discussing their own dieting behaviors with students.
Health care	Healthcare providers should discourage dieting, support physical activity, and promote positive body image, helping teenagers feel better about their bodies so that they will nurture themselves through healthy eating.
Society	Legislative efforts that help change societal norms by requiring advertisers improve the messages in the media about size, weight, and beauty.

Neumark-Sztainer D, Larson NI, Fulkerson JA, Eisenberg ME, Story M. Family meals and adolescents: what have we learned from Project EAT (Eating Among Teens)? *Public Health Nutr.* 2010;13(7):1113–1121. doi:10.1017/S1368980010000169.

Pediatric Diabetes

- Three-quarters of all cases of type 1 diabetes are diagnosed in individuals younger than 18 years of age.
- The hallmark symptoms of type 1 diabetes include increased thirst and frequency of urination (polyuria and polydipsia), and weight loss, and about one-third present with diabetic ketoacidosis.
- Type 1 diabetes is the autoimmune destruction of pancreatic islet cells.
- Patients with type 1 diabetes are at increased risk for other autoimmune diseases.
- Treatment of type 1 diabetes includes supplementation of the missing insulin by injections or insulin pump in accordance with the food supply and level of activity.
- The goal of nutrition therapy in diabetes is to promote healthful eating patterns.
- Children and adolescents with type 1 diabetes should learn to be mindful of their eating and adjust the insulin therapy to their eating but, on the other hand, not be afraid of eating or avoid insulin treatment.
- There is no single ideal dietary distribution of calories among carbohydrates, fats, and proteins for people with diabetes.

- Individuals with type 1 diabetes should consume carbohydrates from whole grains, vegetables, fruits, legumes, dairy products, and foods higher in fiber and lower in glycemic load.
- In general, people with type 1 diabetes should avoid sugar-sweetened beverages.
- Type 2 diabetes is characterized by insulin resistance (the demand for insulin rises and there is inadequate insulin secretion and relative insulin deficiency).
- Insulin resistance results from genetic, metabolic, and environmental causes (there is no identified autoimmune process).
- The healthcare team for a child or adolescent with type 2 diabetes includes a pediatric endocrinologist, diabetes nurse educator, nutritionist, and behavioral specialist.
- Treatment should address behavioral changes that will promote a healthy lifestyle and weight reduction.
- Diet changes should include eliminating sugar-containing beverages, increasing the consumption of vegetables and fruits, reducing the consumption of simple carbohydrates and starch, decreasing the consumption of processed foods, changing to whole grains, and controlling food portions.

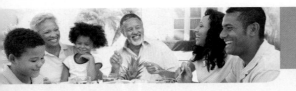

Learning Portfolio (continued)

Fasting plasma glucose ≥ 126 mg/dl
(≥ 7.0 mmol/L)
Fasting = no caloric intake for ≥ 8h

↓

Glucose challenge test of 1.75 g/kg (max
75 g) anhydrous glucose dissolved in water.
Post-challenge plasma glucose ≥ 200 mg/dL
(≥ 11.1 mmol/L)

↓

Symptoms of diabetes (polyuria, polydipsia,
nocturia, unexplained weight loss) and casual
plasma glucose ≥ 200 mg/dL (≥ 11.1 mmol/L)

↓

HbA1c > 6.5% (48 mmol/mol)

- Parental monitoring of healthy habits, including diet and exercise, is recommended.
- Children and adolescents with type 2 diabetes should have their blood pressure, blood lipid levels, eyes, liver, menstrual cycle, and mental health status followed closely.

Nutrition for Young Athletes

- Optimal nutrition is key to maximizing athletic potential.
- Physical activity at an early age has beneficial effects on growth and development as well as morbidity and mortality prevention.

- Physical activity improves bone mass, posture, as well as self-esteem and mood.
- Inadequate nutrition in athletic children and adolescents may cause several complications.
- The nutritional plan for child and adolescent athletes needs to consider the type of sport activity, age, weight, body composition, the amount of training, and seasonal variability.

Table 11.10

Beneficial Effect of Sport Activity in Children and Adolescents

Obesity prevention
Improved body image
Improved self-esteem
Improved mood
Decreased anxiety and depression
Improved bone mass
Improved posture
Improved cognitive function
Improved quality of life
Disease prevention: diabetes, stroke, osteoporosis, cardiovascular disease

- Adolescents should avoid dehydration by drinking adequate amounts of fluid before, during, and after exercise.
- Intense sports require drinking isotonic beverages that include carbohydrates and minerals.
- Carbohydrates are needed to maintain blood glucose levels during exercise and replace muscle glycogen.

Table 11.8

Risk Factors for Type 2 Diabetes

- Being a first- or second-degree relative of family members with type 2 diabetes increases the risk of developing type 2 diabetes.
- Males who are born to mothers who had gestational diabetes and who were born large for gestational age have a higher risk of developing type 2 diabetes than females.[a]
- Youth-onset type 2 diabetes occurs in all races but with higher prevalence among nonwhite adolescents not of European descent (for example, blacks, Native Americans, Hispanics, Asians, and South Asians).
- In the United States and Europe, youth-onset type 2 diabetes is related to obesity, but in Asia type 2 diabetes is often seen in normal-weight adolescents.
- Sex ratio (male:female) of youth-onset type 2 diabetes varies from 1:4 to 1:6 in native North Americans and to 1:1 in Asians.
- In the United States and Europe, youth-onset type 2 diabetes disproportionately affects populations with low socioeconomic and low education levels, whereas in developing countries youth-onset type 2 diabetes is seen in children from higher socioeconomic levels.[a]

[a] Copeland KC, Zeitler P, Geffner M, et al. Characteristics of adolescents and youth with recent-onset type 2 diabetes: the TODAY cohort at baseline. *J Clin Endocrinol Metab.* 2011;96(1):159–167. doi:10.1210/jc.2010-1642.

- Postexercise recovery requires balanced nutrition rich in calories, carbohydrates, protein, vitamins, and minerals.
- Athletes require higher protein intake than the general population.
- Protein needs depend on age, sex, type of sport, and sport intensity.
- Overconsumption of protein may cause an increase in the fat tissue, dehydration, and kidney burden.
- Consumption of fat in the diet is necessary for essential fatty acids and the absorption of fat-soluble vitamins.
- Female athletes and vegetarians are at increased risk for iron deficiency.
- Spreading energy intake over five meals a day (breakfast, lunch, dinner, and two snacks) prevents gastrointestinal overload and provides adequate energy to improve physical performance.
- Pretraining meals should be low fat and eaten at least 3 hours prior to training.
- Snacks such as a low-fat granola bar or a low-fat sandwich can be eaten an hour or two before the training, and a fruit an hour before the training.

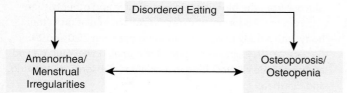

Disordered Eating

Amenorrhea/Menstrual Irregularities ←→ Osteoporosis/Osteopenia

Disordered Eating

The athlete develops one or more harmful eating behaviors in an attempt to lose weight. The result is an energy deficit.

Amenorrhea

Insufficient energy availability, which leads to a decrease in estrogen production, eventually results in menstrual irregularities and amenorrhea.

Osteoporosis/Osteopenia

The lack of estrogen decreases calcium absorption and retention. Dietary deficiency of calcium also is common. Left untreated, this lack of calcium leads to bone loss, stress fractures, and osteoporosis.

- If endurance training lasts longer than 90 minutes, it is recommended athletes schedule a protein and carbohydrate meal posttraining.
- Athletes should be assessed prior to sport participation for female athlete triad.
- Trainers and coaches should be educated to discourage unhealthy weight loss practices.

Adolescent Alcohol and Substance Abuse

- Substance abuse during adolescence can result in physical, psychiatric, and social complications.
- Alcohol and marijuana misuse during adolescence places youth at increased risk for subsequent adult alcohol and drug abuse.
- Alcohol and marijuana use during this crucial time of brain development is associated with increased rates of comorbid mental health disorders and neurocognitive deficits and can negatively influence adolescent academic performance.
- Alcohol is the substance most frequently used by teens.
- White and Hispanic youth have higher rates of alcohol and other drug use initially and increase their use more rapidly over time than nonwhite youth.
- The highest rates of substance use disorders are seen at the ages of 18 to 25 years. Most cases of drug abuse in the United States had their initial onset during adolescence.
- The prevalence of marijuana use has increased, prevalence of cigarette smoking has decreased, but hookah and electronic cigarettes have emerged as a method of nicotine use.
- Alcohol use is strongly influenced by genetics and modeling within the family environment and high levels of parental disapproval of alcohol use and parental monitoring strongly inhibits recent alcohol use.
- Males have higher rates of illicit drug use than females, with the exception that female adolescents have higher rates of nonmedical use of amphetamines, sedatives, and tranquilizers.
- Childhood poverty and socioeconomic stress increase the risk for adult substance use and abuse.
- There are 11 criteria for diagnosis of substance abuse disorders. Meeting 2–3 criteria is diagnosed as a mild disorder. Moderate disorder is diagnosed with the presence of 4–5 symptoms, and the presence of 6 or more symptoms define a severe substance use disorder.

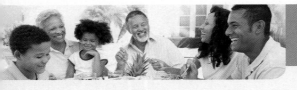

Learning Portfolio (continued)

- Cessation of or reduction in substance use that has been heavy and prolonged may lead to withdrawal syndrome.
- Individual treatments include behavioral interventions, cognitive therapies, and motivational interviewing.
- Family therapy attempts to reduce risk factors for substance use that present in the youth's social environment and family. Parental monitoring for alcohol and drug abuse is recommended.
- Teachers, dietitians, physicians, and any care providers should be encouraged to use the routine meetings with the adolescent to screen for drug use or abuse.

Vegetarian Children and Adolescents

- Vegetarianism is a dietary lifestyle that avoids intake of meat, poultry, or fish.

- Veganism is the avoidance of all animal products and any food products derived from animals or that may include animal by-products.
- Children and adolescents may follow a vegetarian or vegan diet because of religious beliefs, cultural influence, or family or personal preferences.
- A well-planned vegetarian or vegan diet can supply all nutrients needed to maintain adequate nutrition status.
- Low intakes of vitamin B_{12}, vitamin D, calcium, and omega-3 fatty acids are potential risks with the avoidance of dairy products and meat.
- Lower iron status in vegetarians and vegans may be a result of lower iron bioavailability in plant foods when compared to animal foods.
- Research suggests that vegetarians and especially vegans who avoid calcium-rich dairy products may be at greater risk of low bone mineral density and fracture than nonvegetarians.

Key Terms

aphthous stomatitis: common oral mucosal ulcers also known as canker sores.

binge eating: The consumption of large quantities of food in a short period of time, typically as part of an eating disorder.

body dissatisfaction: Negative subjective assessment of one's weight and body image; may be closely related to onset, severity, and treatment outcomes of eating disorders.

glycemic control: Achievement and maintenance of an optimal blood glucose level.

insulin resistance: A condition characterized by the increasing demand for insulin paired with inadequate insulin

secretion and relative insulin deficiency. The diminished ability of cells to respond to the action of insulin in transporting glucose from the bloodstream into muscle and other tissues.

overweight: Abnormal or excessive fat accumulation in the body with a body mass index ranging between 25.0 and 29.

villous atrophy: Inflammation of the small bowel mucosa and atrophy of the villi, resulting in nutrient malabsorption, wasting, and diarrhea.

water intoxication: Excessive intake of water that may lead to diluted minerals in the blood, hyponatremia, renal failure, and even death.

Discussion Questions

1. Discuss the differences in etiology and management of type 1 diabetes mellitus and type 2 diabetes mellitus in adolescents.
2. Explain the key features of in the treatment of eating disorders in adolescents.
3. Describe the unique nutritional considerations for adolescent athletes.

4. Adolescence is a unique time of increased independence in personal lifestyle, physical activity, and food choices. Discuss the influences on food choice during this life stage and how these factors could impact the health and well-being of an adolescent with special health circumstances or nutritional needs such as those mentioned in this chapter.

Activities

1. On the Internet, find three informational websites on celiac disease and provide a summary of the information they provide. Rank each website on how user-friendly it is (with 1 being the most user-friendly, and 3 the least).

2. You've recently been hired by your local department of public health. Your first task is to create a new outreach program aimed at preventing youth obesity. In addition to the youth, what other key people should be involved in the prevention program? What activities might you plan as part of your prevention program?

Study Questions

1. Celiac disease is considered which type of disorder?
   a. Pediatric
   b. Autoimmune
   c. Pancreatic
   d. Cardiac

2. Gluten proteins and related prolamins found in which foods trigger a response in the gut, damaging intestinal villi?
   a. Fruit and vegetables
   b. Fats and oils
   c. Grains such as wheat
   d. Rice

3. Gastrointestinal presentation of celiac disease includes which symptoms?
   a. Abdominal distention
   b. Chronic diarrhea
   c. Constipation and vomiting
   d. All of the above

4. Obesity is the most prevalent pediatric nutritional disorder that affects approximately what proportion of children and adolescents?
   a. Half
   b. One-quarter
   c. One-third
   d. Three-quarters

5. To which conditions can overweight and obesity during childhood and adolescence lead?
   a. Insulin resistance and type 2 diabetes
   b. Hypertension and unfavorable blood lipids
   c. Heart disease and increased risk of adult obesity
   d. All of the above

6. Which is a key factor in the treatment of obesity in preschool- and school-aged children?
   a. Restricting food intake
   b. Parents modeling healthy behaviors
   c. Cutting out all sweets from the diet
   d. Extensive amounts of physical activity

7. Up to which percentage of adolescents with eating disorders do not seek treatment owing to shame, denial, or lack of recognition by the medical system?
   a. 15%
   b. 20%
   c. 30%
   d. 50%

8. Which of the following does the treatment of eating disorders require?
   a. Medical stabilization
   b. The treatment of complications
   c. Refeeding
   d. All of the above

9. Which proportion of all cases of type 1 diabetes is diagnosed in individuals younger than 18 years of age?
   a. Half
   b. One-quarter
   c. Three-quarters
   d. One-eighth

10. Type 1 diabetes is autoimmune destruction of which pancreatic cells?
    a. Islet
    b. Type 1
    c. Alpha
    d. Primary

11. Type 2 diabetes is characterized by which of the following conditions in which the demand for insulin rises, there is inadequate insulin secretion, and there is relative insulin deficiency?
    a. Lack of insulin production
    b. Low blood sugars
    c. Obesity
    d. Insulin resistance

12. Nutritional changes for the treatment of type 2 diabetes include which of the following?
    a. Increasing intake of sugar-containing beverages
    b. Increasing the consumption of vegetables and fruits
    c. Increasing the consumption of simple carbohydrates and starch
    d. All of the above

13. Which symptoms does the female athlete triad include?
    a. Changes in the menstrual cycle, osteoporosis, and low energy availability
    b. Osteoporosis, muscle gain, and fluid overload
    c. Irregular heartbeat, dehydration, and osteoporosis
    d. Anorexia nervosa, mental health problems, and heart disease

14. Adequate amounts of which nutrient are needed to replace muscle glycogen during prolonged exercise?
    a. Fats
    b. Proteins
    c. Carbohydrates
    d. Vitamins

15. Which substance is most often used by teens?
    a. Alcohol
    b. Marijuana
    c. Cocaine
    d. Narcotics

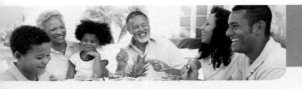

Learning Portfolio (continued)

16. Youths with which racial background have higher rates of alcohol and other drug use initially and increase their use more rapidly over time?
    a. African and Asian
    b. White and Hispanic
    c. Asian and Hispanic
    d. African and white

17. Which factors strongly influence the initiation of alcohol use?
    a. Genetics and family modeling
    b. Peer pressure
    c. Age
    d. Race

18. Vegetarian and vegan diets can supply low intakes of which nutrient?
    a. Vitamin B$_{12}$

    b. Vitamin D
    c. Calcium
    d. All of the above

19. Low iron status in vegetarian and vegan children and adolescents may be a result of which of the following factors?
    a. Lower iron bioavailability from plant foods when compared to animal foods
    b. Polyphenols or phytic acid inhibiting iron absorption
    c. Low amounts of iron in the diet
    d. A and B
    e. B and C

Weblinks

- **Food and Nutrition Center Adolescent and Childhood Obesity**
  https://fnic.nal.usda.gov/weight-and-obesity/adolescent-and-childhood-obesity
  A comprehensive website provided by the U.S. Department of Agriculture that offers web resources on adolescent and childhood obesity, current obesity research, prevention programs, government action to fight obesity, and much more.

- **National Institute of Mental Health: "Most teens with eating disorders go without treatment"**
  http://www.nimh.nih.gov/news/science-news/2011/most-teens-with-eating-disorders-go-without-treatment.shtml
  Learn more about teens with eating disorders from this science update provided by the National Institute of Mental Health.

References

1. Ludvigsson JF, Card T, Ciclitira PJ, et al. Support for patients with celiac disease: a literature review. *United European Gastroenterol J*. 2015;3(2):146–159. doi:10.1177/2050640614562599.
2. Reilly NR, Green PHR. Epidemiology and clinical presentations of celiac disease. *Semin Immunopathol*. 2012;34:473–478. doi:10.1007/s00281-012-0311-2.
3. Kagnoff MF. Celiac disease: pathogenesis of a model immunogenetic disease. *J Clin Invest*. 2007:117(1):41–49. doi:10.1172/JCI30253.
4. Husby S, Koletzko S, Korponay-Szabó IR, et al; European Society for Pediatric Gastroenterology, Hepatology, and Nutrition. European Society for Pediatric Gastroenterology, Hepatology, and Nutrition guidelines for the diagnosis of coeliac disease. *J Pediatr Gastroenterol Nutr*. 2012;54(1):136–160. doi:10.1097/MPG.0b013e31821a23d0.
5. Fasano A, Catassi C. Clinical practice. Celiac disease. *N Engl J Med*. 2012;367(25):2419–2426. doi:10.1056/NEJMcp1113994.
6. Garsed K, Scott BB. Can oats be taken in a gluten-free diet? A systematic review. *Scand J Gastroenterol*. 2007;42(2):171–178. doi:10.1080/00365520600863944.
7. Ogden CL, Carroll MD, Lawman HG, et al. Trends in obesity prevalence among children and adolescents in the United States, 1988–1994 through 2013–2014. *JAMA*. 2016;315(21):2292–2299. doi:10.1001/jama.2016.6361.
8. Crino M, Sacks G, Vandevijvere S, Swinburn B, Neal B. The influence on population weight gain and obesity of the macronutrient composition and energy density of the food supply. *Curr Obes Rep*. 2015;4(1):1–10. doi:10.1007/s13679-014-0134-7.
9. Nielsen SJ, Popkin BM. Patterns and trends in food portion sizes, 1977–1998. *JAMA*. 2003;289(4):450–453.
10. Gordon-Larsen P, Nelson MC, Page P, Popkin BM. Inequality in the built environment underlies key health disparities in physical activity and obesity. *Pediatrics*. 2006;117(2):417–424. doi:10.1542/peds.2005-0058.
11. Seburg EM, Olson-Bullis BA, Bredeson DM, Hayes MG, Sherwood NE. A review of primary care-based childhood obesity prevention and treatment interventions. *Curr Obes Rep*. 2015;4(2):157–173. doi:10.1007/s13679-015-0160-0.

12. Kelsey MM, Zaepfel A, Bjornstad P, Nadeau KJ. Age-related consequences of childhood obesity. *Gerontology*. 2014;60(3):222–228. doi:10.1159/000356023.

13. Stettler N. The global epidemic of childhood obesity: is there a role for the paediatrician? *Obes Rev*. 2004;5(2):91–92. doi:10.1111/j.1467-789X.2004.00138.x.

14. Story MT, Neumark-Stzainer DR, Sherwood NE, et al. Management of child and adolescent obesity: attitudes, barriers, skills, and training needs among health care professionals. *Pediatrics*. 2002;110(1 Pt 2):210–214.

15. DeBar LL, Stevens VJ, Perrin N, et al. A primary care-based, multicomponent lifestyle intervention for overweight adolescent females. *Pediatrics*. 2012;129(3):e611–620. doi:10.1542/peds.2011-0863.

16. Macdonell K, Brogan K, Naar-King S, Ellis D, Marshall S. A pilot study of motivational interviewing targeting weight-related behaviors in overweight or obese African American adolescents. *J Adolesc Health*. 2012;50(2):201–203. doi:10.1016/j.jadohealth.2011.04.018.

17. August GP, Caprio S, Fennoy I, et al. Prevention and treatment of pediatric obesity: an Endocrine Society clinical practice guideline based on expert opinion. *J Clin Endocrinol Metab*. 2008;93(12):4576–4599. doi:10.1210/jc.2007-2458.

18. Centre for Public Health Excellence at NICE (UK); National Collaborating Centre for Primary Care (UK). *Obesity: The Prevention, Identification, Assessment and Management of Overweight and Obesity in Adults and Children*. London, England: National Institute for Health and Clinical Excellence; December 2006. Retrieved from: http://www.nice.org.uk/guidance/Cg43. Accessed September 22, 2016.

19. National Heart, Lung, and Blood Institute. Expert panel on integrated guidelines for cardiovascular health and risk reduction in children and adolescents: summary report. *Pediatrics*. 2011;128(suppl 5):S213–256. doi:10.1542/peds.2009-2107C.

20. Barlow SE. Expert Committee recommendations regarding the prevention, assessment, and treatment of child and adolescent overweight and obesity: summary report. *Pediatrics*. 2007;120(suppl 4):S164–192. doi:10.1542/peds.2007-2329C.

21. Dietz WH, Robinson TN. Clinical practice. Overweight children and adolescents. *N Engl J Med*. 2005;352(20):2100–2109. doi:10.1056/NEJMcp043052.

22. Saelens BE, Sallis JF, Wilfley DE, Patrick K, Cella JA, Buchta R. Behavioral weight control for overweight adolescents initiated in primary care. *Obes Res*. 2002;10(1):22–32. doi:10.1038/oby.2002.4.

23. Doolen J, Alpert PT, Miller SK. Parental disconnect between perceived and actual weight status of children: a meta-synthesis of the current research. *J Am Acad Nurse Pract*. 2009;21(3):160–166. doi:10.1111/j.1745-7599.2008.00382.x.

24. Walker O, Strong M, Atchinson R, Saunders J, Abbott J. A qualitative study of primary care clinicians' views of treating childhood obesity. *BMC Fam Pract*. 2007;8:50. doi:10.1186/1471-2296-8-50.

25. Bloomfield HE, Koeller E, Greer N, MacDonald R, Kane R, Wilt TJ. Effects on health outcomes of a Mediterranean diet with no restriction on fat intake: a systematic review and meta-analysis [published online July 19, 2016]. *Ann Intern Med*. doi:10.7326/M16-0361.

26. Salas-Salvadó J, Guasch-Ferré M, Lee CH, Estruch R, Clish CB, Ros E. Protective effects of the Mediterranean diet on type 2 diabetes and metabolic syndrome [published online March 9, 2016]. *J Nutr*. doi:10.3945/jn.115.218487.

27. Suez J, Korem T, Zeevi D, et al. Artificial sweeteners induce glucose intolerance by altering the gut microbiota. *Nature*. 2014;514(7521):181–186. doi:10.1038/nature13793.

28. National Clinical Guideline Centre (UK). *Obesity: Identification, Assessment, and Management of Overweight and Obesity in Children, Young People and Adults: Partial Update of CG43*. London, England: National Institute for Health and Care Excellence; November 2014. Retrieved from: http://www.nice.org.uk/guidance/Cg189. Accessed September 22, 2016.

29. Wright N, Wales J. (2016). Assessment and management of severely obese children and adolescents [published online June 16, 2016]. *Arch Dis Child*. doi:10.1136/archdischild-2015-309103.

30. Whitlock EP, O'Connor EA, Williams SB, Beil TL, Lutz KW. Effectiveness of weight management interventions in children: a targeted systematic review for the USPSTF. *Pediatrics*. 2010;125(2):e396–418. doi:10.1542/peds.2009-1955.

31. Inge TH, Courcoulas AP, Xanthakos SA. Weight loss and health status after bariatric surgery in adolescents. *N Engl J Med*. 2016;374(20):1989–1990. doi:10.1056/NEJMc1602007.

32. Le Grange D, Lock J. *Eating Disorders in Children and Adolescents: A Clinical Handbook*. New York, NY: Guilford Press; 2011.

33. Smink FR, van Hoeken D, Hoek HW. Epidemiology, course, and outcome of eating disorders. *Curr Opin Psychiatry*. 2013;26(6):543–548. doi:10.1097/YCO.0b013e328365a24f.

34. Espie J, Eisler I. Focus on anorexia nervosa: modern psychological treatment and guidelines for the adolescent patient. *Adolesc Health Med Ther*. 2015;6:9–16. doi:10.2147/AHMT.S70300.

35. Bulik CM, Sullivan PF, Tozzi F, Furberg H, Lichtenstein P, Pedersen NL. Prevalence, heritability, and prospective risk factors for anorexia nervosa. *Arch Gen Psychiatry*. 2006;63(3):305–312. doi:10.1001/archpsyc.63.3.305.

36. Klump KL, Burt SA, McGue M, Iacono WG. Changes in genetic and environmental influences on disordered eating across adolescence: a longitudinal twin study. *Arch Gen Psychiatry*. 2007;64(12):1409–1415. doi:10.1001/archpsyc.64.12.1409.

37. Klump KL, McGue M, Iacono WG. Differential heritability of eating attitudes and behaviors in prepubertal versus pubertal twins. *Int J Eat Disord*. 2003;33(3):287–292. doi:10.1002/eat.10151.

38. Nunn K, Frampton I, Fuglset TS, Törzsök-Sonnevend M, Lask B. Anorexia nervosa and the insula. *Med Hypotheses*. 2011;76(3):353–357. doi:10.1016/j.mehy.2010.10.038.

39. Keys A, Brožek J, Henschel A. *The Biology of Human Starvation*. MINNE ed. St Paul, MN: University of Minnesota Press; 1950.

40. Golden NH, Katzman DK, Sawyer SM, et al. Update on the medical management of eating disorders in adolescents. *J Adolesc Health*. April 2015;56(4)370–375 doi:10.1016/j.jadohealth.2014.11.020.

41. Garber AK, Sawyer SM, Golden NH, et al. A systematic review of approaches to refeeding in patients with\anorexia nervosa. *Int J Eat Disord*. 2016;49(3):293–310. doi:10.1002/eat.22482.

42. Flament MF, Bissada H, Spettigue W. Evidence-based pharmacotherapy of eating disorders. *Int J Neuropsychopharmacol*. 2012;15(2):189–207. doi:10.1017/S1461145711000381.

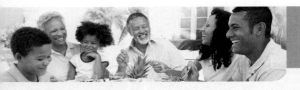

Learning Portfolio (continued)

43. American Diabetes Association. Standard of medical care in diabetes. *Diabetes Care.* 2016;39(1).

44. Miller J, Silverstein JH., Rosenbloom JI. Type 2 diabetes in the child and adolescent. In Lifshitz, F., (ed.), *Pediatric Endocrinology.* 5th ed., Vol. 1. New York, NY: Marcel Dekker; 2007:169–188.

45. Springer SC, Silverstein J, Copeland K,et al; American Academy of Pediatrics. Management of type 2 diabetes mellitus in children and adolescents. *Pediatrics.* 2013;131(2):e648–664. doi:10.1542/peds.2012-3496.

46. Zeitler P, Fu J, Tandon N, et al; International Society for Pediatric and Adolescent Diabetes. ISPAD Clinical Practice Consensus Guidelines 2014. Type 2 diabetes in the child and adolescent. *Pediatr Diabetes.* 2014;15(suppl 20):26–46. doi:10.1111/pedi.12179\.

47. Purcell LK, Section EM. Sport nutrition for young athletes. *Paediatr Child Health.* 2013;18(4):200.

48. Maughan RJ, Burke LM. Practical nutritional recommendations for the athlete. *Nestle Nutr Inst Workshop Ser.* 2011;69:131–149.

49. Rodriguez NR, DiMarco NM, Langley S. Nutrition and athletic performance. *Med Sci Sports Exercise.* 2009;41(3):709–731.

50. Kohl HW III, Cook HD, eds. Committee on Physical Activity and Physical Education in the School Environment; Food Ad Nutrition Board; Institute of Medicine. *Educating the Student Body: Taking Physical Activity and Physical Education to School.* Washington, DC: National Academies Press; 2013.

51. Drake KM, Beach ML, Longacre MR, et al. Influence of sports, physical education, and active commuting to school on adolescent weight status. *Pediatrics.* 2012;130(2):e296–304. doi:10.1542/peds.2011-2898.

52. Hills AP, King NA, Armstrong TP. The contribution of physical activity and sedentary behaviours to the growth and development of children and adolescents: implications for overweight and obesity. *Sports Med.* 2007;37(6):533–545.

53. Kjønniksen L, Torsheim T, Wold B. Tracking of leisure-time physical activity during adolescence and young adulthood: a 10-year longitudinal study. *Int J Behav Nutr Phys Act.* 2008;5:69. doi:10.1186/1479-5868-5-69.

54. Perkins DF, Jacobs JE, Barber BL, Eccles JS. Childhood and adolescent sports participation as predictors of participation in sports and physical fitness activities during young adulthood. *Youth Society.* 2004;35(4):495–520.

55. Casa DJ, Armstrong LE, Hillman SK, et al. National Athletic Trainers' Association position statement: fluid replacement for athletes. *J Athl Train.* 2000;35(2):212–224.

56. Jeukendrup AE, Gleeson M. *Sport Nutrition: An Introduction to Energy Production and Performance.* 2nd ed. Champaign, IL: Human Kinetics; 2010.

57. Petrie HJ, Stover EA, Horswill CA. Nutritional concerns for the child and adolescent competitor. *Nutrition.* 2004;20 (7–8):620–631. doi:10.1016/j.nut.2004.04.002.

58. Tripodi SJ, Bender K, Litschge C, Vaughn MG. Interventions for reducing adolescent alcohol abuse: a meta-analytic review.

Arch Pediatr Adolesc Med. 2010;164(1):85–91. doi:10.1001/archpediatrics.2009.235.

59. Volkow ND, Baler RD, Compton WM, Weiss SR. Adverse health effects of marijuana use. *N Engl J Med.* 2014;370(23):2219–2227. doi:10.1056/NEJMra1402309.

60. D'Amico EJ, Tucker JS, Miles JN, Ewing BA, Shih RA, Pedersen ER. Alcohol and marijuana use trajectories in a diverse longitudinal sample of adolescents: examining use patterns from age 11 to 17 [published online June 14, 2016]. *Addiction.* doi:10.1111/add.13442.

61. Denham BE. Adolescent perceptions of alcohol risk: variation by sex, race, student activity levels and parental communication. *J Ethn Subst Abuse.* 2014;13(4):385–404. doi:10.10 80/15332640.2014.958638.

62. Swendsen J, Burstein M, Case B, et al. Use and abuse of alcohol and illicit drugs in US adolescents: results of the National Comorbidity Survey-Adolescent Supplement. *Arch Gen Psychiatry.* 2012;69(4):390–398. doi:10.1001/archgenpsychiatry.2011.1503.

63. Peiper NC, Ridenour TA, Hochwalt B, Coyne-Beasley T. Overview on prevalence and recent trends in adolescent substance use and abuse. *Child Adolesc Psychiatr Clin N Am.* 2016;25(3):349–365. doi:10.1016/j.chc.2016.03.005.

64. Schulte MT, Ramo D, Brown SA. Gender differences in factors influencing alcohol use and drinking progression among adolescents. *Clin Psychol Rev.* 2009;29(6):535–547. doi:10.1016/j.cpr.2009.06.003.

65. Chan GC, Kelly AB, Connor JP, Hall WD, Young RM, Williams JW. Does parental monitoring and disapproval explain variations in alcohol use among adolescents from different countries of birth? [published online May 24, 2016]. *Drug Alcohol Rev.* doi:10.1111/dar.12413.

66. Wu S, de Saxe Zerden L, Wu Q. The influence of childhood welfare participation on adulthood substance use: evidence from the National Longitudinal Study of Adolescent to Adult Health. *Am J Drug Alcohol Abuse.* 2016;42(6):1–14. doi:10.1080/00952990.2016.1176176.

67. Winters KC, Fahnhorst T, Botzet A, Lee S, Lalone B. Brief intervention for drug-abusing adolescents in a school setting: outcomes and mediating factors. *J Subst Abuse Treat.* 2012;42(3):279–288. doi:10.1016/j.jsat.2011.08.005.

68. Appleby PN, Key TJ. The long-term health of vegetarians and vegans. *Proc Nutr Soc.* 2016;75(3):287–293.

69. Schüpbach R, Wegmüller R, Berguerand C, M Bui, Herter-Aeberli I. Micronutrient status and intake in omnivores, vegetarians and vegans in Switzerland [published online October 26, 2015]. *Eur J Nutr.*

70. Krivosıkova Z, Krajcovicová-Kudláčková M, Spustová V, et al. The association between high plasma homocysteine levels and lower bone mineral density in Slovak women: the impact of vegetarian diet. *Eur J Nutr.* 2010;49:147–153.

71. Maurer M, Burri S, de Marchi S, et al. (2009) Plasma homocysteine and cardiovascular risk in heart failure with and without cardiorenal syndrome. *Int J Cardiol.* May 14, 2010;141(1):32–38.

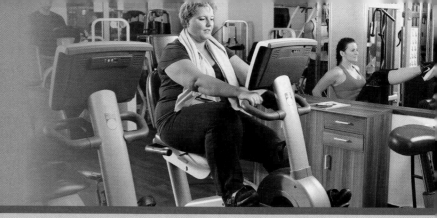

CHAPTER 12

Adult Nutrition

Elizabeth S. Peck, MS, RDN, LD, **and Nancy Munoz**, DCN, MHA, RDN, FAND

Chapter Outline

The Adult Years

Factors Affecting Dietary Intake During the Adult Years

Nutritional Recommendations and Requirements During the Adult Years

Promoting a Healthy Lifestyle

Learning Objectives

1. Describe the physiological changes associated with adulthood and their impact on nutrition.

2. List several factors that affect dietary intake during adulthood.

3. Discuss the unique nutritional needs of adults.

4. Identify how diet and physical activity influence health and wellness during adulthood.

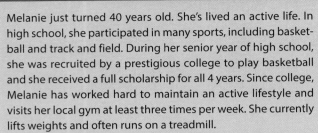
©Creativa Images/Shutterstock

Case Study

Melanie just turned 40 years old. She's lived an active life. In high school, she participated in many sports, including basketball and track and field. During her senior year of high school, she was recruited by a prestigious college to play basketball and she received a full scholarship for all 4 years. Since college, Melanie has worked hard to maintain an active lifestyle and visits her local gym at least three times per week. She currently lifts weights and often runs on a treadmill.

Melanie has always had a voracious appetite and has been able to eat anything she pleases without worrying about weight gain. During a recent doctor's appointment, her doctor expressed concerns about her weight. Throughout college, Melanie, who is 5 feet 11 inches tall, weighed in at a muscular 175 pounds. Now she weighs 200 pounds, with a body mass index (BMI) of 28. Her doctor informs her she considered overweight and encourages her to increase her activity level and modify her diet.

Melanie's physician understands that good nutrition habits along with physical activity in adulthood are key to living long *and* well. Eating the appropriate quantity of nutritious foods along with regular physical activity can prevent debilitating disease later in life.

Questions

1. What factors do you think are contributing to Melanie's weight gain?
2. What are the consequences of being overweight?
3. What can Melanie do to prevent further weight gain and to help keep her healthy for years to come?

The Adult Years

Preview Adulthood, most simply defined, is the life stage occurring after the rapid developmental stages of infancy, childhood, and adolescence and before older adulthood. Human development happens concurrently at biological, psychological, and social levels throughout life. This chapter concentrates primarily on the biological changes that occur during adulthood and how they affect us physically and nutritionally.

Promoting good lifestyle habits is becoming more and more important because adults in the United States are living longer than ever before. In fact, the average life expectancy in the United States is 78.8 years.[1] Men who reach the age of 65 can expect to live until they are almost 83 years of age. Women who reach the age of 65 can expect to live even longer, until they are older than 85 years of age.[2] Healthy habits are key to enjoying a good quality of life in adulthood and old age!

Physiological Changes During the Adult Years

During late adolescence and the early adult years, young men and women complete their physical maturation. Whereas young women are characteristically fully developed by 19 years of age, young men may continue to gain height, weight, muscle mass, and body hair through age 21.[3] Peak physical function and ability occurs in our 20s and early 30s.[4] During this time, our bodies are the strongest, our minds are at their sharpest, and our senses are most acute. After the age of 30, physiological functions begin to deteriorate increasingly, some more rapidly than others.[5] And although we all undergo physical changes related to aging, the rate at which we experience these changes is individual, often based on lifestyle choices, environmental factors, and genetics.

Senescence is a term that refers to the inevitable decline in organ function and physiological function that occurs over time in the absence of injury, illness, or poor lifestyle choices. Senescence is often termed "normal aging." These normal physiological changes can sometimes be self-recognizable during middle adulthood. (See **TABLE 12.1**.) But physiological changes can also go unnoticed. Many of these degenerative age-related changes can be minimized, prevented, and/or reversed by healthy lifestyle practices, including diet. In this chapter, these normal age-related changes and their nutritional implications are discussed.

Body Composition Changes

With increasing age, many physiological changes occur. Starting in the third decade of life, adults experience a progressive decline in lean body mass (LBM), a decline in bone mass, and an increase in the percentage of adipose tissue.[6] Many of these changes are partly related to

Table 12.1

Select Physiological Changes with Age

Affected Organ System	Physiological Change	Clinical Manifestation
Body composition	↓ lean body mass/ muscular mass	↓ strength
	↓ skeletal mass	Weight changes *may* occur
	↑ adipose tissue	
Endocrine system	↓ estrogen and progesterone (menopause)	↑ incidence of diabetes
	↓ testosterone	↓ muscle mass
	↓ vitamin D absorption and activation	↓ bone mass
	↑ incidence of thyroid abnormalities	↑ fracture risk
	↑ insulin resistance and glucose intolerance	
	↑ bone mineral loss	

hormonal changes that occur with age (see the section below on endocrine changes).

Sometimes these body composition changes are noticeable as they occur, for example, when increased fat mass accompanies weight gain, or when usual activities of daily living (ADLs) become more difficult with loss of muscle mass and strength. But it's important to realize that these body composition changes don't always affect weight and aren't always noticeable. Individuals may lose LBM, including muscle and bone, and gain fat mass without changes showing when they step on the scale.

Endocrine Changes

Many of the body composition changes that occur with normal aging in adulthood happen in conjunction with endocrine changes. In general, there is a decline in endocrine function with age. This decline involves both the responsiveness of tissues to particular hormones and reduced hormone secretion from the endocrine glands.[7] For women, a decline in estrogen levels leads to menopause. The fall in estrogen seen with menopause leads to an increased risk for cardiovascular disease and loss of skeletal mass due to estrogen withdrawl.[7] Post-menopausal women experience a decrease in the levels of cardioprotective high-density lipoprotein (HDL) cholesterol, which is thought to be one cause of increased cardiovascular risk in this population. Men experience andropause—a gradual but progressive decline in testosterone levels with age.[7] Reduced testosterone levels in men lead to increased fat mass accumulation (particularly central adiposity), loss of muscle and bone mass, as well as insulin resistance and higher cardiovascular risk.[8]

Growth hormone (GH) secretion and concentrations also fall with age. This change happens in conjunction with a decline in insulin-like growth factor 1 (IGF-1).[9] This reduction in GH secretion is called somatopause and causes a reduction in protein synthesis, decrease in muscle and bone mass, and decline in immune function.[7]

Lean Body Mass Changes

The age-related decline in lean body mass is often called sarcopenia. It's important to distinguish sarcopenia from cachexia. Cachexia is associated with illness or inflammation, whereas sarcopenia is a physiological change

The Big Picture

Body Composition Changes with Aging

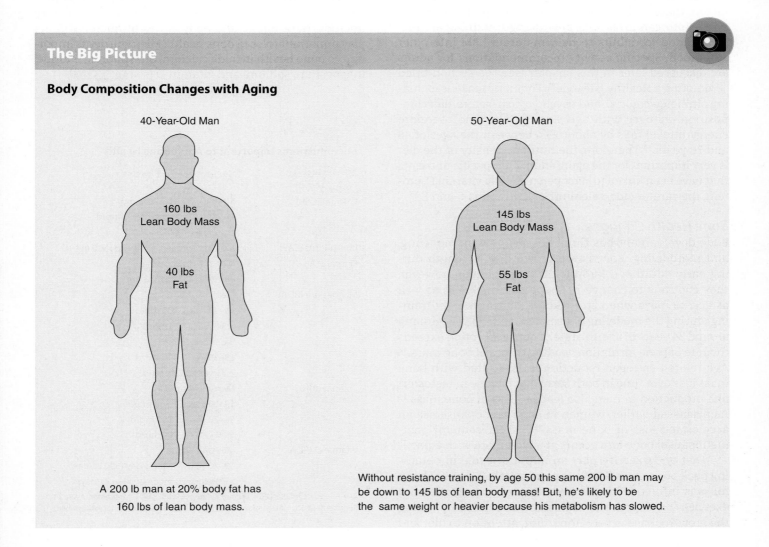

40-Year-Old Man

160 lbs
Lean Body Mass

40 lbs
Fat

A 200 lb man at 20% body fat has
160 lbs of lean body mass.

50-Year-Old Man

145 lbs
Lean Body Mass

55 lbs
Fat

Without resistance training, by age 50 this same 200 lb man may be down to 145 lbs of lean body mass! But, he's likely to be the same weight or heavier because his metabolism has slowed.

associated with aging. The process has been described in three stages: *presarcopenia*, loss of muscle mass; *sarcopenia*, loss of muscle mass and strength; and *severe sarcopenia*, muscle mass loss accompanied by loss of both strength and physical performance.[10]

Although the term LBM refers to total body mass minus fat mass, for the purpose of this text, LBM and muscle mass are used interchangeably. Loss of LBM is thought to begin at some point in the third decade of life. People who are physically inactive can lose as much as 3–5% of their muscle mass per decade after age 30.[11] Although loss of muscle mass starts in early adulthood, it is accelerated in older adulthood.[12] Sarcopenia is thought to be a metabolic consequence of aging.[13] Protein synthesis decreases with aging (in part related to reduced growth hormone production as discussed above), but there is little change in protein degradation. It can be concluded that muscle turnover and repair are likely decreased with age. These changes occur in the setting of increased total body fat mass and an increase in insulin resistance. LBM loss with age may also be related to decreased physical activity and dietary deficiency.

Inactivity and nutritional deficiency are modifiable factors that can be improved with appropriate interventions. Both cardiovascular and strength training are recommended for adults to help maintain LBM into older adulthood. Specific activity recommendations for adults are discussed later in this chapter (see the section titled "Promoting a Healthy Lifestyle"). For many reasons including physiologic, social, and psychological factors, diet composition changes with age. Food intake (and therefore energy intake) falls by about 25% between the ages of 40 and 70 years.[14] Therefore, the nutrient density of the diet is very important for the aging adult. The specific nutrients that have been linked to sarcopenia include vitamin D, protein, the carotenoids, selenium, and vitamins C and E.[15]

Bone Health Changes

Bone development has three phases: growth, modeling, and remodeling. Bones stop growing in in length during early adulthood (around 20 years of age); however, they continue to change in shape and thickness as well as accrue mass when stressed (i.e., during weight training) during the modeling phase (see FIGURE 12.1). Beginning around 34 years of age, the rate of bone resorption exceeds the rate of bone formation, leading to loss of bone mass.[16] Age-related estrogen reduction is associated with bone mass loss over time in both sexes.[17] A decline in testosterone production in men also leads to loss of bone mass.[18] As discussed earlier, women in early menopause see an accelerated loss of bone mass.[16,19,20] Subsequent postmenopausal bone loss occurs at a linear rate with aging.[19]

Diet and exercise play an important role in obtaining peak bone mass (PBM). Approximately 20–40% of bone mass is influenced by lifestyle factors, mainly diet and exercise.[21] Although the acquisition of bone mass during the growth phase is very important, attention to diet and

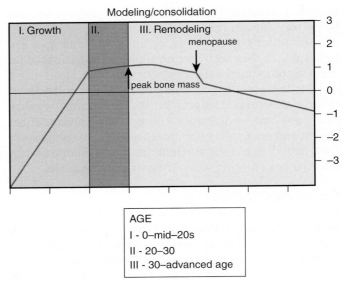

Figure 12.1
General pattern of bone development over time.

physical activity during all phases of bone development is beneficial for bone mass accrual and bone health. Dietary micronutrient intake and body stores of micronutrients play important roles in bone health. Micronutrients important to bone health include calcium, phosphorus, fluoride, magnesium, sodium, and vitamin D (see TABLE 12.2).

Table 12.2	
Micronutrients Important to Adult Bone Health	
Micronutrient (Type of DRI)	**Recommended Intake**
Calcium (EAR)	Men: 19–70 years: 800 mg/d
	Women: 19–50 years: 800 mg/d
	≥ 51 years: 1,000 mg/d
Phosphorus (EAR)	Men and women ≥ 19 years: 580 mg/d
Fluoride (AI)	Men ≥ 19 years: 4 mg/d
	Women ≥ 19 years: 3 mg/d
Magnesium (RDA)	Men:
	19–30 years: 400 mg/d
	≥ 31 years: 420 mg/d
	Women:
	19–30 years: 310 mg/d
	≥ 31 years: 320 mg/d
Sodium (AI)	Men and women:
	19–50 years: 1,500 mg/d
	51–70 years: 1,300 mg/d
	> 70 years: 1,200 mg/d
Vitamin D (RDA)	Men and women:
	19–70 years: 15 mcg/day (600 IU/day)
	> 70 years: 20 mcg/day (800 IU/day)

AI = Adequate Intake; DRI = Dietary Reference Intake; EAR = Estimated Average Requirement; IU = international unit; RDA = Recommended Dietary Allowance.

Case Study

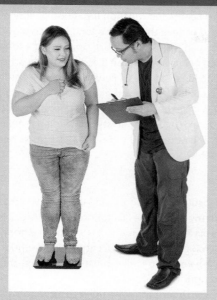

©Creativa Images/Shutterstock

Melanie recently went back to her doctor for a follow-up visit. As part of a routine update to her medical records and family history, her doctor finds out Melanie's sister has osteoporosis. He recommends Melanie undergo bone density scanning, also called dual-energy X-ray absorptiometry (DXA) or bone densitometry. This enhanced form of X-ray technology is used to measure bone loss.

Questions

1. Melanie is in what stage of bone development?
2. What lifestyle factors do you think may contribute (either positively or negatively) to the results of Melanie's DXA scan?
3. How might Melanie's weight loss efforts affect the adequacy of her nutrition?
4. List nutrients and state their function in bone metabolism that Melanie should be consuming in adequate amounts to reduce her risk of bone loss.

Metabolic Changes

There is a reduction in resting metabolic rate (RMR) with age. Studies examining the role of aging on RMR indicate a reduction in RMR that is greater than what can be explained by the simple body composition changes discussed above.[22] Slowing organ metabolic rates with age may lower RMR and lead to changes in body composition, which may in turn have a further impact on RMR. Additional research is needed to examine how RMR changes as individuals age.

The Importance of Nutrition and Physical Activity

It is clear that nutrition along with physical activity are important lifestyle factors that play key roles in health promotion and disease prevention in the adult years. Good nutrition habits and adequate levels of physical activity in the adult years can mean better quality of life as we progress into older adulthood.

The 2015 *Dietary Guidelines for Americans* highlight the importance of following a healthy diet across the life span, emphasizing that all food and beverage choices matter.[23] The guidelines stress that eating a healthy diet, maintaining a healthy weight, and consuming adequate nutrients can reduce risk of chronic disease. *Healthy People 2020* also stresses the importance of a healthy diet and maintaining a healthy weight.[24]

Recap Adults experience a progressive decline in lean body mass (LBM), a decline in bone mass, changes in adipose tissue, and a reduction in resting metabolic rate with aging. These changes are mediated, in part, by hormonal changes that accompany aging. Many of these degenerative age-related changes can be minimized, prevented, or reversed by healthy lifestyle practices, including diet and exercise.

1. How do changes in hormone levels in adulthood influence body composition?
2. What are the physiological changes that occur with aging, and how can lifestyle factors (including diet and physical activity) help to optimize our health in adulthood?

News You Can Use

Is Life Expectancy a Measure of Public Health?

Who among us doesn't want to live a long and healthy life? With the aging population growing exponentially, many businesses, including cosmetic companies, dietary supplement companies, and plastic surgeons, are eager to capitalize on the aging population's desire for everlasting youth. Just take a look in a fashion or fitness magazine. Pay attention when you are browsing the Internet. How many times do you notice an advertisement for an antiaging product?

Antiaging devotees claim that life spans can be prolonged through interventions such as hormone replacement therapy, special exercises, diets, and dietary supplements. Critics, however, including the scientific community, warn that antiaging interventions can be both ineffective and harmful. It remains unlikely that a scientifically proven antiaging complex will be discovered.

Although presently no miracle serum or pill is being developed, those involved in aging research are focusing on ways to improve a person's ability to live a longer life and a healthier life.[a]

Researchers express these objectives in the terms *life span* and *health span*, respectively. Life span is exactly what it seems—the length of time an organism is living. Scientists are currently exploring such factors as genetics, environment, and behavioral traits (including dietary choices) that may contribute to an organism's life span. Changing a factor to see whether it alters life span can provide information on whether that factor affects aging. An organism's ability to resist disease may also be essential to prolonging life span.

Aging research is also concentrating on examining the lives of those who live to old age. This can help to establish patterns of health decline and disease incidence and determine appropriate interventions to help extend life span. The World Health Organization (WHO) is conducting a longitudinal study called the Study on Global AGEing and Adult Health (SAGE). Participants include people aged 50 years and older, plus a smaller comparison sample of adults aged 18–49 years, from nationally representative samples in China, Ghana, India, Mexico, the Russian Federation, and South Africa.[b] The study examines a variety of demographic and socioeconomic characteristics and collects data on risk factors, health exams, and biomarkers of participants.[c] Biomarkers include blood pressure and pulse rate, height and weight, hip and waist circumference, and blood spots from finger pricks. SAGE also collects statistics on grip strength and lung capacity and administers tests of cognition, vision, and mobility to produce objective indicators of respondents' health and ability to carry out basic activities of daily living. Data will continue to be collected during the respondents' later years, which will allow monitoring of health interventions and changes in respondents' well-being.

Something to consider is whether living a long life means living a healthy, enjoyable life. The term *health span* refers to years of good health and function (i.e., good quality of life). Scientists used to believe that living a long life was a good indicator of health span. Think about this: Does living a long life with a high burden of chronic disease (i.e., diabetes, heart disease, or obesity) sound ideal to you? Of course not—it means living with illness and disability, which will negatively affect quality of life. Consequently, life expectancy may no longer be the best indicator of public health. A healthy lifestyle, including regular exercise, healthy diet, and other healthy lifestyle elements, is necessary to increase health span.

References

a. National Institute on Aging. Living long and well: can we do both? Are they the same? Baltimore, MD: NIA/U.S. National Institutes of Health; January 22, 2015. Retrieved from: https://www.nia.nih.gov/health/publication/aging-under-microscope/living-long-and-well-can-we-do-both-are-they-same. Accessed April 1, 2016.

b. World Health Organization. Health statistics and information systems: WHO Study on Global AGEing and Adult Health (SAGE). Geneva, Switzerland: World Health Organization. Retrieved from: http://www.who.int/healthinfo/sage/en. Accessed April 1, 2016.

c. National Institute on Aging. New data on aging and health. Baltimore, MD: NIA/U.S. National Institutes of Health; January 22, 2015. Retrieved from: https://www.nia.nih.gov/research/publication/global-health-and-aging/new-data-aging-and-health. Accessed April 1, 2016.

Factors Affecting Dietary Intake During the Adult Years

Preview Energy balance is key to maintaining a healthy weight. Energy balance can be difficult to achieve because we live in an obesogenic environment. Although guidelines have been developed to help guide us to better nutrition and physical activity habits, many still seek a "quick fix" through fad diets. Pressure to be thin or make healthy dietary changes can lead some to develop disordered eating patterns.

Overweight and obesity remain major concerns for adults in the United States. More than one-third (34.9% or 78.6 million) of U.S. adults are obese.[25] Overweight and obesity stem from a lack of **energy balance**. Energy balance, in simple terms, means that energy in (via beverages and food) equals energy out (the amount of energy burned for breathing, digesting, and being physically active). Many Americans are not physically active and lead a sedentary lifestyle. With the rise of technology and social media, it's not uncommon for many Americans to spend hours in front of the TV or on a computer or other device surfing the Internet. In fact, research shows that more than 2 hours a day of regular TV viewing time is linked to overweight and obesity.[26] Another factor contributing to obesity is the obesogenic environment.

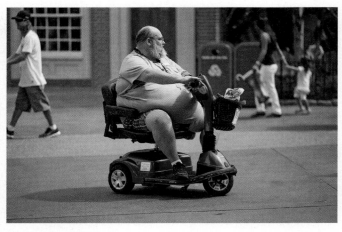
©Mark Waugh/Alamy Stock Photo

Most Americans live in an environment that doesn't support healthy lifestyle habits. Many neighborhoods lack sidewalks and safe places for recreation. Gyms are often expensive to join. Work schedules are demanding, and people often commute hours per day to get to and from work, limiting their spare time. Food portions at restaurants are oversized, and many people lack access to healthy foods. Some people simply can't afford healthy food to eat because of the high price of fresh fruits, vegetables, and other healthy options. Genetics can also affect risk for overweight and obesity. An individual with an overweight or obese parent is more likely to be overweight or obese.[26] Obesity can increase the risk for developing chronic conditions such as heart disease, stroke, type 2 diabetes, and certain types of cancer. These conditions are some of the leading causes of preventable death.[27] Not only is obesity dangerous to our health but also it significantly affects the economy. The estimated annual medical cost of obesity in the United States was $147 billion in 2008.[26]

Healthy People 2020

Healthy People provides 10-year science-based national objectives for improving the health of all Americans.[28] For the past 30 years, Healthy People has established benchmarks and monitored progress over time to help encourage community collaboration, empower individuals to make good health decisions, and monitor and measure the impact of prevention programs. *Healthy People 2020* was launched on December 2, 2010. (See **TABLE 12.3**.)

With overweight and obesity and their health consequences remaining a big concern for our nation, one of the *Healthy People 2020* topics is Nutrition and Weight

Status. Strong scientific evidence supports the health benefits of eating a healthful diet and maintaining a healthy body weight. See **TABLE 12.4** for the Nutrition and Weight Status objectives.

Table 12.3

Healthy People 2020 Vision, Mission, and Goals

Vision

A society in which all people live long, healthy lives

Mission

Healthy People 2020 strives to:

- Identify nationwide health improvement priorities.
- Increase public awareness and understanding of the determinants of health, disease, and disability and the opportunities for progress.
- Provide measurable objectives and goals that are applicable at the national, state, and local levels.
- Engage multiple sectors to take actions to strengthen policies and improve practices that are driven by the best available evidence and knowledge.
- Identify critical research, evaluation, and data collection needs.

Overarching Goals

- Attain high-quality, longer lives free of preventable disease, disability, injury, and premature death.
- Achieve health equity, eliminate disparities, and improve the health of all groups.
- Create social and physical environments that promote good health for all.
- Promote quality of life, healthy development, and healthy behaviors across all life stages.

Reproduced from U.S. Department of Health and Human Services, Office of Disease Prevention and Health Promotion. About Healthy People. Retrieved from: https://www.healthypeople.gov/2020/About-Healthy-People. Accessed September 26, 2016.

Table 12.4

Healthy People 2020 Nutrition and Weight Status Objectives

Healthier Food Access

NWS-1 Increase the number of states with nutrition standards for foods and beverages provided to preschool-aged children in child care.

NWS-2 Increase the proportion of schools that offer nutritious foods and beverages outside of school meals.

NWS-2.1 Increase the proportion of schools that do not sell or offer calorically sweetened beverages to students.

NWS-2.2 Increase the proportion of school districts that require schools to make fruits or vegetables available whenever other food is offered or sold.

NWS-3 Increase the number of states that have state-level policies that incentivize food retail outlets to provide foods that are encouraged by the *Dietary Guidelines for Americans*.

NWS-4 (Developmental) Increase the proportion of Americans who have access to a food retail outlet that sells a variety of foods that are encouraged by the *Dietary Guidelines for Americans*.

Health Care and Worksite Settings

NWS-5 Increase the proportion of primary care physicians who regularly measure the body mass index (BMI) of their patients.

NWS-5.1 Increase the proportion of primary care physicians who regularly assess body mass index (BMI) in their adult patients.

NWS-5.2 Increase the proportion of primary care physicians who regularly assess body mass index (BMI) for age and sex in their child or adolescent patients.

NWS-6 Increase the proportion of physician office visits that include counseling or education related to nutrition or weight.

NWS-6.1 Increase the proportion of physician office visits made by patients with a diagnosis of cardiovascular disease, diabetes, or hyperlipidemia that include counseling or education related to diet or nutrition.

NWS-6.2 Increase the proportion of physician office visits made by adult patients who are obese that include counseling or education related to weight reduction, nutrition, or physical activity.

NWS-6.3 Increase the proportion of physician visits made by all child or adult patients that include counseling about nutrition or diet.

NWS-7 (Developmental) Increase the proportion of worksites that offer nutrition or weight management classes or counseling.

Weight Status

NWS-8 Increase the proportion of adults who are at a healthy weight.

NWS-9 Reduce the proportion of adults who are obese.

NWS-10 Reduce the proportion of children and adolescents who are considered obese.

NWS-10.1 Reduce the proportion of children aged 2 to 5 years who are considered obese.

NWS-10.2 Reduce the proportion of children aged 6 to 11 years who are considered obese.

NWS-10.3 Reduce the proportion of adolescents aged 12 to 19 years who are considered obese.

NWS-10.4 Reduce the proportion of children and adolescents aged 2 to 19 years who are considered obese.

NWS-11 (Developmental) Prevent inappropriate weight gain in youth and adults.

NWS-11.1 (Developmental) Prevent inappropriate weight gain in children aged 2 to 5 years.

NWS-11.2 (Developmental) Prevent inappropriate weight gain in children aged 6 to 11 years.

NWS-11.3 (Developmental) Prevent inappropriate weight gain in adolescents aged 12 to 19 years.

NWS-11.4 (Developmental) Prevent inappropriate weight gain in children and adolescents aged 2 to 19 years.

NWS-11.5 (Developmental) Prevent inappropriate weight gain in adults aged 20 years and older.

Food Insecurity

NWS-12 Eliminate very low food security among children.

NWS-13 Reduce household food insecurity and in doing so reduce hunger.

Food and Nutrient Consumption

NWS-14 Increase the contribution of fruits to the diets of the population aged 2 years and older.

NWS-15 Increase the variety and contribution of vegetables to the diets of the population aged 2 years and older.

NWS-15.1 Increase the contribution of total vegetables to the diets of the population aged 2 years and older.

NWS-15.2 Increase the contribution of dark green vegetables, red and orange vegetables, and beans and peas to the diets of the population aged 2 years and older.

NWS-16 Increase the contribution of whole grains to the diets of the population aged 2 years and older.

NWS-17 Reduce consumption of calories from solid fats and added sugars in the population aged 2 years and older.

NWS-17.1 Reduce consumption of calories from solid fats.

NWS-17.2 Reduce consumption of calories from added sugars.

NWS-17.3 Reduce consumption of calories from solid fats and added sugars.

NWS-18 Reduce consumption of saturated fat in the population aged 2 years and older.

NWS-19 Reduce consumption of sodium in the population aged 2 years and older.

NWS-20 Increase consumption of calcium in the population aged 2 years and older.

Iron Deficiency

NWS-21 Reduce iron deficiency among young children and females of childbearing age.

NWS-21.1 Reduce iron deficiency among children aged 1 to 2 years.

NWS-21.2 Reduce iron deficiency among children aged 3 to 4 years.

NWS-21.3 Reduce iron deficiency among females aged 12 to 49 years.

NWS-22 Reduce iron deficiency among pregnant females.

Reproduced from U.S. Department of Health and Human Services, Office of Disease Prevention and Health Promotion. *Healthy People 2020* topics and objectives: Nutrition and Weight Status. Retrieved from: https://www.healthypeople.gov/2020/topics-objectives/topic/nutrition-and-weight-status/objectives. Accessed September 26, 2016.

These objectives emphasize that efforts to change diet and weight should address individual behaviors as well as the policies and environments that support these behaviors in settings such as schools, worksites, healthcare organizations, and communities.[29]

Fad Diets

With society's ever expanding waistline, it's not surprising millions of people fall prey to fad diets and bogus weight loss products. Even informed consumers can be drawn in by the phony claims made by so-called experts. A fad diet promises quick results for little effort—if it sounds too good to be true, it probably is. Although appealing to many, these diets and products can be harmful to health and set people

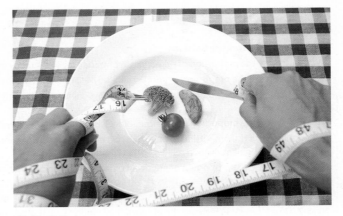

©Pixelbliss/Shutterstock

Table 12.5

Tips for Avoiding Fad Diets

Avoid diet programs, supplements and products that promise:

Substantial and Rapid Weight or Fat Loss

Slow, steady weight loss is more likely to become permeant than rapid changes in body weight. Healthy eating plans target ½ pound to 1 pound per week of weight loss. Quick weight loss leads to more loss of muscle, bone, and water and a higher likelihood of regaining the lost pounds as body fat resulting in undesirable shifts in body composition.

Eliminate or Unlimited

Be wary of diets that eliminate or severely restricts entire foods or food groups and those that promote cleansing or detox drinks, shakes, and specialty bars. Even if you take a multivitamin, you'll still miss some critical nutrients, phytochemicals, and other health-promoting substances.

Diets that allow unlimited quantities of any food can pose health risks and lead to a lack of essential nutrients. It's boring to eat the same thing over and over and hard to stick with monotonous plans.

Food Combining or Blood Type Food Matching

Combining certain foods and eating foods at specific times of day has not been shown to promote weight loss.

Strict Food Plans

Following rigid meal plan may seems like it takes out all the guess work but it does not teach you how to make healthy choices. In addition, it can become boring or overwhelming, and frustrating, if you are missing key foods or want to eat out, go to a party, or indulge in your favorite foods.

Exercise Is Essential

Move more! 30 to 60 minutes a day of physical activity is essential for good health and healthy weight management. Choose activities that you enjoy.

Modified from Academy of Nutrition and Dietetics; January 4, 2016. Staying away from fad diets. Retrieved from: http://www.eatright.org/resource/health/weight-loss/fad-diets/staying-away-from-fad-diets. Accessed September 26, 2016.

up for disappointment. So, what is the truth? There isn't any magic food or supplement that can burn fat. No "super-food" can alter your genetics and make you thin. It all comes down to a healthy lifestyle, including eating well and being physically active. See **TABLE 12.5** for tips from the Academy of Nutrition and Dietetics for avoiding fad diets and products.

Orthorexia: An Unhealthy Obsession

It is well accepted that healthy eating is one key factor to wellness and disease prevention. Because of our nation's concerns with overweight and obesity, and the many

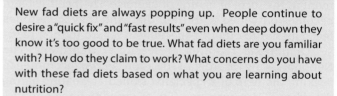

Let's Discuss

New fad diets are always popping up. People continue to desire a "quick fix" and "fast results" even when deep down they know it's too good to be true. What fad diets are you familiar with? How do they claim to work? What concerns do you have with these fad diets based on what you are learning about nutrition?

News You Can Use

Should You Believe Everything You Hear from the "Experts"?

In 2014, the popular TV personality and physician Dr. Mehmet Oz faced scrutiny from Capitol Hill about the promotion of weight loss products on his show, *The Dr. Oz Show*. Dr. Oz was accused of giving consumers false hope by asserting the benefit of products (including green coffee beans and garcinia cambogia) for the promotion of weight loss, despite limited scientific evidence to back up these claims.[a] Senator Claire McCaskill, chair of the Subcommittee on Consumer Protection, Product Safety, and Insurance, commented: "The scientific community is almost monolithic against you in terms of the efficacy of the three products you called 'miracles' … I don't get why you need to say this stuff when you know it's not true. When you have this amazing megaphone, why would you cheapen your show? … With power comes a great deal of responsibility."

Dr. Oz responded by noting that he does use flowery language to describe certain products on his show but added that

he believes in the products so much he has given them to his family.[a]

An example of Dr. Oz's product promotion occurred during a November 2012 airing of his show. "Thanks to brand new scientific research, I can tell you about a revolutionary fat buster." Behind Dr. Oz, the words "No Exercise. No Diet. No Effort" appeared. "It's called garcinia cambogia," he continued.

Interestingly enough, research indicates that garcinia cambogia isn't as beneficial as Dr. Oz claims. In 1998, in a 12-week randomized, double-blind, placebo-controlled trial, garcinia cambogia failed to produce significant weight loss and fat mass loss beyond that observed with placebo.[b] A more recent review of the research concludes that although in some analyzed works there was an observed positive effect on weight loss, appetite reduction, body fat percentage, triglycerides, cholesterol levels, glucose levels, and lipogenesis, other studies showed it had no effect.[c] Therefore, it is necessary to carry out further studies to confirm the efficacy of this fruit in the weight loss process.

So, what's the bottom line? Consumers should be wary of products and the so-called "experts" who are endorsing products as "miracles"!

References

a. Christensen J, Wilson J. Congressional hearing investigates Dr. Oz "miracle" weight loss claims. *CNN*. June 19, 2014. http://www.cnn.com/2014/06/17/health/senate-grills-dr-oz/. Accessed April 1, 2016.

b. Heymsfield SB, Allison DB, Vasselli JR, Pietrobelli A, Greenfield D, Nunez C. Garcinia cambogia (hydroxycitric acid) as a potential antiobesity agent a randomized controlled trial. *JAMA*. 1998;280(18):1596–1600.

c. Fassina P, Scherer Adami F, Terezinha Zani V, et al. The effect of garcinia cambogia as coadjuvant in the weight loss process. *Nutr Hosp*. December 1, 2015;32(6):2400–2408.

health consequences that result, there is societal pressure to make healthy changes to our diet. Being thin is also physically desirable to many. For some, eating healthy has become an "unhealthy obsession." Orthorexia nervosa is a term that means "fixation on righteous eating." Although not currently recognized as a clinical diagnosis in the *Diagnostic and Statistical Manual of Mental Disorders* (*DSM-5*), many people struggle with symptoms associated with this term.[30] Orthorexia typically starts out as an innocent attempt to eat healthy. However, orthorexics quickly become consumed with eating high-quality "pure" food. They become fixated on how much and what to eat and see each day as an opportunity to be "good." If temptation wins, orthorexics often inflict self-punishment in the form of fasting or exercise. Their self-esteem becomes entwined with their diet, and they sometimes feel superior to others, especially in regard to their diet.

Orthorexia requires professional treatment. The National Eating Disorder Association (NEDA) recommends seeking the help of a specialist skilled at treating eating disorders.[30] However, just like other addictions and disorders, the person with orthorexia must first be able to admit there is a problem. The questionnaire in TABLE 12.6

can help determine whether help may be needed for an individual with orthorexia. This questionnaire is not intended to diagnose orthorexia but instead to identify when a more detailed assessment may be needed.

Recap Overweight and obesity are on the rise. Many people live in an environment that promotes unhealthy lifestyle choices, making maintaining a healthy weight challenging. Although fad diets can be tempting because they offer a quick fix, they are rarely successful. The pressure to eat healthy and be "thin" can lead to unhealthy and disordered eating patterns. The key to maintaining health is to consume a balanced diet and be physically active. Efforts to change diet and weight should address individual behaviors as well as the policies and environments that support these behaviors in settings such as schools, worksites, healthcare organizations, and communities.

1. Describe the obesogenic environment and how it affects the health of our nation.
2. How does *Healthy People 2020* aim to promote a healthy lifestyle and fight the obesogenic environment?
3. Explain how to identify a fad diet.
4. What are the symptoms of orthorexia nervosa?

Table 12.6

How Do You Know If You or a Loved One Is Suffering from Orthorexia?

- Do you eliminate entire food groups in attempt for a "clean" or "perfect" diet?
- Do you have severe anxiety regarding how food is prepared?
- Do you avoid family meals and social gatherings involving food for fear of being unable to comply with your diet?
- Do you think critically about others who do not follow strict diets or eat certain foods?
- Do you spend excessive amounts of time and money in meal planning and food choices?
- Do you have feelings of guilt or shame when you are unable to adhere to you diet and food standards?
- Do you feel fulfilled or virtuous from eating "healthy" or "clean" and that you've lost interest in other activities that you once enjoyed?

Modified from: How to Recognize Orthorexia *Article Contributed by Jacquelyn Ekern, MS, LPC and Crystal Karges, MS, RDN, IBCLC of Eating Disorder Hope. https://www.eatingdisorderhope.com/information/orthorexia-excessive-exercise/understand-orthorexia accessed 10/14/16*

Nutritional Recommendations and Requirements During the Adult Years

Preview The energy needed to fuel the body comes from the food consumed as well as energy stored in the body. Energy is needed to perform life-sustaining processes such as respiration and circulation, metabolize food and fluids consumed, support physical activity, and promote growth and body repair.[31] The main sources of energy are carbohydrates, proteins, fats, and, to a smaller amount, alcohol. Micronutrients also play an important role in maintaining health.

Energy

Energy balance depends on each individual's food and fluid intake and energy expenditure. Imbalances between consumption and energy output produce gains or losses resulting in changes in body weight.[31]

Estimated Energy Requirements

The Estimated Energy Requirement (EER) describes the dietary energy intake needed to sustain energy balance and thus promote a healthy weight for individual adults' age, sex, weight, height, and degree of physical activity.

Changes in Energy Expenditure

As people age, the metabolic rate and energy utilization start to decline at a rate of 2.9% for men and 2% for women per decade.[32] The decline in energy utilization and expenditure is influenced by increased sedentary lifestyle and decreased lean muscle mass. During the period between 25 and 65 years of age, an adult's working capacity decreases by 5–10% per decade. The occurrence of musculoskeletal disease, overweight, and obesity and the presence of illnesses can hasten drops in energy expenditure and physical ability.[32]

Assessing Energy Requirements

During an adult's healthy stage of life, energy requirements are equal to energy expenditure. In some clinical circumstances (i.e., pregnancy, lactation, and with certain types of illness or disease), an improved nutritional status is desired, and energy requirements are assessed at a higher level to create a positive energy balance. At the other end of the spectrum, when dealing with obese adults, although energy needs are assessed on the basis of calorie expenditure, a reduction in calorie intake is implemented to create a negative calorie balance to induce weight loss.[33]

The human body needs energy to perform a series of functions that are essential to sustain life. Energy is needed for the synthesis, secretion, and metabolism of enzymes and hormones as well as the transport of protein molecules and other substances. Energy is essential to preserve body temperature, upkeep respiratory muscle, and maintain cardiac and brain function. The amount of energy needed to support these functions is called the basal metabolic rate (BMR). Influenced by age, body composition, body size, sex, and the individual's age and lifestyle, BMR accounts for 45–70% of total daily total energy expenditure.[34]

Dietary-induced thermogenesis or the **thermic effect of food (TEF)** refers to the energy required for the ingestion, digestion, and absorption of food. This metabolic response to food raises energy expenditure by approximately 10% in a 24-hour period for most individuals who consume a mixed diet.[34]

Physical activity level (PAL), also referred to as activity thermogenesis, is the second largest factor of total daily energy expenditure. This is a variable factor that includes both obligatory and discretionary activities. Obligatory activities are actions that are required of individuals in an effort to comply with economic, cultural, and societal requirements. These include activities such as going to work and school and performing activities of daily living. Discretionary activities, although not essential, serve to support health, well-being, and quality of life in individuals. These include activities performed to promote fitness and health.[35] Activity thermogenesis accounts for approximately 20–40% of total energy expenditure.

There are several methods to determine individual energy needs. The Food and Nutrition Board of the Institute of Medicine (IOM) defined Estimated Energy Requirements (EERs) using the data compiled from studies that utilized the doubly labeled water (DLW) technique to measure total daily energy expenditure.[33] The DLW technique has been deemed the best method for assessing energy needs. It consists of labeling the hydrogen and oxygen molecules with isotopes that are uncommon to these elements. Very often, the nonradioactive forms of the elements deuterium and oxygen-18 are used to label the water and determine the metabolic rate measurement.[31] Elimination of isotopes in saliva and urine is used to estimate average energy utilization over several days. The EERs for the reference man and woman are shown in TABLE 12.7 .[23]

Macronutrients

Macronutrients are substances that provide calories (energy) for the body to perform all body functions. The macronutrients, carbohydrates, protein, and fat provide calories per unit consumed. Carbohydrates provide 4 calories per gram, protein provides 4 calories per gram, and fat provide 9 calories per gram.

The Acceptable Micronutrient Distribution Ranges (AMDRs) for total calorie intake from fat, carbohydrates, and protein for adults are as follows:[31]

- Fat: 20–35% of calories
- Carbohydrates: 45–65% of calories
- Protein: 10–35% of calories

Carbohydrates

Carbohydrates (sugars and starches) supply energy to cells in the body, principally the brain, which depends on carbohydrates to function. The Estimated Average Requirement (EAR) for carbohydrate is defined on the basis of the usual amount of glucose needed by the brain. The Recommended Dietary Allowance (RDA) for carbohydrate is set at 130 g/d for adults.[31] The RDA for pregnant women is set higher at 175 g/day, and lactating women have even higher requirements, with the RDA set at 210 g/day.[31]

Dietary fiber is the nondigestible portion of food obtained from plants. **Functional fibers** are sequestered,

Table 12.7

Estimated Energy Requirements per Day, by Age, Sex, and Physical Activity Level

Males				Females[a]			
Age	Sedentary[b]	Moderately Active[c]	Active[d]	Age	Sedentary[b]	Moderately Active[c]	Active[d]
2	1,000	1,000	1,000	2	1,000	1,000	1,000
3	1,000	1,400	1,400	3	1,000	1,200	1,400
4	1,200	1,400	1,600	4	1,200	1,400	1,400
5	1,200	1,400	1,600	5	1,200	1,400	1,600
6	1,400	1,600	1,800	6	1,200	1,400	1,600
7	1,400	1,600	1,800	7	1,200	1,600	1,800
8	1,400	1,600	2,000	8	1,400	1,600	1,800
9	1,600	1,800	2,000	9	1,400	1,600	1,800
10	1,600	1,800	2,200	10	1,400	1,800	2,000
11	1,800	2,000	2,200	11	1,600	1,800	2,000
12	1,800	2,200	2,400	12	1,600	2,000	2,200
13	2,000	2,200	2,600	13	1,600	2,000	2,200
14	2,000	2,400	2,800	14	1,800	2,000	2,400
15	2,200	2,600	3,000	15	1,800	2,000	2,400
16	2,400	2,800	3,200	16	1,800	2,000	2,400
17	2,400	2,800	3,200	17	1,800	2,000	2,400
18	2,400	2,800	3,200	18	1,800	2,000	2,400
19–20	2,600	2,800	3,000	19–20	2,000	2,200	2,400
21–25	2,400	2,800	3,000	21–25	2,000	2,200	2,400
26–30	2,400	2,600	3,000	26–30	1,800	2,000	2,400
31–35	2,400	2,600	3,000	31–35	1,800	2,000	2,200
36–40	2,400	2,600	2,800	36–40	1,800	2,000	2,200
41–45	2,200	2,600	2,800	41–45	1,800	2,000	2,200
46–50	2,200	2,400	2,800	46–50	1,800	2,000	2,200
51–55	2,200	2,400	2,800	51–55	1,600	1,800	2,200
56–60	2,200	2,400	2,600	56–60	1,600	1,800	2,200
61–65	2,000	2,400	2,600	61–65	1,600	1,800	2,000
66–70	2,000	2,200	2,600	66–70	1,600	1,800	2,000
71–75	2,000	2,200	2,600	71–75	1,600	1,800	2,000
76 and older	2,000	2,200	2,400	76 and older	1,600	1,800	2,000

[a] Estimates for females do not include women who are pregnant or breastfeeding.

[b] *Sedentary* means a lifestyle that includes only the physical activity of independent living.

[c] *Moderately active* means a lifestyle that includes physical activity equivalent to walking about 1.5 to 3 miles per day at 3 to 4 miles per hour, in addition to the activities of independent living.

[d] *Active* means a lifestyle that includes physical activity equivalent to walking more than 3 miles per day at 3 to 4 miles per hour, in addition to the activities of independent living.

Reproduced from Institute of Medicine. *Dietary Reference Intakes for Energy, Carbohydrate, Fiber, Fat, Fatty Acids, Cholesterol, Protein, and Amino Acids.* Washington, DC: National Academies Press; 2002; U.S. Department of Health and Human Services and U.S. Department of Agriculture. *2015–2020 Dietary Guidelines for Americans.* 8th ed. Washington, DC: U.S. Department of Health and Human Services and U.S. Department of Agriculture; December 2015. Retrieved from: http://health.gov/dietaryguidelines/2015/guidelines/. Accessed September 6, 2016.

nondigestible forms of carbohydrate that are acquired from starchy foods or are manufactured from starches or sugars. They can possess some of the benefits of natural dietary fiber, for example, helping individuals avoid constipation or reducing postprandial blood glucose levels. Total fiber is the sum of dietary fiber and functional fiber. Viscous fibers decrease gastric emptying (movement of foods from the stomach into the small intestine), thus contributing to a sense of fullness. This delayed emptying effect can contribute to decreased postprandial blood glucose levels. Viscous fibers can also inhibit the absorption of dietary fat and cholesterol and, in addition to the enterohepatic recirculation of cholesterol and bile acids, may create lower concentrations of blood cholesterol in individuals. Adequate Intake (AI) for total fiber is 38 g/d and 25 g/d for men and women ages 19 to 50, respectively.[31]

Protein

Proteins are large molecules made up of one or more chains of amino acids, which are arranged in a precise order defined by the base sequence of nucleotides in the DNA coding for the protein. Proteins form the chief structural components of all the cells in humans and are needed for cell structure, function, and regulation of the body's cells, tissues, and organs. The RDA for both men and women is 0.8 g/kg of body weight per day of protein.[31]

Amino acids (AAs) are the basic structures that make up proteins. Nine AAs are considered essential. Essential AAs (sometimes referred to as indispensable AA) cannot be synthesized by the body and must be supplied via dietary intake. Six amino acids are nonessential (dispensable) in humans, meaning they can be synthesized in the body. Six other AAs are considered conditionally essential: the synthesis of conditionally essential AAs can be limited under special pathophysiological conditions, such as in individuals in severe catabolic distress.[31] See TABLE 12.8 .

Fat

Fat is a chief source of energy for the body. Fat is essential for the absorption of fat-soluble vitamins and carotenoids. There is no established AI or RDA for total fat consumption. Instead, an AMDR of 20–35% of total energy has been assessed for total fat intake. A Tolerable Upper Intake Level (UL) is not set for total fat consumption because there is no distinct level of fat intake at which an adverse effect takes place.[31]

Saturated fatty acids are produced by the body to provide an acceptable level required for their physiological and structural functions. Saturated fatty acids, monounsaturated fatty acids, and cholesterol are produced by the body and do not have an established role in preventing chronic conditions. As a result, there is no AI or RDA set for saturated fatty acids. A UL is not set for saturated fatty acids because, as the consumption of fatty acids increases, so does the risk for coronary heart disease

(CHD).[31] Although there is not AI or RDA set for saturated fatty acids, the *Dietary Guidelines for Americans* recommend limiting intake to no more than 10% of total kilocalories consumed.[23]

Linoleic acid is an n-6 polyunsaturated fatty acid that is classified as an essential fatty acid. It serves as a precursor to eicosanoids. A lack of dietary linoleic acid is associated with rough and scaly skin, dermatitis, and a raised eicosatrienoic acid to arachidonic acid ratio. The AI for linoleic acid is based on the median consumption in the United States where an n-6 fatty acid insufficiency does not exist in healthy persons. The AI has been set at 17 g/d for young men and 12 g/d for young women. There is insufficient evidence to set a UL for n-6 polyunsaturated fatty acids.[31]

Linolenic acid, an n-3 polyunsaturated fatty acid, is essential in maintaining cell structure, particularly in nerve tissue and the retina. It is also a precursor to eicosanoids. Lack of linolenic acid in the diet can result in signs and symptoms of a deficiency such as scaly dermatitis. An AI is set for linolenic acid based on median intakes in the United States where an n-3 fatty acid deficiency does not exist in healthy individuals. The AI is 1.6 g/d for men and 1.1 g/d for women.[31]

Micronutrients of Concern in Adults

Micronutrients are dietary components that include vitamins (organic compounds and phytochemicals) and minerals (trace elements). Although these nutrients are required in the body in small amounts, frequently less than 100 milligrams per day, their presence is essential to normal development, disease prevention, and promotion of overall well-being. Micronutrients are not produced in the body and must be consumed via dietary intake.[36]

Globally, more than 2 billion people are affected by one or more micronutrient deficiencies.[37] Pregnant women from low-income countries are at especially high risk of the health consequences of micronutrient deficiencies.[38]

Underconsumed Micronutrients

In the United States, the majority of the population consumes sufficient amounts of most micronutrients; however, some micronutrients are commonly consumed at levels below the Estimated Average Requirement or Adequate Intake levels.[23] These micronutrients include potassium, choline, magnesium, calcium, and vitamins A, D, E, and C. Iron is also underconsumed by adult women ages 19–50 years. Unhealthy eating patterns resulting from low intake of specific food groups, including vegetables, fruits, whole grains, and dairy, lead to low intake of these specific micronutrients.[23]

Of these underconsumed micronutrients, calcium, potassium, and vitamin D are considered nutrients of public health concern because low intakes are associated with health concerns.[23] For women who are capable of becoming pregnant and women who are pregnant, low intake of iron is also considered a public health concern.[23]

Table 12.8

Amino Acids

Essential AAs	Nonessential AAs	Conditionally Essential AAs
Histidine	Alanine	Arginine
Isoleucine	Aspartic acid	Cysteine
Leucine	Asparagine	Glycine
Lysine	Glutamic acid	Glutamine
Methionine	Selenocysteine	Proline
Phenylalanine	Serine	Tyrosine
Threonine		
Tryptophan		
Valine		

Vitamin A

Vitamin A encompasses a cluster of fat-soluble retinoids that include retinol, retinal, and retinyl esters.[39] Vitamin A is essential for immune function, vision, reproduction, cell differentiation, and cellular communication.[39,40]

Vitamin A is a necessary component of rhodopsin, a protein that absorbs light in the retinal receptors and functioning of the conjunctival membranes and cornea. Vitamin A also plays a vital role in the development and preservation of organs such as the heart, kidneys, and lungs.[40]

RDAs for vitamin A are measured as micrograms of retinol activity equivalents (RAEs) in efforts to account for the different bioactivities of retinol and pro–vitamin A carotenoids. See **TABLE 12.9**.

True vitamin A deficiency is rare in the United States. Yet, vitamin A deficiency is frequently seen in numerous developing countries. The limited access to foods that are high in preformed vitamin A from animal sources that is associated with poverty level is a contributor to vitamin A deficiency.[41] Foods rich in vitamin A in the U.S. diet include dairy products, liver, fish, and fortified cereals. Food items such as carrots, broccoli, cantaloupe, and squash are rich sources of pro–vitamin A carotenoids.[42]

Vitamin C

Vitamin C, a water-soluble vitamin, is also known as ascorbic acid. Unlike most mammals and other animals, humans do not have the ability to make ascorbic acid and must obtain vitamin C from the diet.

Vitamin C functions as an essential cofactor in numerous enzymatic reactions, including the biosynthesis of collagen, carnitine, and catecholamines, and as a potent antioxidant.[43] Vitamin C protects essential molecules in the body (i.e., proteins, fats, carbohydrates, and nucleic acids) from damage by free radicals and reactive oxygen species (ROS) that are generated during normal metabolism, by active immune cells, and through exposure to toxins and pollutants (e.g., certain chemotherapy drugs and cigarette smoke).[43] Vitamin C is also known to regenerate vitamin E from its oxidized form.[44,45]

The RDA for vitamin C is based on the amount of vitamin C intake necessary to maintain neutrophil

Table 12.10

Recommended Dietary Allowance for Vitamin C

Life Stage	Age	Males (mg/d)	Females (mg/d)
Adults	19 years and older	90	75
Smokers	19 years and older	125	110
Pregnancy	18 years and younger	—	80
Pregnancy	19 years and older	—	85
Breastfeeding	18 years and younger	—	115
Breastfeeding	19 years and older	—	120

Data from National Institutes of Health. Office of Dietary Supplements. Fact Sheet for Professionals: Vitamin C. Retrieved from: https://ods.od.nih.gov/factsheets/VitaminC-HealthProfessional/

concentration with minimal urinary excretion of ascorbic acid, presumed to provide sufficient antioxidant protection.[46] See **TABLE 12.10**.

Severe vitamin C deficiency results in the potentially fatal disease scurvy. Symptoms of scurvy include subcutaneous bleeding, poor wound healing, easy bruising, hair and tooth loss, and joint pain and swelling.[43] It is thought these symptoms are related to weakening of blood vessels, connective tissue, and bone, which all contain collagen. The early symptoms of scurvy (for example, fatigue) may result from diminished levels of carnitine, which is needed to derive energy from fat, or from decreased synthesis of the catecholamine norepinephrine.[43] Scurvy is rare in developed countries because it can be prevented by as little as 10 mg of vitamin C daily.[47] However, cases have occurred in children and elderly persons on very restricted diets.[48,49]

Fruits and vegetables are the best sources of vitamin C. Citrus fruits, tomatoes and tomato juice, and potatoes are major contributors of vitamin C to the American diet.[46] Other good food sources include red and green peppers, kiwifruit, broccoli, strawberries, brussels sprouts, and cantaloupe.

Vitamin D

Vitamin D is a fat-soluble vitamin that is naturally present in a very limited number of foods; it is added to some foods and is available as a dietary supplement. It can be produced endogenously when ultraviolet rays from sunlight raid the skin and trigger vitamin D production. Vitamin D acquired from sun exposure, food, and supplements is naturally inactive and must go through two hydroxylations in the body for activation. The first hydroxylation takes place in the liver and changes vitamin D to 25-hydroxyvitamin D (25[OH]D), also identified as calcidiol. The second happens mainly in the kidney and forms the physiologically active 1,25-dehydroxyvitamin D (1,25[OH]$_2$D), also known as calcitriol.[50]

Vitamin D promotes calcium absorption in the gastrointestinal tract and sustains sufficient serum calcium and phosphate concentrations to support normal bone

Table 12.9

Recommended Dietary Allowances (RDAs) for Vitamin A

Age	Male	Female	Pregnancy	Lactation
19–50 y	900 mcg RAE	700 mcg RAE	770 mcg RAE	1,300 mcg RAE
51+ years	900 mcg RAE	700 mcg RAE		

RAE = retinol activity equivalent

Data from Institute of Medicine, Food and Nutrition Board. *Dietary Reference Intakes for Vitamin A, Vitamin K, Arsenic, Boron, Chromium, Copper, Iodine, Iron, Manganese, Molybdenum, Nickel, Silicon, Vanadium, and Zinc*. Washington, DC: National Academies Press; 2001.

mineralization and to avert hypocalcemic tetany. It is also required for bone growth and bone remodeling by osteoblasts and osteoclasts. Insufficient vitamin D in the body allows bones to become thin, brittle, or misshapen. Maintaining adequate levels of vitamin D contributes to the prevention of rickets in children and osteomalacia in adults. Together with calcium, vitamin D helps protect older adults from osteoporosis.[50]

The RDA for vitamin D represents a daily intake that is adequate to preserve bone health and normal calcium metabolism in healthy people. RDAs for vitamin D are defined in both international units (IU) and micrograms (mcg); the biological activity of 40 IU is equal to 1 mcg.[50] See TABLE 12.11.

A vitamin D deficiency can happen when dietary intake is less than recommended levels over a long period of time, sunlight exposure is inadequate, the kidneys cannot convert 25(OH)D to its active form, or absorption of vitamin D from the gastrointestinal tract is impaired. Vitamin D deficiency is common in individuals with lactose intolerance or milk allergy, people who follow an ovo-vegetarian diet, and adults who follow a vegan lifestyle.[50]

Very few foods in nature contain vitamin D. The flesh of fatty fish, such as salmon, tuna, and mackerel, as well as fish liver oils are among the best sources. Small amounts of vitamin D are found in beef liver, cheese, and egg yolks. The vitamin D found in these foods is mainly in the form of vitamin D_3 and its metabolite 25(OH)D_3.[51] Fortified foods provide most of the vitamin D for individuals who live in the United States.[50]

Vitamin E

Vitamin E occurs naturally in food, is used to enrich some foods, and is available as a dietary supplement. Vitamin E is a fat-soluble compound with distinguishing antioxidant qualities. Naturally occurring vitamin E exists in eight distinct chemical forms. Alpha-tocopherol is the only form known to meet human requirements.[46]

As an antioxidant, vitamin E helps to protect cells from the harmful effects of free radicals, which are molecules that contain an unshared electron. Free radicals damage cells and might contribute to the development of cardiovascular disease and cancer.[52] The RDA for vitamin E has been established at 15 mg for individuals 14 years and older. Needs during breastfeeding are higher, at 19 mg/d. See TABLE 12.12.

Table 12.11

RDAs for Vitamin D

Age	Male	Female	Pregnancy	Lactation
19–50 years	600 IU (15 mcg)	600 IU (15 mcg)	600 IU (15 mcg)	600 IU (15 mcg)

Data from National Institutes of Health. Office of Dietary Supplements. Fact Sheet for Professionals: Vitamin D. Retrieved from: https://ods.od.nih.gov/factsheets/VitaminD-HealthProfessional/

Table 12.12

RDAs for Alpha-Tocopherol

Life Stage	Age	Males		Females	
		mg/d	IU/d	mg/d	IU/d
Adults	19 years and older	15	22.5	15	22.5
Pregnancy	All ages	—	—	15	22.5
Breastfeeding	All ages	—	—	19	28.5

Note: One milligram of *2R*-alpha-tocopherol is equivalent to 1.5 IU, and 1 IU is equivalent to 0.67 mg of *2R*-alpha-tocopherol.

Data from National Institutes of Health. Office of Dietary Supplements. Fact Sheet for Professionals: Vitamin E. Retrieved from: https://ods.od.nih.gov/factsheets/VitaminE-HealthProfessional/

True vitamin E deficiency is very rare in the United States, and overt signs and symptoms have not been observed in healthy adults who consume small amounts of vitamin E in their diet. Deficiency symptoms include peripheral neuropathy, ataxia, skeletal myopathy, retinopathy, and impaired immune system.[46]

Nuts, seeds, and vegetable oils are good sources of alpha-tocopherol. Significant amounts of vitamin E are also available in green leafy vegetables and fortified cereals.[53]

Calcium

Calcium, the most abundant mineral in the body, is found in some foods, added to others, available as a dietary supplement, and present in some medications such as antacids. Calcium is vital for vascular contraction and vasodilation, muscle function, nerve transmission, intracellular signaling, and hormonal secretion. Overall, less than 1% of total body calcium is needed to perform these important metabolic roles.[50] Serum calcium is very tightly controlled and does not respond to quick changes in dietary intake. Instead, the body uses bone tissue as a pool for and source of calcium to preserve a continuous concentration of calcium in blood, muscle, and intercellular fluids.[50] Ninety-nine percent of the body's calcium is stored in the bones and teeth. Short-term poor calcium intake will go unnoticed. Long-term poor calcium intake results in hypocalcemia. Signs and symptoms of hypocalcemia include muscle cramps, convulsions, lethargy, anorexia, and abnormal heart rhythm.[54] If left untreated, hypocalcemia can result in death.

The RDA for calcium was established on the basis of the amount of calcium needed to promote bone health and calcium retention in healthy adults. See TABLE 12.13 for calcium RDAs. Milk, yogurt, and cheese are the major sources of calcium in the American diet.

Iron

Iron is an essential component of hemoglobin and myoglobin. Hemoglobin and myoglobin are transport proteins that carry oxygen to the lungs, tissues, and muscles. Iron

Table 12.13

RDAs for Calcium

Age	Male	Female	Pregnancy	Lactating
14–18 years	1,300 mg	1,300 mg	1,300 mg	1,300 mg
19–50 years	1,000 mg	1,000 mg	1,000 mg	1,000 mg

Data from National Institutes of Health. Office of Dietary Supplements. Fact Sheet for Professionals: Calcium. Retrieved from: https://ods.od.nih.gov/factsheets/Calcium-HealthProfessional/

supports metabolism and is needed for growth, development, normal cellular functioning, and synthesis of some hormones and connective tissue.[55]

Dietary iron consists of two main forms: heme and nonheme.[55] Plants and iron-fortified foods contain nonheme iron only. Foods like meat, seafood, and poultry contain both heme and nonheme iron.[56] Heme iron supplies approximately 10–15% of total iron ingestion in Western populations.[42]

The RDA for nonvegetarian individuals is listed in TABLE 12.14. For people following a vegetarian lifestyle, the RDAs for iron are 1.8 times greater than for individuals who consume meat products. Nonheme iron available through plant-based food is less bioavailable than that form in meat products. Food items from animal sources increase the absorption of nonheme iron.[42]

Iron deficiency, as a single-nutrient deficiency, is rare in the United States. Iron deficiency is linked with poor diet, malabsorption, and blood loss. Individuals with iron deficiency typically have other nutrient insufficiencies.[56] The WHO reports that almost one-half of the 1.62 billion cases of anemia worldwide occur as a result of iron deficiency.[57] In developing countries, iron deficiency frequently is an outcome of enteropathies and blood loss related to gastrointestinal parasites.[56]

During pregnancy, plasma volume and red cell mass enlarge as a result of the increases in maternal red blood cell (RBC) production.[56] The increased production of RBCs as well as the needs of the fetus and the placenta contribute to increased iron requirements during pregnancy. Iron deficiency through pregnancy increases the risk of maternal and infant mortality, premature birth, and low birth weight.[58]

Table 12.14

RDAs for Iron

Age	Male	Female	Pregnancy	Lactation
14–18 years	11 mg	15 mg	27 mg	10 mg
19–50 years	8 mg	18 mg	27 mg	9 mg

Data from National Institutes of Health. Office of Dietary Supplements. Fact Sheet for Professionals: Iron. Retrieved from: https://ods.od.nih.gov/factsheets/Iron-HealthProfessional/

Lean meats and seafood are the richest sources of heme iron in the U.S. diet.[23] Food sources of nonheme iron include nuts, beans, vegetables, and fortified grain products. In the United States, approximately 50% of dietary iron comes from bread, cereal, and other grain products.[42,56] Breastmilk has highly bioavailable iron in sufficient amounts to meet the needs of infants up to 4–6 months of age.[56] In the United States as well as many other countries around the world, wheat products and flour are fortified with iron.[59] Infant formulas are fortified with 12 mg of iron per liter.[60]

Potassium

Potassium is an essential major mineral and electrolyte. Normal body function depends on tight regulation of potassium concentrations both inside and outside of cells.[61]

Potassium is a positively charged intracellular ion (cation), whereas sodium is the principal extracellular cation. The concentration differences between potassium and sodium across cell membranes create an electrochemical gradient known as the membrane potential.[62] The membrane potential is maintained by ion pumps located in the cell membrane, especially the sodium–potassium ATPase pump. These pumps use ATP (adenosine triphosphate); energy to pump sodium out of the cell in exchange for potassium. This tight control of cell membrane potential is important for nerve impulse transmission, muscle contraction, and heart function. Potassium plays a role in the management of blood pressure. Data from the Third National Health and Nutrition Examination Survey (NHANES III), which included more than 17,000 adult participants, indicated that higher dietary potassium intakes were associated with significantly lower blood pressures.[63] In the Dietary Approaches to Stop Hypertension (DASH) trial, consumption of a diet including 8.5 servings/day of fruit and vegetables and 4,100 mg/d of potassium (compared to a control diet providing only 3.5 servings/day of fruit and vegetables and 1,700 mg/d of potassium) lowered blood pressure by an average of 2.8/1.1 mm Hg (systolic BP/diastolic BP) in all subjects and by an average of 7.2/2.8 mm Hg in those with hypertension.[64]

Potassium deficiency is most commonly results from excessive loss of potassium. This can occur from prolonged vomiting, the use of certain medications like potassium-wasting diuretics, some forms of kidney disease, or other metabolic disturbances. The symptoms of low potassium are related to alterations in membrane potential and cellular metabolism and include fatigue, muscle weakness and cramps, and intestinal paralysis, which may lead to bloating, constipation, and abdominal pain. Severely low potassium can result in muscular paralysis or abnormal heart rhythms (cardiac arrhythmias) that can lead to heart attack and be fatal.

Dietary sources of potassium include leafy greens, such as spinach and collards, bananas, fruit from vines, such as grapes and blackberries, root vegetables, such as

Table 12.15			
Adequate Intake for Potassium			
Life Stage	Age	Males (mg/d)	Females (mg/d)
Adults	19 years and older	4,700	4,700
Pregnancy	14–50 years	—	4,700
Breastfeeding	14–50 years	—	5,100

Data from Institute of Medicine, Food and Nutrition Board. Potassium. In *Dietary Reference Intakes for Water, Potassium, Sodium, Chloride, and Sulfate*. Washington, DC: National Academies Press; 2005:186–268.

Table 12.16			
RDAs for Magnesium			
Life Stage	Age	Males (mg/d)	Females (mg/d)
Adults	19–30 years	400	310
Adults	31 years and older	420	320
Pregnancy	18 years and younger	—	400
Pregnancy	19–30 years	—	350
Pregnancy	31 years and older	—	360
Breastfeeding	18 years and younger	—	360
Breastfeeding	19–30 years	—	310
Breastfeeding	31 years and older	—	320

Data from Institute of Medicine, Food and Nutrition Board. Magnesium. In *Dietary Reference Intakes: Calcium, Phosphorus, Magnesium, Vitamin D, and Fluoride*. Washington, DC: National Academies Press; 1997:190–249.

carrots and potatoes, and citrus fruits, such as oranges and grapefruit.[65] The Adequate Intake for potassium is listed in **TABLE 12.15**.

Magnesium

Magnesium, an essential mineral and cofactor for hundreds of enzymes, is involved in many physiologic pathways, including energy production, nucleic acid and protein synthesis, ion transport, and cell signaling.[66] It also has structural functions.

Magnesium deficiency in healthy individuals who are consuming a balanced diet is rare because magnesium is abundant in both plant and animal foods. Magnesium levels are also well regulated by healthy kidneys. Healthy kidneys are able to limit urinary excretion of magnesium when intake is low. Conditions that increase the risk of magnesium deficiency include gastrointestinal disorders, renal disorders, and chronic alcoholism. Aging can also negatively affect magnesium levels because older adults tend to have decreased magnesium intake,[67,68] reduced absorption, and increased excretion. Magnesium deficiency can also impede vitamin D and calcium homeostasis.[66]

Magnesium deficiency has been associated with increased risk of cardiovascular disease, osteoporosis, and metabolic disorders, including hypertension and type 2 diabetes mellitus.[66]

The Food and Nutrition Board of the Institute of Medicine increased the RDA for magnesium in 1997 on the basis of results of tightly controlled balance studies that utilized more accurate methods of measuring magnesium (see **TABLE 12.16**).[69]

A large U.S. national survey indicated that average magnesium intake is about 350 mg/d for men and about 260 mg/d for women—significantly below the current RDA. Magnesium intakes were even lower in men and women older than 50 years.[69] These findings suggest that marginal magnesium deficiency may be relatively common in the United States, and magnesium remains on the list of underconsumed nutrients as indicated by the 2015–2020 *Dietary Guidelines for Americans*.[23]

Consuming adequate magnesium through the diet is preferable. Magnesium is part of chlorophyll (the green pigment in plants); therefore, green leafy vegetables are rich in magnesium. Whole grains and nuts also have high magnesium content. Meats and milk have intermediate to moderate amounts of magnesium, whereas refined foods generally have the lowest amounts.[66]

Sodium: An Essential Mineral Consumed in Excess

Several dietary components are of particular public health concern in the United States and should be limited to help individuals achieve a healthier eating pattern. Sodium (Na) is a micronutrient mineral that is essential in supporting blood pressure and fluid in the body. It is also needed for nerve transmission. Sodium and chloride (Cl) are essential to preserve extracellular volume and plasma osmolality. Sodium and chloride are typically found in most foods in the form of sodium chloride, best known as salt.[70]

Healthy Sodium Consumption

Experts including the Health and Medicine Division (HMD) of the National Academies of Science, Engineering, and Medicine, the American Heart Association, and Dietary Guidelines Advisory Committees agree that the average amount of sodium consumed by the U.S. population (3,440 mg/d) is excessive and needs to be reduced. Healthy eating patterns recommended in the 2015 *Dietary Guidelines* support a sodium intake of less than 2,300 mg per day for adults and children 14 years of age and older. Children 1–3 years old should consume 1,500 mg/d and children from 4 to 14 years of age, 1,900 mg/d. Sodium is an essential nutrient and is required by the body in moderately small amounts.[70]

The limits for sodium are the age- and sex-appropriate Tolerable Upper Intake Level (UL). The UL is the highest daily nutrient intake level that is likely to pose no risk of adverse health effects to most individuals in the general population. The sodium recommendation for adults and children older than the age of 14 years, that of limiting consumption to less than 2,300 mg per day, is grounded in evidence demonstrating that increased sodium intake contributes to increased blood pressure in adults. Additionally, moderate evidence indicates that there is a link between increased sodium intake and increased risk of cerebrovascular disease (CVD) in adults. The results of this research are not as consistent as the evidence supporting the relationship between sodium and blood pressure, an indicator of CVD risk.[70]

There seems to be a linear relationship between calories and sodium. The more calories consumed in the form of foods and beverages, the greater the sodium intake. Because children consume fewer calories than adults, the HMD defined lower ULs for children 1–14 years of age centered on median intake of calories. As for their adult counterparts, moderate evidence also suggests that increased sodium consumption increases the risk for high blood pressure.[70]

Adults with prehypertension and hypertension especially benefit from blood pressure lowering. For these individuals, sodium intake should be limited to 1,500 mg per day. Because of the nature of the association between sodium intake and blood pressure, every small reduction in sodium intake that moves toward recommended limits is encouraged. Research suggests adults who are in need of reducing their blood pressure should combine the Dietary Approaches to Stop Hypertension (DASH) dietary pattern with lower sodium intake.[70]

Recap Healthy adults are in a state of energy balance—energy requirements are equal to energy expenditure. The macronutrients carbohydrates, protein, and fat provide our bodies with energy. Although required in smaller amounts, micronutrients are essential to normal development, disease prevention, and promotion of overall well-being. Some micronutrients are underconsumed in the American diet. These include potassium, magnesium, calcium, vitamins A, D, E, and C, and iron. Sodium, on the other hand, is a nutrient that American adults commonly overconsume. During pregnancy and lactation, the need for certain nutrients changes to support the mother and growing baby.

1. How does energy expenditure change with aging?
2. Describe methods for assessing energy requirements in adults.
3. How are the macronutrient and micronutrient needs of adults unique?
4. List nutrients that are commonly inadequate in the diet of adults in the U.S.
5. Identify nutrients that are commonly over consumed by adults in the US and state the consequences.

Promoting a Healthy Lifestyle

Preview Promoting healthy lifestyles can be a challenge for healthcare professionals. Although the majority of individuals recognize the connections among being physically active, nutrition, and health, they appear to be incapable of changing their damaging activities that interfere with securing a healthy weight that could help to improve chronic illnesses. Even though research supports the fact that lifestyle changes can significantly decrease the morbidity and mortality rate of most chronic conditions, many individuals rely on medication use as the main source of controlling chronic illness symptoms.[71]

Healthy Eating Patterns

The *2015–2020 Dietary Guidelines* suggests five main guidelines to promote healthy eating patterns. These guidelines acknowledge the fact that a healthy eating pattern is not a strict prescription; instead, it is a flexible outline that allows individuals to consume foods that meet their personal, cultural, and traditional predilections and that fit within their budget.[23] See **TABLE 12.17** .

Table 12.17

The 2015–2020 Dietary Guidelines for Americans

Follow a healthy eating pattern cross the life span. All food and beverage choices matter. Choose a heathy eating pattern at an appropriate calorie level to help achieve and maintain a healthy body weight, support nutrient adequacy, and reduce risk of chronic disease.

Focus on variety, nutrient density, and amount. To meet nutrient needs within calorie limits, choose a variety of nutrient-dense foods across and within all food groups in recommended amounts.

Limit calories from added sugars and saturated fats and reduce sodium intake. Consume an eating pattern low in added sugars, saturated fats, and sodium. Cut back on foods and beverages higher in these components to amounts that fit within healthy eating patterns.

Shift to healthier food and beverage choices. Choose nutrient-dense foods and beverages across and within all food groups in place of less healthy choices. Consider cultural and personal preferences to make these shifts easier to accomplish and maintain.

Support healthy eating patterns for all. Everyone has a role in helping to create and support healthy eating patterns in multiple settings nationwide, from home to school to work to communities.

U.S. Department of Health and Human Services and U.S. Department of Agriculture. *2015–2020 Dietary Guidelines for Americans*. 8th ed. Washington, DC: U.S. Department of Health and Human Services and U.S. Department of Agriculture; December 2015. Retrieved from: http://health.gov/dietaryguidelines/2015/guidelines/. Accessed September 27, 2016.

Healthy eating patterns help to maintain a healthy body weight and can help to avert and decrease the risk of chronic disease throughout periods of growth, development, and aging as well as during pregnancy. An eating pattern consists of the sum of all foods and beverages consumed and also considers those foods that are eaten minimally or avoided by individuals. For example, The Mediterranean Eating pattern contains more fruits and seafoods and less dairy than the typical US Diet. The foods and beverages consumed as part of a healthy diet work together to meet the nutritional needs of individuals without exceeding the limits defined for saturated fats, added sugars, sodium, and total calories. A healthy eating pattern can include all forms of foods, such as fresh, canned, dried, and frozen. Individuals should strive to meet their nutritional needs using nutrient-dense foods. Nutrient-dense foods are foods that contain essential vitamins and minerals as well as dietary fiber and other naturally occurring ingredients that may have positive health effects. When individuals are not able to meet their nutritional needs for one or more nutrients, fortified foods and dietary supplements may be needed. See TABLE 12.18 for a list of the USDA-recommended meal patterns.

In recent years, restaurants and grocery store shelves have been placing symbols on food items to advertise healthier, nutrient-dense choices. Although the purpose of the labels is to simplify choices for consumers, by promoting the selection of healthier products, these labels, referred to as "front of the package" labels, can create confusion among consumers. To alleviate this confusion, the Institute of Medicine (IOM) appointed a committee to evaluate the current nutrition rating system and recommend a single food guidance system that could be used on the front of all packages to best promote ease in selecting healthy choices. The IOM endorses a single, standardized front-of-packaging system that most consumers can easily understand and that would appear on every product. The amount of calories, saturated and trans fats, added sugars, and sodium will be highlighted.[72]

Table 12.18

Food Intake Amounts for Adults: Healthy U.S.-Style Eating Pattern: Recommended Amounts of Food from Each Food Group

Calorie Level of Pattern Food Groups	1,600	1,800	2,000	2,200	2,400
	Daily Amount of Food from Each Group (vegetable and protein food subgroup amounts are per week)				
Vegetables	2 c-eq	2½ c-eq	2½ c-eq	3 c-eq	3 c-eq
Dark green vegetables (c-eq/wk)	1½	1½	1½	2	2
Red and orange vegetables (c-eq/wk)	4	5½	5½	6	6
Legumes (beans and peas) (c-eq/wk)	1	1½	1½	2	2
Starchy vegetables (c-eq/wk)	4	5	5	6	6
Other vegetables (c-eq/wk)	3½	4	4	5	5
Fruits	1½ c-eq	1½ c-eq	2 c-eq	2 c-eq	2 c-eq
Grains	5 oz-eq	6 oz-eq	6 oz-eq	7 oz-eq	8 oz-eq
Whole grains (oz-eq/day)	3	3	3	3½	4
Refined grains (oz-eq/day)	2	3	3	3½	4
Dairy	3 c-eq	3 c-eq	3 c-eq	3 c-eq	3 c-eq
Protein foods	5 oz-eq	5 oz-eq	5½ oz-eq	6 oz-eq	6 ½ oz-eq
Seafood (oz-eq/wk)	8	8	8	9	10
Meats, poultry, eggs (oz-eq/wk)	23	23	26	28	31
Nuts seeds, soy products (oz-eq/wk)	4	4	5	5	5
Oils	22	24	27	29	31
Limit on calories for other uses	130	170	270	280	350
% total calories for other uses	8%	9%	14%	13%	15%

Notes: Patterns from 1,600 to 3,200 calories are designed to meet the nutritional needs of children 9 years and older and adults.

Food group amounts are shown in cup-(c-eq) or ounce-equivalents (oz-eq). Oils are shown in grams (g).

All foods are assumed to be in nutrient-dense forms, lean or low-fat, and prepared without added fats, sugars, refined starches, or salt. If all food choices to meet food group recommendations are in nutrient-dense forms, a small number of calories remain within the overall calorie limit of the pattern (i.e., limit on calories for other uses).

For additional information and technical tables, see U.S. Department of Agriculture. Center for Nutrition Policy and Promotion. USDA Food Patterns. Available at: http://www.cnpp.usda.gov/USDAFoodPatterns.

U.S. Department of Health and Human Services and U.S. Department of Agriculture. *2015–2020 Dietary Guidelines for Americans.* 8th ed. Washington, DC: U.S. Department of Health and Human Services and U.S. Department of Agriculture; December 2015. Retrieved from: http://health.gov/dietaryguidelines/2015/guidelines/. Accessed September 27, 2016.

Case Study

Good news! Melanie recently received the results of her DXA scan. Her doctor tells her she has satisfactory bone health and attributes this to Melanie's active lifestyle and adequate micronutrient intake based on Melanie's diet history.

However, Melanie is still struggling with weight loss. She continues to exercise often and thinks she's made positive changes in her diet. She no longer eats two donuts in the morning for breakfast, has changed to eating whole-wheat bread, and isn't going to fast-food restaurants daily for lunch. Below is Melanie's diet recall.

Breakfast: Oatmeal with 2 T brown sugar, 12 ounces of orange juice, 2 slices of whole wheat toast with 1 T butter
Lunch: Sandwich with turkey, cheddar cheese, mayonnaise, mustard, and tomato on wheat bread, 1 small bag of potato chips, and 12 oz of regular soda
Dinner: 6 ounces of baked chicken, 1 cup of mashed potatoes made with milk and butter, 1 cup of corn, and 8 ounces of 2% milk
Evening snack: Carrots with 2 T ranch dressing

Questions

1. What positive changes has Melanie made in her diet?
2. Why do you suspect Melanie is having a difficult time losing weight?
3. On the basis of her diet recall, list three suggestions you have for Melanie to help her improve her diet.

Consuming a nutrient-dense diet can be achieved in many ways to meet cultural and personal taste preferences. The *2015 Dietary Guidelines* report scientific evidence that highlights the benefits of consuming a plant-based, low-sodium diet pattern. Current research findings support the adoption of the DASH diet, the Mediterranean diet, and vegetarian diets in efforts to positively influence the risk for developing heart disease, cancer, and diabetes.[23] See **TABLE 12.19**.

Table 12.19

Healthy Diet Patterns

Diet	Items to Consume
DASH diet	Features the consumption of fruits and vegetables, low-fat dairy products, and low-sodium food items
Mediterranean diet	Promotes the consumption of vegetables, fish, and seafood as well as olive oil
Vegetarian diets	Encourages the consumption of fruits and vegetables and meat alternatives

Physical Activity Recommendations for Adults

Being physically active is of benefit for healthy adults, individuals at risk for developing chronic illnesses, and persons with current chronic conditions and disabilities.[73] Regardless of sex and ethnicity, physically active adults have better fitness, including a healthier weight and body composition.[73] **TABLE 12.20** lists some of the health benefits associated with being physically active.

Physical Activity Guidelines for Adults

The *Physical Activity Guidelines* for adults emphasize two types of activity: aerobic activity and muscle-strengthening activity. Aerobic activities, also referred to as endurance activities, are physical events in which people move their large muscles in a rhythmic manner for a continuous period. Some examples of aerobic activities are running, brisk walking, bicycling, playing basketball, dancing, and swimming. Over time, regular aerobic activity contributes to a stronger and fitter cardiovascular system. **TABLE 12.21** provides a summary of key guidelines for adults based on the Physical Activity Guidelines Advisory Committee report. The *Physical Activity Guidelines* are currently in the process of being updated and a new edition is expected to be released in 2018.

Table 12.20

Health Benefits Associated with Regular Physical Activity

Level of Evidence	Health Benefits
Strong evidence	• Lower risk of early death • Lower risk of coronary heart disease • Lower risk of stroke • Lower risk of high blood pressure • Lower risk of adverse blood lipid profile • Lower risk of type 2 diabetes • Lower risk of metabolic syndrome • Lower risk of colon cancer • Lower risk of breast cancer • Prevention of weight gain • Weight loss, particularly when combined with reduced calorie intake • Improved cardiorespiratory and muscular fitness • Prevention of falls • Reduced depression • Better cognitive function (for older adults)
Moderate to strong evidence	• Better functional health (for older adults) • Reduced abdominal obesity
Moderate evidence	• Lower risk of hip fracture • Lower risk of lung cancer • Lower risk of endometrial cancer • Weight maintenance after weight loss • Increased bone density • Improved sleep quality

U.S. Department of Health and Human Services, Office of Disease Prevention and Health Promotion; updated September 27, 2016. *Physical Activity Guidelines for Americans*. Retrieved from: https://health.gov/paguidelines/. Accessed September 27, 2016.

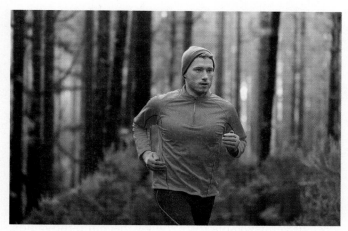
©Maridav/Shutterstock

Engaging in a moderate-intensity aerobic activity for 150 minutes per week can contribute to substantial health benefits. Decreased risk of premature death, coronary heart disease, stroke, and hypertension are a few of the benefits of this type of activity. As adults increase the time spent exercising to 300 minutes per week, benefits such as decreased risk for colon cancer, breast cancer, and weight gain are observed. Aerobic physical activity should occur at last three times per week to promote maximum benefit. Moderate- and vigorous-intensity aerobic exercise should occur in episodes of at least 10 minutes. Events of this length are known to contribute to cardiovascular fitness and the reduction of risk factors associated with heart disease and type 2 diabetes.[74]

Moderate-intensity and vigorous-intensity activities are the recommended intensity activity levels for adults. To comply with the guidelines, adults are required to engage in either moderate-intensity or vigorous-intensity aerobic activities or a combination of both. It takes less time to achieve health benefits from vigorous-intensity activities then from moderate-intensity activities.[74]

Muscle-strengthening activities deliver supplementary benefits that are not provided with performing aerobic activity alone. The benefits of muscle-strengthening activity involve improved bone strength and muscular fitness. Muscle-strengthening activities are also helpful in maintaining muscle mass throughout weight loss phases.[74]

Muscle-strengthening exercises force the muscles to complete activities not normally performed. Resistance training, such as weight training, is an example of a muscle-strengthening activity. Working with resistance bands, calisthenics that use body weight for resistance (such as push-ups, pull-ups, and sit-ups), carrying heavy loads, and heavy gardening (such as digging or hoeing) are other examples of muscle-resistance exercise.[74]

The development of muscle strength and endurance is progressive over time. Increasing the amount of weight used or the days a week the activity is performed will yield stronger muscles. Adults should engage in muscle-strengthening activities for all the major muscle groups minimally 2 days per week.[74]

Promoting Physical Activity

One of the goals for *Healthy People 2020* is to "Improve health, fitness, and quality of life through daily physical activity."[24] This goal will be accomplished through operationalizing two main objectives:

1. Reducing the proportion of adults who engage in no leisure-time physical activity.
2. Increasing the proportion of adults who meet current federal *Physical Activity Guidelines* for aerobic physical activity and for muscle-strengthening activity.

Healthy People 2020 further encourages the development of access to physical activity and fitness programs in the workplace and in community settings. Healthcare providers are encouraged to regularly assess the physical activity level of the patients under their care.

Table 12.21

Key Physical Activity Guidelines for Adults

1. All adults should avoid inactivity. Some physical activity is better than none, and adults who participate in any amount of physical activity gain some health benefits.
2. For substantial health benefits, adults should do at least 150 minutes (2 hours and 30 minutes) a week of moderate-intensity, or 75 minutes (1 hour and 15 minutes) a week of vigorous-intensity aerobic physical activity, or an equivalent combination of moderate- and vigorous-intensity aerobic activity. Aerobic activity should be performed in episodes of at least 10 minutes, and preferably, it should be spread throughout the week.
3. For additional and more extensive health benefits, adults should increase their aerobic physical activity to 300 minutes (5 hours) a week of moderate-intensity, or 150 minutes a week of vigorous-intensity aerobic physical activity, or an equivalent combination of moderate- and vigorous-intensity activity. Additional health benefits are gained by engaging in physical activity beyond this amount.
4. Adults should also do muscle-strengthening activities that are moderate or high intensity and involve all major muscle groups on 2 or more days a week because these activities provide additional health benefits.

U.S. Department of Health and Human Services, Office of Disease Prevention and Health Promotion. Physical Activity Guidelines for Americans. Retrieved from:https://health.gov/paguidelines/. Updated September 27, 2016. Accessed September 27, 2016.

A number of factors influence the level of activity of each adult person. Time motivation level, being overweight and obese, and initial baseline level of inactivity can be barriers to achieving a successful activity level. As discussed earlier, our obesogenic environment is not conducive to weight loss and can serve as a barrier to initiating and maintaining an exercise program. On the other hand, walking groups, exercise buddies, and structural environment changes that include walking trails can be conducive to a more active lifestyle.[75]

Nutrition Interventions for Risk Management

Being physically active is vital to promote health and enhance the quality of life for people of all ages. Individuals with a sedentary lifestyle are almost twice as likely to acquire coronary heart disease as are adults who are physically active.[76] A sedentary lifestyle can contribute almost as much risk for heart disease as cigarette smoking, high blood pressure, or high cholesterol level.[74]

The prevalence of obesity among adults has increased nationally, in every state, and in all segments of the population over the last 10 years.[77] Obesity leads to many health complications, involving hypertension, dyslipidemia, type 2 diabetes, coronary heart disease, stroke, gall bladder disease, osteoarthritis, sleep apnea, respiratory problems, and some cancers. Although the obesity epidemic is multifactorial, prevention needs to focus on helping people decrease their calorie intake and become more physically active.

Prevention Opportunities

Because inadequate dietary patterns and a sedentary lifestyle are linked with many adverse health outcomes, most adults could benefit from interventions intended to improve their eating patterns and promote an active lifestyle. Such intervention platforms can be classified into one of three categories: health promotion, primary prevention, and secondary prevention. The objective of health promotion is to assist people in creating an active lifestyle and healthy eating patterns early in life and preserving these actions throughout their lives. The aim of primary prevention is to aid adults who have risk factors for chronic illness avert or postpone the onset of disease by creating more active lifestyles and healthier eating patterns. The purpose of secondary prevention is to help individuals who already have a chronic disease manage and control disease symptoms and avoid further disability by increasing their physical activity and establishing healthier eating patterns.

Reducing risk and improving the nutritional and health status of adults requires strategies that focus on promoting an active lifestyle and consuming healthy foods. Strategies such as the ones listed below, for example, should be evaluated for implementation.

- Promote increases in physical activity. Being physically active offers numerous health benefits. Health

benefits associated with physical activity should be promoted to sedentary groups of the population.[78]
- Increase fruit and vegetable intake. Higher consumption of fruits and vegetables is linked with decreased occurrence of some chronic diseases, including cardiovascular disease and some cancers.[29]
- Decrease television viewing time. A decrease in the quantity of time that children and adolescents spend watching television may lessen the risk for obesity among young adults.[79]

Community-engaging programs such as "Shape up Somerville" (http://www.somervillema.gov/departments/health/sus) and the Guide to Community Preventive Services in Pennsylvania (http://www.thecommunityguide.org/pa/index.html) provide information on the importance of being physically active. To increase fruit and vegetable consumption, the CDC is collaborating with the Produce for a Better Health Foundation to promote the consumption of fruits and vegetables via the Fruits and Veggies—More Matters (http://www.fruitsandveggiesmorematters.org) program. This campaign encourages people to make 50% of their plate fruits and vegetables at mealtime.

Promoting a healthy lifestyle that encourages optimum nutritional status and an active lifestyle requires strategies that involve individuals and social, organizational, and public policy entities.

Let's Discuss

You've learned that leading an active lifestyle and consuming healthy foods are key prevention opportunities. However, living in an obesogenic environment can make it challenging to follow through with these recommendations. Take some time to consider the community where you live. What challenges does your community face that prevents all people from living a healthy lifestyle? What ideas do you have that might help promote healthy eating and exercise?

Health Promotion

Low household income is associated with undesirable health outcomes as well as higher obesity rates and decreased diet quality.[80] Food insecurity is a reality for approximately 15% of U.S. households. For black and Hispanic homes, the rate of food insecurity is higher than the national average, 26% and 27%, respectively.[81]

A number of federal programs facilitate the consumption of a healthier diet. The Supplemental Nutrition Assistance Program (SNAP) provides food purchasing assistance to many eligible, low-income and no-income individuals and families. This federal program is administered by the

USDA, under the Food and Nutrition Service (FNS). The benefits are dispersed by the state's division of Social Services or Children and Family Services.[82] Programs, other than the SNAP program, help families gain food security. These include food banks, soup kitchens, government extension programs, and meals on wheels.

Sisters Together: Move More, Eat Better (https://www.niddk.nih.gov/health-information/health-topics/weight-control/sisters-together-program-guide/Pages/sisters-together.aspx) is an example of a health awareness program that inspires black women 18 years and older to sustain a healthy weight by being more physically active and eating healthy foods. This program is a project of the National Institute of Diabetes and Digestive and Kidney Diseases (NIDDK), part of the National Institutes of Health (NIH), through the Weight-Control Information Network (WIN). This program is managed locally by committed persons or groups. Anyone who sees a need in their community and wishes to help can start a Sisters Together program.

Recap Healthy eating patterns help to maintain a healthy body weight and can decrease the risk of chronic disease throughout periods of growth, development, and aging as well as during pregnancy. In addition to healthy eating, being physically active benefits healthy adults, individuals at risk for developing chronic illnesses, and persons with current chronic conditions and disabilities. Current guidelines, including the Dietary Guidelines for Americans, Healthy People 2020, and the Physical Activity Guidelines, provide lifestyle recommendations and promote healthy living. Local and federal programs and health professionals can use these guidelines to create wellness activities and teach healthy habits to the community.

1. How does *Healthy People 2020* aim to promote physical activity in adults?
2. Discuss key prevention activities that can improve adult health.
3. Describe a program that engages the community and encourages health awareness.

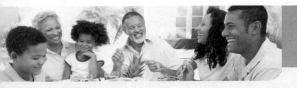

Learning Portfolio

Visual Chapter Summary

The Adult Years

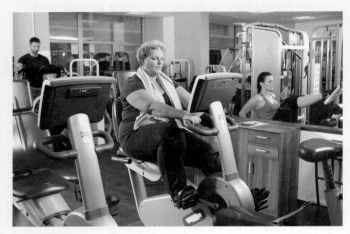

©StockLite/Shutterstock

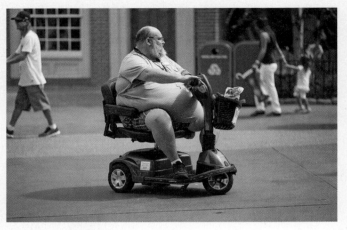

©Mark Waugh/Alamy Stock Photo

- During late adolescence and the early adult years, young men and women complete their physical maturation.
- Peak physical function and ability occurs in the 20s and early 30s. After the age of 30, physiological functions begin to deteriorate increasingly, some more rapidly than others.
- *Senescence* is a term that refers to the inevitable decline in organ function and physiological function that occurs over time in the absence of injury, illness, or poor lifestyle choices.
- Adults experience a progressive decline in lean body mass (LBM), a decline in bone mass, and an increase in the percentage of adipose tissue through age 60.
- Many physiological changes are related to hormonal changes that occur with aging.
- Many age-related changes can be minimized, prevented, or reversed by healthy lifestyle practices, including diet.

Factors Affecting Dietary Intake During the Adult Years

- A big factor contributing to obesity is the obesogenic environment. More than one-third (34.9% or 78.6 million) of U.S. adults are obese.

- *Healthy People 2020* objectives emphasize that efforts to change diet and weight should address individual behaviors, policies, and environments.
- A fad diet promises quick results for little effort—if it sounds too good to be true, it probably is.
- *Orthorexia nervosa* is a term that means "fixation on righteous eating."
- Orthorexia typically starts out as an innocent attempt to eat healthy. However, orthorexics quickly become consumed with eating high-quality, "pure" food.
- The National Eating Disorder Association (NEDA) recommends that people suffering with orthorexia seek the help of a specialist skilled at treating eating disorders.

Nutritional Recommendations and Requirements During the Adult Years

- As we age, the adult's metabolic rate and energy utilization start to decline at a rate of 2.9% for men and 2% for women per decade.
- For a healthy adult, energy requirements equal energy expenditure.
- Obese adults require a reduction in calorie intake to create a negative calorie balance to induce weight loss.
- Energy is needed for the synthesis, secretion, and metabolism of enzymes and hormones; the transport of proteins, molecules, and substances; preservation of body temperature; and upkeep of respiratory muscle, cardiac, and brain function.

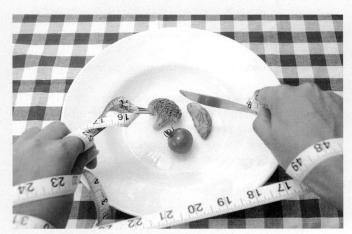

©Pixelbliss/Shutterstock

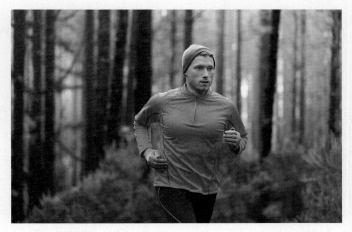

©Maridav/Shutterstock

- The amount of energy needed to support physiologic functions is called the basal metabolic rate (BMR).
- The IOM defines Acceptable Micronutrient Distribution Ranges (AMDRs) as 45–65% carbohydrates, 20–35% fat, and 10–35% protein in the diet.
- The RDA for carbohydrate is set at 130 g/d for adults and children.
- An AI for total fiber is defined at 38 and 25 g/d for men and women ages 19 to 50, respectively.
- The RDA for protein for both men and women is 0.8 g/kg of body weight/d.
- Fat is an important source of energy for the body and is essential in the absorption of fat-soluble vitamins and carotenoids.
- Deficiencies in micronutrients such as iron, iodine, vitamin A, folate, and zinc can have harmful results.
- Pregnant and lactating females have higher nutritional needs than their nonpregnant/nonlactating counterparts.

Promoting a Healthy Lifestyle

- The *2015–2020 Dietary Guidelines for Americans* reflects the latest research supporting healthy eating habits and being physically active.
- The information provided in the Dietary Guidelines is intended as a resource for policymakers and healthcare professionals to use in creating federal food, nutrition, and health policies and programs.

- A healthy eating pattern includes limiting the amount of saturated fats and trans fats, added sugars, and sodium.
- Healthy eating patterns help to maintain a healthy body weight and can help avert and decrease the risk of chronic disease throughout life.
- The *Physical Activity Guidelines* for adults emphasize two types of activity: aerobic and muscle-strengthening.
- One of the goals for *Healthy People 2020* is to "Improve health, fitness, and quality of life through daily physical activity."
- Individuals with a sedentary lifestyle are almost twice as likely to acquire coronary heart disease as are adults who are physically active.
- Health promotion aims to assist people in creating an active lifestyle and healthy eating patterns early in life and to preserve these actions throughout their lives.
- The aim of primary prevention is to help adults who have risk factors for chronic illness to avert or postpone the onset of disease by creating more active lifestyles and healthier eating patterns.
- The purpose of secondary prevention is to help individuals who already have a chronic disease manage and control disease symptoms and avoid further disability by increasing their physical activity and establishing healthier eating patterns.
- Programs that engage the community and encourage health awareness are key to health promotion and disease prevention.

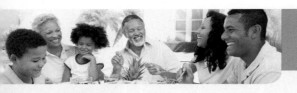

Learning Portfolio (continued)

Key Terms

activities of daily living (ADLs): Daily activities that people tend to do every day without needing assistance, such as eating, bathing, dressing, toileting, transferring (walking), and continence (holding their bowels and bladder).

andropause: A gradual but progressive decline in testosterone levels with age.

energy balance: When calories consumed equal calories burned.

functional fibers: Isolated, nondigestible forms of carbohydrate that have been extracted from starchy foods or manufactured from starches or sugars. They may have some of the benefits of naturally occurring dietary fiber, such as helping to prevent constipation or lowering blood glucose levels after meals.

menopause: A natural biological process in women that involves a decline in estrogen production. It typically occurs 12 months after the last menstrual period and marks the end of menstrual cycles.

orthorexia nervosa: An obsession with eating foods that one considers healthy and pure; a fixation on righteous eating.

resting metabolic rate (RMR): The number of calories needed to support basic functions, including breathing and circulation.

sarcopenia: Age-associated loss of skeletal muscle mass (lean body mass) and function. The causes of sarcopenia are multifactorial and can include disuse, altered endocrine function, chronic diseases, inflammation, insulin resistance, and nutritional deficiencies. Sarcopenia is associated with muscle weakness, functional limitations, and disability, as well as impairments in cardiovascular capacity and metabolic health.

senescence: The inevitable decline in organ function and physiological function that occurs over time in the absence of injury, illness, or poor lifestyle choices. The process of growing old; senescence involves the accumulation of deleterious changes in cells that cause them to die more rapidly than they are replaced.

thermic effect of food (TEF): The increase in energy expenditure in response to the digestion, absorption, and storage of food.

Discussion Questions

1. The physiological changes that occur during adulthood are inevitable. Choose one physiological change discussed in the chapter, and discuss healthy lifestyle habits that can help prevent or slow the decline in physical health that often accompanies aging.

2. Discuss the many factors contributing to obesity. By what means is *Healthy People 2020* aiming to promote healthy nutrition and weight?

3. Outline a healthy adult's macro- and micronutrient needs and discuss how Estimated Energy Requirements can be calculated.

4. You've just been hired as an intern with the Department of Public Health. Your manager asks you to write an overview of healthy eating and physical activity recommendations. What key recommendations would you include?

Activities

1. **Health Promotion: Create Your Own Awareness Program.** Based on the needs of your community, create plans for an awareness program that promotes healthy habits. Create a slideshow presentation using the following items to guide your presentation.

   a. The name of your program (be creative!)
   b. Why this program is needed (what are the issues?)
   c. What will this program aim to do (how can the issues be solved/helped?)
   d. What activities/programming will this program provide?

   e. How will you measure the outcomes of the program?
   f. What barriers might you face?

2. **Fad Diets: Debunking Bad Advice!** Find a fad diet or herbal/nutritional supplement of interest to you, and be prepared to answer the following questions:

   a. What is product/diet, and what benefits does it claim to have?
   b. What does the scientific evidence say about this product/diet? Is there any scientific evidence?
   c. What possible harm can this product/diet cause?

Study Questions

1. Physiological functions begin to deteriorate increasingly after which age?
   a. 25 years
   b. 30 years
   c. 35 years
   d. 40 years

2. *Senescence* is a term that refers to a decline in organ function and physiological function caused by injury, illness, or poor lifestyle choices.
   a. True
   b. False

3. Which physiological changes occur with aging?
   a. Increase in LBM and increase in fat mass
   b. Decrease in LBM and decrease in bone mass
   c. Increase in bone mass and increase in estrogen
   d. Increase in fat mass and increase in testosterone

4. What is bone mass affected by?
   a. Dietary micronutrient intake
   b. The body's micronutrient stores
   c. Level of physical activity
   d. All of the above

5. Factors that contribute to the obesogenic environment include all of the following *except* which one?
   a. Lack of sidewalks
   b. Expensive gym memberships
   c. Reduced portion sizes at restaurants
   d. Long commutes to and from work

6. Healthy People has established benchmarks and monitored progress over time to help encourage community collaboration and empower individuals to make good health decisions.
   a. True
   b. False

7. A "superfood" can help you lose weight.
   a. True
   b. False

8. What is a characteristic of people who struggle with orthorexia nervosa?
   a. They are focused on eating only vegan food.
   b. They want to lose weight and be thin.
   c. They vomit when they eat unhealthy foods.
   d. They can feel superior to others in regard to their food habits.

9. What is the Estimated Energy Requirement?
   a. The additional calories needed by the body to support weight gain
   b. The needed dietary energy intake to sustain energy balance

   c. The number of calories needed to promote weight loss in obese adults
   d. The energy required to promote health

10. What is the basal metabolic rate?
    a. The energy needed to support main body functions
    b. The energy required to support activities of daily living
    c. The energy required daily to support an exercise program
    d. The energy required to metabolize the food consumed

11. What is the thermic effect of food?
    a. The energy required to facilitate exercise
    b. The reaction that occurs when food is consumed
    c. The energy required for the ingestion, digestion, and absorption of food
    d. The energy required for the synthesis and secretion of hormones

12. What are macronutrients?
    a. Substances that provide vitamins and minerals to the body
    b. Substances such as vitamin B_6, B_{12}, and zinc
    c. Substances such as carbohydrates, protein, and fat
    d. Substances that help the body preserve body temperature and cardiac output

13. What is a function of carbohydrates?
    a. Help repair cells in the body
    b. Supply energy to the cells in the body
    c. Maintain proper GI tract functioning
    d. Promote heart function

14. What are amino acids?
    a. The basic structures of proteins
    b. The basic structures of carbohydrates
    c. The basic structures of fat
    d. Substances needed for vitamin absorption

15. What are micronutrients?
    a. Substances such as carbohydrates, protein, and fat
    b. Vitamins and minerals
    c. Substances essential for the absorption of fat-soluble vitamins and carotenoids
    d. Structural components of all the cells in humans

16. Mrs. Jones is a 24-year-old woman who is breast-feeding her 2-month-old child. What are her caloric needs?
    a. The same as the calorie needs of other 24-year-old females with the same level of activity, height, and weight.

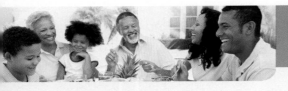

Learning Portfolio (continued)

b. Lower than the needs of other 24-year-old females with the same level of activity, height, and weight.

c. There is no accurate way to determine the caloric needs for Mrs. Jones.

d. Higher than the needs of other 24-year-old females with the same level of activity, height, and weight.

17. What is a key role of the Dietary Guidelines?
a. To help professionals guide individuals to consume a healthy, nutritionally adequate diet
b. To help individuals develop nutrition education materials
c. To facilitate the development of public health policies
d. To assist teachers in teaching 6- to 8-year-olds proper nutrition

18. To decrease the risk of many chronic conditions, how long should individuals strive to exercise?
a. 60 minutes per day
b. 180 minutes per week
c. 150 minutes per week
d. 40 minutes per day

19. Which of the following is an aerobic activity?
a. Running
b. Walking
c. Biking
d. All of the above

20. The objective of primary prevention is to assist people in creating an active lifestyle and healthy eating patterns early in life and to preserve these actions throughout their lives.
a. True
b. False

Weblinks

- **Minnesota Public Radio, "The Salt": Fad Diets Will Seem Even Crazier After You See This**
http://www.npr.org/sections/thesalt/2013/08/23/214912007/fad-diets-will-seem-even-crazier-after-you-see-this
Visit this provoking website to see a unique photo series visually representing fad diets!

- **Baylor College of Medicine Calorie Needs Calculator**
https://www.bcm.edu/cnrc-apps/caloriesneed.cfm
Use this tool to estimate how many calories you need.

- **Choose MyPlate Interactive Tools: SuperTracker**
http://www.choosemyplate.gov/supertracker-other-tools

Do you want to plan a healthy diet and track your physical activity? Use the Chose MyPlate SuperTracker to help you achieve your health and fitness goals.

- **USDA Choose MyPlate: Pregnancy and Lactation**
http://www.choosemyplate.gov/moms-pregnancy-breastfeeding
Learn more about nutrition needs during pregnancy and lactation.

- **Interactive DRI Tool for Healthcare Professionals**
http://fnic.nal.usda.gov/fnic/interactiveDRI/
Use this tool to calculate daily nutrient recommendations to assist you with planning your diet based on the Dietary Reference Intakes (DRIs).

References

1. Center for Disease Control and Prevention; updated June 13, 2016. Life expectancy. Hyattsville, MD: National Center for Health Statistics. Retrieved from: http://www.cdc.gov/nchs/fastats/life-expectancy.htm. Accessed October 13, 2016.

2. Center for Disease Control and Prevention; updated July 16, 2016. Older persons' health. Hyattsville, MD: National Center for Health Statistics. Retrieved from: http://www.cdc.gov/nchs/fastats/older-american-health.htm. Accessed February 22, 2016.

3. Head Start, Administration for Children and Families Early Childhood Education Learning and Knowledge Center. Stages of adolescent development. Washington, DC: U.S. Department of Health and Human Services. Retrieved from: http://eclkc.ohs.acf.hhs.gov/hslc/tta-system/ehsnrc/docs/_34_Stages_of_adolescence1.pdf. Accessed February 22, 2016.

4. Center for Aging with Dignity. *Aging: Age-Related Physical Changes*. Cincinnati, OH: University of Cincinnati College of Nursing; 2011. Retrieved from: http://nursing.uc.edu/content/dam/nursing/docs/CFAWD/Aging%20Series/Part%202%20Aging%20Physical%20Changes.pdf. Accessed February 21, 2016.

5. Shock NW. The science of gerontology. In Jeffers BC, ed. *Proceedings of Seminars 1959–61*. Durham, NC: Duke University Press; 1962: 123–140.

6. Besdine RW. Physical changes with aging: Selected physiologic age-related changes. Merck Manual Professional Version; reviewed July 2013. Retrieved from: http://www.merckmanuals.com/professional/geriatrics/approach-to-the-geriatric-patient/physical-changes-with-aging#v1130874. Accessed February 21, 2016.

7. Chahal HS, Drake WM. The endocrine system and ageing. *J Pathol.* 2007;211:173–180.

8. Hak AE, Witteman JC, de Jong FH, Geerlings MI, Hofman A, Pols HA. Low levels of endogenous androgens increase the risk of atherosclerosis in elderly men: the Rotterdam study. *J Clin Endocrinol Metab.* 2002;87(8):3632–3639.

9. Corpas E, Harman SM, Blackman MR. Human growth hormone and human aging. *Endocr Rev.* 1993;14(1):20–39.

10. Mitchell WK, Williams J, Atherton P, Larvin M, Lund J, Narici M. Sarcopenia, dynapenia, and the impact of advancing age on human skeletal muscle size and strength; a quantitative review. *Front Physiol.* July 11, 2012;3:260.

11. DerSarkissian C Sarcopenia with aging. WebMD; reviewed July 6, 2016. Retrieved from: http://www.webmd.com/healthy-aging/sarcopenia-with-aging?print=true. Accessed February 23, 2016.

12. Siparsky PN, Kirkendall DT, Garrett WE. Muscle changes in aging: understanding sarcopenia. *Sports Health.* 2014;6:36–40.

13. Evans WJ. Skeletal muscle loss: cachexia, sarcopenia, and inactivity. *Am J Clin Nutr.* 2010;91:1123S–1127S.

14. Nieuwenhuizen WF, Weenen H, Rigby P, Hetherington MM. Older adults and patients in need of nutritional support: review of current treatment options and factors influencing nutritional intake. *Clin Nutr.* 2010;29(2):160–169.

15. Kaiser M, Bandinelli S, Lunenfled B. Frailty and the role of nutrition in older people. A review of the current literature. *Acta Biomedica.* 2010;81(1):37–45.

16. Krolner B, Pors Nielsen S. Bone mineral content of the lumbar spine in normal and osteoporotic women: cross-sectional and longitudinal studies. *Clin Sci (Lond).* 1982;62:329–336.

17. Khosla S, Oursler MJ, Monroe DG. Estrogen and the skeleton. *Trends Endocrinol Metab.* 2012;23:576–581.

18. Gray A, Fledman HA, McKinlay JB, Longcope C. Age, disease, and changing sex hormone levels in middle-aged men: results of the Massachusetts Male Aging Study. *J Clin Endocrinol Metab.* 1991;73(5):1016–1025.

19. Nordin BE, Need Ag, Chatterton BE, Horowitz M, Morris HA. The relative contributions of age and years since menopause to postmenopausal bone loss. *J Clin Endocrinol Metab.* 1990;70:83–88.

20. Gallagher JC, Goldgar D, Moy A. Total bone calcium in normal women: effect of age and menopause status. *J Bone Miner Res.* 1987;2:491–496.

21. Krall EA, Dawson-Hughes B. Heritable and lifestyle determinants of bone mineral density. *J Bone Miner Res.* 1993;8:1–9.

22. St.-Onge M, Gallagher D. Body composition changes with aging: the cause or result of alterations in metabolic rate and macronutrient oxidation? *Nutrition.* 2010;26(2):152–155.

23. U.S. Department of Health and Human Services and U.S. Department of Agriculture. *2015–2020 Dietary Guidelines for Americans.* 8th ed. Washington, DC: U.S. Department of Health and Human Services and U.S. Dept of Agriculture; December 2015. http://health.gov/dietaryguidelines/2015/guidelines/. Accessed August 13, 2016.

24. U.S. Department of Health and Human Services, Office of Disease Prevention and Health Promotion. *Healthy People 2020* topics and objectives: objectives A–Z. Retrieved from: https://www.healthypeople.gov/2020/topics-objectives. Accessed February 21, 2016.

25. Ogden CL, Carroll MD, Kit BK, Flegal KM. Prevalence of childhood and adult obesity in the United States, 2011–2012. *JAMA.* 2014;311(8):806–814.

26. National Heart, Lung, and Blood Institute; updated July 13, 2012. What causes overweight and obesity? Retrieved from: http://www.nhlbi.nih.gov/health/health-topics/topics/obe/causes. Accessed February 21, 2016.

27. Center for Disease Control and Prevention; updated September 1, 2016. Adult obesity facts. Retrieved from: http://www.cdc.gov/obesity/data/adult.html. Accessed February 22, 2016.

28. U.S. Department of Health and Human Services, Office of Disease Prevention and Health Promotion. About Healthy People. Retrieved from: https://www.healthypeople.gov/2020/About-Healthy-People. Accessed February 22, 2016.

29. U.S. Department of Health and Human Services, Office of Disease Prevention and Health Promotion. *Healthy People 2020* topics and objectives: Nutrition and weight status. Retrieved from: https://www.healthypeople.gov/2020/topics-objectives/topic/nutrition-and-weight-status. Accessed February 22, 2016.

30. Kratina K. Orthorexia nervosa. National Eating Disorders Association. Retrieved from: https://www.nationaleatingdisorders.org/orthorexia-nervosa. Accessed February 24, 2016.

31. Institute of Medicine, Food and Nutrition Board. *Dietary Reference Intakes for Energy, Carbohydrate, Fiber, Fat, Fatty Acids, Cholesterol, Protein, and Amino Acids.* Washington, DC: National Academies Press; 2005.

32. *Human Energy Requirements. Report of a Joint FAO/WHO/UNU Expert Consultation.* FAO Food and Nutrition Technical Report Series 1, Rome, Italy: Food and Agriculture Organization, World Health Organization, and United Nations University; 2004. ftp://ftp.fao.org/docrep/fao/007/y5686e/y5686e00.pdf. Accessed February 3, 2016.

33. Otten JJ, Pitzi Hellwig J, Meyers LD, eds; Institute of Medicine. *Dietary Reference Intakes: The Essential Guide to Nutrient Requirements.* Washington, DC: National Academies Press; 2006. http://www.nap.edu/catalog/11537.html. Accessed February 4, 2016.

34. Food and Agriculture Organization of the United Nations (FAO). *Food Energy—Methods of Analysis and Conversion Factors. Report of a Technical Workshop.* Food and Nutrition Paper No. 77. Rome, Italy: Food and Agriculture Organization; 2003. http://www.fao.org/uploads/media/FAO_2003_Food_Energy_02.pdf. Accessed February 4, 2016.

35. Food and Agriculture Organization of the United Nations. *Energy and Protein Requirements: Report of a joint FAO/WHO/UNU Expert Consultation.* WHO Technical Report Series No. 724. Geneva, Switzerland: World Health Organization; 1985. http://www.fao.org/docrep/003/aa040e/aa040e00.htm. Accessed February 4, 2016.

36. DSM Nutritional Products. *Micronutrients, Macro Impact: The Story of Vitamins and a Hungry World.* Basel, Switzerland: Sight and Life Press; 2011. http://www.sightandlife.org/fileadmin/data/Books/Micronutrients_Macro_Impact.pdf. Accessed February 9, 2016.

37. Micronutrient Initiative. *Investing in the Future: A United Call to Action on Vitamin and Mineral Deficiencies.* Ottawa, ON, Canada: Micronutrient Initiative; 2009. http://www.unitedcalltoaction.org. Accessed February 9, 2016.

38. World Health Organization. Nutrition: micronutrients. Geneva, Switzerland: World Health Organization. Retrieved from: http://www.who.int/nutrition/topics/micronutrients/en/. Accessed February 9, 2016.

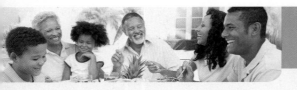

Learning Portfolio (continued)

39. Johnson EJ, Russell RM. Beta-carotene. In: Coates PM, Betz JM, Blackman MR, et al., eds. *Encyclopedia of Dietary Supplements*. 2nd ed. London, England: Informa Healthcare; 2010:115–120.

40. Solomons NW. Vitamin A. In: Bowman B, Russell R, eds. *Present Knowledge in Nutrition*. 9th ed. Washington, DC: International Life Sciences Institute; 2006:157–183.

41. Ross CA. Vitamin A. In: Coates PM, Betz JM, Blackman MR, et al., eds. *Encyclopedia of Dietary Supplements*. 2nd ed. London, England: Informa Healthcare; 2010:778–791.

42. Institute of Medicine, Food and Nutrition Board. *Dietary Reference Intakes for Vitamin A, Vitamin K, Arsenic, Boron, Chromium, Copper, Iodine, Iron, Manganese, Molybdenum, Nickel, Silicon, Vanadium, and Zinc*. Washington, DC: National Academies Press; 2001.

43. Oregon State University, Linus Pauling Institute Micronutrient Information Center. Vitamin C. Corvallis, OR: Oregon State University; updated January 1, 2014. Retrieved from: http://lpi.oregonstate.edu/mic/vitamins/vitamin-C. Accessed August 7, 2016.

44. Carr AC, Frei B. Toward a new recommended dietary allowance for vitamin C based on antioxidant and health effects in humans. *Am J Clin Nutr*. 1999;69(6):1086–1107.

45. Bruno RS, Leonard SW, Atkinson J, et al. Faster plasma vitamin E disappearance in smokers is normalized by vitamin C supplementation. *Free Radic Biol Med*. 2006;40(4):689–697.

46. Institute of Medicine, Food and Nutrition Board. *Vitamin C. Dietary Reference Intakes for Vitamin C, Vitamin E, Selenium, and Carotenoids*. Washington, DC: National Academies Press; 2000:95–185.

47. Sauberlich HE. A history of scurvy and vitamin C. In Packer L, Fuchs J, eds. *Vitamin C in Health and Disease*. New York, NY: Marcel Decker; 1997:1–24.

48. Stephen R, Utecht T. Scurvy identified in the emergency department: a case report. *J Emerg Med*. 2001;21(3):235–237.

49. Weinstein M, Babyn P, Zlotkin S. An orange a day keeps the doctor away: scurvy in the year 2000. *Pediatrics*. 2001;108(3):E55.

50. Institute of Medicine, Food and Nutrition Board. *Dietary Reference Intakes for Calcium and Vitamin D*. Washington, DC: National Academies Press; 2010.

51. Ovesen L, Brot C, Jakobsen J. Food contents and biological activity of 25-hydroxyvitamin D: a vitamin D metabolite to be reckoned with? *Ann Nutr Metab*. 2003;47:107–113.

52. Verhagen H, Buijsse B, Jansen E, Bueno-de-Mesquita B. The state of antioxidant affairs. *Nutr Today*. 2006;41:244–250.

53. Dietrich M, Traber MG, Jacques PF, Cross CE, Hu Y, Block G. Does gamma-tocopherol play a role in the primary prevention of heart disease and cancer? A review. *Am J Coll Nutr*. 2006;25:292–299.

54. Weaver CM, Heaney RP. Calcium. In: Shils ME, Shike M, Ross AC, Caballero B, Cousins RJ, eds. *Modern Nutrition in Health and Disease*. 10th ed. Baltimore, MD: Lippincott Williams & Wilkins; 2006:194–210.

55. Wessling-Resnick M. Iron. In: Ross AC, Caballero B, Cousins RJ, Tucker KL, Ziegler RG, eds. *Modern Nutrition in Health and Disease*. 11th ed. Baltimore, MD: Lippincott Williams & Wilkins; 2014:176–188.

56. Aggett PJ. Iron. In: Erdman JW, Macdonald IA, Zeisel SH, eds. *Present Knowledge in Nutrition*. 10th ed. Washington, DC: Wiley-Blackwell; 2012:506–520.

57. World Health Organization. *Worldwide Prevalence of Anemia 1993–2005: WHO Global Database on Anemia*. Geneva, Switzerland: World Health Organization; 2008.

58. World Health Organization. *Iron Deficiency Anemia: Assessment, Prevention, and Control*. Geneva, Switzerland: World Health Organization; 2001.

59. Whittaker P, Tufaro PR, Rader JI. Iron and folate in fortified cereals. *J Am Coll Nutr*. 2001;20:247–254.

60. Baker RD, Greer FR. Diagnosis and prevention of iron deficiency and iron-deficiency anemia in infants and young children (0–3 years of age). *Pediatrics*. 2010;126:1040–1050.

61. Peterson LN. Potassium in nutrition. In: O'Dell BL, Sunde RA, eds. *Handbook of Nutritionally Essential Minerals*. New York, NY: Marcel Dekker; 1997:153–183.

62. Oregon State University, Linus Pauling Institute Micronutrient Information Center. Potassium. Corvallis, OR: Oregon State University; reviewed December 2010. Retrieved from: http://lpi.oregonstate.edu/mic/minerals/potassium#references. Accessed August 7, 2016.

63. Hajjar IM, Grim CE, George V, Kotchen TA. Impact of diet on blood pressure and age-related changes in blood pressure in the US population: analysis of NHANES III. *Arch Intern Med*. 2001;161(4):589–593.

64. Appel LJ, Moore TJ, Obarzanek E, et al. A clinical trial of the effects of dietary patterns on blood pressure. DASH Collaborative Research Group. *N Engl J Med*. 1997;336(16):1117–1124.

65. U.S. National Library of Medicine. Potassium. MedlinePlus. Retrieved from: https://medlineplus.gov/potassium.html. Accessed August 7, 2016.

66. Oregon State University, Linus Pauling Institute Micronutrient Information Center. Magnesium. Corvallis, OR: Oregon State University; last reviewed May 2014. Retrieved from: http://lpi.oregonstate.edu/mic/minerals/magnesium. Accessed August 7, 2016.

67. Sebastian RS, Cleveland LE, Goldman JD, Moshfegh AJ. Older adults who use vitamin/mineral supplements differ from nonusers in nutrient intake adequacy and dietary attitudes. *J Am Diet Assoc*. 2007;107(8):1322–1332.

68. Moshfegh A, Goldman J, Ahuja J, Rhodes D, LaComb R. What we eat in America, NHANES 2005–2006: usual nutrient intakes from food and water compared to 1997 Dietary Reference Intakes for vitamin D, calcium, phosphorus, and magnesium. Washington, DC: U.S. Department of Agriculture, Agricultural Research Service; 2009.

69. Institute of Medicine, Food and Nutrition Board. Magnesium. In *Dietary Reference Intakes: Calcium, Phosphorus, Magnesium, Vitamin D, and Fluoride*. Washington, DC: National Academies Press; 1997:190–249.

70. Institute of Medicine, Food and Nutrition Board. *Dietary Reference Intakes for Water, Potassium, Sodium, Chloride, and Sulfate (2005)*. Washington, DC: National Academies Press; 2005.

71. Elmer PJ, Obarzanek E, Vollmer WM, et al. Effects of comprehensive lifestyle modification on diet, weight, physical fitness, and blood pressure control: 18-month results of a randomized trial. *Ann Intern Med*. 2006;144:485–495.

72. Committee on Examination of Front-of-Package Nutrition Rating Systems and Symbols (Phase II), Food and Nutrition Board; Wartella EA, Lichtenstein AH, Yaktine A, Nathan R, eds. *Front-of-Package Nutrition Rating Systems and Symbols Promoting*

Healthier Choices. Washington, DC: National Academies Press; 2011. http://www.nap.edu/read/13221/chapter/1. Accessed February 15, 2016.

73. U.S. Department of Health and Human Services. *2008 Physical Activity Guidelines for Americans.* Washington, DC: U.S. Department of Health and Human Services; 2008. ODPHP Publication No. U0036.

74. Centers for Disease Control and Prevention. Physical activity and the prevention of coronary heart disease. *MMRW.* 1993;42:669–672.

75. Heath GW, Parra DC, Sarmiento OL, et al; Lancet Physical Activity Series Working Group. Evidence-based intervention in physical activity: lessons from around the world. *Lancet.* 2012;380(9838):272–281.

76. U.S. Department of Health and Human Services. *Physical Activity and Health: A Report of the Surgeon General.* Atlanta, GA: U.S. Department of Health and Human Services, Centers for Disease Control and Prevention; 1996.

77. Center for Disease Control and Prevention; updated September 1, 2016. Adult obesity facts: obesity is common, serious and costly. Retrieved from: http://www.cdc.gov/obesity/data/adult.html. Accessed February 17, 2016.

78. U.S. Department of Health and Human Services, Office of Disease Prevention and Health Promotion; updated September 26, 2016. *Physical Activity Guidelines.* Retrieved from: http://health.gov/paguidelines/. Accessed February 19, 2016.

79. Andersen R, Crespo C, Bartlett S, Cheskin L, Pratt M. Relationship of physical activity and TV watching with body weight and level of fatness among children: results from the Third National Health and Nutrition Examination Survey. *JAMA.* 1998;279(12):938–942.

80. Brennan Ramirez LK, Baker EA, Metzler, M. Promoting health equity: a resource to help communities address social determinants of health. Atlanta, GA: U.S. Department of Health and Human Services, Centers for Disease Control and Prevention; 2008.

81. Centers for Disease Control and Prevention. *State Indicator Report on Physical Activity, 2010.* Atlanta, GA: U.S. Department of Health and Human Services; 2010. Retrieved from: http://www.cdc.gov/physicalactivity/PS_State_Indicator_Report_2010.pdf. Accessed February 19, 2016.

82. U.S. Department of Agriculture, Food and Nutrition Service. Supplemental Nutrition Assistance Program (SNAP). Retrieved from: http://www.fns.usda.gov/snap/supplemental-nutrition-assistance-program-snap. Accessed February 19, 2016.

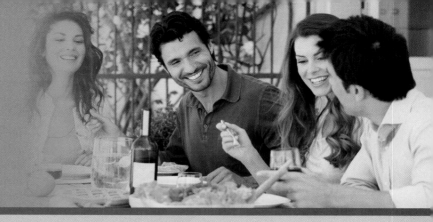

CHAPTER 13

Nutrition for Health and Disease in Adults

Chris Wellington, RD, MS, BSc

Chapter Outline

Overweight and Obesity

Gastrointestinal Conditions

Endocrine and Metabolic Conditions

Cardiovascular Disease and Hypertension

Cancer

Immune Disorders: HIV and AIDS

Learning Objectives

1. Explain the key features for the dietary management of overweight and obesity.

2. Discuss dietary guidance to prevent gastrointestinal conditions, including GERD, IBS, IBD, gall bladder disease, and diverticular disease.

3. Explain the key features of dietary management and dietary management of diabetes and metabolic syndrome.

4. Summarize the dietary management of cardiovascular disease and its risk factors.

5. Describe how diet affects risk factors for cancer.

6. Discuss the role of diet in protecting bone health.

7. List the key features of nutrition in immune disorders.

©NightAndDayImages/E+/Getty

Case Study

Jasmine R. and Annie M. are two typical people suffering from chronic diseases. Currently, Jasmine R., a divorced woman in her mid-60s with three children and five grandchildren, lives in the midwestern United States. As a child, Jasmine R. was above average in terms of her body mass index, but she thinned out during puberty. She was married at an early age and only worked for a short time as a sales clerk in a retail store. She developed obesity after her first pregnancy and, with subsequent pregnancies following, she was unable to lose the weight. She went back to work after her divorce and works full time as a cashier in a local grocery store. She found it difficult to work and run the household as a single mom. She did not receive regular financial support from her husband and took on an extra job cleaning homes on weekends. As her life progressed, she developed a number of other serious chronic diseases often associated with obesity, including hypertension, type 2 diabetes, and osteoporosis.

In contrast to Jasmine R., Annie M., a married young woman in her mid-20s with no children, grew up in the midwestern United States but now resides in California. She suffers with ulcerative colitis, a serious and chronic disease that was first diagnosed when she was 10 years of age. Her disease is currently stable and has been treated with drug therapy and dietary management so far. There is a family history of ulcerative colitis, with her grandmother having developed

the disease later in life. Annie M.'s grandmother was treated with medications and diet, but ultimately she had to have an ileostomy. Neither of Annie M.'s parents or her siblings have manifested the disease. She comes from an upper-middle-class family, and both her parents are health professionals. As such, Annie M. was exposed to an environment with good nutrition. In addition, she has constant access to informed advice.

As a professional performer who puts on athletic demonstrations, she must maintain a high level of fitness at all times and must maintain an attractive appearance. In addition, her work and lifestyle are nonroutine, involving training, traveling, and auditioning at odd hours of the day. Her work may involve many consecutive hours of rehearsal followed by short and intense performances. The jobs she gets are generally short duration, and even steady work generally lasts less than a year. As such, she is challenged to have a consistent routine with regular meals and healthy dietary choices available. The requirement to continually audition for much of her work and the lack of stability create considerable pressure and tension for her.

As we go through this chapter, we will discuss serious and chronic diseases and their impact on people like Jasmine R. and Annie M. The chapter illustrates how dietary management can play a role in the prevention, treatment, and management of these diseases.

Lifestyle factors that contribute to the development of chronic diseases include diet, physical inactivity, overweight, tobacco use, and alcohol and drug abuse. A balanced diet is a key consideration in both the prevention and management of serious and chronic diseases.

The focus of this chapter is on the dietary management of a number of frequently encountered disease conditions that may be either serious or chronic or both. These disease conditions include overweight and obesity; gastrointestinal (GI) conditions such as gastroesophageal reflux disease (GERD), irritable bowel syndrome (IBS), inflammatory bowel disease (IBD), diverticular disease, and gallbladder disease; endocrine and metabolic conditions such as metabolic syndrome and type 2 diabetes; cardiovascular disease; hypertension; cancers; skeletal health concerns such osteoporosis, arthritis, and gout; and immune disorders such as human immunodeficiency virus (HIV) infection and acquired immune deficiency syndrome (AIDS).

In some cases, these disease conditions may be primarily associated with poor dietary habits and lifestyle choices. Other times, the disease conditions arise from genetic predispositions or environmental exposure. Most often, though, these disease conditions are associated with a combination of poor dietary habits and lifestyle choices in addition to genetic predispositions and

environmental exposures. This chapter focuses on the dietary relationships associated with these disease conditions and their prevention and also discusses the dietary management once a disease or condition has been diagnosed and a treatment regime has been instituted.

The chapter presents each disease condition and discusses its prevalence and etiology. Next, the risk factors associated with each disease condition are discussed. The methods and goals for the prevention of disease are then provided. Finally, the nutritional management of the disease is presented, including the cases where prevention has failed or may not be feasible, for example, in congenital conditions.

Overweight and Obesity

Preview Overweight and obesity are complex diseases that involve many factors. Overweight and obesity are rapidly becoming a threat to the health of populations in many countries around the world. This section defines overweight and obesity, discusses the prevalence of this condition, identifies its risk factors, and then discusses the prevention and management of overweight and obesity.

The Big Picture

A chronic disease affecting over a third of Americans: Obesity is a key risk factor in almost every other chronic disease.

Since 1980, obesity worldwide has more than doubled. In 2014, more than 1.9 billion adults 18 years and older were overweight. Of these, more than 600 million were obese. **FIGURE 13.1** shows a map of obesity prevalence around the world.

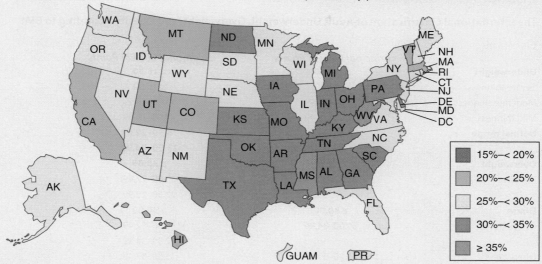

Figure 13.1a

Map of obesity prevalence in the United States in 2013.

Reproduced from Centers for Disease Control and Prevention Obesity prevalence maps. Atlanta, GA: Centers for Disease Control and Prevention; updated July 1, 2016. Retrieved from: http://www.cdc.gov/obesity/data/prevalence-maps.html. Accessed August 31, 2016.

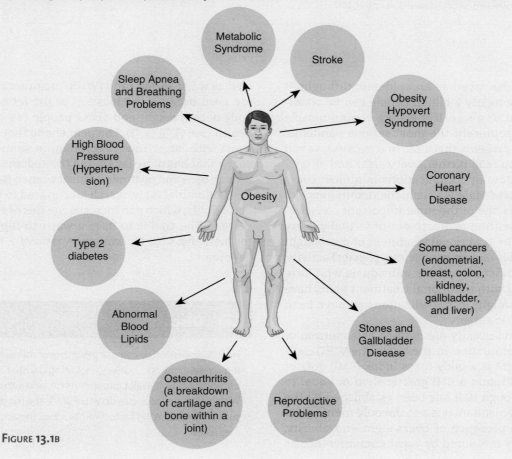

FIGURE **13.1B**

Body mass index (BMI) is a simple index of weight-for-height that is commonly used to classify underweight, overweight, and obesity in adults (see **TABLE 13.1**). It is defined as the weight in kilograms divided by the square of the height in meters (kg/m²). For example, an adult who weighs 70 kg and whose height is 1.75 m has a BMI of 22.9.

$$BMI = 70 \text{ kg} \div (1.75 \text{ m})^2 = 70 \div 3.06 = 22.9$$

Table 13.1

The International Classification of Adult Underweight, Overweight, and Obesity According to BMI

Classification	BMI (kg/m²)	
	Principal Cut-Off Points	*Additional Cut-Off Points*
Underweight	**< 18.50**	**< 18.50**
Severe thinness	< 16.00	< 16.00
Moderate thinness	16.00–16.99	16.00–16.99
Mild thinness	17.00–18.49	17.00–18.49
Normal range	**18.50–24.99**	**18.50–22.99**
		23.00–24.99
Overweight	**≥ 25.00**	**≥ 25.00**
Pre-obese	25.00–29.99	25.00–27.49
		27.50–29.99
Obese	**≥ 30.00**	**≥ 30.00**
Obese class I	30.00–34.99	30.00–32.49
		32.50–34.99
Obese class II	35.00–39.99	35.00–37.49
		37.50–39.99
Obese class III	≥ 40.00	≥ 40.00

Reproduced from World Health Organization. BMI classification; Table 1. The International Classification of adult underweight, overweight, and obesity according to BMI. Geneva, Switzerland: WHO; updated November 14, 2016. Retrieved from: http://apps.who.int/bmi/index.jsp?introPage=intro_3.html. Accessed November 11, 2016.

Obesity could be described as an epidemic throughout the world because nearly 2 billion people can be classified as overweight or obese. If it were a communicable disease, it would represent the most serious pandemic ever! This chapter presents this topic first because, as you will discover as you read further, overweight and obesity represent risk factors or complications in almost every other chronic disease state. As such, the maintenance of a healthy weight is one of the most important considerations in the prevention or treatment of virtually every chronic disease. The traditional treatment of overweight and obesity includes dietary counseling, physical activity, and behavior modification. Obese individuals who have been unsuccessful with traditional treatment plans have been prescribed weight loss medications or have been referred for bariatric surgery.

Overweight and obesity are defined as abnormal or excessive fat accumulation in the body. The WHO definition of overweight is a body mass index (BMI) greater than or equal to 25, and a BMI greater than or equal to 30 is obesity. Although BMI has been established by the World Health Organization, it is not the only metric used to determine the presence of overweight and obesity. Abdominal obesity measured by waist circumference as well as waist-to-hip ratio (WHR) are other measures that are used because the location of the fat on the human body in overweight and obese people can also influence health (see **TABLE 13.2**). The pear shape that has a smaller waist with larger hips is common in women. The apple shape that has more fat around the abdomen area is common in men and postmenopausal women (see **FIGURE 13.2**). The abdominal fat (visceral) fat can lead to increased levels of lipids, which can increase the risk of cardiovascular disease. The goal is to have a waist-to-hip ratio of ≤ 0.9 for men and ≤ 0.8 for women. A ratio of ≥ 1.0 is the danger area.[1]

Let's Discuss

Health professionals can use a number of methods for measuring overweight and obesity, including a visual assessment of body shape, BMI, waist circumference, and waist-to-hip ratio. Which of these measures do you think is the most reliable measure of obesity? What factors might affect the accuracy of these measures?

Table 13.2		
Waist Circumference and Obesity by Ethnicity		
Country or Ethnic Group	Central Obesity as Defined by Waist Circumference *Women, inches*	Central Obesity as Defined by Waist Circumference *Men, inches*
Caucasian	≥ 35 inches	≥ 40 inches
European, sub-Saharan African, Eastern Mediterranean, and Middle Eastern (Arab)	≥ 32 inches	≥ 37.6 inches
South Asian, Chinese, Japanese, South and Central American	≥ 32 inches	≥ 36 inches

Data from Canadian Diabetes Association. Managing weight and diabetes: body mass index and waist circumference. Toronto, CA: Canadian Diabetes Association; 2013. Retrieved from: http://guidelines.diabetes.ca/CDACPG/media/documents/patient-resources/body-mass-index-and-waist-circumference.pdf. Accessed August 31, 2016.

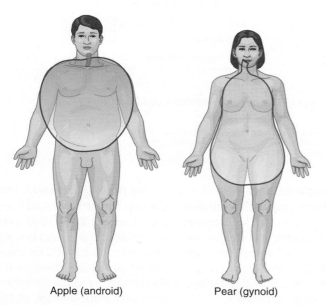

Apple (android)   Pear (gynoid)

Figure 13.2
Pear- versus apple-shaped body types.

Prevalence and Etiology of Overweight and Obesity

Since 1980, obesity worldwide has more than doubled. In 2014, more than 1.9 billion adults 18 years and older were overweight. Of these, more than 600 million were obese. In the United States, the prevalence of overweight and obesity has increased (see **FIGURE 13.3**).[2] The southern states had the highest prevalence of obesity (30.2%), followed by the Midwest (30.1%), the Northeast (26.5%), and the West (24.9%) (see Figure 13.1).

Obesity represents a large cost to the healthcare system and is a cause of reduced work productivity. Currently, estimate places the cost of obesity in the U.S. to be $147 to $210 billion dollars annually.[3,4] Aside from the medical costs, the loss of productivity associated with absenteeism associated with obesity is estimated at $8.65 billion.[5] In addition to the social costs, obesity and overweight are a tremendous business for the weight loss industry. In 2012, an estimated 108 million dieters in the United States spent $61.6 billion on products, programs, and supplements to lose weight.[6] Many individuals are unable to attain their desired weight loss levels, and even for those who do, almost all of them regain their weight.

Risk Factors of Overweight and Obesity

Many risk factors are involved in the development of overweight and obesity. These factors are very complex, and many mechanisms are involved (**TABLE 13.3**). In general, a combination of diet, physical inactivity, and other risk factors contribute to the onset and sustained excess body weight prevalent in the United States.

A vast majority of American adults are overweight or obese. For example, 69% of Americans aged 20 years and older are overweight or obese, with BMIs over 25. By age cohort, the percentages of people with a BMI over 25 are as follows: 20–39 years, 60%; 40–59 years, 75.3%; and 60 years and older, 71.6%.[6] It is common for men and women to gain most of their excess weight between the ages of 25 and 34 years. Weight gain continues slowly throughout the rest of the life cycle except for women during menopause, which is a time of quick weight gain because women have decreases in the hormone estrogen. A major reason for weight gain associated with aging is the combination of a natural slowing of metabolism and a decrease in vigor of physical activity as a person ages. People tend to maintain the same caloric intake while their output of energy declines, their metabolism naturally slows, and their activity level decreases, thus leading to weight gain.

Race and Ethnicity

In the United States, obesity rates (BMIs over 30) differ significantly according to race and ethnic background. For example, the obesity rate among Asian adults is 10.8%, the lowest of all the ethnic groups. Among whites, the obesity rate is 32.6%, and Hispanics have a higher rate of 42.5%. In black people, the rate climbs to 47.8%. When sex is considered, the rates are as follows: Asian males, 10%; Asian females, 11.4%; white men, 32.4%; white women, 32.8%;

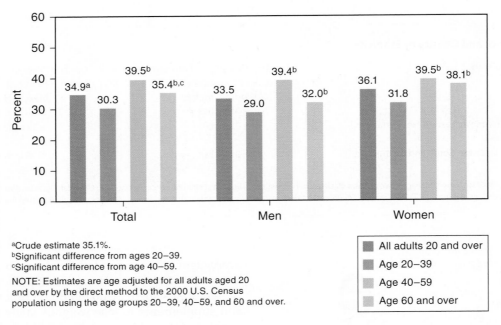

aCrude estimate 35.1%.
bSignificant difference from ages 20–39.
cSignificant difference from age 40–59.

NOTE: Estimates are age adjusted for all adults aged 20 and over by the direct method to the 2000 U.S. Census population using the age groups 20–39, 40–59, and 60 and over.

Figure 13.3
Age-adjusted prevalence of obesity, by sex and age group, among adults aged 20 and older: United States 2011–2012.

Reproduced from Ogden CL, Carroll MD, Kit BK, Flegal KM. Prevalence of obesity among adults: United States, 2011–2012. NCHS Data Brief No. 131. Hyattsville, MD: National Center for Health Statistics, Centers for Disease Control and Prevention; October 2013. Retrieved from: http://www.cdc.gov/nchs/data/databriefs /db131.htm. Accessed August 31, 2016.

Table 13.3

Risk Factors for Overweight and Obesity

Age
Race and ethnicity
Education
Income
Family history
Physical activity
Environment
Alcohol
Smoking
Sleep deprivation

Hispanic men, 40.1%; Hispanic women, 44.4%; black men, 37.1%; and black women, 56.6%. (See **FIGURE 13.4** .) When rates of obesity by sex are compared while controlling for ethnicity and race, the only group in which the obesity rate differs between men and women is for blacks. Black men have a lower rate of obesity than black women, and this difference is statistically significant.[7]

Education

In the United States, obesity rates increased among all adults regardless of level of education. From 1988–1994 to 2007–2008, obesity levels among adults at all levels of education increased. Among men with a college degree, the prevalence of obesity increased from 15.6% to 27.4%

between 1988–1994 and 2005–2008. Among those with less than a high school diploma, the prevalence increased from 22.6% to 32.1%. A comparison of recent 2005–2008 data indicates that the lowest rates of obesity are found among men and women who are college educated: 27.4% for men, and 23.4% for women. As level of education changes for women, the rates of obesity also change as follows: women college graduates, 23.4%; women with some college, 38.4%; women who have completed high school, 39.8%; and women who have not completed high school, 42.1%. For men, obesity associated with level of education is as follows: men college graduates, 27.4%; men with some college, 36.2%; men who have completed high school, 34.8%; and men who have not completed high school, 32.1%.[8]

Income

Between 1988–1994 and 2007–2008, the prevalence of obesity increased among adults at all income levels. Approximately 33% of men who live in households with income at or above 350% of the poverty level are obese, and 29.2% of men who live below 130% of the poverty level are obese. Approximately 29.0% of women who live in households with income at or above 350% of the poverty level are obese, and 42.0% of those with income below 130% of the poverty level are obese. Obesity and income in men varies by race and ethnicity.[8]

Family History of Obesity

Many researchers believe that a combination of genes and behavior are needed for a person to become overweight.

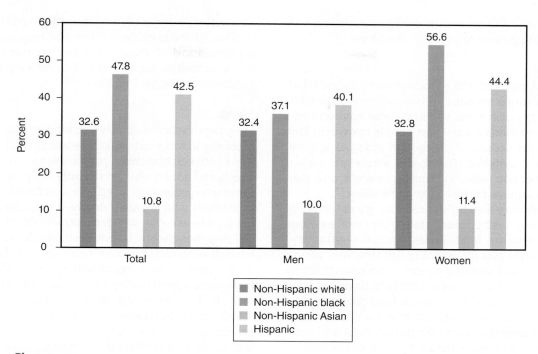

Figure 13.4

Obesity prevalence by race and sex in the United States.

Reproduced from Ogden CL, Carroll MD, Kit BK, Flegal KM. Prevalence of obesity among adults: United States, 2011–2012. NCHS Data Brief No. 131. Hyattsville, MD: National Center for Health Statistics, Centers for Disease Control and Prevention; October 2013. Retrieved from: http://www.cdc.gov/nchs/data/databriefs/db131.htm. Accessed August 31, 2016.

In some individuals, multiple genes may increase their susceptibility to obesity, but an abundance of food or inactivity or both is also needed for an individual's weight to increase. Obesity risk is two to eight times higher for a person with a family history of obesity. Weight gain and adiposity increase with age, an effect also influenced by heredity. A 2014 study found that consumption of fried food could interact with genes related to obesity, which finding stresses the importance of reducing fried food consumption in individuals who might be genetically predisposed to obesity.[9,10]

Physical Activity

Physical activity has been shown to have a number of health benefits, including helping to manage weight; reducing the risks of type 2 diabetes, heart disease, and some cancers; strengthening bones and muscles; and improving mental health.[11] To achieve weight loss and prevent weight regain in adults, greater amounts of physical activity are needed.

Obesity and sedentary behavior co-occur, and both are associated with cardiovascular disease (CVD) in women. The Centers for Disease Control and Prevention (CDC) has shown that in areas of the United States where rates of obesity are higher than 30%, the prevalence of adults who report minimal leisure-time physical activity is also higher than 30%.

The American College of Sports Medicine (ACSM) published a position paper stating that "overweight and obese individuals will most likely experience greater weight reduction and prevent weight regain with 250+ minutes/week of moderate-intensity physical activity."[12] In addition, the ACSM recommends incorporating strength training to increase fat-free mass to further reduce health risks (see TABLE 13.4).

Table 13.4

American College of Sports Medicine Physical Activity Recommendations

Prevent weight gain:	Weight loss:	For weight maintenance after weight loss:
• 150–250 minutes/week of moderate-intensity physical activity is associated with prevention of weight gain. • More than 150 minutes/week of moderate-intensity physical activity is associated with modest weight loss.	• 150–250 minutes/week of moderate-intensity physical activity provides only modest weight loss. • Greater amounts (i.e., > 250) provide clinically significant weight loss.	• There is some evidence that > 250 minutes/week of moderate-intensity physical activity will prevent weight regain.

Data from Donnelly JE, Blair SN, Jakicic JM, et al. American College of Sports Medicine position stand: appropriate physical activity intervention strategies for weight loss and prevention of weight regain for adults. *Med Sci Sports Exerc.* 2009;41:459–471.

Physical activity combined with energy restriction will increase weight loss as compared to diet alone.

Environment

Physical, social, political, and economic surroundings that influence how much we eat and how active we are have changed over the past several years. These environmental changes have made it easier for people to overeat and more difficult for people to get enough physical activity. Healthy foods (vegetables, fruits, and whole grains) are more expensive than refined grains and sweets, and they may be too expensive for low-income families.[13]

Time availability also influences how we eat. It takes longer to prepare healthy meals, and busy families often purchase convenience foods or fast food. Lower-income households, single parents working full time and taking care of children, and working parents who have children in many after-school activities are likely to have less time for meal preparation and other household chores.[14,15]

People living in neighborhoods that are zoned exclusively for residential use must take transportation to work because it is almost always too far to walk. Communities that lack full-service grocery stores and neighborhood food markets also have less access to fresh fruits and vegetables. Inner cities often lack full-service grocery stores or specialty stores with a wide variety of fresh fruits and vegetables.

Certain types of public amenities (e.g., public parks and recreational facilities, sidewalks, streetlights, and interconnectivity of streets) encourage physical activity and help to reduce the risk of obesity and related health problems. Lack of parks and recreational facilities, busy roads with high-speed traffic, and automobile-focused transportation tend to discourage activity and ultimately increase obesity risk. These factors have contributed to the increasing rate of overweight and obesity in our society.[16,17]

Alcohol Intake

The high level of caloric intake associated with alcohol consumption may be a significant contributor to the rise in obesity. Regular consumption of alcohol, through its effects in suppressing fat oxidation, is considered to be a significant risk factor for weight gain and hypertriglyceridemia. Alcoholic beverages are energy dense and often are not substituted in place of food but rather added to the total daily energy intake. In fact, people are often advised to take food and not drink on an empty stomach to reduce the rate of absorption of alcohol and avoid becoming inebriated.[18–20]

Smoking

Some studies indicate that heavy smoking could be associated with a greater risk of obesity.[21,22] Some researchers have suggested that this could be because of the fact that heavy smokers often adopt behaviors that lead to weight gain (minimal physical activity, unhealthy diet, and high alcohol intake) compared with light smokers or nonsmokers. Smokers eat less fruit and vegetables and also adopt unhealthy patterns of nutrient intake in relation to food choices. There is evidence that smoking leads to greater accumulation of visceral fat and greater insulin resistance as well as increased risk of developing metabolic syndrome and type 2 diabetes.[23–25]

Sleep

Sleep deprivation could play a significant role in the etiology of obesity in some individuals. Research studies have shown a link between how much people sleep and how much they weigh, and adults who get too little sleep weigh more than those who get enough sleep. A reason for this might be that individuals who are sleep deprived may complain of being too tired to exercise, which decreases "calories burned."

Another theory is that individuals who do not get enough sleep may consume more calories than those who do get enough sleep because they are awake longer and have more opportunities to eat. The lack of sleep can disrupt the balance of the hormones that control appetite, which could then cause more hunger than in those who get enough rest each night.[26–30] Evidence suggests that the lack of sleep may affect the metabolic balance and cause obesity and other metabolic disorders.[31]

A relatively new factor that is contributing to sleep deprivation is the use of multimedia (e.g., television, computer, and Internet), which may aggravate sedentary behavior and increase caloric intake. In addition, shift work, long working hours, and increased time commuting to and from work have also been hypothesized to favor weight gain and obesity-related metabolic disorders because of their strong link to shorter sleep times.[32,33]

Prevention of Overweight and Obesity

Obesity is a preventable condition, but prevention needs to begin early in life. Families should encourage lifelong habits of healthy eating along with regular exercise. Following a healthy lifestyle can help prevent overweight and obesity. With adults, it is important to focus on prevention of further weight gain for everyone. The World Health Organization (WHO) recommends taking the following three steps:

1. Universal public health prevention that is aimed at the entire population
2. Selective prevention that is aimed at those individuals who have a higher risk of developing obesity
3. Targeted prevention that is aimed at those high-risk individuals who already have weight problems and who are at risk for becoming obese[34]

Obesity prevention incorporates many behaviors, as listed in TABLE 13.5 .

Management of Overweight and Obesity

There is no single or simple solution to the overweight/obesity epidemic happening around the globe. It is a complex problem that requires a multifaceted approach.

Table 13.5

Obesity Prevention Behaviors

- Individuals are encouraged to follow a healthy eating plan. It is important to look at energy in versus energy out when choosing food items.
- Avoid skipping meals.
- Focus on portion size is to be encouraged both at home and while eating out.
- Consume at least "5 a day" fruits and vegetables.
- Increase consumption of whole-grain foods.
- Consume "nutrient-dense" foods more often than "energy-dense" foods. Limit consumption of refined grains, sweets, high-fat foods, and high-salt foods.
- People should be encouraged to pay attention to their behaviors when eating: where they are eating (at the computer, in front of the TV, at their desk), with whom they are eating (coworkers, friends, family, alone), why they are eating (habit, lonely, angry, stressed), what they are eating (sweets, fatty foods, salty foods). Behavior plays a large role in our eating patterns.
- Daily physical activity is necessary for everyone of all ages and offers many benefits. All individuals should exercise for at least 30 minutes a day.
- Screen time in our society takes up a lot of our time. It is important to reduce screen time or to be creative and "move" when watching TV (walk on a treadmill/elliptical machine while watching a show or movie).
- Pay attention and keep track of behaviors. Keeping a food diary of what was consumed, where food was consumed, and how a person felt before and after eating may help. Recording exercise on a calendar and using a quick checklist to record every time a fruit or vegetable is consumed can help to achieve the 5-a-day recommendations.
- Get at least 6 hours of sleep each night.
- Reduce stress or find ways to deal with stressful situations.

What works for one individual may not work for another. Some individuals are overweight as a result of a genetic or biological tendency to gain weight in a specific environment. Perhaps early identification of these genes can assist individuals early in life and help set them on the path of healthy eating and exercise. Many individuals worldwide are overweight owing to an environment that promotes a sedentary lifestyle along with an energy-rich, high-fat diet. Neighborhoods and communities are working to improve their local environments to encourage more physical activity by including areas that are more conducive to walking and biking, including green space for outdoor gatherings, and offering safe parks that promote physically active play for children and their families.

The first goal of a treatment plan for overweight individuals is to prevent further weight gain. The basic treatment plan for obese individuals should include weight maintenance followed by a small, gradual weight loss (5–10%) over a 6-month period and management of comorbidities. The specific management strategy should incorporate dietary adjustments, physical activity, and lifestyle changes with continued support for each individual. Medication and surgery are options for obese individuals who are not successful with the first line of treatment.

Because obesity is a complex issue, society must play a role in its treatment. Government, food industry, and media all must assist in changing the environment so that further weight gain around the world is avoided. The federal and local governments must create and disseminate simple, clear, and effective dietary guidelines with targeted consumer education and intervention programs, and ensure the safety of foods and strict adherence to marketing, production, and labeling of food products. The food industry will need to genuinely put the health of consumers first by producing healthy and affordable foods that are widely available and honestly marketed. The media must commit to accurate and reliable reporting on nutrition and healthy lifestyles.[35]

Obesity management programs should be set up both in community and healthcare settings with easy accessibility for all individuals. The programs should be designed to allow for modest weight loss, weight maintenance, and management strategies for obesity comorbidities.

Dietary Treatment

Overweight and obese patients often have concomitant medical problems such as diabetes, heart disease, and hypertension, and these conditions must be accounted for in a recommended dietary composition for weight loss. A counseling session with a registered dietitian nutritionist (RDN) for medical nutrition therapy is recommended. Collaborative care and self-management of chronic diseases must be emphasized in the treatment of obesity for any success to be expected.

To start with, it is important for everyone to have a healthy diet that is low in fat, high in complex carbohydrates, high in fruits, and high in vegetables.[36,37] Meal replacements, which are foods designed to take the place of a meal or snack, that provide nutrients within a fixed caloric limit may be beneficial in the weight loss process. A RDN can create a low-calorie diet that includes an energy deficit of 500–1,000 kcal/day, which should cause a weight loss of 0.5–1 kg/week. For example, RDNs will often start with a diet of 1,000–1,200 kcal/day for most overweight women and a diet of 1,200–1,600 kcal/day for overweight men and for some women who exercise regularly. The majority of weight loss diets are self-managed, and obese individuals often underestimate their intake by approximately 30–50%. RDNs, therefore, need to teach patients how to read food labels, measure portion sizes, and record their food intake after eating.

Choose MyPlate (www.choosemyplate.gov) is a great website that offers tools and information to promote healthy eating habits, which are key for maintaining a healthy weight. It provides nutrition information about foods plus tools that enable users to track calorie intake, plan meals, and find healthy recipes.

News You Can Use

The Hottest Fad Diet Product: *Caralluma*

Weight loss products are big business in the United States, and this business is constantly growing. In 2012, an estimated 108 million dieters in the United States spent $61.6 billion on products, programs, and supplements to lose weight.[a] "Lose weight fast and keep it off" is one of the miracle promises these fad products make. The miracle product is *Caralluma*, a simple pill that helps people lose weight—no need to make any lifestyle changes except the simplest: Remember to take a pill and the weight problem is solved almost immediately! Of course, people are skeptical about miracles, so a seductive marketing pitch supported by a credible source offering a credible explanation is required.

The marketing pitch begins with the popular Dr. Oz commenting, "This thing is lightning in a bottle; it's a miracle flower to fight your fat." This is exactly what people want to hear: a former practicing physician who has his own TV show and who can explain the miracle. According to Dr. Oz, *Caralluma* "goes in and causes the body to burn fat from within 'like a furnace,' literally melting the fat away. The second feature, and the most important one, is that after *Caralluma* has burnt the fat, you're left with the sleek, lean muscle that was buried underneath. The third feature is its ability to strengthen not only the muscles but the bones as well."[b]

With the credible source provided, the marketing pitch continues with a testimonial from a person who has used *Caralluma*. Enter Rachael Ray, who took the product every day for 4 weeks and who makes the following claim: "I Lost 25 Pounds in 4 Weeks, No Special Diet, No Intense Exercise."[b] The third element of the marketing effort involves directing people to an information website where the makers of *Caralluma* present the following claims:

> Based on the results of a 12-week clinical study published in the U.S. National Library of Medicine (National Institutes of Health):

- *Caralluma* contains no stimulants.
- *Caralluma* contains 10% pure *Caralluma*, the active ingredient in pure natural *Caralluma*.
- *Caralluma* has been found to burn belly fat from within your body, boosting weight loss by more than 33.77%.
- Studies have shown that daily *Caralluma* intake can increase lean muscle and bone density.[b]

As the orders pour in, the makers of *Caralluma* are happy, but what about their clients who are taking the product and who still need medical advice? When they go to see a health practitioner and tell the practitioner they are taking *Caralluma* or some other miracle supplement to lose weight, what does the health practitioner do?

It is very important for health practitioners to be well informed and have access to credible sources of information to advise their patients. According to WebMD—a more credible source than the Dr. Oz show, a patient like Rachael, and a promotional website—"*Caralluma* is a succulent plant (cactus) from India where it grows wild. Traditionally, Indian tribes chewed chunks of *Caralluma* to keep from being hungry during a long hunt. These days, a solution that contains chemicals taken from the plant (extract) is used to decrease appetite for weight loss.[d-f] It is also used to quench thirst and to increase endurance."[c] The Natural Medicines Comprehensive Database states: "There is insufficient reliable evidence to rate this product for weight loss. Developing evidence suggests that taking a *Caralluma* extract that is 500 mg for 60 days might decrease waistline, feelings of hunger, and fat and calorie intake. However it does not decrease weight, body mass index (BMI), body fat, or hip measurements. More evidence is needed before it can be used for weight loss."[d]

According to these sources, *Caralluma* seems to be safe for most people when 500 mg of the extract is taken twice daily for up to 60 days but the long-term safety is not known. *Caralluma* might cause some mild side effects such as gastrointestinal issues, bloating, constipation, flatulence, gastritis, and stomach pain.

Chemicals contained in the *Caralluma* plant are thought to decrease appetite.[d] Specifically, the pregnane glycoside elements that are contained in *Caralluma* are thought to have a role in the decrease of appetite. A study of 50 adult men and women published in 2007 in *Appetite* reported that the experimental group showed a trend toward greater decreases in body weight, body mass index, hip circumference, body fat, and energy intake between assessment time points than did the placebo group, but the differences were not significant.[e] Another study from Australia involved a small sample of adults aged 29–59 years found that supplementation with *Caralluma* extract for 12 weeks in combination with controlling dietary intake and physical activity may potentially aid in the reduction of waist circumference.[f]

An informed health practitioner can comment that *Caralluma* is an interesting supplement with some scientific evidence for effectiveness and safety in weight loss. However, further research must be done on this supplement (or any other that comes up for discussion) and it has not yet been approved as a weight loss product by the U.S. Food and Drug Administration. Therefore, a discussion of tried and true methods of weight loss management must ensue.

References

a. Marketdata. Weight loss market in U.S. up 1.7% to $61 billion. PRWeb; April 16, 2013. Retrieved from: http://www.prweb.com/releases/2013/4/prweb10629316.htm. Accessed August 23, 2015.

b. Truth in Advertising. *How Rachael Dropped 25 Pounds and 4 Dress Sizes.* Everyday Health and Wellness Report. Retrieved from: https://www.truthinadvertising.org/wp-content/uploads/2015/09/CLA-Safflower-Oil-website.pdf. Accessed August 31, 2016.

c. WebMD. Caralluma. Retrieved from: http://www.webmd.com/vitamins-supplements/ingredientmono-1160-caralluma.aspx?activeingredientid=1160&.

d. Natural Medicines Comprehensive Database. Stockton, CA: Therapeutic Research Faculty. Retrieved from: http://naturaldatabase.therapeuticresearch.com/home.aspx?cs=&s=ND. Accessed August 29, 2015.

e. Kurivana R, Raja T, Srinivasb SK, et al. Effect of *Caralluma fimbriata* extract on appetite, food intake and anthropometry in adult Indian men and women. *Appetite.* May 2007;48(3):338–344.

f. Astell KJ, Mathai ML, McAinch AJ, Stathis CG, Su XQ. A pilot study investigating the effect of *Caralluma fimbriata* extract on the risk factors of metabolic syndrome in overweight and obese subjects: a randomised controlled clinical trial. *Complement Therap Med.* June 2013;21(3):180–189.

Physical Activity

Physical activity that is sustained over time is another important factor in weight loss and weight maintenance. The benefits of physical activity include inducing negative energy balance (by increasing calorie expenditure), sparing fat-free mass during weight loss, and improving cardiovascular fitness. Physical activity produces minimal weight loss by itself and is more effective when combined with a calorie-restricted diet. For this reason, it is important to encourage the combination of dietary changes along with physical activity.[12,38–40]

Self-Monitoring

Self-monitoring is a strategy used in achieving lifestyle goals, where individuals track their food intake, physical activity, and weight throughout the treatment process. Tracking data is beneficial for both the individual and the healthcare provider because it provides information on dietary intake that can be evaluated to reflect and plan the diet. It also provides information to the individual, who can then apply techniques of restraint. Tracking physical activity by recording time or steps is also beneficial in this process.[41]

Activity Monitors

The American College of Sports Medicine (ACSM) recently announced in its annual fitness trend forecast that wearable technology will be the number one trend in fitness in 2016.[42] Wearable technology started out as step counters and devices that measured the duration and intensity of physical activity and progressed to more advanced systems that provide quantitative and qualitative information on an individual's activity behavior. Devices now include fitness trackers, smartwatches, heart rate monitors, and GPS tracking devices.[43]

One recent study of overweight and obese adults examined the effectiveness of TECH (BodyMedia Fit) used alone and in combination with an in-person behavioral weight loss intervention. Participants who used the technology and participated in regular in-person meetings showed greater weight loss compared with that of participants in the standard program.[44] It is expected that the trend in wearable technology will continue and that new devices will be used in the weight loss process.[45]

Behavior Modification

Common techniques of behavior modification include self-monitoring food intake and activity level; controlling stimuli, such as altering the environment that activates eating to avoid overeating; slowing eating, which allows signals of fullness to be recognized; setting goals; and building social support. Internet and telephone communication also allows individuals to have continuous and extended contact with a health team to promote weight loss maintenance. These interventions have the potential to reach large numbers of adults and to improve the cost-effectiveness of intervention.[46]

Medication

In 2011, approximately 2.74 million patients in the United States used obesity drugs.[47] Pharmacotherapy is approved for patients with a BMI $\geq$ 30 kg/m^2 or $\geq$ 27 kg/m^2 when complicated by an obesity comorbidity. Drugs regularly used to treat obesity in the United States include phentermine and diethylpropion, which have a similar adverse-effect and weight loss profile to phentermine, phendimetrazine, and benzphetamine, the latter two less commonly prescribed for obesity treatment. The profiles and sides effects of these drugs are presented in **TABLE 13.6**. The gastrointestinal lipase inhibitor orlistat, when taken three times a day during or up to 1 hour after meals, leads to the excretion of approximately 30% of ingested fat. Orlistat, however, often causes uncomfortable gastrointestinal side effects. Many individuals do not

Table 13.6

Drugs Used to Treat Obesity

Generic Drug	Proprietary Name		Common Adverse Effects
Short-term approval[a]	*Noradrenergics causing appetite suppression*		
Phentermine	Adiplex-P		Information about 1-year weight change not included.
	Fastin		
	Oby-Cap, Ionamin		
Diethypropion	Tenuate		Common adverse effects include:
	TenuateDospan		Insomnia, elevation in heart rate, dry mouth, taste alterations, dizziness, tremors, headache. diarrhea, constipation, vomiting, gastrointestinal distress, anxiety, and restlessness[c]
	Tepanil		
Phendimetrazine	Bontril		
Benzphentamine	Didrex		
Long-term approval[a]	*Mechanism of Action*		
Orlistat[d]	Alli	Lipase inhibitor causing excretion of approximately 30% of ingested triglycerides in stool	Oily spotting, flatus with discharge, fecal urgency, fatty oily stool, increased defecation, fecal incontinence[e]
	Xenical		
Lorcaserin[b]	Belviq	Highly selective serotonergic 5-HT2C receptor agonist causing appetite suppression	Headache, dizziness, fatigue, nausea, dry mouth, cough, and constipation; and in patients with type 2 diabetes, back pain, cough, and hypoglycemia[e]
Phentermine plus topiramate-ER[b]	Qysmia	Noradrenergic + GABA-receptor activator, kainite/AMPA glutamate receptor inhibitor causing appetite suppression	Paresthesias, dizziness, taste alterations, insomnia, constipation, dry mouth, elevation in heart rate, memory or cognitive changes[e]

AMPA = alpha-amino-3-hydroxy-5-methyl-4-isoxazole propionic acid; ER = extended release; GABA = gamma-aminobutyric acid.

[a] Food and Drug Administration–approved for short-term (i.e., a few weeks) or long-term use.

[b] Medications listed on Drug Enforcement Administration Schedule IV are associated with a lower risk of abuse than medications on Schedule III.

[c] Common adverse events for noradrenergic agents include those listed as common in Prescription Medications for the Treatment of Obesity because adverse event frequency is not available in drug package inserts for these agents.

[d] Orlistat is a non–Drug Enforcement Administration–scheduled drug.

[e] For orlistat, lorcaserin, and phentermine plus topiramate-ER, common adverse events are those listed in the drug package inserts that are reported to occur more frequently than placebo and with more than 5% prevalence. See full prescribing information for all adverse effects, cautions, and contraindications.

Modified from: Yanovski SZ, Yanovski JA. Long-term drug treatment for obesity: a systematic and clinical review. *JAMA*. January 1, 2014;311(1):74–86.

reduce their fat intake and therefore discontinue therapy owing to negative side effects.[48]

Additional studies are needed to determine the long-term health effects of obesity medications. Only orlistat, lorcaserin, and phentermine/topiramate-ER are U.S. Food and Drug Administration (FDA)-approved for long-term use; the others are approved only for short-term use.

Surgical Treatment

Individuals with a BMI of 40 or above and those with a BMI of 35 and above who have cardiopulmonary disease or type 2 diabetes may be considered as candidates for surgery. Bariatric surgery, which focuses on reducing the amount of food the stomach can hold, is the most common intervention for obese patients. Research has shown an improvement in type 2 diabetes, hypertension, dyslipidemia, and obstructive sleep apnea in patients after bariatric surgery. Individuals who are candidates for weight loss surgery must undergo a comprehensive assessment by a multidisciplinary team of healthcare providers that includes a physician, registered dietitian, and mental health professional.[49]

Morbidly obese individuals often have preexisting nutritional deficiencies possibly due to higher intake of high-calorie processed foods with poor nutritional. Before surgery, RDNs, exercise physiologists, and social workers instruct individuals on healthy eating and physical activity patterns, behavioral strategies to implement the lifestyle changes, and the importance of stress reduction and social support for long-term success.[50]

Bariatric surgery patients are at increased risk of developing nutrient deficiencies because of vomiting, decreased food intake, food intolerance, reduction of gastric secretions, and bypass of absorption surface areas.[51] The longer the length of bypassed proximal intestine the higher the risk of developing protein and vitamin deficiencies.[52] Long-term vitamin and mineral supplementation and nutrition monitoring are required after bariatric surgery.

One recent study reports a link between vitamin D status, season of the year, geographical location, and surgery outcomes. Researchers report that patients who had bariatric surgery in the United States during the winter months (January to March), the time of lowest vitamin D levels, had worse outcomes than those who underwent procedures in the summer. They also noted that patients who had surgery in the northern United States had more complications than those who had surgery in the southern United States.[53]

Obesity is a serious and highly prevalent disease that is associated with increased morbidity and mortality. Healthcare providers must take an active role in the identification, evaluation, and treatment of high-risk individuals. The interprofessional healthcare team must be comfortable discussing the topic of weight and conducting an obesity-focused treatment plan. Patients who are obese should be encouraged to participate in lifestyle therapy. Pharmacotherapy and bariatric surgery are options when indicated. Primary treatment should be directed at preventing further weight gain for overweight patients and achieving a modest 10% weight loss for obese patients.

Recap Overweight and obesity are defined as abnormal or excessive fat accumulation in the body. A person with a BMI greater than or equal to 25 is overweight, and a person with a BMI greater than or equal to 30 is obese. In 2014, more than 1.9 billion adults 18 years and older around the world were overweight, and of these, more than 600 million were obese. There is no single or simple solution to the world's overweight/obesity epidemic. The basic goal of a treatment plan for overweight individuals is to prevent further weight gain. The programs should be designed to allow for modest weight loss, weight maintenance, and management strategies for obesity comorbidities.

1. Discuss what you believe to be the most significant underlying causes for obesity.
2. Describe the treatments available for overweight and obesity. Identify which one(s) you think are most promising and discuss why you think this way.

Gastrointestinal Conditions

Preview Gastrointestinal diseases such as gastroesophageal reflux disease, irritable bowel syndrome, inflammatory bowel disease, gall bladder disease, and diverticular disease are common GI conditions affecting millions of Americans with varying levels of disease and complications that influence nutritional health and quality of life. This section defines each of these gastrointestinal diseases, discusses their prevalence, identifies their risk factors, and discusses prevention and management.

Gastroesophageal reflux disease (GERD), irritable bowel syndrome (IBS), inflammatory bowel disease (IBD), gall bladder disease, and diverticular diseases account for substantial morbidity and mortality and contribute heavily to direct healthcare costs along with indirect costs such as loss of work time and reduced worker productivity.[54] An estimated 60 to 70 million Americans are affected by these diseases every year with varying levels of severity.[55]

Gastroesophageal Reflux Disease

Gastroesophageal reflux disease (GERD) is a chronic condition in which the stomach contents reflux into the esophagus and upward, causing symptoms and complications. GERD is usually graded as mild, moderate, and severe. The most common symptoms of GERD are heartburn described as burning pain in the center of the chest behind the breastbone and regurgitation. Inflammation, erosion of the esophageal mucosa, and bleeding are also symptoms that some individuals experience.

Prevalence and Etiology of GERD

The prevalence of reflux symptoms has been steadily rising throughout the industrialized world. An estimated 20–40% of Western adult populations report chronic heartburn or regurgitation symptoms.[56] **FIGURE 13.5** provides an illustration of the worldwide levels of GERD. The incidence of GERD increases after the age of 40, and many individuals wait years before seeking medical treatment.[57]

Over 9 million primary care visits are attributed to GERD each year, and it is the most common gastroenterology-related outpatient diagnosis.[54] GERD is characterized by symptoms of gastrointestinal reflux that occurs more than twice a week and is increasingly being associated with reports of restricted activity and missed work, causing a financial burden for both employer and healthcare systems.[58,59]

Risk Factors for GERD

Current thinking is that GERD is caused by a combination of factors, both lifestyle and physiological. The most common belief is that it is a physiological problem that occurs in people with dysfunction of the lower esophageal sphincter (LES), a ring of muscle located at the bottom of the esophagus. The LES allows food to enter the stomach and then closes to prevent stomach acid from leaking back into the esophagus. In GERD, the sphincter does not always close properly, and thus allows acid to leak out of the stomach into the esophagus. GERD is associated with known risk factors such as pregnancy, alcohol consumption, poor posture, consuming large meals, eating just before bedtime, and diabetes. Factors that can lower LES pressure and lead to GERD include increased secretion of hormones (gastrin, estrogen, and progesterone), some medications (morphine, dopamine, theophylline), hiatal hernia, obesity, smoking, a high-fat diet, and consumption of specific foods, notably, spearmint, peppermint, caffeine (coffee, tea, and cola drinks), and some spices but this varies among individuals.

Percent of Population	Countries in this Criteria
15.1-30%	USA
	Argentina
	UK
	Sweden
	Turkey
	Israel
10.1%-15.0%	Iran
	Australia
5.1-10.0%	Spain
	China
0.1-5.0%	South Korea

Figure 13.5
Global distribution of the burden of gastroesophageal reflux disease. Sample-size weighted mean estimates of the prevalence of at least weekly heartburn or regurgitation in each country.

Data from El-Serag HB, Sweet S, Winchester CC, Den J. Update on the epidemiology of gastro-esophageal reflux disease: a systematic review. *Gut*. 2014;63(6):871–880. Retrieved from: http://www.ncbi.nlm.nih.gov/pmc/articles/PMC4046948/figure/F2/. Accessed August 31, 2016.

Prevention of GERD

Reducing risk factors is the primary means by which GERD can be prevented. The risk of heartburn increases as a person's BMI increases, suggesting that it is important for health professionals to encourage patients with above-average BMIs to lose weight. Even a sustained loss of just 3% to 5% of body weight can lead to health benefits.[60]

A common dietary suggestion is to avoid fatty foods. RDNs should encourage individuals with GERD to choose lean meats, poultry, fish, and beans as protein sources to reduce symptoms. Limiting the amount of fats added during cooking and at the table and choosing baked dishes instead of fried foods also reduce dietary fat. Low-fat dairy foods are a great source of calcium and vitamin D that also help prevent GERD symptoms when substituted for high-fat options.

Management of GERD

It is important for individuals diagnosed with GERD to know what and when to eat to prevent GERD flare-ups. In general, the goals of treatment are to, first, reduce the reflux, second, relieve symptoms, and, third, prevent damage to the esophagus. A common recommendation for the treatment of mild GERD is to have a trial of lifestyle modification combined with over-the-counter medications such as antacids or antisecretory agents. These strategies may provide additional health benefits along with an improvement in GERD.

Control of gastric acid secretion using pharmacologic or surgical methods should be considered. Proton pump inhibitors (PPIs) are considered the most effective medical therapy for esophagitis. GERD can cause a number of nutrition issues and poor food intake for a variety of reasons such as decreased appetite, abdominal pain, restricted eating, and intolerance of certain foods.[61–64] If vomiting occurs, electrolyte problems can develop, and if bleeding is present, iron deficiency can occur. Also, if a patient uses medications over a long period of time, calcium, iron, and vitamin B_{12} can become deficient owing to a change in stomach acid. Until controlled studies are available, diet and lifestyle modification should be used as an adjunct to medication rather than as primary treatment.[65] Surgical therapy is indicated when there is a failure of lifestyle and medical management and the symptoms persist. Surgery for GERD is called fundoplication. The goal of this surgery is to "reinforce the LES to recreate the barrier that stops reflux from occurring. This is done by wrapping a portion of the stomach around the bottom of the esophagus in an effort to strengthen, augment, or recreate the LES valve."[66] **TABLE 13.7** lists recommendations for the management of GERD.

Irritable Bowel Syndrome

Irritable bowel syndrome (IBS) is a chronic condition with symptoms that come and go. IBS comprises a group of symptoms that include discomfort and pain in the abdominal area and a change in bowel patterns that involves changes in colon rhythm. There can be alternating bouts of diarrhea and constipation.[67] IBS is one of the most common disorders diagnosed and treated by physicians and nurse practitioners.[68]

There are four types of IBS: IBS with constipation, IBS with diarrhea, mixed IBS, and unsubtyped IBS.[69] The key characteristics of each are listed in **TABLE 13.8**.

Table 13.7

Dietary and Lifestyle Modifications for the Management of GERD

- Achieve and maintain a healthy weight. Diets should be tailored to the specific patient.
- Quit smoking.
- Limit or avoid beverages that contain alcohol.
- Limit or avoid drinks with caffeine (coffee, tea, or cola drinks).
- Remain sitting upright during meals and for 45 to 60 minutes after eating.
- Avoid eating 2 to 3 hours before bedtime.
- Avoid eating large amounts of food at one time.
- Raise the head of the bed 6 to 8 inches when sleeping.
- "Bed blocks," special foam wedges, or a hospital bed may be beneficial. Pillows are not adequate because they only raise the head. (Esophagus should be higher than the stomach.)
- Avoid tight-fitting clothing.
- Limit or avoid foods that may trigger symptoms such as spices, peppermint, chocolate, citrus juices, onions, garlic, and tomato products.
- Reduce consumption of black and red pepper.
- Eat small frequent meals.

Data from: McQuaid, K. R. (2013). Gastrointestinal disorders. In M. A. Papadakis & S. J. McPhee (Eds.), 2013 *Current medical diagnosis & treatment*. (52nd ed., pp.593–597). New York, NY: McGraw-Hill Medica.; and Nowak M, Buttner P, Harrison S, and McCutchan, C. How do dietitians treat symptoms of gastro-oesophageal reflux disease in adults? Nutrition & Dietetics. 2010;67: 224–230.

Table 13.8

IBS Classifications

IBS Classification	Symptoms
IBS with constipation (IBS-C)	• Hard or lumpy stools at least 25% of the time • Loose or watery stools less than 25% of the time
IBS with diarrhea (IBS-D)	• Loose or watery stools at least 25% of the time • Hard or lumpy stools less than 25% of the time
Mixed IBS	• Hard or lumpy stools at least 25% of the time • Loose or watery stools at least 25% of the time
Unsubtyped IBS, or IBS-U	• Hard or lumpy stools less than 25% of the time • Loose or watery stools less than 25% of the time

Reproduced from National Institute of Diabetes and Digestive and Kidney Diseases. Retrieved from: https://www.niddk.nih.gov/health-information/health-topics/digestive-diseases/irritable-bowel-syndrome/Pages/definition-facts.aspx

Prevalence and Etiology of IBS

It is estimated that IBS affects 10% to 15% of U.S. adults. However, only 5% to 7% of U.S. adults have received an official diagnosis of IBS. IBS affects about twice as many women as men and most often occurs in people younger than age 45.[69] Individuals living with IBS have decreased work productivity and a diminished quality of life. Total healthcare costs for people with IBS are between 35% and 59% higher than those of patients without this condition. In the United States, the cost of IBS is estimated at $1.56 billion in indirect costs and $1.35 billion in direct costs. On a global basis, the prevalence of IBS is estimated at approximately 11%, although this estimate can vary depending on the diagnostic criteria used by the health professional.[70–75]

Analyses of gut motility on individuals living with IBS show variable transit times. Some individuals have very strong, rapid peristaltic contractions, and others have less powerful contractions.[76] The rhythm of these contractions may result from several factors such as hereditary genetics, psychosocial factors, and postinflammatory changes after a GI infection. Ingestion of enteropathogens (*Campylobacter* and *Salmonella*) from contaminated food and water can also cause acute gastroenteritis. Most individuals improve postinfection, but chronic IBS can develop in some individuals.[77–79] IBS is not associated with bowel tissue mutations or the risk of colorectal cancer. Recent research has examined hypersensitivities and allergies to certain foods. The results of this research suggest that these conditions may cause symptoms or increase the severity of symptoms by activating the immune system. Other researchers are looking at intolerances to poorly absorbed carbohydrates (e.g., fructose, lactose, sorbitol along with other sugar alcohols).[80,81]

In 2006, the Rome III diagnostic criteria were designed to enable medical practitioners to diagnose IBS. "The Rome criteria is a system developed to classify the functional gastrointestinal disorders (FGIDs) of the digestive system in which symptoms cannot be explained by the presence of structural or tissue abnormality, based on clinical symptoms."[82] A comparison table of the ROME II and III diagnostic criteria is available at http://www.romecriteria.org/assets/pdf/20_RomeIII_apB_899-916.pdf.

Risk Factors for IBS

The cause of IBS is unknown, but many factors may play a role in the development of this condition (see TABLE 13.9).

Stress has been associated with exacerbations of IBS symptoms, and anxiety and depression are also noted in some individuals who suffer with IBS. Corticotrophin-releasing hormone (CRH) moderates the stress response of the gut–brain axis. CRH can increase the colonic motility and contribute to inflammation in some IBS individuals. It may also change the gut microbiota, alter secretions, cause visceral sensitivity, and affect mucosal blood flow. Women diagnosed with IBS often suffer with symptoms during their menstrual cycle, which could suggest that reproductive hormones can have some effect.

Some patients with IBS have alterations in gut microbiota; increased ratio of Firmicutes to Bacteroidetes and a reduction in *Lactobacillus* or *Bifidobacterium* species. IBS symptoms may be caused by these bacteria. Increased Firmicutes may cause abdominal pain because they secrete large amounts of proteases that can stimulate sensory afferents in the gut. *Lactobacillus* and *Bifidobacterium* have anti-inflammatory effects in the gut, and a decrease in their numbers in the body could contribute to low-grade inflammation.[83–88]

Table 13.9

Risk Factors for IBS

- Stress
- Intestinal motility disorders
- Diet
- Menstrual cycle
- Low-fiber diets
- Consumption of suspected irritating foods
- Genetics

Data from Dinan TG, Quigley EM, Ahmed SM, et al. Hypothalamic-pituitary-gut axis dysregulation in irritable bowel syndrome: plasma cytokines as a potential biomarker? *Gastroenterology.* 2006;130(2):304–311; O'Malley D, Quigley EM, Dinan TG, Cryan JF. Do interactions between stress and immune responses lead to symptom exacerbations in irritable bowel syndrome? *Brain Behav Immun.* 2011;25(7):1333–1341; Fukudo S. Role of corticotropin-releasing hormone in irritable bowel syndrome and intestinal inflammation. *J Gastroenterol.* 2007;42(suppl 17):48–51; Konturek PC, Brzozowski T, Konturek SJ. Stress and the gut: pathophysiology, clinical consequences, diagnostic approach and treatment options. *J Physiol Pharmacol.* 2011;62(6):591–599.

Vitamin D deficiency has been found to be strongly correlated with IBS. A study of 51 adults found that 82% of participants had vitamin D levels considered insufficient. Further, the study reported that the severity of IBS symptoms was related to the level of vitamin D insufficiency. The implications of the study—whether vitamin D deficiency is a direct cause or an effect of IBS— are not fully established, but these findings do suggest that attention to maintaining adequate levels of vitamin D in patients diagnosed with IBS is warranted.[89]

Prevention of IBS

Because the cause of IBS is unknown, it is extremely difficult to prevent this disease. A focus on the controllable risk factors of stress, diet, and avoidance of irritating foods is the only means by which IBS might be prevented. In essence, stress management and eating a balanced diet are key considerations in preventing a wide variety of diseases, including IBS. In contrast, genetic predispositions, menstrual cycles, and intestinal motility disorders are not controllable factors that can enable prevention of IBS.

Management of IBS

The medical management of IBS may include diet therapy, stress management, drug therapy, and consumption of probiotics. Probiotics are live strains of bacteria and yeasts that are normally found in the digestive system and that contribute to keeping the gut healthy. All individuals should be encouraged to record a diet/symptom log (see FIGURE 13.6).

Diet Therapy

The foods or substances most commonly identified as causing symptoms in individuals with IBS include fatty foods, gas-producing foods, wheat, red meats, eggs, alcohol, caffeine, lactose, and fiber. The dietary restriction of specific foods needs to be individualized based on symptom management. To identify foods that may exacerbate symptoms, it is recommended that patients complete a detailed dietary intake of food and symptom chart for at least 7 days. Healthcare professionals need to recognize that complete restrictions of food groups can be more harmful than helpful. Many individuals start eliminating entire groups of foods (e.g., all proteins), and this can lead to a severely unbalanced nutritional intake or an obsessive preoccupation with diet.

It has been suggested that individuals with IBS may have an intolerance to certain carbohydrates. Dietitians may recommend a trial diet using the **FODMAP diet** (low fermentable oligosaccharides, disaccharides, monosaccharides, and polyol) strategy. These short-chain carbohydrates are not completely absorbed in the gastrointestinal tract and are fermented by the gut bacteria. This fermentation is a cause of the pain, gas, and diarrhea symptoms of IBS. FODMAPs are found in a variety of foods, including those containing lactose, fructose in excess of glucose, fructans, galactooligosaccharides, and polyols (sorbitol, mannitol, xylitol, and maltitol) (see FIGURE 13.7). Symptoms associated with a high-FODMAP diet include pain, bloating, distension, flatulence, and diarrhea. Luminal distension by unabsorbed or fermented FODMAPs has been considered the cause of many of the symptoms of IBS. Low-FODMAP diets have been shown to reduce GI symptoms compared with high-FODMAP diets and unrestricted diets.[90–94]

Unabsorbed fructose that reaches the colon provides a prebiotic substrate for some of the existing bacteria, which then increases the production of short-chain fatty acids (SCFAs) and gases, which include hydrogen. This can produce the IBS symptoms of excessive flatulence, bloating, and loose stools.[95–97]

Fermentable carbohydrates: Fructooligosaccharides (FOS) are carbohydrates made out of a short chain of fructose molecules. Galactooligosaccharides (GOS) are produced through the action of β-galactosidases on lactose. FOS and GOS are classified as sources of dietary fiber and are now being added to common foods for their beneficial prebiotic (food for the probiotics) effect. They are not digestible and are fermented in the colon by the gut

Fill in the log to keep track of your symptoms.
Discuss with your doctor to help identify triggers and determine how foods affects your symptoms.

Date	Time	Foods and Beverages	Symptoms Experienced	Actions Taken

Figure 13.6
GI food and symptom log.

F	Formentable: Formentable carbohydrates are sugars that are broken download digested by bacteria in our intestines, producing gas and other by-products.
O	Oligo saccharides: Oligo saccharides are short chains of carbohydrate molecules linked to gether.
	Fructans(a chain offructo semolecules) and galacto-oligosaccharides (a chain of galacto semolecules) are oligo saccharides that humans cannot break down and properly absorb in the small intestine
D	Disaccharides: Disaccharides are two carbohydrate molecules linked to gether.
	Lactose, the sugar found in milk and dairy products, is a disaccharide composed of glucose and galactose. Lactose must be broken down by the digestive enzyme lactase before it can be absorbed in the small intestine. In people with lactose intolerance, the level of lactaseenzymeis insufficient to properly digest lactose and lactose travels to the colon where fermentation occurs.
M	Monosaccharides: Monosaccharides are single carbohydrate molecules.
	Fructose, the sugar found in many fruits and some vegetables, is a monosaccharide and does not require any digestion before it is absorbed. When foods containing equl amounts of fructose and glucoseare eaten, glucose helps fructose to be completely absorbed. However, when fructose is present in greater quantities than glucose, fructose absorption depends upon the activity of sugar transporters located in the intestinal wall. Theability to absorb excess fructose varies from person to person. In people with fructose malabsorption, the capacity of sugar transporters is limited excess fructose travels to the colon where fermentation occurs.
A	And
P	Polyols: Polyols, or sugar alcohols, are a type of carbohydrate that humans can only partially digest and absorb in the small intestine.
	Polyols, such as sorbitol, mannitol, xylitol, maltitol and isomalt, mimic the sweetness of sucrose (table sugar), however, because their absorption is much slower, only a small amount of what is eaten is actually absorbed. Polyols are often used as low-calorie sweeteners in sugar-free and diet products.

Figure 13.7

What does FODMAP mean?

Reproduced from Canadian Digestive Health Foundation. Understanding FODMAPs. Oakville, ON: Canadian Digestive Health Foundation. Retrieved from: http://www.cdhf.ca/bank/document_en/32-fodmaps.pdf#zoom=100. Accessed August 30, 2016.

microbiota, stimulating growth of the resident microbiota (e.g., *Bifidobacteria*). GOS have been shown to improve pain, bloating, and constipation in patients with IBS.[98],[99] Polyols are sugar alcohols such as sorbitol, mannitol, xylitol, maltitol, and isomalt. Some polyols are too large to diffuse through intercellular spaces and they remain unabsorbed, which leads to flatulence, abdominal pain, and osmotic diarrhea. Lactose is a disaccharide that is hydrolyzed by the enzyme lactase. When a person lacks the lactase enzyme, the result is that unabsorbed lactose passes into the colon, where it undergoes bacterial fermentation that produces SCFAs and gases, leading to flatulence, diarrhea,

bloating, and nausea. Examples of specific foods that contain FODMAPS are presented in TABLE 13.10.

To reduce the symptoms associated with FODMAPs, researchers recommend limiting fructose to less than 0.2 g per serving, GOS and fructans to less than 0.2 g (less than 0.3 g for breads/cereals) per serving, and sugar polyol to less than 0.3 g per individual polyol or less than 0.5 g total polyols per serving.[100]

The FODMAP diet is fairly restrictive, and a RDN should be consulted to assist individuals with menu planning to ensure the diet provides adequate nutrients. For example, an RDN can assist individuals with lactose

Table 13.10

Foods that Contain FODMAPs

Fructans	Galactooligosaccharides	Lactose	Fructans	Polyols
Vegetables:	*Legumes:*	*Milk Products:*	*Fruits:*	*Fruits:*
Artichokes, asparagus, beets, garlic, leeks, onions	Beans: baked kidney, chickpeas, lentils, soy products	Milk and milk products such as custard, dairy desserts, ice cream, margarine, yogurt	Apples, figs, mangoes, pears, watermelon	Apples, apricots, blackberries, cherries, nectarines, peaches, pears, plums, prunes
Grains:		*Cheese:*	*Sweeteners:*	*Vegetables:*
Barley, rye, and wheat in large amounts, fructooligosaccharides, inulin		Ricotta cheese, cottage cheese, cream cheese	Agave, corn syrup, high-fructose corn syrup, honey	Avocado, cauliflower, green pepper, mushrooms, pumpkin, snow peas
Nuts:			*Alcohol:*	*Sweeteners:*
Cashews, pistachios			Rum	Sorbitol, mannitol, isomalt, maltitol, xylitol

Modified from Canadian Digestive Health Foundation. Understanding FODMAPs. Oakville, ON: Canadian Digestive Health Foundation. Retrieved from: http://www.cdhf.ca/bank /document_en/32-fodmaps.pdf. Accessed August 30, 2016.

intolerance who have difficulty meeting the daily requirements for calcium and vitamin D.

It is also important for any person who experiences IBS to realize that fluid intake is extremely important to alleviate and deal with symptoms. If individuals are constipated, then adequate fluid is needed so that stools are not so hard. Conversely, with diarrhea, a person suffers considerable fluid loss that needs to be replaced. In both situations, adequate fluid intake can help reduce symptoms.

Probiotics have been shown to be of help in some individuals living with IBS. However, replicable scientific evidence is limited owing to the differences in the strain and species of probiotics studied and the duration of therapy. A decrease in bacterial fermentation through the introduction of probiotics may decrease the gas-related symptoms of IBS and alter colonic transit. *Bifidobacterium infantis* 35624, for example, was shown to result in alleviation of symptoms in patients with IBS in two clinical trials and also has been shown to exert potent anti-inflammatory effects.[101–107]

Inflammatory Bowel Disease

Inflammatory bowel disease (IBD) is a chronic condition with periodic immune responses combined with inflammation in the gastrointestinal tract. The two most common forms of IBD are ulcerative colitis (see **FIGURE 13.8**) and Crohn's disease. Crohn's disease affects the entire digestive tract and all three of the mucosal layers. In ulcerative colitis, the symptoms are restricted to the large intestine, and the mucosa is affected. The clinical presentation of both of these diseases often involves similar symptoms such as diarrhea, abdominal discomfort, and other symptoms involving the skin, joints, and eyes.

Prevalence and Etiology of IBD

Current research studies suggest there has been an increase in the number of people with IBD. The most recent data indicate that approximately 1.6 million Americans have IBD, an increase of about 200,000 since 2011. Annually, nearly 70,000 new cases of IBD are diagnosed in the United States.[108–111]

Individuals with IBD experience a variety of symptoms and complications that change over time, ranging from mild to severe (see **TABLE 13.11**). IBD can go into remission for a time and then flare up again. Symptoms of IBD that are specifically related to inflammation of the GI tract often include diarrhea, rectal bleeding, an urgent need to move bowels, abdominal cramps and pain, sensations of incomplete evacuation, and constipation that can lead to bowel obstruction. Other general symptoms can occur with IBD such as fever, loss of appetite, weight loss, fatigue, night sweats, and, in women, loss of normal menstrual cycle.

Risk Factors for IBD

At this time, there is no known direct cause of IBD, but linkages that involve an interaction between genes, the immune system, and environmental factors are suspected. A number of risk factors, both modifiable and nonmodifiable, have been identified and are listed in **TABLE 13.12**. Approximately 10% to 25% of individuals with

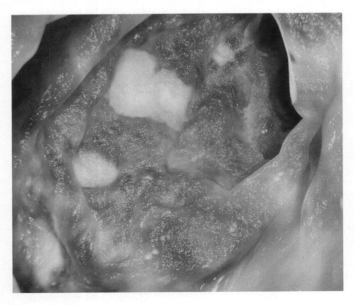

Figure 13.8
Ulcerative colitis.

©Juan Gartner/Science Photo Library/Getty

Table 13.11		
Complications of IBD		
Complications Inside the GI Tract		Complications Outside the GI Tract
Crohn's Disease	*Ulcerative Colitis*	*Crohn's Disease and Ulcerative Colitis*
Fistula	Diarrhea	Eyes: sore, red, itchy
Stricture	Rectal bleeding	Mouth: sores
Abscess	Rectal pain	Joints: swelling and pain
Perforated bowel	Perforated bowel	Skin: sores, rash, erythema nodosum, pyoderma gangrenosum
Ulcers	Toxic megacolon	Bones: osteopenia/ osteoporosis
Colon cancer		Kidney stones—common side effect of Crohn's disease that often require restriction of oxalate in the meal plan
Dietary complications: malabsorption/ malnutrition		

Data from: Crohn's and Colitis Foundation of America; May 11, 2011. Facts about inflammatory bowel diseases. Retrieved from: http://www.ccfa.org/resources/facts-about-inflammatory.html. Accessed August 31, 2016.

Table 13.12
Risk Factors for IBD
Age and gender
Race and ethnicity
Genetics
Smoking
Diet
Physical activity
Infections
Antibiotics
Appendectomy
Psychosocial factors
Sleep deprivation

IBD have a first-degree relative with either Crohn's disease or ulcerative colitis.[112,113] The most common age of diagnosis is between 15 and 40 years for both males and females. There can be a second wave of diagnosis between 50 and 80 years of age. The cause of the second wave is unclear, but some researchers suggest that it could result from a higher susceptibility as individuals age or that IBD may occur later in life owing to environmental exposure earlier in life.

Slightly more females than males are diagnosed with Crohn's disease, and it is suspected that a hormonal factor increases the incidence of the disease in women later in life. There is a slightly higher incidence of ulcerative colitis in males. Both ulcerative colitis and Crohn's disease are more common in individuals of Jewish heritage. The incidence of IBD is lower in black and Hispanic populations as compared with Caucasian populations.

Smoking is associated with an increased risk of Crohn's disease. Cigarette smoking may have a different effect in ulcerative colitis: The administration of nicotine may alleviate the signs and symptoms of ulcerative colitis in ex-smokers. Smoking cessation in patients with ulcerative colitis is associated with an increase in the disease activity and hospitalization.[114,115]

At this time, data suggest that a "North American" diet (high in processed, fried, and sugary foods) is associated with an increased risk of developing Crohn's disease and possibly ulcerative colitis. Hypersensitivity to cow's milk protein in infancy has been discussed as a cause of IBD, especially ulcerative colitis. A survey of IBD patients noted that cow's milk hypersensitivity was more common in patients diagnosed with ulcerative colitis and Crohn's disease when compared with controls. Refined sugar intake has also been linked to the development of IBD, especially Crohn's disease. Long-term intake of dietary fiber, particularly from fruit, has been associated with a decrease in the risk of Crohn's disease, but not ulcerative colitis. An increased dietary intake of total fat, animal fat,

polyunsaturated fatty acids, and milk protein has been correlated with an increased incidence of ulcerative colitis and Crohn's disease and also relapses in patients previously diagnosed with ulcerative colitis. A higher intake of omega-3 fatty acids and a lower intake of omega-6 fatty acids have been associated with a lower risk of developing Crohn's disease.[116,117] In addition to diet, physical activity has been identified as a modifiable risk factor associated with a decrease in risk of Crohn's disease, but not of ulcerative colitis.[118]

An imbalance in the gut microbiome may contribute to the development of IBD. Several observational studies suggest an association between acute gastroenteritis and the development of IBD.[119] The change in gut flora from overuse of antibiotics may be a risk factor for IBD. So far, antibiotic use has been associated with IBD, but conclusive evidence in this area is not available and more research is needed.[120] A number of studies suggest that appendectomy may protect against the development of ulcerative colitis, but the reason for this is unknown.[117]

Stress may have a role in the exacerbation of symptoms in patients with IBD. Stress is associated with changes in both the systemic immune and the inflammatory functions, which may be relevant to the pathogenesis of IBD.[121] Sleep deprivation has been associated with an increased risk of ulcerative colitis and disease flares in patients previously diagnosed with IBD.[122]

Case Study

Annie M. did not have incidences of sleep deprivation prior to diagnosis at the age of 10 years. However, her current lifestyle, which involves travel and performing, does lead to some incidences of sleep deprivation, thus putting her at higher risk.

Questions:

1. What suggestions can you make for Annie M. to improve her eating pattern while traveling?
2. What effects does sleep deprivation have on diet and food intake?

Prevention of IBD

As is the case with IBS, the cause of IBD is unknown, making it very difficult to prevent this disease. Like IBS, the best approach is to focus on the controllable risk factors of stress, diet, smoking, physical activity, and sufficient sleep. Stress management, eating a balanced diet, and leading a healthy lifestyle, as well as many other choices related to lifestyle, are key to preventing IBD. In contrast, a genetic predisposition is not a controllable factor that can enable prevention of IBS.

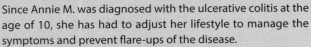

Case Study

Since Annie M. was diagnosed with the ulcerative colitis at the age of 10, she has had to adjust her lifestyle to manage the symptoms and prevent flare-ups of the disease.

Her disease is currently stable and has been treated with drug therapy and dietary management so far. Always athletic, as an adult Annie has become a professional performer who puts on athletic demonstrations that require her to maintain a high level of fitness and an attractive appearance. Her lifestyle and profession pose challenges for having a regular routine with regular meals and healthy dietary choices. Annie M.'s athletic and performance skills are the focus of her life at this time. Because of a mild learning disability, Annie M. has always found academic pursuits very challenging, so a career change is not something that would be either welcome or easy. Lately, however, Annie M has felt tired and lack of ability to concentrate, which concerns her with an upcoming busy performance and travel schedule.

Questions

1. Discuss some of the complications that could develop over time, both inside and outside the GI tract, in individuals like Annie M., who are living with IBD.
2. Identify the key risk factors for IBD and discuss how they relate to the case of Annie M.
3. Describe some of the prevention strategies that people with family histories can employ for IBD once they have been diagnosed.
4. Offer Annie M. some dietary suggestions to increase her energy and improve her concentration.

Management of IBD

The goal of medication use for people with IBD is to suppress the enhanced immune response to induce or to maintain remission. Commonly used medications for IBD treatment include corticosteroids, aminosalicylates, and immune suppressants such as methotrexate and azathioprine. The recent development of biological agents (monoclonal antibodies against tumor necrosis factor [TNF]-alpha) that target the adaptive immune system has improved the quality of life of many patients living with IBD. Approximately one-third of patients will achieve remission, however, many of the individuals who initially respond to this treatment will eventually lose their response over time.[123]

Diet Therapy

A regular evaluation of nutrient status is recommended because malnutrition is present in up to 85% of patients with IBD and weight loss occurs in up to 80% of patients with Crohn's disease. Between 18% and 62% of patients diagnosed with ulcerative colitis also experience weight loss.[124–126] Consequently, patients who have been diagnosed with IBD should routinely have their BMI measured. As such, every individual with IBD needs ready access to the services of a dietitian. Regular measurement helps the dietitian develop a long-term assessment of each individual's nutritional status. In addition to BMI, an assessment of muscle function provides useful information.

Registered dietitian nutritionists (RDNs) often ask individuals with IBD to complete a food and symptom record (see Figure 13.6). Individuals are also asked to complete a symptom diary that can help with the identification of foods that may trigger or exacerbate events and symptoms. The typical time frame for record keeping for an initial assessment is 3 days that includes one weekend day.

Nutrition intervention depends on the status of the gastrointestinal tract. During acute exacerbations, the level of nutrition intervention is determined by the amount of diarrhea, amount of vomiting, presence of obstructions, use of surgical procedures, and amount of bleeding. Enteral nutrition or parenteral nutrition is used as supportive therapy when an oral diet cannot meet nutritional needs. During exacerbations or when an individual has a stricture, fiber intake is restricted. It is recommended that individuals eat small, frequent meals; drink adequate fluids; avoid caffeine and alcohol; take vitamin and mineral supplements as recommended by a RDN; eliminate dairy foods if lactose intolerant; limit excess fat; and reduce carbohydrates. Special supplemental food formulas have been developed and marketed for use during Crohn's or ulcerative colitis flares. These formulas are often elemental or semielemental preparations and are usually not consumed for long periods of time owing to cost, taste, smell, and texture. The overall goal is to slowly add all foods back to the diet as tolerated.[127–130]

Calorie and Protein Intake

Consumption of appropriate energy and protein is required for patients who need to gain weight or if weight was lost during a flare or as a result of surgery or who need to prevent weight loss. The goal is to replenish nutrient stores, and an RDN needs to provide customized counseling to each individual because of the varying gastrointestinal functions. A well-balanced, complete, and nutrient-dense diet is the ultimate goal for IBD patients who are in remission. Patients with IBD may have increased protein needs because of excessive loss from inflammation of the intestinal tract or catabolism resulting from an infection. In addition, protein may assist with the healing process in both pre- and post-surgery circumstances. RDNs often recommend protein intakes of 1.0–1.5 g/kg body weight as long as the individual has normal kidney function.

Energy
Protein
Fluid
Electrolytes
Iron
Magnesium (in those with increased intestinal losses)
Calcium
Vitamin D
Vitamin B$_{12}$
Folate
Copper (in those with excessive diarrhea, fistulas, or ostomies)
Zinc (in those with excessive diarrhea, fistulas, or ostomies)
Vitamin A

Figure 13.9
Nutrient deficiencies observed in IBD.

Vitamins and Minerals

Nutrient deficiencies are a major concern in patients with IBD (see FIGURE 13.9), and the patient's dietitian may decide to focus on specific areas of nutrition, depending on the individual's nutritional status. Iron deficiency occurs in about 60–80% of patients with IBD, and anemia manifests in approximately one-third of patients. Poor dietary intakes of iron-rich foods resulting from food aversions or intolerances can contribute to anemia. Individuals often cannot tolerate oral iron supplements because of gastrointestinal side effects, and they may require an intravenous administration. Anemia in IBD may also be caused by folate or vitamin B$_{12}$ deficiency that can result from increased nutritional requirements, poor dietary intake, malabsorption, or the medication sulfasalazine that is used in the treatment of inflammatory bowel disease.[131–134]

B vitamins: Serum vitamin B$_{12}$ and folate deficiencies are more common in patients with Crohn's disease compared with patients with ulcerative colitis. Previous surgery on the small intestine is a risk factor for having a low serum vitamin B$_{12}$ level in Crohn's disease patients; vitamin B$_{12}$ deficiency can occur in patients who have had surgical resections of the stomach where intrinsic factor is produced or the terminal ileum the site of absorption.[135] Some medications used to treat IBD such as methotrexate, a folate antagonist, and sulfasalazine, for example, block folate absorption and therefore increase folate requirements.[136]

Calcium and vitamin D: Patients with IBD have up to a 40% increased risk of fractures compared with the general population's risk. The research shows that osteopenia in ulcerative colitis is found in about 35% of patients, and osteoporosis in about 15%, based on dual-energy X-ray absorptiometry (DXA) scans. Few studies have been completed on the prevalence of osteopenic and osteoporotic fractures in patients with ulcerative colitis. Poor calcium and

vitamin D intake, aging, weight loss over 10% of body weight, a BMI less than 20, malabsorption, corticosteroid use, and inflammation all contribute to the development of osteoporosis. RDNs examine the dose and duration of corticosteroids, assess dietary intake of calcium and vitamin D, and then recommend supplements if needed.[137–139]

Nutrition Recommendations During Remission in IBD

Following are suggestions for nutrition management during IBD remission:

Low-FODMAP diet: As previously discussed in the section on IBS, FODMAPs are poorly digested short-chain carbohydrates that increase fluid and gas production in the gastrointestinal tract. In IBD patients, increases in gas and fluid may lead to abdominal bloating, pain, flatulence, and diarrhea. A low-FODMAP diet is complex, avoids a wide range of foods, and requires several dietary counseling sessions with detailed written information to support the dietary advice.[140] Some individuals in remission with IBD but who experience IBS symptoms respond well to a low-FODMAP diet.[141]

Probiotics: Probiotics are live strains of bacteria and yeasts normally found in the digestive system that contribute to keeping the gut healthy. Only a few randomized controlled trials have been completed using probiotics in patients with IBD. Probiotic therapy with *Escherichia coli* Nissle 1917 has been found to be as effective as drug therapy with aminosalicylate (5-ASA) in maintaining IBD remission. More research is needed to determine efficacy, recommended use, and dosing for patients with IBD. TABLE 13.13 summarizes information on the probiotics used in patients with IBD.[142–146]

Table 13.13

Probiotic Use for IBD

Form of IBD	Probiotics Used
Ulcerative colitis	*E. coli* Nissle 1917
	VSL#3
	A blend of bacteria, including *Bifidobacterium breve, B. longum, B. infantis, Lactobacillus acidophilus, L. plantarum, L. casein, L. bulgaricus, Streptococcus thermophile, L. boulardi,* and *L. rhamnosis GG.*
Crohn's disease (probiotics haven't shown significant benefit in Crohn's disease)	*L. boulardi*
	L. rhamnosis GG
	L. johnsonii
	VSL#3
Pouchitis	VSL#3
	L. rhamnosis GG

Diverticular Disease

As a person ages it is common for the walls in the colon to develop bulging pockets of tissue, or sacs. A single sac that has an outward bulge is referred to as a diverticulum (see **FIGURE 13.10**). Multiple sacs are referred to as diverticula. A person who has diverticula in the colon is diagnosed with **diverticulosis**. However, the mere presence of diverticula alone does not mean a person exhibits symptoms or develops diverticular disease.

Prevalence and Etiology of Diverticular Disease

Diverticular disease is a common problem and is a very costly disease. Each year, complications from diverticular disease account for over 300,000 hospital admissions, 1.5 million inpatient days, and $2.4 billion in healthcare costs.[147] Individuals older than 60 years often have colonic diverticula, with 10% to 25% developing complications such as diverticulitis. Diverticular disease has been considered a "Western disease." The highest prevalence is in the United States, Europe, and Australia, where approximately 50% of the population 60 years of age and older have diverticulosis. In the United States, its prevalence increases with age, and about 70% of people 80 years and older show diverticulosis. The incidence of diverticular disease and its complications is increasing, and the number of patients suffering from diverticular disease is expected to expand in the following years as a result of the increase in the number of older adults in the U.S. population.[148–151] There are some racial differences in the manifestation of the disease.[152]

Diverticular disease starts with herniation of the colonic mucosa and muscularis mucosa through the intestinal wall, which is more often seen in the sigmoid colon. A herniation seen as a saccular protrusion or outpouching of the colon is called a diverticulum, and more than one are called diverticula. The presence of diverticula is called diverticulosis. **Diverticulitis** occurs when there is inflammation of one or more diverticula. Diverticulitis complications include intestinal obstruction, bleeding, abscess, fistula, and perforation. The location of colonic diverticula can lead to different complications: left diverticulosis shows higher risk of inflammatory complications (mainly diverticulitis), and right diverticulosis has a higher risk of bleeding.[153,154] The majority of people with diverticular disease do not have any symptoms, however, apporximately 25% of those with diverticulosis experience symptoms such as occasional bloating, flatulence, pain, nausea, vomiting, fever, and a problem with their intestinal motility, which results in either diarrhea or constipation. Diverticulitis most commonly is diagnosed when an acute attack results in an emergency hospital admission.[155]

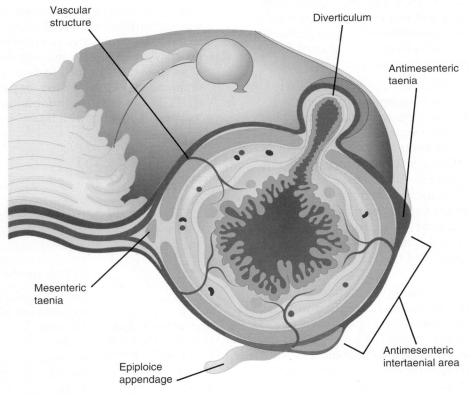

Figure 13.10
Diverticular disease.

Risk Factors for Diverticular Disease

Some researchers propose that a low-fiber diet causes segmentation to occur more frequently, which can result in higher localized intraluminal pressure. Higher intraluminal pressure along with a weakened colonic musculature, which naturally occurs with aging, can favor the development of diverticular disease. A number of well-known factors such as aging, genetics, body weight, and other GI disorders affect the risk of developing diverticular disease.

With advancing age there is an increase in collagen in the colonic wall and a reduction in tensile strength that can result in herniation. Further, as individuals age, intestinal motility slows, meaning stool stays in the colon a longer time, putting pressure on the colonic wall and increasing time of exposure to intestinal wastes.[156] There is an association between certain rare genetic disorders and predisposition toward diverticula formation and a familial component has been suggested.[157–160] One theory concerning the link between obesity and diverticular disease is that obesity alters the gut microbiota, which might be contributory to the development of diverticular disease. Researchers have proposed that microflora may affect the development of diverticular disease.[161–163] Inflammation has been observed in people who are obese. It is known that adipose tissue secretes various cytokines and proinflammatory compounds that have local and systemic effects.[164,165] People who already suffer from IBS appear to have significantly increased risk for diverticular disease.[156,166,167]

Physical inactivity, a history of constipation, red meat consumption, meat-based versus plant-based diets, higher socioeconomic status, and hypertension have been suggested as risk factors of diverticular disease, but so far studies in these areas are limited. More research on the influence of these factors on the development and progression of diverticular disease is needed.[168,169]

Prevention of Diverticular Disease

To prevent diverticular disease, it is recommended that individuals meet the daily recommended fiber intakes of 38 g/day for men 19–50 years of age, 30 g/day for men 51 years of age and older, 25 g/day for women 19–50 years of age, and 21 g/day for women 51 years of age and older. Many people do not get enough fiber in their diet, and experts suggest an increase of 5 g per week until recommended levels are reached. For people who are adding fiber to their diet, it is important that they increase fiber intake gradually and consume plenty of fluid as fiber intake increases.

Regular exercise, especially aerobic exercise, is also recommended. Exercise speeds the movement of food through the colon, reducing the risk of constipation and the formation of hard, dry stools. Both fiber and exercise assist in obesity prevention. Obesity has been linked in several reports to the development of diverticulitis and diverticular bleeding.

Management of Diverticular Disease

As described earlier, diverticulosis is simply the presence of small bulging sacs in the colon. However, if one or more of these diverticula become infected, the patient develops diverticulitis. The treatment for diverticulitis involves oral antibiotics, anti-inflammatory medication, and a low-fiber diet when symptoms are acute. When abdominal pain and tenderness are more severe, a fever is present, and the patient is unable to consume food, the individual must be hospitalized and treatment involves bowel rest, IV fluids, and antibiotics. Surgery may be required if there is obstruction, major perforations, abscesses, or fistulas.[170]

Dietary Recommendations for Diverticulitis

If diverticulitis is suspected, the individual will be given nothing by mouth before medical tests are conducted. The goal is to rest the bowel until the bleeding and diarrhea resolve. The next step is to add clear fluids. Enteral nutrition may be needed if bowel obstruction occurs or if the ileocecal valve is inefficient and there is distension in the small intestine. The medical nutrition therapy (MNT) for acute diverticulitis consists of a low-fiber diet (10 to 15 g/day) for a short time after the attack and then very gradual increases in fiber.

Dietary Recommendations for Diverticulosis

The goal is to reach and maintain a high-fiber diet and include enough fluids on a daily basis. The fiber recommendation for Americans is 25 g for most adult women and up to 38 g for men. The restriction of nuts, seeds, corn, and popcorn, once a hallmark of MNT for this disease, is now no longer considered necessary.[170] RDNs will assess dietary intake and nutritional status and may recommend folic acid, vitamin B_{12}, or iron if anemia is present from gastrointestinal bleed or poor nutritional status. Dietitians may also recommend adding into the meal plan a probiotic food such as yogurt or kefir daily.[143,144,152,171–178]

Gallbladder Disease

The gallbladder plays an important role in the human digestive system. It stores bile produced by the liver until it is needed for digestion of fats in the small intestine. The gallbladder is directly connected to the small intestine via the common bile duct. As food passes from the stomach into the small intestine, the hormone cholecystokinin is released, causing the gallbladder to contract and secrete bile into the small intestine. Bile is composed of bile salts, fatty compounds, cholesterol, and other substances. These bile salts act as emulsifiers and surfactants to reduce the size of the fat droplets, thus breaking up fats. **Gallbladder disease** is any impairment of the normal function of the gallbladder that leads to abdominal discomfort and the inability to digest fatty foods.

Prevalence and Etiology of Gallbladder Disease

More than 25 million Americans have gallstones, and a million are diagnosed each year (see FIGURE 13.11). A small percentage (1–3%) of the population complain of symptoms. Approximately 60% of patients with acute cholecystitis are women; however, the disease tends to be more severe in men.[179]

Gallstones form when the bile becomes concentrated in the gallbladder and transforms into a stone-like material. There are three types of stones: cholesterol, pigment, and primary bile duct. Although most gallstones do not cause any symptoms, they can cause problems if they obstruct the bile ducts, which can then cause inflammation, infection, and pancreatitis. Common symptoms observed in gallbladder disease include fever, jaundice, abdominal pain after eating high-fat foods, abdominal bloating, gas, indigestion, and clay-colored stools.

Risk Factors for Gallbladder Disease

A number of well-recognized risk factors for gallbladder disease are listed in TABLE 13.14 .

Females have a greater risk of developing gallstones if they become pregnant because gallbladder motility is decreased. In addition, females on hormone therapy or birth control pills are at higher risk because estrogen increases cholesterol and its saturation in bile and promotes slow motility of the gallbladder.[180,181]

People who are older than 60 years of age have an increased risk of gallbladder disease. Individuals who develop complex symptomatic cholelithiasis are often older in age as well. Females who develop gallstones are typically in their 40s. American Indians have the highest prevalence of cholelithiasis. Gallstone disease is also prevalent in Hispanics of Chilean and Mexican

Table 13.14
Risk Factors for Gallbladder Disease
Gender
Age
Ethnicity
Obesity
Weight loss
Diabetes
High-carbohydrate diet

descent.[180,182] A diet high in fats and carbohydrates predisposes a patient to obesity, which increases cholesterol synthesis and biliary secretion of cholesterol. Some individuals who lose weight very quickly, who lose a large amount of weight, or who follow a very-low-kilocalorie diet can develop gallbladder problems. This is because when the body metabolizes fat as an individual loses weight quickly, the liver secretes extra cholesterol into the bile, changing its consistency, which can lead to gallstones. A very-low-calorie diet or fasting can decrease the movement of bile in the gallbladder, which can then cause the bile to become overconcentrated with cholesterol, thus leading to the development of gallstones. People with diabetes are at higher risk for gallstones, and when stones develop, individuals with diabetes are at higher risk of developing infection. A high intake of sugar and carbohydrates has been associated with an increased risk for gallstones.

Prevention and Management of Gallbladder Disease

Achieving a healthy weight and consuming a healthy diet that incorporates fiber and fruit and vegetables has been shown to decrease risk for gallstones.

A cholecystectomy (surgical removal of the gall bladder) is the primary method of treating gallstones when there is a problem. This surgery is done either by laparoscopy or by open technique. Diarrhea can occur in some individuals after a cholecystectomy as a result of an increased amount of bile in the large bowel. Dietary intervention is very important both pre- and postsurgery. Typically, an RDN instructs patients to consume a healthy diet with moderate amounts of fat—20–35% of calories as fat—before surgery. A diet too low in fat may lead to decreased cholecystokinin secretion and inadequate bile production, which can lead to stone formation. Small, frequent meals may be better tolerated than large meals. After surgery, patients should be able to tolerate a normal diet that provides 20–35% of calories from fat.[183]

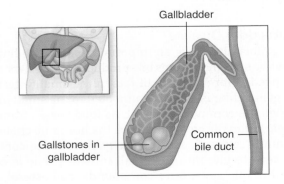

Figure 13.11
Gallstones in the gallbladder.

Recap Gastroesophageal reflux disease (GERD) is a chronic condition in which stomach contents reflux into the esophagus and upward, causing symptoms and complications. An estimated 20–40% of Western adult populations report chronic heartburn or regurgitation symptoms. Diet and lifestyle modification are used as an adjunct to medication rather than as primary treatment for GERD.

Irritable bowel syndrome (IBS) is a chronic condition comprising a group of symptoms that include discomfort and pain in the abdominal area and a change in bowel patterns. Globally, the prevalence of IBS is estimated to be approximately 11% of the population. RDNs may suggest using the FODMAP diet (a diet low in fermentable oligosaccharides, disaccharides, monosaccharides, and polyols) for treatment.

Inflammatory bowel disease (IBD) is a chronic condition with periodic immune responses combined with inflammation in the gastrointestinal tract. Approximately 1.6 million Americans have IBD. The two most common forms are ulcerative colitis and Crohn's disease. A regular evaluation of nutrient status is recommended because malnutrition is often present.

Diverticular disease is common in the population because as individuals age the walls of the colon often develop bulging pockets of tissue or sacs known as diverticula. In the United States, approximately 50% of the population 60 years of age and older have diverticulosis. If these sacs become inflamed and infected, diverticulitis occurs and is usually treated with oral antibiotics, anti-inflammatory medication, and a low-fiber diet.

Gallbladder disease is an impairment of the normal function of the gallbladder usually caused by gallstones blocking the bile duct. Gallstones form when the bile becomes concentrated in the gallbladder, transforming into a stone-like material. More than 25 million Americans have gallstones, and aside from surgical removal, patients are usually instructed to consume a healthy diet with moderate amounts of fat (20–35% of calories from fat).

1. Identify the risk factors associated with GERD and the primary physiological cause of GERD.
2. Discuss the dietary recommendations that might be suggested for patients who have been diagnosed with GERD.
3. List some ways to help people with IBS manage their symptoms.
4. Name five important nutritional deficiencies associated with IBD and discuss how they can be managed.
5. Explain the key preventive measures a person can take to avoid diverticular disease.
6. Identify the symptoms of gallbladder disease.

Endocrine and Metabolic Conditions

Preview The two most significant endocrine and metabolic conditions are metabolic syndrome and type 2 diabetes mellitus, which are both chronic diseases. This section discusses the prevalence and etiology, identifies key risk factors, and then discusses methods of prevention and management.

Metabolic syndrome has a high rate of incidence throughout the world, and the rate continues to rise. Lifestyle changes accompanied by proper dietary management can positively influence the outcome of metabolic syndrome. Type 2 diabetes mellitus may develop in people who first exhibit metabolic syndrome. It is a condition in which the pancreas fails to produce enough insulin for normal body function or the insulin that is produced does not work properly in the body. Type 1 diabetes mellitus is the most common form of diabetes, and proper dietary management is an essential component in successful management of this chronic disease.

Metabolic Syndrome

Metabolic syndrome is not a disease but rather a combination of risk factors that include high cholesterol level, high blood sugar level, high blood pressure, and excess abdominal fat. In combination, these risk factors predispose an individual to higher risks of heart attack, stroke, and type 2 diabetes mellitus.

Prevalence and Etiology of Metabolic Syndrome

The incidence of metabolic syndrome among adults has risen dramatically around the world. Approximately one-third of the adult population in the United States has metabolic syndrome.[184] The occurrence of metabolic syndrome increases with age and increases in relation to higher BMI levels. Nearly 35% of all U.S. adults and 50% of those 60 years of age or older were estimated to have metabolic syndrome in 2011–2012. Prevalence increased by age groups, from 18.3% among those 20 to 39 years of age to 46.7% among people 60 years or older. Within the 60-plus age group, more than 50% of women and Hispanics had metabolic syndrome.

The prevalence of metabolic syndrome in the United States is highest among Hispanic adults and blacks. Genetic and environmental factors may contribute to the progression of metabolic syndrome, but the close relationship between abdominal obesity and insulin resistance may be another factor in the increasing rate of diagnosis.[185–187]

Risk Factors for Metabolic Syndrome

Lifestyle is a key factor in the cause and management of metabolic syndrome. Metabolic syndrome is defined by a group of physiological, biochemical, clinical, and metabolic factors, namely, insulin resistance, visceral adiposity, dyslipidemia, endothelial dysfunction, and elevated blood pressure, that increase the risk of cardiovascular disease and type 2 diabetes.[188]

The National Cholesterol Education Program Adults Treatment Panel III identified six areas of metabolic syndrome that are related to cardiovascular disease. They are central abdominal obesity, dyslipidemia (elevated triglycerides, low high-density lipoprotein [HDL] cholesterol, elevated low-density lipoprotein [LDL] cholesterol), high blood pressure, insulin resistance, proinflammatory state (elevations of C-reactive protein [CRP]), and prothrombotic state (increased plasma plasminogen activator inhibitor as well as fibrinogen). Fibrinogen is an acute-phase reactant like CRP and increases in response to a high-cytokine state.[189]

The National Cholesterol Education Program Adult Treatment Panel III Report (**ATP III**) recommends that the diagnosis of metabolic syndrome be made when three or more of the following risk determinants are present: abdominal obesity, high levels of triglycerides, low levels of HDL cholesterol, high blood pressure, and high fasting plasma glucose (see **TABLE 13.15**).[190,191]

Prevention of Metabolic Syndrome

Prevention of metabolic syndrome is a foremost goal for the American population. The focus of efforts is to prevent or decrease abdominal obesity. Lifestyle modification with diet and increased physical activity is recommended. Another goal for Americans is to prevent insulin resistance and hyperglycemia. Lifestyle modification and weight loss are recommended to assist in the prevention of insulin resistance. Insulin resistance is a condition in which the tissues of the body have lowered response levels to the hormone insulin. Blood pressure should be lowered to achieve a goal of < 140/90 mm Hg. Lifestyle modifications and following the DASH (Dietary Approaches to Stop Hypertension) diet can assist with this process.[192–194] *Healthy People 2020* includes dietary

Table 13.15

ATP III Clinical Identification of Metabolic Syndrome

Risk Factor	Defining Level
Abdominal obesity, given as waist circumference[a]	
Men[b]	> 102 cm (> 40 inches)
Women	> 88 cm (> 35 inches)
Triglycerides	≥ 150 mg/dL
HDL cholesterol	
Men	< 40 mg/dL
Women	< 50 mg/dL
Blood pressure	≥ 130/≥ 85 mm Hg
Fasting glucose	≥ 110 mg/dL[c]

[a] Overweight and obesity are associated with insulin resistance and metabolic syndrome. However, the presence of abdominal obesity is more highly correlated with the metabolic risk factors than is an elevated BMI. Therefore, the simple measure of waist circumference is recommended to identify the body weight component of metabolic syndrome.

[b] Some male patients can develop multiple metabolic risk factors when the waist circumference is only marginally increased, for example, 94 to 102 cm (37 to 39 inches). Such patients may have a strong genetic contribution to insulin resistance. They should benefit from changes in life habits similar to men with categorical increases in waist circumference.

[c] The American Diabetes Association has recently established a cut point of ≥ 100 mg/dL, above which persons have either prediabetes (impaired fasting glucose) or diabetes. This new cut point should be applied to identify the lower boundary of elevated glucose level as one criterion for establishing metabolic syndrome.

Data from Alberti KGMM, Eckel RH, Grundy SM, et al. Joint scientific statement: harmonizing the metabolic syndrome. *Circulation*. October 20, 2009;120: 1640–1645. doi:http://dx.doi.org/10.1161/CIRCULATIONAHA.109.192644.

Table 13.16

Healthy People 2020 Dietary Recommendations for Chronic Disease Prevention

- Consume a variety of nutrient-dense foods within and across the food groups, especially whole grains, fruits, vegetables, low-fat or fat-free milk or milk products, and lean meats and other protein sources.
- Limit the intake of saturated and trans fats, cholesterol, added sugars, sodium (salt), and alcohol.
- Increase the contribution of dark green vegetables, red and orange vegetables, and beans and peas to the diets of the population.
- Increase consumption of calcium.
- Limit caloric intake to meet caloric needs.

Reproduced from U.S. Department of Health and Human Services, Office of Disease Prevention and Health Promotion. *Healthy People 2020*: nutrition and weight status. Retrieved from: http://www.healthypeople.gov/2020/topics-objectives/topic/nutrition-and-weight-status. Accessed August 31, 2016.

recommendations for chronic disease prevention (**TABLE 13.16**). Another way to prevent metabolic syndrome is for patients to follow the *Physical Activity Guidelines* for American as listed in **TABLE 13.17** .

Adults who spend 60 minutes or more each day in moderate-to-vigorous physical activity are less likely to have abdominal obesity, hypertriglyceridemia, and low HDL cholesterol as compared to individuals who spend less than 30 minutes each day performing moderate- to vigorous physical activity, independent of sex, age, education, smoking, alcohol consumption, and total sedentary time.[195] Some specific examples of moderate and vigorous physical activities are presented in **TABLE 13.18** .

Management of Metabolic Syndrome

Lifestyle changes are the first line of therapy for both prevention and treatment of metabolic syndrome. It is important for health practitioners to work with individuals to reduce their risk of heart disease by managing blood pressure, lowering LDL cholesterol, increasing HDL cholesterol, and lowering elevated triglycerides. **Triglycerides** are the main constituents of natural fats and oils and are composed of three fatty acid chains linked to a glycerol molecule. The second goal of treatment is to prevent the onset of type 2 diabetes. Individuals must focus on managing the modifiable risk factors: body weight, physical activity, dietary intake, and smoking. If lifestyle changes do not produce results, then medications may be added to the treatment plan.[196]

Physical Activity

Individuals are encouraged to participate in regular physical activity, which assists in weight loss, improves blood lipid levels, decreases blood pressure, and helps with insulin resistance. Recent research examines the type of physical activity that assists in preventing and managing metabolic syndrome.[197] Studies show that moderate to intense physical activity reduces the risk for metabolic

Table 13.17

Physical Activity Guidelines for Americans

- All adults should avoid inactivity. Some physical activity is better than none, and adults who participate in any amount of physical activity gain some health benefits.
- For substantial health benefits, adults should do at least 150 minutes (2 hours and 30 minutes) a week of moderate-intensity or 75 minutes (1 hour and 15 minutes) a week of vigorous-intensity aerobic physical activity or an equivalent combination of moderate- and vigorous-intensity aerobic activity. Aerobic activity should be performed in episodes of at least 10 minutes, and preferably, it should be spread throughout the week.
- For additional and more extensive health benefits, adults should increase their aerobic physical activity to 300 minutes (5 hours) a week of moderate-intensity or 150 minutes a week of vigorous-intensity aerobic physical activity or an equivalent combination of moderate- and vigorous-intensity activity. Additional health benefits are gained by engaging in physical activity beyond this amount.
- Adults should also include muscle-strengthening activities that involve all major muscle groups on 2 or more days a week.

Modified from U.S. Department of Health and Human Services. *2008 Physical Activity Guidelines for Americans.* Washington (DC): U.S. Department of Health and Human Services; 2008. Retrieved from: http://www.health.gov/paguidelines. Accessed November 15, 2016.

Table 13.18

Examples of Moderate and Vigorous Physical Activities

Moderate-Intensity Physical Activity	Vigorous-Intensity Physical Activity
• Walking briskly (3 miles per hour or faster, but not race walking)	• Race-walking, jogging, or running
• Water aerobics	• Swimming laps
• Bicycling slower than 10 miles per hour	• Tennis (singles)
• Tennis (doubles)	• Aerobic dancing
• Ballroom dancing	• Bicycling 10 miles per hour or faster
• General gardening	• Jumping rope
	• Heavy gardening (continuous digging or hoeing)
	• Hiking uphill or with a heavy backpack

syndrome in middle-aged and older women.[198,199] Vigorous physical activity reduces the risk of metabolic syndrome by one-third in both males and females. Participation in only moderate activity has not shown any improvement in women and very little improvement in men. Regular long-term participation in resistance training improved metabolic syndrome in both men and women with impaired glucose tolerance.[200]

Nutrition Therapy

No single diet plan has been specifically recognized for the management of metabolic syndrome. The principal concept is to incorporate lifestyle changes to initiate metabolic changes. Meal plans should be individualized and designed by a registered dietitian nutritionist. The goal is to decrease energy intake. Diets low in saturated and trans fat, balanced in carbohydrate intake throughout the day, high in dietary fiber, high in fruit and vegetable intake, and inclusive of low-fat dairy foods are protective against metabolic syndrome. Individuals need to reduce their intake of foods with simple sugars and refined grains such as soda, juices, white bread, sweetened cereals, desserts, and candy. Individuals should also be encouraged to increase their servings of whole grains and high-fiber

foods, for example, whole-grain bread, oatmeal, fruits and vegetables, and legumes. Consuming foods such as fish and flax that are good sources of omega-3 fatty acids two times a week may also help to improve insulin action.[201]

Evidence suggests that a Mediterranean-style diet is also associated with a reduced risk of metabolic syndrome. The Mediterranean diet traditionally includes fruits, vegetables, grains, beans, and nuts. Olive oil and olives are used liberally, and sweets are limited and incorporated for special occasions only. Overall 40–50% of the total daily energy intake should be from carbohydrates, 30–35% from fats (emphasizing unsaturated fats), and the remainder of energy from protein.[202]

Weight Management

Losing only 5–7% of body weight can help reduce insulin levels. The development of a healthful lifestyle with behavior modification is important for overall fitness and health. The American Academy of Nutrition recommends that individuals develop healthy lifestyles and work on behavior modification.[203]

Smoking

Smokers are at greater risk than nonsmokers of becoming insulin resistant and developing cardiovascular disease. In smokers, a hormone imbalance can promote the accumulation of abdominal fat, which can lead to insulin resistance. Cessation of smoking decreases the risk of developing metabolic syndrome. Treatments for smoking cessation that have been shown to be effective include physician support; individual, group, or telephone counseling; cognitive behavior therapy (CBT); and nicotine replacement medications.[204–207]

Current Metabolic Syndrome Research

Emerging data suggest that metabolic syndrome may be linked to sleep deprivation through a variety of pathways.[208] Some evidence supports an association between **nonalcoholic fatty liver disease (NAFLD)** and metabolic syndrome.[209,210]

Gallstone disease has been shown in some studies to be strongly associated with metabolic syndrome.[211]

Lifestyle modification programs that include improving the overall quality of the diet and promoting physical activity are main approaches for the prevention and treatment of metabolic syndrome. The high prevalence of metabolic syndrome signifies that population-level interventions are needed to address the cardiovascular disease risks. The focus has been on providing calorie labeling in chain restaurants, decreasing the levels of sodium in foods, eliminating the use of trans fats in food establishments, increasing the availability of fresh produce at reasonable costs, and creating environments conducive to physical activity.[212]

Type 2 Diabetes Mellitus

Type 2 diabetes is a condition in which the pancreas does not produce enough insulin for normal functioning or the insulin that is produced does not work properly in the body. The key to avoiding diabetes is that the pancreas has some functional ability to produce insulin and that target cells are receptive to the presence of insulin.

Prevalence and Etiology of Type 2 Diabetes

Type 2 diabetes is the most prevalent form of diabetes, accounting for approximately 90–95% of all diagnosed cases of diabetes.[184] It is estimated that 29.1 million people, or 9.3% of the U.S. population, have diabetes, but only 21.0 million have actually been diagnosed, while 8.1 million people have the disease but are undiagnosed.[213] In 2013, diabetes was the seventh leading cause of death in the United States (see 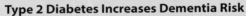 **TABLE 13.19**).

Prediabetes is defined as when blood glucose levels are higher than normal, but not yet high enough to be

Table 13.19
Number of Deaths from the Top 10 Leading Causes of Death in the United States in 2014
1. Heart disease: 614,348
2. Cancer: 591,699
3. Chronic lower respiratory diseases: 147,101
4. Accidents (unintentional injuries): 136,053
5. Stroke (cerebrovascular diseases): 133,103
6. Alzheimer's disease: 93,541
7. Diabetes: 76,488
8. Influenza and pneumonia: 55,227
9. Nephritis, nephrotic syndrome, and nephrosis: 48,146
10. Intentional self-harm (suicide): 42,773
National Center for Health Statistics. Leading causes of death. Hyattsville, MD: National Center for Health Statistics, Centers for Disease Control and Prevention; updated April 27, 2016. Retrieved from: http://www.cdc.gov/nchs/fastats/leading-causes-of-death.htm. Accessed August 31, 2016.

diagnosed as type 2 diabetes. Not everyone with prediabetes develops type 2 diabetes, although many people do over time.

Type 2 diabetes is associated with insulin resistance along with defects in insulin secretion. Type 2 diabetes is often undiagnosed for many years because hyperglycemia develops gradually and in the early stages is often not serious enough for the individual to recognize the typical symptoms of diabetes. **Hyperglycemia** is a high concentration of glucose in the bloodstream. Individuals with hyperglycemia are at an increased risk of developing macrovascular and microvascular complications.[214] For this

News You Can Use

Type 2 Diabetes Increases Dementia Risk

A recent review of 14 published studies involving more than 2 million individuals, including 100,000 dementia patients, shows that individuals living with type 2 diabetes are at a higher risk for dementia than those people who do not have diabetes. Vascular dementia is caused by impaired blood flow to the brain, usually resulting from many small, undetected strokes. Diabetes causes a higher risk for vascular dementia in women than in men. In fact, women living with diabetes have higher risk for also developing heart disease and stroke.

The review reported the following: "People with diabetes were 60 percent more likely to develop any dementia than people without diabetes…. Women with diabetes were more than twice as likely as those without it to develop vascular dementia, compared to a smaller increase in risk for men with diabetes."

R.R. Huxley, a researcher for this study, states, "There needs to be more research into how sugar in the blood interacts with the blood vessels and whether that process is different in women than in men." Huxley also comments "that women can be undertreated for vascular risks relative to men. We can't definitively say whether

the relationship is causal or not because the studies were all observational (rather than randomized trials) and therefore there always remains the possibility that the relationship is confounded."

Huxley also mentions that a third factor, such as obesity, could have played a role in the relationship between diabetes and dementia.

The message is that a focus on keeping fit, maintaining a healthy diet, quitting smoking, and undertaking both daily physical exercise and regular brain exercises can help decrease the risk of dementia for people with diabetes.

Reference

Chatterjee S, Peters S, Woodward W, et al. Type 2 diabetes as a risk factor for dementia in women compared with men: a pooled analysis of 2.3 million people comprising more than 100,000 cases of dementia [published online ahead of print]. *Diabetes Care.* December 17, 2015. Retrieved from: http://care.diabetesjournals.org/content/early/2015/12/09/dc15-1588.abstract. Accessed August 31, 2016.

reason, it has been suggested that screening programs to diagnose and treat individuals at an earlier stage of their disease are needed to decrease cardiovascular risks and improve long-term health.[215,216]

Risk Factors for Type 2 Diabetes

The cause of type 2 diabetes is unknown, but genetic and environmental factors may contribute to its development. The risk factors for developing type 2 diabetes are increased age, obesity, family history of diabetes, history of gestational diabetes, impaired glucose metabolism, physical inactivity, and ethnicity. Risk factors that individuals can modify to lower risk for diabetes are elevated blood glucose, overweight and obesity, hypertension, abnormal lipids, smoking, and physical inactivity. American Indians, some Asians, Hispanics/Latinos, blacks, Native Hawaiians, and Pacific Islanders are high risk groups for developing type 2 diabetes with complications (see FIGURE 13.12).

A large waist circumference is often a marker of insulin resistance. Health professionals should encourage measurement of BMI at each checkup (see Table 13.1) and encourage patients to achieve and maintain a healthy BMI.

High blood sugar is a strong risk factor for diabetes, heart disease, and stroke. Individuals should be screened regularly by their primary care physician. Hypertension leads to increased risk for stroke, kidney disease, eye problems, and myocardial infarction. Hypertension is a chronic condition in which a person's blood pressure is consistently elevated above the population average. Blood pressure should be measured at each visit. The goal is to have a blood pressure less than 140/80 mm Hg and to avoid high LDL cholesterol levels, low HDL cholesterol levels, and high triglycerides.[217] Smokers are 30–40% more likely to develop type 2 diabetes than nonsmokers. Individuals living with type 2 diabetes who smoke are more likely than nonsmokers to have difficulty with insulin dosing and managing their disease.[218,219]

Prevention of Type 2 Diabetes

Diabetes and obesity are linked: Obesity increases the risk of diabetes and contributes to the disease progression as well as to the development of cardiovascular disease. Many patients with type 2 diabetes are obese, which contributes to insulin resistance. There are many benefits of weight loss for the prevention and management of diabetes, but weight reduction is difficult for individuals with type 2 diabetes.[220] Some patients who are not obese by traditional weight measurement standards may have a higher percentage of body fat distributed mainly in the abdominal region.

A waist circumference of 40 inches or more in men and 35 inches or more in women is associated with the following health issues: type 2 diabetes, heart disease, and high blood pressure.[221] The Canadian Diabetes Association 2013 Clinical Practice Guidelines created waist circumference targets based on sex and ethnicity (see TABLE 13.20).

Weight reduction using intensive lifestyle intervention has been shown to reduce the incidence of diabetes by 58%.[222] The Diabetes Prevention Trial sponsored by the National Institutes of Health found that people at increased risk for type 2 diabetes could prevent or delay the onset of the disease by losing 5–7% of their body weight through increased physical activity and a reduced-fat and lower-calorie diet. In the Diabetes Prevention Trial, modest weight loss proved effective in preventing or delaying type 2 diabetes in all groups at high risk for the disease.[223] The Standards of Medical Care in Diabetes 2015 changed the BMI cut point for screening overweight or obese Asian Americans for prediabetes and type 2 diabetes to 23 (from 25) because this population is at a higher risk for developing diabetes at lower BMI levels compared with the general population.[224]

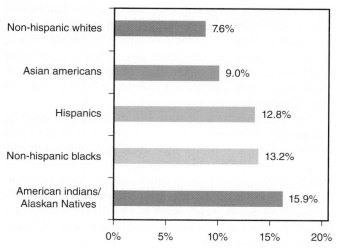

Age-adjusted* percentage of people aged 20 years or older with diagnosed diabetes, by race/ethnicity, United States, 2010–2012

Non-hispanic whites	7.6%
Asian americans	9.0%
Hispanics	12.8%
Non-hispanic blacks	13.2%
American indians/ Alaskan Natives	15.9%

*Based on the 2000 U.S. standard population.

Figure 13.12
Rates of diagnosed diabetes by ethnicity.

Reproduced from Centers for Disease Control and Prevention. Retrieved from: http://www.cdc.gov/diabetes/pubs /statsreport14/national-diabetes-report-web.pdf

Table 13.20

Ethnicity-Specific Values for Waist Circumference

Country or Ethnic Group	Women	Men
South Asian, Chinese, Japanese, South and Central American	32 inches or greater	36 inches or greater
European, sub-Saharan African, Eastern Mediterranean, and Middle Eastern (Arab)	32 inches or greater	37.6 inches or greater

Data from Canadian Diabetes Association. Waist circumference. Toronto, CA: Canadian Diabetes Association. Retrieved from: http://www.diabetes. ca/diabetes-and-you/healthy-living-resources/weight-management/waist-circumference. Accessed August 31, 2016.

1. Testing should be considered in all adults who are overweight (BMI ≥25 kg/m2 or ≥23 kg/m2 in Asian Americans) and have additional risk factors:
   - physical inactivity
   - first-degree relative with diabetes
   - high-risk race/ethnicity (e.g., African American, Latino, Native American, Asian American, Pacific Islander)
   - women who delivered a baby weighing >9 lb or were diagnosed with GDM
   - hypertension (≥140/90 mmHg or on therapy for hypertension)
   - HDL cholesterol level <35 mg/dL (0.90 mmol/L) and/or a triglyceride level >250 mg/dL (2.82 mmol/L)
   - women with polycystic ovary syndrome
   - A1C ≥5.7%, IGT, or IFG on previous testing
   - other clinical conditions associated with insulin resistance (e.g., severe obesity, acanthosis nigricans)
   - history of CVD

2. For all patients, particularly those who are overweight or obese, testing should begin at age 45 years.

3. If results are normal, testing should be repeated at a minimum of 3-year intervals, with consideration of more frequent testing depending on initial results (e.g., those with prediabetes should be tested yearly) and risk status.

Figure 13.13

Criteria for testing for diabetes or prediabetes in asymptomatic adults.

Data from American Diabetes Association. Standards of medical care in diabetes 2015. *Diabetes Care*. 2015;38 (Suppl. 1):S8–S16.

The American Diabetes Association recommendations for diabetes screening in asymptomatic adults are shown in **FIGURE 13.13**.

Management of Type 2 Diabetes

The goal of treatment is to maintain blood glucose levels within a range that prevents or reduces the risk of complications. Home blood glucose monitoring provides feedback to both the patient and the health professional. Type 2 diabetes is treated and managed by regular physical activity, healthy dietary intake, loss of excess weight, and medications, with the overall goal to lower blood glucose levels. Medications need to be adjusted as the disease progresses. It is important to reduce cardiovascular disease risk factors, which include high blood pressure, elevated lipids, and tobacco use (e-cigarettes are not recommended as a replacement for smoking or for use with smoking cessation therapy). The success of treatment depends on the individual's ability to accept the diagnosis and actively manage the disease. Unfortunately, adherence in patients with type 2 diabetes is often poor.[225,226]

Physical Activity

Physical activity can help people with diabetes increase cardiorespiratory fitness, improve glycemic control, decrease insulin resistance, improve lipid profile, decrease blood pressure, and assist with weight loss and weight maintenance.[227–230] Health professionals should encourage everyone to limit their sedentary activity, and it is recommended that all adults "move" after 90 minutes of sitting.[231] The immediate effects of exercise are related to improvements in insulin action, with most individuals experiencing a decrease in their blood glucose levels during both mild and moderate-intensity exercise; this can continue for 2–7 hours postexercise. It is recommended that health professionals promote regular exercise as a key component of therapy.

Diet

Nutrition therapy is important for preventing diabetes, managing existing diabetes, and preventing or decreasing diabetes complications. All individuals diagnosed with diabetes should be referred to an RDN for medical nutrition therapy. The RDN will create an individual meal plan that addresses culture, personal preferences, financial status, access to healthy foods, food-related values readiness for change, and other factors. The goals of medical nutrition therapy focus on promoting healthy eating habits, encouraging consumption of nutrient-dense foods, managing portion size, maintaining healthy body weight, and improving blood glucose and lipid levels. The key features of dietary treatment of diabetes are outlined in **TABLE 13.21**.

Routine monitoring of glucose, lipids, blood pressure, body weight, and renal function in patients diagnosed with type 2 diabetes can ensure successful health outcomes.[232] Nutrition therapy that a registered dietitian individualizes includes developing an eating pattern designed to lower glucose, lower blood pressure, and alter lipid profiles. This approach is important in the management of diabetes and lowers the risk for CVD, coronary heart disease, and stroke.[233]

When a patient with type 2 diabetes is classified as overweight or obese, it is recommended that the individual achieve a 5–10% weight loss. Behavior modification, exercise, and diet are necessary for a comprehensive weight management program. Recently, meal replacements have been used once or twice daily to replace self-prepared meals. This can result in significant weight loss for some individuals, but they must be monitored closely by the healthcare team.[234]

Treatment often requires the use of oral medications, unique noninsulin injectable drugs, and insulin. Monotherapy and combination therapy can assist in achieving glycemic control. Dosages are adjusted depending on the results of blood glucose monitoring.

Table 13.21

Key Features of Dietary Treatment of Diabetes

Energy balance	For overweight or obese individuals, reducing energy intake that incorporates food choices from all of the food groups is a focus of dietary management.
Carbohydrate	The amount of carbohydrates and available insulin is a key factor in influencing glycemic response after eating and should be considered when developing the eating plan.
	Monitoring carbohydrate intake using the carbohydrate counting method can be valuable in achieving glycemic control. Carbohydrate intake from vegetables, fruits, whole grains, legumes, and dairy products is preferred over intake from other carbohydrate sources, especially those that contain added fats, sugars, or sodium. Substituting low-glycemic-load foods for higher-glycemic-load foods may assist in improving glycemic control.
Fiber	People with diabetes should consume at least the same amount of fiber and whole grains as that recommended for the general public. High-fiber foods should be increased slowly over time, and individuals should be encouraged to increase their fluid intake to avoid intestinal discomfort. The focus of the diet should be on choosing nutrient-dense foods.
Fat	Individuals living with diabetes are at a higher risk for developing cardiovascular problems. The recommended guidelines are similar to those for the general population in that saturated fat should be less than 7% of total kilocalories and trans fat should be minimal; many professionals also encourage the consumption of trans fat to be less than 1% of total kilocalories.
Protein	The intake recommendations are similar to those for the general population. Lean protein choices are recommended because they contain less fat.
Micronutrients	The intake recommendations are the same as those for the general population.
Sodium	The recommendation for the general population is to reduce sodium to less than 2,300 mg/day, and this recommendation is also appropriate for people with diabetes.

Case Study

In the opening of the chapter you met Jasmine R., a woman in her sixties who has been overweight from early childhood. Recently, she had her annual medical checkup, after which her physician sent her for a number of laboratory tests and arranged for her to meet with a dietitian for a nutrition consultation.

At the nutrition consultation, the registered dietitian nutritionist asked her about her personal and family medical and dietary history. The RDN learned that Jasmine has three children and five grandchildren. Her parents were overweight their whole life, and her brother developed obesity after college. Two of her children are also struggling with weight problems, although the third, her oldest child, has a normal weight. During her three pregnancies, Jasmine gained 40 lb or more. Jasmine and her husband divorced about 3 years after the birth of her third child, and this forced Jasmine to go back to work as a grocery clerk and to find a second job house cleaning. After her divorce, Jasmine found that cooking meals every night was a struggle because she was so tried from working and she had no energy to cook meals. She often prepared quick and easy meals for the children, and instead of sitting down with the children and eating, she would snack. Later in the evening, after everyone was in bed, Jasmine would watch TV and snack on potato chips, ice cream, and chocolate. Jasmine made lunches for the children to take to school, but she didn't take time to make lunch for herself and would grab a hamburger, Coke, and fries at McDonalds or eat Chinese food from the restaurant across the street from the supermarket.

Eventually, her children grew up, got married, and left home, leaving Jasmine by herself. Now that she lives on her own, she no longer takes part-time cleaning jobs but still has to work at the grocery store to make ends meet. Jasmine does not feel the need to cook full meals and often has canned soup and a sandwich for supper. She still snacks in the evenings on the "treats" she keeps in the cupboard for when her grandchildren visit. She does not eat many dairy products because they "upset her stomach." She does not exercise owing to exhaustion and pain in her knees from standing at work all day long. When the RDN asked Jasmine about the medications she was taking, she admitted to forgetting to take her evening metformin along with her blood pressure medication at least three times a week. She only meets with her family physician once a year because she doesn't have a good medical plan and cannot take time off work to go to physician appointments. She rarely tests her blood glucose level, but the recent lab results showed an HbA$_{1c}$ level of 13. She just had her first DXA scan and was diagnosed with osteoporosis.

Questions

1. What specific food and nutrition recommendations would you suggest to Jasmine?
2. Discuss the linkages between diabetes and obesity.
3. What type of physical activity would you recommend for Jasmine, knowing that her knees hurt on a daily basis and explain how the exercise affects blood glucose levels?

Recap Metabolic syndrome is not a disease but rather a combination of risk factors, including high cholesterol levels, high blood sugar levels, high blood pressure, and excess abdominal fat. Approximately one-third of the adult population in the United States has metabolic syndrome. The occurrence increases with age and increases in relation to higher BMI levels. Diets that are low in saturated and trans fat, have balanced carbohydrate intakes throughout the day, are high in dietary fiber, have high fruit and vegetable intakes, and include low-fat dairy foods are protective against metabolic syndrome. Type 2 diabetes is a condition in which the pancreas does not produce enough insulin for normal functioning or the insulin that is produced is not working properly in the body. It is estimated that 9.3% of the U.S. population has diabetes. Type 2 diabetes is treated and managed by regular physical activity, healthy dietary intake, loss of excess weight, and medication, with the overall goal to lower blood glucose levels.

1. Discuss metabolic syndrome and its etiology.
2. Name and describe the prevailing means of treatment for metabolic syndrome.
3. Identify a number of the key risk factors associated with type 2 diabetes.
4. State the prevalence of type 2 diabetes and then describe some of the preventive measures that can be taken to reduce the prevalence of type 2 diabetes.

Cardiovascular Disease and Hypertension

Preview This section presents cardiovascular disease (CVD) and hypertension (HTN). It defines both of these chronic diseases, discusses the prevalence of each condition, identifies their risk factors, and then discusses the prevention and management of both cardiovascular disease and hypertension.

Cardiovascular disease (CVD) includes any disease or injury of the heart and its blood vessels as well as the blood vessels throughout the body and in the brain. It presents in a number of forms, including coronary heart disease (CHD); cerebrovascular disease (CVD), a group of conditions that affect the circulation of blood to the brain; peripheral artery disease (PAD); aortic atherosclerosis; and thoracic or abdominal aortic aneurysm. Hypertension (HTN) is a chronic condition in which a person's blood pressure is consistently elevated above the population average.

Prevalence and Etiology of Cardiovascular Disease

Heart disease is the leading cause of death in the United States (See Table 13.19 in the Diabetes section). Coronary heart disease (CHD), which includes myocardial infarction, angina pectoris, heart failure, and coronary death, is the most common type of heart disease, leading to over 370,000 deaths annually. Approximately 735,000

Americans have a heart attack each year; of these, 525,000 are a first heart attack, and approximately 210,000 occur in people who have already had a heart attack.[235,236]

The risk of cardiovascular disease increases with age (see **FIGURE 13.14**). With increased longevity and decreases in age-specific death rates from CVD, CHD, and stroke, the incidence of cardiovascular disease complications remains high and they are very costly to the medical system.

Coronary Heart Disease
Coronary heart disease (CHD) includes myocardial infarction (MI), angina pectoris, heart failure, and coronary death. Nearly one-third of all deaths worldwide result from cardiovascular diseases, the greatest proportion of which are from CHD.[237] The main cause of CHD is atherosclerosis, which is a buildup of cholesterol and atherosclerotic plaques in the coronary artery walls. The symptoms of heart disease can include angina, shortness of breath, fatigue, arrhythmia, light-headedness, and peripheral edema. Some individuals may have no signs or symptoms, and often the disease is not diagnosed until a myocardial infarction or heart failure occurs.

Cerebrovascular Disease
Cerebrovascular disease (CVD) is a group of conditions that affect the circulation of blood to the brain and that cause limited or no blood flow to certain areas of the brain, which is known as stroke or transient ischemic attack. Often, CVD has a sudden onset, and it may be stable, progressive, or completely resolved. The most common cause of ischemic stroke is atherosclerotic disease. High cholesterol levels along with inflammation in arteries in the brain can cause the cholesterol to build up in the blood vessel in the form of a thick, waxy plaque. This plaque affects blood flow to the brain, causing a stroke or transient ischemic attack, or even dementia.[238]

Peripheral Artery Disease
Peripheral artery disease (PAD) is a narrowing of the peripheral arteries to the legs, stomach, arms, and head. Individuals with PAD have a much higher risk of heart attack or stroke than the general population. PAD is usually caused by atherosclerosis in the peripheral arteries.[239]

Aortic Atherosclerosis and Thoracic or Abdominal Aortic Aneurysm
Atherosclerosis is one of the major causes of aneurysms in the descending thoracic aorta. The aortic wall is made up of cells that require oxygen and nutrients that are carried by the blood vessels and that seep into the walls. If the lining of the aorta becomes covered with plaque, oxygen and nutrients can't get through to the cells, cells die, and the aortic wall weakens. The pressure in the blood vessels eventually causes the walls of the blood vessel to expand in the area of the plaque, and the wall dilates to the point where an aneurysm occurs.[240]

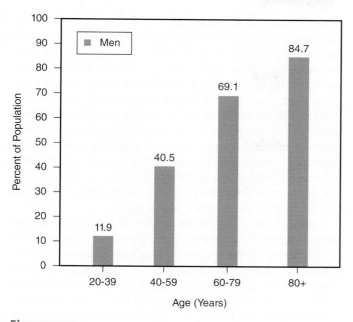

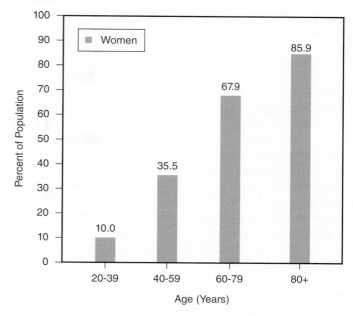

Figure 13.14

Prevalence of cardiovascular disease in adults ≥ 20 years of age by age and sex.

Data from Mozaffarian D, Benjamin EJ, Go AS, et al. Heart disease and stroke statistics--2015 update: a report from the American Heart Association. *Circulation*. 2015;131:e29–e322. Retrieved from: http://www.heart.org/idc/groups/heart-public/@wcm/@sop/@smd/documents/downloadable/ucm_449847.pdf. Accessed August 31, 2016.

Risk Factors for Cardiovascular Disease

Similar to other chronic diseases and conditions, there are two types of risk factors associated with cardiovascular disease: unmodifiable and modifiable. Those that cannot be changed are family history, ethnicity, and age, and those that can be treated or changed are tobacco exposure, high blood pressure, high cholesterol, obesity, physical inactivity, diabetes, unhealthy diets, and harmful use of alcohol.[241]

Obesity

As BMI increases, the risk of heart disease and stroke increases, with 21% of ischemic heart disease being attributable to a BMI over 21.[242] Intra-abdominal fat plays a significant role in the body's metabolism. This type of fat affects blood pressure and blood lipid levels and can affect the body's ability to use insulin.

Diabetes and High Blood Pressure

Diabetes increases the risk of developing cardiovascular disease. Even if blood glucose levels are under control, diabetes increases the risk of heart disease and stroke. The risks are greater if blood sugar is not under control. Most people with diabetes die of some form of heart or blood vessel disease.

Hypertension (HTN) is another risk factor for coronary heart disease and the most important risk factor for stroke. Hypertension causes about 50% of ischemic strokes and also increases the risk of hemorrhagic stroke. Hypertension can lead to atherosclerosis and narrowing of the blood vessels. Damage to the arteries can also create weak spots that can rupture or thin spots that can

balloon out, resulting in an aneurism.[243] Elevated blood pressure in people younger than 50 years of age is associated with increased cardiovascular risk. Hypertension is called the "silent" disease because it often has no signs or symptoms. Sometimes individuals complain of headaches with high blood pressure. When high blood pressure exists with obesity, smoking, high blood cholesterol levels, or diabetes, the risk of heart attack or stroke is increased several times.

Blood Cholesterol

As blood cholesterol level rises, the risk of coronary heart disease increases. When high blood pressure and tobacco smoking are present, this risk increases even more. A person's cholesterol level is affected by age, sex, heredity, and diet. The goal is to have total cholesterol levels of less than 180 mg/dL. Total cholesterol and HDL cholesterol are used to predict risk for heart attack or stroke. **High-density lipoprotein (HDL)** is synthesized primarily in the liver and small intestine and carries cholesterol out of the bloodstream. Low HDL cholesterol levels increase the risk for heart disease. Individuals with high blood triglyceride levels commonly have lower HDL cholesterol levels. Risk factors such as genetics, type 2 diabetes, some medications (beta blockers and anabolic steroids), smoking, overweight and obesity, and lack of physical activity can all result in lower HDL cholesterol levels.

High levels of HDL can reduce the risk of atherosclerosis because HDLs aid in reverse transport of cholesterol from the bloodstream to the liver, where they are removed from the bloodstream and then excreted in the bile.[244] Activity level and moderate alcohol consumption increase HDL levels. It is recommended that HDL levels in men be ≥ 40 mg/dL and in women, ≥ 50 mg/dL.[245]

High levels of LDL cholesterol are an important risk factor for coronary heart disease and can contribute to the formation of plaque, buildup of plaque, and destabilization and rupture of atherosclerotic plaque. **Low-density lipoprotein (LDL)** cholesterol transports cholesterol to the cells of the body. LDLs circulate in the bloodstream and deliver cholesterol to the cells. The American Heart Association recommends all adults age 20 or older have their cholesterol checked every 4 to 6 years. Maintaining a low LDL cholesterol level is important for heart health. For those individuals taking statins, the newest guidelines suggest that they need not reach a specific target number for LDL. A diet high in saturated and trans fats raises LDL cholesterol.[246–249]

A high triglyceride level combined with low HDL cholesterol or high LDL cholesterol is associated with atherosclerosis, which increases the risk for heart attack and stroke. High triglyceride levels (200–499 mg/dL) and very high triglyceride levels (>500 mg/dL) can be caused by obesity, high-carbohydrate diets, and lack of physical activity.

Smoking

Smoking is estimated to cause approximately 10% of cardiovascular disease and is the second leading cause of CVD after hypertension. Smoking can result in disturbances to the endothelium, the thin layer of cells that line the interior surface of blood vessels. There is evidence to show that injury to the endothelium plays an important role in the development of atherosclerosis, which leads to higher blood pressure.[250] Tobacco decreases the amount of oxygen that the blood carries and increases the chance for blood to clot. The risk of coronary heart disease is 25% higher in females who smoke than in male smokers. Chewing tobacco more than doubles the risk of a heart attack. Nonsmokers who breathe second-hand smoke have a 25–30% increased risk of developing CVD.[248,251–255]

Diet

A diet that's high in fat, salt, sugar, and cholesterol can contribute to the development of heart disease. Dietary saturated fats have the greatest negative effect on LDL cholesterol (LDL-C) concentrations, and dietary trans fatty acids (TFAs) are the most dangerous type of fat relative to increased risk for CHD. Some studies show that, in addition to increasing plasma LDL-C, trans fatty acids also decrease plasma HDL cholesterol (HDL-C) and may increase lipoprotein(a).[256] Lipoprotein(a) is a subclass of lipoproteins. High lipoprotein predicts risk of early atherosclerosis independent of other cardiac risk factors.

Excessive alcohol consumption can increase blood pressure and contribute to the development of heart disease and stroke. Research has demonstrated that excessive consumption can lead to alcoholic cardiomyopathy (failure of the heart muscle resulting from damage by ethanol).[257,258]

Age, Gender, and Genetics

The majority of people who die of coronary heart disease are older than 65 years. Men have a greater risk than women of having a heart attack earlier in life. Yet older, postmenopausal women who have heart attacks are more likely than men to die from the attack within a few weeks.[259] A decrease in the hormone estrogen may be a factor in the increased incidence of heart disease among postmenopausal women because estrogen is thought to have a protective effect on the inner layer of artery walls, helping to keep blood vessels flexible. After menopause, the death rate from heart disease for women increases, but the death rate for men is still higher.

Children whose parents developed heart disease also have a higher likelihood of developing heart disease later in life. Blacks have more serious high blood pressure problems than whites and, as such, have a higher risk of heart disease. Heart disease risk is also higher among Mexican Americans, American Indians, native Hawaiians, and some Asian Americans. The higher rates of the key risk factors obesity and diabetes among these ethnic groups are the major reason for these findings.[260]

Physical Inactivity

An inactive lifestyle is a risk factor for coronary heart disease. Over the long term, individuals who engage in regular physical activity at moderate to vigorous levels have lower risks of heart and blood vessel disease. Physical activity can help control blood cholesterol, diabetes, and obesity as well as help lower blood pressure in some people. Inactive individuals tend to develop obesity and have higher levels of cholesterol and thus are more likely to develop heart disease.[261]

Prevention of Cardiovascular Disease

Most chronic disease states are prevented or their impact is minimized with healthy choices. A healthy lifestyle is the best way to prevent cardiovascular disease. Diet, healthy body weight, and regular physical activity are modifiable risk factors important for the prevention of CVD.

Diet

Choosing healthy meals and snacks can help avoid heart disease and its complications. Nutrient-dense foods as well as plenty of fresh fruits and vegetables should be included in the daily meal plan. Eating foods low in saturated fat and cholesterol and high in fiber can help prevent high blood cholesterol. Replacing saturated fats with monounsaturated and polyunsaturated fats improves lipid profiles and decreases CVD risk. Current recommendations to prevent CVD are to consume 20–35% of energy from fats with saturated fat limited to < 7% of energy, trans fat limited to < 1% of energy, and the balance of fat as unsaturated (monounsaturated and polyunsaturated) fat.

Eating high-fiber foods and half of grain consumption as whole grains is also protective. Two servings per week of fish are recommended as a source of long-chain omega-3 fatty acids for CVD risk reduction. Limiting salt or sodium to less than 2,300 mg/day can also lower blood pressure. Less than 300 mg/day of cholesterol is also recommended. Foods high in sugar such as pastries, candy bars, cookies, and sweetened cereals along with beverages that are high in sugar should be limited. Drinking excessive amounts of alcohol can raise blood pressure, and therefore alcohol should be consumed in moderation to reduce risk.[262]

Body Weight

Overweight and obesity increase the risk for heart disease. BMI is used to determine whether an individual's weight is in the healthy range (18.5–24.9). The waist measurement (88 cm in females; 102 cm in males) and waist-to-hip ratio (< 0.85 in females; < 0.90 in males) are also used to assess a person's excess body fat. Physical activity helps to maintain and decrease weight and lowers cholesterol and blood pressure.

Management of Cardiovascular Disease

Once diagnosed, dietary and lifestyle changes can reduce high LDL-C by 20–40%. The treatment goals are to reduce the heart's workload by controlling blood pressure and using beta blockers or calcium channel blockers to decrease the intensity of heart pumping. Other medications prescribed may include anticoagulants, aspirin, antiplatelet drugs, angiotensin-converting enzyme (ACE) inhibitors, and statins. Procedures such as angioplasty or coronary artery bypass grafting (CABG) can improve coronary blood flow, and coronary artery blood clots can sometimes be dissolved by medications. Dietary treatment goals are designed to lower LDL cholesterol and raise HDL cholesterol. Smoking cessation is encouraged because cigarette smoking greatly increases the risk for heart disease.

Weight loss can assist in reducing LDL-C and triglyceride levels and is desirable for overweight and obese individuals. Energy intake needs to be designed by a registered dietitian so that individuals can maintain a healthy weight and avoid any further weight gain.

Physical activity prevents the development of coronary artery disease and reduces symptoms in patients with established cardiovascular disease. Several meta-analyses have shown that comprehensive, exercise-based cardiac rehabilitation reduces mortality rates in patients after myocardial infarction.[263–265] The Surgeon General recommends adults engage in moderate-intensity exercise for a number of daily sessions totaling up to 150 minutes each week. To lower the risk for heart attack and stroke adults should aim for 40 minutes of aerobic exercise of moderate to vigorous intensity three to four times a week. (see **FIGURE 13.15**).

Factors that Lower Lipoprotein and Triglyceride Levels

Dietary fiber recommendations to prevent CVD aim for individuals to include 5–10 g of soluble viscous fiber per

Adults need at least:

 2 hours and 30 minutes (150 minutes) of moderate-intenisty aerobic activity (i.e., brisk walking) every week **and**

 muscle-strengthening activities on 2 or more days a week that work all major muscle groups (legs, hips, back, abdomen, chest, shoulders, and arms).

OR

 1 hour and 15 minutes (75 minutes) of vigorous-intensity aerobic activity (i.e., jogging or running) every week **and**

 muscle-strengthening activities on 2 or more days a week that work all major muscle groups (legs, hips, back, abdomen, chest, shoulders, and arms).

OR

 An equivalent mix of moderate-and vigorous-intensity aerobic activity **and**

 muscle-strengthening activities on 2 or more days a week that work all major muscle groups (legs, hips, back, abdomen, chest, shoulders, and arms).

Figure 13.15
CDC recommendations for physical activity in adults.
Reproduced from the Centers for Disease Control. How Much Physical Activity do Adults Need? Retrieved from: https://www.cdc.gov/physicalactivity/basics/adults/.

day. Soluble fiber and resistant starch molecules are fermented by bacteria in the large intestine, producing short-chain fatty acids that help reduce circulating cholesterol levels. Total fiber intake should meet the daily recommendations of 25 g for women ages 19–50 years and 21 g for women 51 years and older. For men, the fiber intake recommendation is 38 g for ages 19–50 years and 30 g for men 51 years and older.[266] Whole grains that contain the entire grain—the bran, germ, and endosperm—include whole wheat, oats/oatmeal, rye, barley, corn, popcorn, brown rice, wild rice, buckwheat, triticale, bulgur, millet, quinoa, and sorghum and are important for total health.

Evidence is mounting that consumption of soy protein (25–50 g/day) in place of animal protein lowers blood cholesterol levels by approximately 4–8%. The beneficial effects of soy are even greater in people with hypercholesterolemia.[267–269] It is recommended that individuals consume 2 g/day of plant stanols and plant sterols, which can be found in nuts, seeds, and vegetable oils, and they have been added to some margarines and yogurts. Flavonoid compounds are found in fruits and vegetables, wine, and tea and have been noted to play a role in improving heart health. Fish that live in cold waters (salmon, mackerel, Atlantic herring, sardines, and trout) are high in omega-3 fatty acids, which can help prevent blood clots and lower blood pressure.[270–272]

Elevated triglycerides may contribute to hardening of the artery walls, which increases risk for stroke, heart attack, and heart disease. High triglycerides are a sign of other medical conditions such as obesity, poorly controlled diabetes, low thyroid hormones, and liver or kidney disease. The dietary recommendation for reducing triglycerides suggests limiting sugar consumption. Excess alcohol consumption can raise triglycerides, provide extra calories, and raise blood pressure. Reducing alcohol consumption or even stopping alcohol consumption is another recommendation for lowering triglycerides. Therapeutic dietary approaches that include probiotics such as *L. reuteri* NCIMB 30242 can be among the potential options to manage LDL-C.[273] Probiotics have been added to food products such as yogurt and are also available as capsules. *L. reuteri* NCIMB 30242 capsules may be useful as an adjunctive therapy for treating hypercholesterolemia.[274–280]

Hypertension

Hypertension is a major independent risk factor for coronary artery disease (CAD), stroke, and kidney failure. HTN is a chronic condition in which a person's blood pressure is consistently elevated above the population average. The typical cutoff value used to determine high blood pressure is a systolic pressure consistently 140 mm Hg or a diastolic pressure consistently 90 mm Hg.

Prevalence and Etiology of Hypertension

Twenty-nine percent of adults in the United States have hypertension (see **FIGURE 13.16**).[281] The Joint National Committee on Prevention, Detection, Evaluation, and Treatment of High Blood Pressure classification of blood pressure for adults ages 18 and older is listed in **TABLE 13.22**. Hypertension can be considered primary or essential hypertension, which accounts for 90–95% of adult cases resulting from environmental or genetic causes,

Table 13.22

The Classification of Blood Pressure for Adults

Blood Pressure Classification	Systolic Blood Pressure	Diastolic Blood Pressure
Normal	< 120 mm Hg	< 80 mm Hg
Prehypertension	120–139 mm Hg	80–89 mm Hg
Stage 1	140–159 mm Hg	90–99 mm Hg
Stage 2	≥ 160 mm Hg	≥ 100 mm Hg

Reproduced from National Heart, Lung, and Blood Institute. *The Seventh Report of the Joint National Committee on Prevention, Detection, Evaluation, and Treatment of High Blood Pressure.* Bethesda, MD: U.S. Department of Health and Human Services, National Institutes of Health, National Heart, Lung, and Blood Institute, and National Blood Pressure Education Program; August 2004:Table 3. Retrieved from: http://www.nhlbi.nih.gov/files/docs/guidelines/jnc7full.pdf. Accessed August 31, 2016.

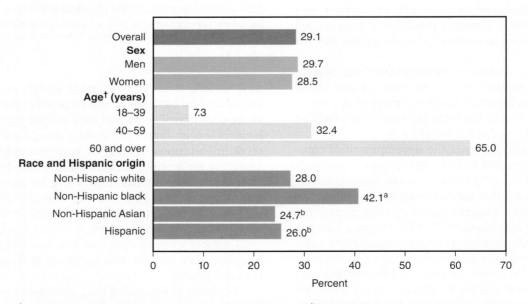

†Significant linear trend [a]Sgnificantly different from non-Hispanic white. [b]Significantly different from non-Hispanic black.
NOTE : Estimates were age adjusted by the direct method to the Census 2000 populatuion, using the age groups 18–39, 40–59, and 60 and over.

Figure 13.16
Age-specific and age-adjusted prevalence of hypertension among adults ages 18 and older: United States, 2011–2012.

Reproduced from Nwankwo T, Yoon SS, Burt V, Gu Q. Hypertension among adults in the United States: National Health and Nutrition Examination Survey, 2011–2012. *NCHS Data Brief.* October 2013;(133:4). Retrieved from: http://www.cdc.gov/nchs/data/databriefs/db133.pdf. Accessed August 31, 2016.

or secondary, which has multiple etiologies, including renal, vascular, and endocrine causes and accounts for 2–10% of cases.[282]

Risk Factors for Hypertension

The main risk factors for hypertension include family history and ethnicity, advanced age, lack of physical activity, poor diet, overweight and obesity, and alcohol consumption. Family history is a major predictor of hypertension. Individuals whose parents or other close relatives have had high blood pressure have an increased risk of developing hypertension. Hypertension is more common in black adults. More than 40% of black men and women have hypertension.[283] Hypertension has an additive effect on other independent risk factors of CVD (see FIGURE 13.17). Increased age increases the risk for developing high blood pressure and cardiovascular disease because blood vessels lose flexibility with age, which can contribute to the increased pressure.

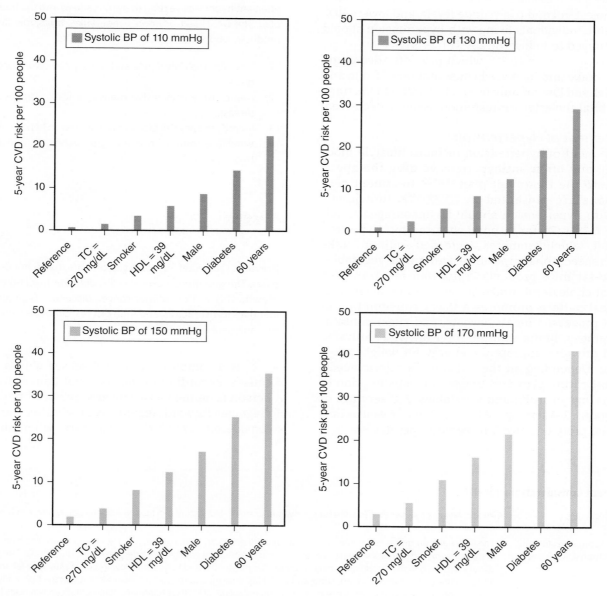

Figure 13.17

Additive effects of risk factors on cardiovascular disease at 5 years. Cumulative absolute risk of CVD at 5 years according to systolic blood pressure and specified levels of other risk factors. The reference category is a nondiabetic, nonsmoking 50-year-old woman with a serum total cholesterol of 154 mg/dL (4.0 mmol/L) and HDL cholesterol of 62 mg/dL (1.6 mmol/L). The CVD risks are given for systolic blood pressure levels of 110, 130, 150, and 170 mm Hg. In the other categories, the additional risk factors are added consecutively. As an example, the diabetes category is a 50-year-old diabetic man who is a smoker and who has a total cholesterol of 270 mg/dL (7 mmol/L) and HDL cholesterol of 39 mg/dL (1 mmol/L).

CVD = cardiovascular disease; TC = total cholesterol.

Modified from: Jackson R, Lawes CM, Bennett DA, et al. Treatment with drugs to lower blood pressure and blood cholesterol based on an individual's absolute cardiovascular risk. *Lancet*. 2005;365:434-441.

Physical activity is necessary to keep the heart and circulatory system healthy. An inactive lifestyle increases the chances of high blood pressure, heart disease, blood vessel disease, and stroke. A diet that is high in calories, fats, sugar, and salt and low in essential nutrients contributes directly to poor health, obesity, and hypertension. Heavy and regular use of alcohol can increase blood pressure. It can also lead to heart failure and stroke and produce irregular heartbeats. Overweight and obesity increase the risk of developing high blood pressure. Excess weight increases the strain on the heart, raises blood cholesterol and triglyceride levels, and lowers HDL cholesterol. Individuals living with hypertension should be encouraged to follow the **DASH (Dietary Approaches to Stop Hypertension) diet**, which promotes decreased sodium intake and increased consumption of fruits and vegetables and low-fat milk products. Saturated fat, trans fat, and total cholesterol intake should also be decreased.

Management of Hypertension

The treatment of hypertension includes lifestyle modification, and often antihypertensive drug therapy is added into the treatment plan.[284–292] Treatment considerations are presented in TABLE 13.23 . Individuals living with hypertension should be encouraged to follow the DASH (Dietary Approaches to Stop Hypertension) diet, which promotes decreased sodium intake and increased consumption of fruits and vegetables and low-fat milk products. Saturated fat, trans fat, and total cholesterol intake should also be decreased. This meal pattern promotes a lower consumption of red and processed meats, sweets, and sugar-containing beverages; limits sodium, total fat, and saturated fat; and provides appropriate energy for weight management. Depending on the individual's caloric needs, the DASH eating plan encourages the consumption of 8–10 servings of fruits and vegetables, 7–8 servings of whole grains, 2–3 servings of low-fat dairy, as well as limits animal protein to two 3-oz servings per day.[289]

Recap Cardiovascular disease (CVD) includes any disease or injury of the heart and blood vessels. Coronary heart disease is the most common type of heart disease, leading to over 370,000 deaths annually. The treatment goals are to reduce the heart's workload by controlling blood pressure and using beta blockers or calcium channel blockers to decrease the intensity of heart pumping. Approximately 29% of the adults in the United States have hypertension, a chronic condition in which a person's blood pressure is consistently elevated above the population average. The treatment of hypertension includes lifestyle modification, and often antihypertensive drug therapy is added into the treatment plan. The DASH diet promotes vegetables, fruits, low-fat dairy products, whole grains, poultry, fish, and nuts.

1. Describe the prevalence and etiology of cardiovascular disease.
2. Name three preventive measures for cardiovascular disease.
3. Identify the key risk factors associated with hypertension.
4. What are some of the key approaches to managing hypertension?

Cancer

Preview Cancer refers to a group of more than a hundred diseases. The growth of a cancer cell is different from normal cell growth. This section defines cancer, discusses its prevalence, identifies its risk factors, and then discusses the prevention and management of cancer.

Cancer is a complex group of diseases with a variety of causes. According to the National Cancer Institute, "A person is defined as a cancer survivor from the time of diagnosis forward, regardless of whether the person is considered cured."[293] Cancer starts when abnormal

Table 13.23
Treatment Considerations for HTN

Weight loss	Weight loss approaches as discussed for overweight or obese individuals can lead to a significant decrease in blood pressure.
Dietary Approaches to Stop Hypertension (DASH) diet	The DASH diet promotes vegetables, fruits, low-fat dairy products, whole grains, poultry, fish, and nuts. The plan discourages sweets, sugar-sweetened beverages, and red meats. It encourages a decrease in sodium intake. The DASH dietary pattern is high in potassium, magnesium, calcium, protein, and fiber, with a low intake of saturated fat, total fat, and cholesterol. The National Heart, Lung, and Blood Institute funded the DASH trial in 1995. It was the first study "to provide convincing scientific evidence that a non-pharmaceutical lifestyle treatment could significantly reduce blood pressure."[a]
Exercise	Aerobic exercise, along with resistance training, can decrease systolic and diastolic pressures by an average of 4 to 6 mm Hg and 3 mm Hg, respectively. Most studies that demonstrated a decrease in blood pressure have required three to four sessions of moderate-intensity aerobic exercise lasting 40 minutes for a period of 12 weeks.
Limited alcohol intake	Women who consume two or more alcoholic beverages per day and men who have three or more drinks per day have an increased incidence of hypertension compared with nondrinkers. Decreasing alcohol intake in individuals who drink excessively significantly lowers blood pressure.

[a] Forman JP, Stampfer MJ, Curhan GC. Diet and lifestyle risk factors associated with incident hypertension in women. *JAMA*. 2009;302:401–411.

- In 2016, an estimated 1,685,210 new cases of cancer will be diagnosed in the United States and 595,690 people will die from the disease.

- The most common cancers in 2016 are projected to be breast cancer, lung and bronchus cancer, prostate cancer, colon and rectum cancer, bladder cancer, melanoma of the skin, non-Hodgkin lymphoma, thyroid cancer, kidney and renal pelvis cancer, endometrial cancer, leukemia, and pancreatic cancer.

- The number of cancer deaths (cancer mortality) is 171.2 per 100,000 men and women per year (based on 2008–2012 deaths).

- The number of new cases of cancer (cancer incidence) is 454.8 per 100,000 men and women per year (based on 2008–2012 cases).

- Cancer mortality is higher among men than among women (207.9 per 100,000 men and 145.4 per 100,000 women). It is highest in black men (261.5 per 100,000) and lowest in Asian/Pacific Islander women (91.2 per 100,000). (Based on 2008–2012 deaths.)

- The number of people living beyond a cancer diagnosis reached nearly 14.5 million in 2014 and is expected to rise to almost 19 million by 2024.

- Approximately 39.6% of men and women will be diagnosed with cancer at some point during their lifetimes (based on 2010–2012 data).

- In 2014, an estimated 15,780 children and adolescents ages 0 to 19 were diagnosed with cancer and 1,960 died of the disease.

- National expenditures for cancer care in the United States totaled nearly $125 billion in 2010 and could reach $156 billion in 2020.

Figure 13.18
The burden of cancer in the United States.

Reproduced from National Cancer Institute. Cancer statistics. Rockville, MD: National Cancer Institute, National Institutes of Health, U.S. Department of Health and Human Services; updated March 14, 2016. Retrieved from: http://www.cancer.gov/about-cancer/what-is-cancer/statistics. Accessed November 18, 2016.

cells grow out of control. Instead of dying, cancer cells grow and form new cells that are abnormal, and these cells can invade other tissues.[294] More than 1.5 million new cases of cancer are diagnosed each year. Dietary, lifestyle, and health-related behavioral strategies are important for both the prevention and the treatment of cancer.

Prevalence and Etiology of Cancer

Fundamentally, cancer is caused by a mutation in the DNA of a body's cells that causes cells to alter their normal functions. As a result of mutations, cells may exhibit rapid and uncontrolled growth. In addition, damaged DNA is not properly repaired in cells, which also impairs cell functions.[295] Cancer does not manifest in the same way typical hereditary diseases do. It has been postulated that living organisms actually have cancer-causing genes called proto-oncogenes, which are inactive. Throughout their lives, people can be exposed to carcinogens—physical, chemical, or biological agents that mutate and activate proto-oncogenes into active, cancer-causing oncogenes. A normal control mechanism is lost resulting from altered gene activity, and the abnormal cell growth and cell division are then permitted to occur.[296] Gene mutations may be caused by a variety of factors, for example, smoking, radiation, viruses, cancer-causing chemicals, obesity, hormones, chronic inflammation, and lack of exercise.[295]

The National Cancer Institute has reported on the burden of cancer in the United States (see FIGURE 13.18). Some of the most prominent statistics reported are that "in 2016, an estimated 1,685,210 new cases of cancer will be diagnosed in the United States and 595,690 people will die from the disease; the most common types of cancer are: breast cancer, lung and bronchus cancer, prostate cancer, colon and rectum cancer, bladder cancer, melanoma of the skin, non-Hodgkin lymphoma, thyroid cancer, kidney and renal pelvis cancer, endometrial cancer, leukemia, and pancreatic cancer; and the cost for cancer in the United States totaled nearly $125 billion in 2010 and could reach $156 billion in 2020."[297] The top body sites where cancer is found include breasts, prostate, lungs, colon, uterus, bladder, skin, lymph glands, kidneys, and pelvis (see FIGURE 13.19).

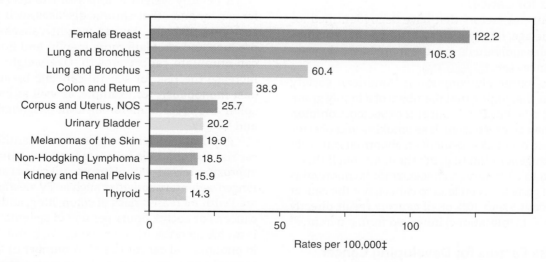

Figure 13.19
Top 10 human cancer sites in the United States.

Reproduced from U.S. Cancer Statistics Working Group. *United States Cancer Statistics: 1999–2013 Incidence and Mortality Web-Based Report.* Atlanta, GA: U.S. Department of Health and Human Services, Centers for Disease Control and Prevention, and National Cancer Institute; 2016. Retrieved from: https://nccd.cdc.gov/uscs/toptencancers.aspx. Accessed August 31, 2016.

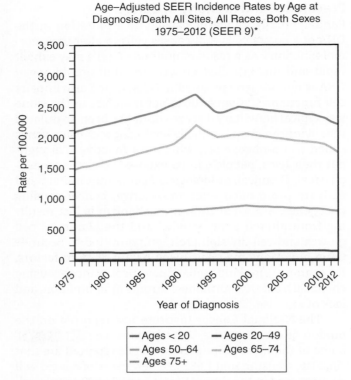

Age–Adjusted SEER Incidence Rates by Age at Diagnosis/Death All Sites, All Races, Both Sexes 1975–2012 (SEER 9)*

Year of Diagnosis

— Ages < 20   — Ages 20–49
— Ages 50–64   — Ages 65–74
— Ages 75+

*Cancer sites include invasive cases only unless otherwise noted.
Rates are per 100,000 and are age adjusted to the 2000 US Standard Population (19 age groups - Census P25–1130).
Regression lines are calculated using the Joinpoint Regression Program Version 4.2.0, April 2015,
National Cancer Institute.
Incidence source: SEER 9 areas (San Franciso, Connecticut, Detroit, Hawaii, Iowa, New Mexico, Seattle, Utah, and Atlanta).

Figure 13.20
Incidence of cancer by age.

Reproduced from National Cancer Institute. Compare statistics by age. Rockville, MD: National Cancer Institute. Surveillance, Epidemiology, and End Results Program; 2015. Retrieved from: http://seer.cancer.gov/faststats /selections.php?#Output. Accessed August 29, 2015.

Risk Factors for Cancer

The prominent risk factors that have been identified for cancer include age, family history, lifestyle, and environment. The older individuals are, the more likely they are to develop cancer (see **FIGURE 13.20**).

Cancer is extremely common in American society and, therefore, the finding that members of a family group with relatives who have had cancer is expected. Common risk factors may be present, such as smoking and obesity. Cancer can also occur as a result of an abnormal gene that is passed from generation to generation. Although this is often referred to as inherited cancer, what is inherited is the abnormal gene that can lead to cancer, not the cancer itself. Only about 5% to 10% of all cancers result directly from gene defects (mutations) inherited from a parent.[298]

Lifestyle Risk Factors for Developing Cancer

The major lifestyle consideration associated with the risk of developing cancer is level of exposure to carcinogens on a daily basis. Carcinogens are substances or agents that are known to be or are strongly suspected of being causes of cancer. One of the most significant lifestyle choices related to cancer is the use of tobacco products, and in particular smoking cigarettes and cigars, because of the known carcinogens associated with tobacco. The Surgeon General of the United States reported in 2015, "Tobacco use in the United States is the cause for nearly 1 in 5 deaths; equivalent to approximately 480,000 early deaths each year."[219]

In addition to smoking, dietary factors are also related to cancer. The World Health Organization reports that dietary factors account for at least 30% of all cancers in Western countries and up to 20% in developing countries. A key dietary factor identified as increasing risk of cancer is a high intake of red meat and processed meat. Meat is low in fiber and is often high in saturated fat. The carcinogenic compounds heterocyclic amines and polycyclic aromatic hydrocarbons form during the processing and cooking of meat.[299]

Another carcinogen associated with food consumption is acrylamide. Frying, baking, broiling, or roasting at high temperatures causes a chemical reaction between specific sugars and the amino acid asparagine in the food that creates acrylamide. Boiling, steaming, and microwaving do not produce acrylamide. Acrylamide is found in plant foods, potato products, grain products, and coffee. French fries and potato chips have a very high amount of acrylamide.[300] One estimate indicates that Americans eat an average of 29 pounds of french fries each year, which means there is very widespread exposure to this carcinogen.[301]

Alcohol abuse can damage the liver, which can lead to liver cancer. Alcohol consumption has been associated with risk of primary cancer in the mouth, pharynx, larynx, esophagus, liver, breast, and colon.[302,303] Alcohol intake can increase the risk for new primary cancers of these sites in individuals who have already received a diagnosis of cancer.[304]

A healthy weight is important to decrease the risk for cancer and other chronic diseases such as heart disease and diabetes. Excess weight causes the body to produce and circulate more insulin and hormones that can stimulate cancer growth. Overweight and obesity increase the risk for several cancers: breast in women past menopause, for example, as well as cancers of the colon and rectum, endometrium, esophagus, pancreas, and kidney.[305]

Physical inactivity has also been identified as a cancer risk factor and is estimated to be the main cause for approximately 21–25% of breast and colon cancers.[306] Prolonged sedentary activities such as TV viewing are associated with increased risks of colon, lung, and endometrial cancer. For each 2 hours per day of sedentary time there is an 8% increase in colon cancer risk and 10% increase in endometrial cancer risk.[307] A number of factors in the general environment can also increase the risk of cancer, for example, ultraviolet (UV) ionizing radiation (radon, X-rays, gamma rays) and exposure to carcinogens in the general and working environments, such as asbestos, formaldehyde, herbicides, and coal tars.

Prevention of Cancer

It is important to note that although a number of risk factors have been associated with cancer, the majority of cancers occur in people who do not have a known risk factor for their cancer.[308] As such, it is very hard to protect any individual from this disease. However, people can increase their odds of avoidance by minimizing controllable risk factors. To some extent, environmental factors may not be controllable because of where one lives or works.

One of the best preventive actions a person can take is to abstain from tobacco use and avoid exposure to second-hand tobacco smoke. The next major action is to modify lifestyle to minimize the other controllable cancer risks with diet and physical activity. Up to one-third of the cancer deaths that occur each year are in some way related to diet and physical activity. Lifestyle choices such as eating healthy, increasing physical activity, maintaining a low intake of alcohol, and quitting smoking can significantly reduce cancer risk.[309]

Early detection and effective treatments have contributed to 65.8% of cancer survivors reaching a 5-year survival marker, and 40% have survived 10 years or more.[310] Cancer survivors often face a variety of nutrition-related conditions. For example, many individuals have long-lasting side effects from cancer and its treatment or they can develop negative effects that appear months or years after their initial treatment.[311]

The consumption of fruits and vegetables may protect against the development of cancer. Fruits and vegetables contain phytochemicals and antioxidants that may reduce the oxidative reaction and enhance immune function. Fruits and vegetables along with fiber may protect against colon cancer. Consumption of lean meats, avoidance of sugar and sugar-sweetened beverages, and limited intake of alcohol and salty foods also protect against cancer.

Often obese individuals have increased inflammation, which has been linked to an increased risk for cancer.[312] People can undertake a wide variety of activities to stay fit to prevent cancer and other chronic diseases (see TABLE 13.24). Staying at a healthy weight is a way to protect against cancer.

Management of Cancer

The three main approaches to treating cancer are: (1) surgery, (2) radiation therapy, and (3) chemotherapy. The general goal of treatment is to prevent further growth of cancer or to remove tissue that can develop into cancer. Sometimes the specific objective is to cure the cancer, and other times the objective is to stop the cancer from growing, spreading, or recurring. Treatment objectives may be designed to decrease pain and symptoms and improve quality of life.

Table 13.24

Examples of Moderate and Vigorous Activities for Keeping Fit

Moderate Activities[a]	Vigorous Activities[b]
Ballroom and line dancing	Aerobic dance
Biking on level ground or with few hills	Biking faster than 10 miles per hour
Canoeing	Fast dancing
General gardening (raking, trimming shrubs)	Heavy gardening (digging, hoeing)
Sports where you catch and throw (baseball, softball, volleyball)	Hiking uphill
Tennis (doubles)	Jumping rope
Using your manual wheelchair	Martial arts (such as karate)
Using hand cyclers (also called ergometers)	Race walking, jogging, or running
Walking briskly	Sports with a lot of running (basketball, hockey, soccer)
Water aerobics	Swimming fast or swimming laps
	Tennis (singles)

[a] Activities that *I can talk while I do them, but I can't sing.*

[b] Activities that *I can only say a few words without stopping to catch my breath.*

Reproduced from US Department of Health and Human Services. *Be Active Your Way: A Fact Sheet for Adults.* Washington, DC: US Department of Health and Human Services; 2008. http://www.health.gov/PAGuidelines/factSheetAdults.aspx.

Regardless of treatment regimen, cancer treatments tend to be very physically demanding. A number of commons side effects of cancer and its treatment are relevant to nutritional status and physical fitness, including anorexia, nausea, vomiting, weight loss, fever, night sweats, muscle wasting, tiredness, peripheral neuropathy, changed sense of taste, difficulty chewing and swallowing, difficulty in replenishing lean body mass, and persistent bowel changes such as diarrhea or constipation.

The effect of the cancer itself must be considered. Cancer can cause a marked weight loss in patients that cannot be reversed by normal nutritional support. This is called *cancer cachexia*, also known as "wasting syndrome." Cancer cachexia is characterized by the following set of associated symptoms: progressive weight loss, anorexia, and persistent erosion of host body cell mass in response to a malignant growth. It can develop in the early stages of tumor growth even before there are any signs or symptoms of malignancy. Cancer cachexia is mainly associated with preterminal patients bearing disseminated disease. A decline in food intake in relation to energy expenditure is a major factor leading to cancer-associated weight loss.[313]

Ensuring patients have good nutritional status and a reasonable level of physical fitness can support the success of treatment and recovery and help reduce or deal with the side effects of treatment.[309] The American Institute for Cancer Research (AICR) recommends survivors aim to follow the organization's cancer prevention recommendations for diet, physical activity, and healthy weight

Table 13.25

Recommendations to Reduce Cancer Risk Before and After Treatment

1. Achieve a healthy body weight.
2. Aim for at least 30 minutes of moderate physical activity every day.
3. Choose nutritious wholesome foods and limit sugar-sweetened beverages and processed foods that are low in fiber and high in calories added sugar or fat.
4. Eat a variety of vegetables, fruits, whole grains, and legumes such as beans.
5. Eat less red meat and processed meat products.
6. If you drink alcoholic beverages, they should be limited to two a day for men and one for women a day.
7. Eat less foods processed with salt such as salty snacks and ready to eat meals.
8. Food first—its best to meet your nutritional requirements with food as much as possible and use dietary supplements to fill in the gaps.
9. Do not smoke or chew tobacco.

Data from American Institute for Cancer Research. AICR's guidelines for cancer survivors. Washington, DC: American Institute for Cancer Research; May 22, 2012. Retrieved from: http://www.aicr.org/patients-survivors/aicrs-guidelines-for-cancer.html. Accessed August 9, 2015.

Table 13.26

Guidelines for Dietary Supplement Use in Cancer Patients

- **"Food First":** Before taking dietary supplements, try to get all your needed nutrients with foods and beverages.
- **Consult your doctor and a registered dietitian nutritionist** before taking a dietary supplement to replace a deficient nutrient.
- **More is not always better**, especially in consideration of emerging data that suggest higher nutrient intakes, especially from sources other than foods, could be harmful instead of helpful.

Data from Rock CL, Doyle C, Demark-Wahnefried W, et al. Nutrition and physical activity guidelines for cancer survivors. *CA Cancer J Clin.* July/August 2012;62(4):242–274.

maintenance (see TABLE 13.25). Weight gain is a frequent complication of treatment and a concern when individual already have a high BMI.[314]

Nutritional Treatment of Cancer

Cancer can cause metabolic and physiological changes that affect an individual's requirements for macro- and micronutrients.[315] Side effects of cancer and its treatment include anorexia, early satiety, alterations in taste and smell, and bowel issues and can lead to inadequate nutrient intake and eventually cause malnutrition. Weight loss and poor nutritional status can occur at the beginning stages of some cancers. Therefore, it is important for individuals to consume enough calories to prevent additional weight loss.[316] Surgery, radiation, and chemotherapy can affect nutritional needs and adversely affect how the body digests, absorbs, and utilizes food.

A registered dietitian nutritionists should conduct a nutritional assessment right after diagnosis. A nutritional assessment requires the RDN to consider the treatment plan and goals (cure, control, or palliation); to evaluate the current nutritional status; and to anticipate symptoms occurring from treatment that could compromise the patient's nutritional status. The overall goals during the treatment phase are to prevent or resolve nutrient deficiencies, achieve or maintain a healthy weight, preserve lean body mass, minimize nutrition-related side effects, and maximize the quality of life.[317,318]

The use of vitamins, minerals, and other dietary supplements during cancer treatment is controversial. Some evidence shows negative effects from the use of dietary supplements in cancer patients, and therefore most primary care providers advise against patients taking supplements during and after treatment unless the supplements are used in consultation with a registered dietitian to treat a particular nutrient deficiency (see TABLE 13.26). Nutritional supplements (nutrient-dense beverages and foods) may be recommended to those who cannot eat or drink enough to maintain sufficient energy intake. The use of enteral nutrition and parenteral nutrition support should be individualized and work in conjunction with the overall treatment goals.[319]

Exercise

Recent studies have looked at the value of exercise during primary cancer treatment.[320,321] Cancer patients should be encouraged to maintain activity as much as possible. Exercise is safe and can improve physical functioning, fatigue, and multiple aspects of quality of life.[322] The decisions about when to start exercise and how to maintain physical activity should be individualized in consideration of the patient's condition and preferences. Exercise during cancer treatment improves posttreatment adverse effects on bone health and muscle strength.[323,324]

Recommendations for Long-Term Disease-Free Individuals

Goals for weight management, physical activity, and healthy eating are necessary to promote overall health, quality of life, and longevity. Individuals who have been diagnosed with cancer are at a higher risk of developing second primary cancers as well as chronic diseases.[325,326] Family members of cancer survivors may also be at a higher risk of developing cancer, and healthcare providers should encourage families to follow the guidelines listed in TABLE 13.27.

Long-term dietary therapy must be individualized, reviewed, and adjusted on a regular basis. The RDN will focus on preventing weight loss and nutrient deficiencies, maintaining lean body mass, and preventing unintentional weight gain. In addition, it is important for the dietitian to identify and manage adverse effects individuals suffer from the various cancer treatments. Additional

Table 13.27

Summary of the American Cancer Society Guidelines on Nutrition and Physical Activity for Cancer Survivors

Achieve and maintain a healthy body weight.

To aid in weight loss limit consumption of high-calorie foods and sugar-sweetened beverages and increase physical activity.

To aid in weight gain, eat nutritious calorie-dense foods, frequent small meals, and well-balanced snacks.

Be physically active 3-5 times weekly and avoid inactivity as much as possible.

Limit sedentary behavior and attempt to return to normal daily activities as soon as possible following diagnosis.

Try to exercise at a moderate intensity at least 30 minutes per day.

To preserve muscle and lean body mass, perform strength-training exercises at least 2 days per week.

Eat more plant foods such as vegetables, fruits, and whole grains and limit red meat and processed meats and foods made with refined grains.

Data from Summary of the ACS guidelines on nutrition and physical activity. Dallas, TX: American Cancer Society; updated February 5, 2016. Retrieved from: http://www.cancer.org/healthy/eathealthygetactive/acsguidelinesonnutritionphysicalactivityforcancerprevention/acs-guidelines-on-nutrition-and-physical-activity-for-cancer-prevention-summary. Accessed November 16, 2016.

into the daily meal plan. Individuals should be encouraged to choose whole grains and whole-grain foods as their source of fiber rather than relying on fiber supplements. Foods high in sugar can replace nutrient-dense food choices and increase the caloric content of the diet and therefore should be limited. Many healthcare providers recommend that individuals receiving chemotherapy or biological therapy avoid alcohol consumption during treatment.

Vegetables and fruits contain essential vitamins, minerals, phytochemicals, and fiber that can possibly inhibit cancer progression. These foods are nutrient dense, increase satiety, and may assist with healthy weight management. Some studies suggest that omega-3 fatty acids have specific benefits for cancer survivors to alleviate cachexia and improve quality of life. More research is needed in this area before recommendations can be made. In the meantime, foods that are high in omega-3 fatty acids can be incorporated into the diet plan.[327] Cured, processed meats are the primary source of nitrites in the average American diet. Research has shown a link between nitrite/nitrate intake and the risk of gastrointestinal cancer and colorectal cancer; experts recommend that people avoid processed meats.[328]

Food Safety

Although always important, food safety can be critical for individuals during episodes of treatment-related immunosuppression that occur with certain cancer treatment regimens.[329] During any immunosuppressive cancer treatment, patients should take extra precautions to prevent infection and avoid eating foods that may contain unsafe levels of pathogenic microorganisms **TABLE 13.29** .

considerations for the long-term dietary treatment of cancer patients are listed in **TABLE 13.28** .

Adequate protein intake is important at all stages of cancer treatment. The best choices to meet protein needs are foods that are also low in saturated fat such as fish, lean meat, skinless poultry, eggs, nonfat and low-fat dairy products, and legumes. Healthy carbohydrates from vegetables, fruits, whole grains, and legumes that are rich in phytochemicals and fiber should be incorporated

Table 13.28

Dietary Considerations for the Long-Term Treatment of Cancer Patients

- Small, frequent snacks may be better tolerated than the consumption of three large meals.
- Food choices will need to adapt to the individual's changing needs.
- The diet must contain protein, carbohydrate, and fat to provide energy, and each is available from a wide variety of food choices.
- Food choices should be easy to chew, swallow, digest, and absorb.
- Supplements and nutrient-dense snacks may need to be added to assist in providing adequate nutrient intake.
- If oral nutrition support is inadequate to meet nutritional requirements or when severe malnutrition is diagnosed, enteral or parenteral support should be considered as well.
- Because many cancer survivors are at a higher risk of developing other chronic diseases, the recommended amounts and types of fat, protein, and carbohydrate associated with reducing cardiovascular disease risk are also appropriate for cancer survivors.
- The Institute of Medicine recommends the following balance of fat, carbohydrate, and protein in the diet to provide energy: fat, 20–35% of energy; carbohydrate, 45–65% of energy; and protein, 10–35% of energy.

U.S. Department of Agriculture and U.S. Department of Health and Human Services. *Dietary Guidelines for Americans, 2010.* 7th ed. Washington, DC: U.S. Government Printing Office; December 2010. Retrieved from: https://health.gov/dietaryguidelines/dga2010/DietaryGuidelines2010.pdf. Accessed August 26, 2016; American Heart Association Nutrition Committee, Lichtenstein AH, Appel LJ, et al. Diet and lifestyle recommendations revision 2006: a scientific statement from the American Heart Association Nutrition Committee. *Circulation.* 2006;114:82–96; Kushi LH, Doyle C, McCullough M, et al. American Cancer Society Guidelines on nutrition and physical activity for cancer prevention: reducing the risk of cancer with healthy food choices and physical activity. *CA Cancer J Clin.* 2012;62:30–67; National Research Council. *Dietary Reference Intakes for Energy, Carbohydrate, Fiber, Fat, Fatty Acids, Cholesterol, Protein, and Amino Acids (Macronutrients).* Washington, DC: National Academies Press; 2002.

Table 13.29

General Guidelines for Food Safety

Wash hands with soap and warm water thoroughly before handling foods or eating.

Keep raw meats, fish, poultry, and egg separate from ready-to-eat foods, fresh produce, and cooked foods.

Clean all utensils, countertops, cutting boards, and sponges that have contact with raw meat in hot soapy water.

Cook all foods thoroughly especially meats to 145°F, ground meat to 160°F, poultry to 165°F, and fish and seafood to 145°F. Beverages (milk and juices) should be pasteurized.

Store foods promptly at 40°F or below to minimize bacterial growth.

Drink clean water.

Data from Rock CL, Doyle C, Demark-Wahnefried W, et al. Nutrition and physical activity guidelines for cancer survivors. *CA Cancer J Clin*. July/August 2012;62(4):242–274; and Partnership for Food Safety Education. Fight BAC! Retrieved from: http://www.fightbac.org/. Accessed November 16, 2016.

Potentially Protective Foods

A number of foods have been studied for their cancer-protective effects, including tea, garlic, cruciferous vegetables, and soy foods/isoflavones. Studies that looked at tea intake and lung cancer show that tea is significantly protective on lung cancer risk, for example.[330,331] Also, preliminary data suggest that components of garlic may play a role in lung cancer prevention.[332,333] Some evidence suggests that cruciferous vegetable intake may decrease the risk of lung cancer.[334] Recently, it was found that women who consumed soy foods before their diagnosis of lung cancer had better overall survival rates.[335]

Recap *Cancer* refers to a group of more than a hundred diseases. Cancer cells grow and form new cells that are abnormal, and these cells can invade other tissues. Annually, more than 1.6 million new cases of cancer are diagnosed in the United States. Ensuring patients have good nutritional status and a reasonable level of physical fitness can support the success of treatment and recovery and help reduce or deal with the side effects of cancer treatment.

1. Discuss the incidence and etiology of cancer.
2. What are some of the key approaches for preventing cancer?
3. Describe why nutritional status is important for the successful treatment of cancer.

Immune Disorders: HIV and AIDS

Preview This section presents infection with HIV and the disease that develops from it, AIDS. Most people fear HIV and AIDS and highly misunderstand them. This section defines HIV and AIDS, discusses their prevalence, identifies risk factors, and then discusses their prevention and management.

HIV (human immunodeficiency virus) is an incurable retrovirus that attacks the immune system. The **acquired immune deficiency syndrome (AIDS)** is an infectious disease that develops from HIV. HIV destroys the immune cells, in particular, the T helper cells, tissue macrophages, and blood monocytes, and some cells of the central nervous system can be affected. HIV and its treatment can affect the metabolism and thus energy expenditure, lipid metabolism, hormonal balance, and immune function can be altered. Both macronutrient and micronutrient requirements change throughout the course of the disease. Protein-energy malnutrition, anemia, and status of other micronutrients are altered.[336]

Prevalence and Etiology of HIV and AIDS

Once considered a death sentence, HIV infection, and the death rate from AIDS, has declined in recent years. Part of the reason for this is that the progression from HIV to AIDS has decreased.[337,338] In the United States, 1.2 million people live with the HIV infection; approximately 12.8% of people with HIV are unaware that they have it, which increases the risk of transmission and causes treatment delays. In 2010, men who had sex with men accounted for 78% of new HIV infections among males, representing 63% of new infections overall. Over the past few years, the incidence of HIV has remained approximately the same, with an estimated 50,000 new HIV infections diagnosed annually. The prevalence of HIV infection and AIDS is increasing in women who live in underserved populations in both the United States and Canada. An individual who is well nourished is more likely to handle the effects of HIV infection, which can in turn delay the progression of the disease. A BMI in the normal range predicts survival in individuals with HIV infection.[339] Several studies show that weight loss is associated with increased morbidity and mortality.[340]

Statistically, minority populations experience higher percentages of new cases and regional variations arise in terms of ethnicity of people diagnosed with AIDS (see **FIGURE 13.21**). The Centers for Disease Control and Prevention reports that the number of HIV infections progressing to AIDS has decreased since 1996 owing to the use of combination antiretroviral drugs that assist in keeping the viral load under control and that help to improve T cell counts and immune function.[341,342] **FIGURE 13.22** presents the estimated numbers of new HIV infections in the United States by the most affected populations.

The symptoms of HIV infection include fever, tiredness, swollen lymph nodes, sore throat, skin rashes, muscle and joint pain, and diarrhea. If the HIV infection is not treated, the number of T cells decreases and a person becomes susceptible to opportunistic infections. AIDS is diagnosed during the advanced stages of HIV infection, when the body is unable to fight illness (see **FIGURE 13.23**).

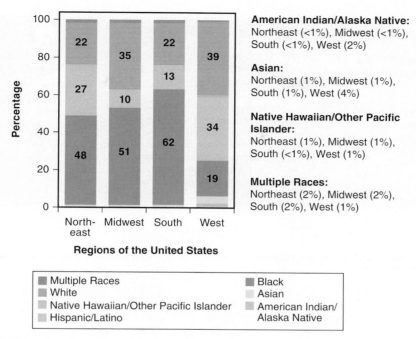

American Indian/Alaska Native:
Northeast (<1%), Midwest (<1%),
South (<1%), West (2%)

Asian:
Northeast (1%), Midwest (1%),
South (1%), West (4%)

Native Hawaiian/Other Pacific
Islander:
Northeast (1%), Midwest (1%),
South (<1%), West (1%)

Multiple Races:
Northeast (2%), Midwest (2%),
South (2%), West (1%)

Figure 13.21
Race/ethnicity of persons diagnosed with AIDS in 2010 in the 50 states and District of Columbia, by region of residence.

Reproduced from Centers for Disease Control and Prevention. HIV/AIDS: HIV and AIDS in the United States by geographic distribution. Atlanta, GA: Centers for Disease Control and Prevention; updated May 25, 2016. Retrieved from: http://www.cdc.gov/hiv/statistics/basics/geographicdistribution. html. Accessed November 18, 2016\.

Acute Infection Stage

Often, between 2 and 4 weeks after being infected with HIV, flu-like symptoms develop (fever, swollen glands, rash, muscle and joint pain, headache, and tiredness). This is referred to as the acute retroviral syndrome (ARS) or primary HIV infection. The disease then progresses into the clinical latency stage when the virus is not producing symptoms; however, during this stage HIV continues to reproduce at very low levels. Many factors affect the time between infection with HIV and development of AIDS. These factors, listed in TABLE 13.30, may shorten or lengthen the time frame.

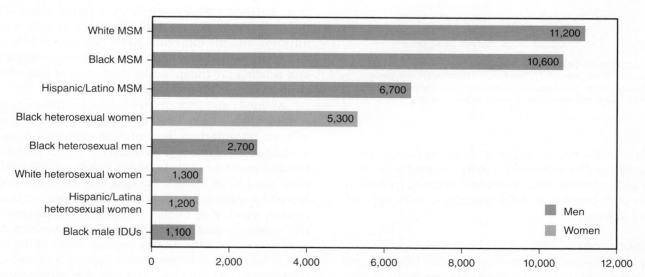

Figure 13.22
Estimated new HIV infections in the United States, 2010, for the most affected subpopulations.

IDUs = injected drug users; MSM = men who have sex with men.

Reproduced from Centers for Disease Control and Prevention. HIV/AIDS: HIV in the United States: at a glance. Atlanta, GA: Centers for Disease Control and Prevention; updated June 2016. Retrieved from: http://www.cdc .gov/hiv/statistics/basics/ataglance.html. Accessed November 18, 2016.

1 **ACUTE INFECTION:**	**2** **CLINICAL LATENCY:**	**3** **AIDS:**
During this time, large amounts of the virus are being produced in your body.	During this stage of the disease, HIV reproduces at very low levels, although it is still active.	As your CD4 cells fall below 200 cells/mm^3, you are considered to have progressed to AIDS.
Many, but not all, people develop flu-like symptoms often described as the "worst flu ever."	During this period, you may not have symptoms. With proper HIV treatment, people may live with clinical latency for several decades. Without treatment, this period lasts an average of 10 years, but some people may progress through this stage faster.	Without treatment, people typically survive 3 years.

Figure 13.23
Stages of HIV infection.

Reproduced from U.S. Department of Health and Human Services. Stages of HIV infection. Washington, DC: U.S. Department of Health and Human Services. Retrieved from: https://www.aids.gov/hiv-aids-basics/just-diagnosed-with-hiv-aids/hiv-in-your-body/stages-of-hiv/. Accessed August 31, 2016.

Table 13.30

Factors that Affect the Time Between HIV Infection and AIDS

Factors that may shorten the time between HIV infection and AIDS	• Older age • HIV subtype • Coinfection with other viruses • Poor nutrition • Severe stress • Genetic background
Factors that may delay the time between HIV infection and AIDS	• Taking antiretroviral therapy • Staying in HIV care • Closely adhering to physician's or nurse practitioner's recommendations • Eating healthy foods • Taking care of oneself • Genetic background

Reproduced from U.S. Department of Health and Human Services. Stages of HIV infection. Washington, DC: U.S. Department of Health and Human Services. Retrieved from: https://www.aids.gov/hiv-aids-basics/just-diagnosed-with-hiv-aids/hiv-in-your-body/stages-of-hiv/. Accessed August 31, 2016.

Once AIDS develops, the immune system is badly damaged and the individual is more vulnerable to infections and infection-related cancers. Without treatment, people who progress to AIDS typically survive approximately 3 years.[343]

Complications of HIV

Many complications can develop with HIV infection, but the most notable are HIV lipodystrophy syndrome, weight loss, anorexia and poor dietary intake, metabolic changes, and food insecurity.

HIV lipodystrophy syndrome can develop in some individuals who use highly active antiretroviral therapy

(HAART) medication to suppress the HIV infection. In these cases, problems can develop with glucose and fat metabolism. With this syndrome, body fat redistributes centrally, insulin resistance can occur, and blood lipid levels can become abnormal (see **FIGURE 13.24**).[344]

Aggressive treatment plans have reduced "wasting syndrome" (see Figure 13.25), but this complication still affects many people with AIDS. Wasting syndrome is defined as a loss of at least 10% of body weight within 12 months. A small amount of weight loss (5%) is associated with an increased risk of mortality and increased risk of infection. Wasting syndrome is often caused by anorexia, poor diet, changes in metabolism and nutrient absorption, diarrhea, and diet–medication interactions. When the body breaks down protein tissues in response to an infection and the individual has a decrease in food consumption, weight loss and wasting develop. Weight loss and wasting are independent predictors of mortality in patients with HIV infection.[345,346]

Anorexia and poor dietary intake contribute to malnutrition, which can lead to immune dysfunction even without HIV infection; malnutrition continues to be the leading cause of immune dysfunction. It is important for medical practitioners to be aware that some HIV medications need to be taken with food, but when the patient has no appetite, they may not adhere to their medication regime, which may further compromise their health. If HIV enters the gastrointestinal tract, it can become damaged very early in the disease process. Some of the treatments for HIV lead to nutritional changes and metabolic alterations. Hypertension, cardiovascular disease, insulin resistance and diabetes, liver dysfunction, renal dysfunction, and bone mineral density loss are some conditions that affect individual nutritional management.[347–350] Elevated blood lipid levels, insulin sensitivity or glucose

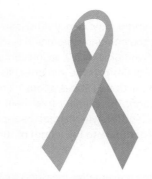

As HIV disease progresses in your body,

YOU MAY NOTICE PHYSICAL CHANGES.

— Some changes may occur —

as side effects of medical treatment for HIV.

WHILE THIS IS OFTEN A SIGN OF LATE STAGE
DISEASE, WASTING SYNDROME CAN BE TREATED BY:

Proper diet

Medications to stimulate appetite

Medications to control diarrhea

Hormonal therapy to build muscle

**YOUR BODY CAN GAIN EXTRA FAT
OR LOSE FAT IN THESE PLACES:**

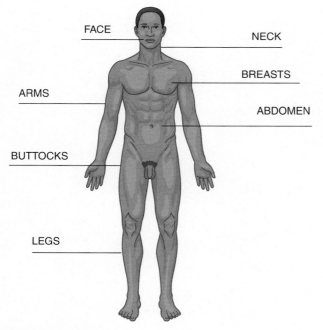

Figure 13.24
Physical changes that can occur with AIDS.

Reproduced from U.S. Department of Health and Human Services. Physical changes. Washington, DC: U.S. Department of Health and Human Services. Retrieved from: https://www.aids.gov/hiv-aids-basics/just-diagnosed-with-hiv-aids/hiv-in-your-body/physical-changes/index.html. Accessed August 31, 2015.

intolerance, mitochondrial toxicity, and lactic acidosis have been reported in some individuals living with HIV.[351]

A situation in which a person lacks money or the resources to acquire food is known as food insecurity. Many individuals living with HIV are impoverished, socially isolated, ostracized, and often face many barriers to acquiring healthy food.

Risk Factors for HIV Infection

A number of factors are well recognized risks for exposure and infection with HIV leading to AIDS, including unprotected sex, sexually transmitted infections, intravenous drug use, uncircumcised males, and blood transfusions. According to the National Heart, Lung, and Blood Institute, only about 1 in 2 million blood donations might carry HIV and transmit HIV if given to a patient.[352]

Prevention and Treatment of HIV/AIDS

Because there is no cure for AIDS, the best course of action is prevention. HIV is most often sexually transmitted and can be spread by contaminated body fluids (blood, semen, vaginal secretions, and breast milk). It is important that individuals at risk be tested for HIV antibodies because many individuals are unaware that they have been infected.

HIV/AIDS is not a curable disease at this time. The primary treatment for HIV/AIDS involves medications and lifestyle changes to support the health of the patient and contribute to the length of survival and the quality of life.

Antiretroviral (ARV) medications are recommended for all HIV-infected individuals. By suppressing the amount of virus in the body, people infected with HIV can lead longer and healthier lives. ARVs also help to reduce the risk of disease progression. The medication must be continued throughout the patient's life.

Some of the common side effects of ARVs, such as nausea, diarrhea, fatigue, headache, and myalgia, can interfere with proper nutrition and food intake. These side effects typically resolve 1–2 months after initiating therapy. Some adverse effects associated with ARVs are dyslipidemia, insulin resistance, glucose intolerance, and anemia. ARVs suppress the virus, but they do not completely eliminate HIV from the body; therefore not a cure.

In addition to taking medications to directly fight and manage HIV infection, patients also may take medications for symptom management or nutritional rehabilitation. Many of the medications that are prescribed for HIV have adverse effects that affect the nutritional status of the patient. RDNs should be consulted in treatment to minimize the negative nutritional impact of medications and their side effects.[353]

Nutritional Considerations

A registered dietitian should create meal plans and nutrition strategies for each individual. Nutritional repletion that provides adequate calories has been shown to improve the immune function and should begin right after diagnosis. Both macronutrient and micronutrient requirements can change throughout the course of the disease. Energy requirements vary for each individual and depend on the person's levels of malabsorption, nutrient depletion, complications, and infections. Protein needs increase for individuals with loss of lean body mass, and can range from 1.2 g/kg/day to 2.0 g/kg/day. There is no difference in fat requirements compared with the general population's. The intake of B vitamins, vitamins A, E, and D, as well as selenium and zinc should be carefully monitored.[354–356] Sometimes malabsorption and medications can require a change in treatment with numerous complications. Individuals living with HIV are more susceptible to foodborne illnesses.

Sores in the mouth, taste changes, and nausea can affect eating and food preference. Frequent small meals may be helpful. Dietitians may recommend liquid nutrition supplements. If the individual is unable to tolerate oral feedings, a tube feeding may be suggested. If there are problems with the tube or presence of diarrhea or malabsorption, parenteral nutrition may be suggested.

Prolonging health also involves keeping food safe to avoid foodborne illness and regular physical activity (see

Recap HIV (human immunodeficiency virus) is an incurable retrovirus that attacks the immune system and leads to acquired immune deficiency syndrome (AIDS), an infectious disease that develops from HIV. HIV destroys the immune cells, in particular, the T helper cells. In the United States, about 1.2 million people live with HIV infection. The primary treatment for HIV/AIDS involves medications and lifestyle changes to support the health of the patient and contribute to the length of survival and the quality of life.

1. Identify all of the preventative measures for HIV/AIDS.
2. Discuss the nutritional considerations for someone with HIV/AIDS.

Table 13.29, General Guidelines for Food Safety, in the section on cancer). Many of these illnesses can be prevented with safe food handling. Exercise at low to moderate intensities does not increase the risk for developing other infections. Both aerobic exercise and resistance training can improve strength and muscle and cardiovascular endurance in those suffering from muscle wasting.[357]

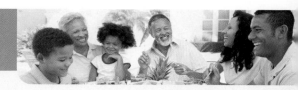

Learning Portfolio

Visual Chapter Summary

Overweight and Obesity

- Overweight and obesity are defined as abnormal or excessive fat accumulation in the body.
- A person with a BMI greater than or equal to 25 is overweight, and a person with a BMI greater than or equal to 30 is obese.
- In 2014, more than 1.9 billion adults 18 years and older were overweight throughout the world, and of these, more than 600 million were obese.
- The basic goal of a treatment plan for overweight individuals is to prevent further weight gain. The programs should be designed to allow for modest weight loss, weight maintenance, and management strategies for obesity comorbidities.
- Excess abdominal fat can lead to increased levels of blood lipids, which can increase the risk of cardiovascular disease.

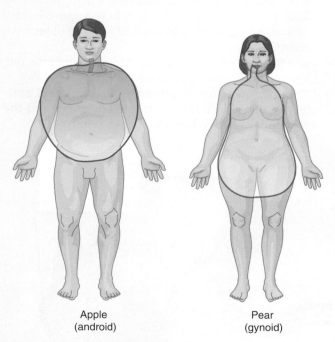

Apple
(android)

Pear
(gynoid)

Pear- versus apple-shaped body types.

Gastrointestinal Conditions

- Gastroesophageal reflux disease (GERD) is a chronic condition in which stomach contents reflux into the esophagus and upward, causing symptoms and complications.

- The prevalence of reflux symptoms has been steadily rising throughout the industrialized world, with an estimated 20–40% of Western adult populations reporting chronic heartburn or regurgitation symptoms.
- Diet and lifestyle modification should be used as adjuncts to medication rather than as primary treatment for GERD.

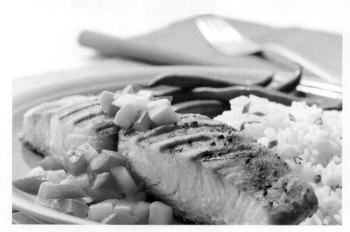

©NightAndDayImages/E+/Getty

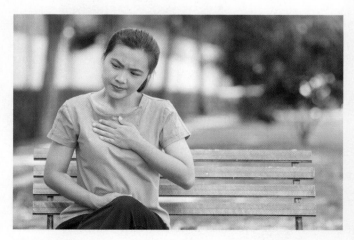

©CHAjAMP/Shutterstock

- Irritable bowel syndrome (IBS) is a chronic condition comprising a group of symptoms that include discomfort and pain in the abdominal area and a change in bowel patterns that involves changes in the colon's rhythm.

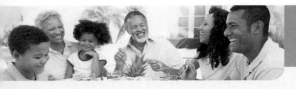

Learning Portfolio (continued)

- On a global basis, the prevalence of IBS is estimated at approximately 11%.
- Individuals with IBS have an intolerance to certain carbohydrates, so dietitians may suggest a trial diet using the FODMAP diet (low in fermentable oligosaccharides, disaccharides, monosaccharides, and polyols) strategy.

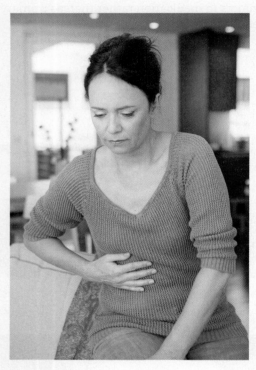

©Image Point Fr/Shutterstock

- Inflammatory bowel disease is a chronic condition with periodic immune responses combined with inflammation in the gastrointestinal tract.
- The two most common forms of IBD are ulcerative colitis, whose symptoms are restricted to the large intestine, and Crohn's disease, which affects the entire digestive tract.
- Approximately 1.6 million Americans have IBD.
- A regular evaluation of nutrient status is recommended because malnutrition is present in up to 85% of patients with IBD and weight loss occurs in up to 80% of patients with Crohn's disease.
- As a person ages, it is common for the walls in the colon to develop bulging pockets of tissue or sacs known as diverticula.

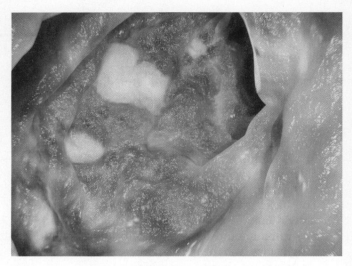

Ulcerative colitis.
©Andrew Gentry/Shutterstock

- Diverticular disease has been considered a "Western disease." The highest prevalence is in the United States, Europe, and Australia, where approximately 50% of the population 60 years of age and older have diverticulosis.
- The diverticula sacs become inflamed and infected, a person has developed diverticulitis.
- The treatment for diverticulitis involves oral antibiotics and anti-inflammatory medication, and the patient needs to follow a low-fiber diet.

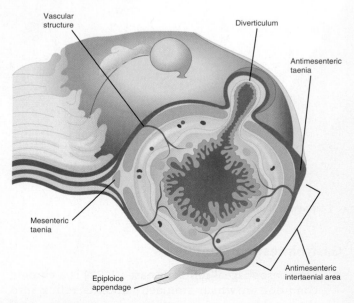

Diverticular disease.

- Gallbladder disease is an impairment of the normal function of the gallbladder that leads to abdominal discomfort and the inability to digest fatty foods.
- Gallstones form when bile becomes concentrated in the gallbladder and becomes a stone-like material. Gallstones can cause problems if they obstruct the bile ducts, which then causes inflammation, infection, and pancreatitis.
- More than 25 million Americans have gallstones, and a million are diagnosed with gallstones each year.
- Typically, a registered dietitian instructs patients to consume a healthy diet with moderate amounts of fat: 20–35% of calories as fat.

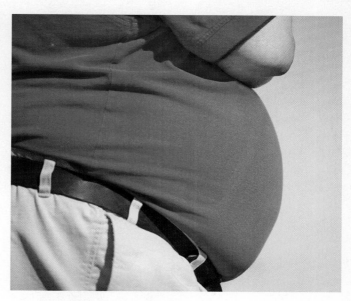

©Suzanne Tucker/Shutterstock

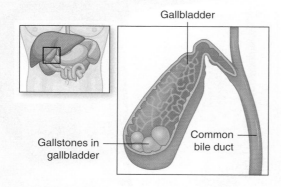

Gallstones in the gallbladder.

Endocrine and Metabolic Conditions

- Metabolic syndrome is not a disease of its own but rather a combination of risk factors, including high cholesterol levels, high blood sugar levels, high blood pressure, and excess abdominal fat.
- Approximately one-third of the adult population in the United States has metabolic syndrome.
- The occurrence of metabolic syndrome increases with age and in relation to higher BMI levels.
- Diets that are low in saturated and trans fats, balanced in carbohydrate intake throughout the day, high in dietary fiber, high in fruit and vegetable intake and that include low-fat dairy foods are protective against metabolic syndrome.
- Type 2 diabetes mellitus is a condition in which the pancreas does not produce enough insulin for

normal functioning or the insulin that is produced is not working properly in the body.
- It is estimated that 29.1 million people, or 9.3% of the U.S. population, have diabetes, but only 21.0 million have actually been diagnosed.
- Type 2 diabetes is treated and managed by regular physical activity, healthy dietary intake, loss of excess weight, and medications, with the overall goal to lower blood glucose levels.

Cardiovascular Disease and Hypertension

- Cardiovascular disease (CVD) includes any disease or injury of the heart and blood vessels. Coronary heart disease is the most common type of heart disease, leading to over 370,000 deaths annually.
- A healthy lifestyle is essentially the best way to prevent cardiovascular disease.
- Dietary and lifestyle changes can reduce high LDL-C by 20–40%.
- The treatment goals for CVD are to reduce the heart's workload by controlling blood pressure and using beta blockers or calcium channel blockers to decrease the intensity of heart pumping.
- About 29% of the adults in the United States have hypertension (HTN), a chronic condition in which a person's blood pressure is consistently elevated above the population average.

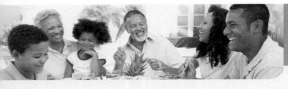

Learning Portfolio (continued)

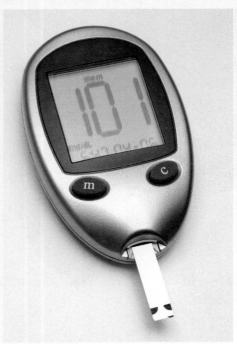

©Andrew Gentry/Shutterstock

- The typical cut-off values used to determine high blood pressure is a consistent systolic pressure of 140 mm Hg and a consistent diastolic pressure of 90 mm Hg.
- The treatment of hypertension includes lifestyle modification, and often antihypertensive drug therapy is added into the treatment plan.
- The DASH (Dietary Approaches to Stop Hypertension) diet promotes consumption of vegetables, fruits, low-fat dairy products, whole grains, poultry, fish, and nuts. The plan discourages sweets, sugar-sweetened beverages, and red meats.

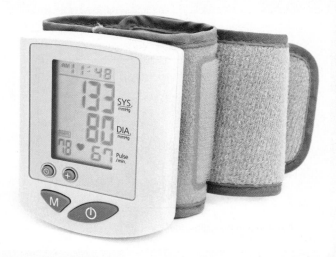

©Andrei Shumskiy/Shutterstock

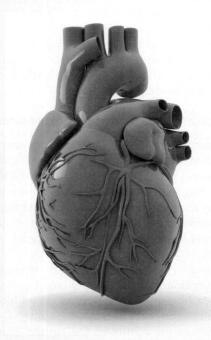

©Science Photo Library-PASIEKA/Brand X Pictures/Getty

Cancer

- Cancer refers to a group of more than a hundred diseases.
- Cancer cells grow and form new cells that are abnormal, and these cells can invade other tissues.
- Annually, more than 1.6 million new cases of cancer are diagnosed in the United States, and about 600,000 people die from this disease.
- Ensuring patients have good nutritional status and a reasonable level of physical fitness can support the success of treatment and recovery and help reduce or deal with the side effects of cancer treatment.

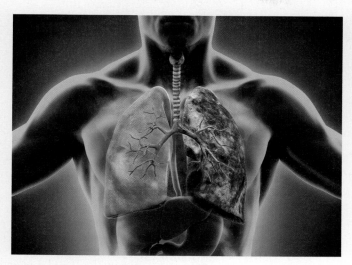

©Nerthuz/Shutterstock

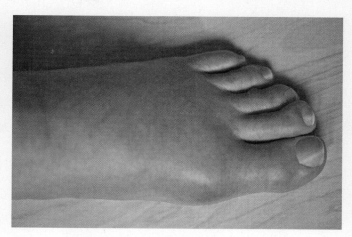

©BSIP/Universal Images Group/Getty

Immune Disorders: HIV and AIDS

- HIV (human immunodeficiency virus) is an incurable retrovirus that attacks the immune system and leads to acquired immune deficiency syndrome (AIDS), an infectious disease that develops from HIV.
- HIV destroys the immune cells, in particular, the T helper cells.
- In the United States, about 1.2 million people live with an HIV infection.

- The primary treatment for HIV/AIDS involves medications and lifestyle changes to support the health of the patient and contribute to the length of survival and quality of life.
- Prolonging health involves regular physical activity and keeping food safe to avoid foodborne illness, which would stress the immune system.

① **ACUTE INFECTION:**	② **CLINICAL LATENCY:**	③ **AIDS:**
During this time, large amounts of the virus are being produced in your body.	During this stage of the disease, HIV reproduces at very low levels, although it is still active.	As your CD4 cells fall below 200 cells/mm^3, you are considered to have progressed to AIDS.
Many, but not all, people develop flu-like symptoms often described as the "worst flu ever."	During this period, you may not have symptoms. With proper HIV treatment, people may live with clinical latency for several decades. Without treatment, this period lasts an average of 10 years, but some people may progress through this stage faster.	Without treatment, people typically survive 3 years.

Stages of HIV infection.

Reproduced from U.S. Department of Health and Human Services. Stages of HIV infection. Washington, DC: U.S. Department of Health and Human Services. Retrieved from: https://www.aids.gov/hiv-aids-basics/just-diagnosed-with-hiv-aids/hiv-in-your-body/stages-of-hiv/. Accessed August 31, 2016.

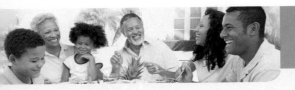

Learning Portfolio (continued)

Key Terms

acquired immune deficiency syndrome (AIDS): An infectious disease that develops from human immunodeficiency virus (HIV) infection.

ATP III: The National Cholesterol Education Program Adult Treatment Panel III Report, which recommends the diagnosis of metabolic syndrome be made when three or more of the following risk determinants are present: abdominal obesity, high levels of triglycerides, high levels of high-density lipoprotein (HDL), high blood pressure, and high fasting plasma glucose.

cancer: A group of more than a hundred diseases. Cancer starts when abnormal cells grow out of control. Instead of dying, cancer cells grow and form new cells that are abnormal, and these cells can also invade other tissues.

carcinogen: Substance or agent that is known to be or that are strongly suspected to be causes of cancer.

cardiovascular disease (CVD): Any disease or injury of the heart and its blood vessels as well as the blood vessels throughout the body and the brain.

cerebrovascular disease: Disease of the blood vessels and, especially, the arteries that supply the brain that affects the circulation of blood to the brain, causing limited or no blood flow to certain areas of the brain known as stroke or transient ischemic attacks.

coronary heart disease (CHD): Disease or injury of the heart that includes myocardial infarction (MI), angina pectoris, heart failure, and coronary death.

DASH (Dietary Approaches to Stop Hypertension) diet: A dietary pattern promoted by the U.S.-based National Heart, Lung, and Blood Institute (part of the National Institutes of Health, an agency of the U.S. Department of Health and Human Services) to prevent and control hypertension. It involves decreased sodium intake and increased consumption of fruit and vegetables and low-fat dairy products.

diverticular disease: The presence of bulging pockets of tissue or sacs in the walls of the colon.

diverticulitis: Inflammation and/or infection of one or more diverticula, especially in the colon, causing pain and disturbance of bowel function.

diverticulosis: A condition in which diverticula (small, bulging sacs) are present in the intestine without signs of inflammation.

FODMAP diet: A diet consisting of foods containing low fermentable oligosaccharides, disaccharides, monosaccharides, and polyols.

food insecurity: Limited or uncertain availability of nutritionally adequate and safe foods or limited or uncertain ability to acquire acceptable foods in socially acceptable ways, such as when a person lacks the money or the resources to acquire food. Food insecurity manifests as difficulty providing enough food for all family members at some time during the year as a result of a lack of resources.

gallbladder disease: Any impairment of the normal function of the gallbladder that leads to abdominal discomfort and the inability to digest fatty foods.

gallstone: A calculus (as of cholesterol) formed in the gallbladder or biliary passages; also called biliary calculus or cholelith. Gallstones occur when the bile becomes concentrated in the gallbladder and becomes a stone-like material that can potentially block the flow of bile in the bile duct.

high-density lipoprotein (HDL): A blood lipoprotein that contains low levels of triglycerides and high levels of protein. HDL is synthesized primarily in the liver as well as in the small intestine. HDL carries cholesterol out of the bloodstream. HDL is called the good cholesterol.

hyperglycemia: High concentration of glucose in the bloodstream.

hypertension: A chronic condition where a person's blood pressure is consistently elevated above the population average. Resting blood pressure exceeds 140 mm Hg systolic or 90 mm Hg diastolic.

hyperuricemia: Chronic elevated serum uric acid levels.

low-density lipoprotein (LDL): Composed primarily of cholesterol transports cholesterol to the cells of the body.

lower esophageal sphincter (LES): A ring of smooth muscle fibers at the junction of the esophagus and stomach.

metabolic syndrome: A cluster of at least three biochemical and physiological abnormalities that are risk factors for heart disease and type 2 diabetes: hypertriglyceridemia, low HDL cholesterol, hyperglycemia, hypertension, or excess abdominal fat.

nonalcoholic fatty liver disease (NAFLD): A term used to describe the accumulation of fat in the liver of people who drink little or no alcohol.

nutritional supplement: Nutrient-dense beverage and food.

peripheral artery disease (PAD): A narrowing of the peripheral arteries to the legs, stomach, arms, and head.

Rome III diagnostic criteria: A system developed to classify the functional gastrointestinal disorders (FGIDs) of the digestive system in which symptoms cannot be explained by the presence of structural or tissue abnormality, based on clinical symptoms.

triglycerides: The main constituents of natural fats and oils. They are fats composed of three fatty acid chains linked to a glycerol molecule.

type 2 diabetes: A form of diabetes in which the body does not use insulin properly.

Discussion Questions

1. Describe the prevalence and etiology of IBD and then describe the methods of treatment for this disease and whether it can be cured.

2. Summarize the prevalence and etiology of obesity. It would seem that the formulation for treating obesity is quite simple: Decrease calorie intake from food and increase calorie output through exercise and activity. Discuss the reasons why this simple formulation is so difficult to apply in the treatment of obesity.

3. Define type 2 diabetes mellitus and its dietary treatment.

4. Tobacco consumption is a key preventable cause of cardiovascular disease. Yet with all the facts and information available, tobacco consumption persists. Discuss why you think this is the case and then discuss methods by which tobacco consumption could be reduced or eliminated. Make some recommendations you would enact if you had the authority to do so.

5. Why is food safety a critical consideration in the treatment of both cancer and HIV/AIDS? Discuss the importance of food safety and describe the food safety procedures that people who are being treated for cancer or HIV/AIDS should follow.

6. Of all the chronic diseases, HIV/AIDS most often calls for the services of a professional registered dietitian nutritionist in its treatment. Explain the approach to nutritional management and why it is so important in the treatment of this disease.

Activities

1. **Family History Case Study.** Virtually every family has one or more members who have suffered from or manifested one or more chronic diseases. Develop your own chronic disease case study based on your family history. Pick a person from your family tree who has suffered from one of the chronic diseases listed in the chapter. Identify the disease condition, define it, and then present information on its symptoms, causes, risk factors, complications, treatments, and prevention. Discuss your family experience of the disease. Be sure to "disguise" the person in some fashion to maintain confidentiality.

2. **Myth or Miracle?** In the past, near miracle cures have been found for some diseases. For example, vitamin C as a cure and preventative for scurvy, cimetidine for stomach ulcers, and penicillin for serious infections. Medical research is ongoing, and this provides hope for all disease sufferers. Many of your patients will have access to the Internet and will seek information on their diseases. They will ask you what you know. Perhaps the next miracle cure is at hand for one of the diseases presented in this chapter. Select one of the chronic diseases presented in this chapter. Go online and search for websites or articles that promise "miracle" cures or preventions for the disease you have chosen. Investigate the sources of these articles and then see whether there is any scientific support or proof behind these claims. Prepare a report on the claims and then present your own research to either support or debunk these claims.

3. **Flipped Classroom Report.** Select one of the chronic diseases presented in this chapter. Using the links at the end of the chapter research the disease by investigating at least two reports or articles from each link. Prepare a PowerPoint presentation report on the disease for the class and then deliver it.

Study Questions

1. Factors that can lower the LES pressure and lead to GERD include all of the following *except* which one?
   a. Apples
   b. Smoking
   c. Obesity
   d. High-fat diets

2. Luminal distension by unabsorbed or fermented _____ has been considered as the cause of many of the symptoms of IBS.
   a. FODMAPs
   b. Meats
   c. Fish
   d. Fats

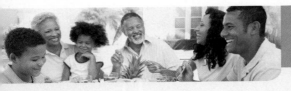

Learning Portfolio (continued)

3. Some medications used to treat IBD (methotrexate, sulfasalazine), block the production of which nutrient?
   a. Folate
   b. Vitamin C
   c. Vitamin E
   d. Vitamin B$_{12}$

4. How is a BMI of 36.2 classified?
   a. Obese class 2
   b. Obese class 1
   c. Normal class
   d. Preobese

5. Dumping syndrome is a common occurrence in approximately 50% of gastric bypass patients. This results from which factor?
   a. The absence of the pylorus, pyloric valve, and duodenum
   b. A side effect of diabetes
   c. Loss of appetite
   d. The presence of inflamed diverticulum

6. Risk factors of metabolic syndrome include all of the following *except* which one?
   a. Fasting blood glucose ≤ 90 mg/dL
   b. Abdominal waist circumference for a male > 40 inches
   c. HDL cholesterol for a male < 40 mg/dL
   d. Triglycerides ≥ 150 mg/dL

7. Losing only _____ of body weight can help reduce insulin levels.
   a. 5–7%
   b. 1–2%
   c. 3–4%
   d. 4–4.5%

8. In the management of cardiovascular disease, how much saturated fat should a person consume?
   a. < 7% of total caloric intake
   b. 15% of total caloric intake
   c. 20% of total caloric intake
   d. 25% of total caloric intake

9. The DASH diet promotes intake of vegetables, fruit, low-fat dairy products, whole grains, lean meat, and which other item?
   a. Nuts
   b. Sodium intake of 3,500 mg/day
   c. Red meat four times a week
   d. Fish intake once a week

10. Which of the following dietary factors are related to cancers?
    a. High intake of red meat
    b. Potatoes cooked at high temperatures
    c. Daily consumption of green vegetables
    d. Both A and B

11. The Institute of Medicine recommends which balance of fat, carbohydrate, and protein?
    a. 20–35%; 45–65%; 10–35%
    b. 10–25%; 40–50%; 25–35%
    c. 40–50%; 25–35%; 35–40%
    d. 15–19%; 35–39%; 5–50%

12. Which factor may delay the time between HIV infection and AIDS?
    a. Eating a healthy balanced diet
    b. Consuming high-fat foods
    c. Experiencing daily stress
    d. Being older

13. An individual living with HIV/AIDS can be susceptible to many types of infection, including those brought on by disease-causing bacteria and other pathogens that cause foodborne illness. Which major pathogen can cause a foodborne illness?
    a. *Campylobacter*
    b. Purine
    c. Lysine
    d. Leucine

Weblinks

- **Academy of Nutrition and Dietetics**
  http://www.eatright.org
  An organization of food and nutrition professionals devoted to helping the public make better nutrition choices. The website provides articles on chronic diseases and conditions, including diabetes, HIV/AIDS, and many others.

- **Centers for Disease Control and Prevention**
  http://www.cdc.gov

The CDC is an important division of the U.S. federal government's Department of Health and Human Services. The website offers a number of key reports on the health status of Americans, a number of links to other health organizations, and a wealth of statistical information on chronic diseases, including cancer, heart disease, diabetes, overweight and obesity, and many others.

- **World Health Organization**
  http://www.who.int

An agency of the United Nations. The WHO website offers information broken down into distinct health topics such as cancer, cardiovascular diseases, diabetes, HIV/AIDS, nutrition disorders, obesity, and many others.

■ **The Mayo Clinic**
http://www.mayoclinic.org/

An internationally renowned healthcare organization based in Rochester, Minnesota. The website provides a set of guides and information about hundreds of disease conditions on its Patient Care and Health Info tab. Virtually every chronic disease condition is defined along with its symptoms, causes, risk factors, complications, treatments, home remedies, and prevention.

References

1. BMI calculator. Retrieved from: http://www.bmi-calculator.net/waist-to-hip-ratio-calculator/. Accessed August 26, 2016.
2. World Health Organization. Obesity and overweight fact sheet. Geneva, Switzerland: World Health Organization; updated June 2016. Retrieved from: http://www.who.int/mediacentre/factsheets/fs311/en/. Accessed August 26, 2016.
3. Cawley J, Meyerhoefer C. The medical care costs of obesity: an instrumental variables approach. *Journal of J Health Economics*. 2012;31:219–230.
4. Finkelstein EA, Trogdon JG, Cohen JW, Dietz W. Annual medical spending attributable to obesity: payer-and service-specific estimates. *Health Aff* (Millwood). September-October 2009;28(5):w822-831. doi: 10.1377/hlthaff.28.5.w822.
5. Andreyeva T, Luedicke J, Wang YC. State-level estimates of obesity-attributable costs of absenteeism. *J Occup Environ Med*. 2014;56(11):1120.
6. Marketdata. Weight loss market in U.S. up 1.7% to $61 billion. PRWeb; April 16, 2013. Retrieved from: http://www.prweb.com/releases/2013/4/prweb10629316.htm. Accessed August 23, 2015.
7. Ogden CL, Carroll MD, Kit BK, Flegal KM. Prevalence of childhood and adult obesity in the United States, 2011–2012. *JAMA*. 2014;311(8):806–814.
8. Ogden CL, Lamb MM, Carroll MD, Flegal KM. Obesity and socioeconomic status in adults: United States, 2005–2008. *NCHS Data Brief* No. 50; December 2010. Retrieved from: http://www.cdc.gov/nchs/data/databriefs/db50.pdf. Accessed August 20, 2015.
9. Qi L, Cho YA. Gene–environment interaction and obesity. *Nutr Rev*. 2008;66:684–694.
10. Qi Q, Chu AY, Kang JH, et al. Fried food consumption, genetic risk, and body mass index: gene–diet interaction analysis in three US cohort studies. *BMJ*. 2014;19;348:g1610.
11. Centers for Disease Control and Prevention. Physical activity and health: the benefits of physical activity. Atlanta, GA: Centers for Disease Control and Prevention; updated June 4, 2015. Retrieved from: http://www.cdc.gov/physicalactivity/basics/pa-health/. Accessed August 26, 2016.
12. Donnelly JE, Blair SN, Jakicic JM, et al. American College of Sports Medicine position stand: appropriate physical activity intervention strategies for weight loss and prevention of weight regain for adults. *Med Sci Sports Exerc*. 2009;41:459–471.
13. Darmon N, Drewnowski A. Does social class predict diet quality? *Am J Clin Nutr*. 2008;87:1107–1117.
14. Dubowitz T, Acevedo-Garcia D, Salkeld J, et al. Lifecourse, immigrant status and acculturation in food purchasing and preparation among low-income mothers. *Public Health Nutr*. 2007;10:396–404.
15. Larson N, Story M. A review of environmental influences on food choices. *Ann Behav Med*. 2009;38:S56–73.
16. Lopez RP, Hynes HP. Obesity, physical activity, and the urban environment: public health research needs. *Environ Health*. 2006,5:25.
17. Christakis NA, Fowler JH. The spread of obesity in a large social network over 32 years. *N Engl J Med*. July 2007;357:370–379.
18. Suter PM. Is alcohol consumption a risk factor for weight gain and obesity? *Crit Rev Clin Lab Sci*. 2005;42(3):197–227.
19. Shelton NJ, Knott CS. Association between alcohol calorie intake and overweight and obesity in English adults. *Am J Pub Health*. April 2014;104(4):629–631.
20. Risérus U, Ingelsson E. Alcohol intake, insulin resistance, and abdominal obesity in elderly men. *Obesity*. July 2007;15(7):1766–1773.
21. John U, Hanke M, Rumpf HJ, Thyrian JR. Smoking status, cigarettes per day, and their relationship to overweight and obesity among former and current smokers in a national adult general population sample. *Int J Obes Relat Metab Disord*. 2005;29:1289–1294.
22. Chiolero A, Jacot-Sadowski I, Faeh D, et al. Association of cigarettes daily smoked with obesity in a general European adult population. *Obes Res*. 2007;15(5):1311–1318.
23. Kvaavik E, Meyer HE, Tverdal A. Food habits, physical activity and body mass index in relation to smoking status in 40–42 year old Norwegian women and men. *Prev Med*. 2004;38:1–5.
24. Chiolero A, Wietlisbach V, Ruffieux R, et al. Clustering of risk behaviors with level of cigarette consumption: a population-based survey. *Prev Med*. 2006;42(5):348–353.
25. Mizuno O, Okamoto K, Sawada M, et al. Obesity and smoking: relationship with waist circumference and obesity-related disorders in men undergoing a health screening. *J Atheroscler Thromb*. 2005;12(4):199–204.
26. Patel SR, Hu FB. Short sleep duration and weight gain: a systematic review. *Obesity* (Silver Spring). 2008;16:643–653.
27. Patel SR, Malhotra A, White DP, et al. Association between reduced sleep and weight gain in women. *Am J Epidemiol*. 2006;164:947–954.
28. Gangwisch JE, Malaspina D, Boden-Albala B, Heymsfield SB. Inadequate sleep as a risk factor for obesity: analyses of the NHANES I. *Sleep*. 2005;28(10):1289–1296.
29. Pannain S, Miller A, Van Cauter E. Sleep loss, obesity and diabetes: prevalence, association and emerging evidence for causation. *Obes Metab-Milan*. 2008;4:28–41.
30. Knutson KL, Van Cauter E. Associations between sleep loss and increased risk of obesity and diabetes. *Ann N Y Acad Sci*. 2008;1129:287–304.

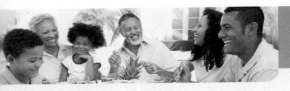

Learning Portfolio (continued)

31. Anic GM, Titus-Ernstoff L, Newcomb PA, et al. Sleep duration and obesity in a population-based study. *Sleep Med.* 2010;11:447–451.

32. Brum MC, Filho FF, Schnorr CC, et al. Shift work and its association with metabolic disorders. *Diabetol Metab Syndr.* May 17, 2015;7:45.

33. Bayon V, Leger D, Gomez-Merino D, et al. Sleep debt and obesity. *Ann Med.* 2014;46(5):264–272.

34. World Health Organization. Global strategy on diet, physical activity and health. Geneva, Switzerland: World Health Organization; May 2004. Retrieved from: http://www.who.int/dietphysicalactivity/strategy/eb11344/strategy_english_web.pdf. Accessed August 23, 2015.

35. World Health Organization. Part V: Challenges for the new millennium. In Obesity: preventing and managing the global epidemic. Report of a WHO Consultation (WHO Technical Report Series 894). Geneva, Switzerland: World Health Organization; 2000. Retrieved from: http://www.who.int/nutrition/publications/obesity/WHO_TRS_894/en/. Accessed July 15, 2015.

36. Seagle HM, Strain GW, Makris A, Reeves RS; American Dietetic Association. Position of the American Dietetic Association: weight management. *J Am Diet Assoc.* 2009;109(2):330–346.

37. Bodenheimer T, Lorig K, Holman H, Grumbach K. Patient self-management of chronic disease in primary care. *JAMA.* 2002;288:2469–2475.

38. U.S. Department of Agriculture and U.S. Department of Health and Human Services. *Dietary Guidelines for Americans, 2010.* 7th ed. Washington, DC: U.S. Government Printing Office; December 2010. Retrieved from: https://health.gov/dietaryguidelines/dga2010/DietaryGuidelines2010.pdf. Accessed August 26, 2016.

39. Jakicic JM. The effect of physical activity on body weight. *Obesity.* 2009;17(suppl 3):S34– S38.

40. Saks FM, Bray GA, Carey VJ, et al. Comparison of weight-loss diets with different compositions of fat, protein, and carbohydrates. *N Engl J Med.* 2009;360:859–873.

41. Burke LE, Wang J, Sevick MA. Self-monitoring in weight loss: a systematic review of the literature. *J Am Diet Assoc.* 2011;111:92–102.

42. Thompson W. Worldwide survey of fitness trends for 2016: 10th anniversary edition. *ACSM'S Health Fitness J.* November/December 2015;19(6):9–18.

43. Bonomi AG, Westerterp KR. Advances in physical activity monitoring and lifestyle interventions in obesity: a review. *Int J Obes.* 2012;36(2):167–177.

44. Pellegrini C, Verba S., Otto A. et al. The comparison of a technology-based system and an in-person behavioral weight loss intervention. *Obesity* (Silver Spring). 2012;20(2):356–363.

45. Lewis ZH, Lyons EJ, Jarvis JM, Baillargeon J. Using an electronic activity monitor system as an intervention modality: a systematic review. *BMC Public Health.* 2015;15:585.

46. Butryn ML, Webb V, Wadden TA. Behavioral treatment of obesity. *Psychiatr Clin North Am.* 2011;34(4):841–859.

47. Hampp C, Kang EM, Borders-Hemphill V. Use of prescription antiobesity drugs in the United States. *Pharmacotherapy.* 2013;33(12):1299–1307.

48. Yanovski, SZ, Yanovski JA. Long-term drug treatment for obesity: a systematic and clinical review. *JAMA.* January 1, 2014;311(1):74–86.

49. Keidar, A. Bariatric surgery for type 2 diabetes reversal: the risks. *Diabetes Care.* May 2011;34(suppl 2):S361–S366.

50. Kushner RF. Clinical assessment and management of adult obesity circulation. *Obesity.* 2012;126:2870–2877.

51. Schweiger C, Keidar A. Nutritional deficiencies in bariatric surgery patients: prevention, diagnosis and treatment [article in Hebrew]. *Harefuah.* 2010;149:715–720,748.

52. Gracia JA, Martinez M, Aguilella V. Postoperative morbidity of biliopancreatic diversion depending on common limb length. *Obes Syrg.* 2007;17:1306–1311.

53. Peterson LA, Canner JK, Cheskin LJ, et al. Proxy measures of vitamin D status—season and latitude—correlate with adverse outcomes after bariatric surgery in the Nationwide Inpatient Sample, 2001–2010: a retrospective cohort study. *Obes Sci Pract.* December 2015;1(2):88–96. doi:10.1002/osp4.15.

54. Peery AF, Dellon ES, Lund J, et al. Burden of gastrointestinal disease in the United States: 2012 update. *Gastroenterology.* 2012;143(5):1179–1187.

55. Everhart JE, Ruhl CE. Burden of digestive diseases in the United States part I: overall and upper gastrointestinal diseases. *Gastroenterology.* 2009;136:376–386.

56. El-Serag HB. Time trends of gastroesophageal reflux disease: a systematic review. *Clin Gastroenterol Hepatol.* 2007;5:17–26.

57. Vakil N, van Zanten SV, Kahrilas P, Dent J, Jones R; Global Consensus Group. The Montreal definition and classification of gastroesophageal reflux disease: a global evidence-based consensus. *Am J Gastroenterol.* 2006;101(8):1900–1920.

58. International Foundation for Functional Gastrointestinal Disorders. GERD costs America nearly $2 billion each week in lost productivity [media release]. Milwaukee, WI: International Foundation for Functional Gastrointestinal Disorders; updated August 3, 2015. Retrieved from: http://www.iffgd.org/site/news-events/press-releases/2005-1125-gerd-costs. Accessed August 26, 2016.

59. Fedorak RN, Veldhuyzen van Zanten S, Bridges R. Canadian Digestive Health Foundation public impact series: gastroesophageal reflux disease in Canada: incidence, prevalence, and direct and indirect economic impact. *Can J Gastroenterol.* 2010;24:431–443.

60. Jensen MD, Ryan DH, Apovian CM, et al. 2013 AHA/ACC/TOS guideline for the management of overweight and obesity in adults: a report of the American College of Cardiology/American Heart Association Task Force on Practice Guidelines and the Obesity Society. *Circulation.* 2014;129(25 suppl 2):S102–138.

61. Yang YX, Lewis JD, Epstein S, Metz, DC. Long-term proton pump inhibitor therapy and risk of hip fracture. *JAMA.* 2006;296(24):2947–2953.

62. O'Connell MB, Madden DM, Murray AM, et al. Effects of proton pump inhibitors on calcium carbonate absorption in women: a randomized crossover trial. *Am J Med.* 2005;118(7):778–781.

63. Fox M, Barr C, Nolan S, et al. The effects of dietary fat and calorie density on esophageal acid exposure and reflux symptoms. *Clin Gastroenterol Hepatol.* 2007;5(4):439–444.

64. Shapiro M, Green C, Bautista JM, et al. Assessment of dietary nutrients that influence perception of intra-oesophageal acid reflux events in patients with gastro-oesophageal reflux disease. *Aliment Pharmacol Therapeut.* 2007;25(1):93–101.

65. Vemulapalli R. Diet and lifestyle modifications in the management of gastroesophageal reflux disease. *Nutr Clin Pract.* 2008;23:293–298.

66. International Foundation for Functional Gastrointestinal Disorders. Surgical treatments. Milwaukee, WI: International Foundation for Functional Gastrointestinal Disorders; updated February 18, 2016. Retrieved from: http://www.aboutgerd.org/surgery/surgical-treatments.html. Accessed June 26, 2016.

67. Camilleri M. Peripheral mechanisms in irritable bowel syndrome. *N Engl J Med.* 2012;367:1626–1635.

68. National Institute of Diabetes and Digestive and Kidney Diseases. Irritable bowel syndrome (IBS). Bethesda, MD: U.S. Department of Health and Human Services, NIH, National Institute of Diabetes and Digestive and Kidney Diseases. Retrieved from: https://www.niddk.nih.gov/health-information/health-topics/digestive-diseases/irritable-bowel-syndrome/Pages/overview.aspx. Accessed August 26, 2016.

69. Grundmann O, Yoon SL. Irritable bowel syndrome: epidemiology, diagnosis, and treatment: an update for health-care practitioners. *J Gastroenterol Hepatol.* 2010;25:691–699.

70. Dean BB, Aguilar D, Barghout V, et al. Impairment in work productivity and health-related quality of life in patients with IBS. *Am J Manag Care.* 2005;11(1 suppl):S17–26.

71. Longstreth GF, Wilson A, Knight K, et al. Irritable bowel syndrome, health care use, and costs: a US managed care perspective. *Am J Gastroenterol.* 2003;98(3):600–607.

72. Lovell RM, Ford AC. Global prevalence of and risk factors for irritable bowel syndrome: a meta-analysis. *Clin Gastroenterol Hepatol.* 2012;10(7):712–721.

73. Sandler RS, Everhart JE, Donowitz M, et al. The burden of selected digestive diseases in the United States. *Gastroenterology.* 2002;122(5):1500–1511.

74. Longstreth GF, Thompson WG, Chey WD, et al. Functional bowel disorders. *Gastroenterology.* 2006;130(5):1480–1491.

75. Mearin F, Lacy BE. Diagnostic criteria in IBS: useful or not? *Neurogastroenterol Motil.* 2010;24:791–801.

76. Lesbros-Pantoflickova D, Michetti P, Fried M, Beglinger C, Blum AL. Meta-analysis: the treatment of irritable bowel syndrome. *Aliment Pharmacol Ther.* 2004;20:1253–1269.

77. Marshall JK, Thabane M, Garg AX, et al. Incidence and epidemiology of irritable bowel syndrome after a large waterborne outbreak of bacterial dysentery. *Gastroenterology.* 2006;131(2):445–450.

78. Okhuysen PC, Jiang ZD, Carlin L, et al. Post-diarrhea chronic intestinal symptoms and irritable bowel syndrome in North American travelers to Mexico. *Am J Gastroenterol.* 2004;99(9):1774–1778.

79. Dunlop SP, Jenkins D, Spiller RC. Distinctive clinical, psychological, and histological features of postinfective irritable bowel syndrome. *Am J Gastroenterol.* 2003;98(7):1578–1583.

80. Harvey RF, Mauad EC, Brown AM. Prognosis in the irritable bowel syndrome: a 5-year prospective study. *Lancet.* 1987;1:963–965.

81. Lied GA, Lillestøl K, Lind R, et al. Perceived food hypersensitivity: a review of 10 years of interdisciplinary research at a reference center. *Scand J Gastroenterol.* 2011;46(10):1169–1178.

82. Rome Foundation. *Rome III: The Functional Gastrointestinal Disorders.* 3rd ed. Raleigh, NC: Rome Foundation; 2006. Retrieved from: http://www.romecriteria.org/assets/pdf/20_RomeIII_apB_899–916.pdf. Accessed August 26, 2016.

83. Rajilić-Stojanović M, Biagi E, Heilig HG, et al. Global and deep molecular analysis of microbiota signatures in fecal samples from patients with irritable bowel syndrome. *Gastroenterology.* 2011;141(5):1792–1801.

84. Buhner S, Li Q, Vignali S, et al. Activation of human enteric neurons by supernatants of colonic biopsy specimens from patients with irritable bowel syndrome. *Gastroenterology.* 2009;137(4):1425–1434.

85. Steck N, Mueller K, Schemann M, Haller D. Republished: bacterial proteases in IBD and IBS. *Postgrad Med J.* 2013;89(1047):25–33.

86. Vizoso Pinto MG, Rodriguez Gómez M, Seifert S, et al. Lactobacilli stimulate the innate immune response and modulate the TLR expression of HT29 intestinal epithelial cells in vitro. *Int J Food Microbiol.* 2009;133(1–2):86–93.

87. Kim G, Deepinder F, Morales W, et al. *Methanobrevibacter smithii* is the predominant methanogen in patients with constipation-predominant IBS and methane on breath. *Dig Dis Sci.* 2012;57(12):3213–3218.

88. Hayes PA, Fraher MH, Quigley EM. *Gastroenterol Hepatol.* 2014;10(3):164–174.

89. Tazzyman S, Richards N, Trueman AR, et al. Vitamin D associates with improved quality of life in participants with irritable bowel syndrome: outcomes from a pilot trial. *BMJ Open Gastroenterol.* 2015;2(1) e000052 doi:10.1136/bmjgast-2015-000052.

90. Gibson PR. Shepherd SJ. Evidence-based dietary management of functional gastrointestinal symptoms: the FODMAP approach. *J Gastroenterol Hepatol.* 2010;25(2):252–258.

91. Staudacher HM, Lomer MC, Anderson JL, et al. Fermentable carbohydrate restriction reduces luminal bifidobacteria and gastrointestinal symptoms in patients with irritable bowel syndrome. *J Nutr.* 2012;142(8):1510–1518.

92. Staudacher HM, Whelan K, Irving PM, Lomer MC. Comparison of symptom response following advice for a diet low in fermentable carbohydrates (FODMAPs) versus standard dietary advice in patients with irritable bowel syndrome. *J Hum Nutr Diet.* 2011;24(5):487–495.

93. Barrett JS, Gearry RB, Muir JG, et al. Dietary poorly absorbed, short-chain carbohydrates increase delivery of water and fermentable substrates to the proximal colon. *Aliment Pharmacol Ther.* 2010;31(8):874–882.

94. de Roest RH, Dobbs BR, Chapman BA, et al. The low FODMAP diet improves gastrointestinal symptoms in patients with irritable bowel syndrome: a prospective study. *Int J Clin Pract.* 2013;67(9):895–903.

95. Roberfroid M, Gibson GR, Hoyles L, et al. Prebiotic effects: metabolic and health benefits. *Br J Nutr.* 2010;104(suppl 2):S1–S63.

96. Silk DB, Davis A, Vulevic J, et al. Clinical trial: the effects of a trans-galactooligosaccharide prebiotic on faecal microbiota and symptoms in irritable bowel syndrome. *Aliment Pharmacol Ther.* 2009;29(5):508–518.

97. Shepherd SJ, Gibson PR. Fructose malabsorption and symptoms of irritable bowel syndrome: guidelines for effective dietary management. *J Am Diet Assoc.* 2006;106(10):1631–1639.

98. Shephard SJ, Halmos E, Glance S. The role of FODMAPS in irritable bowel syndrome. *Curr Opin Clin Nutr Metab Care.* 2014;17(6):605–609.

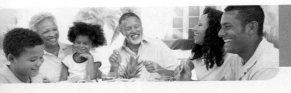

Learning Portfolio (continued)

99. Barboza L, Talley N, Moshiree BJ. Current and emerging pharmacotherapeutic options for irritable bowel syndrome. *Drugs*. 2014;74:1849–1870.

100. Monash University Medicine, Nursing and Health Sciences. Low FODMAP diet for irritable bowel syndrome. Melbourne, Australia: Monash University Medicine, Nursing and Health Sciences. Retrieved from: http://www.med.monash.edu/cecs/gastro/fodmap/. Accessed August 26, 2016.

101. Moayyedi P, Ford AC, Talley NJ, et al. The efficacy of probiotics in the therapy of irritable bowel syndrome: a systematic review [published online December 17, 2008]. *Gut*. 2010;59(3):325-332.

102. Nikfar S, Rahimi R, Rahimi F, et al. Efficacy of probiotics in irritable bowel syndrome: a meta-analysis of randomized, controlled trials. *Dis Colon Rectum*. 2008;51(12):1775–1780.

103. Kim HJ, Vazquez Roque MI, Camilleri M, et al. A randomized controlled trial of a probiotic combination VSL# 3 and placebo in irritable bowel syndrome with bloating. *Neurogastroenterol Motil*. 2005;17(5):687–696.

104. Kajander K, Myllyluoma E, Rajilic-Stojanovic M, et al. Clinical trial: multispecies probiotic supplementation alleviates the symptoms of IBS and stabilizes intestinal microbiota [published online October 6, 2007]. *Aliment Pharmacol Ther*. January 1, 2008;27(1):48–57.

105. O'Mahony L, McCarthy J, Kelly P, et al. *Lactobacillus* and *Bifidobacterium* in irritable bowel syndrome: symptom responses and relationship to cytokine profiles. *Gastroenterology*. 2005;128(3):541–551.

106. Whorwell PJ, Altringer L, Morel J, et al. Efficacy of an encapsulated probiotic *Bifidobacterium infantis* 35624 in women with irritable bowel syndrome. *Am J Gastroenterol*. 2006;101(7):1581–1590.

107. Konieczna P, Groeger D, Ziegler M, et al. *Bifidobacterium infantis* 35624 administration induces Foxp3 T regulatory cells in human peripheral blood: potential role for myeloid and plasmacytoid dendritic cells. *Gut*. 2012;61(3):354–366.

108. Molodecky NA, Soon IS, Rabi DM, et al. Increasing incidence and prevalence of the inflammatory bowel diseases with time, based on systematic review. *Gastroenterology*. 2012;142(1):46–54.

109. Khalili H, Huang ES, Ananthakrishnan AN, et al. Geographical variation and incidence of inflammatory bowel disease among US women. *Gut*. 2012;61:1686–1692.

110. Kappelman MD, Rifas-Shiman SL, Kleinman K, et al. The prevalence and geographic distribution of Crohn's disease and ulcerative colitis in the United States. *Clin Gastroenterol Hepatol*. 2007;5:1424–1429.

111. Loftus EV Jr, Shivashankar R, Tremaine WJ, et al. Updated incidence and prevalence of Crohn's disease and ulcerative colitis in Olmsted County, Minnesota (1970–2011). Paper presented at: ACG 2014 Annual Scientific Meeting; October 2014; Philadelphia, PA.

112. Russell RK, Satsangi J. Does IBD run in families? *Inflamm Bowel Dis*. 2008;14(S2):S20–S21.

113. Moller FT, Andersen V, Wohlfahrt J, Jess T. Familial risk of inflammatory bowel disease: a population-based cohort study 1977–2011. *Am J Gastroenterol*. 2015;110:564–571.

114. Ananthakrishnan AN. Environmental triggers for inflammatory bowel disease. *Curr Gastroenterol Rep*. 2013;15(1):302–309.

115. Calabrese E, Yanai H, Shuster D, et al. Low-dose smoking resumption in ex-smokers with refractory ulcerative colitis. *J Crohns Colitis*. 2012;6(7):756–762.

116. Hou JK, Abraham B, El-Serag H. Dietary intake and risk of developing inflammatory bowel disease: a systematic review of the literature. *Am J Gastroenterol*. April 2011;106:563–573.

117. Molodecky NA, Kaplan GG. Environmental risk factors for inflammatory bowel disease. *Gastroenterol Hepatol*. May 2010;6(5):339–346.

118. Khalili H, Ananthakrishnan AN, Konijeti GG, et al. Physical activity and risk of inflammatory bowel disease: prospective study from the Nurses' Health Study cohorts. *BMJ*. 2013;347:f6633.

119. García Rodríguez LA, Ruigómez A, Panés J. Acute gastroenteritis is followed by an increased risk of inflammatory bowel disease. *Gastroenterology*. 2006;130(6):1588–1594.

120. Kronman MP, Zaoutis TE, Haynes K, et al. Antibiotic exposure and IBD development among children: a population-based cohort study. *Pediatrics*. 2012;130(4):e794–e803.

121. Mawdsley JE, Rampton DS. Psychological stress in IBD: new insights into pathogenic and therapeutic implications. *Gut*. 2005;54(10):1481–1491.

122. Peppercorn MA, Cheifetz AS. Definition, epidemiology, and risk factors in inflammatory bowel disease. Up To Date; updated May 7, 2015. Retrieved from: http://www.uptodate.com/contents/definition-epidemiology-and-risk-factors-in-inflammatory-bowel-disease. Accessed May 7, 2015.

123. Machiels K, Joossens M, Sabino J, et al. Bacterial dysbiosis in ulcerative colitis patients differs from Crohn's disease patients. *Gastroenterology*. 2012;142:S46.

124. Vagianos K, Bector S, McConnell J, Bernstein CN. Nutrition assessment of patients with inflammatory bowel disease. *J Parenter Enteral Nutr*. July–August 2007;31(4):311–319.

125. Valentini L, Schaper L, Buning C, et al. Malnutrition and impaired muscle strength in patients with Crohn's disease and ulcerative colitis in remission. *Nutrition*. 2008;24:694–702.

126. Gassull MA, Cabre E. Nutrition in inflammatory bowel disease. *Curr Opin Clin Nutr Metab Care*. 2001;4:561–569.

127. Brown AC, Rampertab SD, Mullin GE. Existing dietary guidelines for Crohn's disease and ulcerative colitis. *Expert Rev Gastroenterol Hepatol*. 2011;5(3):411–425.

128. Prince A, Moose A, Whelan K, et al. Patients with Crohn's disease and ulcerative colitis have similar food and nutrition problems and share views on research priorities in inflammatory bowel disease. *J Hum Nutr Diet*. 2010;23:460–461.

129. Chapman-Kiddell CA, Davies PS, Gillen L, et al. Role of diet in the development of inflammatory bowel disease. *Inflamm Bowel Dis*. 2010;16:137–151.

130. Jowett SL, Seal CJ, Pearce MS, et al. Influence of dietary factors on the clinical course of ulcerative colitis: a prospective cohort study. *Gut*. 2004;53:1479–1484.

131. Dignass JS. Management of iron deficiency anemia in inflammatory bowel disease—a practical approach. *Ann Gastroenterol*. 2013;26(2):104–113.

132. Gasche C, Lomer MC, Cavill I, et al. Iron, anaemia, and inflammatory bowel diseases. *Gut.* 2004;53:1190–1197.

133. Gasche C, Berstad A, Befrits R, et al. Guidelines on the diagnosis and management of iron deficiency and anemia in inflammatory bowel diseases. *Inflamm Bowel Dis.* 2007;13:1545–1553.

134. Lomer MC, Cook WB, Jan-Mohamed HJ, et al. Iron requirements based upon iron absorption tests are poorly predicted by haematological indices in patients with inactive inflammatory bowel disease. *Br J Nutr.* 2012;107(12):1806–1811.

135. Yakut M, Ustün Y, Kabaçam G, Soykan I. Serum vitamin B12 and folate status in patients with inflammatory bowel diseases. *Eur J Intern Med.* 2010;21(4):320–323.

136. Eiden KA. Nutritional considerations in inflammatory bowel disease. In Parrish CR, ed. *Nutrition Issues in Gastroenterology.* Series 5. *Prac Gastroenterol.* May 2003:33–54. https://med.virginia.edu/ginutrition/wp-content/uploads/sites/199/2015/11/eidenarticle-May-03.pdf. Accessed August 15, 2015.

137. Ali T, Lam D, Bronze MS, Humphrey MB. Osteoporosis in inflammatory bowel disease. *Am J Med.* 2009;122(7):599–604.

138. Goodhand JR, Kamperidis N, Nguyen H, et al. Application of the WHO fracture risk assessment tool (FRAX) to predict need for DEXA scanning and treatment in patients with inflammatory bowel disease at risk of osteoporosis. *Aliment Pharmacol Ther.* 2011;33:551–558.

139. van Staa TP, Cooper C, Brusse LS, Leufkens H, Javaid MK, Arden NK. Inflammatory bowel disease and the risk of fracture. *Gastroenterology.* 2003;125:1591–1597.

140. Gearry RB, Irving PM, Barrett JS, et al. Reduction of dietary poorly absorbed short-chain carbohydrates (FODMAPs) improves abdominal symptoms in patients with inflammatory bowel disease. *J Crohns Colitis.* 2009;3:8–14.

141. Joyce T, Staudacher H, Whelan K, et al. Symptom response following advice on a diet low in short-chain fermentable carbohydrates (FODMAPs) for functional bowel symptoms in patients with IBD. *Gut.* 2014;63:A164.

142. Calafiore A, Gionchetti P, Calabrese C, et al. Probiotics, prebiotics and antibiotics in the treatment of inflammatory bowel disease. *J Gastroenterol Hepatol.* 2012;1(6):97–106.

143. Jonkers D, Penders J, Masclee A, Pierik M. Probiotics in the management of inflammatory bowel disease: a systematic review of intervention studies in adult patients. *Drugs.* 2012;72(6):803–823.

144. Douglas LC, Sanders ME. Probiotics and prebiotics in dietetics practice. *J Am Diet Assoc.* 2008;108(3):510–521.

145. Mimura T, Rizzello F, Helwig U, et al. Once daily high dose probiotic therapy (VSL#3) for maintaining remission in recurrent or refractory pouchitis. *Gut.* 2004;53:108–114.

146. Kruis W, Fric P, Pokrotnieks J, et al. Maintaining remission of ulcerative colitis with the probiotic *Escherichia coli* Nissle 1917 is as effective as with standard mesalazine. *Gut.* 2004;53:1617–1623.

147. Tursi A. The role of colonoscopy in managing diverticular disease of the colon. *J Gastrointestin Liver Dis.* March 2015;24(1):85–93.

148. Vikram BR, Longo WE. The burden of diverticular disease on patients and healthcare systems. *Gastroenterol Hepatol* (NY). 2013;9(1):21–27.

149. Shaheen NJ, Hansen RA, Morgan DR, et al. The burden of gastrointestinal and liver diseases, 2006. *Am J Gastroenterol.* 2006;101:2128–2138.

150. Weizman AV, Nguyen GC. Diverticular disease: epidemiology and management. *Can J Gastroenterol.* 2011;25(7):385–389.

151. Everhart JE, Ruhl CE. Burden of digestive diseases in the United States part III: liver, biliary tract, and pancreas. *Gastroenterology.* 2009;136:1134–1144.

152. Tursi A, Papagrigoriadis S. Review article: the current and evolving treatment of colonic diverticular disease. *Aliment Pharmacol Ther.* 2009;30(6):532–546.

153. Shahedi K, Fuller G, Bolus R, et al. Long-term risk of acute diverticulitis among patients with incidental diverticulosis found during colonoscopy. *Clin Gastroenterol Hepatol.* 2013;11:1609–1613.

154. Aucheron JL, Roblin X, Bichard P, Heluwaert F. The prevalence of right-sided colonic diverticulosis and diverticular haemorrhage. *Colorectal Dis.* 2013;15:e266–e270.

155. Martel J, Raskin JB. History, incidence, and epidemiology of diverticulosis. *J Clin Gastroenterol.* 2008;42(10):1125–1127.

156. Orr WC, Chen CL. Aging and neural control of the GI tract IV. Clinical and physiological aspects of gastrointestinal motility and aging. *Am J Physiol Gastrointest Liver Physiol.* 2002;283(6):G1226–G1231.

157. Bristow J, Carey W, Egging D, et al. Tenascin-X, collagen, elastin, and the Ehlers-Danlos syndrome. *Am J Med Genet C Semin Med Genet.* 2005;139c(1):24–30.

158. Lindor NM, Bristow J. Tenascin-X deficiency in autosomal recessive Ehlers-Danlos syndrome. *Am J Med Genet A.* 2005;135:75–80.

159. Deshpande AV, Oliver M, Yin M, et al. Severe colonic diverticulitis in an adolescent with Williams syndrome. *J Paediatr Child Health.* 2005;41:687–688.

160. Lederman ED, McCoy G, Conti DJ, Lee EC. Diverticulitis and polycystic kidney disease. *Am Surg.* 2000;66:200–203.

161. National Task Force on the Prevention and Treatment of Obesity. Overweight, obesity, and health risk. *Arch Intern Med.* 2000;160(7):898–904.

162. Korzenik JR. Case closed? Diverticulitis: epidemiology and fiber. *J Clin Gastroenterol.* 2006;40(suppl 3):S112–S116.

163. Floch MH, White JA. Management of diverticular disease is changing. *World J Gastroenterol.* 2006;12(20):3225–3228.

164. Cildir G, Akıncılar SC, Tergaonkar V. Chronic adipose tissue inflammation: all immune cells on the stage. *Trends Mol Med.* 2013;19(8):487–500.

165. Sun S, Ji Y, Kersten S, Qi L. Mechanisms of inflammatory responses in obese adipose tissue. *Annu Rev Nutr.* 2012;32:261–286.

166. Jung HK, Choung RS, Locke GR, et al. Diarrhea-predominant irritable bowel syndrome is associated with diverticular disease: a population-based study. *Am J Gastroenterol.* 2010;105(3):652–661.

167. Hall KE, Proctor DD, Fisher L, Rose S. American Gastroenterological Association future trends committee report: effects of aging of the population on gastroenterology practice, education, and research. *Gastroenterology.* 2005;129(4):1305–1338.

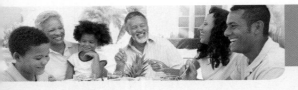

Learning Portfolio (continued)

168. Lin OS, Soon MS, Wu SS, et al. Dietary habits and right-sided colonic diverticulosis. *Dis Colon Rectum.* 2000;43(10):1412–1418.

169. Crowe FL, Appleby PN, Allen NE, Key TJ. Diet and risk of diverticular disease in Oxford cohort of European Prospective Investigation into Cancer and Nutrition (EPIC): prospective study of British vegetarians and non-vegetarians. *BMJ.* 2011;343:d4131.

170. Feingold D, Steele SR, Lee S, et al. Prepared by the Clinical Practice Guideline task force of the American Society of Colon and Rectal surgeons. Practice parameters for the treatment of sigmoid diverticulitis. *Dis Colon Rectum.* 2014;57:284–294.

171. Strate LL, Liu YL, Syngal S, et al. Nut, corn, and popcorn consumption and the incidence of diverticular disease. *JAMA.* August 27, 2008;300(8):907–914.

172. Sheth AA, Longo W, Floch MH. Diverticular disease and diverticulitis. *Am J Gastroenterol.* 2008;103(6):1550–1556.

173. Eglash A, Lane CH, Schneider DM. Clinical inquiries. What is the most beneficial diet for patients with diverticulosis? *J Fam Pract.* 2006;55(9):813–815.

174. Decher N, Krenitsky JS. Medical nutrition therapy for lower gastrointestinal tract disorders. In Mahan LK, Escott-Stump S, Raymond JL, eds. *Krause's Food and the Nutrition Care Process.* 13th ed. St. Louis, MO: Saunders; 2012:636.

175. U.S. Department of Agriculture Agricultural Research Service. Dietary intake data: what we eat in America, NHANES 2009–2010. Washington, DC: US DA Agricultural Research Service; June 2012. Retrieved from: http://www.ars.usda.gov/SP2UserFiles/Place/80400530/pdf/0910/wweia_2009_2010_data.pdf. Accessed August 26, 2016.

176. Panel on Macronutrients, Panel on the Definition of Dietary Fiber, Subcommittee on Upper Reference Levels of Nutrients, Subcommittee on Interpretation and Uses of Dietary Reference Intakes, and the Standing Committee on the Scientific Evaluation of Dietary Reference Intakes. *Dietary Reference Intakes for Energy, Carbohydrate, Fiber, Fat, Fatty Acids, Cholesterol, Protein, and Amino Acids (Macronutrients).* Washington, DC: National Academies Press; 2002. http://www.nap.edu/read/10490/chapter/1. Accessed August 26, 2016.

177. Boynton W, Floch M. New strategies for the management of diverticular disease: insights for the clinician. *Therap Adv Gastroenterol.* 2013;6(3):205–213.

178. Tursi A. Preventing recurrent acute diverticulitis with pharmacological therapies. *Ther Adv Chronic Dis.* 2013;4(6):277–286.

179. Strasberg SM. Acute calculous cholecystitis. *N Engl J Med.* 2008;358:2804–2811.

180. Cuevas A, Miquel JF, Reyes MS, et al. Diet as a risk factor for cholesterol gallstone disease. *J Am Coll Nutr.* 2004;23:187–196.

181. Mills JC, Stappenbeck TS, Bunnett NW. Gastrointestinal disease. In: McPhee SJ, Hammer GD, eds. *Pathophysiology of Disease: An Introduction to Clinical Medicine.* 6th ed. New York, NY: McGraw-Hill Medical; 2010.

182. Marschall HU, Einarsson C. Gallstone disease. *J Intern Med.* 2007;261:529–542.

183. Williams EJ, Green J, Beckingham I, et al. Guidelines on the management of common bile duct stones (CBDS). *Gut.* 2008;57(7):1004–1021.

184. Centers for Disease Control and Prevention. *National Diabetes Statistics Report: Estimates of Diabetes and Its Burden in the United States, 2014.* Atlanta, GA: U.S. Department of Health and Human Services; 2014. Retrieved from: http://www.cdc.gov/diabetes/pubs/statsreport14/national-diabetes-report-web.pdf. Accessed August 26, 2016.

185. Heiss G, Snyder ML, Teng Y, et al. Prevalence of metabolic syndrome among Hispanics/Latinos of diverse background: the Hispanic Community Health Study/Study of Latinos. *Diabetes Care.* 2014;37(8):2391–2399.

186. Aguilar M, Bhuket T, Torres S, et al. Prevalence of the metabolic syndrome in the United States, 2003–2012. *JAMA.* 2015;313(19):1973–1974.

187. Crist LA, Champagne CM, Corsino L, et al. Influence of change in aerobic fitness and weight on prevalence of metabolic syndrome. *Prev Chronic Dis.* 2012;9:110–171.

188. Ervin RB. Prevalence of metabolic syndrome among adults 20 years of age and over, by sex, age, race and ethnicity, and body mass index: United States, 2003–2006. *National Health Statistics Reports.* May 5, 2009;(13):1–7. http://www.cdc.gov/nchs/data/nhsr/nhsr013.pdf. Accessed July 15, 2015.

189. Huang PL. A comprehensive definition for metabolic syndrome. *Dis Model Mech.* May–June 2009;2(5–6):231–237.

190. Cleeman JI, Daniels SR, Donato KA, et al. Diagnosis and management of the metabolic syndrome: an American Heart Association/National Heart, Lung, and Blood Institute scientific statement. *Circulation.* 2005;112:2735–2752.

191. Kaur J. A comprehensive review on metabolic syndrome. *J Cardiol Res Pract.* 2014;2014:943162.

192. U.S. Department of Health and Human Services, National Institutes of Health, National Heart, Lung, and Blood Institute. *Your Guide to Lowering Blood Pressure.* Washington, DC: National Institutes of Health; May 2003. Retrieved from: http://www.nhlbi.nih.gov/files/docs/public/heart/hbp_low.pdf. Accessed July 15, 2015.

193. Ebrahimof S, Mirmiran P. Nutritional approaches for prevention and treatment of metabolic syndrome in adults. *J Paramed Sci.* Spring 2013;4(2):123–134.

194. Cornier MA, Dabelea D, Hernandez TL, et al. The metabolic syndrome. *Endocrine Rev.* 2008;29(7):777–822.

195. Scheers T, Philippaerts R, Lefevre J. SenseWear-determined physical activity and sedentary behavior and metabolic syndrome. *Med Sci Sports Exerc.* 2013;45(3):481–489.

196. National Heart, Lung, and Blood Institute. How is metabolic syndrome treated? Washington, DC: National Institutes of Health, National Heart, Lung, and Blood Institute; updated June 22, 2016. Retrieved from: https://www.nhlbi.nih.gov/health/health-topics/topics/ms/treatment. Accessed August 26, 2016.

197. Ford ES, Kohl HW, Mokdad AH, Ajani UA. Sedentary behavior, physical activity, and the metabolic syndrome among U.S. adults. *Obes Res.* 2005;13(3):608–614.

198. Lin CH, Chiang SL, Yates P, et al. Moderate physical activity level as a protective factor against metabolic syndrome in middle-aged and older women. *J Clin Nurs.* 2015;24(9–10):1234–1245.

199. Mostafavi F, Ghofranipour F, Feizi A, Pirzadeh A. Improving physical activity and metabolic syndrome indicators in women: a transtheoretical model-based intervention. *Int J Prev Med.* April 1, 2015;6:28.

200. Ilanne-Parikka P, Laaksonen DE, Eriksson JG, et al. Leisure-time physical activity and the metabolic syndrome in the Finnish Diabetes Prevention Study. *Diabetes Care.* July 2010;33(7):1610–1617.

201. De Caterina R, Madonna R, Bertolotto A, et al. n-3 fatty acids in the treatment of diabetic patients. *Diabetes Care.* 2007:30(4):1012–1026.

202. Feldeisen SE, Tucker KL. Nutritional strategies in the prevention and treatment of metabolic syndrome. *Appl Physiol Nutr Metab.* 2007;32(1):46–60.

203. American Dietetic Association. Position of the American Dietetic Association: weight management. *J Am Diet Assn.* 2009;109(2):330–346.

204. Kawada T, Otsuka T, Endo T, Kon Y. Number of components of the metabolic syndrome, smoking and inflammatory markers. *Int J Endocrinol Metab.* 2013;11(1):23–26.

205. Cena H, Maria Fonte ML, Turconi G. Relationship between smoking and metabolic syndrome. *Nutr Rev.* December 2011;69(12):745–753.

206. Fiore MC, Jaén CR, Baker TB, et al. *Treating Tobacco Use and Dependence: 2008 Update—Clinical Practice Guidelines.* Rockville, MD: U.S. Department of Health and Human Services, Public Health Service, Agency for Healthcare Research and Quality; 2008.

207. Cena H, Tesone A, Niniano R, Cerveri I, Roggi C, Turconi G. Prevalence rate of metabolic syndrome in a group of light and heavy smokers. *Diabetol Metab Syndr.* 2013;5(1):28.

208. Calvin AD, Albuquerque FN, Lopez-Jimenez F, Somers VK. Obstructive sleep apnea, inflammation, and the metabolic syndrome. *Metab Syndr Relat Disord.* 2009;7(4):271–277.

209. Paschos P, Paletas K. Non alcoholic fatty liver disease and metabolic syndrome. *Hippokratia.* January–March 2009;13(1):9–19.

210. Almeda-Valdés P, Cuevas-Ramos D, Aguilar-Salinas CA. Metabolic syndrome and non-alcoholic fatty liver disease. *Ann Hepatol.* 2009;8(suppl 1):S18–24.

211. Mendez-Sanchez N, Chavez-Tapia NC, Motola-Kuba D, et al. Metabolic syndrome as a risk factor for gallstone disease. *World J Gastroenterol.* 2005;11:1653–1657.

212. Jahangiry L, Shojaeizadeh D, Montazeri A, et al. Modifiable lifestyle risk factors and metabolic syndrome: opportunities for a web-based preventive program. *J Res Health Sci.* Autumn 2014;14(4):303–307.

213. American Diabetes Association. Statistics about diabetes. Framingham, MA: American Diabetes Association; updated April 1, 2016. Retrieved from: http://www.diabetes.org/diabetes-basics/statistics/. Accessed August 26, 2016.

214. American Diabetes Association. Classification and diagnosis of diabetes. Sec. 2. In Standards of Medical Care in Diabetes—2015. *Diabetes Care.* 2015;38(suppl 1):S8–S16. http://care.diabetesjournals.org/content/38/Supplement_1/S8.full. Accessed July 12, 2015.

215. Borch-Johnsen KLT. Screening for type 2 diabetes: should it be now? *Diabet Med.* 2003:20:175–181.

216. Engelgau MM, Nayan KM, Herman WH. Screening for type 2 diabetes. *Diabetes Care.* 2000;23:1563–1580.

217. American Heart Association. Understand your risk for diabetes. Dallas, TX: American Heart Association. Retrieved from: http://www.heart.org/HEARTORG/Conditions/More/Diabetes/UnderstandYourRiskforDiabetes/Understand-Your-Risk-for-Diabetes_UCM_002034_Article.jsp#.WC9P-morK00. Accessed November 18, 2016.

218. Canadian Diabetes Association. Smoking and diabetes. Toronto, CA: Canadian Diabetes Association. Retrieved from: http://www.diabetes.ca/diabetes-and-you/healthy-living-resources/heart-health/smoking-diabetes. Accessed July 15, 2015.

219. U.S. Department of Health and Human Services. *The Health Consequences of Smoking—50 Years of Progress: A Report of the Surgeon General.* Atlanta, GA: U.S. Department of Health and Human Services, Centers for Disease Control and Prevention, National Center for Chronic Disease Prevention and Health Promotion, Office on Smoking and Health; 2014. Retrieved from: http://www.surgeongeneral.gov/library/reports/50-years-of-progress/. Accessed July 15, 2015.

220. Van Gaal L, Scheen A. Weight management in type 2 diabetes: current and emerging approaches to treatment. *Diabetes Care.* 2015;38:1161–1172.

221. Canadian Diabetes Association. Waist circumference. Toronto, CA: Canadian Diabetes Association. Retrieved from: http://www.diabetes.ca/diabetes-and-you/healthy-living-resources/weight-management/waist-circumference. Accessed July 15, 2015.

222. Knowler WC, Barrett-Connor E, Fowler SE, et al. Diabetes Prevention Program Research Group. Reduction in the incidence of type 2 diabetes with lifestyle intervention or metformin. *N Engl J Med.* 2002;346:393–403.

223. National Institute of Diabetes and Digestive and Kidney Diseases Small Steps. Big Rewards. Prevent type 2 diabetes campaign overview. Bethesda, MD: U.S. Department of Health and Human Services, NIH, National Institute of Diabetes and Digestive and Kidney Diseases. Retrieved from: https://www.niddk.nih.gov/health-information/health-communication-programs/ndep/partnership-community-outreach/campaigns/small-steps-big-rewards/Pages/smallstepsbigrewards.aspx. Accessed August 26, 2016.

224. American Diabetes Association. Standards of medical care in diabetes 2015. *Diabetes Care.* 2015;38(suppl 1):S8–S16.

225. Peyrot M, Rubin RR, Lauritzen T, et al. The International DAWN Advisory Panel: psychosocial problems and barriers to improved diabetes management: results of the cross-national Diabetes Attitudes, Wishes and Needs (DAWN) study. *Diabetes Care.* 2005;28(11):2673–2679.

226. García-Pérez LE, Álvarez M, Dilla T, et al. Adherence to therapies in patients with type 2 diabetes. *Diabetes Ther.* 2013;4(2):175–194.

227. Chudyk A, Petrella RJ. Effects of exercise on cardiovascular risk factors in type 2 diabetes: a meta-analysis. *Diabetes Care.* 2011;34:1228–1237.

228. Colberg SR, Sigal RJ, Fernhall B, et al. Exercise and type 2 diabetes: the American College of Sports Medicine and the American Diabetes Association: joint position statement. *Diabetes Care.* 2010;33(12):2692–2696.

229. Snowling NJ, Hopkins WG. Effects of different modes of exercise training on glucose control and risk factors for complications in type 2 diabetic patients: a meta-analysis. *Diabetes Care.* 2006;29:2518–2527.

230. Wing RR, Goldstein MG, Acton KJ, et al. Behavioral science research in diabetes: lifestyle changes related to

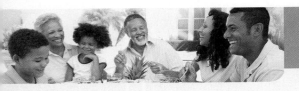

Learning Portfolio (continued)

obesity, eating behavior, and physical activity. *Diabetes Care.* 2001;24(1):117–123.

231. Henson J, Yates T, Biddle SJH, et al. Associations of objectively measured sedentary behaviour and physical activity with markers of cardiometabolic health. *Diabetologia.* 2013;56(5):1012–1020.

232. Karmally W. Nutrition therapy for diabetes and lipid disorders. In Franz M, Evert A, eds. *American Diabetes Association Guide to Nutrition Therapy for Diabetes.* Alexandria, VA: American Diabetes Association; 2012:265–294.

233. Suckling RJ, He FJ, Macgregor GA. Altered dietary salt intake for preventing and treating diabetic kidney disease. *Cochrane Database Syst Rev.* 2010;(12):CD006763.

234. Keogh JB, Clifton PM. Meal replacements for weight loss in type 2 diabetes in a community setting. *J Nutr Metab.* 2012;2012:918571.

235. Xu J, Murphy SL, Kochanek KD, Bastian BA; Division of Vital Statistics. 2013 mortality multiple cause microdata files [detailed tables released ahead of full report]. In Deaths: final data for 2013. *Natl Vital Stat Rep.* February 16, 2016;64(2):1–119. http://www.cdc.gov/nchs/data/nvsr/nvsr64/nvsr64_02.pdf. Accessed July 16, 2015.

236. Mozaffarian D, Benjamin EJ, Go AS, et al. Heart disease and stroke statistics—2015 update. *Circulation.* January 2015;131(4):e29–e322.

237. Wong ND. Epidemiological studies of CHD and the evolution of preventive cardiology. *Nature Rev Cardiol.* 2014;11:276–289.

238. Kraft S. What is cerebrovascular disease? What causes cerebrovascular disease? Medical News Today; updated September 26, 2014. Retrieved from: http://www.medicalnewstoday.com/articles/184601.php. Accessed July 16, 2015.

239. American Heart Association. About peripheral artery disease (PAD). Dallas, TX: American Heart Association; updated August 5, 2014. Retrieved from: http://www.heart.org/HEARTORG/Conditions/More/PeripheralArteryDisease/About-Peripheral-Artery-Disease-PAD_UCM_301301_Article.jsp. Accessed July 16, 2015.

240. University of Michigan Frankel Cardiovascular Center. Arteriosclerotic aortic disease. Ann Arbor, MI: University of Michigan Frankel Cardiovascular Center. Retrieved from: http://www.umcvc.org/conditions-treatments/arteriosclerotic-aortic-disease. Accessed August 26, 2015.

241. World Health Federation. Cardiovascular disease risk factors. Geneva, Switzerland: World Heart Federation website. http://www.world-heart-federation.org/cardiovascular-health/cardiovascular-disease-risk-factors/. Accessed August 26, 2015.

242. World Health Federation. Obesity. Geneva, Switzerland: World Heart Federation. Retrieved from: http://www.world-heart-federation.org/cardiovascular-health/cardiovascular-disease-risk-factors/obesity/. Accessed July 16, 2015.

243. World Health Federation. Hypertension. Geneva, Switzerland: World Heart Federation. Retrieved from: http://www.world-heart-federation.org/cardiovascular-health/cardiovascular-disease-risk-factors/hypertension/. Accessed July 16, 2015.

244. Assman G, Gotto A. Atherosclerosis: evolving vascular biology and clinical implications HDL cholesterol and protective factors in atherosclerosis. *Circulation.* 2004;109:III-8–III-14.

245. Riwanto M, Landmesser U. High density lipoproteins and endothelial functions: mechanistic insights and alterations in cardiovascular disease. *J Lipid Res.* 2013;54(12):3227–3243.

246. Roger VL, Go AS, Lloyd-Jones DM, et al. Heart disease and stroke statistics—2012 update: a report from the American Heart Association. *Circulation.* 2012;125:e2–e220.

247. National Cholesterol Education Program Expert Panel on Detection, Evaluation, and Treatment of High Blood Cholesterol in Adults (Adult Treatment Panel III). Third report of the National Cholesterol Education Program (NCEP) Expert Panel on Detection, Evaluation, and Treatment of High Blood Cholesterol in Adults (Adult Treatment Panel III) final report. *Circulation.* 2002;106:3143–3421.

248. Mendis S, Puska P, Norrving B; World Health Organization, eds. *Global Atlas on Cardiovascular Disease Prevention and Control.* Geneva, Switzerland: World Health Organization with World Heart Federation, World Stroke Organization; 2011.

249. Grundy SM. Promise of low-density lipoprotein-lowering therapy for primary and secondary prevention. *Circulation.* 2008;117:569–573.

250. Pittilo RM. Cigarette smoking, endothelial injury and cardiovascular disease. *Int J Exp Pathol.* 2000; 81(4):219–230.

251. World Health Federation. Tobacco: totally avoidable risk factor of CVD. Geneva, Switzerland: World Heart Federation; 2012. Retrieved from: http://www.world-heart-federation.org/fileadmin/user_upload/documents/Fact_sheets/2012/Tobacco_avoidable_risk_factor_of_CVD.pdf. Accessed July 16, 2015.

252. Huxley R, Woodward M. Cigarette smoking as a risk factor for coronary heart disease in women compared with men: a systematic review and meta-analysis of prospective cohort studies. *Lancet.* 2011;378(9799):1297–1300.

253. Vollset SE, Tverdal A, Gjessing HK. Smoking and deaths between 40 and 70 years of age in women and men. *Ann Intern Med.* 2006;144(6):381–389.

254. Centers for Disease Control and Prevention. Smoking and tobacco use: health effects of cigarette smoking. Atlanta, GA: Centers for Disease Control and Prevention; updated October 1, 2015. Retrieved from: http://www.cdc.gov/tobacco/data_statistics/fact_sheets/health_effects/effects_cig_smoking/index.htm. Accessed July 16, 2015.

255. World Health Organization. Tobacco. Geneva, Switzerland: World Health Organization; updated June 2016. Retrieved from: www.who.int/mediacentre/factsheets/fs339/en/index.html. Accessed August 26, 2016.

256. Mensink RP, Zock PL, Kester ADM, Katan MB. Effects of dietary fatty acids and carbohydrates on serum lipids and apolipoproteins: a meta-analysis of 60 controlled trials. *Am J Clin Nutr.* 2003;77:1146–1155.

257. Centers for Disease Control and Prevention. Million hearts: strategies to reduce the prevalence of leading cardiovascular disease risk factors. *Morb Mortal Wkly Rep.* September 16, 2011;60(36):1248–1251.

258. Piano MR. Alcoholic cardiomyopathy: incidence, clinical characteristics, and pathophysiology. *Chest.* 2002;121:1638–1650.

259. Texas Heart Institute. Women and heart disease. Texas Heart Institute; updated July 2015. Retrieved from: http://

www.texasheart.org/HIC/Topics/HSmart/women.cfm. Accessed July 16, 2015.

260. American Heart Association. Understand your risks to prevent a heart attack. Dallas, TX: American Heart Association; reviewed June 2016. Retrieved from: http://www.heart.org/HEARTORG/Conditions/HeartAttack/UnderstandYourRiskofHeartAttack/Understand-Your-Risk-of-HeartAttack_UCM_002040_Article.jsp?appName=MobileApp. Accessed July 16, 2016.

261. American Heart Association. Coronary artery disease—coronary heart disease. Dallas, TX: American Heart Association; reviewed July 2015. Retrieved from: http://www.heart.org/HEARTORG/Conditions/More/MyHeartandStrokeNews/Coronary-Artery-Disease---Coronary-Heart-Disease_UCM_436416_Article.jsp. Accessed July 16, 2015.

262. Yusuf S, Hawken S, Ôunpuu S, et al. Obesity and the risk of myocardial infarction in 27,000 participants from 52 countries: a case-control study. *Lancet*. 2005;366(9497):1640–1649.

263. O'Connor GT, Buring JE, Yusuf S, et al. An overview of randomized trials of rehabilitation with exercise after myocardial infarction. *Circulation*. 1989;80:234–244.

264. Oldridge NB, Guyatt GH, Fischer ME, et al. Cardiac rehabilitation after myocardial infarction: combined experience of randomized clinical trials. *JAMA*. 1988;260:945–950.

265. Seal CJ. Whole grains and CVD risk. *Proc Nutr Soc*. 2006;65(1):24–34.

266. National Academies of Sciences, Engineering, Medicine. Dietary Reference Intakes tables and applications. Washington, DC: National Academies of Sciences, Engineering, Medicine. Retrieved from: http://iom.nationalacademies.org/Activities/Nutrition/SummaryDRIs/DRI-Tables.aspx. Accessed July 17, 2015.

267. Erdman JW Jr. AHA Science Advisory: Soy protein and cardiovascular disease: a statement for healthcare professionals from the Nutrition Committee of the AHA. *Circulation*. 2000;102(20):2555–2559.

268. Lichtenstein A. Soy protein, isoflavones, and cardiovascular disease risk. *J Nutr*. 1998;128:1589–1592.

269. Allen JK, Becker DM, Kwiterovich PO, et al. Effect of soy protein-containing isoflavones on lipoproteins in postmenopausal women. *Menopause*. 2007;14:106–114.

270. De Backer G, Catapano AL, Chapman J, et al. Guidelines on CVD prevention: confusing or complementary? *Atherosclerosis*. 2013;226:299–300.

271. Goff DC, Lloyd-Jones DM, Bennett G, et al. ACC/AHA guideline on the assessment of cardiovascular risk: a report of the American College of Cardiology/American Heart Association Task Force on Practice Guidelines. *Circulation*. June 24, 2014;129(25 suppl 2):S49–73.

272. Slavin JL, Martini MC, Jacobs DR Jr, Marquart L. Plausible mechanisms for the protectiveness of whole grains. *Am J Clin Nutr*. 1999;70(3 suppl):459S–463S.

273. DiRienzo DB. Effect of probiotics on biomarkers of cardiovascular disease: implications for heart-healthy diets. *Nutr Rev*. 2014;72(1):18–29.

274. Guo Z, Liu XM, Zhang QX, et al. Influence of consumption of probiotics on the plasma lipid profile: a meta-analysis of randomised controlled trials. *Nutr Metab Cardiovasc Dis*. 2011;21:844–850.

275. Agerholm-Larsen L, Raben A, Haulrik N, et al. Effect of 8 week intake of probiotic milk products on risk factors for cardiovascular diseases. *Eur J Clin Nutr*. 2000;54:288–297.

276. Fabian E, Elmadfa I. Influence of daily consumption of probiotic and conventional yoghurt on the plasma lipid profile in young healthy women. *Ann Nutr Metab*. 2006;50:387–393.

277. Ataie-Jafari A, Larijani B, Alavi Majd H, et al. Cholesterol-lowering effect of probiotic yogurt in comparison with ordinary yogurt in mildly to moderately hypercholesterolemic subjects. *Ann Nutr Metab*. 2009;54:22–27.

278. Sadrzadeh-Yeganeh H, Elmadfa I, Djazayery A, et al. The effects of probiotic and conventional yoghurt on lipid profile in women. *Br J Nutr*. 2010;103:1778–1783.

279. Jones ML, Martoni CJ, Parent M, et al. Cholesterol-lowering efficacy of a microencapsulated bile salt hydrolase-active *Lactobacillus reuteri* NCIMB 30242 yoghurt formulation in hypercholesterolaemic adults. *Br J Nutr*. 2012;107:1505–1513.

280. Jones ML, Martoni CJ, Prakash S. Cholesterol lowering and inhibition of sterol absorption by *Lactobacillus reuteri* NCIMB 30242: a randomized controlled trial. *Eur J Clin Nutr*. 2012;66:1234–1241.

281. Nwankwo T, Yoon SS, Burt V, Gu, Q. Hypertension among adults in the United States: National Health and Nutrition Examination Survey, 2011–2012. *NCHS Data Brief*. October 2013:(133). http://www.cdc.gov/nchs/data/databriefs/db133.pdf. Accessed July 15, 2015.

282. Madhur MS. Hypertension. Medscape. Retrieved from: http://emedicine.medscape.com/article/241381-overview. Accessed August 27, 2015.

283. American Heart Association. High blood pressure and African Americans. Dallas, TX: American Heart Association; updated August 13, 2014. Retrieved from: http://www.heart.org/HEARTORG/Conditions/HighBloodPressure/UnderstandYourRiskforHighBloodPressure/High-Blood-Pressure-and-African-Americans_UCM_301832_Article.jsp. Accessed July 17, 2015.

284. James PA, Oparil S, Carter BL, et al. 2014 evidence-based guideline for the management of high blood pressure in adults: report from the panel members appointed to the Eighth Joint National Committee (JNC 8). *JAMA*. 2014;311:507–520.

285. Forman JP, Stampfer MJ, Curhan GC. Diet and lifestyle risk factors associated with incident hypertension in women. *JAMA*. 2009;302:401–411.

286. Carnethon MR, Evans NS, Church TS, et al. Joint associations of physical activity and aerobic fitness on the development of incident hypertension: coronary artery risk development in young adults. *Hypertension*. 2010;56:49–55.

287. Eckel RH, Jakicic JM, Ard JD, et al. 2013 AHA/ACC guideline on lifestyle management to reduce cardiovascular risk: a report of the American College of Cardiology/American Heart Association Task Force on Practice Guidelines. *J Am Coll Cardiol*. 2014;63:2960.

288. Schaeffer J. Eat to lower blood pressure—nutrition strategies for counseling patients. *Today's Dietitian*. January 2012;14(1):18.

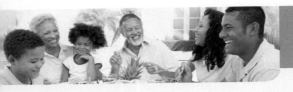

Learning Portfolio (continued)

289. Appel LJ, Brands MW, Daniels SR, et al. Dietary approaches to prevent and treat hypertension: a scientific statement from the American Heart Association. *Hypertension.* 2006;47:296–308.

290. Elmer PJ, Obarzanek E, Vollmer WM, et al. Effects of comprehensive lifestyle modification on diet, weight, physical fitness, and blood pressure control: 18-month results of a randomized trial. *Ann Intern Med.* 2006;144:485–495.

291. National Heart, Lung, and Blood Institute. *Your Guide to Lowering Your Blood Pressure with DASH.* NIH Publication No. 06-5834. Washington, DC; National Heart, Lung, and Blood Institute; updated August 2015. https://www.nhlbi.nih.gov/files/docs/public/heart/dash_brief.pdf. Accessed July 16, 2015.

292. National Heart, Lung, and Blood Institute. Description of the DASH eating plan. Washington, DC: National Heart, Lung, and Blood Institute; updated September 16, 2015. Retrieved from: https://www.nhlbi.nih.gov/health/health-topics/topics/dash. Accessed November 18, 2016.

293. American Cancer Society. What is cancer? A guide for patients and families. Dallas, TX: American Cancer Society; updated December 8, 2015. Retrieved from: http://www.cancer.org/cancer/cancerbasics/what-is-cancer. Accessed July 21, 2015.

294. Twombly R. What's in a name: who is a cancer survivor? *J Natl Cancer Inst.* 2004;96(19):1414–1415.

295. Mayo Clinic. Diseases and conditions: cancer. Rochester, MN: Mayo Clinic; May 23, 2015. Retrieved from: http://www.mayoclinic.org/diseases-conditions/cancer/basics/causes/con-20032378. Accessed August 29, 2015.

296. CancerWebPage. Etiology of cancer. Retrieved from: http://www.cancerwebpage.com/etiology-of-cancer. Accessed August 29, 2015.

297. National Cancer Institute. Cancer statistics. Bethesda, MD: National Cancer Institute; updated March 14, 2016. Retrieved from: https://www.cancer.gov/about-cancer/understanding/statistics. Accessed November 16, 2015.

298. American Cancer Society. Family cancer syndromes. Dallas, TX: American Cancer Society; updated June 25, 2014. Retrieved from: http://www.cancer.org/cancer/cancercauses/geneticsandcancer/heredity-and-cancer. Accessed July 25, 2015.

299. National Cancer Institute. Chemicals in meat cooked at high temperatures and cancer risk. Bethesda, MD: National Cancer Institute. Retrieved from: https://www.cancer.gov/about-cancer/causes-prevention/risk/diet/cooked-meats-fact-sheet. Accessed November 18, 2016.

300. American Cancer Society. Acrylamide and cancer risk: what is acrylamide? Dallas, TX: American Cancer Society; updated March 10, 2016. Retrieved from: http://www.cancer.org/cancer/cancercauses/othercarcinogens/athome/acrylamide. Accessed August 10, 2016.

301. MindBodyGreen. What are we eating? What the average American consumes in a year. MindBodyGreen; August 2, 2010. Retrieved from: http://www.mindbodygreen.com/0-1198/What-Are-We-Eating-What-the-Average-American-Consumes-in-a-Year-Image.html. Accessed August 29, 2015.

302. Colditz GA, DeJong W, Hunter DJ, et al. Harvard report on cancer prevention. Vol 1. Causes of human cancer. *Cancer Causes Control.* 1996;7(suppl):S3–59.

303. Bellizzi KM, Rowland JH, Jeffery DD, McNeel T. Health behaviors of cancer survivors: examining opportunities for cancer control intervention. *J Clin Oncol.* 2005;23:8884–8893.

304. Nielsen SF, Nordestgaard BG, Bojesen SE. Associations between first and second primary cancers: a population-based study. *CMAJ.* 2012;184:E57–E69.

305. National Cancer Institute. Obesity and cancer risk. Bethesda, MD: National Cancer Institute; reviewed January 3, 2012. Retrieved from: http://www.cancer.gov/about-cancer/causes-prevention/risk/obesity/obesity-fact-sheet. Accessed August 11, 2015.

306. Brennan SF, Cantwell MM, Cardwell CR, et al. Dietary patterns and breast cancer risk: a systematic review and meta-analysis. *Am J Clin Nutr.* 2010;91(5):1294–1302.

307. Schmid D, Leitzmann MF. Television viewing and time spent sedentary in relation to cancer risk: a meta-analysis. *J Natl Cancer Inst.* 2014;106(7):dju098.

308. Mayo Clinic staff. Diseases and conditions: cancer. Rochester, MN: Mayo Clinic; May 23, 2015. Retrieved from: http://www.mayoclinic.org/diseases-conditions/cancer/basics/causes/con-20032378. Accessed August 29, 2015.

309. World Cancer Research Fund International/American Institute for Cancer Research. *Food, Nutrition, Physical Activity, and the Prevention of Cancer: A Global Perspective.* Washington, DC: American Institute for Cancer Research; 2007. http://www.aicr.org/assets/docs/pdf/reports/Second_Expert_Report.pdf. Accessed July 22, 2015.

310. de Moor JS, Mariotto AB, Parry C, et al. Cancer survivors in the United States: prevalence across the survivorship trajectory and implications for care. *Cancer Epidemiol Biomarkers Prev.* 2013;22(4):561–570.

311. Howlader N, Noone AM, Krapcho M, et al, eds. *SEER Cancer Statistics Review, 1975–2010.* Bethesda, MD: National Cancer Institute; 2013.

312. Friedenreich CM, Orenstein MR. Physical activity and cancer prevention: etiologic evidence and biological mechanisms. *J Nutr.* 2002;132(11 suppl):3456S-3464S.

313. Jatoi A. Anorexia and cachexia. CancerNetwork; June 1, 2015. Retrieved from: http://www.cancernetwork.com/cancer-management/anorexia-and-cachexia. Accessed June 26, 2016.

314. Chlebowski RT, Aiello E, McTiernan A. Weight loss in breast cancer patient management. *J Clin Oncol.* 2002;20:1128–1143.

315. Schattner M, Shike M. Nutrition support of the patient with cancer. In Shils ME, Shike M, Ross AC, Cabellero B, Cousins RJ, eds. *Modern Nutrition in Health and Disease.* 10th ed. Philadelphia, PA: Lippincott Williams & Wilkins; 2006:1290–1313.

316. Fearon K, Strasser F, Anker SD, et al. Definition and classification of cancer cachexia: an international consensus. *Lancet Oncol.* 2011;12:489–495.

317. Ravasco P, Monteiro-Grillo I, Vidal PM, Camilo ME. Dietary counseling improves patient outcomes: a prospective, randomized, controlled trial in colorectal cancer patients undergoing radiotherapy. *J Clin Oncol.* 2005;23:1431–1438.

318. Rock CL. Dietary counseling is beneficial for the patient with cancer. *J Clin Oncol.* 2005;23:1348–1349.

319. August DA, Huhmann MB; American Society for Parenteral and Enteral Nutrition (A.S.P.E.N.) Board of Directors. A.S.P.E.N. clinical guidelines: nutrition support therapy

during adult anticancer treatment and in hematopoietic cell transplantation. *J Parenter Enteral Nutr*. 2009;33:472–500.

320. Galvao DA, Taaffe DR, Spry N, et al. Combined resistance and aerobic exercise program reverses muscle loss in men undergoing androgen suppression therapy for prostate cancer without bone metastases: a randomized controlled trial. *J Clin Oncol*. 2010;28:340–347.

321. Speck RM, Courneya KS, Masse LC, et al. An update of controlled physical activity trials in cancer survivors: a systematic review and meta-analysis. *J Cancer Surviv*. 2010;4:87–100.

322. Schmitz KH, Courneya KS, Matthews C, et al; American College of Sports Medicine. American College of Sports Medicine roundtable on exercise guidelines for cancer survivors. *Med Sci Sports Exerc*. 2010;42:1409–1426.

323. Winters-Stone KM, Dobek J, Nail L, et al. Strength training stops bone loss and builds muscle in postmenopausal breast cancer survivors: a randomized, controlled trial. *Breast Cancer Res Treat*. 2011;127:447–456.

324. Schwartz AL, Winters-Stone K. Effects of a 12-month randomized controlled trial of aerobic or resistance exercise during and following cancer treatment in women. *Phys Sportsmed*. 2009;37:62–67.

325. Coward DD. Supporting health promotion in adults with cancer. *Fam Community Health*. 2006;29(suppl 1):52S–60S.

326. Ng AK, Travis LB. Second primary cancers: an overview. *Hematol Oncol Clin North Am*. 2008;22:271–289.

327. Hardman WE. (n-3) fatty acids and cancer therapy. *J Nutr*. 2004;134(suppl 12):3427S–3430S.

328. American Institute for Cancer Research. Recommendations for cancer prevention. Washington, DC: American Institute for Cancer Research; updated September 12, 2014. Retrieved from: http://www.aicr.org/reduce-your-cancer-risk/recommendations-for-cancer-prevention. Accessed August 9, 2015.

329. Moe G. Low-microbial diets for patients with granulocytopenia. In Bloch AS, ed. *Nutrition Management of the Cancer Patient*. Rockville, MD: Aspen Publishers; 1990:125.

330. Arts IC. A review of the epidemiological evidence on tea, flavonoids, and lung cancer. *J Nutr*. 2008;138(8):1561S–1566S.

331. Xu X, Cai L. A case-control study on tea consumption and the risk of lung cancer. *Wei Sheng Yan Jiu*. 2013;42(2):211–216.

332. American Institute for Cancer Research. Foods that fight cancer: garlic. Washington, DC: American Institute for Cancer Research; updated July 1, 2011. Retrieved from: http://www.aicr.org/foods-that-fight-cancer/foodsthatfightcancer_garlic.html. Accessed August 9, 2015.

333. Jin ZY, Han RQ, Zhang XF, et al. [The protective effects of green tea drinking and garlic intake on lung cancer, in a low cancer risk area of Jiangsu province, China] [article in Chinese]. *Zhonghua Liu Xing Bing Xue Za Zhi*. 2013;34(2):114–119.

334. Wu QJ, Xie L, Zheng W, et al. Cruciferous vegetables consumption and the risk of female lung cancer: a prospective study and a meta-analysis. *Ann Oncol*. 2013;24(7):1918–1924.

335. Yang G, Shu XO, Li HL, et al. Prediagnosis soy food consumption and lung cancer survival in women. *J Clin Oncol*. 2013;31(12):1548–1553.

336. Kruzich LA, Marquis GS, Carriquiry AL, et al. US youths in the early stages of HIV disease have low intakes of some micronutrients for optimal immune function. *J Am Diet Assoc*. 2004;104:1095–1101.

337. Slama L, LeCamus C, Serfaty L, et al. Metabolic disorders and chronic viral disease: the case of HIV and HCV. *Diabetes Metab*. 2009;35:1–11.

338. Llibre JM, Falco V, Tural C, et al. The changing face of HIV/AIDS in treated patients. *Curr HIV Res*. 2009;7:365–377.

339. Mocroft A, Ledergerber B, Zilmer K, et al. Short-term clinical disease progression in HIV-1–positive patients taking combination antiretroviral therapy: The EuroSIDA risk-score. *AIDS*. 2007;21:1867–1875.

340. Siddiqui J, Phillips AL, Freedland ES, et al. Prevalence and cost of HIV-associated weight loss in a managed care population. *CurrMed Res Opin*. 2009;25(5):1307–1317.

341. Centers for Disease Control and Prevention. HIV in the United States: at a glance. Atlanta, GA: Centers for Disease Control and Prevention; June 2016. Retrieved from: http://www.cdc.gov/hiv/statistics/basics/ataglance.html. Updated July 11, 2016. Accessed August 27, 2016.

342. Centers for Disease Control and Prevention. Prevention benefits of HIV treatment. Atlanta, GA: Centers for Disease Control and Prevention; February 9, 2016. Retrieved from: http://www.cdc.gov/hiv/prevention/research/tap/. Accessed August 12, 2016.

343. U.S. Department of Health and Human Services. Stages of HIV infection. Washington, DC: U.S. Department of Health and Human Services; updated August 27, 2015. Retrieved from: https://www.aids.gov/hiv-aids-basics/just-diagnosed-with-hiv-aids/hiv-in-your-body/stages-of-hiv/. Updated August 27, 2015. Accessed August 31, 2015.

344. Cofrancesco J Jr, Freedland E, McComsey G. Treatment options for HIV-associated central fat accumulation. *AIDS Patient Care STDS*. 2009;23(1):5–18.

345. Grinspoon S, Mulligan K. Weight loss and wasting in patients infected with human immunodeficiency virus. *Clin Infect Dis*. 2003;36(suppl 2):S69–S78.

346. Mangili A, Murman DH, Zampini AM, Wanke CA. Nutrition and HIV infection: review of weight loss and wasting in the era of highly active antiretroviral therapy from the nutrition for healthy living cohort. *Clin Infect Dis*. March 15, 2006;42(6):836–842.

347. Duggal S, Chugh TD, Duggal AK. HIV and malnutrition: effects on immune system. *Clin Development Immunol*. 2012;2012:1–8.

348. Crum-Cianflone NF. HIV and the gastrointestinal tract. *Infect Dis Clin Pract*. 2010;18(5):283–285.

349. El-Sadr WM, Mullin CM, Carr A, et al. Effects of HIV disease on lipid, glucose and insulin levels: results from a large antiretroviral-naive cohort. *HIV Med*. 2005;6(2):114–121.

350. Ferrando SJ, Rabkin JG, Lin SH, McElhiney M. Increase in body cell mass and decrease in wasting are associated with increasing potency of antiretroviral therapy for HIV infection. *AIDS Patient Care STDS*. 2005;19(4):216–223.

351. Gelato MC. Insulin and carbohydrate dysregulation. *Clin Infect Dis*. 2003;36(suppl 2):91–95.

352. National Heart, Lung, and Blood Institute. What are the risks of a blood transfusion? Washington, DC: National Heart, Lung and Blood Institute updated January 30, 2012. Retrieved from: https://www.nhlbi.nih.gov/health/health-topics/topics/bt/risks. Accessed August 31, 2015.

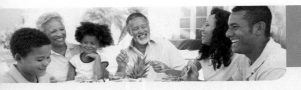

353. Mahan LK, Raymond JL, Escott-Stump S. *Krause's Food and the Nutrition Care Process*. 13th ed. St. Louis, MO: Elsevier Saunders; 2012:868–869.

354. Berneis K, Battegay M, Bassetti R, et al. Nutritional supplements combined with dietary counseling diminish whole body protein catabolism in HIV-infected patients. *Eur J Clin Invest*. 2000;30:87–94.

355. Bogden JD, Kemp FW, Han S, et al. Status of selected nutrients and progression of human immunodeficiency virus type 1 infection. *Am J Clin Nutr*. 2000;72(3):809–815.

356. Hadigan C, Jeste S, Anderson EJ, et al. Modifiable dietary habits and their relation to metabolic abnormalities in men and women with human immunodeficiency virus infection and fat redistribution. *Clin Infect Dis*. 2001;33(5):710–717.

357. Perry AC, LaPerriere A, Klimas N. Acquired immune deficiency syndrome (AIDS). In Durstine JL, Moore GE, Painter PL, Roberts SO, eds. *ACSM's Exercise Management for Persons with Chronic Diseases and Disabilities*. 3rd ed. Champagne, IL: Human Kinetics; 2009.

CHAPTER 14

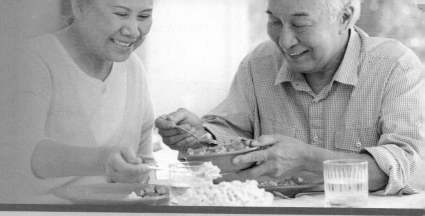

Older Adult Nutrition

Melissa Bernstein, PhD, RD, LD, FAND

Chapter Outline

Physiology of Aging

Dietary Intake of Older Adults

Nutritional Recommendations and Requirements for Older Adults

Promoting Healthy Lifestyles

Learning Objectives

1. Explain the key changes that occur with age in each body system.

2. List the main factors that affect food intake of older adults.

3. Describe the nutritional recommendations for older adults.

4. Discuss ways to encourage older adults to lead a healthy lifestyle.

©jwblinn/Shutterstock

Case Study

Sherry is a vibrant 95-year-old woman who lives alone in her own apartment in a residential area with other seniors and middle-aged professionals. Sherry does her own cooking, shopping, and housekeeping. She still drives, although in the past few years has limited her driving to daytime only because her night vision is deteriorating. Since her husband died about 10 years ago, Sherry enjoys a quiet breakfast at home and usually goes out for lunch to a local restaurant or senior center with friends. If she is not going out with friends for dinner, Sherry eats at home with family or friends or in front of the television. Aside from the "normal aches and pains of being 95," Sherry is otherwise healthy. She makes an effort to walk daily and attends a fitness class twice weekly. Sherry has never smoked and tries to eat healthy, unprocessed foods, although she admits to having a weakness for chocolates. She does not regularly drink alcohol. Sherry is at a normal body mass index (BMI) and has always been conscientious about her weight and physical appearance.

Older adults are the largest growing segment of the population in the United States. For the first time in U.S. history, the total number of older adults in the U.S. is unparalleled. The older population in 2030 is anticipated to double, increasing from 35 million in 2000 to 72 million and representing almost 20% of the total U.S. population.[1] By 2050, the number of adults 65 years and older is forecasted to reach 89 million people.[1] Ethnic and racial diversity are characteristics of this shift in the population. This trend will continue in the United States as minority populations continue to grow and are estimated to account for 43% of older adults by 2050 (**FIGURE 14.1**).[1]

Throughout the life span, successful aging depends on the interaction of a variety of factors, including health behaviors, genetics, environment and lifestyle, and medical conditions. To reduce the burden of chronic disease and maximize quality of life and healthy aging, all older adults must adopt healthy lifestyle practices and dietary habits. Healthy eating and an active lifestyle are essential to maintaining a functional quality of life and preventing chronic health problems. Ensuring adequate nutritional intake is an indispensable factor in promoting health and well-being, maintaining functional independence, and preventing malnutrition and related comorbidities such as increased susceptibility to acute and chronic illness and impaired immune function. This chapter provides an overview of some of the biologic and physiological changes of aging and introduces the nutritional implication of these changes in generally healthy older adults.

Physiology of Aging

Preview Nutrition is well recognized as one of the major determinants of successful aging. From early in life, eating a nutritious diet, maintaining a healthy body weight, and leading a physically active lifestyle are key influential factors in helping individuals

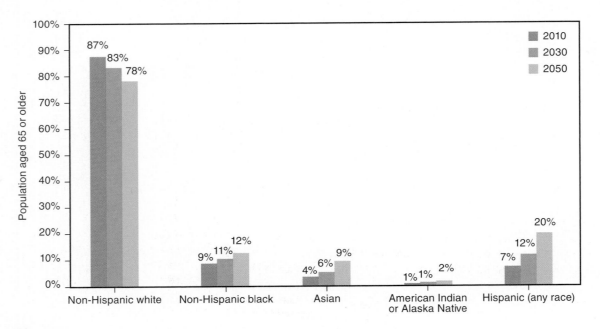

Figure 14.1
The U.S. population ages 65 years and older.

Reproduced from Centers for Disease Control and Prevention. *The State of Aging and Health in America 2013*. Atlanta, GA: Centers for Disease Control and Prevention, U.S. Department of Health and Human Services; 2013: Fig. 1: U.S. population aged 65 years or older and diversity, 2010–2050. Retrieved from: http://www.cdc.gov/aging/pdf/state-aging-health-in-america-2013.pdf. Accessed July, 11, 2016.

avoid the physical and mental deteriorations associated with aging. Aging and life expectancy are dynamic processes influenced by genetics, the environment, and lifelong choices. Age-related changes in body systems influence and are influenced by disease risk and development. Distinguishing normal age-related changes from those associated with disease and disuse can be complicated in older adults because of dynamic and interdependent causes and consequences.

Older adults experience numerous physiological changes and medical conditions that either lead to or require a change in nutritional requirements and food intake. Efforts to consume a healthy diet can be influenced by health status, changes in taste perception, decreased olfactory ability, difficulty chewing and swallowing, and changes in digestion and absorption and nutrient metabolism. These factors may occur naturally with aging or as a result of illness or medication side effects. Changes in body composition or physiological function that occur with age may also influence nutritional requirements. Declines in muscle mass and bone density and functional status, changes in gastrointestinal functioning, immune function, nutrient absorption, and metabolism may interfere with the capability of older adults to meet nutritional needs especially when calorie needs are reduced.

Defining Aging

Beginning before conception, nutrition is dynamic in its effect on human development and growth and, then ultimately, the aging process. Aging is characterized by a gradual decline in organ function beginning as early as 30 to 40 years of age. In the absence of disease, aging alone does not lead to overt disease; however, physiologic changes that occur as part of aging can make the occurrence of disease more likely. Alterations to the skeletal system, such as changes in bone turnover and loss of bone mass, for example, make osteoporosis and associated fractures more likely. Therefore, it can be difficult to separate alterations related to aging from those related to disease.[2]

Life Expectancy

A child born in 2011 could expect to live until approximately the age of 79 years—almost 30 years longer than a child born in 1900.[3] Today, adults who reach the age of 65 have a life expectancy of an additional 19.2 years, to an average old age of 83.6 years.[3] Along with general trends in the U.S. population, Hispanic, American Indian, Alaska Native, African American (or black), Asian, Hawaiian, and Pacific Islander populations are also living longer.[4]

Aging is a multifactorial consequence of the interactions between genes and environment. Aging cannot be reversed; however, it may be altered through nutrition, physical activity, and other healthy lifestyle choices. The

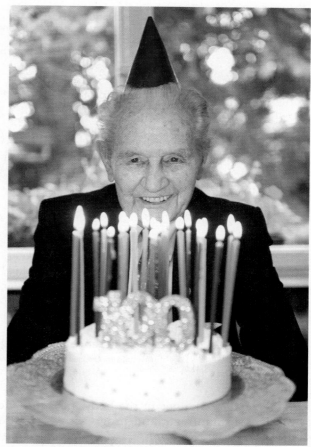
©Claudia Paulussen/ShutterStock, Inc

presence and rate of progression of age-related changes differ significantly among individuals and may influence how a disease manifests and its severity as well as consequences. Some of these changes can be slowed with good health habits, including diet and exercise and appropriate medical interventions, whereas others are thought to be part of normal aging (**FIGURE 14.2**). Ultimately, the combination of changes can lead to a decline in health and functional capacity and can contribute to an increase in susceptibility to injury and vulnerability to disease.

Aging Systems

Throughout the years, numerous aging theories have been proposed, for example, evolutionary theories of aging, such as apoptosis, the theory of mutation accumulation, and the antagonistic pleiotropy hypothesis.[5,6] There does appear to be a genetic predisposition to longevity for some genes or combination of genes. Genes may function to improve longevity by offering disease protection, whereas others may function in combination with environment and lifestyle choices. Despite the genetic predisposition to long life for some individuals, of critical importance to longevity and quality of life are environmental factors and lifelong health-related behaviors such as physical activity, smoking, and body weight maintenance.[7]

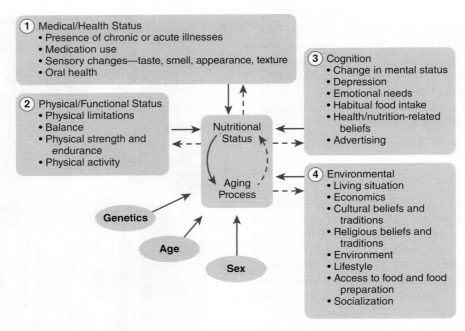

Figure 14.2
Factors that influence aging and quality of life.

Modified from American Dietetic Association. Position paper of the American Dietetic Association: nutrition across the spectrum of aging. *J Am Diet Assoc.* 2005;105(4):616–633.

Aging-related changes in the body may influence how a disease manifests and progresses as well as the severity of the disease (TABLE 14.1). Most disability of old age is associated with age-dependent conditions such as coronary heart disease, adult-onset diabetes, and Alzheimer's disease, which are ultimately the main causes of death in persons older than the age of 65.[8] Distinguishing normal age-related changes from changes related to disease, medication use, and physical disuse can be complicated because of overlapping and interdependent consequences. In older adults, whether changes are associated with normal aging or diseases, medication use, and physical disuse, if the initiating factors can be determined and then prevented or treated, the disease or the consequences can be averted.

Table 14.1

Selected Physiologic and Metabolic Changes with Age and the Effects on Body Systems, Nutrition, and Health

Physiologic or Metabolic Change	Impact on Nutrition	Health-Related Consequence
Decreased total energy expenditure	Decreased energy requirements	Increased risk of obesity
	Increased importance of nutrient-dense food choices	
Decreased muscle mass and strength	Functional impairment could limit food access	Increased risk for sarcopenia and functional dependency
	Decreased need for energy	
	Increased need for high-quality protein	
Reduced skin synthesis of vitamin D (cholecalciferol)	Increased requirement for vitamin D and calcium	Decreased bone density and skeletal mass
		Increased risk for bone fractures and osteoporosis
Decreased kidney function	Reduced ability to concentrate urine contributes to increased fluid needs	Increased risk for dehydration
		Alterations in drug metabolism
Decreased immune function	Increased needs for high-quality proteins, antioxidants, vitamin B_6, vitamin E, and zinc	Increased susceptibility to illness and disease
Gastrointestinal changes: atrophic gastritis and increased gastric pH	Increased requirements for folate, calcium, vitamin K, vitamin B_{12}, and iron	Increased risk for pernicious anemia and vitamin B_{12} deficiency
Slowed gastric motility	Increased need for fluids and fiber	Increased risk for constipation

Gastrointestinal Changes

Gastrointestinal changes affect older adults along the length of the gastrointestinal (GI) tract, beginning with oral health in the mouth and continuing to the anus. Changes that occur along the length of the GI tract are important in determining nutritional requirements, medication dosing, and medical nutritional therapy to treat chronic diseases and conditions (TABLE 14.2).

Upper GI Changes

Impairments in the oral cavity and changes in taste and smell with age, disease, and medication use can contribute to inadequate intake, lead to malnutrition, and worsen disease and health outcomes. These changes are of particular concern in this group. Swallowing disorders are common in older adults; however, research suggests that conditions of impaired swallowing such as dysphagia result from disease rather than aging. Any disruption in normal swallowing can be considered dysphagia, and the prevalence among older adults ranges from 15% to 35%.[9,10] Nutritional status may be compromised in older adults who have difficulty chewing and swallowing if they avoid meats, fresh fruits, and fresh vegetables because these foods are difficult to chew and swallow.

Delays in stomach emptying and declines in gastric output have been found to occur with age. Whether **gastroparesis** is a result of age or other underlying conditions, such as atrophic gastritis, is unclear. **Atrophic gastritis** results in a decreased secretion of acid and **intrinsic factors** in the stomach, which contribute to vitamin B_{12} malabsorption in pernicious anemia. The prevalence of atrophic gastritis has been reported as more than 40% in adults older than age 80 years. Declines in liver, gall bladder, and pancreas function can have profound effects on the digestion and absorption of fat, protein, and carbohydrates as well as some vitamins and minerals. A decline in the production of enzymes necessary to digest foods also occurs with age. Impaired ability to digest dietary fat, for example, may result in inadequate energy and malabsorption of some nutrients.

Lower GI Changes

The small intestine is where the digestion of protein, fat, and nearly all carbohydrate is completed and where most nutrients are absorbed. Disruption in normal functioning of the small intestine can have a profound effect on nutritional well-being. The colon, for many older adults, is a source of discomfort, symptoms, and disease predominantly associated with disorders in motility such as constipation. Constipation, one of the most common gastrointestinal conditions of older adults, is most frequently attributed to diet, behavior, and inactivity; however, there are multiple factors in its etiology.[11] Dehydration, dementia, functional limitations, chronic disease, and neurologic

Table 14.2

Changes Along the GI Tract with Age

Oral cavity changes	• The first signs of micronutrient deficiencies and malnutrition often appear in the oral tissues. • Chronic diseases and medications in older adults can lead to complications in the oral cavity that result in pain, tooth loss, xerostomia, and problems with chewing and swallowing, which contribute to poor appetite and impaired ability to eat and drink.
Esophageal changes	• Dysphagia is associated with advancing age because of age-related physiologic changes in swallowing. • Dysphagia is common in older adults with neurodegenerative diseases such as dementia or stroke and psychiatric diseases. • Medications that can cause confusion, decrease alertness, or affect consciousness or swallowing may contribute to delays in swallowing response. • Gastroesophageal reflux disease (GERD) and peptic ulcer disease are common causes of dyspepsia in older adults. • Delayed emptying of gastric contents, reduced lower esophageal sphincter functioning, reduced peristalsis, hiatal hernia, and frequently used medications to treat conditions common in older adults all affect esophageal functioning.
Changes in gastric function	• In the stomach and small intestine of older adults, digestive secretions are reduced, resulting in decreased capacity for nutrient absorption from foods. • Atrophic gastritis interferes with normal absorption of vitamin B_{12} and leads to a deficiency of this vitamin.
Pancreas, gall bladder, liver changes	• Pancreatic and gall bladder secretions and liver function all decline with age. • Changes in liver function could influence the effectiveness of medications, side effects of medications, and nutrient digestion, absorption, and metabolism.
Small intestine changes	• Nutrient digestion and absorption are affected by changes that occur along the small intestine.
Large intestine changes	• The primary functions of the colon are to act as a reservoir for fecal matter and to reabsorb water, electrolytes, bile salts, and short-chain fatty acids. • Slowing of gastrointestinal motility with age along with a low-fiber diet, low fluid intake, and medication use contribute to constipation.

Bernstein MA. The Physiology of Aging in Nutrition for the Older Adult. 2e. Bernstein MA and Munoz N.eds. 2016 Burlington, MA. Jones and Bartlett Learning.

disease such as multiple sclerosis and Parkinson's are additional factors that may play a role in constipation in elderly persons. The many myths and misinformation about gastrointestinal effects of various foods among older adults and even the medical community can lead to unnecessary dietary restrictions and inadequate nutrient intake. Optimizing GI health is fundamental to maximizing older patients' ability to consume a healthful and varied diet.

Changes in Body Composition with Age

Body weight generally increases until the sixth decade of life, after which adults experience a loss of muscle mass and increase in body fat. These changes in body composition can interfere with the ability to maintain independence in daily activities and result in increased frailty, declining physical functioning, and worsening health.[12] Loss of skeletal muscle mass and strength, termed sarcopenia, is widespread among older adults, affecting 8–40% of those older than age 60 years and more than 50% of adults older than 75 years.[13] Sarcopenia has many interrelated causes and is part of a complex cycle that includes

worsening of disease burden and illness, nutritional inadequacy, increased disability, and functional dependence.[12] Optimizing nutritional intake, adequate high-quality protein and antioxidants in particular, and progressive resistance strength training are the most effective interventions to prevent and reverse sarcopenia.[14–16]

Overweight and Obesity

The burden of poor health from excess body weight and body fat will continue to increase in the older adult population with the rising number of older adults and their longer life expectancy. Similar to younger age groups, currently more than 30% of adults age 65 and older are classified as obese as a result of poor food choices, primarily consumption of a low-quality diet with too many calories and an inactive lifestyle.[17] Older adults who are overweight have an increased risk of chronic diseases such as heart disease, diabetes, metabolic syndrome, and cancer.

Unintentional weight loss, on the other hand, and low body mass index (BMI) in elderly adults often are suggestive of underlying disease associated with poor health outcomes and are markers for deterioration in

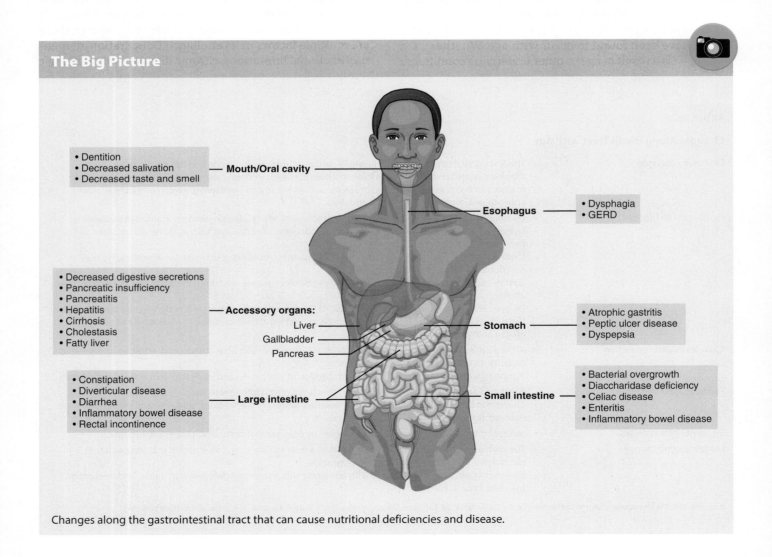

The Big Picture

- Dentition
- Decreased salivation
- Decreased taste and smell
— **Mouth/Oral cavity**

Esophagus
- Dysphagia
- GERD

- Decreased digestive secretions
- Pancreatic insufficiency
- Pancreatitis
- Hepatitis
- Cirrhosis
- Cholestasis
- Fatty liver
— **Accessory organs:**
Liver
Gallbladder
Pancreas

Stomach
- Atrophic gastritis
- Peptic ulcer disease
- Dyspepsia

- Constipation
- Diverticular disease
- Diarrhea
- Inflammatory bowel disease
- Rectal incontinence
— **Large intestine**

Small intestine
- Bacterial overgrowth
- Diaccharidase deficiency
- Celiac disease
- Enteritis
- Inflammatory bowel disease

Changes along the gastrointestinal tract that can cause nutritional deficiencies and disease.

well-being.[12] When sarcopenia and obesity occur simultaneously, the condition is termed sarcopenic obesity. Sarcopenic obesity is detrimental to physical functioning and the health of older adults and contributes to worsening of health status.[18]

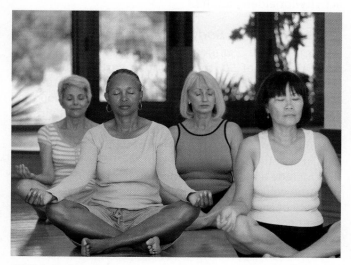

©Ariel Skelley/Blend Images/Getty

Cardiovascular and Respiratory System Changes with Age

Decline in cardiovascular function is a major physical impairment associated with aging. More than 70% of adults older than age 60 and more than 83% of adults ages 80 and older have coronary heart disease (CHD).[19] Age-associated changes in cardiovascular performance are observed beginning in middle age; however, an increasingly sedentary lifestyle contributes significantly to a progressive deconditioning of the cardiorespiratory system. Normal aging leads to progressive wear and tear on the structure and function of the heart; however, these atherosclerotic changes are strongly influenced by environmental factors, especially diet. Modifiable lifestyle choices such as dietary habits, body weight, smoking, and physical activity determine risk for atherosclerosis and heart disease in older adults. TABLE 14.3 lists some dietary factors associated with risk of heart disease.

Dietary guidance from the American Heart Association to lower cardiovascular risk emphasizes increasing food items such as fruits and vegetables, fish, nuts and legumes, and fiber-rich whole grains and reducing consumption of such foods as sodium, sugar, processed meats, and trans fats.[20] Older adults are recommended to follow the same nutritional principles as younger adults for the general treatment of hypertension with the objective of reducing cardiovascular and renal morbidity and mortality. Efforts to reduce low-density lipoprotein (LDL) cholesterol, by increasing dietary fiber, for example, can also prove to be beneficial in the management of body weight, diabetes, and constipation.

Older adults, particularly those who are frail or malnourished, are more susceptible to pulmonary infections such as pneumonia, bronchitis, and tuberculosis as well as aspiration pneumonia. In addition to physiological changes in the lung tissue, age-related changes in the

Table 14.3

Dietary Risk Factors for Coronary Heart Disease

Dietary Component	Role in Cardiovascular Health
Dietary fat (especially dietary trans fat)	Plays a role in the regulation of circulating lipoprotein levels.
Omega-3 fatty acids	Decrease the risk of arrhythmias that can lead to sudden death; decrease triglycerides; slow the rate of atherosclerotic plaque; and slightly lower blood pressure.
Dietary sugar	Excess dietary sugar provides added calories and may lead to weight gain, overweight, and obesity and contribute to metabolic syndrome and risk factors for diabetes, CVD, and cancer.
Energy intake	Is central to the management of body weight, which affects lipoprotein levels, insulin sensitivity, plasma glucose, and blood pressure.
Dietary sodium	Plays a role in the development and management of HTN.
Dietary antioxidants (especially vitamin E)	Protective effects against CHD risk.
Vitamin B_6, vitamin B_{12}, and folate	May lower plasma HCY levels (moderate elevations in HCY increase the risk of CHD by promoting platelet activation, oxidative stress, endothelial dysfunction, hypercoagulability, vascular smooth muscle cell proliferation, and endoplasmic reticulum stress).
Alcohol	Drinking too much alcohol can raise triglycerides and lead to high blood pressure, heart failure, and stroke. Other problems of excessive alcohol are cardiomyopathy, cardiac arrhythmia, and sudden cardiac death.
Dietary fiber	Aids in lowering LDL cholesterol.

CHD = coronary heart disease; CVD = cerebrovascular disease; HCY = homocysteine; HTN = hypertension; LDL = low-density lipoprotein.

Data from American Heart Association. The American Heart Association's diet and lifestyle recommendations. Dallas, TX: AHA; updated January 20, 2016. Retrieved from: http://www.heart.org/HEARTORG/HealthyLiving/HealthyEating/Nutrition/The-American-Heart-Associations-Diet-and-Lifestyle-Recommendations_UCM_305855_Article.jsp#. V6q5tPmAOkr. Accessed August 10, 2016.

bones and muscles of the chest, nervous system, and immune system can all have effects on the lungs.

Renal System Changes with Aging

It is estimated that by age 60, the average person has lost approximately 25% of kidney function. Kidney changes and loss of renal function can affect the older adult's ability to maintain fluid and electrolyte balance. Reduced ability of the kidneys to concentrate urine also can be an important factor contributing to dehydration in older adults. Chronic kidney disease is most common in adults older than age 70, and more than half of the adults on dialysis in the United States are older than age 65.[21,22]

Kidneys are affected by the aging process and also by illness, medications, and other conditions that influence kidney function such as diabetes, cardiovascular disease, hypertension, and obesity. Chronic kidney disease itself increases the risk of heart disease, heart attacks, and strokes and is related to other health problems such as high blood pressure and edema, anemia, weakened immunity, depression, osteoporosis, and malnutrition. In older adults with kidney disease, functional declines, unintentional weight loss, and sarcopenia are undesirable consequences that contribute to frailty, worsen disease burden, and have profound effects on health and quality of life.

Changes in Skeletal Health with Aging

Although peak bone mass is largely determined by genetics, modifiable factors play a significant role in the maintenance of bone health with advancing age. The rate at which an adult loses bone is highly dependent on lifestyle factors, such as diet, exercise, body weight, hormonal status, medication, tobacco and alcohol use, and illness.[23]

Fat-soluble vitamin D functions as one of several hormones responsible for safeguarding bone health as well as maintaining calcium and phosphorus concentrations at physiologically desirable levels.[24] Older adults often have poor vitamin D status because their skin cells are less effective in synthesizing vitamin D when exposed to sunlight, and tissues are less efficient in absorbing dietary vitamin D from the blood.[25] Many older adults limit their time in direct sunlight, further reducing the opportunity for adequate vitamin D synthesis and negatively affecting calcium absorption and ultimately bone quality. Low levels of circulating sex hormones in both men and women can also contribute to declining bone mass with age.

Osteoporosis

Osteoporosis, the most common bone disease in humans, results when there is a loss of bone mass and strength that predisposes an individual to bone fracture (FIGURE 14.3). In addition to appropriate amounts of calcium, vitamin D, phosphorus, vitamin K, magnesium, and fluoride, other nutrients such as iron, zinc, copper, several B vitamins, carotenoids, protein, and the essential fatty acids are important for bone health.[26] Individuals at risk for osteoporosis should avoid regularly overconsuming protein, phosphorus, sodium, alcohol, vitamin A, and caffeine in amounts that exceed recommended levels because overconsumption may have a negative impact on bone health.[27] According to the surgeon general, reducing the risk of falls may be the biggest benefit of physical activity for elderly adults.[27]

Changes in Other Body Systems

Immune System Changes

After the age of 50, the functions carried out by the immune system begin to deteriorate, termed **immunosenescence**. Age-related declines in immune function may cause a reduction in the body's ability to combat viruses, bacteria, and other infections, contributing to increased morbidity and mortality from infectious disease and cancer in older adults. Age-related changes in immunity include a reduction in the number or functioning of immune cells and their receptors, which decreases the capacity of the immune system to respond normally. The clinical consequence of these changes is increased susceptibility to pneumonia, upper respiratory tract infections such as influenza, urinary tract infections, pressure sores, and foodborne illnesses.

Chronic poor nutrition contributes to declines in the immune system seen in older adults. Currently, much research is focused on the role of overall nutrition status, antioxidants, probiotics, omega fatty acids, caloric restriction, and the role of physical activity in countering immunologic aging.[28]

Nervous System Changes

The number of nerve cells and the total weight of the brain and the spinal cord are reduced, and message processing time increases with advancing age. This latter change can have a profound impact on food sensation, can contribute to reduced food intake, and can affect GI function in the digestion of food and absorption of nutrients. Nutrients affect cerebral functioning, including cognitive and intellectual abilities. For example, folic acid has been found to preserve memory in aging, and vitamins B_6 and B_{12}, among others, are directly involved in the synthesis of certain neurotransmitters. Vitamin B_{12} delays the onset of signs of dementia.[29] Vitamin D has recently gained the interest of investigators for its potential role in the prevention of depression in older adults as well as various other neurodegenerative and neuroimmune diseases.[30] Additionally, the physical and functional consequences of neurologic declines can negatively affect the ability of older adults to secure and consume a nutritious diet.

Endocrine System Changes

Hormones play a significant role in the regulation of nutrient intake and utilization; conversely, nutritional status markedly affects circulating hormone levels. The aging process is characterized by widespread changes in hormone production and activity. Alterations in circulating

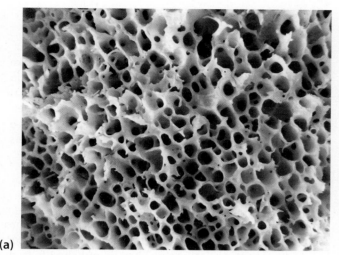

(a)

© Dr. Alan Boyde/Getty Images   © Dr. Alan Boyde/Getty Images

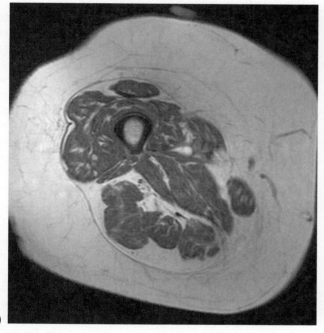

(b)

Courtesy of Professor Maria A. Flatarone Singh.   Courtesy of Professor Maria A. Flatarone Singh.

Figure 14.3
(a) Healthy bone and osteoporotic bone (b) MRI Scan of a sedentary woman and an active woman.

hormone levels and function can be a result of the normal aging process or secondary to disease. Age-related changes in hormone levels affect many of the body's metabolic functions, can cause alterations in energy and nutrient metabolism, and play a role in the development of frailty and sarcopenia.[31]

Hematologic Changes: Anemia
Almost 10% of today's older adult population suffer from some type of anemia;[32] this rate approaches 20% in individuals older than age 85.[33] Anemia is associated with substantial morbidity, including functional impairment and physical decline, increased rates of hospitalization, reduced mobility, and decreased quality of life; therefore, understanding the pathophysiology of anemia in older adults is important when working with this population.[34]

Evaluation of nutritional status in the older adult plays an important role in the diagnostic approach to anemia. Identifying issues such as inadequate dietary folate, vitamin B_{12}, or iron; alcohol use or abuse; and reduction of cobalamin absorption secondary to atrophic gastritis, *Helicobacter pylori* infection, chronic bleeding from the GI tract, and use of gastric-acid-suppressing agents can help to determine whether a nutritional approach will affect the underlying anemia.

Case Study

Just following her 95th birthday, Sherry started having some tingling in her hands and feet, forgetfulness, and trouble with her balance. Her only medication change recently was the addition of an antacid for mild reflux. These changes are making her anxious; she likes to think of herself as very "with it," and she is worried that she is "getting old." She has not been going out as much for fear of falling and misses her previously busy social schedule of eating out with friends, playing cards, going to her exercise class, and taking a weekly girls' trip to the casino.

Questions

1. List the physiologic changes that could account for some of Sherry's symptoms.
2. What questions would you ask Sherry to help identify the cause of these changes?
3. What suggestions would you make for her at this time?

Recap Older individuals have an increased susceptibility to gastrointestinal complications of comorbid illnesses. Alterations in gut function with aging have particular implications in the esophagus, stomach, and colon. The most prevalent clinical manifestations are dysphagia, gastroesophageal reflux disease, constipation, and fecal incontinence. The presence of obesity in older adults that results from dietary excesses, poor food choices, and physical inactivity magnifies a significant number of health problems. Changes in body composition in older adults favor loss of lean mass and increases in body fat, contributing to poor health, functional impairment, and disease comorbidities. As in younger adults, obesity in older adults is a complex problem that contributes to increased morbidity and reduced quality of life. Years of interaction among genetics, normal aging processes, and environmental factors such as diet, physical activity, and stress determine the development of CVD in older adults. Age-related changes and diseases affect the functioning of the kidneys, skeletal system, immune system, nervous system, and endocrine system. Careful diagnosis of any underlying diseases and conditions and appropriate medical nutrition therapy are crucial to the successful nutritional management of older adults. Dietary interventions for older adults should be prioritized to maximize treatment and mitigate additional insult to aging body systems while preserving quality of life and overall well-being.

1. Describe the main changes in each body system that occur with age.
2. Discuss the nutritional implications of physiologic aging.
3. Explain the challenges in meeting the nutritional needs of older adults with changes in body composition and health status.

Dietary Intake of Older Adults

Preview A poor-quality diet can result in inadequate intake of energy and essential nutrients, resulting in malnutrition and worsening of health status. Medical, physical, and social barriers to eating a healthy diet affect older adults. Consideration of the unique factors influencing food intake should be individualized for each older adult to help overcome barriers to a healthy diet.

Eating a nutritious diet is essential to sustain life and promote wellness. Nutritional health and the aging process have a synergistic relationship throughout the life cycle. The desire to eat well-liked foods and the amount of food eaten are strong influences on chronic disease risk and management. Each adult arrives at old age with dramatically different nutritional as well as health and social requirements built on lifelong eating behaviors and patterns for food choices and preferences. Older adults are a heterogeneous group, and challenges in meeting their nutritional requirements are as different as the older adults themselves. It can be difficult for older adults to meet their nutritional needs because of their increased requirements for some nutrients, lower energy needs, numerous barriers to adequate food intake, and health and lifestyle barriers.

Factors That Affect Diet

Unlike genetics, sex, and age, diet can be changed positively or negatively to influence health and risk of disease. Nutrition can influence how a person will age; in turn, the process of aging affects nutrition. Food contributes to a sense of security, meaning, and structure to the day, often providing the older adult with something to look forward to, not only for physical nourishment but also as an opportunity for socialization and psychological well-being (**FIGURE 14.4**).

A variety of medical and social factors have all been shown to influence the eating habits and nutritional status of both institutionalized and noninstitutionalized older adults. (See **TABLE 14.4** .) A lifetime of food choices and dietary intake is influenced by physiological, behavioral, social, environmental, and psychological factors, which in older adults are compounded by functional and health factors that also influence food intake (**FIGURE 14.5**). These and other age-related complications that interfere with food intake underscore the need for a multidisciplinary approach to increase dietary quality and variety and maximize nutritional well-being. The goals for nutrition intervention in the older population should ultimately be to maintain health and quality of life across the continuum of the aging process.

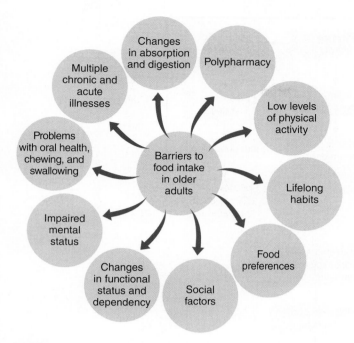

Figure 14.4
Barriers to food intake in older adults.

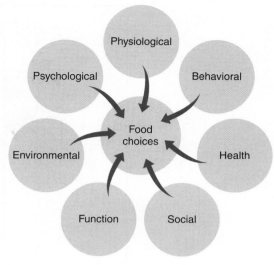

Figure 14.5
Factors that impact food choices of older adults.

Health and Medical Factors that Influence Diet

Chronic diseases are common among older adults. The majority of older adults have one or more chronic health conditions that could be improved with proper nutrition, and many of these illnesses limit activity and diminish quality of life (FIGURE 14.6). Malnourished older adults are more prone to infections and diseases, their injuries take longer to heal, surgery is riskier, and their hospital stays are longer and more expensive.

Table 14.4

Selected Factors that Affect Food Intake and Nutritional Status of Older Adults

Medical and physical	• Chronic and acute illnesses • Polypharmacy • Changes in absorption and digestion • Impaired mental status, memory loss, and depression • Problems with oral health, such as difficulty chewing, and swallowing • Functional decline, disability, and physical limitations • Inability to self-feed due to functional and medical limitations • Anorexia of aging
Social, cultural, and economic	• Living arrangement, transportation, proximity to a grocery store • Socioeconomic status and finances • Support of friends, family, and caregivers • Lifelong dietary habits and food preferences, spiritual and religious beliefs

A number of acute and chronic health conditions affect food intake and the nutritional status of older adults. Arthritis, cardiovascular disease, diabetes, cancer, obesity, osteoporosis, gastroesophageal reflux disorder, food intolerances, alcoholism, poor oral health, pressure injuries, anorexia of aging and malnutrition, constipation, and dehydration are just some of the more common conditions in older adults that can result from chronic dietary inadequacies and also require dietary modifications as part of their treatment. Mentioned earlier, age-related changes in gastrointestinal function, specifically, nutrient digestion and absorption, can influence nutrient status and requirements.

Restrictive medical diets can become unpalatable and unenjoyable for an older adult, thus worsening food intake and nutritional status.[35] Additionally, medication use and **polypharmacy** can cause side effects that affect food intake. Changes in taste and smell or medications that affect appetite can lower food intake; other medications can influence the absorption or metabolism of nutrients, leading to alterations in nutrient needs.

For many older adults, illness and depression are common factors that can reduce the willingness to cook and eat meals. Changes in mental status are common in older adults and can have a profound effect on food intake. Conditions such as Alzheimer disease, depression, dementia, and changes in mental status and cognition can have a profound effect on an older adult's ability to eat a healthy diet. Often overlooked are changes in vision, oral health, and dentition, as well as declines in taste and smell that can affect an older person's ability to prepare enjoyable and tasty meals.

Physical and Functional Factors that Affect Diet

Maintaining health, independence, and functional status is related to an individual's ability to shop, cook,

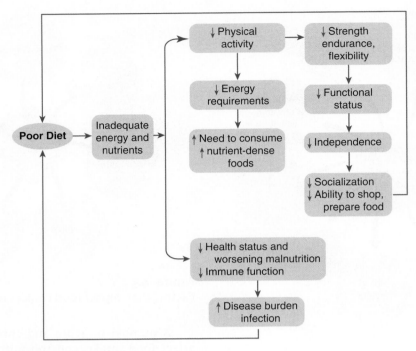

Figure 14.6
Effects of a poor-quality diet in older adults.

and eat independently, which is directly related to food intake and nutritional status. Physical limitations, such as muscle weakness, diminished endurance, loss of strength and flexibility, and poor balance, resulting from physical inactivity and chronic conditions, can make the simple tasks of shopping and cooking meals overwhelming.

Disability is defined as limited ability to conduct activities of daily living (ADLs) or instrumental activities of daily living (IADLs). Challenges with physical performance and independence become increasingly common as a result of changes in body composition and health conditions with advancing age. These functional declines

and limitations make obtaining healthy and nutritious foods more challenging, leading to progressive worsening of nutritional status, which further impairs health and well-being.

Environmental, Social, and Cultural Factors that Affect Diet

Living alone and limited socialization can influence the older adult's appetite, resulting in decreased food intake and poor dietary choices. Living arrangements; presence of a spouse, family member, or caregiver; availability of transportation to a local grocery as well as finances have an impact on the ability to buy food. These factors alone or in combination with medical and physical factors may contribute to dietary inadequacies and lead to the consumption of a low-quality diet, thus affecting the health and well-being of older adults. Having a family member or caregiver present, for example, can influence diet quality because the person can assist with food shopping and preparation, encourage healthy foods and medical dietary compliance, and provide socialization during mealtime.

Older individuals are more likely than younger individuals to maintain traditional food choices because their food preferences are well established. For many individuals, food is selected, prepared, served, and eaten based on culture. Limited information is available about culture and food choices among older adults. In the United States, individuals from different ethnic groups start replacing traditional foods from the first to the second generation.

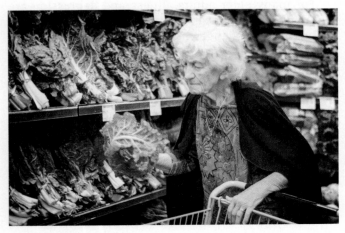

For some groups, acculturation improves nutrient intake and dietary diversity, whereas for others nutrient intake is negatively affected by acculturation.[36]

Older adults have a strong attachment to their food-related behaviors that is multidimensional. Their connection to food includes cultural beliefs about appropriate food use in the presence of health and disease, beliefs about healing properties of foods, and attitudes as gatekeepers of cultural traditions. Foodways may include categorizations of core and secondary foods that orient food choices, such as religious beliefs and practices; healthy and unhealthy foods; and foods of opposing categories, such as the hot/cold system observed by some Hispanic groups or the yin–yang Chinese principles. Some factors that may contribute to changes in food choices include, among others, access and availability of cultural foods. Rarely does nutrition motivate changes in cultural food patterns. It is of utmost importance that healthcare providers address the uniqueness of each older adult. This includes their cultural and ethnic behaviors regarding food preferences and disease prevalence to promote overall healthy aging.

For many older adults, limited finances, lack of transportation, and social isolation are common factors that can reduce their ability and willingness to cook and eat nutritious meals. For community-dwelling adults, living in food deserts, dependency on transportation, and limited finances affect their ability to purchase fresh, wholesome foods and can be significant contributors to food insecurity for this age group. Participation in organized nutrition programs can improve food and nutrient intake, increase fruit and vegetable consumption, and stimulate the desire to consume healthy foods.

Case Study

Sherry has always been very independent. Even when her husband of 69 years died after a long illness, she managed on her own and relied very little on friends or family for help with her daily activities or self-care, something, in fact, on which she prided herself. Lately, however, she is finding that even the smallest activity really wears her out. Yesterday, for example, she wanted to cook dinner for her friend, who just lost her husband, but just the thought of going to the store, shopping, and then coming home to prepare the meal was exhausting to her, so she ordered delivery from the local Italian restaurant.

Questions

1. List some of the barriers to eating a healthy diet that could be affecting Sherry.
2. What suggestions would you give her to overcome these barriers?

Recap Numerous factors affect adequate food intake and complicate the task of maximizing nutrition in older adults. Multiple chronic and acute illnesses, changes in absorption and digestion, polypharmacy, low levels of physical activity, lifelong habits and food preferences, social factors, changes in functional status and dependency, impaired mental status, and problems with oral health, chewing, and swallowing have all been shown to influence the eating habits and nutritional status of older adults. Social, economic, and cultural practices have a significant impact on food choice and preparation and provide an opportunity to individualize food programs to promote healthy diets.

1. Discuss factors that influence the eating patterns of older adults.
2. Describe the challenges faced by older adults who live in an area with limited access to fresh, healthy food choices.

Nutritional Recommendations and Requirements for Older Adults

Preview Macronutrient needs for older adults are similar to those for younger adults as a percentage of total calories; however, total calorie requirements tend to decline with advancing age, requiring the selection of more nutritious foods to meet individual nutrient needs. Certain vitamins and minerals as well as aspects of their metabolism in relation to the aging process and chronic diseases require special consideration for older adults.

Older adults are particularly vulnerable to compromised nutritional status. With advancing age, the consumption of a high-quality, nutritionally dense diet is increasingly essential to optimal health and well-being. Poor nutritional status and nutrient inadequacies can interfere with health and the ability to remain independent and lead to other complications such as increased burden of poor health, polypharmacy, and reduced socialization and physical activity. The nutritional status and needs of older people are multifactorial and related to age-associated biological changes as well as to socioeconomic changes. Decreased food intake, sedentary lifestyle, and reduced energy expenditure commonly seen in older adults make meeting nutritional requirements a challenge and place older adults at risk for malnutrition and worsening health status. Persistent chronic health conditions impose difficulty on older adults and may result in altered requirements for some nutrients because of changes in digestion, absorption, and metabolism or because of therapeutic alterations to dietary intake to manage disease.

Dietary Guidance for Older Adults

Maintaining a nutrient-dense diet in old age is essential to well-being and preventing nutrition-related complications that could contribute to declining health, increased functional dependency, and frailty. Healthy older adults may benefit from the same dietary recommendations as those provided for the general adult population; however, the appropriateness of and ability to adhere to these recommendations may be more challenging as an individual becomes increasingly functionally dependent, frail, and ill.

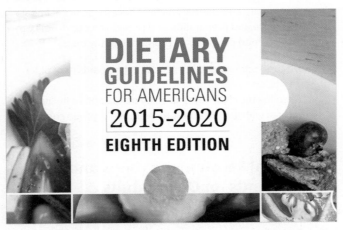

U.S. Department of Health and Human Services and U.S. Department of Agriculture. *2015–2020 Dietary Guidelines for Americans*. 8th ed. Washington, DC: U.S. Department of Health and Human Services and U.S. Department of Agriculture; December 2015. Retrieved from: http://health.gov/dietaryguidelines/2015/guidelines/. Accessed August 13, 2016.

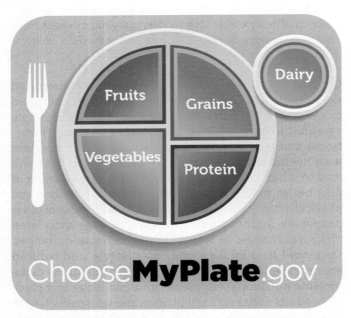

U.S. Department of Agriculture. MyPlate. ChooseMyPlate.gov. Retrieved from: http://www.choosemyplate.gov/MyPlate. Accessed September 28, 2016.

2015 Dietary Guidelines for Americans and MyPlate

The *Dietary Guidelines for Americans* encourage Americans at every age to balance caloric intake with physical activity and make small shifts in food choices to include more vegetables, fruits, whole grains, fat-free

and low-fat dairy products, and seafood. The *Dietary Guidelines for Americans* and MyPlate offer dietary guidance for whole foods and food groups rather than individual nutrients.

Selecting foods that are less processed and lower in sodium, trans fats, added sugars, and refined grains is increasingly important with advancing age. It is challenging for older adults to consume a nutrient-dense diet that meets nutritional requirements without too many calories. This task that can be really difficult because age-related problems present unique challenges to achieving a healthy diet as defined by the 2015 *Dietary Guidelines for Americans*.

To optimize the nutrient intake of those older than 70 years, some modifications of MyPlate are appropriate, as shown in **FIGURE 14.7**. While maintaining MyPlate's emphasis on vegetables and fruits, whole grains, and low-fat dairy choices, MyPlate for Older Adults highlights the unique dietary needs of adults older than 70 by emphasizing nutrient-dense food choices and the importance of drinking plenty of fluids, choosing healthy oils and a variety of protein-rich foods, and seasoning with herbs and spices to enhance the flavor of food. MyPlate for Older Adults also provides guidance about foods that could best meet the unique needs of older adults and stresses the importance of staying physically active.

Current food guidelines continue to emphasize the recommendation that the majority if not all of the nutrients an older adult consumes should come from food rather than supplements.[12] The topic area of "older adults" is new for *Healthy People 2020* and was developed in response to the rapidly aging population. The aim of the older adult initiative is to "improve the health, function, and quality of life of older adults."[37]

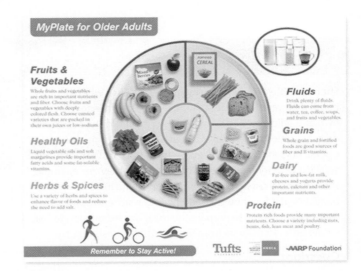

Figure 14.7
Updated MyPlate for Older Adults.

"My Plate for Older Adults" Copyright 2016 Tufts University, all rights reserved. "My Plate for Older Adults" graphic and accompanying website were developed with support from the AARP Foundation. "Tufts University" and "AARP Foundation" are registered trademarks and may not be reproduced apart from their inclusion in the "My Plate for Older Adults" graphic without express permission from their respective owners.

The Dietary Reference Intakes

The Dietary Reference Intakes (DRIs) are quantitative estimates of nutrient intakes for healthy individuals; therefore, additional interpretation may be necessary when applying them to older adults who have multiple medical conditions. The aging process has an impact on nutrient requirements, and although an understanding of the nutritional needs of older adults is increasing, the specific needs of this group is an area of ongoing investigation. Changes in body composition, for example, along with chronic and degenerative health conditions and limited ability for physical activity may affect caloric and nutrient requirements. Dietary recommendations for calories and some essential nutrients and food components, such as dietary fiber, have been identified in the DRIs, including the Acceptable Macronutrient Distribution Ranges (AMDRs) for carbohydrate, protein, and fat (TABLE 14.5). The precise nutrient needs of an older adult at any age are, however, multifactorial owing to the diversity of this population group. Changes in nutrient requirements and nutrients of particular concern for older adults are reviewed in TABLE 14.6 .

Energy

With advancing age, energy requirements frequently decline. This causes a unique problem for many older individuals; in general, they require less energy to maintain their weight, but nutrient needs stay the same and in some cases increase.[38,39] Lower energy requirements with age are the result of decreased energy expenditure, losses in lean body mass, and decreased physical activity.[12] Meeting nutrient recommendations while staying within energy needs is fundamental to dietary guidance for older adults, and those who do not reduce their caloric intake to balance a decrease in energy expenditure may become overweight. This underscores the importance of older adults making nutritious foods choices. A variety of nutrient-dense foods selected from all of the food groups is associated with better nutritional status and should be an important goal for older individuals.

Carbohydrates

For health promotion and disease prevention, the *Dietary Guidelines for Americans* currently emphasize that carbohydrate requirements be met with nutritious whole grains, fruits, and vegetables and recommend limiting daily intake of sugar. This guidance is particularly relevant for older adults who need to monitor their caloric intake and in particular limit sugar intake. Simple sugars are low in nutrient content and can contribute to excess calories and inadequate intake of essential nutrients; therefore, lowering intake of sugars and sweets helps to ensure sufficient intake of nutrients without ingesting excess empty calories. For individuals, especially older adults who need to maximize their nutrient intake while keeping energy intake at a level for weight maintenance, whole grains and fiber-rich carbohydrates are better, more nutritious choices.

Dietary Fiber

Dietary fiber plays a beneficial role in numerous medical conditions that affect many older people. Consumption of high-fiber-containing foods is recommended by the American Diabetes Association for the management of diabetes mellitus, as well as by the American Heart Association to reduce the risk of cardiovascular disease, and the National Cancer Institute to reduce the risk of various types of cancer. Both insoluble and soluble, including nonviscous and viscous, fibers are important for the health of older adults. Nonviscous fiber slows glucose absorption and reduces postprandial blood glucose concentrations and therefore has been shown to be beneficial for the management of diabetes mellitus. Foods that contain high amounts of insoluble fiber increase fecal bulk and decrease transit time in the colon, helping to lower the incidence of constipation and formation of diverticula, conditions common in older adults. Fiber also delays gastric emptying of ingested foods into the small intestine, which can result in the sensation of fullness, and is therefore helpful for weight management in older adults; however, fiber can be detrimental for frail elders who need to consume extra calories.

The *Dietary Guidelines for Americans* and MyPlate recommend choosing fiber-rich foods for a health-promoting diet. Recommendations for older adults range from 25 to

Table 14.5

Dietary Reference Intakes (DRIs) for Older Adults

Nutrient	Value	Recommendation
Carbohydrates	AMDR	45–65% total daily calories
	DRI	130 g/day
	EAR	100 g/day
Fiber	AI: Men	30 g/day
	AI: Women	21 g/day
Fat	AMDR	20–35% total daily calories
n-6 PUFA (linoleic acid)	AMDR	5–10% total daily calories
	AI: Men	14 g/day
	AI: Women	11 g/day
n-3 PUFA (alpha-linolenic acid)	AMDR	0.6–1.2% total daily calories
	AI: Men	1.6 g/day
	AI: Women	1.1 g/day
Protein	AMDR	10–35% total daily calories
	RDA	0.8 g/kg/day
	EAR	0.66 g/kg/day
	RDA: Men	56 g/day
	RDA: Women	46 g/day
Water	AI: Men	3.7 L/day
	AI: Women	2.7 L/day

AI = Adequate Intake; AMDR = Acceptable Macronutrient Distribution Range; EAR = Estimated Average Requirement; PUFA = polyunsaturated fatty acid; RDA = Recommended Dietary Allowance.

Modified from Institute of Medicine, Food and Nutrition Board. *Dietary Reference Intakes for Energy, Carbohydrate, Fiber, Fat, Fatty Acids, Cholesterol, Protein and Amino Acids (Macronutrients)*. Washington, DC: National Academies Press; 2005.

Table 14.6	

Nutrients of Concern in Older Adults

Nutrient	Considerations for the Older Adult
Water	Sufficient fluids must be provided in efforts to prevent dehydration.
	Adequate fluids sustain homeostasis in the body and aid in moving nutrients to cells, metabolizing medications, and eliminating waste products.
Fiber	Fiber is important for gastrointestinal health, improves lipoprotein levels, reduces risk factors for coronary heart disease, and aids in weight management and the maintenance of normal blood glucose levels.
	Consuming too much fiber can cause gastrointestinal distress, and too little fiber can lead to constipation.
Calcium	Calcium is essential in promoting healthy bones and teeth.
	Calcium also has an important role in blood clotting, muscle contraction, and nerve transmission.
Vitamin D	Vitamin D is essential in promoting bone health.
	Vitamin D has a well-established function in bone metabolism, calcium homeostasis, and the prevention of osteoporosis.
	Higher levels of vitamin D have been found to be associated with a reduction in cancer risk.
	Vitamin D has also been found to exert a protective effect against cardiovascular disease, arthritis, multiple sclerosis, and diabetes mellitus.
Zinc	Zinc is a functional component of many enzymes and proteins and is involved in the regulation of gene expression.
	Zinc deficiency can contribute to conditions common in the older adult such as loss of appetite, hair loss, delayed wound healing, skin abnormalities, impaired taste, and depression.
Folate	Adequate folate functions with vitamins B_6 and B_{12} in the metabolism of methionine and homocysteine.
	Deficiency can cause megaloblastic anemia and hyperhomocysteinemia.
	High consumption of folic acid can mask a serious vitamin B_{12} deficiency.
Vitamin B_{12}	Vitamin B_{12} is a coenzyme in nucleic acid metabolism.
	A deficiency causes megaloblastic anemia.
	Older adults may have suboptimal levels of vitamin B_{12} due to inadequate diet or poor absorption resulting from a lack of intrinsic factor or atrophic gastritis.
	Vitamin B_{12} deficiency can lead to changes in mental status, peripheral neuropathy, balance disturbances, and high homocysteine.
Iron	Iron is a structural component of hemoglobin.
	Iron deficiency leads to microcytic hypochromic anemia.
	Iron deficiency in older adults is frequently caused by a GI bleed, poor nutrition intake, and medication side effects.
Carotenoids	Carotenoids with vitamin A activity such as lutein and zeaxanthin are found in the macula of the eye and may help to prevent the onset and progression of age-related macular degeneration (AMD).
	Carotenoids with antioxidant activity can help reduce the risk of cataracts.

Data from Institute of Medicine, Food and Nutrition Board. *Dietary Reference Intakes: The Essential Guide to Nutrient Requirements.* Washington, DC: National Academies Press; 2006. Retrieved from: https://fnic.nal.usda.gov/sites/fnic.nal.usda.gov/files/uploads/DRIEssentialGuideNutReq.pdf. Accessed September 27, 2016; Institute of Medicine, Food and Nutrition Board. *Dietary Reference Intake: Calcium and Vitamin D.* Washington, DC: National Academies Press; 2011. Retrieved from: https://fnic.nal.usda.gov/sites/fnic.nal.usda.gov/files/uploads/FullReport.pdf. Accessed September 27, 2016.

35 g/d, with the Adequate Intake (AI) for total fiber set at 30 g/d and 21 g/d for men and women older than the age of 51, respectively (based on 14 g fiber per 1,000 kcal). Data from national studies for mean nutrient intake by older adults show that average fiber consumption is consistently lower than recommended levels for women and men of all ages, including those older than 50 years.[40,41] Choosing a variety of fiber-rich foods from a variety of fruits, vegetables, legumes, whole grains, and breakfast cereals is the best way to increase fiber consumption. Selecting fewer processed foods and more natural and whole-grain products is sound advice for those trying to improve their nutritional intake. Care needs to be taken, however, when planning the diet of *frail* older adults with regard to foods high in dietary fiber. Fiber-rich foods may increase the feeling of satiety and cause overall food intake to decrease, thereby limiting intake of necessary nutrients from food sources and contributing to difficulties in maintaining an appropriate body weight. When choosing a diet high in fiber, it is particularly important that older adults meet fluid and water recommendations to prevent constipation and fecal impaction.

Fats

For healthy older adults, keeping fat and carbohydrate intake within the recommended ranges helps to lower the risk for heart disease, obesity, and diabetes. Older adults should choose dietary fats in similar distributions to those recommended for younger adults, including limiting trans fats and deriving a minimum of 10% of total energy from fats to ensure adequate energy and essential fatty acid intake. Fat provides a valuable source of concentrated energy for frail older individuals who may be struggling to consume enough calories to maintain an appropriate body weight, and limiting fat too much can lead to weight loss and nutrient deficiencies.

Essential Fatty Acids

Foods high in dietary fat provide a necessary source of the essential fatty acids linoleic acid (n-6), an omega-6 fatty acid, and linolenic acid (n-3), an omega-3 fatty acid. Deficiency of linoleic and linolenic acids leads to reduced production of the eicosanoids arachidonic acid, eicosapentaenoic acid (EPA), and docosahexaenoic acid (DHA). Higher circulating omega-3 levels are associated with lower total mortality, particularly from heart disease, in older adults.[42,43] Evidence indicates that both omega-3 and omega-6 fatty acids may have beneficial effects on inflammation markers.[44,45]

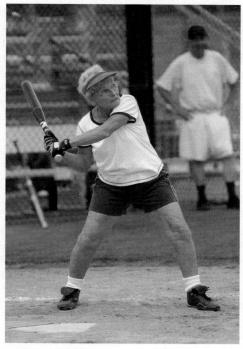

©Glenda M. Powers/Shutterstock

Protein

Age-related changes in body composition and decreases in the amount of skeletal muscle, along with other physiologic changes, contribute to loss of total body protein and sarcopenia.[15] Increased frailty, skin fragility, impaired wound healing, and impaired immune function are all consequences of reduced body proteins.[46] Limited information is available to establish clear evidence-based dietary protein recommendations for older adults; therefore, the requirements for dietary protein for older adults continue to be a topic of vigorous debate.[47] The current Recommended Dietary Allowance (RDA) for men and women is set at 56 g/d for males and 46 g/d for females, or 0.80 g/kg body weight/day of protein based on nitrogen balance studies.[40] Some experts propose that the RDA for protein may not be adequate to meet the metabolic and physiologic needs even as a minimum level for older adults. Moderate increases in protein intake above 0.80 g/protein/d may contribute to enhanced muscle protein metabolism as well as provide a mechanism for reducing progressive muscle loss that commonly accompanies

aging.[46] Higher levels of dietary protein may be needed to meet additional demands of physiologic stress.

Getting enough high-quality dietary protein may be challenging for older adults, many of whom have reduced appetite, functional and social limitations, and economic hardship. Inadequate protein consumption likely contributes to an acceleration of sarcopenia and other morbidities. Additionally, protein undernutrition worsens diseases and conditions common in older adults and can contribute to increased susceptibility to disease and poor clinical outcomes. Dietary protein with a high biological value, such as proteins from animal sources, provides high-quality protein and essential amino acids along with iron, vitamin B_{12}, and other vital nutrients, and it should be regularly included in the diet of older adults.

To ensure older adults are eating enough protein, some experts suggest an even distribution of protein-rich foods throughout the day. To meet this recommendation, older adults should aim to consume 25–30 g of high-quality protein with each meal. Encouraging increased dietary protein intake with protein-rich foods has numerous advantages over supplementation with protein and amino acid products, including cost, accessibility, socialization, and dietary variety.

Water

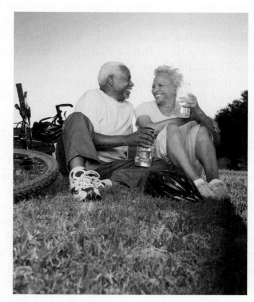

©Jupiterimages/Thinkstock

Water is an essential nutrient that requires special consideration for older adults. Water constitutes approximately 55% of an older adult's body weight, 10% to 15% less than in younger adults.[48] This lower percentage of body water is a result of the losses in lean body mass, which is higher in water than fat. A number of other changes affect the ability of older adults to maintain water balance. A decrease in the sensation of thirst and alterations in the ability of the kidneys to concentrate urine as well as illness and limitations in activities of daily living that may limit fluid intake contribute to a decrease in total body water with advancing age.[49] Endocrine changes, hemodynamic factors, environmental factors, medication use, and voluntary restriction can also reduce intake and affect fluid balance and make older adults more vulnerable to fluid imbalance. Water imbalance is more likely during times of metabolic stress, such as illness or hospitalization, as well as in extreme weather conditions.

Changes in mental status, cognitive abilities, and depression can lead to dehydration as a result of forgetfulness or deliberate fluid restriction. Older adults with limited strength and functional independence and those who are at risk for falling may also voluntarily restrict fluid intake in an attempt to reduce bathroom trips and manage incontinence. Many medications, both prescription and over the counter, also influence fluid balance, requirements, and hydration status or have side effects that interfere with fluid intake, such as nausea, confusion, or alterations in gastrointestinal status. Many medications require adequate fluid for proper metabolism, so poor fluid status and dehydration can actually alter medication function and effectiveness.

Dehydration is the most common fluid and electrolyte disturbance in older adults and can be life threatening.[50] The AI for total water is set at 2.7 and 3.7 liters daily for women and men ages 51 and older, respectively;[51] this amount is intended to prevent dehydration. Fluid intake should compensate for normal physiologic losses. Additional fluid is needed to compensate for losses associated with illness. Daily fluid intake can come from food and beverages. The Tufts University MyPlate for Older Adults (as shown in Figure 14.7) emphasizes the importance of adequate fluid intake for older adults and of including a variety of sources.[52]

Micronutrients: Vitamins and Minerals

Age-related changes in nutrient absorption, use, or activation contribute to higher dietary requirements for many vitamins and minerals. Vitamin D and vitamin B_{12} status, for example, are affected by physiological changes that occur with age. In some instances, vitamin requirements stay unchanged, underscoring the need for older adults to consume nutrient-dense foods. Recommended intakes of vitamins and minerals for older adults attempt to take into consideration the variability among older adults by offering recommendations for those ages 51 to 70 years and for those ages 70 and older.[53] Adequate intake of these essential nutrients becomes increasingly important with advancing age, but attainment of these goals becomes an increasing challenge.

The B Vitamins

The vitamins B_{12}, B_6, and folate are of special interest in the older population. As a group, vitamin B_{12}, vitamin B_6, and folate function as coenzymes involved in one-carbon metabolism.

Normal changes in the stomach and small intestine that occur with aging and common disorders of older adults can have significant negative influences on the absorption of vitamin B_{12}. The prevalence of vitamin B_{12} deficiency increases with age. An estimated 6% of adults aged 60 or older are vitamin B_{12} deficient, and approximately 20% have borderline low levels.[54] A compromised vitamin B_{12} status is, therefore, a significant concern in older adults.

Despite sufficient intake of vitamin B_{12}, 10% to 30% of older adults do not absorb protein-bound vitamin B_{12} from foods owing to a decrease in gastric acid, lack of intrinsic factor, atrophic gastritis with accompanying small bowel bacterial overgrowth, and medication use that can negatively affect vitamin B_{12} digestion and absorption.[12] Confusion, forgetfulness, and other changes in mental status and disturbances in balance should not be dismissed as "old age" but should prompt further assessment. Vitamin B_{12} deficiency is characterized by sensory disturbances and neurologic abnormalities, including cognitive decline, peripheral neuropathy, decreased muscle strength, and functional disability.[55] Low vitamin B_{12} is also linked to an increased risk of a number of other age-related conditions, including cardiovascular disease, cognitive dysfunction, dementia, and osteoporosis.[56]

A daily consumption of 2.4 mg of vitamin B_{12} is suggested for all adults 51 years and older;[53] however, dietary intake of vitamin B_{12}–rich foods may be inadequate in older adults and should be assessed. Often vitamin supplements and fortified foods are recommended as sources of vitamin B_{12} in the older population because it is easier to absorb synthetic vitamin B_{12} than food-bound vitamin B_{12}.

One of the important combined roles of vitamins B_{12}, B_6, and folate is their function as coenzymes in the metabolism of homocysteine, a nonessential sulfur-containing amino acid. Approximately 14% of older persons have elevated homocysteine levels.[57] Elevated serum homocysteine (hyperhomocysteinemia) is an independent risk factor for cardiovascular diseases and mortality and plays an important role in atherosclerosis, neurodegenerative and cognitive impairment and dementia, diabetes mellitus, decreased skeletal health, gastrointestinal disorders, and immune responses.[58,59] High folic acid consumption in excess of recommended levels can mask a vitamin B_{12} deficiency. The vitamin B_{12} status of at-risk older adults in countries such as the United States, where there is mandatory fortification of food with folic acid, should be regularly monitored.

Calcium and Vitamin D

Calcium and vitamin D are well known for their primary role in bone health. Calcium has other essential roles in the blood and extracellular fluid and in vasodilation and vasocontraction, muscle contraction, blood clotting, and nerve transmission.[39] Vitamin D increases intestinal calcium uptake, and a greater need for calcium stimulates greater absorption. Vitamin D plays a significant role in bone health and prevention of osteoporosis and has a direct effect on skeletal muscle formation by promoting protein synthesis. Evidence suggests that older adults deficient in vitamin D are more likely to have limitations in mobility and physical performance and function, whereas adequate vitamin D has been found to reduce the risk of falling by more than 20%.[60,61] Low levels of vitamin D have recently been associated with developing symptoms of depression in older adults, possibly through a biologic role in the brain affecting memory, motor control, and social behaviors.[62] Vitamin D has also been found to exert a protective effect against cardiovascular disease, arthritis, multiple sclerosis, cancer, and diabetes mellitus.[25]

National surveys find that calcium and vitamin D intake is frequently lower than recommended levels in older men and women. For women aged 51 to 70 years, the RDA for calcium has been established at 1,200 mg/d. The RDA for men in this age group is 1,000 mg/d. In adults older than the age of 70, the RDA for calcium is 1,200 mg/d, regardless of sex.[39] Low-fat dairy products are good sources of calcium, vitamin D, and protein and are low in calories and fat, making them a good food choice for older adults. Reduced acid secretion in the stomach occurs often in older adults and may reduce calcium absorption.

Vitamin D insufficiency or deficiency is common in the older population because of reduced dietary intake and skin synthesis and decreased renal production. Older adults have a tendency to spend more time indoors, limiting exposure to sunlight, and those with lactose intolerance avoid dairy products, posing further challenge to vitamin D status. In addition to direct sunlight exposure, the Institute of Medicine has set vitamin D requirements at 600 IU for men and women ages 51 to 70 years and 800 IU for men and women older than 70 years to support bone health. Some reasearch suggests a need for a minimum of 1,000–2,000 IU/d for adults to achieve adequate serum vitamin D levels.[63] It can be challenging for older adults to consume the recommended amount of calcium and vitamin D from food alone. Vitamin D supplementation, providing between 1,000 and 2,000 IU daily, may be recommended for older adults with poor milk intake or limited sunlight exposure.[39] Ensuring adequacy of other nutrients involved in bone health such as protein, vitamins A and K, magnesium, and phytoestrogens is also advisable when working with older adults.

Sodium, Iron, Zinc
Sodium
Usual intake of sodium for women and men ages 51 to 70 is 2,600 mg and 3,800 mg/d, and for women and men older than 70 is 2,400 mg and 3,200 mg/d, respectively.[51] Mixed dishes that contain grains, meats, sauces, vegetables, and other processed items contribute the largest proportion to total sodium intake. Meat, poultry, fish, and eggs contribute 19%, about half of that coming from deli and cured meats.[64] Other high-sodium foods include processed foods and meats, packaged meals, canned soups, cheese, smoked or canned fish, and snack foods with visible salt such as chips and crackers; these are foods older adults commonly consume owing to their convenience and shelf life.[65] High sodium intake is associated with hypertension and low-bone-mineral-density conditions common in older adults. The Tolerable Upper Intake Level (UL) for sodium is 2.3 g/d (2,300 mg) for adults ages 51 and older.

FIGURE 14.8 is a pie chart that shows the percentage of sodium in the diet of the U.S. population ages 2 years and older that comes from different food categories: mixed dishes, 44%; protein foods, 14%; grains, 11%; vegetables, 11%; snacks and sweets, 8%; dairy, 5%; condiments, gravies, spreads, salad dressings, 5%; beverages (not milk or 100% fruit juice), 3%; fruits and fruit juice, 0%. The inset bar chart expands the mixed dishes category to show the percentage of sodium in the diet from different types of mixed dishes: burgers, sandwiches, 21%; rice, pasta, grain dishes, 7%; pizza, 6%; meat, poultry, seafood dishes, 6%; soups, 4%.

Older adults can have a reduced ability to excrete sodium and may be more sensitive to sodium intake with respect to their blood pressure.[51,66] *Salt sensitivity* refers to the response of blood pressure to changes in dietary salt intake. The percentage of those who are salt sensitive seems to increase with age. Advice to follow a healthy eating pattern that is low in sodium and to cut back on foods and beverages that are high in sodium is part of the 2015 *Dietary Guidelines for Americans*.[67] For adults who need to lower their blood pressure, the Dietary Guidelines suggest following the Dietary Approaches to Stop Hypertension (DASH) dietary plan, which is high in vegetables, fruits, low-fat dairy products, whole grains, poultry, fish, beans, and nuts and is low in sweets, sugar-sweetened beverages, and red meats. It is also low in saturated fats and rich in potassium, calcium, and magnesium, as well as dietary fiber and protein. DASH is lower in sodium than the typical American diet and has been found to reduce CVD risk factors.[67,68] Frequent monitoring of older adults prescribed a low-sodium diet is recommended because the sodium restriction has been shown to lower blood pressure but may also contribute to a less palatable diet, causing poor food intake and decreased calorie, protein, and calcium consumption.[69]

Iron
Reduced meat consumption associated with taste changes, medication use, economics, and poor dentition can contribute to poor iron intake. Important dietary sources of iron for older adults are those that are well absorbed, such as beef, fish, pork, tofu, legumes, and fortified breakfast cereals. Iron deficiency is not prevalent in older adults because iron losses due to menstruation in women ceases with menopause and average dietary iron

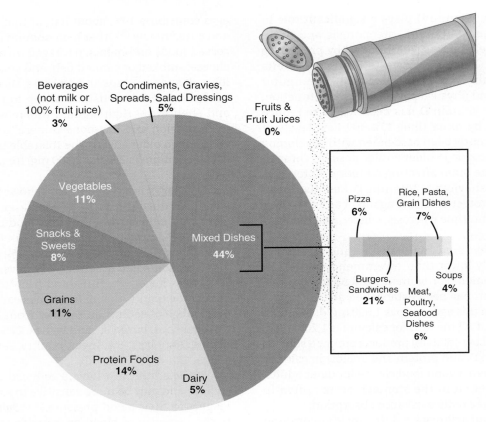

Figure 14.8
Food category sources of sodium in the U.S. population ages 2 years and older.

Reproduced from U.S. Department of Health and Human Services and U.S. Department of Agriculture. *2015–2020 Dietary Guidelines for Americans*. 8th ed. Washington, DC: U.S. Department of Health and Human Services and U.S. Department of Agriculture; December 2015:Fig. 2-14. Retrieved from: http://health.gov /dietaryguidelines/2015/guidelines/chapter-2/a-closer-look-at-current-intakes-and-recommended-shifts/#figure-2-14-food-category-sources-of-sodium-in -the-us-population. Accessed September 27, 2016.

intake for older adults is usually above the RDA of 8 mg/d for men and women ages 51 and older. Iron deficiency, however, can occur with poor intake over a long period of time, gastrointestinal bleeding, prolonged malabsorption, or because of medical conditions.[70] Most dietary iron is absorbed in the small intestine; therefore, gastrointestinal conditions that result in inflammation of the small intestine can reduce dietary iron absorption. A reduction in stomach acidity, **achlorhydria**, occurs in about one-third of elderly people and may decrease absorption of iron.[71] Low iron levels can lead to anemia and symptoms such as decreased energy, episodes of syncope, pale skin, irregular heartbeat, cold extremities, and headaches. For older adults with anemia, iron supplementation is considered appropriate.

Zinc

There is no consistent evidence that aging affects zinc absorption or that requirements are higher in older adults. Zinc supplementation in older adults could be of benefit to immune function if zinc deficiency exists.[70] Zinc supplementation for the prevention or treatment of age-related macular degeneration remains questionable, but it may slow the progression of age-related macular degeneration

to an advanced stage.[72] Although zinc deficiency is rare, the average zinc intake for older adults tends to be below the RDA. Stress, particularly in hospitalized older adults, may increase the risk for low zinc levels and impaired immune function. Multivitamin (MVI) supplementation is recommended for patients with pressure injuries with diagnosed or suspected deficiencies. Zinc supplementation has not been demonstrated to improve wound healing.[73] Excess zinc may actually inhibit healing, affect immune function, alter the absorption of other minerals, and may lower high-density lipoprotein (HDL) cholesterol and therefore should be used with medical supervision.

Antioxidants

Antioxidants, specifically, vitamins A, E, and C, have been identified as nutrients involved in reducing disease rates through several protective mechanisms. Both higher serum antioxidants and intake of fruits and vegetables are associated with lower mortality and better health outcomes. Adequate intake of antioxidants is important for older adults because of the health-promoting effects of these substances and the overwhelming benefits of a dietary pattern high in these nutrients, one that includes generous amounts of fruits and vegetables and healthy fats.

A diet pattern that contains generous amount of **antioxidants** is associated with lower prevalence of degenerative diseases and maintenance of physiological functions in older adults. These health-protective effects are attributed to the role of antioxidant nutrients and phytochemicals in reducing oxidative stress that contributes to aging and disease pathogenesis. High fruit and vegetable intakes have been associated with lower incidences of cardiovascular disease, age-related macular degeneration, and cancer. Antioxidants may have a protective effect against the impairment to the brain that may result in Alzheimer disease and other deteriorations in cognition that are common in aging.[74]

Vitamin E functions primarily as a chain-breaking antioxidant, maintaining cell integrity by preventing lipid peroxidation; it also plays a role in immune function and the blood clotting process. Vitamin C is a potential preventive agent against cognitive impairment; serves a vital role in collagen synthesis, wound healing, and immune function; and facilitates iron absorption.[75–77] Good sources of vitamin E include vegetable oil, nuts, seeds, whole grains, and dark green leafy vegetables. Vitamin C is found mainly in fruits and vegetables. Higher mortality, however, has been associated with high-dose nutrient supplements, suggesting that there is a threshold level for these nutrients and toxic effects can occur at higher supplement intakes.[78] Therefore, older adults should aim to boost dietary sources of antioxidants and supplement when necessary with medical supervision.

Carotenoids

Carotenoids have antioxidant properties and, like other antioxidants, carotenoids protect against oxidative reactions that produce free radicals that lead to tissue damage and increased risk of age-related diseases. Aging results in greater oxidative stress, which increases further with most chronic diseases. Carotenoids have been found to provide protection against various cancers, age-related macular degeneration (AMD), dementia, cardiovascular disease, and arthritis.[76] In these situations when demand for antioxidants is high, low blood levels may occur, which could affect disease progression and the aging process.[79] Determining the appropriate time to assess carotenoid function over the life span, recommended intakes, disease states, and duration of particular intakes is currently under investigation. Older adults considering supplementation with vitamin A or carotenoids to protect or improve their vision should consult with their physician. TABLE 14.7 lists some foods that are good sources of dietary carotenoids to help boost intake for older adults.

Nutrient Supplementation

More than half of older adults in a recent survey reported using complementary and alternative medicine (CAM), and more than a third, including almost 25% of those aged 85 years and older, take some type of herbal product or dietary supplement (FIGURE 14.9).[80]

Table 14.7

Suggested Foods Sources of Dietary Carotenoids for Older Adults

Dietary Carotenoid	Food Sources[a]
Alpha-carotene	Pumpkin, carrots, winter squash, tangerines
Beta-carotene	Carrots, spinach, kale, cantaloupe, apricots
Lutein and zeaxanthin	Turnips, collard and mustard greens, spinach, kale, broccoli, kiwi, honeydew melon
Lycopene	Tomatoes, pink grapefruit, watermelon
Beta-cryptoxanthin	Papaya, mango, peaches, oranges, bell peppers, corn, watermelon

[a] Fresh, frozen, or canned are all good options for older adults.

Data from Institute of Medicine, Food and Nutrition Board. Dietary Reference Intakes: *The Essential Guide to Nutrient Requirements.* Washington, DC: National Academies Press; 2006. Retrieved from: https://fnic.nal.usda.gov/sites/fnic.nal.usda.gov/files/uploads/DRIEssentialGuideNutReq.pdf. Accessed September 27, 2016; Institute of Medicine, Food and Nutrition Board. *Dietary Reference Intake: Calcium and Vitamin D.* Washington, DC: National Academies Press; 2011. Retrieved from: https://fnic.nal.usda.gov/sites/fnic.nal.usda.gov/files/uploads/FullReport.pdf. Accessed September 27, 2016.

News You Can Use

Adults use complementary and alternative medicine, including taking dietary supplements, for a few main reasons, such as to prevent illness and for overall wellness, to reduce pain and treat painful conditions, to treat a specific health condition, and to supplement conventional medical treatments. More than two-thirds of adults do not discuss their supplement use with a healthcare provider, often because they do not consider herbs or dietary supplements medications.[a] This is alarming because some dietary supplements can affect the absorption of other nutrients, interfere with the absorption and metabolism of prescription medications, contribute to polypharmacy, and, in large amounts, have toxic or other negative effects on health. St. John's wort, for example, an herb used in the treatment of mild to moderate depression, can interfere with the action of many prescription medications.[a]

References

a. National Center for Complementary and Integrative Health, National Institutes of Health, U.S. Department of Health and Human Services. Complementary and alternative medicine: what people aged 50 and older discuss with their health care providers. Bethesda, MD: National Center for Complementary and Integrative Health; updated December 15, 2015. Retrieved from: https://nccih.nih.gov/research/statistics/2010. Accessed May 18, 2016.

b. National Center for Complementary and Integrative Health, National Institutes of Health, U.S. Department of Health and Human Services. St. John's wort. Bethesda, MD: National Center for Complementary and Integrative Health; updated June 13, 2016. Retrieved from: https://nccih.nih.gov/health/stjohnswort/ataglance.htm. Accessed May 18, 2016.

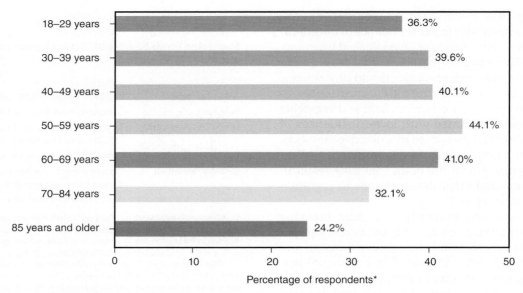

Figure 14.9

CAM use in the past 12 months among U.S. adults, by age category.

Reproduced from National Center for Complementary and Integrative Health, National Institutes of Health, U.S. Department of Health and Human Services. Complementary and alternative medicine: what people aged 50 and older discuss with their health care providers. Bethesda, MD: National Center for Complementary and Integrative Health; updated December 15, 2015. Retrieved from: https://nccih.nih.gov/research/statistics/2010. Accessed May 18, 2016.

A large number of older adults find it difficult to eat enough nutrient-dense foods to meet the recommended amounts of many nutrients from foods alone, necessitating the use of nutritional and dietary supplements to support health. Nutritional supplements may be useful for older adults who need additional calories or protein to maintain health and body weight. When dietary variety is limited, a multivitamin/mineral supplement can help older adults meet recommended nutrient intake levels. In particular, fiber, antioxidants, calcium, vitamin D, and vitamin B_{12} are nutrients that are often low in the diets of older adults and that should be considered for supplementation. Medical professionals working with older adults should ask about complementary medicine and dietary supplement use, including herbal supplements, carotenoids, and phytochemicals, during healthcare visits.

Case Study

At her annual appointment with her primary care physician, Sherry mentioned her lack of energy and increasing forgetfulness. Her primary care doctor told her that she should begin taking a multivitamin/multimineral supplement and should not worry about it because, "after all, you are 95 years old." He did some routine blood work and told her that he would call with the results in about a week.

Questions

1. What do you think about the physician's suggestion that Sherry's symptoms are due to her advancing age?
2. What questions about her diet would you ask Sherry?

Recap Age-related changes in health influence digestion, absorption, and metabolism of foods and nutrients, translating to changes in nutritional requirements. The decreased food intake, sedentary lifestyle, and reduced energy expenditure commonly seen in this population place older adults at risk for malnutrition, especially protein and micronutrient deficiencies. Persistent, chronic conditions create additional challenges for older adults for carrying out their activities of daily living, including food-related tasks. For older adults, meeting caloric and macronutrient recommendations requires consideration of numerous factors that are influenced by changes in health and physical well-being and social environment. Older adults should be encouraged to consume a variety of nutrient-dense foods. Maintaining adequate dietary intake is essential in preserving health and independence, along with controlling healthcare costs. Supplementation should be considered when dietary intake is inadequate.

1. Review the key features of the dietary recommendations for older adults.
2. Choose three nutrients and describe how the requirements for each change with advancing age.
3. Explain the importance of choosing nutrient-dense foods for older adults and give some examples.

Promoting Healthy Lifestyles

Preview Food not only is critical to one's physiological well-being but also contributes to quality of life. Older adults may require specialized nutrition services aimed at maintaining independence and health. Participation in federal, state, and local food and nutrition programs can improve dietary quality and health indicators for older adults. Food restrictions should be liberalized for older adults who cannot maintain appropriate body weight to ensure adequate calorie, protein, and nutrient intake. The role of nutrition in health promotion and disease prevention is an evolving practice with guidelines that need to be tailored to meet the needs of the aging individual.

Although many adults are living longer and more healthfully, for many the aging process represents a continued decline in health and well-being. Approximately 37 million older adults will have more than one chronic condition by 2030.[37] Evidence suggests that numerous physiological changes associated with the leading chronic diseases and even death are often avoidable or can be delayed. The role nutrition plays in the prevention and modulation of chronic disease in older adults is of special interest to the aging population because lifelong diet influences healthy aging. Dietary shifts to include low-fat dairy products, lean meats, adequate fiber, whole grains, fruits, and vegetables while also limiting sugar, trans fatty acids, sodium, and excess calories are priorities to improve and maintain health for individuals of any age. Older adults with barriers to eating a healthy diet may find nutritional recommendations difficult to achieve, especially as medical nutrition therapy may further limit choices.

The goal of nutrition recommendations in the aging population is one not only of disease management but also of health protection so that individuals can live long and enjoy good health. Older adults often have numerous medical conditions that require a change in nutrient intake as well as the use of various prescriptions and over-the-counter medications that can decrease food intake or modify digestion, absorption, metabolism, and excretion. Efforts to consume a healthy diet can be negatively affected by these physiologic and medical factors as well as social factors, economic hardships, and physical and functional limitations that impair shopping for or preparing foods. Decreased food intake in an older adult can have undesirable consequences. In addition to the functional ability to obtain food and prepare meals, geographic location, access to transportation, and the economic resources to purchase wholesome foods influence the nutritional component of the aging process.

Nutrition Considerations for the Older Adult: Nutritional Risk Factors

Older adults require specialized nutrition services aimed at maintaining independence and health. The ability to consume the appropriate quality and quantity of foods is influenced by food accessibility, availability, acceptability and preference, preparation, and the eating process itself. Whether healthful foods are accessible and available, for example, can depend on social and economic factors such as marital status and household roles, health behaviors, financial status, housing, neighborhood and community factors, geographic location and neighborhood resources, transportation, and social/caregiver support. The act of eating can be challenging in older adults who are unable to feed themselves or those with poor dentition, difficulty chewing and swallowing, or, for example, individuals who have diminished sense of taste and smell, and those with anorexia of aging, for whom food is not appetizing. Older adults are at nutritional risk as a result of numerous factors that contribute to poor dietary intake, as illustrated in FIGURE 14.10 . Psychological factors that have a strong influence on an individual's nutritional well-being include food security, education, literacy, and language along with cultural beliefs.

Acceptability of Food Choices

Food acceptability may be the result of a variety of psychosocial factors such as lifelong food habits, culture, ethnic background, food faddism, food temperature, food texture or appearance, perceived intolerance, personal motivation, mental status and cognitive function, depression, and life stresses. Physiological factors that influence acceptability of food include health, individual and multiple diseases, medication use, and altered sense of taste, smell, or oral status resulting from medication side effects or disease processes.[81] Medications may decrease appetite, diminish taste, alter salivation, or impair swallowing. Preparation and eating food can also be affected by physiological factors such as mobility, balance, nutritional status, sight and hearing, cognitive deficits, or physical limitations, such as difficulty opening containers or packages. The location and number of meal

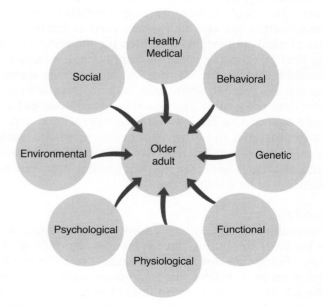

Figure 14.10
Catagories of Nutritional risk factors for older adults.

occasions, meal size, and food choice can also influence food intake. Almost 20% of older adults do not usually eat breakfast, which is usually a nutrient-dense meal, meaning that older adults who do not regularly eat breakfast have lower nutrient intake than those older adults who do eat breakfast.[82]

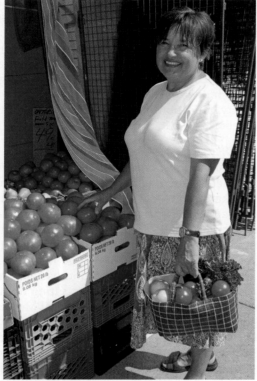

©Elena Elisseeva/Shutterstock

Food Insecurity

Unfortunately, far too many older adults face food insecurity, the risk of not having enough food. Food-insecure individuals might adopt strategies such as limiting the size of meals or portions to stretch the money available for food or choosing between competing demands for limited resources, for example, choosing among spending money on medications, bills, or food. Smaller meals may limit the quality and quantity of food and put an individual at risk for low nutrient intake. Food assistance programs and other community programs, such as meal-delivery programs, may be inadequate or may not be available because of lack of funding or volunteer resources or long waiting lists.

Food Deserts

Community factors such as unsafe neighborhoods, lack of business community involvement, geographic isolation, absence of sidewalks, and minimal or no transportation make it difficult for some older adults to shop. The situation is exacerbated in food deserts, which are geographic areas, especially rural or impoverished urban locations, lacking accessible supermarkets or grocery stores. Healthy food options are limited and expensive at convenience stores, which generally stock few or no fresh fruits or vegetables and limited low-fat or fat-free dairy products and more snack items, processed meats, and canned foods.[83] Convenience store foods are usually more expensive than foods in larger grocery stores, so older adults with limited finances who are forced to rely on convenience stores have higher average food costs, reducing their food-purchasing power.[83] When an older adult has to travel farther to a grocery store, it can be exhausting and greater transportation costs further lower the amount of money available to purchase food. The home environment may pose additional challenges, such as inadequate refrigeration or lack of safe and appropriate cooking appliances. Inadequate refrigeration or storage means that some older adults must shop more frequently for fresh groceries.

Food Safety and Preventing Foodborne Illnesses

Foodborne illnesses are potentially serious and life-threatening concerns for older adults. Older adults are at particular risk for suffering extreme consequences and even death from foodborne illnesses for several reasons, including comorbidities and immunosenescence.

Older adults should take extra precautions to ensure foods are stored and prepared according to safety standards. Food safety experts recommend that consumers follow four rules (**FIGURE 14.11**)—clean, separate, cook, and chill—to help ensure food safety. Hand washing is the single most important means of preventing the spread of infection. Older adults or individuals with a compromised immune system should be discouraged from using recipes in which eggs, any animal products, or fish remain raw or only partially cooked. Providing practical advice on food safety can help prevent sickness or even death. Increased awareness of the dangers associated with foodborne illnesses and preventive guidance to older adults helps to protect them.

Nutrition Programs for Older Adults

Nutrition plays a central role in the primary, secondary, and tertiary prevention of disease. Prevention occurs in a variety of settings for older adults, from those who are independent and living in the community to those who are frail and in the community, hospitalized, in adult day

CLEAN   SEPARATE   COOK   CHILL

Figure 14.11
Fight Bac.

Reproduced from USDA. Check Your Steps: Food Safe Families. Retrieved from: https://www.fsis.usda.gov/wps/portal/fsis/topics/food-safety-education/teach-others/fsis-educational-campaigns/check-your-steps

care, or institutionalized. Overall good nutrition helps to promote health, function, independence, and the prevention of nutrition-related disease. Nutrition is a primary component in the management of disease conditions and for prevention against worsening morbidity and disability.

Health and Well-Being

When asked to rate their health as excellent, very good, good, fair, or poor, 76% of people 65 years and older rated their health as very good or excellent.[3] Self-reported health score diminishes with age, however: 67% of older adults ages 85 and older report very good or excellent health. Health and well-being are influenced by numerous interrelated factors that accumulate over a lifetime, and nutrition is a major determinant of successful aging (FIGURE 14.12). Eighty-five percent of noninstitutionalized older adults, for example, have at least one chronic health condition that could be improved with proper nutrition, and up to half may present with clinical evidence of malnutrition.[8] TABLE 14.8 lists chronic diseases that are the leading cause of death among older adults. Many older adults can live for years with these chronic conditions that limit their activity and diminish quality of life.

Nutrition Services for Older Adults

Older adults in the United States are living longer, healthier, and more functionally fit lives than ever before. Although many older persons have at least one or more chronic health conditions, approximately four in every five older adults are healthy and independent enough to engage in their normal activities. The achievement and maintenance of good nutritional health and a longer and

Table 14.8
Chronic Diseases that Are the Leading Causes of Death Among U.S. Adults Aged 65 and Older
Heart disease
Cancer
Stroke
Chronic lower respiratory diseases
Influenza and pneumonia
Alzheimer disease
Diabetes
Data from Centers for Disease Control and Prevention. *The State of Aging and Health in America 2013*. Atlanta, GA: Centers for Disease Control and Prevention, U.S. Department Health and Human Services; 2013. Retrieved from: http://www.cdc.gov/aging/pdf/state-aging-health-in-america-2013.pdf. Accessed May19, 2016.

healthier life requires efforts at the individual, family, organization, community, and policy levels. Public nutrition policy with regard to older adults takes many forms, including national goals, the development and dissemination of nutritional recommendations, and nutrition assistance programs.

The Administration on Aging

The Administration on Aging (AoA) plays a central role in federal efforts to promote health and wellness and to eliminate health disparities among older adults, in particular, older minority adults. The AoA supports prevention and wellness programs designed to support community-based services, ensuring that services are provided to economically and socially vulnerable older adults.

About 28% of noninstitutionalized older persons live alone, and almost half of older women (46%) ages 75 years and older live alone; however, the number of institutionalized adults increases with age, and 10% of persons older than the age of 85 live in institutional settings.[84] AoA programs and services are successful in helping older adults remain in their communities and homes and in providing services to needy older adults in an effective manner.[81]

Medicare and the Affordable Care Act

Care for the nation's older population falls under several systems. One is the healthcare system, which is composed of individual private health insurance, health maintenance organizations, and Medicare. Nearly all older adults over the age of 65 (93.5%) are covered, in part, by Medicare.[84] The focus of this system is the promotion of health through the treatment of disease. The Affordable Care Act (ACA) increases access to no- or low-cost preventive services that may result in improvements to health, disease prevention, and decreased long-term healthcare costs. Despite the link between nutrition and health in older persons, however, Medicare provides limited coverage for nutrition services.

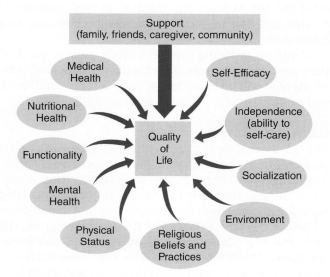

Figure 14.12

Many factors influence quality of life in older adults.

Modified from the Position Paper of the American Dietetic Association: nutrition across the spectrum of aging. *J Am Diet Assoc.*2005;105(4):616–633.

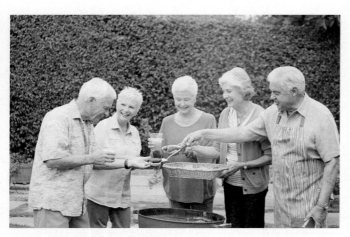

©Ronnie Kaufman/Larry Hirshowitz/Blend Images/Getty

Home and Community-Based Long-Term Care

Enabling older adults to stay at home and in their community is replacing institutional care in an effort to preserve higher quality of life and reduce long-term healthcare costs.[85] With the Home and Community-Based Services (HCBS) Waiver program under the Social Security Act, states can allow community-based services to be care providers by waiving certain Medicaid statutes and regulations. This allows individuals at risk of being placed in long-term care facilities to receive care at home, preserving their independence and ties to family and friends.[86] Approved nutrition services include home-delivered meals, nutrition risk-reduction counseling, and nutritional supplements, as appropriate. Each state determines and implements its own benefits package. The objective of the home and community-based long-term care system is to promote health through an array of services, including nutrition, that help maintain the quality of life and independence of older adults and prevent or delay institutionalization.

The Older Americans Act

In 1961, the first White House Conference on Aging was established to highlight the problems facing older Americans and to make policy recommendations on how best to improve the lives of the growing group of older adults. The AoA, a branch of the U.S. Department of Health and Human Services (HHS), is responsible for administering nutrition services to America's older adults. The AoA was established to carry out the Older Americans Act (OAA) of 1965. The OAA "promotes the well-being of older individuals by providing services and programs designed to help them live independently in their homes and communities. The Act also empowers the federal government to distribute funds to the states for supportive services for individuals over the age of 60."[84]

The passage of the OAA established a national goal to promote better health through improved nutrition and to help older adults remain independent in their own homes. The OAA Nutrition program is the largest national food and nutrition program specifically designed to serve older adults; however, currently the Older Americans Act Nutrition Programs (OAANPs) reach less than 5% of all older individuals.[85] The Office of Nutrition and Health Promotion Programs (ONHPP) manages health, prevention, and wellness programs for older adults. These include behavioral health information, chronic disease self-management education programs, diabetes self-management, disease prevention and health promotion services ("Title IIID"), falls prevention programs; HIV/AIDS education, nutrition services, and oral health promotion.[84]

Title IIIC

Title IIIC of the OAA includes congregate and home-delivered meals. *Congregate meals* are served at community centers such as senior dining centers, religious-based settings, schools, and adult day centers. Initially designed to provide nutritious meals in a social setting, congregate sites also provide an opportunity for socialization, mental stimulation, and community involvement. Congregate meals provide an estimated 40% to 50% of daily nutrients and calories. Many older adults eat more nutritious food at congregate sites than they would eat at home.

In 1978, the nutrition program was expanded to include a home-delivered meals component for the growing number of frail and homebound older adults unable to travel to a congregate site. Commonly known as *Meals on Wheels*, this home-delivered meal program offers more than just food: volunteers who deliver meals provide social interaction, especially for older adults who live alone. Despite participating in food assistance programs, many older adults still consume less than adequate diets, and many experience food insufficiency and worsening health and nutritional status over time. All OAANP meals must provide at least one-third of dietary recommendations and use the *Dietary Guidelines for Americans* as a framework.

Challenges facing OAANP include greater demand than allocated resources, an increasing numbers of older adults who will be living longer with chronic conditions, and waiting lists for nutrition services (**FIGURE 14.13**).

USDA Nutrition Programs

The U.S. Department of Agriculture (USDA) has several programs designed to fight hunger that serve older adults, including the Federal Supplemental Nutrition Assistance Program (formerly the Food Stamp Program), Food Stamp Nutrition Education, Commodity and Supplemental Foods, the Emergency Food Assistance Program, the Child and Adult Care Food Program, and the Senior Farmers' Market Nutrition Program. The Supplemental Nutrition Assistance Program (SNAP) is the largest USDA food assistance program and provides electronic benefit transfer (EBT) cards or coupons to eligible low-income individuals and families. This is an entitlement program, and participants who meet the requirements set by law are

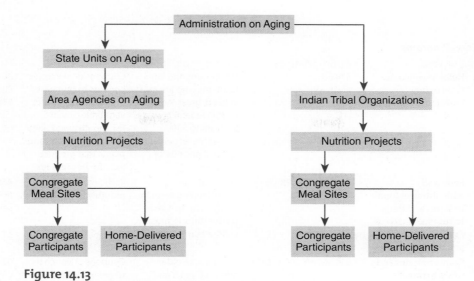

Figure 14.13

Title III and IV nutrition programs.

guaranteed program benefits. There are few restrictions on food purchases, and the purchase of alcohol, tobacco, and other nonfood items is not permitted.[87] **TABLE 14.9** provides a summary of HHS Administration on Aging and USDA Food and Nutrition Service programs.

The Commodity Supplemental Food Program (CSFP) works to improve the health of low-income Americans by supplementing their diets with nutritious USDA commodity foods. Targeted populations include adults older than age 60 with incomes less than 130% of the federal poverty

Table 14.9

HHS Administration on Aging and USDA Food and Nutrition Service Programs

US Department of Health and Human Services Administration of Aging Programs

Program	Purpose	Appropriations	Target Population	Services	Participation
Older Americans Act: Titles I–VII	Grants to state, tribal, and community programs on aging; research, demonstration projects, etc.	$1.42B (FY 2008)	Age 60+ in greatest economic need and/or social need, with particular attention to low-income minorities, those in rural areas, and those with limited English proficiency	Nutrition services, supportive and health services, protection of vulnerable older Americans	9.5M older adults (FY 2006)
Older Americans Act: Title III	Nutrition services to older adults	$816.3M (FY 2012)	Age 60+, < 60 years and disabled who live in elderly housing, disabled living at home, and those who eat at congregate sites or who receive home-delivered meals	Congregate and home-delivered meals; nutrition screening, assessment, education, counseling	2.6M older adults, 238.3M meals (FY 2006)
Office of the Assistant Secretary for Planning and Evaluation: Title VI	Tribal and Native organizations for aging programs and services	$33.4M (FY 2012)	Age requirement determined by tribal organizations or Native Hawaiian program	Congregate and home-delivered meals; nutrition screening, education, counseling; array of other supportive and health services	70,000 older adults, 4M meals (FY 2006)
Nutrition Services Incentive Program (NSIP)	Provides proportional shares to states and tribes based on number of meals served in prior year	$160.4M (FY 2012)	Same as Title III	Cash and/or commodities to supplement meals	

USDA Programs

UDSA Food and Nutrition Programs

Program	Purpose	Appropriations	Target Population	Services	Participation
Supplemental Nutrition Assistance Program (SNAP)	Helps low-income families buy nutritionally adequate food	$74.6B (FY 2012)	U.S. citizens and legal residents who are most in need, gross income <130% federal poverty level; up to $2000 countable resources, $3000 if age 60+ or disabled	Coupons or electronic benefits to purchase breads, cereals, fruits, vegetables, meats, fish, poultry, and dairy products or seeds and plants that produce food for households	46.6M monthly, 51% children, 41% adults, 8% age 60+
Commodity Supplemental Food Program	Food and administrative funds to states and tribes to supplement diets. Available in 33 states and through 2 tribes	$140M (FY 2008)	Pregnant and breastfeeding women, mothers up to 1 year postpartum, infants, children up to age 6	Participants receive a monthly food package	466,180 participants (FY 2007); 92% of those served are 60+
Senior Farmers' Market Nutrition Program	Grants to states and tribes to provide fresh foods and nutrition services while providing the opportunity for farmers to enhance their business	$19.5M (FY 2008–2013)	Low-income older adults 60 years and older who have household incomes of not more than 185% federal poverty	Coupons or vouchers to be exchanged for fresh fruits, vegetables, herbs, and honey at local farmers markets	52 agencies (FY 2012); 885,116 older adults (FY 2012)
The Emergency Food Assistance Program	Provides food to local agencies that serve the public directly	$189.5M (FY 2008), plus $67M worth of surplus commodity foods $250M annually in Farm Bill	Adults aged 60+ who meet state criteria based on income, including homeless, low-income older adults	Emergency food for low-income needy persons, including older adults. States provide food to local agencies, usually food banks, which, in turn, distribute food to soup kitchens and food pantries that serve the public directly	3.8M households
Child and Adult Care Food Program	Healthy, nutritious meals for children and adults in day centers	$2.8B (FY 2012)	Children younger than 12 years, homeless children, migrant children younger than 15 years. Disabled citizens regardless of age. Age 60+; functionally impaired; reside with family members	Nutritional meals and snacks	1.9B meals served (FY 2012) 2.9M children, 86,000 older adults (FY 2007)

guidelines. Local agencies determine eligibility, distribute the foods, and provide nutrition education. CSFP food packages do not provide a complete diet, but they may be good sources of nutrients typically lacking in diets.

The Emergency Food Assistance Program (TEFAP) is a commodity-food distribution program in which the USDA buys food, including processed and packaged items, and ships it to states based on its low-income and unemployed population. States provide the food to local agencies, usually food banks, which, in turn, distribute the food to soup kitchens and food pantries that serve the public.

The Child and Adult Care Food Program (CACFP) serves nutritious meals that meet minimum nutrition requirements and snacks to eligible adults in participating adult day centers. The number of meals served in adult day centers is growing faster than the number served in child care centers.[88]

The Senior Farmers' Market Nutrition Program (SFMNP) awards grants to states, U.S. territories, and federally recognized Indian tribal governments to provide low-income older adults with coupons that can be exchanged for eligible foods at farmers' markets, roadside stands, and community-supported agriculture programs. The program is designed to improve health and stimulate community-supported agriculture by providing access to locally grown fresh and unprocessed fruits, vegetables, honey, and herbs. Annual benefits, however, are modest and are available only during the local growing season.[89]

Health Promotion

The World Health Organization refers to 'active ageing' and defines it as:

> the process of optimizing opportunities for health, participation and security in order to enhance quality of life as people age. Active ageing allows people to realize their potential for physical, social, and mental well-being throughout the life course and to participate in society, while providing them with adequate protection, security and care when they need.... "Health" refers to physical, mental and social well-being.... Maintaining autonomy and independence for the older people is a key goal in the policy framework for active ageing.[90]

It is never too late to make small shifts toward improving health and quality of life. Although not all diseases can be prevented or reversed, considerable evidence supports health promotion activities even for the oldest adults. Although an individual may demonstrate attributes of healthy aging, alterations in wellness can occur that result in disease, functional limitation, or disability. Aging should be considered as the individual existing along a continuum—from healthy aging to unhealthy aging.

Health promotion is a broad term used to describe actions that are deliberately taken with the intent of moving an individual to a higher level of wellness. Eating a healthy diet, exercising, quitting smoking, obtaining appropriate levels of sleep/rest, reducing stress, and participating in leisure time activities help shift the older adult toward healthy aging.

One of the myths of aging is that health promotion activities will have little benefit or that older adults have no interest in health promotion activities. These myths, however, are not supported by the scientific evidence; instead, it is well accepted that health and well-being can be improved at any age. Disease prevention, alternatively, is considered to be those activities that an individual deliberately takes to prevent illness or disease. Whereas not all diseases can be prevented, a considerable body of literature supports the efficacy of health promotion activities for older adults. It is of high importance when working with older adults to consider individualized strategies through dietary, lifestyle, and physical activity interventions while simultaneously giving special attention to comorbidities.

Nutrition guidance aimed at promoting health in older adults should be integrated into the overall healthcare plan. State and local governments as well as private sources provide a large number of programs and resources. The nutritionist is part of the interprofessional healthcare team responsible for assessing and implementing activities aimed at health promotion and disease prevention.

Physical Activity and Exercise

Evidence supports the idea that a substantial portion of what historically has been thought of as "normal aging," especially with regard to changes in muscle, fat, and bone, are in fact related to an energy imbalance resulting from either excess or insufficient energy consumption, decreased energy expenditure from physical activity, or both factors in combination.[91] Physical fitness and habitual activity levels in old age have been shown to be directly related with functional limitations as well as indirectly related with functional limitations through diseases associated with inactivity. It is well accepted that physical activity and exercise are central in the promotion of health and prevention of disease for individuals regardless of age.

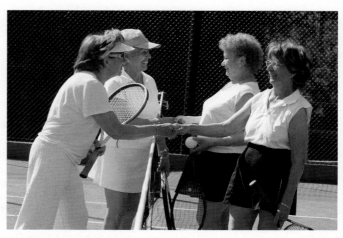
©Carme Balcells/Shutterstock

Physical activity is essential to long-term health and maintenance of functional well-being. Even small changes in daily activity levels have been shown to be extremely important to improving health, and Americans of all ages, including older adults, are encouraged to meet the *Physical Activity Guidelines for Americans* to help promote health and reduce the risk of chronic disease.[67] The benefits of regular physical activity and exercise are far-reaching in older adults and include not only disease risk reduction and weight management but also maintenance of functional independence and improved quality of life.

Health Benefits of Physical Activity and Exercise for Older Adults

Regular physical activity and exercise have consistently been linked with lower mortality rates; chronic disease prevention, reduction, and management; and improved mental and cognitive capability, depressive states, psychological health, independence, balance, bone and muscular strength, and overall quality of life across the life span.[92,93] Regular physical activity has been associated with reduced risk of the following chronic diseases: cardiovascular disease, type 2 diabetes, obesity, osteoporosis, hypertension, thromboembolic stroke, colon cancer, breast cancer, depression, and anxiety. Increased physical functioning has also been related to regular physical activity by reducing the risk of falls and injuries from falls. Physical activity is also used in therapeutic and disease management roles for numerous conditions that affect older adults, including hypertension, type 2 diabetes, obesity, cholesterol, osteoarthritis, peripheral vascular disease, coronary heart disease, chronic obstructive pulmonary disease, claudication, dementia, pain, congestive heart failure, stroke, back pain, depression and anxiety disorders, syncope, constipation, balance disorders, insomnia, and physical disability.[92] Despite these recognized beneficial effects, older adults remain some of our nation's least physically active individuals.[94,95]

Guidelines to Physical Activity and Exercise

All ages benefit from integrating more exercise into their lives, and the majority of older adults should be physically active.[96] The American College of Sports Medicine (ACSM), the Centers for Disease Control and Prevention (CDC), and the American Heart Association (AHA) joined together to update recommendations regarding physical activity for adults ages 65 and older and adults ages 50–64 with clinically significant chronic disease or functional limitations that affect movement ability, fitness, or physical activity, stating, "*Regular physical activity, including aerobic activity and muscle-strengthening activity, is essential for healthy aging.*"[96] The ACSM/CDC/AHA's recommendations for healthy adults older than age 65 have been shown to have benefits for disease prevention and treatment as well as maintenance of cardiovascular and musculoskeletal fitness (TABLE 14.10). Approximately 30 minutes per day is sufficient to meet the requirements for all four modes of exercise: aerobic, strengthening, balance, flexibility, and is feasible for most individuals of retirement age. The ACSM/CDC/AHA's recommendations are similar to those made in the 2008 *Physical Activity Guidelines for Americans* and the World Health Organization's *Global Recommendations on Physical Activity for Health* for individuals 65 years and older. The comprehensive *Physical Activity Guidelines* by the U.S. Department of Health and Human

---

Table 14.10

Exercise Recommendations for Older Adults

The ACSM/CDC and AHA basic recommendation is that older adults:

1. "Do moderately intense aerobic exercise for 30 minutes a day, five days a week."

or

2. "Do vigorously intense aerobic exercise for 20 minutes a day, 3 days a week."

Notes: *Aerobic activity.* Aerobic exercise increases oxygen use to improve heart and lung function. These activities are important for their cardiovascular benefits such as strengthening of the heart and lungs as well as lowering blood pressure and cholesterol. Aerobic activities have also been shown to improve mood and sleep. Walking, swimming, dancing, aerobic exercise classes, climbing stairs, pushing a lawn mower, biking to the store, playing with children, gardening, and even heavy housework are also types of activity that count, as long as activity is moderate or vigorous for at least 10 minutes at a time.

Intensity. Intensity is how hard the body is working during an activity. Older adults should aim to include 150 minutes of moderate-intensity physical activity each week.

Moderate-intensity aerobic exercise means working at a 5 or 6 on a 10-point scale, with 0 = sitting, and 10 = as hard as possible. As a rule of thumb the exerciser should still be able to carry on a brief conversation but not sing a song. For those with a higher level of fitness and limited time to be active, older adults could include 75 minutes of vigorous activity weekly or an equivalent amount of time by combining moderate and intense activities.

Vigorous-intensity activity produces larger increases in breathing and heart rate. The activity should rate a 7 or 8 on the 10-point scale. Breathing will be hard enough so that the exerciser cannot say more than a few words without catching his or her breath.

and

3. "Do 8–10 strength-training exercises, 10–15 repetitions of each exercise twice–three times per week."

Notes: *Muscle-strengthening activities* are strength-training exercises designed to increase muscle strength and endurance. These activities prevent loss of muscle and bone and thereby help to maintain health and physical independence. To gain the health benefits of muscle-strengthening exercises, the activities need to be done to the point where it becomes difficult to finish the repetitions without help. There are many ways older adults can strengthen their muscles such as lifting weights, working with resistance bands, doing exercises that use body weight for resistance such as sit-ups and push-ups and yoga. The activities should work all the major muscle groups in the body including the chest, shoulders, arms, legs, hips, abdomen, and the muscles of the back.

An additional bonus for older adults is the beneficial effects of physical activity for their *functional health*. Improvements in functional health contribute to the ease of performing everyday activities such as walking, grocery shopping, food preparation, and housekeeping.

and

4. "If you are at risk of falling, perform balance exercises."

Notes: *Balance exercises* are recommended for community-dwelling adults with a history of falling or trouble walking. The activity plan for these adults should include exercise specifically designed to maintain or improve balance.

Flexibility activities such as stretching large muscle groups are also recommended. Stretching helps to maintain the necessary range of motion for the performance of everyday activities.

and

5. "Have a physical activity plan."

Notes: Experts also recommend that older adults have an *activity plan* developed with a health professional. This plan should be designed to maximize physical activity while managing risks, taking therapeutic needs into account, and ensuring safety.

Data from American College of Sports Medicine. Exercise and physical activity for older adults. *Med Sci Sports Exerc.* July 2009;41(7):1510-30. doi: 10.1249/MSS.0b013e3181a0c95c.

Nelson ME, Rejeeski WJ, Blair SN, et al. Physical activity and public health in older adults: recommendations from the American College of Sports Medicine and the American Heart Association. *Med Sci Sports Exerc.* August 2007;39(8):1435-45; Centers for Disease Control and Prevention. Physical activity: how much physical activity do adults need? Atlanta, GA: CDC. Retrieved from: http://www.cdc.gov/physicalactivity/everyone/guidelines/adults.html. Accessed May 12, 2014.

Services include a chapter specific to older adults.[97] The four main components of fitness; strength, endurance, flexibility, and balance, should all be incorporated into an exercise plan for older adults.

Although more activity is usually better, at the very least, all adults should strive to avoid being inactive. Being sedentary is bad for health regardless of someone's age or physical condition. Individual barriers to physical activity should be addressed when starting or maintaining a physical activity plan. Common obstacles to physical activity for older adults include medical problems, disabilities, caregiving role, disinterest, fear of injury, finances, geographical constraints, environmental constraints, lack of social support, lack of equipment, lack of healthcare provider education about exercise, psychological issues, transportation, perception of few benefits, and societal norms/expectations of older adulthood being sedentary.[94]

Of people age 65 and older, 36% reported some type of disability (i.e., difficulty in hearing, vision, cognition,

ambulation, self-care, or independent living) in 2013 (**FIGURE 14.14**). Some of these disabilities may be relatively minor, but others cause people to require assistance to meet important personal needs. Older adults often have medical problems that do not preclude exercise; however, these conditions may place them at higher risk for exercise-related adverse events. Visual impairment, balance disorders, osteoarthritis of the shoulder or weight-bearing joints, low thresholds for ischemia or bronchospasm, peripheral vascular disease, and peripheral neuropathy may not be obvious conditions that could make it more challenging for older adults to safely participate in exercise programs. With careful monitoring, these conditions need not be a contraindication to exercise and, in fact, could actually be considered a primary indication for beginning an exercise program.

Using limitations in activities of daily living (ADLs) and instrumental activities of daily living (IADLs) to measure disability, in 2012, 33% of community-resident Medicare beneficiaries age 65 years and older reported

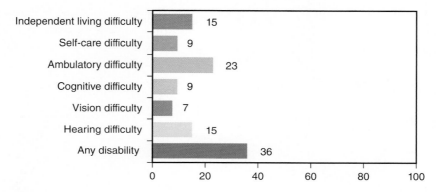

Figure 14.14

Percentage of persons 65 years and older with a disability.

U.S. Census Bureau, American Community Survey.

difficulty in performing one or more ADLs and an additional 12% reported difficulty with one or more IADLs. In contrast, 96% of institutionalized Medicare beneficiaries had difficulties with one or more ADLs and 83% of them had difficulty with three or more ADLs. (ADLs include bathing, dressing, eating, and getting around the house. IADLs include preparing meals, shopping, managing money, using the telephone, doing housework, and taking medication.) Limitations in activities because of chronic conditions increase with age. Approximately 1.3 million older adults are living in nursing homes and almost half are age 85 and older. These individuals often need care with their ADLs and/or have severe cognitive impairment due to Alzheimer disease or other dementias.

The ability of exercise training to slow the progression or even reverse some of the commonly accepted "signs of aging" suggests that a proportion of what we regard as "aging" is not an inevitable biologic process. Physical activity, exercise, and physical fitness are not merely medical prescriptions or treatments; they are lifestyle choices that minimize and delay what is still considered by some as "normal aging." Healthcare practices and policies for older adults must promote fitness, activity, and independence to the fullest extent possible as an important component of quality of life.

Case Study

Sherry's granddaughter was getting more and more worried about her grandmother's declining health and social withdrawal. Having just finished learning about nutrition for older adults, her granddaughter, who is a vegetarian, asked whether her grandmother's vitamin B_{12} levels had been checked recently and whether the blood work showed any signs of anemia. The granddaughter also suggested that they look into local congregate meal sites and Meals on Wheels until Sherry is feeling more like herself. Sherry and her granddaughter also made some calls to other older ladies in the apartment complex and started a small daily walking group that will walk around the lake on the property, and they contacted a local fitness expert to lead group classes in the building recreation room.

Questions

1. Do you agree with the granddaughter's theory of anemia?
2. What other food and nutrition programs would you suggest for Sherry?
3. What barriers may Sherry face to benefiting from their plan to increase her physical activity?

Recap Aging populations are increasing in number rapidly, requiring more and better care and services. Healthful eating relies on making the right food selections. Food selection is influenced by personal factors, individual and community resources, social context, and the food environment and involves decisions made on the basis of convenience and quality. Individual and community resources may be inadequate for older adults to be able to choose the foods that are optimal for nutritional health. Federal food and nutrition assistance programs provide a critical source of nutrition support for many older adults. Encouraging regular physical activity improves functional status and allows for higher energy consumption, thereby providing an important vehicle for meeting nutritional requirements. Physical activity and age-appropriate exercise interventions have the potential to increase and preserve skeletal muscle mass, improve physical functioning, and prevent disability across the life span.

1. What barriers exist for older adults who are trying to improve their food intake?
2. What obstacles exist for older adults who are trying to increase their physical activity?
3. Describe food and nutrition programs that are available to improve the nutritional status of older adults.

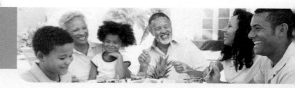

Learning Portfolio

Visual Chapter Summary

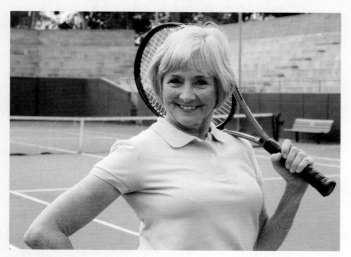

©jwblinn/Shutterstock

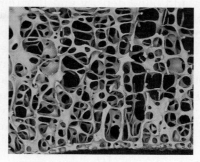

© Dr. Alan Boyde/Getty Images

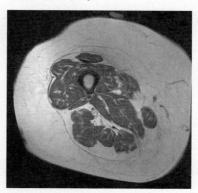

Courtesy of Professor Maria A. Flatarone Singh.

- Older adults are the largest growing segment of the population in the United States, and their proportion of the population is expected to reach more than 20% of the total population (over 72 million) by 2030.
- Successful aging depends on the interaction of a variety of factors, including health behaviors, genetics, environment and lifestyle, and medical conditions.
- Ensuring adequate nutritional intake is essential for promoting health and well-being, maintaining functional independence, and preventing malnutrition and related comorbidities such as increased susceptibility to acute and chronic illness and impaired immune function for all older adults.

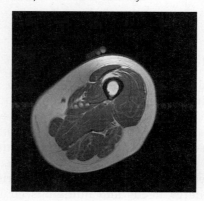

Courtesy of Professor Maria A. Flatarone Singh.

Physiology of Aging

- Physiological changes and medical conditions can either lead to or require a change in nutritional requirements and food intake with advancing age.
- Health status, alterations in taste perception, decreased olfactory ability, difficulty chewing and swallowing, and changes in digestion, absorption and nutrient metabolism can affect an older person's ability to consume a healthy diet.

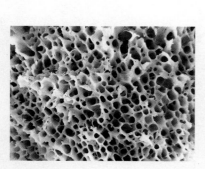

©Dr. Alan Boyde/Getty Images

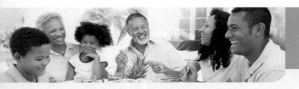

Learning Portfolio (continued)

■ Unfavorable alterations to body composition, changes in physiological function, declines in muscle mass and bone density and functional status, changes in major body systems (cardiovascular, respiratory, renal, skeletal, nervous, endocrine) and in gastrointestinal functioning, immune function, nutrient absorption, and metabolism may interfere with older adults' abilities to meet nutritional needs and may influence nutritional requirements.

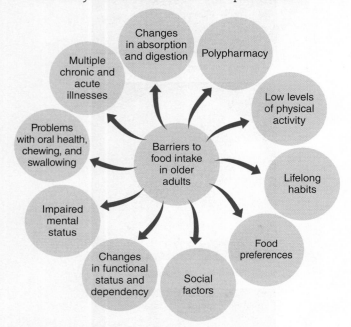

Dietary Intake of Older Adults

■ Older adults are a heterogeneous group, and challenges in meeting their nutritional requirements are as different as the older adults themselves. They have dramatically different nutritional, health, and social requirements built on lifelong eating behaviors and patterns for food choices and preferences.

■ Increased requirements for some nutrients with lower energy needs and numerous challenges to adequate food intake along with health and lifestyle barriers can make it difficult for older adults to meet their nutritional needs.

■ Multiple chronic and acute illnesses, changes in absorption and digestion, polypharmacy, low levels of physical activity, lifelong habits and food preferences, social factors, changes in functional status and dependency, impaired mental status, and problems with oral health, chewing, and swallowing along with social, economic, and cultural practices have a significant impact on food choice and preparation and influence the eating habits and nutritional intake of older adults.

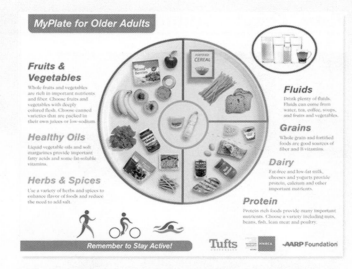

Nutritional Recommendations and Requirements for Older Adults

■ Poor nutritional status and nutrient inadequacies lead to increased burden of poor health, polypharmacy, reduced socialization and physical activity and interfere with health and the ability to remain independent.

■ Decreased food intake, sedentary lifestyle, and reduced energy expenditure make meeting nutritional requirements a challenge and place older adults at risk for malnutrition and worsening health status.

■ Age-related changes in health influence digestion, absorption, and metabolism of foods and nutrients, which translates into changes in nutritional requirements.

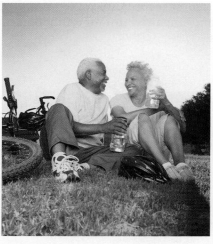

©Jupiterimages/Thinkstock

Promoting Healthy Lifestyles

■ Decreased food intake in an older adult can have undesirable consequences. Age-related factors that might contribute to decreased intake are the functional ability to obtain food and prepare meals, geographic location, access to transportation, and the economic resources to purchase wholesome foods.

■ Dietary shifts to include low-fat dairy products, lean meats, adequate fiber, whole grains, fruits, and vegetables and that also limit sugar, trans fatty acids, sodium, and excess calories are priorities to improve and maintain health for individuals of any age.

■ Individual and community resources may be inadequate to enable older adults to choose the foods that are optimal for nutritional health; therefore, federal food and nutrition assistance programs provide a critical source of nutrition support for many older adults.

■ Physical activity and age-appropriate exercise interventions have the potential to increase and preserve skeletal muscle mass, improve physical functioning, and prevent disability, and they allow for higher energy consumption, thereby providing an important vehicle for meeting nutritional requirements at all ages.

Key Terms

acculturation: The process whereby a group's or individual's culture is modified while adapting to another culture. Diet acculturation can be seen with immigrants who after years (and generations) of living in a new country begin to adopt food patterns similar to those of the host country.

achlorhydria: The absence of hydrochloric acid in the gastric juice.

antagonistic pleiotropy hypothesis: Known as the "pay later" theory, William's theory on aging proposes that some genes are beneficial at earlier ages but harmful at later ages. These genes with age-related opposite effects are called pleiotropic genes. This theory assumes that a particular gene can have an effect on several of an organism's traits (pleiotropy), which can affect the organism in antagonistic ways.

apoptosis: Preprogrammed cell death, which occurs when a cell is no longer viable and its mechanisms for fixing errors in DNA, for example, are unable to keep up. This is a naturally occurring phenomenon experienced by all living creatures.

atrophic gastritis: Also known as type A or type B gastritis; chronic inflammation of the stomach lining (mucosa) that can lead to loss of gastric glandular cells, which produce important substances such as the carrier for vitamin B_{12} known as intrinsic factor or enzymes and hydrochloric acid; that leads to their eventual replacement by intestinal and fibrous tissues. Occurs more frequently in older adults and is often associated with pernicious anemia or gastric carcinoma.

coenzyme: Organic compounds often B-Vitamin derivatives that combine with an inactive enzyme to form an active one. Coenzymes associate closely with these enzymes allowing them to catalyze certain metabolic reactions in a cell.

disease prevention: The deferral or elimination of medical illnesses and conditions through appropriate interventions for an individual or group with the goal of improving health and quality of life.

food desert: Geographic neighborhoods and communities that are characterized by limited access to fresh, affordable, healthy, and nutritious foods.

foodways: Food customs or traditions of a group of people that involve how foods are obtained, prepared, served, and consumed. Foodways encompass beliefs about food, food preferences, and customs and have cultural, social, and economic components.

gastroparesis: A condition where the muscles in the stomach do not function normally, limiting stomach motility and leading to delays in gastric emptying. Gastroparesis can interfere with normal digestion and cause symptoms such as nausea, vomiting, blood sugar dysregulation, and altered nutrition.

health promotion: Deliberate actions that are taken with the intent of moving an individual to a higher level of wellness.

immunosenescence: The gradual deterioration and impairment of the immune system that results from age-related changes in innate and adaptive immunity and an imbalance between them; results in decreased function and ability to respond to infections.

intrinsic factor: A substance secreted by the stomach that enables the body to absorb vitamin B_{12}. It is a glycoprotein. Deficiency results in pernicious anemia.

polypharmacy: The simultaneous use of multiple prescribed or over-the-counter medications by a single patient for one or more conditions. Major polypharmacy involves the use of five or more drugs per day.

sarcopenia: Loss of skeletal muscle mass and strength.

sarcopenic obesity: When an obese person has little muscle mass. Sarcopenic obesity is the simultaneous occurrence of sarcopenia and obesity, which results from excess body fat and reduction of muscle mass.

theory of mutation accumulation: Medawar's theory of aging that suggests that aging is due to an accumulation of harmful mutations over time.

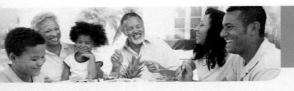

Learning Portfolio (continued)

Discussion Questions

1. Describe age-related changes that commonly occur in older adults and how these changes affect food intake and nutritional status.
2. Suggest diet and health interventions to slow the progression of disease and aging.
3. Explain how aging affects nutritional requirements and nutrient intake.
4. Discuss the food and nutrition programs and services available to older adults.
5. Explain how barriers to food intake affect nutritional well-being and health of older adults; include medical, physical, functional, and social factors and offer solutions for each.

Activities

1. List and discuss the diet and nutrition challenges facing older adults. Give specific examples and then as a group offer suggestions for recommendations you would suggest to overcome these challenges.
2. Role Play: Imagine you are part of a interprofessional healthcare team assigned to improve the quality of life in community dwelling older adults. Choose the role of family member, physician, dietitian, social worker, pharmacist, physical therapist or psycologist and from your perspective list the most important factors in maintaining a high quality of life for adults as they age. Describe how your team will prioritize steps and design interventions to address these factors.
3. Using the *Dietary Guidelines for Americans* food plans and the Tufts MyPlate for Older Adults, suggest a 1-day menu for an older adult with a chronic condition. What alterations would you make to that menu with a different or additional condition? What further suggestions would you have for homebound older adults?
4. Older adults often live alone and have medical and physical challenges that make meal preparation difficult. Suggest three to five easy-to-prepare meals and snacks for older adults and discuss how these can be made ahead of time and kept on hand for easy access.

Study Questions

1. Which body composition changes occur with aging?
   a. Decreased lean body mass
   b. Increased creatinine production
   c. Increased skeletal mass
   d. Increased total body water
2. Which of the following factors contributes to constipation in the older adult?
   a. Increased gastric motility
   b. Functional limitations
   c. Dehydration
   d. Over-the-counter medication use
   e. Chronic disease
   f. A high-fiber diet
   g. Dementia
3. Which changes that occur with aging place an older adult at risk for malnutrition?
   a. Decreased food intake
   b. Sedentary lifestyle
   c. Decreased energy expenditure
   d. Persistent chronic conditions
   e. All of the above
4. What does decreased energy expenditure in older adults mean?
   a. Maintaining body weight is more difficult because energy intake must also decrease to prevent weight gain.
   b. Meeting nutritional needs becomes easier because less energy expenditure means lower nutrient requirements.
   c. Older adults do not have to make healthy foods choices as often as younger adults.
   d. Energy expenditure does not decrease in sedentary older adults.
   e. All of the above.
5. Which of the following choices defines sarcopenia?
   a. A side effect of lipid-lowering medication that causes patients to have swelling in the extremities
   b. Age-related decline in visual acuity and cataract development
   c. Age-associated loss of muscle mass

d. Loss of mental status that leads to a decline in functional independence

e. Mouth pain related to ill-fitting dentures that can result in poor food intake

6. Symptoms and indicators of dehydration include all of the following *except* which one?
   a. Thirst
   b. Dry mouth
   c. Confusion
   d. Falls
   e. Weight gain

7. Which physiological change that occurs with aging does not influence nutrient metabolism?
   a. Decreased lean body mass
   b. Increased proportion of body fat
   c. Decreased body water
   d. Decreased height

8. Water is an essential nutrient that requires special attention for older adults for which reason?
   a. Total body water decreases with age as a result of loss of lean mass.
   b. The desire to drink often declines in older adults.
   c. Renal function declines with age.
   d. Forgetfulness and changes in mental status can cause low water intake.
   e. All of the above.

9. On what is the AMDR for essential fatty acids for older adults based?
   a. Average body weight of adults older than the age of 65
   b. DRI for protein
   c. Long-term studies showing the beneficial health effects of essential fatty acid consumption
   d. UL for essential fatty acids
   e. All of the above

10. What protein guideline is suggested for older adults?
    a. Consume 75% of their daily protein before noon so that the amino acids are available to be incorporated into proteins eaten later that day.
    b. Consume twice to three times the DRI for protein if their calorie intake declines below 1,000 kcal/d.
    c. Choose half of their protein sources from meat products and the other half from plant sources.
    d. Consume 25–30 g of high-quality protein with each meal to stimulate muscle protein synthesis.
    e. Do not eat too many high-protein foods because they are hard for the aging kidneys to metabolize.

11. Which of the following statements characterizes protein recommendations for older adults?
    a. Are more challenging to meet for sedentary individuals because of their low energy requirements.
    b. They are based on nitrogen balance studies.
    c. They may be too low to meet metabolic and physiologic needs.
    d. Moderate increases above the current RDA may enhance muscle protein metabolism.
    e. All of the above.

12. By what is deficiency of vitamin B_{12} in older adults commonly caused?
    a. Malabsorption
    b. Medication interactions
    c. Alcoholism
    d. Disease

13. Which of the following statements is *not* correct regarding vitamin D for older adults?
    a. Skin conversion of vitamin D increases with advancing age.
    b. Absorption of dietary vitamin D is approximately 50%.
    c. Fortified foods are the largest dietary source of vitamin D in this population.
    d. Decreased vitamin D intake contributes to deficiency in older adults.

14. Which of the following is true regarding vitamin E in older adults?
    a. It functions as a pro-oxidant to prevent lipid peroxidation.
    b. Dietary recommendations are based on alpha-tocopherol, the most biologically active form of the vitamin.
    c. In this population, dietary intake often exceeds recommended levels.
    d. No adverse effects have been found for older adults who take supplemental vitamin E.
    e. All of the above.

15. What is an important function of vitamin K in older adults?
    a. Coenzyme in fat metabolism
    b. Bone formation
    c. Antioxidant
    d. Visual acuity
    e. All of the above

16. What does vitamin D do?
    a. Helps to prevent osteoporosis.
    b. Helps to promote protein synthesis in skeletal muscle.
    c. Increases apoptosis of malignant cells.

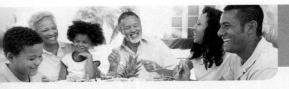

Learning Portfolio (continued)

d. Plays a role in blood glucose levels and insulin secretion.
e. All of the above.

17. Supplemental folate can hide a deficiency of which nutrient?
a. Vitamin B_{12}
b. Vitamin B_2
c. Vitamin B_1
d. Pantothenic acid
e. All of the above

18. Vitamin C found in fruits and vegetables may help to lower the risk of which condition for older adults?
a. Cognitive declines
b. Cardiovascular disease
c. Cancer
d. Age-related macular degeneration
e. All of the above

19. Which vitamin is *least* likely to be deficient in the diet of an older adult?
a. Niacin
b. Vitamin D
c. Vitamin B_{12}
d. Folate

20. Which of the following statements characterizes absorption of vitamin B_{12}?
a. Requires hydrochloric acid and pepsin.
b. Requires intrinsic factor.
c. Is reduced in older adults with atrophic gastritis.
d. All of the above.

21. Iron deficiency is characterized by an increase in _____ and a decrease in _____.
a. Total iron binding capacity; hemoglobin and hematocrit
b. Ferritin; transferrin
c. Hemoglobin; hematocrit
d. Hematocrit and hemoglobin; iron

22. The RDA for which of the following minerals increases in the older adult?
a. Magnesium
b. Phosphorus
c. Sodium
d. Chloride
e. All of the above

23. The dietary restriction of which of the following minerals is most likely to lead to malnutrition in elderly persons?
a. Potassium
b. Chromium

c. Molybdenum
d. Sodium
e. All of the above

24. From the list below, which nutrient is not included in bone metabolism of older adults?
a. Calcium
b. Iron
c. Magnesium
d. Phosphorus
e. Fluoride

25. Reduced dietary intake of _____ can lead to a reduced intake of calcium, calories, and protein.
a. Sodium
b. Phosphorus
c. Potassium
d. Magnesium
e. None of the above

26. Medications may cause _____, which can lead to reduced food acceptability in the older adult population.
a. Decreased appetite
b. Diminished taste
c. Altered salivation
d. Impaired swallowing
e. All of the above

27. Congregate meals provide what percentage of daily nutrients and calories?
a. 30%
b. 40%
c. 40–50%
d. 50–60%
e. 65%

28. Which of the following are considered aspects of "health promotion"?
a. Eating a healthy diet
b. Exercising
c. Quitting smoking
d. Reducing stress
e. All of the above

29. Which of the following is true in regard to assessing calorie needs in the older adult as compared to the general population?
a. Older adults need higher calorie intake because of malabsorption.
b. Older adults need lower calorie intake because of decreased metabolic demand.
c. Older adults need higher calorie intake because of their sedentary lifestyle.
d. Older adults need about the same number of calories but require a higher percentage of calories from fat.

30. What percentage of adults older than the age of 65 reported using complementary or alternative medicine (CAM)?
    a. 33%
    b. 55%
    c. 70%
    d. 88%
    e. > 90%

31. Older adults over the age of 65 should aim to be physically active for how many hours per week?
    a. 1–2 hours/wk.
    b. 3–3.5 hours/wk.
    c. 5 hours/wk.
    d. There is no standardized recommendation for older adults.

32. Which of the following are risk factors for dehydration?
    a. Weight loss
    b. Electrolyte abnormalities
    c. Confusion
    d. Difficulty chewing or swallowing
    e. All of the above

33. Which of the following is a consequence of malnutrition in the older adult?
    a. Increased risk for infection
    b. Increased length of hospital stay
    c. Increased mortality
    d. All of the above

34. Which of the following is *not* a psychological or social risk factor that could affect the nutritional status of the older adult?
    a. Food security, income, resources for food preparation
    b. Education level, literacy level, language barriers, lack of ability to communicate needs
    c. Cultural factors, religious beliefs, food preferences
    d. Caregiver, neighborhood, community resources or social support system
    e. Transportation to obtain food, mobility
    f. Stressful employment, getting along with coworkers

Weblinks

- **Tufts University MyPlate for Older Adults**
  http://hnrca.tufts.edu/myplate/

- **Administration on Aging**
  http://www.aoa.gov/

- **National Aging Network**
  http://www.aoa.acl.gov/AoA_Programs/OAA/Aging_Network/Index.aspx

- **National Association of States United for Aging and Disabilities**
  http://www.nasuad.org/

- **Nutrition Programs for Seniors**
  https://www.nutrition.gov/food-assistance-programs/nutrition-programs-seniors

References

1. Centers for Disease Control and Prevention. *The State of Aging and Health in America 2013*. Atlanta, GA: Centers for Disease Control and Prevention, U.S. Department of Health and Human Services; 2013. Retrieved from: http://www.cdc.gov/aging/pdf/state-aging-health-in-america-2013.pdf. Accessed January 26, 2014.

2. Knapowski J, Wieczorowska-Tobis K, Witowski K. Pathophysiology of aging. *J Physiol Pharmacol*. 2002;53(2):135–146.

3. Administration for Community LIving. Administration on Aging: Aging Statistics. Profile of older Americans: 2012. Washington, DC: Administration for Community Living, U.S. Department of Health and Human Services; 2013. Retrieved from: http://www.aoa.gov/Aging_Statistics/Profile/2012/3.aspx. Accessed February 24, 2014.

4. Administration for Community LIving. Administration on Aging: Aging Statistics. Projected future growth of older population. Washington, DC: Administration for Community Living, U.S. Department of Health and Human Services. Retrieved from: http://www.aoa.gov/aging_statistics/future_growth/future_growth.aspx. Accessed February 26, 2014

5. Gavrilov LA, Gavrilova NS. Evolutionary theories of aging and longevity. *Sci World J*. February 7, 2002;2:339–356.

6. Ljubunic P, Reznick AZ. The evolutionary theories of aging-revisited—a mini review. *Gerontology*. 2009;55(2):205–216.

7. Zeng Y, Cheng L, Chen H, et al. Effects of FOXO genotypes on longevity: a biodemographic analysis. *J Gerontol A Biol Sci Med Sci*. 2010;65(12):1285–1299.

8. Chernoff R. *Geriatric Nutrition: The Health Professional's Handbook*. 4th ed. Burlington, MA: Jones & Bartlett Learning; 2013.

9. Sura L, Madhavan A, Carnaby G, Crary MA. Dysphagia in the elderly: management and nutritional considerations. *Clin Interv Aging*. 2012;7:287–298.

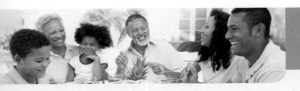

Learning Portfolio (continued)

10. Serra-Prat M, Hinojosa G, López D, et al. Prevalence of oropharyngeal dysphagia and impaired safety and efficacy of swallow in independently living older persons. *J Am Geriatr Soc.* 2011;59:186–187.

11. Ravindrin NC, Moskovitz DN, Kim YI. The aging gut. In: Chernoff R, ed. *Geriatric Nutrition: A Health Professional's Handbook.* 4th ed. Burlington, MA: Jones & Bartlett Learning; 2013.

12. Bernstein M, Munoz N; Academy of Nutrition and Dietetics. Position of the Academy of Nutrition and Dietetics: food and nutrition for older adults: promoting health and wellness. *J Acad Nutr Diet.* 2012;112:1255–1277.

13. Kim J, Wilson J, Lee S. Dietary implications on mechanisms of sarcopenia: roles of protein, amino acids and antioxidants. *J Nutr Biochem.* 2010;21(1):1–13.

14. Boire Y. Physiopathological mechanisms of sarcopenia. *J Nutr Health Aging.* 2009;13(8):717–723.

15. Paddon-Jones D, Short KR, Campbell WW, et al. The role of dietary protein in sarcopenia and aging. *Am J Clin Nutr.* 2008;87(suppl):1562s–1566s.

16. Chaput J, Lord C, Coutier M, et al. Relationship between antioxidant intakes and class l sarcopenia in elderly men and women. *J Nutr Healthy Aging.* July–August 2007;11(4):363–369.

17. Federal Interagency Forum on Aging-Related Statistics. *Older Americans 2010: Key Indicators of Well-Being.* Washington, DC: U.S. Government Printing Office; July 2010. Retrieved from: http://agingstats.gov/docs/PastReports/2010/OA2010.pdf. Accessed January 2, 2014.

18. Houston DK, Nicklas BJ, Zizza CA. Weighty concerns: the growing prevalence of obesity among older adults. *J Am Diet Assoc.* 2009;109(11):1886–1895.

19. Go AS, Mozaffarian D, Roger VL, et al; on behalf of the American Heart Association Statistics Committee and Stroke Statistics Subcommittee. Heart disease and stroke statistics—2013 update: a report from the American Heart Association. *Circulation.* 2013;127(1):e6–e245. doi:10.1161/CIR.0b013e31828124ad.

20. Lloyd-Jones DM, Hong Y, Labarthe D, et al., on behalf of the American Heart Association Strategic Planning Task Force and Statistics Committee. Defining and setting national goals for cardiovascular health promotion and disease reduction. The American Heart Association's strategic impact goal through 2020 and beyond. *Circulation.* 2010;121(4):586–613. doi:10.1161/CIRCULATIONAHA.109.192703.

21. Centers for Disease Control and Prevention. *National Chronic Kidney Disease Fact Sheet, 2014.* Atlanta, GA: U.S. Department of Health and Human Services, Centers for Disease Control and Prevention; 2014. Retrieved from: http://www.cdc.gov/diabetes/pubs/pdf/kidney_factsheet.pdf. Accessed February 17, 2014.

22. United States Renal Data System. *2013 Atlas of CKD and ESRD.* Bethesda, MD: National Institutes of Health, National Institute of Diabetes and Digestive and Kidney Diseases; 2013. Retrieved from: http://www.usrds.org/atlas.aspx. Accessed April 28, 2014.

23. U.S. Department of Health and Human Services. *The Surgeon General's Report on Bone Health and Osteoporosis: What It Means to You.* Washington, DC: U.S. Department of Health and Human Services, Office of the Surgeon General; 2012. http://www.niams.nih.gov/health_info/bone/SGR/surgeon_generals_report.asp. Accessed September 27, 2016.

24. Jones G. Vitamin D. In: Ross AC, Caballero B, Cousins RJ, et al, eds. *Modern Nutrition in Health and Disease.* 11th ed. Philadelphia, PA: Lippincott Williams and Wilkins; 2014.

25. National Institutes of Health, Office of Dietary Supplements; updated February 11, 2016. Health information: vitamin D fact sheet for health professionals. Retrieved from: http://ods.od.nih.gov/factsheets/VitaminD-HealthProfessional/. Accessed February 20, 2014.

26. Tucker KL, Rosen CJ. Prevention and management of osteoporosis. In: Ross AC, Caballero B, Cousins RJ, Tucker KL, Ziegler TR, eds. *Modern Nutrition in Health and Disease.* 11th ed. Philadelphia, PA: Lippincott Williams & Wilkins; 2014.

27. Office of the Surgeon General. *Bone Health and Osteoporosis: A Report of the Surgeon General.* Rockville, MD: Office of the Surgeon General; 2004. Retrieved from: http://www.ncbi.nlm.nih.gov/books/NBK45513/pdf/TOC.pdf. Accessed April 28, 2014.

28. Pae M, Meydani SN, Wu D. The role of nutrition in enhancing immunity in aging. *Aging Dis.* February 2012;3(1):91–129.

29. Bourre JM. Effects of nutrients (in food) on the structure and function of the nervous system: update on dietary requirements for brain. Part 1: micronutrients. *J Nutr Health Aging.* September–October 2006;10(5):377–385.

30. Anglin RE, Samaan Z, Walter SD, McDonald SD. Vitamin D deficiency and depression in adults: systematic review and meta-analysis. *Br J Psychiatry.* February 2013;202:100–107.

31. Morley JE, Malmstrom TK. Frailty, sarcopenia, and hormones. *Endocrinol Metab Clin North Am.* June 2013;42(2):391–405.

32. American Society of Hematology. Anemia and older adults. Washington, DC: American Society of Hematology. Retrieved from: http://www.hematology.org/Patients/Blood-Disorders/Anemia/5226.aspx. Accessed February 24, 2014.

33. Guralnik JM, Eisenstaedt RS, Ferrucci L, Klein HG, Woodman RD. Prevalence of anemia in persons 65 years and older in the United States: evidence for a high rate of unexplained anemia. *Blood.* 2004;104:2263–2268.

34. Woodman R, Ferrucci L, Guralnik J. Anemia in older adults. *Curr Opin Hematol.* 2005;12:123–128.

35. Dorner B1, Friedrich EK, Posthauer ME; American Dietetic Association. Position of the American Dietetic Association: individualized nutrition approaches for older adults in health care communities. *J Am Diet Assoc.* 2010;110:1549–1553.

36. Arandia G, Nalty C, Sharkey JR, Dean WR. Diet and acculturation among Hispanic/Latino older adults in the United States: a review of the literature and recommendations. *J Nutr Gerontol Geriatr.* 2012;31:16–37.

37. U.S. Department of Health and Human Services, Office of Disease Prevention and Health Promotion. *Healthy People 2020 topics and objectives: older adults.* Retrieved from: http://www.healthypeople.gov/2020/topicsobjectives2020/overview.aspx?topicid=31. Accessed August 1, 2016.

38. Otten JJ, Pitzi Hellwig J, Meyers LD, eds; Institute of Medicine. *Dietary Reference Intakes: The Essential Guide to Nutrient Requirements.* Washington, DC: National Academies Press; 2006. https://fnic.nal.usda.gov/sites/fnic.nal.usda.gov/files/uploads/DRIEssentialGuideNutReq.pdf. Accessed September 27, 2016.

39. Institute of Medicine, Food and Nutrition Board. *Dietary Reference Intakes: Calcium and Vitamin D.* Washington, DC: National Academies Press; 2011. https://fnic.nal.usda.gov/sites/fnic.nal.usda.gov/files/uploads/FullReport.pdf. Accessed September 27, 2016.

40. Institute of Medicine, Food and Nutrition Board. *Dietary Reference Intakes for Energy, Carbohydrate, Fiber, Fat, Fatty Acids, Cholesterol, Protein and Amino Acids (Macronutrients)*. Washington, DC: National Academies Press; 2005.

41. King DE, Mainous AG III, Lambourne CA. Trends in dietary fiber intake in the United States, 1999–2008. *J Acad Nutr Diet*. May 2012;112(5):642–648. doi:10.1016/j.jand.2012.01.019.

42. Mozaffarian D, Lemaitre RN, King IB, et al. Plasma phospholipid long-chain ω-3 fatty acids and total and cause-specific mortality in older adults: a cohort study. *Ann Intern Med*. 2013;158(7):515–525.

43. Wilk JB, Tsai MY, Hanson NQ, Gaziano JM, Djoussé L. Plasma and dietary omega-3 fatty acids, fish intake, and heart failure risk in the Physicians' Health Study. *Am J Clin Nutr*. 2012;96(4):882–888.

44. Johnson GH, Fritsche K. Effect of dietary linoleic acid on markers of inflammation in healthy persons: a systematic review of randomized controlled trials. *J Acad Nutr Diet*. 2012;112(7):1029–1041.

45. Chiuve SE, Rimm EB, Sandhu RK, et al. Dietary fat quality and risk of sudden cardiac death in women. *Am J Clin Nutr*. September 2012;96(3):498–507.

46. Paddon-Jones D, Rasmussen BB. Dietary protein recommendations and the prevention of sarcopenia. *Curr Opin Clin Nutr Metab Care*. 2009;12(1):86–90.

47. Volpi E, Campbell WW, Dwyer JT, et al. Is the optimal level of protein intake for older adults greater than the Recommended Dietary Allowance? *J Gerontol A Biol Sci Med Sci*. June 2013;68(6):677–681.

48. Popkin BM, D'Anci KE, Rosenburg IH. Water, hydration, and health. *Nutr Rev*. 2010;68(8):439–458.

49. Bernstein MA, Plawecki KL. Macronutrient and fluid recommendations and alcohol in older adults. In Bernstein MA, Munoz N, eds. *Nutrition for the Older Adult*. 3rd ed. Burlington, MA: Jones & Bartlett Learning; 2016.

50. Weinberg AD, Minaker KL. Dehydration: evaluation and management in older adults. *JAMA*. 1995;274:1552–1556.

51. Institute of Medicine, Food and Nutrition Board. *Dietary Reference Intakes for Water, Potassium, Sodium, Chloride, and Sulfate*. Washington, DC: National Academies Press; 2004.

52. Tufts University. Tufts University nutrition scientists provide updated MyPlate for Older Adults. Medford, MA: Tufts University; March 7, 2016. Retrieved from: http://now.tufts.edu/news-releases/tufts-university-nutrition-scientists-provide-updated-myplate-older-adults. Accessed September 27, 2016.

53. Institute of Medicine, Food and Nutrition Board. Dietary Reference Intakes: vitamins. Washington, DC: National Academies Press. Retrieved from: https://www.nationalacademies.org/hmd/~/media/Files/Activity%20Files/Nutrition/DRIs/DRI_Vitamins.pdf. Accessed May 7, 2014.

54. Allen LH. How common is vitamin B-12 deficiency? *Am J Clin Nutr*. 2009;89(2):693S–696S.

55. Oberlin BS, Tangney CC, Gustashaw KAR, Rasmussen HE. Vitamin B12 deficiency in relation to functional disabilities [published online November 12, 2013]. *Nutrients*. 2013;5(11):4462–4475. doi:10.3390/nu5114462.

56. Hughes CF, Ward M, Hoey L, McNulty H. Vitamin B12 and ageing: current issues and interaction with folate. *Ann Clin Biochem*. 2013;50(Pt 4):315–329. doi:10.1177/0004563212473279.

57. Pfeiffer CM, Caudill SP, Gunter EW, et al. Analysis of factors influencing the comparison of homocysteine values between the Third National Health and Nutrition Examination Survey (NHANES) and NHANES 1999. *J Nutr*. 2000;130:2850–2854.

58. Ganguly P, Alam SF. Role of homocysteine in the development of cardiovascular disease. *Nutr J*. 2015;14:6. doi:10.1186/1475-2891-14-6.

59. Schalinske KL, Smazal AL. Homocysteine imbalance: a pathological marker. *Adv Nutr*. November 1, 2012;3(6):755–762. doi:10.3945/an.112.002758.

60. Sohl E, van Schoor NM, de Jongh RT, Visser M, Deeg DJH, Lips P. Vitamin D status is associated with functional limitations and functional decline in older individuals. *JCEM*. September 1, 2013;98(9). doi:http://dx.doi.org/10.1210/jc.2013-1698.

61. Houston DK, Neiberg RH, Tooze JA, et al. Low 25-hydroxyvitamin D predicts the onset of mobility limitation and disability in community-dwelling older adults: the Health ABC Study. *J Gerontol A Biol Sci Med Sci*. 2013;68(2):181–187.

62. Milaneschi Y, Hoogendijk W, Lips P, et al. The association between low vitamin D and depressive disorders [published online April 9, 2013]. *Mol Psychiatry*. 2014;19(4):444–451. doi:10.1038/mp.2013.36.

63. Boucher BJ. The problems of vitamin D insufficiency in older people. *Aging Dis*. 2012;3(4):313–329.

64. Hoy MK, Goldman JD, Murayi T, Rhodes DG, Moshfegh AJ. Sodium intake of the U.S. population: what we eat in America, NHANES 2007–2008. Food Surveys Research Group Dietary Data Brief No. 8; October 2011. Retrieved from: https://www.ars.usda.gov/ARSUserFiles/80400530/pdf/DBrief/8_sodium_intakes_0708.pdf. Accessed September 27, 2016.

65. DeSimone JA, Beauchamp GK, Drewnowski A, Johnson GH. Sodium in the food supply: challenges and opportunities. *Nutr Rev*. 2013;71(1):52–59.

66. Meneton P, Jeunemaitre X, de Wardener HE, MacGregor GA. Links between dietary salt intake, renal salt handling, blood pressure, and cardiovascular diseases. *Physiol Rev*. 2005;85(2):679–715.

67. U.S. Department of Health and Human Services and U.S. Department of Agriculture. *2015–2020 Dietary Guidelines for Americans*. 8th ed. Washington, DC: U.S. Department of Health and Human Services and U.S. Department of Agriculture; December 2015. Retrieved from: http://health.gov/dietaryguidelines/2015/guidelines/. Accessed September 27, 2016.

68. National Heart, Lung, and Blood Institute. Description of the DASH eating plan. Bethesda, MD: National Heart, Lung, and Blood Institute; updated September 16, 2015. Retrieved from: http://www.nhlbi.nih.gov/health/health-topics/topics/dash. Accessed August 3, 2016.

69. Gunn JP, Barron JL, Bowman BA, et al. Sodium reduction is a public health priority: reflections on the Institute of Medicine's report, Sodium Intake in Populations: Assessment of Evidence. *Am J Hypertens*. 2013;26(10):1178–1180.

70. Institute of Medicine. *Dietary Reference Intakes for Vitamin A, Vitamin K, Arsenic, Boron, Chromium, Copper, Iodine, Iron, Manganese, Molybdenum, Nickel, Silicon, Vanadium, and Zinc*. Washington, DC: National Academies Press; 2001.

71. Umbreit J. Iron deficiency: a concise review. *Am J Hematol*. 2005;78:225–231.

72. Vishwanathan R, Chung M, Johnson EJ. A systematic review on zinc for the prevention and treatment of age-related macular degeneration. *Invest Ophthalmol Vis Sci*. 2013;54(6):3985–3998.

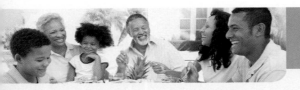

Learning Portfolio

73. Posthauer ME, Banks M, Dorner B, Schols J. The role of nutrition for pressure ulcer management: National Pressure Ulcer Advisory Panel, European Pressure Ulcer Advisory Panel, and Pan Pacific Pressure Injury Alliance white paper. *Adv Skin Wound Care.* 2015;28(4):175–188.

74. Devore E, Kang J, Stampfer M, Grodstein F. (2010). Total antioxidant capacity of diet in relation to cognitive function. *Am J Clin Nutr.* 2010;92:1157–1164.

75. National Institutes of Health, Office of Dietary Supplements. Health information: vitamin C fact sheet for health professionals. Bethesda, MD: National Institutes of Health, Office of Dietary Supplements; updated February 11, 2016. Retrieved from https://ods.od.nih.gov/factsheets/VitaminC-HealthProfessional/. Accessed May 18, 2016

76. National Institutes of Health, Office of Dietary Supplements. Health information: vitamin A fact sheet for health professionals. Bethesda, MD: National Institutes of Health, Office of Dietary Supplements; updated February 11, 2016. Retrieved from: https://ods.od.nih.gov/factsheets/VitaminA-HealthProfessional/. Accessed September 27, 2016.

77. National Institutes of Health, Office of Dietary Supplements. Health information: vitamin E fact sheet for health professionals. Bethesda, MD: National Institutes of Health, Office of Dietary Supplements; updated August 31, 2016. Retrieved from: https://ods.od.nih.gov/factsheets/VitaminE-HealthProfessional/. Accessed September 27, 2016.

78. Goyal A, Terry MD, Siegel AB. Serum antioxidant nutrients, vitamin A, and mortality in US adults. *Cancer Epidemiol Biomarkers Prev.* 2013;22(12):2202–2211.

79. Saffel-Shrier S. Vitamin requirements of the older adult. In Bernstein M, Munoz N, eds. *Nutrition for the Older Adult.* 2nd ed. Burlington, MA: Jones & Bartlett Learning; 2016.

80. National Center for Complementary and Integrative Health, National Institutes of Health, U.S. Department of Health and Human Services. Complementary and alternative medicine: what people aged 50 and older discuss with their health care providers. Bethesda, MD: National Center for Complementary and Integrative Health; updated December 15, 2015. Retrieved from: https://nccih.nih.gov/research/statistics/2010. Accessed May 18, 2016.

81. Sharkey JR, Bustillos BD, Ustattd Meyer MR, Legg TJ. Nutrition services for older adults. In Bernstein MA, Munoz MN, eds. *Nutrition for the Older Adult.* 2nd ed. Burlington, MA: Jones & Bartlett Learning; 2016.

82. Sharkey JR, Branch LG, Giuliani C, Haines PS, Zohoori N. Nutrient intake and BMI as predictors of severity of ADL disability over 1 year in homebound elders. *J Nutr Health Aging.* 2004;8:131–139.

83. Sharkey JR, Dean WR, Nalty C. Convenience stores and the marketing of foods and beverages through product assortment. *Am J Prev Med.* 2012;43(3S2):S109–S115.

84. Administration on Aging, Administration for Community Living. *A Profile of Older Americans: 2014.* Washington, DC: U.S. Department of Health and Human Services; 2014. Retrieved from: http://www.aoa.acl.gov/Aging_Statistics/Profile/2014/docs/2014-Profile.pdf. Accessed May 22, 2016.

85. Kamp BJ, Wellman NS, Russell C. Position of the American Dietetic Association, American Society for Nutrition, and Society for Nutrition Education: food and nutrition programs for community-residing older adults. *J Am Diet Assoc.* 2010;110:463–472.

86. Centers for Medicare & Medicaid Services. Home and community-based services 1915(c). Baltimore, MD: Centers for Medicare & Medicaid Services. Retrieved from: http://www.medicaid.gov/Medicaid-CHIP-Program-Information/By-Topics/Long-Term-Services-and-Supports/Home-and-Community-Based-Services/Home-and-Community-Based-Services-1915-c.html. Accessed May 19, 2016.

87. U.S. Department of Agriculture, Food and Nutrition Service. Supplemental Nutrition Assistance Program (SNAP). Washington, DC: U.S. Department of Agriculture, Food and Nutrition Service; updated August 11, 2016. Retrieved from: http://www.fns.usda.gov/SNAP/. Accessed September 1, 2016.

88. U.S. Department of Agriculture, Food and Nutrition Service. Child and Adult Care Food Program (CACFP). Washington, DC: U.S. Department of Agriculture, Food and Nutrition Service; updated September 22, 2014. Washington, DC: U.S. Department http://www.fns.usda.gov/cacfp/why-cacfp-important. Accessed May 19, 2016.

89. U.S. Department of Agriculture, Food and Nutrition Service. Senior Farmers' Market Nutrition Program (SFMNP). Washington, DC: U.S. Department of Agriculture, Food and Nutrition Service; updated April 15, 2015. Retrieved from: http://www.fns.usda.gov/sfmnp. Accessed May 19, 2016

90. World Health Organization. Ageing and life-course: what is "active ageing"? Geneva, Switzerland: World Health Organization. Retrieved from: http://www.who.int/ageing/active_ageing/en/. Accessed June 19, 2016.

91. Homer MJ. *Healthy Aging: Lessons from the Baltimore Longitudinal Study of Aging.* Washington, DC: National Institutes of Health, National Institute of Aging, and U.S. Department of Health and Human Services; 2010. Retrieved from: http://www.nia.nih.gov/sites/default/files/healthy_aging_lessons_from_the_baltimore_longitudinal_study_of_aging.pdf. Accessed May 16, 2016

92. Sun F, Norma IJ, White AE. Physical activity in older people: a systematic review. *BMC Public Health.* 2013;13:449.

93. World Health Organization. Global Strategy on Diet, Physical Activity and Health: global recommendations on physical activity for health. Geneva, Switzerland: World Health Organization. Retrieved from: http://www.who.int/dietphysicalactivity/factsheet_recommendations/en/. Accessed November 13, 2013.

94. Moran M, Van Cauwenberg J, Hercky-Linnewiel R, Cerin E, Deforche B, Plaut P. Understanding the relationships between the physical environment and physical activity in older adults: a systematic review of qualitative studies. *Int J Behav Nutr Phys Act.* July 17, 2014;11:79. doi:10.1186/1479-5868-11-79.

95. Centers for Disease Control and Prevention. Prevalence of physical activity, including lifestyle activities among adults—United States, 2001 and 2005. *MMWR.* 2007;56(46);1209–1212.

96. Nelson ME, Rejeski WJ, Blair SN, et al. Physical activity and public health in older adults: recommendations from the American College of Sports Medicine and the American Heart Association. *Med Sci Sports Exerc.* 2007;39(8):1435–1445.

97. U.S. Department of Health and Human Services. *2008 Physical Activity Guidelines for Americans.* Washington, DC: U.S. Department of Health and Human Services; 2008. Retrieved from: http://www.health.gov/paguidelines. Accessed May 19, 2016.

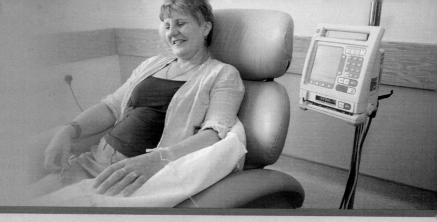

CHAPTER 15

Geriatric Nutrition

Roschelle A. Heuberger, PhD, RD

Chapter Outline

Senescence

Factors That Affect Dietary Intake in Later Life

General Nutrition Guidelines in the Geriatric Population

Polypharmacy in Geriatrics

End-of-Life Considerations

Nutrition Care Process

Learning Objectives

1. Describe the physiologic factors affecting aging that influence dietary intake in late life.

2. Delineate the nutritional recommendations and requirements in geriatrics, as well as the nutritional considerations of supplementation.

3. Explain the implications of declining cognition, polypharmacy, alcohol interactions, and frailty.

4. Discuss the controversies and issues in end-of-life decision making, artificial nutrition, and hydration, and the ethics of feeding and hydrating persons near death.

5. Synthesize the nutritional management of compromised older adults.

6. Evaluate the Nutrition Care Process and model for the assessment, diagnosis, intervention, and monitoring of compromised older adults.

7. Describe comorbidities in the compromised older adult population.

Case Study

Mr. Xi is a 94-year-old male. He is married to a disabled 84-year-old woman who cannot care for him at home any longer. He is suffering from frailty and severe cognitive decline due to vascular dementia; Mr. Xi has multiple signs and symptoms of late-stage dementia and frailty. Yesterday, a neighbor stopped by in the late afternoon to find food burning in the oven and determined that Mr Xi had forgotten about the chicken and potatoes he was baking for lunch.

Senescence

Preview Many factors influence the aging process. Genetic, behavioral, and environment factors all play a significant role in how we grow old.

In this chapter, an overview of special topics with aging is introduced. It begins with senescence and geriatric nutrition and then discusses factors affecting nutritional status, frailty, dependence, cognitive decline, polypharmacy, alcohol, and end-of-life considerations. Senescence, or the process of growing old, involves the accumulation of deleterious changes in cells that cause them to die more rapidly than they are replaced. Apoptosis, or preprogrammed cell death, occurs when the cells are no longer viable and the mechanisms for fixing errors in DNA, for example, are unable to keep up. There are also other definitions of aging that have to do with chronological age, or the number of years of life; physiological age, which has to do with the cell's innate ability to function properly; and phenotypical or functional age, which is the characterization of the expression of DNA under particular environmental constraints. The latter explains how someone who is genetically predetermined to be long lived and who has had the proper environment to prevent accumulation of damage to cells can be very physically and mentally fit despite being chronologically in their eighties or nineties.

Factors That Influence the Aging Process

There are multiple influences on the aging process and the rate with which the process occurs. Primary aging occurs as a function of time alone. The increased number of years of life results in increased loss of functional cells and increased vulnerability to stressors. Cells are not replaced so that tissues and organs experience the irreversible loss of viability over time. Secondary aging results from the effects of disease on the cell's abilities to function or be replaced. Disease can be either acute or chronic and may affect one or more cell types, tissues, organs, or systems. Primary aging results in a susceptibility to disease, or secondary aging.

Immunosenescence, or the failure of the immune system to perform due to age-related declines in function, has long been shown to occur.[1] Pro-inflammatory cytokines (chemical messengers) and circulating levels of inflammatory mediators are the hallmarks of these age-related changes; aging in and of itself decreases the numbers and the functionality of T cells, B cells (white blood cells), and other immunomodulators (proteins or glycolipids).[2] Tertiary aging occurs as a result of the interaction of the environment with the individual.

Multiple influences of financial status, social isolation, loss, cognitive changes, and other factors affect the aging process, accelerating pathophysiologic changes occurring in the older adult.[3] The oldest old have the greatest likelihood of having all three processes occurring simultaneously.[4] Geriatrics takes into consideration the unique medical and social factors of older adults to promote health and well-being with advancing age.

Case Study

Mr. Xi has had repeated urinary tract infections (UTIs) because he is unable to perform the activities of daily living (ADLs) involving proper hygiene, and, as a result, fecal bacteria have made their way up the urethra and caused severe infections. Because he is unable to mount an immune response, he becomes septic, meaning the infections spread to the blood and through the body, causing delirium, fainting, fever, pain, and difficulty breathing. He has been repeatedly admitted to the emergency room for administration of intravenous (IV) antibiotics, fluids, and electrolytes. He had been discharged to the home several times on multiple medications, with instructions to drink plenty of fluids.

Questions

1. How does decreased immunity ultimately further the frailty syndrome in Mr. Xi?
2. What are the factors that play into dehydration in Mr. Xi's case?

Recap This section provides some key definitions and concepts about senescence. Multiple factors influence the aging process. Primary aging is a result of time alone, with cells dying more rapidly than they are replaced by new ones. Secondary aging occurs because primary aging makes the individual more susceptible to disease. Tertiary aging occurs as a result of environmental impact on the individual.

1. What are the three tiers of aging?
2. How does apoptosis affect aging?
3. How do inflammatory mediators affect vulnerability to stressors?
4. How does a person's environment affect his or her nutritional status?
5. What other interrelated factors may affect senescence?

Factors That Affect Dietary Intake in Later Life

> **Preview** Pathophysiological and other changes that occur late in life can vastly affect nutritional status.

The deterioration of motor input, impaired cellular function, and cumulative damage result in overt changes that can limit food intake or alter food preferences. Availability or palatability of food items may not be conducive to increased intake. Furthermore, changes occurring from the presence of disease or disability may also decrease and deleteriously affect food consumption and food intake patterns.

Effects of Aging on Nutritional Status

Individuals vary in what they experience in terms of the effect of aging on their nutritional status. Older adults, a heterogeneous population, may have none, some, or all of the factors that influence overall nutriture (TABLE 15.1).

Physical and Health-Related Factors

As age increases and sensory input and motor function declines, persons may experience a loss of appetite known as **anorexia of aging** and a decrease in nutritious food consumption. The swallow reflexes are a complex cascade of neuronal impulses and muscular actions. Aging and pathophysiological changes can affect the person's ability to swallow properly, resulting in dysphagia (abnormal swallowing). There are varying degrees of swallow deficiency as well as different types of swallow reflex deterioration. Diets with varied thicknesses are prescribed, along with positioning techniques and other adaptions for dysphagia. Dysphagia has been associated with deficits in nutrition.[5]

Dysphagia is also associated with choking, drooling, and aspiration. Aspiration is the abnormal inhalation of food particles during an eating event. This results in blocked airways and increases the chance for pneumonia, a bacterial infection of the lungs, with associated inflammatory changes. Aspiration pneumonia may prove deadly to an older adult who already has a compromised immune system.[6]

Case Study

Mr. Xi also has recently been diagnosed with dysphagia and xerostomia. His dysphagia is due to his frailty and the loss of musculoskeletal function and neurological input. He is on a dysphagia diet, but it is hard to keep him hydrated with the thickened liquids, which he doesn't like. He has to be repeatedly reminded to drink over the course of the day and night. His wife cannot cope with caring for him and gets angry that he doesn't remember to drink thickened liquids, which increases his level of agitation and confusion.

Questions

1. What are some of the dementia symptoms that affect Mr. Xi's nutritional status?

There may be deficits in sensory perception, leading to symptoms such as **dysgeusia** or **ageusia** (abnormal taste or absence of taste); **dysosmia** or **anosmia** (abnormal smell or absence of smell), edentulousness (loss of teeth), periodontal disease (gum disease), ill-fitting dentures (causing pain when rubbing on the gums), or **xerostomia** (a condition causing dry mouth due to impaired salivary gland activity).[7–9] All these would influence the consumption of nutritious foods, from inability to chew and swallow properly, to the inability to taste or

---

Table 15.1				
Conditions that Impact the Nutritional Status of Older Adults				
Physiologic Conditions				
Ageusia	Atrophic gastritis	Dentures	Gastroesophageal reflux	Insomnia
Anosmia	Cognitive declines	Depression	Immunocompromise	Nausea
Anxiety	Confusion	Dysgeusia	Inactivity	Sleep–wake reversal
Aspiration	Constipation	Dysosmia	Incontinence	Tremor
Ataxia	Poor dentition	Dysphagia	Inflammation	Xerostomia
Psychosocial Conditions				
Agoraphobia	Geographic limitation	Loss—memory	Loss—control	
Medical and dental insurance coverage (uninsured)	Grief	Loss—peer group	Neglect/ elder abuse	
Falls	Inability to drive	Loss—separation	Social isolation	
Fiscal hardship	Insurance costs	Loss—independence	Vulnerability/safety	

smell food normally, which is an enormous factor influencing what and how much is eaten or whether food is enjoyed.

Abnormal walking, ataxia, dizziness, inner ear changes in equilibrium, falls, and fear of falling or lack of confidence in going outside may lead to an older person's inability to shop or obtain food.[10]

Gastrointestinal Factors

Gastrointestinal disturbances and lactose intolerance increase with age, limiting food choices and eating patterns and behaviors. Conditions, such as nausea, heartburn (gastrointestinal reflux), and constipation, are common in the oldest old. In addition, decreased activity of the parietal cells lining the stomach that occurs in advanced age can lead to achlorohydria (absence of hydrochloric acid, HCL), diminution of intrinsic factor (IF) production (IF is responsible for picking up vitamin B_{12}), and inability to digest and absorb proteins owing to decreased protein denaturation by HCL and proteolysis in the stomach.[11] The digestion and absorption of protein is dependent on the functionality of the gut; absorption depends on the ability of enzymes, transporters, and other factors to work properly or to be produced in appropriate amounts. Failure to obtain, digest, transport, utilize, and remove waste is a significant factor in nutritional status and the advent of frailty syndrome in the older adult.[12]

Mental and Neurological Factors

Depressed isolated persons are less likely to eat a nutritious diet. Other conditions, such as Parkinson's disease, with its hallmark tremors, or wandering, as seen in dementia patients, may increase nutritional needs, such as the need for energy and protein.[13] Cognitive changes and neuromuscular disease may cause increases in muscle wasting, leading to further frailty. Conditions that affect sleep–wake cycles, such as early-onset Alzheimer disease (AD), are associated with increased energy needs due to wandering and wakefulness at night.[14] "Sun-downing," or the agitation seen at the end of the day among early AD patients, may increase energy needs as well. Insomnia, sleep–wake disorders, and mental status changes such as confusion, memory loss, or agitation may also limit food intake. Persons may forget to eat, be afraid to eat, have a fear of being fed, become increasingly agitated with feeding, or may not be fed when they are awake in the middle of the night.[15–18] Vascular dementia is the cumulative loss of brain function due to the changes associated with aging and vascular narrowing of vessels to the brain, leading to loss of oxygen and nutrients and resulting in cell death.

Social/Environmental Factors

Persons who are frail and who can no longer participate in their own care or in social activities are less likely to be independent, to be active, to perform activities of daily

Case Study

Mr. Xi has fallen repeatedly over the past year, not breaking any bones, but becoming bruised, and he has had at least one documented concussion. This leads to further dizziness and falling. His wife tries to keep him sedated to prevent his wandering at night, and falling down the stairs, while she is sleeping. Mr. Xi continues to wander during the night and sleep most of the day. His dementia has features of abnormal circadian rhythm when the sleep–wake cycle is disturbed. He becomes very frightened and agitated when woken during the day to eat meals or take medication.

Questions

1. How do Mrs. Xi's older age, mobility problems, and health problems affect Mr. Xi's nutritional status?
2. What are some significant contributory factors in falls among the oldest old adult population?

living (ADLs) and are more likely to experience anxiety, depression, and isolation.[19,20] Other factors are retirement, fiscal hardship, or economic circumstances that impair the person's ability to purchase nutritious foods.[21] The burgeoning oldest old population is likely to be poor and have limitations on what they eat. Many may be using a social service program, such as Meals on Wheels or congregate meals, where food is prepared and either served at a community center or delivered to the person's home. Those who are homebound and receive Meals on Wheels and other government subsidies have no control over the food that is brought, or, if they are institutionalized, what meals are served. This loss of control is also a pervasive factor in depression and decline. Having no choice in what you eat can be detrimental to nutritional status.[22–24] More care facilities are moving to menus with options to improve intake.[25]

Advanced age also implies the loss of peer groups, spouses, friends, and family, and grief. Eating alone is considered a factor in the evaluation of older adults because it has been correlated with poor appetite, withdrawal, and lower intake of key macro- and micronutrients.[26] Loss is a great stressor, and the physical losses are as varied as the emotional ones. Loss implies loss of control over one's environment.[27] This alone can be a contributing factor to poor nutritional status in institutionalized older adults.

Persons in rural areas or inner cities may not be able to get to locations that serve meals or to go shopping for food. Cognitive decline may also impair a person's ability to shop, prepare, or eat safely. Caregivers may not be careful or educated in nutrition, and thus may not provide or assist the older adult with feeding appropriate items, thus secondarily contributing to malnutrition. Older adults requiring caregiving at higher levels and caregivers of those persons often perceive their own health and quality of life as being poor.[28–31]

Case Study

Mr. Xi cannot leave the home without chaperones. He also becomes very upset if restrained. He has not received general medical or dental care for many months, nor has he been involved in any social activities. His wife is hard of hearing and often yells when she doesn't understand what he is doing or what he wants. Mr. Xi has mild agnosia, a particular form of cognitive deficit, where he has lost his ability to recognize people's faces and places and to communicate effectively. He also has intermittent aphasia, an inability to speak or process language. Mr. Xi has a long history of dental and gastrointestinal problems, for which he has not been treated in recent months.

Mr. Xi had complained of pins and needles in his feet for some time. He also perceives a loss of sensation in his legs but cannot express what it is he feels. This results in an unsteady gait, ataxia, and a propensity to fall. Mr. Xi holds the wall when he walks. He has tried to go to the kitchen and make himself tea on multiple occasions during the night, neglecting to shut off the stove, put thickener into the beverage, or sit forward while drinking. This leads to choking and aspiration. The geriatrician told Mr. Xi that all of these are important to risk factors in persons with dysphagia and dementia. He has also fallen at night. This has resulted in accidents that have led to emergency room visits.

Question

1. How do age, genetics, comorbid conditions, and environment play into Mr. Xi's current nutritional status?

Malnutrition

Malnutrition, in conjunction with either inactivity or hyperactivity and aging itself, may lead older adults to becoming frail.[32-34] Frailty has been designated a "syndrome" or a composite of signs, symptoms, and the presence of multiple pathogenic processes or diseases. The frailty syndrome is characterized by the presence of multiple indicators of decline in function due to decreased lean body mass and total body water and increased total fat mass.

Frailty syndrome is diagnosed with the presence of two or more indicator groups:

- Impairment in physical functioning
- Impaired nutritional status
- Impaired cognitive abilities
- Impaired sensory abilities

The FRAIL Scale and other rating scales focus on different measurements for the assessment of frailty syndrome. (See TABLE 15.2.) In an effort to distinguish frailty from *disability*, or "being physically unable to perform activities that are required for specific purposes,"

Table 15.2

The International Academy of Nutrition and Aging: FRAIL Scale*

F	Fatigue (self-reported)
R	Resistance
A	Ambulation (slow walking speed)
I	Illness
L	Loss (5% or more in the past year)

*An older person is classified as frail when three or more components are present.

Dent E, Kowal P, Hoogendikl EO. Frailty measurement in research and clinical practice: a review. Eur J Intern Med. 2016; 31:3-10.

additional measures were included: self-reported exhaustion, weakness as measured by the loss of grip strength (See FIGURE 15.1) over time, reduction in the speed with which the person could walk, and decline in physical activities. (See TABLE 15.3.) Weight loss, including loss of total body weight and of lean body mass, or other measures, such as a 10-pound or more total weight loss within the last year, are also featured.[35-37] There is lack of standardization regarding the definitions and symptoms to define frailty and for measurement of the "frailty syndrome."

Sarcopenia

Because of the increasing rates of obesity in this country, another term was coined: "sarcopenic obesity." This is when an obese person has very little muscle mass and is therefore frail and weak. The person is classified as overweight or obese when measured by body weight alone for their height. Central or abdominal obesity is common in this population. This form of obesity is also known to cause metabolic syndrome in older age groups. Persons who are older and who have sarcopenic central obesity are more prone to having complications and a rapid deterioration in their physical functioning. In addition to the inflammation caused by the central obesity, there are increased inflammatory processes

Table 15.3

Grip Strength Measurements Derived from Cardiovascular Health Study Data

Weakness as Determined by Measurements of Grip Strength

Females	*Males*
≤ 17 kg for BMI ≤ 23	≤ 29 kg for BMI ≤ 24
≤ 17.3 kg for BMI = 23.1 – 26	≤ 30 kg for BMI = 24.1 – 26
≤ 18 kg for BMI = 26.1 – 29	≤ 30 kg for BMI = 26.1 – 28
≤ 21 kg for BMI > 29	≤ 32 kg for BMI > 28

Pel-Little RE, Schuurmans MJ, Emmelot-Vonk MH, Verhaar HJ. Frailty: defining and measuring of a concept. *J Nutr Health Aging*. 2009;13(4):390–394.

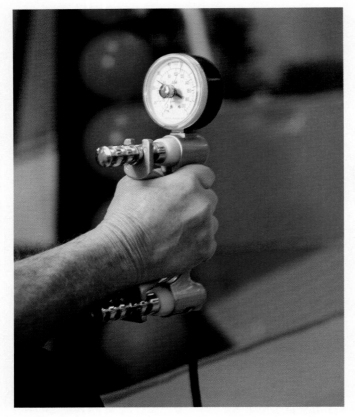

Figure 15.1
Grip strength is a reliable measure of the amount of static force the hand can squeeze around a dynamometer. When following standardized methods and compared to normative data, grip strength is related to physical frailty and disability, bone mineral density and risk of osteoporosis, and is predictive of mortality from some diseases.

©John Foxx/Stockbyte/Getty Images

from comorbid diseases and from aging itself. Therefore, a heightened state of inflammation results in the rapid decline in function among this population.[38–40] Risk for disease advancement and death increases for the individual who is frail, abdominally obese, and sarcopenic.

Recap There are many factors, such as physical or health-related factors like swallowing problems or infections, and social and environmental factors such as financial hardship or geographic location that impact nutrition. Malnutrition and sarcopenia, or the loss of lean muscle mass, are important concerns. Frailty is a syndrome that is very common in older persons. Frailty implies the loss of muscle mass and impaired overall functioning.

1. Are all older persons equally affected in terms of their nutritional status?
2. How does dysphagia complicate the ability to be well nourished?

3. What oral health factors or sensory changes might affect consumption of nutritious food?
4. What is frailty and why should this be of concern for older person?
5. What social or environmental considerations must be assessed when it comes to older adults and their nutrition?

Case Study

Mr. Xi is becoming increasingly frail. He is significantly sarcopenic and meets the criteria for the frailty syndrome. While he has lost a significant amount of weight, and only his belly appears to be large, he has lost height as he has aged as a result of kyphosis (stooping of the posture related to degeneration of the discs and their cushions along the spine) and osteoporosis (loss of bone mineral and bone strength). This causes his body mass index (BMI) calculation to classify him as overweight. He still sleeps most of the day and is now unable to walk long distances or climb stairs. His grip strength is poor. He weighs 155 pounds and is 65 inches tall. His grip strength is 25 kg.

Question

1. What are the key indicators of frailty in older adults and which of those are relevant to Mr. Xi?

News You Can Use

You don't need to be thin to be frail! According to the British Geriatrics Society, there are plenty of people who are overweight but still considered frail. Why? Because they don't have muscle mass and are often very sedentary. Their health, mobility, and level of strength are poor, and sometimes they are even bedbound and prone to bedsores owing to their fat mass. The signs and symptoms of frailty include decreased walking speed, poor hand grip strength, and declining lean muscle mass. Obese persons often have these signs and symptoms. In addition, once you take into account the diseases a person has, people who are either extremely thin or who are considered overweight have greater risk for deterioration and death. This is called a U-shaped relationship. Several research studies have concluded that the development and maintenance of a BMI > 30 in late adulthood and advanced age predispose an older person to becoming frail and having more disability as well as disease.

Reference

Sheehan K. You don't need to be thin to be frail. London, UK: British Geriatrics Society; November 21, 2013. Retrieved from: https://britishgeriatricssociety.wordpress.com/2013/11/21/you-dont-need-to-be-thin-to-be-frail/. Accessed September 29, 2016.

Case Study

Mr. Xi has been declining for almost 2 years. He no longer reads the newspaper or watches the news, which were his hobbies. He doesn't know what year it is or what month or day. He doesn't recognize his daughter, who lives in another state and can only visit occassionally. Mr. Xi's wife doesn't want to worry her daughter, so she doesn't tell her about the cognitive decline, the falls, and the emergency room visits. Mr. Xi used to take care of all the finances and bills. Because he can't do this any longer, the couple have had the electricity turned off because Mrs. Xi didn't think she had to pay the bill right away. Mr. Xi spent several nights in very cold temperatures, and because he has poor thermoregulation due to poor circulation, his body temperature dipped below normal and he has suffered mild hypothermia.

Mr. Xi is depressed and anxious. When he is lucid, he realizes that he is no longer able to do things or take care of himself. He becomes more agitated and doesn't want to eat. The couple receives Meals on Wheels, and the food is very unappetizing in but because of his choking, the food is placed into a blender all at once and comes out smelling and looking unappealing. Mr. Xi doesn't really taste or smell anything that hasn't been sprinkled with a great deal of sugar or salt. Mr. Xi has had a slow but steady rise in his average blood pressure, from the normal 120/80 to 160/100 mm Hg in the past year. His blood sugar levels have also greatly fluctuated from very high to very low. His hyper- and hypoglycemia have also caused him to feel dizzy and become more dehydrated, which has contributed to his falls. His wife would rather that he sleep than wander at night and has started to give him brandy along with his 11 different nightly medications.

Questions

1. Explain how lack of sensory input affects Mr. Xi's nutritional status
2. Describe the relationships between cognitive decline and impaired nutritional status, using physiological, biochemical, and cellular mechanisms to illustrate the relationships.

The Big Picture

The progression of clinical frailty in the older adult.

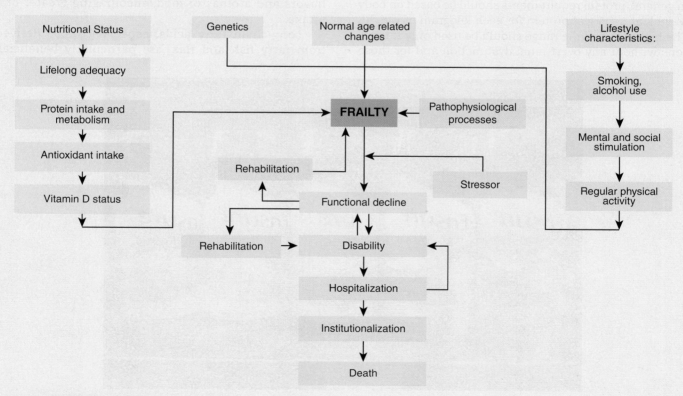

The progression of clinical frailty in the older adult.

Modified from: Abellan van Kan G, Rolland YM, Morley JE, Vellas B. Frailty: towards a clinical definition. *J Am Med Direct Assoc*. 2008;9(2):71–72; Bortz W. Understanding frailty. *J Gerontol A Biol Sci Med Sci*. 2010;65A(3):255–256; Morley JE, Haren MT, Rolland Y, Kim MJ. Frailty. *Med Clin N Am*. 2006;90(5):837–847.

General Nutrition Guidelines in the Geriatric Population

Preview The need to individualize nutritional and lifestyle recommendations is of utmost importance to successfully promote health and well-being with advancing age becomes increasingly crucial as older adults experience multiple and simultaneous health conditions, become more frail and shift from healthy to ill and infirmed. Few nutritional needs change with chronological age alone; this section reviews the influences that failing health and declining functional status have on nutrient requirements and intake for frail older adults.

For many older adults there is no clear demarcation from independent and free living to dependence but rather a continuum of deteriorating health and function. It is necessary to provide an individualized nutrition plan for older persons, particularly if they have one or more disease states that require dietary modifications, such as hypertension and decreasing the sodium content of the diet or atrophic gastritis that requires monitoring vitamin B$_{12}$.[41–43]

Protein

In general, protein requirements should be based on body weight, at 1–1.5 g of protein for each kilogram of weight. The higher end of the range should be used only for persons without any overt renal dysfunction and for those with impaired absorption and hypercatabolic conditions, such as infections, decubitus ulcers, and cancer, among others. The protein should be of high biological quality such as eggs, meat, fish, or poultry and should contain the complete array of needed amino acids. Oral nutrition supplement products contain protein sources (caseinates or soy protein isolates) and are ready to eat and convenient for older adults. Oral nutrition supplements may be an easier alternative to increasing intake of protein from food sources for someone who is eating poorly.[44] (see **FIGURE 15.2**)

Fats

Similar to younger adults, fats in particular, trans and saturated fats, should be kept low in the diet, as should cholesterol sources. Fats should comprise less than 30% of total calories, with saturated fat sources comprising less than 10%. Total cholesterol ingestion should be below 300 mg per day from all animal sources. Trans fats should not be included in the diet, or if they are, they should remain below 0.5% of total calories. Total calories should be based on ideal body weight, at 30–35 calories per kilogram ideal body weight. However, if the person has a poor appetite, the use of fats increase energy (kilocalories) and increase taste perception because fats carry odor molecules and taste molecules better than other macronutrients. This may enhance flavors and aromas of food, encouraging greater oral intake.

Long-chain fatty acids, especially those derived from fatty fish and flax, are particularly beneficial,

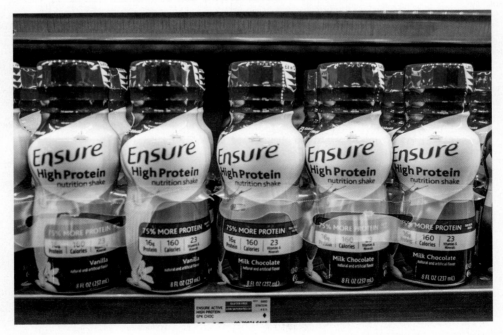

Figure 15.2
Oral nutrition supplements are an easy and convenient option for older adults that are having difficulty meeting their nutritional needs with food alone.

©Sara Stathas/Alamy Stock Photo

with known heart health benefits as well as evidence to suggest that they slow cognitive decline over time. (see FIGURE 15.3A and B) Many of these fish oils can be obtained through supplementation if oral ingestion is not sufficient.[45]

Carbohydrates

Carbohydrates are a group of compounds that include simple sugars, starches, complex carbohydrates (such as whole grains), and fiber. Recommendations regarding the consumption of carbohydrates in the adult population focus on limiting the intake of simple sugars because the foods and drinks that contain high levels of simple sugars often don't have as many vitamins and minerals, and thus are "empty" calories are even more imperative in frail older adults. Examples of these foods and drinks include the following:

- Regular soda
- Products containing high-fructose corn syrup, such as salad dressings and condiments
- Sweets such as candy or snack bars
- Baked goods, such as cakes or doughnuts
- Canned fruits in syrup

In addition, sugars may dysregulate blood glucose levels in those persons prone to insulin resistance and may contribute to obesity, dental caries, gingivitis, and oral disease. Carbohydrates that are complex, like whole grains that have soluble and insoluble fibers, are best. Choosing whole-grain breads, pasta, brown rice, cereals, and tortillas, wraps, or pitas is important. Older adults need an average of 3 "ounce equivalents" of whole grains per day. Examples of whole-grain ounce equivalents are these:

- Whole-grain slice of bread
- 1 cup of whole-grain ready-to-eat cereal
- ½ cup of cooked brown rice
- 1 whole-wheat tortilla
- 1 whole-grain pita
- 5 whole-wheat crackers

Fiber

Fiber is also extremely important in geriatric nutrition. Fiber sources may not be easily chewed if there are dental problems. Fresh fruits and vegetables may be more costly or not accessible to those who can't shop any longer. Fiber, both soluble and insoluble, is important for colonic health and populates the colon with friendly bacteria that produce short-chain fatty acids, vitamin K, and vitamin B_{12}. Short-chain fatty acids fuel the intestinal cells, which are rapidly sloughed and replaced. They also help in the control of metabolic processes. Vitamin B_{12} is important in many metabolic reactions, and long-term deficiencies result in irreversible nerve damage or neuropathy. Vitamin K is involved in normal blood clotting.[46,47]

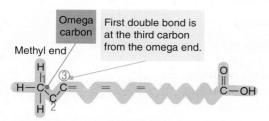

Alpha-linolenic, an omega-3 fatty acid

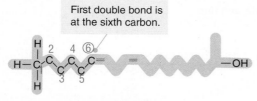

Linoleic, an omega-6 fatty acid

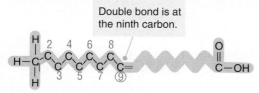

A   **Oleic, an omega-9 fatty acid**

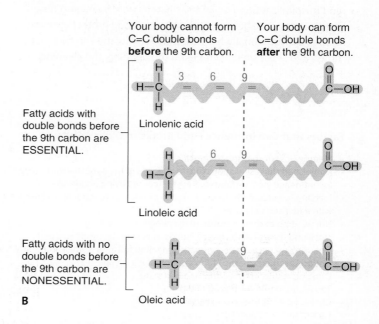

B

Figure 15.3

(A) Omega-3, omega-6, and omega-9 fatty acids. Unsaturated fatty acids can be classified by counting from the omega carbon to the location of the first double bond. (B) Essential and nonessential fatty acids. The human body makes some types of fatty acids, but others are essential to obtain from the diet.

Fiber intake also requires fluid intake to relieve constipation and improve gut function. Persons with age-related changes in their gastrointestinal tract may not be able to handle the quantities of fiber that are recommended. Bloating, flatulence, cramping, and stomach upset may keep an older person from consuming fiber. High-fiber diets cause feelings of fullness, early satiety, and other symptoms that decrease overall food intake, which could be problematic for those struggling to meet their target caloric and nutrition requirements. Fiber does, however, decrease cholesterol available from foods, decreases cancer risk, improves heart health, and helps relieve constipation. The recommendations of 35 g per day may not be achievable for an older adult especially those with poor appetite. Formulas are now routinely fortified with fiber, so older

adults can get more than they would if they were eating a high-fiber diet.[48,49]

Hydration

Hydration is one of the most important issues in geriatric nutrition. Fluid intake may be hampered by many factors, such as those listed in TABLE 15.4.

An older adult has diminished capacity to store body water because of decreased muscle mass. Older persons also get dehydrated more easily resulting from decreased thermoregulation (ability to adjust to changing temperatures), the use of diuretic medications (medications that cause increased urination or diuresis), and an inability to transfer water efficiently from tissues to the bloodstream without excretion through sweat, breath, urine, and feces. Water intake

Case Study

Calculation

Mr. Xi weighs 70 kg. He only drinks 8 ounces of thickened liquids per day. He doesn't like the texture of the thickened liquids. It is also expensive to buy the thickener at the store, so his wife tries to conserve the amounts that she uses. Mr. Xi is mostly awake during the night and his wife is sleeping. He doesn't remember that he is not supposed to drink anything without the Thick-It product. He often chokes on the water he tries to drink. One ounce of liquid is equal to approximately 30 mL. He drinks approximately 240 mL/day, when he should be drinking 10 times that amount, (35 mL × 70 kg = 2,450 mL) of liquid per day. His dehydration has contributed to his repeated urinary tract infections, followed by delirium and hospitalizations. His wife has had trouble managing his urinary incontinence because he won't wear adult protective undergarments. Additionally has soiled the couch and the bed many times, and she is tired of changing the bedding and cleaning. As

a result, his wife prefers not having him drink too much fluids. He also has a long-standing history of constipation and obstruction, owing to gastrointestinal transit deficit, with weakened gastrointestinal tract muscles, dehydration, and the constipating effects of his medications.

Questions

1. Calculate the recommendation for the following for Mr. Xi:
BMI (kg/m²)
Energy needs (total kcal/day)
Protein needs (g/d)
Fluid needs (ml/d)
Fiber recommendation (g/d)

2. State the DRIs value and rationale for the following nutrients Iron, vitamin D, calcium, sodium, potassium, vitamin B12, folate, and zinc

Table 15.4

Factors that Can Influence Fluid Intake in Older Adults

- Memory loss (forgetting to drink)
- Diminished thirst sensations due to changes in the hypothalamus (a part of the brain responsible for hunger and thirst control)
- Incontinence (not wanting to drink for fear of having accidents)
- Inability to get and drink liquids due to physical or functional declines (can't get up to get a drink, can't hold a cup because of tremors, such as with Parkinson's disease)
- Not wanting to drink because of dysphagia and choking
- Not liking the use of thickened liquids as part of the dysphagia diet
- Not drinking because of early satiety (feeling full after a small amount of food or liquid is ingested)
- Not accustomed to consuming enough fluids
- Drinking results in dysgeusia, or a bad taste
- Too fatigued to drink enough fluids
- Gastric upset with drinking certain beverages
- Lack of taste or appeal of beverages
- Fear of drinking, due to dementia or agitation, or fear of the person offering the beverage
- Attitudes and beliefs regarding drinking (only will drink hot or cold beverages, only drink with meals)

Table 15.5

Summary Table: Dietary Reference Intakes (DRIs) for Carbohydrate, Fiber, Fat, Protein, and Water for Adults Aged 51 Years and Older

Nutrient	Value	Recommendation
Carbohydrates	AMDR	45–65% total daily calories
	DRI	130 g/day
	EAR	100 g/day
Fiber	AI: Men	30 g/day
	AI: Women	21 g/day
Fat	AMDR	20–35% total daily calories
n-6 PUFA (linoleic acid)	AMDR	5–10% total daily calories
	AI: Men	14 g/day
	AI: Women	11 g/day
n-3 PUFA (alpha-linolenic acid)	AMDR	0.6–1.2% total daily calories
	AI: Men	1.6 g/day
	AI: Women	1.1 g/day
Protein	AMDR	10–35% total daily calories
	RDA	0.8 g/kg/day
	EAR	0.66 g/kg/day
	RDA: Men	56 g/day
	RDA: Women	46 g/day
Water	AI: Men	3.7 L/day
	AI: Women	2.7 L/day

AI = Adequate Intake; AMDR = Acceptable Macronutrient Distribution Range; EAR = Estimated Average Requirement; PUFA = polyunsaturated fatty acid; RDA = Recommended Dietary Allowance.

Modified from Institute of Medicine, Food and Nutrition Board. *Dietary Reference Intakes for Energy, Carbohydrate, Fiber, Fat, Fatty Acids, Cholesterol, Protein and Amino Acids (Macronutrients)*. Washington, DC: National Academies Press; 2005.

should parallel calorie intake with 35 mL per kilogram of body weight per day.[50–52] (**TABLE 15.5**)

Micronutrients

Dietary recommendations for frail older adults should be liberalized if possible to promote intake. Stringent restrictions on compounds such as salt, for example may actually deter eating because of lack of taste. Keeping sodium below 2 g per day and potassium high at 5 g per day is a rule of thumb, except if the older person is taking potassium-sparing diuretics, such a spironolactone and triamterene, in which case potassium-containing salt substitutes and supplements with high levels of potassium and phosphorus should be avoided.

Iron

Iron deficiency and anemia of chronic disease are also issues in the older adult population. Because iron has the potential to act as a free radical, iron status should be closely monitored. Ferrous gluconate is the most easily absorbed and most effective, even under conditions such as the loss of HCL secretion in the gastric lumen.

Acid enhances iron absorption by changing its redox state. Animal sources of iron, the use of acidic foods to enhance iron absorption, and the use of supplements that are balanced for optimal iron absorption should be considered. The average requirements for iron are 8 mg per day.[53–55]

Calcium and Vitamin D

Calcium and vitamin D are important nutrients to consider in particular with older adults that are institutionalized or homebound. The requirements for calcium are to exceed 1,200 mg a day and exceed 800 IU for vitamin D. It is estimated that a majority of older adults are deficient in vitamin D if they have not been supplemented. Because of the issues with osteoporosis, cancer, musculoskeletal, cognitive, and neurological disease, among others, that are associated with vitamin D deficit and abnormalities resulting in calcium homeostasis, there has been a push to monitor older persons for active vitamin D levels, using blood assays for 1,25 dihydroxycholecalciferol over time. Vitamin D production from skin declines with age; older adults do not get large amounts of vitamin D from foods, such as oily fish, and do not go outdoors much in wintertime. In addition, the kidneys and liver must perform hydroxylation of the vitamin to produce the active form, which is a superhormone and responsible for turning on and off multiple genes for the synthesis of important proteins and cytokines and for controlling systemic functions, in addition to calcium homeostasis. (see **FIGURE 15.4**)[56–59]

Vitamin K

Vitamin K is a nutrient required in small amounts but is essential for normal blood clotting. Recommendations have been made to avoid vitamin K–containing foods, such as leafy greens, if an older adult is taking blood thinners such as warfarin. This is not actually the case. The vitamin K–containing foods are to be taken in at a constant rate so that the medication can remain at a constant blood level without any complications. As long as intake of high vitamin K–containing foods is regularly eaten in the same amounts, there should not be restrictions on those foods.

Vitamin B$_{12}$

Older adults with atrophic gastritis or impaired synthesis of the transporters for vitamin B$_{12}$, either due to lack of intrinsic factor, transcobalamin, or other proteins, may be at risk for deficiency. Liver impairment or poor protein intake may also become contributing factors. Because vitamin B$_{12}$ is stored in the liver and is recycled, usually pathological conditions contribute to the deficiency, which may lead to irreversible nerve damage. Vitamin B$_{12}$ comes from animal products, but supplementation or administration either sublingually or via a nasal spray is very effective.[60,61]

VITAMIN D: FROM SOURCE TO DESTINATION

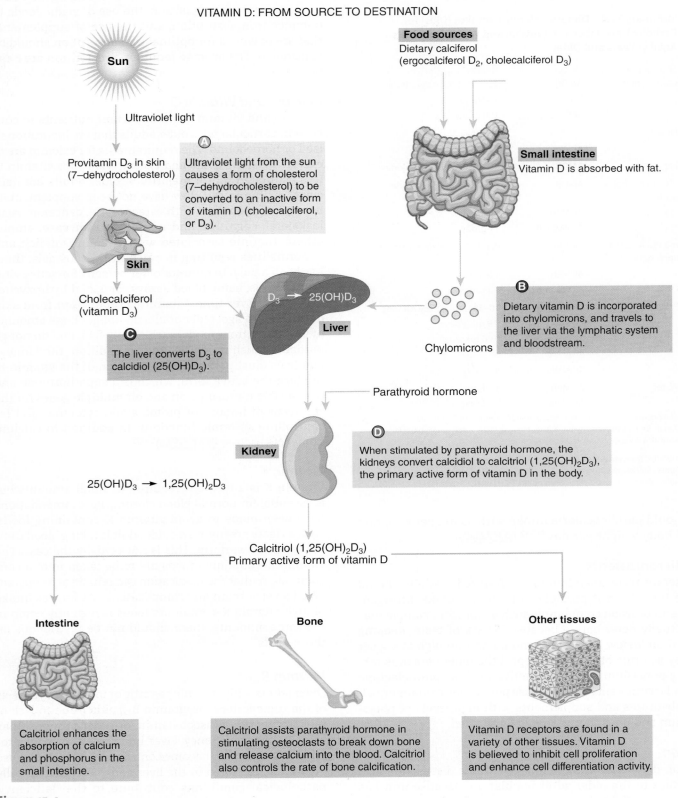

Food sources
Dietary calciferol
(ergocalciferol D$_2$, cholecalciferol D$_3$)

Ultraviolet light

Provitamin D$_3$ in skin
(7–dehydrocholesterol)

A Ultraviolet light from the sun
causes a form of cholesterol
(7–dehydrocholesterol) to be
converted to an inactive form
of vitamin D (cholecalciferol,
or D$_3$).

Small intestine
Vitamin D is absorbed with fat.

Skin

Cholecalciferol
(vitamin D$_3$)

D$_3$ → 25(OH)D$_3$

Liver

C The liver converts D$_3$ to
calcidiol (25(OH)D$_3$).

B Dietary vitamin D is incorporated
into chylomicrons, and travels to
the liver via the lymphatic system
and bloodstream.

Chylomicrons

Parathyroid hormone

Kidney

25(OH)D$_3$ → 1,25(OH)$_2$D$_3$

D When stimulated by parathyroid hormone, the
kidneys convert calcidiol to calcitriol (1,25(OH)$_2$D$_3$),
the primary active form of vitamin D in the body.

Calcitriol (1,25(OH)$_2$D$_3$)
Primary active form of vitamin D

Intestine

Bone

Other tissues

Calcitriol enhances the
absorption of calcium
and phosphorus in the
small intestine.

Calcitriol assists parathyroid hormone in
stimulating osteoclasts to break down bone
and release calcium into the blood. Calcitriol
also controls the rate of bone calcification.

Vitamin D receptors are found in a
variety of other tissues. Vitamin D
is believed to inhibit cell proliferation
and enhance cell differentiation activity.

Figure 15.4
Vitamin D: from source to destination. Vitamin D is unique because given sufficient sunlight, the human body can
synthesize all it needs. Both dietary and endogenous vitamin D must be activated by reactions in the kidneys and liver.
Active vitamin D [1,25(OH)2D3, or calcitriol] is important for calcium balance and bone health and may have a role in
cell differentiation. Highlighted areas maybe affected in older adults.

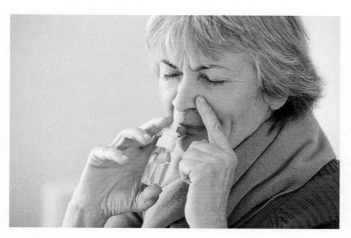

©Image Point Fr/Shutterstock

Other B Vitamins

Folic acid along with vitamins B_{12} and B_6 function as coenzymes in the metabolism of one carbon units and homocysteine. Homocysteine is a nonessential sulfur containing amino acid produced in the metabolism of methionine or transsulfuration of cysteine (see FIGURE 15.5). Hyperhomocystenemia, which can result from low levels of vitamins B_6, B_{12}, or folate, is an independent risk factor for vascular disease. The fortification of the food supply with folic acid although intended primarily to lower the incidence of neural tube defects has been beneficial in raising serum folate levels. However, serum folate should be monitored in older adults because fortification of foods in combination with supplementation could lead to masking a vitamin B_{12} deficiency. The other B vitamins are not often problematic in terms of deficiency for older persons as a result of fortification of the food supply. There are some considerations with niacin and thiamin. Niacin in high doses had previously been used to regulate hypertension and is known to mediate blood vessel responsiveness. A minimum of 15 mg per day is required. Because it is involved in so many reactions as a cofactor throughout the body, thiamin status may become problematic in persons who overconsume ethanol or drinking alcohol. The tolerable upper intake levels of micronutrients for older adults are listed in TABLE 15.6 .

Alcohol dehydrogenase and acetaldehyde dehydrogenase are just a two of the enzymes required for the detoxification of alcohols, and they require thiamin to perform. The body is required to handle many other types of alcohols. An alcohol is anything with an OH group. Retinol, or preformed vitamin A, is an example of an alcohol. Certain medications have a marked impact on alcohol modification or reduction in the body, and thus older adults, who frequently take these medications, may have increased needs for thiamin-dependent enzymes and thus have increased dietary requirements for thiamin.[62,63]

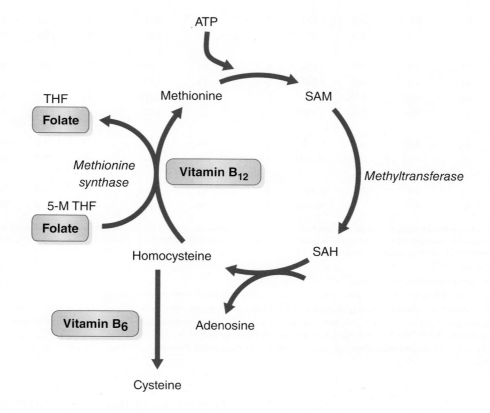

Figure 15.5

Folate, Vitamin B12, and Vitamin B6 Metabolism. ATP = adenosine triphosphate; SAM=S-adenosyl-methionine; SAH=S-adenosyl-homocysteine; 5-M THF=5-methyl tetrahydrofolate; THF=tetrahydrofolate.

Table 15.6

Tolerable Upper Intake Levels (ULs[1])

Life stage group	Vitamin A[2] (µg/d)	Vitamin D (µg/d)	Vitamin E[3,4] (mg/d)	Niacin[4] (mg/d)	Vitamin B6 (mg/d)	Folate[4] (µg/d)	Vitamin C (mg/d)	Choline (g/d)	Calcium (g/d)	Phosphorus (g/d)	Magnesium[5] (mg/d)	Sodium (g/d)
Infants												
0-6 mo	600	25	ND[7]	ND	ND	ND	ND	ND	ND	ND	ND	ND
7-12 mo	600	25	ND	ND	ND	ND	ND	ND	ND	ND	ND	ND
Children												
1-3 y	600	50	200	10	30	300	400	1.0	2.5	3	65	1.5
4-8 y	900	50	300	15	40	400	650	1.0	2.5	3	110	1.9
Males, females												
9-13 y	1,700	50	600	20	60	600	1,200	2.0	2.5	4	350	2.2
14-18 y	2,800	50	800	30	80	800	1,800	3.0	2.5	4	350	2.3
19-70 y	3,000	50	1,000	35	100	1,000	2,000	3.5	2.5	4	350	2.3
>70 y	3,000	50	1,000	35	100	1,000	2,000	3.5	2.5	3	350	2.3
Pregnancy												
≤18 y	2,800	50	800	30	80	800	1,800	3.0	2.5	3.5	350	2.3
19-50 y	3,000	50	1,000	35	100	1,000	2,000	3.5	2.5	3.5	350	2.3
Lactation												
≤18 y	2,800	50	800	30	80	800	1,800	3.0	2.5	4	350	2.3
19-50 y	3,000	50	1,000	35	100	1,000	2,000	3.5	2.5	4	350	2.3

Life stage group	Iron (mg/d)	Zinc (mg/d)	Selenium (µg/d)	Iodine (µg/d)	Copper (µg/d)	Manganese (mg/d)	Fluoride (mg/d)	Molybdenum (µg/d)	Boron (mg/d)	Nickel (mg/d)	Vanadium[6] (mg/d)	Chloride (g/d)
Infants												
0-6 mo	40	4	45	ND	ND	ND	0.7	ND	ND	ND	ND	ND
7-12 mo	40	5	60	ND	ND	ND	0.9	ND	ND	ND	ND	ND
Children												
1-3 y	40	7	90	200	1,000	2	1.3	300	3	0.2	ND	2.3
4-8 y	40	12	150	300	3,000	3	2.2	600	6	0.3	ND	2.9
Males, females												
9-13 y	40	23	280	600	5,000	6	10	1,100	11	0.6	ND	3.4
14-18 y	45	34	400	900	8,000	9	10	1,700	17	1.0	ND	3.6
19-70 y	45	40	400	1,100	10,000	11	10	2,000	20	1.0	1.8	3.6
>70 y	45	40	400	1,100	10,000	11	10	2,000	20	1.0	1.8	3.6
Pregnancy												
≤18 y	45	34	400	900	8,000	9	10	1,700	17	1.0	ND	3.6
19-50 y	45	40	400	1,100	10,000	11	10	2,000	20	1.0	ND	3.6
Lactation												
≤18 y	45	34	400	900	8,000	9	10	1,700	17	1.0	ND	3.6
19-50 y	45	40	400	1,100	10,000	11	10	2,000	20	1.0	ND	3.6

[1] UL = The maximum level of daily nutrient intake that is likely to pose no risk of adverse effects. Unless otherwise specified, the UL represents total intake from food, water, and supplements. Due to lack of suitable data, ULs could not be established for vitamin K, thiamin, riboflavin, vitamin B12, pantothenic acid, biotin, or carotenoids. In the absence of ULs, extra caution may be warranted in consuming levels above recommended intakes.

[2] As preformed vitamin A (retinol) only.

[3] As α-tocopherol; applies to any form of supplemental α-tocopherol.

[4] The ULs for vitamin E, niacin, and folate apply to synthetic forms obtained from supplements, fortified foods, or a combination of the two.

[5] The ULs for magnesium represent intake from a pharmacological agent only and do not include intake from food and water.

[6] Although vanadium in food has not been shown to cause adverse effects in humans, there is no justification for adding vanadium to food and vanadium supplements should be used with caution. The UL is based on adverse effects in laboratory animals and these data could be used to set a UL for adults but not children or adolescents.

[7] ND = Not determinable due to lack of data on adverse effects in this age group and concern with regard to lack of ability to handle excess amounts. Source of intake should be from food only to prevent high levels of intake.

Trace Minerals

Some trace elements are also very important in geriatric nutrition. Zinc is an example. Because zinc is important to sensory and neurological function, zinc is important in taste and smell. It is also important in immune function. Zinc is not easily obtained from foods, because foods that are very high in zinc, such as shellfish, are not readily available or provided. The transporters for zinc,

Table 15.7

Sources of Zinc and Selenium from Foods

Zinc Sources: High-Zinc Foods		Selenium Sources: High-Selenium Foods	
Food	*Milligrams/serving*	*Food*	*Micrograms/serving*
Oysters	200	Brazil nuts	500
Enriched cereals	35	Oysters	130
Crab	16	Tuna fish	90
Baked beans and pork	12	Whole-wheat bread toasted (fortified)	13

such as metallothionein, are also not produced effectively by the body at oldest age or with any decrease in liver functionality. Zinc recommendations are set for approximately 10 mg/d. There are genetic differences among individuals in terms of their capacity to absorb and utilize minerals like zinc and selenium. Selenium is very important to the synthesis of glutathione, a potent antioxidant, made in the liver through the methionine cycle. Selenium recommendations are 55 mcg per day.[64,65] (See TABLE 15.7 .)

Alcohol

Alcohol intake in moderation has been shown to have health effects in younger persons. The baby boomer generation, now entering older adult life, was brought up with this belief. However, alcohol use in the older adult population should be strongly discouraged. FIGURE 15.6A–D shows the progression of liver damage that can result from alcohol overuse. Geriatric populations are at increased risk from adverse events related to alcohol, including but not limited to falls, accidents, drug–ethanol

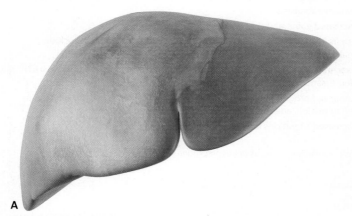

A

©Sebastian Kaulitzki/Alamy Stock Photo

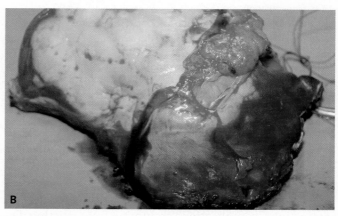

B

©Chaikom/Shutterstock

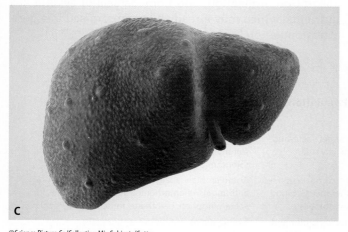

C

©Science Picture Co/Collection Mix Subjects/Getty

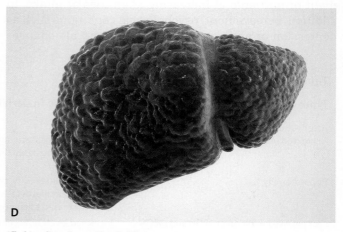

D

©The Science Picture Company/Alamy Stock Photo

Figure 15.6
(A) Healthy (B) Fatty (C) Fibrotic (D) Cirrhotic

Table 15.8

Age-Related Changes Negatively Influencing Tolerance to Ethanol in the Older Adult

Age-Related Change	Effect
Decreased alcohol dehydrogenase (gastric)	Decreased first-pass metabolism.
Decreased alcohol dehydrogenase (hepatic)	Decreased second-pass metabolism.
Decreased acetaldehyde dehydrogenase	Increased circulating levels of acetaldehyde.
Decreased catalase production	Increased circulation of ethanol and by-products of detoxification.
Decreased efficiency C-p450E-1	Increased circulation of ethanol and by-products of detoxification.
Decreased microsomal ethanol oxidizing system function (general)	Decreased metabolism.
Inefficient excretion (decrements in renal capabilities)	Increased retention of ethanol and by-products.
Increased passage of ethanol across blood–brain barrier	Increased intoxication, lengthened inebriation, increased accumulation of ethanol in the CNS.
Alterations in the HPA axis	Increased vulnerability to CNS effects of ethanol.
Alterations in cortisol secretion	Increased vulnerability to hormonal effects of ethanol.
Alterations in neurotransmission, sensitivity to neurotransmitters, and changes in synaptic architecture	Increased vulnerability to CNS effects of ethanol.
Sarcopenia leading to decrements in total body water	Decreased dilution and distribution of ethanol, leading to increased levels in circulation.
Poorer defense against reactive oxygen species	Increased ethanol damage to viable cells.
Prescribed medication usage requiring cytochrome metabolism (e.g., CYP2E1 binding site interactions)	Interactions with ethanol that may either decrease the drug's metabolism or enhance it, depending on the drug, or allow alcohol to circulate while drug metabolism occurs.
Vulnerability to drug–nutrient–ethanol cellular damage (vitamin A–aspirin–ethanol)	Damage to gastric mucosa increases absorption of ethanol, decreases first-pass metabolism.
Excessive alcohol to brain cell ratio associated with neuronal losses	Increased vulnerability to CNS effects of ethanol.
Displacement of nutrient-dense foods with alcohol	Ethanol entry into circulation is rapid, and long-term outcomes include malnutrition.
Increased incidence of depressive, anxiolytic, and cognitive disorders	Exacerbation of existing mental status changes; ethanol is classified as a CNS depressant.
Increased incidence of periodontal, salivary, and other orofacial changes	Enhanced progression of pathophysiological changes leading to infection, inflammation, edentulousness, poor nutritional intake.
Alterations in sensory perception (dysosmia, dysgeusia), hypothalamic changes, alterations in appetitive behavior	Increased alterations in perception.

Note: Age-related changes vary widely depending on genetic predisposition, environmental and lifestyle factors, as well as preexisting disease states and comorbid conditions.
CNS = central nervous system; HPA = hypothalamic–pituitary–adrenal.

interactions, complications stemming from existing disease states and comorbid conditions, as well as displacement of nutrients at increasing quantities of intake. In addition, bereavement, psychological conditions such as depression or anxiety, social isolation, and life changes such as with retirement may precipitate late-onset heavy drinking or alcohol abuse. Alcohol interferes with the absorption, utilization, and homeostasis of several key nutrients, which may already be compromised in a geriatric population.[66–68] (See **TABLE 15.8** and **TABLE 15.9**.)

Table 15.9

Types of Drug–Alcohol Interactions Commonly Found in Geriatric Populations

Interaction	Effect	Drug or Class of Drug
Decreased or competitive drug metabolism	Enhanced drug effects, longer effect, increased blood levels, increased drug toxicity risk	Opioids, benzodiazepines, anticoagulants, sulfonylureas (morphine, diazepam, warfarin, tolbutamide)
Hepatotoxicity	Increased drug toxicity, decreased conversion to active metabolite, decreased therapeutic blood level, decreased tolerance to xenobiotics	Antimicrobials, analgesics, anesthetics, antifungals, chemotherapeutic agents (isoniazid, acetaminophen, halothane, imidazoles, pyrozoles)
Competitive inhibition of ALDH and MEOS pathways	Increased levels of, accumulation of, prolonged circulation of acetaldehyde (disulfiram reaction—nausea, vomiting, headache, shortness of breath, postural hypotension, convulsions)	Sulfonylureas, antibiotics, antifungals, antihelminthics (chlorpropamide, ceftriaxone, griseofulvin, mebendazole)

Interaction	Effect	Drug or Class of Drug
Inhibition of first-pass gastric ADH metabolism	Increased ethanol blood levels, longer circulation time	Histamine H_2 antagonists (cimetidine, ranitidine)
Enhanced gastric irritation	Mucosal irritation, bleeding, slow healing, rebleeding risk	Analgesics, anti-inflammatory, antiplatelet (aspirin, NSAIDs, clopidogrel)
Activation of $GABA_A$ receptors (GABA is an amino butyric acid, a neurotransmitter in the central nervous system.)	Induction of CNS depression, sedative-hypnotic effects via inhibition of excitatory neuronal activity. Drowsiness, slurred speech, decreased motor function, cognitive disturbances, blurred vision, vertigo, hypotension	Sedating antidepressants, antihistamines, anticonvulsants, barbiturates, muscle relaxants, neuroleptics (nortriptyline, diphenhydramine, phenobarbital, pentobarbital, cyclobenzaprine, gabapentin)
Alterations in norepinephrine signals within the rostral ventrolateral medulla (brain)	Hypotension, respiratory depression	Vasodilators, antihypertensives (nitrates, doxazosin, clonidine)
Induction of CYP2D6 and CYP3A4 (cytochrome P450 subtypes)	Increase metabolism and excretion of drug, leading to failure to achieve therapeutic blood levels of drug; treatment failure	Anti-Alzheimer's, antiretroviral drugs for HIV (donepezil, nevirapine)

Note: This is a noncomprehensive listing of potential drug–ethanol interactions, mechanistic considerations, and adverse clinical consequences.

AHD = alcohol dehydrogenase; ALDH = aldehyde dehydrogenase; CNS = central nervous system; GABA = gamma-aminobutyric acid; HIV = human immunodeficiency virus; MEOS = microsomal ethanol oxidizing system; NSAIDs = nonsteroidal anti-inflammatory drugs.

Older persons are far more likely to experience negative outcomes with any alcohol use. Because of the age-related pathophysiological changes that occur in late life, the harmful effects outweigh any benefits of alcohol consumption in this group. Recommendations should exclude ethanol consumption as a general rule.

Comorbid conditions such as diabetes, vascular disease, gastrointestinal or liver disease, dental disorders, bone health and falls, and neurological, cognitive, and musculoskeletal diseases are all worsened by heavy alcohol consumption in an older person. This may be the cumulative effect of age-related changes, pathophysiological changes associated with the comorbid conditions, or environmental factors. Alcohol consumption in an older diabetic, for example, may alter glucose homeostasis and result in the need for either more or less insulin. Alcohol may replace food intake in someone who is already malnourished. Alcohol has no appreciable nutrient profile, with the exception of the 7 kilocalories per gram of ethanol. Significant empty calories can come from alcohol consumption. The body interrupts the metabolism of other substrates, such as important nutrients like vitamin A and fatty acids, to reduce, detoxify, metabolize, and excrete ethanol by-products. (see **FIGURE 15.7** and **FIGURE 15.8**) Alcohol ingestion also affects appetite and may alter intake. Because alcohol is also diuretic, there may be additional dehydration stemming from increased alcohol consumption.

A large number of older adults take one or more over-the-counter, herbal, or prescription medications. The number of drugs taken increases with advancing age, until it plateaus or sharply declines in the last year of life. One of the most concerning negative outcomes is the combined use of alcohol with multiple medications.[69–71] (see Table 15.9)

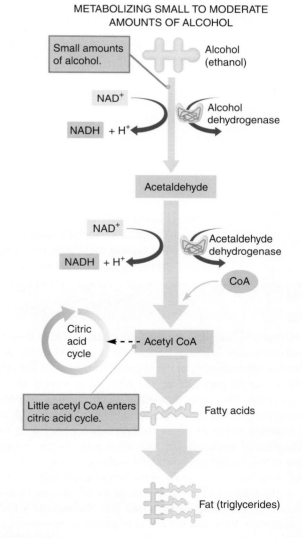

Figure 15.7
Metabolizing alcohol. The metabolism of alcohol inhibits the citric acid cycle and primarily forms fat.

THE MEOS OVERFLOW PATHWAY

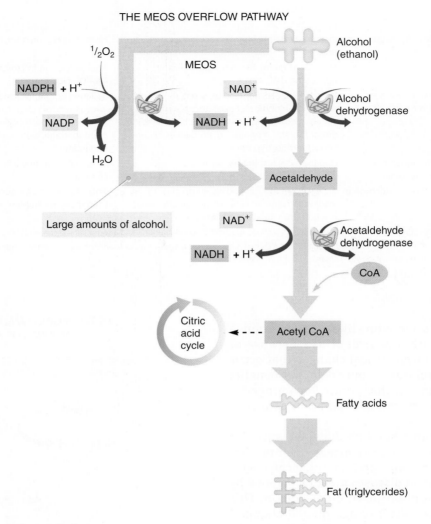

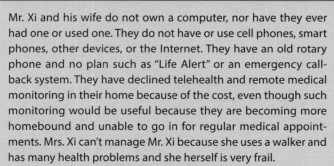

Figure 15.8
The MEOS overflow pathway. Large amounts of alcohol can overwhelm the typical metabolic route, so excess alcohol enters an overflow pathway called the microsomal ethanol-oxidizing system (MEOS).

Case Study

Mr. Xi and his wife do not own a computer, nor have they ever had one or used one. They do not have or use cell phones, smart phones, other devices, or the Internet. They have an old rotary phone and no plan such as "Life Alert" or an emergency call-back system. They have declined telehealth and remote medical monitoring in their home because of the cost, even though such monitoring would be useful because they are becoming more homebound and unable to go in for regular medical appointments. Mrs. Xi can't manage Mr. Xi because she uses a walker and has many health problems and she herself is very frail.

The Xi's do not have what is called "health literacy," meaning the ability to sort out research-based, accurate and reliable health information. They read the ads in newspapers, magazines, and on TV and believe that these claims are always truthful. Mrs. Xi always listens to the health advice of her friends and her general practitioner doctor, but not her daughter or any healthcare pro-

vider that is not an MD. Mrs. Xi also relies on remedies that were passed down over the generations from her great-grandmother. She swears that these work better than any new treatment ever could. Examples include using brandy and warm milk for insomnia, castor oil and a hot compress for pain, and drinking olive oil for constipation. Although as he gets older, Mr Xi is showing more signs of lactose intolerance, such as severe cramps, bloating, gas, and gastrointestinal motility problems, Mrs. Xi doesn't believe it is related to his dairy intake and continues to give Mr. Xi brandy, warm milk, and all his medications simultaneously before bed.

Questions

1. Describe how herbals, OTC, and other remedies could potentially complicate Mr. Xi's already complex medical situation.
2. Explain how environmental and familial situations contribute to Mr. Xi's overall decline.

Recap Nutrition guidelines for older adults present problems because this population is so heterogeneous. In general, bioavailable sources for protein should be used, and there should be a decrease in fat and an increase in fiber consumption. Hydration is the most important area to consider because older persons are at greater risk for dehydration. In terms of micronutrients, making sure that the need for iron, calcium, vitamins D and K, as well as B_{12}, are met should be emphasized because malnutrition with these nutrients is more prevalent in frail elderly persons. Trace minerals such as zinc and selenium should also be monitored because of their importance in immune function and wound healing. Alcohol consumption should be minimal because of adverse effects.

1. Which fats should be limited in the diet of an older person?
2. What roles does fiber play in health?
3. Why is hydration such an important issue for geriatric persons?
4. Which micronutrients need to be checked more closely in geriatric persons?
5. Why does limiting alcohol consumption in general constitute a good recommendation for health in the older adult population?

Polypharmacy in Geriatrics

Preview Older adults utilize more than 33% of all prescribed medications, supplements, and over-the-counter (OTC) preparations sold. The risk for adverse drug events is a significant health concern for older adults. Side effects of frequently used medications can have profound nutritional consequences.

Out-of-pocket drug-related expenditures are greater than $10 billion per year. Any drug could have an effect on nutritional status, and the use of many different medications simultaneously is known to have a negative impact on nutrition in the geriatric patient.[72-78] The risk for polypharmacy is higher with advancing age as is the risk of drug–drug and drug–nutrient interactions. Age and disease may change the efficacy and metabolism of drugs, which also complicate the issues of interaction. A drug's ability to effectively perform is its therapeutic index. The therapeutic index is a ratio of how much drug or specific nutrient is needed to get the desired effect versus how much is toxic. This is also known as a window or index of safety and is usually measured by administering drugs and nutrient to animals in LD_{50} (lethal dose 50%) and NCDR (normal curve versus dose response) studies.

Defining Polypharmacy

Polypharmacy is defined as the use of five or more drugs. Drugs include things like alcohol, herbals, and over the counter (OTC) items. Geriatric persons living in the community take, on average, six different compounds. Those in an institution take an average of nine different medications, and those hospitalized for acute treatment average 11 different compounds simultaneously. Each unique combination has interactions, which is magnified exponentially when there are several different classes of drugs being used. (See TABLE 15.10.) All these interactions affect nutrient digestion, absorption, trafficking, metabolism, utilization, and waste excretion. Potentially inappropriate medication (PIM) use has been attributed to polypharmacy and polyprescribing, the use of multiple doctors, pharmacies, and other venues to get drugs.

Magnitude of the Problem

The risk for adverse drug events (ADEs), reactions, and interactions increases proportionally with the number of drugs taken, such that the use of five or more compounds increases risk for ADEs to more than 50%, and the use of seven or more drugs results in a risk of more than 80%. More than 30% of all hospital admissions in the

Table 15.10

Drug–Nutrient Interaction Classification

Type I: Ex Vivo Bioinactivation	Reactions that occur prior to the compound's entry into the system.
Type IIA: Absorption Phase Interaction	Administration of compounds change the function of a key enzyme, thus precipitating an adverse event, such as toxicity.
Type IIB: Absorption Phase Interaction	Administration of compounds change the function of a key transporter, thus precipitating an adverse event, such as malabsorption, or decreased ability to reach the target tissue.
Type IIC: Absorption Phase Interaction	Administration of compounds that interact, bind, or deactivate one another in the gut, thus precipitating an adverse event, such as deficiency or inadequate levels of drug, leading to treatment failure.
Type III: Physiologic Interaction	Administration of compounds leads to adequate absorption, but interactions occur during distribution to target tissues, during first-pass metabolism to active metabolite or alteration of receptor functionality needed for therapeutic efficacy.
Type IV: Elimination Interactions	Administration of compounds, absorption, distribution, trafficking, and first-pass metabolism are unaffected, but the renal or hepatic clearance of the drug is impaired because of interaction, leading to adverse consequences such as treatment failure or toxicity, with increased levels of circulating metabolites.

Data from Chan L. Drug nutrient interactions. *J Paren Enter Nutr.* 2013;37(4):450–459.

Case Study

Mr. Xi has been taking many different medications his whole life. He has been treated by many different doctors and has used many different pharmacies. Over the years, he has been given unlimited refills on several of his medications. One of them is the benzodiazapine group. These are antianxiety drugs, like Valium (diazepam) and Xanax (alprazolam). They are addictive, and Mr. Xi has required a higher and higher dosage to obtain the desired effects. Benzodiazapine withdrawal is very dangerous for an older person when not done correctly. The drugs must be withdrawn slowly and steadily over time. Mr. Xi's wife has been giving him high doses to keep him sedated, but they are not effective anymore because of his tolerance. Benzodiazapines and ethanol are a very bad combination, especially in the oldest old. And as discussed previously, Mrs Xi often gives him brandy to take with his medications. This has contributed to his delerium and agitation, dizziness, fainting, falls, and trouble breathing and shortness of breath. This combination depresses the respiratory center and may result in death from respiratory failure. Mr. Xi also takes a blood thinner called warfrin for his poor circulation and clots in the legs; peripheral atherscleriosis and narrowing of the very small vessels of the legs, plus inactivty, can cause thickened blood to form clots that cut off circulation to the surrounding tissues.

Mr. Xi has also been given three different medications for his constipation: Colace, a stool softener, Miralax, a polyethylene glycol, and Bisacodyl, a stimulant laxative. All three are addictive in terms of the gut, and if the gut becomes dependent on laxatives it loses its own motility. In addition, these are designed to be ingested with plenty of fluids to avoid dehydration and obstruction. Obstruction occurs when there is a large, hard mass that blocks the colon that can't be pushed out.

Mr. Xi has also been taking blood pressure medicine. One is a diuretic, called hydrochlorothiazide (HCTZ). It is an older medication and has been widely used in the past, but there are newer drugs that have more pronounced effects, so the number of blood pressure drugs can be decreased. Mr. Xi hasn't been prescribed newer drugs, so he takes the HCTZ and furosemide. These medications are dehydrating and cause frequency and urgency of urination. Many of the drugs Mr. Xi is taking are on the "do not use" list for older persons, or what is known as the updated Beers Criteria.

Question

1. Explain the dangers of polypharmacy in the older adult from a pathophysiological standpoint.

---

older age groups are for ADEs, at a cost of more than $77 billion annually.

Adverse Effects of Polypharmacy

Because so many medications pose harm to older adults, the Beers Criteria were developed and are updated regularly. This is a list of medications that should not be prescribed or that could be prescribed and very closely monitored in older persons. Adverse drug events and inappropriate prescribing pose a significant threat to older persons' nutritional status. Many of these adverse events compromise already impaired function and directly or indirectly affect appetite, digestion, absorption, utilization, metabolism, and excretion of nutrients. This furthers frailty and may decrease immunity. Combinations of these drugs also cause dysgeusia, gastrointestinal distress, nausea, cramping, and early satiety. Many combinations of drugs also cause anorexia, dehydration, and constipation.[79–82]

Medication class has been found to be highly correlated to polypharmacy and ADEs in studies, with anticoagulants (e.g. warfarin) or psychoactive agents such as the benzodiazepines (e.g., Valium) of particular concern. Polypharmacy has been strongly related to functional decline, dizziness, poor balance and coordination, falls, and fractures in a variety of settings among older persons.[83–85]

Polypharmacy is very costly and is so much of a concern that the Beers Criteria is thought to be insufficient for addressing PIMs in older persons. It should be used in conjunction with other criteria and screening tools, such as the Medication Appropriateness Index (MAI), Screening Tool of Older Persons' Prescriptions (STOPP), Assessing Care of Vulnerable Elders (ACOVE), Comprehensive Geriatric Assessment (CGA), and other measures.[86–88]

Case Study

Mr. Xi takes OTC compounds and herbal remedies in addition to his prescribed medications. He takes melatonin for sleeping, St. John's wort for depression, and naproxen for aches and pains. He takes Prilosec (omeprazole) for his heartburn and Pepto-Bismol (bismuth subsalicylate) for his gastrointestinal distress of bloating, gas, cramps, and belching. His wife prefers using these because prescription medications are so expensive, and they have high copayments on Medicare.

Questions

1. How would you explain to Mr. and Mrs. Xi the benefits and risks of complementary medicine and dietary supplements?

Supplement Use Contributes to Polypharmacy

The use of nutritional and herbal products or supplements is common among older persons. Data support an upward trend in utilization among this demographic.

The Big Picture

Relationships between morbidity, polypharmacy, and nutritional status.

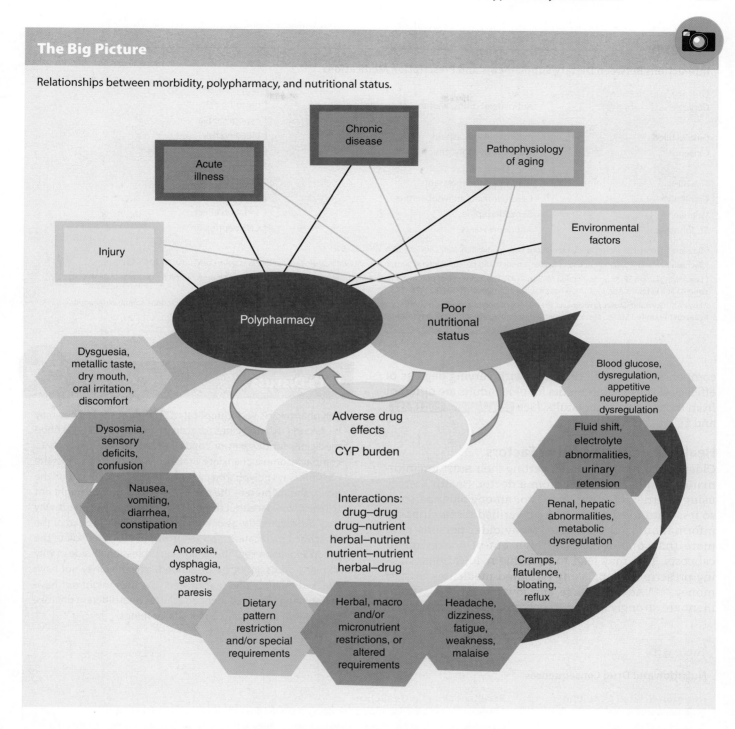

Supplements, OTC products, and "natural" products is a $40 billion industry in the United States, with more than 40% of the population taking dietary supplements, vitamins, minerals, herbals, and mixed compounds. Herbals, despite having pharmacologic applications, are still considered a "supplement," and there are more than 100,000 different OTC products available in U.S. markets. Supplements are not tightly regulated or subject to federally mandated stringent safety and efficacy testing, and approximately a thousand new products are introduced annually. Many of these products are marketed to older adults using advertising slots geared to this specific demographic.[89–94] Natural compounds, herbal medicines, and many OTC preparations act as drugs and affect drug metabolism and utilization as well as nutrient metabolism and utilization. (See TABLE 15.11.) Compounds are largely handled by detoxification first-pass metabolism in the liver, and others are handled exclusively by the kidney. A few are metabolized and excreted through the skin or lungs. Because all senescent organs and systems process

Table 15.11

Interactions Between Dietary Supplements and Prescription Medications

Dietary Supplement	Drug	Effect
Garlic[a,b,c]	Antiplatelet drugs, warfarin, glyburide	↑ bleeding risk
		↑ hypoglycemia
Gingko biloba[b,d]	Anticoagulants, aspirin	↑ bleeding risk
Ginseng[a,b]	Warfarin, hypoglycemic agents	↓ effect
		↑ hypoglycemia
Fish oil[a]	Warfarin, antidepressants	↑ effect
Carnitine[a,c]	Levothyroxine, anticholinergics	↓ effect
Valerian[a]	Benzodiazepine	↑ sedation effect
St. John's wort[a,b]	Antidepressants	↑ CNS depression

[a] Boullata J. Natural health product interactions with medication. *Nutr Clin Prac*. 2005;20(1):33–51.

[b] Tachjian A, Maria V, Jahangir A. Use of herbal products and potential interactions in patients with cardiovascular diseases. *J Am Coll Cardiol*. 2010;55(6):515–525.

[c] Lee AH, Ingraham SE, Kopp M, Foraida MI, Jazieh AR. The incidence of potential interactions between dietary supplements and prescription medications in cancer patients at a Veterans Administration hospital. *Am J Clin Oncol*. 2006;29(2):178–182.

[d] Loya AM, Gonzalez-Stuart A, Rivera JO. Prevalence of polypharmacy, polyherbacy, nutritional supplement use and potential product interactions among older adults living on the United States–Mexico border: a descriptive, questionnaire-based study. *Drugs Aging*. 2009;26(5):423–436.

compounds at altered rates and with varying degrees of efficacy, dosing requirements for older adults are different from those for younger adults. (See TABLE 15.12, TABLE 15.13, and TABLE 15.14.)

Health Literacy and Other Factors

Older adults generally prefer getting their nutrition information and health advice from a doctor. Health literacy using Internet information is poor among older persons, so it is hard for them to look up verified research-based information on the Internet. Many older persons have more than one doctor and high out-of-pocket medical costs. This may lead to hoarding medications, sharing prescriptions, or using outdated medicines to save money.[95–98] Advanced age and low educational attainment are strongly related to polypharmacy and ADEs, as

Let's Discuss

Polypharmacy is very complicated for older people. They may be taking OTC medicines for pain or constipation, prescribed medicines for diseases or conditions, and herbal products to combat insomnia or anxiety. Break into groups and discuss the possible ways polypharmacy can have adverse effects. Half the group should present the patient's side of why they might not tell their provider about the medicines they share or hoard, why they use expired drugs or herbals/supplements instead of the prescribed medication, and so forth, and the other half of the group should present the healthcare professional's side of why so many drugs are being prescribed, why they may not have checked multiple pharmacies, and why they might not have investigated why the patient is seeing several different doctors, all of whom are prescribing for similar things.

Table 15.12

Nutrition and Drug Consequences

Nutrition-Related Condition	Resultant Drug Consequence
Poor nutritional status[a]	Alterations in the intestinal mucosa resulting in limited drug absorption and metabolism.
Sarcopenia or obesity[b–d]	Drug dosage implications; many dosing regimens require average lean body tissue, average fat mass for disposition, distribution, and metabolism.
Alterations in GI function, pH[e]	Increased or decreased absorption dependent on drug class, increased or decreased disposition of drugs and metabolites.
Declining liver and kidney function[e]	Decreased metabolism, clearance, excretion, increased levels, duration of action. Drug dosage implications.
Alterations in circulation and circulating serum proteins[e,f]	Drug disposition, distribution, and dosing implications.

[a] Salazar JA, Poon I, Nair M. Clinical consequences of polypharmacy in elderly: expect the unexpected, think the unthinkable. *Expert Opin Drug Saf*. 2007;6(6):695–704.

[b] Cheymol G. *Clin Pharmacokinet*. Effects of obesity on pharmacokinetics implications for drug therapy 2000;39(3):215–231.

[c] Jacques KA, Erstad BL. Availability of information for dosing injectable medications in underweight or obese patients *Am J Health Syst Pharm*. 2010;67(22):1948–1950.

[d] Green B, Duffull SB. What is the best size descriptor to use for pharmacokinetic studies in the obese? *Br J Clin Pharmacol*. 2004;58(2):119–133.

[e] Bushra R, Aslam N, Khan AY. Food-drug interactions *Oman Med J*. 2011;26(2):77–83.

[f] Akamine D, Filho MK, Peres CM. Drug-nutrient interactions in elderly people. *Curr Opin Clin Nutr Metab Care*. 2007;10(3):304–310.

Table 15.13

Potential Drug–Nutrient Interactions

Nutrient or Food	Drug	Effect
Grapefruit juice[a,b,f]	Statins, calcium channel blockers, cyclosporines	↑ drug effectiveness
Vitamin K[b,f]	Warfarin	↓ drug effect
Fruit juice[c]	Fexofenadine	↓ drug effectiveness
Potassium[b]	ACE inhibitors	↑ hyperkalemia risk
High-fat meal[d]	Not drug specific	Can affect bile flow, splanchnic blood flow, GI pH, gastric emptying, physical/chemical interactions with drugs
High-fiber diet[f]	Digoxin	↓ drug bioavailability
High protein content[e]	Levodopa	↓ drug absorption
Fruit/vegetable phytochemicals[f]	Drugs metabolized by CYP3A4 enzyme	↑ drug effects
Calcium[b]	Tetracyclines	↓ drug absorption
Vitamin D[a]	Anticonvulsants (phenytoin)	↑ vitamin D need
Flavonoids[g]	Drugs metabolized or transported using same pathway as flavonoids	↑ or ↓ effectiveness
Biotin[h,i]	Anticonvulsants	↑ biotin catabolism

[a] Bushra R, Aslam N, Khan AY. Food–drug interactions. *Oman Med J.* 2011;26(2):77–83.

[b] Boullata J. Natural health product interactions with medication. *Nutr Clin Prac.* 2005;20(1):33–51.

[c] Dresser GK, Bailey DG, Leake BF, et al. Fruit juices inhibit organic anion transporting polypeptide-mediated drug uptake to decrease the oral availability of fexofenadine. *Clin Pharmacol Ther.* 2002;71(1):11–20.

[d] Custodio JM, Wu CY, Benet LZ. Predicting drug disposition, absorption/elimination/transporter interplay and the role of food on drug absorption. *Adv Drug Deliv Rev.* 2008;60(6):717–733.

[e] Bonnici A, Ruiner CE, St.-Laurent L, Hornstein D. An interaction between levodopa and enteral nutrition resulting in neuroleptic malignant-like syndrome and prolonged ICU stay. *Ann Pharmacother.* 2010;44(9):1504–1547.

[f] Rodriguez-Fragoso L, Martinez-Arismendi JL, Orozco-Bustos D, Reyes-Esparza J, Torres E, Burchiel SW. Potential risks resulting from fruit/vegetable–drug interactions: effects on drug-metabolizing enzymes and drug transporters. *J Food Sci.* 2011;76(4):R112–124.

[g] Cermak R. Effect of dietary flavonoids on pathways involved in drug metabolism. *Expert Opin Drug Metab Toxicol.* 2008;4(1):17–35.

[h] Said HM, Redha R, Nylander W. Biotin transport in the human intestine: inhibition by anticonvulsant drugs. *Am J Clin Nutr.* 1989;49(1):127–131.

[i] Mock DM, Dyken ME. Biotin catabolism is accelerated in adults receiving long-term therapy with anticonvulsants. *Neurology.* 1997;49(5):1444–1447.

Table 15.14

Age-Related Physiological Alterations that Affect Absorption, Transport, Disposition, Metabolism, Excretion, and Action of Drugs and Other Compounds in the Older Adult

↓ lean body mass/total body water	↓ volume of distribution for hydrophilic drugs with ↑ plasma concentrations and toxicity.
↑ fat mass	↑ volume of distribution with ↓ effect. ↑ accumulation in fatty tissue with continuous dosing.
↓ hepatic blood flow and liver function	Drugs with hepatic first-pass metabolism that liberate active metabolite results in ↓ efficacy. Drugs with metabolism to inactive metabolites show ↑ bioavailability and ↑ onset of action.
↓ hepatic enzyme production or function	↓ cytochrome P450 oxidation, ↑ toxicity of drugs that require the enzyme for catabolism.
↓ renal function	Major excretory route for many drugs, ↑ toxicity. Prolonged duration of drug effect. Clearance is ↓↓ in older women.
↓ serum carriers, such as albumin	↑ free drug levels, drug toxicity.
↓ receptor sensitivity	↓ cellular responsivity to agents, ↓ drug effects.
↑ permeability membranes, blood–brain barrier	↑ cellular damage, vulnerability of CNS to drug effects and damage.
↓ motility, ↓ gastric acid secretion	Variable absorption and bioavailability of drugs requiring ↓ pH.
↓ enzymatic function	↑ action and circulating levels of drug. ↑ among CYP enzymes (warfarin, St. John's wort, vitamin K epoxide reductase).
Alterations in transporter production, function, distribution, catabolism	Changes in absorption, transport, distribution, and efficacy of drugs, ↑ competition for carriers → ↓ transport of compounds with ↓ affinity for carrier proteins (magnesium, zinc, antiprotozoals, diuretics).
Thinning of skin, ↓ subdermal adipose tissue, subdermal layers	Topical and transdermal delivery of drugs is ineffective and may lead to additional harmful changes in fragile skin.
↓ cardiac output, vascular integrity, change in blood pressure/viscosity	↓ distribution of drugs and metabolites, ↓ end organ delivery, ↓ drug efficacy, and ↓ excretion rates.

↓ immunity, ↓ natural killer, T lymphocytes ↓ B lymphocyte production of antibodies	Antibiotics + anti-infective agents ↓ perform as intended, ↑ requirement for extended administration, concentrate in unintended tissues, ↑ adverse events, ↓ therapeutic results.
↓ in lung capacity, elasticity, affinity binding, receptor coupling, second messenger production	↓ levels and delay in responsivity to agents (e.g., beta adrenoreceptor agonists such as inhaled albuterol for asthma, drugs for COPD, or lung fibrosis).
Frailty-induced ↓ esterase glucuronidation and sulfation reactions	↓ in drug metabolism, clearance, excretion and ↑ circulating levels thus ↑ effects and toxicity (opioids, psychotropics).
Alterations in fluid and electrolyte homeostasis	Changes in drug absorption, distribution, metabolism, and excretion, ↑ for renal routes.
↓ sensory capacity and manual dexterity or ↓ cognitive status	↑ noncompliance with dosing or administration, unintentional overdose, or inappropriate dosing or intentional misuse.
↓ resilience, ↑ comorbid chronic diseases, damage due to stressors	↑ need for multiple drugs to treat multiple conditions, ↑ drug–drug, drug–nutrient, drug–environmental interactions.

CNS = central nervous system; COPD = chronic obstructive pulmonary disease; CYP = cytochrome P450.

Shi S, Mörike K, Klotz U. The clinical implications of ageing for rational drug therapy. *Eur J Clin Pharmacol*. 2008; 64(2):183-199.

McLachlan AJ, Bath S, Naganathan V, et al. Clinical pharmacology of analgesic medicines in older people: impact of frailty and cognitive impairment. *Br J Clin Pharmacol*. 2011;71(3):351–364. doi:10.1111/j.1365-2125.2010.03847.x.

Merle L, Laroche ML, Dantoine T, Charmes JP. Predicting and preventing adverse drug reactions in the very old. *Drugs Aging*. 2005;22(5):375–392.

Parikh AO. Principles of geriatric pharmacology. *J Indian Med Assoc*. 2007;105(5):282, 284.

Jesson B. Minimizing the risk of polypharmacy *Nurs Older People*. 2011;23(4):14–20.

Pugh MJV, Vancott AC, Steinman MA, et al. Choice of initial antiepileptic drug for older veterans: possible pharmacokinetic drug interactions with existing medications *J Am Geriatr Soc*. 2010;58(3):465–471.

Ginsberg G, Hattis D, Russ A, Sonawane B. Pharmacokinetic and pharmacodynamic factors that can affect sensitivity to neurotoxic sequelae in elderly individuals. *Environ Health Perspect*. 2005;113(9):1243–1249.

is residence type, institutionalization, and hospital discharge destination such as home versus long-term care.

Older persons are more vulnerable to claims, advertising, and scams. Older persons should be questioned repeatedly about herbal, supplement, and nutritional formula usage, as well as other alternative medicine techniques. This may include dietary regimens, such as "hot" versus "cold" foods or "eating clean foods." Others could include aromatherapy, chiropractic, Reiki, or Chinese medical methods, including acupuncture, reflexology, or herbals. Of particular concern is the use of such modalities by older adults at the end of life. This population is classified as extremely vulnerable to resorting to untested alternative treatments.[99,100]

Recap Polypharmacy is a very complex problem in older persons. The use of multiple prescribed, OTC, and dietary supplements or alcohol has major consequences in terms of both nutrition and overall health. A list of drugs to be avoided called the Beers Criteria is updated every 5 years. Low health literacy, very advanced age, and multiple health conditions all increase adverse events from polypharmacy. The use of herbal supplements and over-the-counter compounds complicates the picture even further because most compounds require a functional liver for metabolism and clearance. Nutritional status is also affected by the use of these compounds.

1. What is the definition of polypharmacy?
2. Why is polypharmacy dangerous for older adults?
3. Why does supplement use influence adverse event risk?
4. How does the liver handle drugs, supplements, and macro- and micronutrients?

End-of-Life Considerations

Preview Older persons at the end of life are vulnerable to inappropriate decision making by others as well as neglect and even abuse.

End-of-life (EOL) considerations have important components, including decisions made in a chaotic, stressful climate; the personal, religious, cultural, and fiscal factors that affect those decisions; and demographics, knowledge, attitudes, and beliefs of both the patient and the caregivers who treat them.[101–105]

Elder Abuse and Neglect

There is a growing concern about elder abuse and neglect, particularly for those persons who require around-the-clock care at the end of their life. Outside caregivers, and even family members, experience caregiver fatigue and burden.[106,107] This may lead to frustration, anger, and loss of control over time. Outside caregivers may also be people who are paid poorly or who may not be skilled enough to get other kinds of jobs. Caring for an elderly or dying person is very stressful, and people who are caregivers may not have appropriate outlets for their tension. Older adults may receive intensive medical care in an institutional setting or a family may choose home health care under the direction of the elder's primary care physician. In long-term care environments, interpersonal violence and aggression by other residents have also been recognized as a serious problem.[108,109] In community-dwelling older adults, who have outside family or home care caregivers, abuse has been correlated with being

News You Can Use

Did you know that elder abuse and neglect are the most under-reported statistics today? It is estimated that the rates are well above 10%, which is the high end of the reported instances of elder abuse and neglect. Because of the increasing numbers of oldest old persons, very-low-income older adults, and older adults with disabilities and cognitive dysfunction, it is thought that the rates of neglect and abuse, whether self-inflicted or not, will continue to skyrocket.

The National Center on Elder Abuse, which is a branch of the National Institute on Aging and the National Institutes of Health, reports that elders who have experienced any abuse or neglect, even in mild cases, have an increased death rate that is almost 300% of those who were never abused or mistreated. Estimates for how much this problem costs in terms of the burden on the healthcare system alone range in excess of $5 billion to almost $10 billion in the United States. There are many global studies of the cost of elder abuse and neglect as well.

Depression, anxiety, and other stress-related consequences are also shown to be much higher in older adults who have been mistreated. Studies have found that close to 50% of dementia patients have been mistreated by their caregivers. Of those, most develop additional problems as a result. Approximately 10% of complaints against institutions, such as long-term care facilities, are brought by loved ones or staff for neglect or outright abuse. Unfortunately, the rates of abuse of one resident by another are on the rise, even though these events are underreported. Because people are reluctant to report instances of abuse, neglect, or violence, authorities believe the rates are substantially higher than those that are disseminated. There are many reasons why people are reluctant to report these crimes. Some of those reasons include fear of retaliation, being unsure about what really constitutes abuse or neglect, and feeling like there is nothing that can be done about it anyway. None of these are good reasons, and you should always report suspicious actions or instances of mistreatment, neglect, and outright abuse or violence against elders.

Reference

https://ncea.acl.gov/whatwedo/research/statistics.html

poor, functionally impaired, and living alone.[110],[111] Elder abuse and neglect are associated with hospitalization, institutionalization, and mortality. Elder self-neglect, a syndrome in which older persons fail to take care of themselves and/or seek assistance, is the most common form of abuse and neglect and has even higher rates for adverse consequences.[112],[113]

End-of-Life Feeding Considerations

One of the most important issues is the feeding of someone who is near death. Food is considered by most to be a palliative measure that is necessary until death. Research has shown, however, that there are many considerations regarding feeding and hydrating someone whose body tissues and cells are shutting down. Experimental and clinical evidence suggests that feeding and hydrating someone who is terminally ill and close to death is unethical, contrary to patients' wishes, and may in fact cause a more uncomfortable death. Persons near death naturally don't want to eat or drink, and forcing nutrients and fluids can result in a number of undesirable consequences. These are listed in **TABLE 15.15**.

Provision of food and fluids gives the appearance of "doing something" to save a family's loved one. Often,

Table 15.15

Undesirable Consequences of Forcing Food and Fluids at the End of Life

Increased secretions, urination, defecation, requiring more mechanical manipulation of the bedbound patient.

Increased disinfection and cleaning of fragile skin.

Increased lung secretions cause coughing, choking, and aspiration.

Increased gastrointestinal contents cause bloating and pain.

Depending on what is fed or given as fluids, there may be obstruction in the gut or edema (accumulation of fluid due to decreased protein content of the blood and immobility, with poor circulation).

Use of a catheter because the person can't get up to use the bathroom causes irritation, inflammation, infection, and sepsis or whole-body infection that can be deadly.

The presence of fluids and food in a gastrointestinal tract that is no longer motile causes greater nausea, vomiting, and ascites (edema in the peritoneum).

Skin breakdown occurs more frequently, leading to decubitus ulcers.

A syndrome known as the "death rattle" occurs when secretions in the lungs vibrate while the person is breathing. It is almost a gargling noise with each breath.

Dehydration is a natural anesthetic, decreasing the firing of pain neurons and nociceptors (pain sensors).

Arguments for nonoral hydration, often using either intravenous fluids or hypodermoclysis (subcutaneous fluids, with a line inserted under the skin, as opposed to in a vein or port), vary from:

a. Increasing the detoxification and removal of wastes from naturally occurring metabolism or ingestion

b. Keeping electrolytes stable in the terminal portion of the illness

family or friends (surrogates) become decision makers, and the burden falls to them, not to the dying older adult. This is difficult when the older adult is not competent to voice wishes and no legal documentation exists delineating the person's preferences. Healthcare providers are mandated to do what the patient would want them to do, but it becomes complicated when the family wants something else and there is no one to advocate for the patient.[104,114–118]

There are many ways to care for the dying. Persons with 6 months left to live, as stated by a physician or practitioner specializing in palliative care, in most states qualify for home hospice care. Alternatively, there are community hospice and hospital hospice centers. Palliative care units exist in many hospitals and skilled facilities. End-of-life care is usually handled by a team interdisciplinary approach. An interdisciplinary team may consist of a variety of professionals, depending on the unique situation.[119,120] A list of professionals can be found in TABLE 15.16 . TABLE 15.17 includes descriptions of care concepts and terms related to end of life services.

Table 15.16

Professionals Involved in Interdisciplinary Healthcare Teams

Doctors	Osteopaths
Nurses	Pharmacists
Social workers	Dietitians
Rehabilitation specialists	Speech-language pathologists
Case managers	Clergy
Caregivers	Psychologists
Alternative-complementary therapists	Physical therapists
Administrators	Persons named as healthcare proxy
Bioethicists	Legal counsel
Aides or ancillary personnel	Hospice or hospital volunteers
Specialists (e.g., cardiologist)	Respiratory therapists
Occupational therapists	Community representatives
Financial advisers	Certified dietary managers
Handler, pet therapist	Recreation therapists

Table 15.17

Description of Care Concepts and Legal Terms Related to End-of-Life Services

Advance Medical Directive[a]	Description
Living will	• A legal document that states what medical and other life-sustaining procedures may or may not be done in the event that a person becomes mentally incompetent, comatose, otherwise incapacitated, or terminally ill. • Documentation should include decisions regarding artificial nutrition and hydration as well as other treatment modalities.
Power of attorney	• A health-care durable power of attorney is documentation that identifies the person who can make healthcare decisions and carry out an individual's wishes in the event that there is an emergent situation, the individual is incapacitated mentally or physically, or the person becomes comatose. This responsibility is also known as healthcare proxy with regard to healthcare matters.
Healthcare proxy	• The right of a legally named person to execute the wishes for treatment or refusal of treatment when an individual is incapacitated.
Last will and testament	• The will is a document that is a legal set of directions for what should be done after a person dies. • The executor of the will is responsible for dealing with the dead person's estate, assets, or other interests.

Other[b]	Description
Resuscitation	• To restore to life or consciousness, usually involving cardiopulmonary efforts, such as mouth-to-mouth breathing or cardiac massage. • Do not resuscitate, or DNR, orders are medically and legally binding.
Pain management	• Management of pain and suffering requires an interdisciplinary approach that uses several branches of medicine and allied health including pharmacotherapy, biofeedback, physical and occupational therapies, and psychotherapeutic approaches. • Several different kinds of analgesic medications, including opioids, can be used.
Persistent vegetative state	• A state of extreme unresponsiveness that lasts for more than 1 month, with no awareness or higher cerebral function. • Midbrain and brainstem functions are preserved, with sleep–wake cycling and autonomic control over functions such as breathing and heart rate. There may be some reflexive movement.
Permanent vegetative state	• The diagnosis is changed to "permanent vegetative state" after approximately 1 year of persistent vegetative state.
Coma	• State of extreme unresponsiveness, with no voluntary movement or behavior, and sometimes normal reflexes may be lost. There is maintenance of autonomic functions. • If the state persists for more than a month, it becomes a persistent vegetative state.
Brain death	• Initial requirements for determination of brain death include neuroimaging or clinical findings that suggest catastrophic cerebral events in which there are no identifiable other conditions that may represent brain death, such as severe metabolic derangement, intoxication, poisoning, or other acute vascular anomaly.

Other[b]	Description
	• There is persistent unresponsiveness, no reflexive responses to pain or any brainstem responses, and there is apnea, with cessation of respiration and circulation.
Uniform Determination of Death Act (UDDA)[c]	• A determination of death must be made in accordance with accepted medical standards." The UDDA states: "An individual who has sustained either (1) irreversible cessation of circulation and respiratory functions, or (2) irreversible cessation of all functions of the entire brain, including the brain stem, is dead."

[a] President and Fellows of Harvard College. A guide to living wills and health care proxies. Harvard Special Health Report. *Harvard Annual Report.* 2008;1:27.

[b] Faymonville ME, Pantke KH, Berre J, et al. Cerebral functions in brain damaged patients: what is meant by coma, vegetative state, minimally conscious state, locked in syndrome and brain death? *Der Anaesthetist.* 2004;53:1195–2003.

[c] Uniform Law Commission. Determination of Death Act summary. Retrieved from: http://www.uniformlaws.org/ActSummary.aspx?title=Determination%20of%20Death%20Act. Accessed September 29, 2016.

Data from Journal of Nutrition for the Elderly. Artificial Nutrition and Hydration at End of Life. Taylor & Francis. Retrieved from: http://www.tandfonline.com/doi/pdf/10.1080/01639366.2010.521020

Artificial Nutrition and Hydration at the End of Life

Several methods exist for feeding a person at the end of life. If the person can still eat orally, then that is the preference. Careful hand feeding and coaching take many hours of staffing time for a terminal older adult. Sometimes a nasogastric tube is used, where the tube is placed up the nose and down the esophagus to the stomach. Feeding this way still utilizes the stomach but is quick and ensures that enough nutrients are being consumed. The problems with tube feeding include irritation of the sensitive skin around the nose, choking, burping, and aspirating and demented patients yanking the tube because they do not understand or forget why it is supposed to be there.[121–123]

Another method is the **percutaneous endoscopic gastrostomy (PEG) tube**. This is placed laparoscopically, and a formula is poured through the tube that has been placed through the skin and muscle to the lumen of the stomach. PEG tubes offer the advantages of decreased time to feed, a variety of formulas that can be obtained, and little to no kinking of the tube or plugging. (See TABLE 15.18 .) The disadvantages are inflammation at the

Table 15.18

Tube Feeding Formulas

Type of Tube Feeding	Key Elements	Product Examples and Manufacturers	Uses	Contraindications
Standard (polymeric)	Fiber free	Osmolite (Abbott), Nutren (Nestlé Nutrition)	Can be used for most standard enteral feedings	Intolerance to feeding, food allergies, inability to digest intact proteins and long-chain triglycerides
	Fiber containing	Jevity (Abbott), Fibersource HN (Nestlé Nutrition), Isosource 1.5 (Nestlé Nutrition)	Should be first choice in tube feeding	
	High protein	Promote (Abbott), Replete (Nestlé Nutrition)	Wound healing, need for increased protein without additional calories	
	Fluid restricted	TwoCal (Abbott), Novasource 2.0 (Nestlé Nutrition), Isosource 1.5 (Nestlé Nutrition)	Conditions requiring fluid restrictions	Normal fluid requirements
Partially hydrolyzed	Elemental	Vivonex (Nestlé Nutrition)	Gastrointestinal impairments	Able to digest intact protein formulas
	Semielemental	Peptamen (Nestlé Nutrition), Vital (Abbott)	Gastrointestinal impairments	
Disease specific	Diabetic	Glucerna (Abbott), Glytrol (Nestlé Nutrition)	Diabetes mellitus	Absence of diabetes mellitus
	Dialysis	Nepro (Abbott)	Chronic kidney disease	Absence of kidney disease
	Nondialysis	Suplena (Abbott), Renalcal (Nestlé Nutrition)	Acute renal failure	Absence of acute renal failure
	Immune enhancing	Impact Peptide 1.5 (Nestlé Nutrition), Pivot (Abbott)	Patients at risk of infection associated with major surgery or critical illness, major elective surgery, trauma, burns, wounds, and early enteral feeding	Severe sepsis*

Data from McClave SA, Taylor BE, Martindale RG, et al. Guidelines for the provision and assessment of nutrition support therapy in the adult critically ill patient: Society of Critical CareMedicine (SCCM) and American Society for Parenteral and Enteral Nutrition (ASPEN). *JPEN J Parenter Enteral Nutr.* 2016;40(2):159–211.

site of tube placement, dislodging of the tube, infection, or damage if the person tries to pull it.

Total parenteral nutrition is also an option for feeding and hydrating but should be considered as a last resort. This feeding method bypasses the gut and is done through a port with an infusion pump. It is too dangerous for frail, demented older persons. A number of methods of restraint are used for older demented patients to keep them from dislodging the apparatus, such as belly bands, tape, and soft collars, but actual "restraints" are illegal.[124–126]

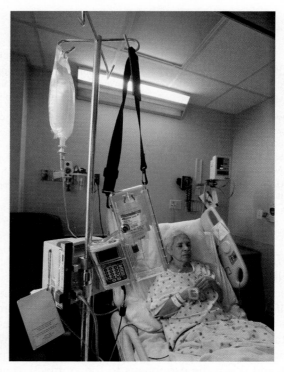

©Marjorie Kamys Cotera/Bob Daemmrich Photography/Alamy Stock Photo

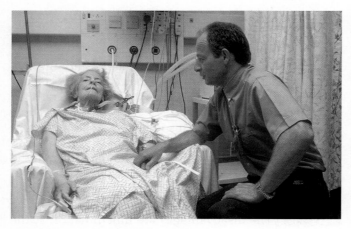

©Photofusion/Universal Images Group/Getty

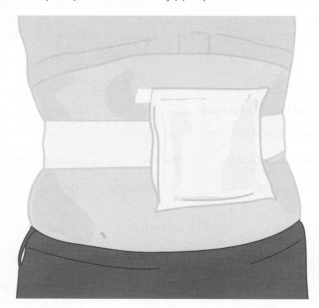

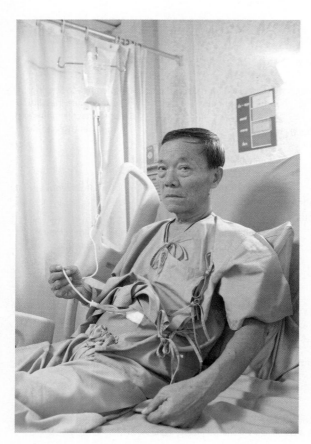

©Stockphoto mania/Shutterstock

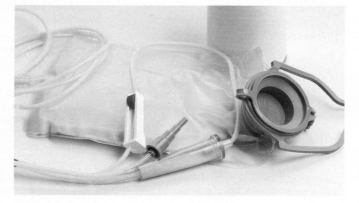

©Sherry Yates Young/Shutterstock

Ethical and Legal Considerations

There are ethical and legal considerations about artificially hydrating and feeding a person at the end of their life. Certain medications can't be used when the patient is being artificially fed and hydrated. Some of these medications include the pain medications, and then a quality-of-life issue arises. Or maybe the person never wanted to be kept alive in this way, religious beliefs may have prevented or promoted artificially feeding and hydrating, or perhaps the financial burden is too great or the quality of life too low. There is a belief that if a demented patient continually pulls the tubes, that is an expression of the person's wishes and should be honored. Alternatively, family members may refuse to remove tubes once they have been inserted, regardless of the quality of life of the patient.[127–135]

Caregivers, family members, and the healthcare providers who must deal with end-of-life and crises situations carry a large burden. Although laws state that it is legal to withdraw or withhold artificial nutrition and hydration in an EOL situation, many are unfamiliar with the legal statutes. Voluntary refusal of food and fluids (also referred to as voluntary stopping of eating and drinking) is a legal and ethical option in which the individual has the right to choose to die through dehydration and starvation as long as the person is competent to make that decision. Physician-assisted suicide is not legal in the United States but is in some European countries. There is a right to die movement in the United States, which does sometimes promote travel to another country to have the services of assisted suicide provided to a patient. Also, a body of literature states that artificial nutrition and hydration does not statistically increase number of days of life from

matched controls. Ethnic and racial differences in which EOL treatment options are available to patients and their families can determine what decisions are ultimately made.[101,103–105,136]

It is best if an individual makes his or her preferences regarding artificial nutrition and hydration, resuscitation, extreme measures, and all other facets of EOL care known, in a legal document, and names a trusted person to carry out those wishes. This document should be on file with the person, physician, family, healthcare proxy, and attorney in the event of a crisis situation.

Let's Discuss

Ethics of Artificial Feeding and Hydration at the End of Life

What do you think about the right to die movement? Should people be allowed voluntary refusal of foods and fluids when they are terminally ill? Break into groups and discuss the issues surrounding right to die and voluntary refusal of foods and fluids. Half the group should take the perspective of the patient and half the perspective of the family, loved ones, or healthcare provider.

Should demented persons be artificially fed and hydrated when they are at the end of their lives? Discuss the pros and cons of feeding and hydrating a person who has advanced dementia and is no longer able to swallow. Break into groups and discuss the key points. Half the group should take the perspective of legal/liability issues, and half the perspective of personal, ethical, and religious convictions that might have an impact on decision making in this population.

Case Study

Mr. Xi has had another urinary tract infection. He is septic and became delirious, paranoid, and aggressive. He tried to stab the home health aide with scissors because he thought she was an intruder. He thought his wife was conspiring against him with the aide and started to become increasingly agitated. The police were called in and he was taken to a hospital that specializes in geriatric psychiatry. He is confused and combative and screams and can no longer express himself coherently. His daughter was called and the time she arrives, the state has filed an Elder Abuse Neglect hold. Mr. Xi can no longer be returned to his home and his wife of 60 years.

Mr. Xi is in a strange, noisy place surrounded by strangers he does not recognize. He has refused to eat or drink. There is no documentation of his wishes, and his wife refuses to come and see him or fill out the paperwork. The daughter was notified, but it takes 72 hours for her to reach the hospital. In the meantime, a port was placed, IV fluids, electrolytes, antibiotics, and macro- and micronutrients were added, and an infusion pump started. Mr. Xi has his right arm immobilized and the port protected by a plastic guard. He has tried to pull out the lines, so a 24-hour-a-day

security measure was put in place, and he has to have one-on-one supervision day and night.

Mr. Xi was taken off many of his prior medications and new ones have been instituted. He is now on 13 different prescription medications, including fluoxetine (Prozac), an antidepressant; clonazepam, an antianxiety medication; quetiapine, an antipsychotic; eszopiclone, a sleep agent; and other drugs known to cause dizziness, sedation, xerostomia, constipation, anorexia, nausea, dyspepsia, and other side effects that affect nutrition status. Mr. Xi is now also hallucinating because of the new medications he takes in combination.

Mr. Xi's daughter arrives after a PEG tube is placed and Mr. Xi has been transferred to a dementia unit very far from his wife and their apartment. He is no longer septic and has moments of lucidity. He chokes and often coughs and drools when the thickened liquids are given to keep his oral cavity moistened. Mr. Xi had informed his daughter years before his dementia that he never wanted to go to a nursing home or have any interventions medically. Now, because the procedures are in place, the nursing home is refusing to remove the PEG tube, claiming they do not have the staffing to try to feed Mr. Xi orally and that the liability for removal is too great.

Because he is no longer restrained, Mr. Xi wanders the dementia unit looking for his wife and his belongings. He cries and asks everyone he sees if he can "go home now," but state will not allow him to return home. Mr. Xi's daughter had to go back home to her family and her job and doesn't know what to do. Mrs. Xi's wife is afraid to travel so far to see him, so he has no visitors. Mr. Xi turns 95 crying out for his wife and daughter. Mr. Xi has developed pneumonia from aspiration, has become septic again and has another serious urinary tract infection. He is hospitalized in terrible pain and moans and cries and flails. He no longer has cognitive capacity, his pupils are fixed, and he doesn't understand what is going on around him. He is being given high doses of morphine and his breathing is poor.

Question

1. What are the primary considerations as the Xi family begins to consider end-of-life care for Mr Xi?

Recap End-of-life care is very important, and decisions should not be made when everything is in chaos. There are many determinants for EOL decision making. Caring for persons at this time is stressful, and there is more risk of elder abuse and neglect. Forcibly feeding and hydrating persons near death has negative consequences. It is common for many different kinds of professionals to be involved in the care and decision making of dying persons. In addition to legal and ethical issues, there are considerable nutritional, feeding, and hydration concerns. The recent popularity of "right to die" and "voluntary refusal of food and fluids" movements indicates the heightened awareness of these issues.

1. What are the consequences of feeding and hydrating a person who is near death?
2. Which professionals might be involved in the caring and decision-making processes for dying persons?
3. What are the concepts of care in EOL services?
4. What are some methods of provision of artificial nutrition and hydration?

Nutrition Care Process

Preview It is necessary to get dietary information on both usual intake and current intake, reliable anthropometric data, biochemical data, neurological assessment, evaluation of oral health, as well as a social history and medication use, including dietary supplements and use of complementary and integrative health approaches. Approaches to study, evaluate, and design interventions should be uniquely designed to meet the challenges of this population.

Assessing a patient for the whole picture is very important. Many factors can contribute to deficits in nutrition, and some of those factors are not always easily recognized. Repetition, repeated measures over time, and using the patient's own information, medical records, and other documents should be used in conjunction with reports from caregivers and family members to get a more complete set of data. This systematic way to collect and disseminate data for outcomes to healthcare providers is the **Nutrition Care Process**.

Nutrition Assessment

For patients who are incapacitated, it is necessary to get dietary information on both usual intake and current intake from a surrogate. A surrogate is someone who cares for the client in such a way that he or she knows what and how much was consumed. Important information like plate waste, method of food item preparation, frequency of eating, and quantity eaten that is valid and reliable must be obtained from a third party. The best way to achieve an increase in the reliability of the information requested is to train the surrogate. It is always best for data accuracy if the information is obtained from only one person and that the information is repeatedly obtained over the course of a longer time period. For example, the primary caregiver always cooks and serves the meals, then clears the dishes after she and the patient have eaten together. This person would be trained to estimate portion sizes and keep a diary or food record over the course of several days or weeks. In this record, not only can dietary data be obtained but also behavior, times of eating, functional limitations, and other important facts can be documented.

Anthropometric Data

Getting anthropometric data is important, but the data should be evaluated for consistency. Geriatric patients have difficulty standing and may have lost height. Bed scales can obtain weight, but it must be dry weight. Fluid and shifting may result in a spurious bed weight, which is why the weight is documented and averaged over time. Longitudinal measurement is extremely important to note shifts. Ideally, body composition could be measured. The use of a dual X-ray absorptiometer would be best because bioelectrical impedance is often invalidated by fluid deficit or edema, and comparative data for the older subpopulations do not exist.

Muscle thickness estimates, either with or without calipers, fat pad deficit measurements, and any accumulation of fluid or dehydration should be monitored. Many professionals use the "depress" test. The depress test involves pushing on the swollen area and seeing how fast it springs back and how far you can push without resistance. A change in skin tone is seen with the depression. Dehydration can be measured by tenting the skin and watching how long it takes to return to its non-tented state.

Biochemical Data

Often, geriatric panels or a series of blood and urine tests specifically chosen to evaluate the geriatric comorbid patient are performed. These encompass several key systems and their indicators of function. In addition to the standard 22 labs that adults are given, geriatric panels can include additional measures. Adults are usually evaluated for albumin, red and white blood cell levels, blood glucose, serum electrolytes, and various lipoproteins and triglycerides. Geriatric panels often include these in addition to liver enzyme function tests, kidney function tests, endocrinology assays, and inflammatory markers. Tests are also available for specific proteins, assays for specific blood levels of vitamins, and tests that can be done to ascertain the level of muscle catabolism under certain conditions.

Neurological Assessment

Neurological and brain function testing is also available. There are many different measures of cognitive decline, and these are usually best when used over a long period with repeated administration. As a result of new technologies, the functionality of the brain and nervous system can now be measured. The use of rating tools such as the Subjective Global Assessment, where physically touching and measuring the patient are critical components of the score, is important in geriatrics. The Subjective Global Assessment, or SGA, has a patient-generated short form, where the patient or the patient's surrogate fills out some of the form and the healthcare provider does the rest. Training for this measurement tool is available at the Academy of Nutrition and Dietetics website.

Social Assessment

Information about socioeconomics, demographics, social interaction, environmental conditions, living situation, past medical history, and family medical history is important to collect, either from the patient who is competent or from a close relative or caregiver. Prior medical records are better sources of information in this population. An assessment of health literacy is important, as is repeated questioning to make sure that the data being gathered are reliable. Forgetfulness or inability to provide information is common, and surrogate information is often unreliable as well.

Complementary and Integrative Approaches and Dietary Supplements

Alternative remedies, herbals, OTC, prescribed, or obtained medications should be inventoried, using the physical bottles if at all possible. Having the bottles brought

in allows the health practitioner to record the name of the patient, the dosing parameters, the dose itself, refills, medical numbers, and expiration dates. Food–drug interactions should be looked up and documented. A pharmacist should be consulted for drug–drug interactions, compliance with Beers Criteria, and any potential for inappropriate prescribing. Other allied health professionals should also double-check medications in this population because of the dangers of adverse drug effects and the high rates of polypharmacy.

Monitoring and Evaluation

Because the oldest old persons are not frequently used in rigorous research studies, there is a dearth of comparative data for the geriatric population. This makes it very difficult to compare what is an essentially heterogeneous population with any known surveillance data. Data that come from smaller groups of subjects may be used, or data widely available for persons older than 70 years will need to be substituted, even if those figures do not represent the individual patient being assessed.

Prioritization of only a few key nutrition diagnoses is very difficult in this population. However, it may be wise to choose the ones that can actually be remedied, thus narrowing down the selections. Older persons usually have only two major intake diagnoses to evaluate: inadequate fluid intake and inadequate nutrient intake; from the clinical domain, drug–nutrient interactions and impaired nutrient utilization; and from the behavioral–environmental domain, there is knowledge deficit and inactivity.

Nutrition Interventions

The interventions that are chosen should be laid out one at a time, and then implemented fully prior to instituting a second intervention. This way, the change is gradual and not frightening to an older person or overwhelming. In certain instances it is not advisable to intervene at all. For example, when a person has dementia and consistently forgets that he or she just ate. The intervention must be tailored to the individual, slowly and gradually implemented, and nothing new added until solidification occurred. Measurements of successful solidification should be made longitudinally. It is always better to measure at the same time of day, on the same day of the week, and using the same techniques. This way, analytical strategies, laboratories, and personnel using identical parameters can minimize measurement error, which can be high in geriatric populations.

Education and Counseling

Education and counseling that are done should be done with both the patient and any caregivers. It is best to provide written materials at a level of literacy consistent with the surrogate's educational level. Instructions should be repeated, and then the surrogate and patient should reiterate what was said to determine whether

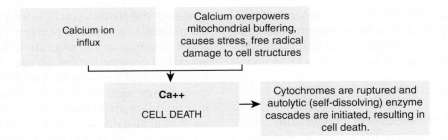

they understood. Under certain circumstances it is also advisable to contact the surrogate or patient later in the week to determine whether any questions have arisen and whether or not they have been able to implement the instructions.

Interprofessionalism

Interdisciplinary teams are now a hallmark of good health care. It is essential that all members of the team are kept abreast of any findings, all information collected, and any changes that occur. The changes are usually slowly progressive, then very rapid toward the end of life. To avoid crisis situations and failure to convey important information, the use of charting in electronic medical records has become very appealing. Persons who are authorized can access the information from anywhere at any time.

The largest loss of data and lack of continuity of health care happen during transfer. Transfer is when a patient goes from his or her home to the hospital and then home again, or from the hospital to a rehabilitation facility. Often, the electronic medical records at different facilities do not talk to one another, and the physical hard copies do not get forwarded in a timely manner. This generates the right environment for making medical mistakes. It is very important to continually monitor patients and not let them "slip through the cracks." This means consistent follow-up with the transfer institution or follow-up to the home. Monitoring and evaluation should occur for an extended time period or until the person in deceased. Monitoring and evaluation over the course of what may be months or years incur large costs. Monitoring and evaluation should track all the parameters set forth initially and correct for any changes in nutritional status or overall health.

Geriatric nutrition is a complex field that must account for several different influences. It is a challenging and rewarding field that recognizes that nutritional status and dietary patterns in the geriatric population require individualization and careful attention to quality of life, mental status, physical and mental capacity, and environmental input, while the changes of aging and those imposed by chronic disease add additional burden to achieving optimal nutrition in the patient. Geriatric nutrition is a growing field for nutrition professionals, due to increases in the aging population and the ability to live more years of life with declining functional status as a result of advances in medicine and technology.

Recap The Nutrition Care Process is fundamental to providing sound nutrition care regardless of age group. It is important to have standardized methods for assessing, recording, interpreting, and disseminating information about a patient. Several components of the process are important for better outcomes for patients. It also allows other health professionals to understand the work that is being done that is outside their discipline and allows for aggregate data to inform practice guidelines. In the older adult population, this process is particularly important to provide good quality care and reduce medical mistakes.

1. List the components of the Nutrition Care Process (NCP).
2. What are good measures to use in the assessment portion of the NCP?
3. Why is longitudinal measurement over time superior than a one-time measure? Why is this so important in NCP?
4. What does the concept of continuity of care mean? How can it be implemented?

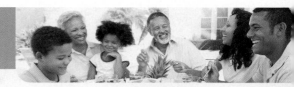

Learning Portfolio

Visual Chapter Summary

Senescence

- Senescence, or the process of growing old, can be seen as a function of apoptosis outweighing new cell production.
- There are three tiers of aging: primary, secondary, and tertiary.
- Inflammation is a hallmark of aging theory.

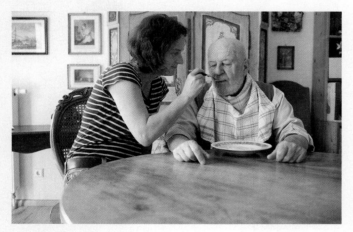

©Ute Grabowsky/photothek images UG/Alamy Stock Photo

Factors that Affect Dietary Intake in Later Life

- Multiple factors affect dietary intake in older age.
- Aging effects on nutritional status are very individual, and every person will be affected differently.
- Factors such as physical disability or disease-related consequences greatly affect feeding and appetite.

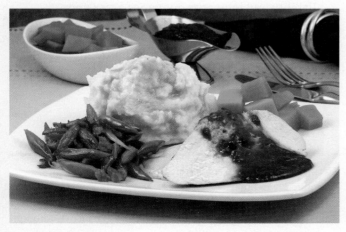

©tacar/Shutterstock

- Social and environmental factors also greatly affect eating and appetite.
- Malnutrition and loss of lean mass are consequences of alterations in feeding and appetite.
- Frailty is a syndrome associated with aging, where strength, lean body mass, mobility, and other parameters are affected.

General Nutrition Guidelines in the Geriatric Population

- Even though older people are a heterogeneous group, there are homogenous dietary intake recommendations for persons 65 years and older.
- Disease states usually result in the need for specifically altering the recommendations for both or either the macronutrients and micronutrients.
- Highly bioavailable protein sources and limits on fats, such as saturated and trans fats, are important.
- Certain micronutrients are especially important to monitor in older people, such as calcium, vitamin D, iron, vitamin B_{12}, zinc, and selenium.
- Water and hydration are the most important nutritional factors to consider in older people.
- Alcohol should be avoided by frail elderly.

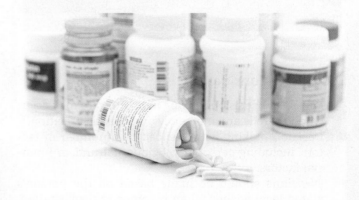

©KoBoZaa/Shutterstock

Polypharmacy in Geriatrics

- Polypharmacy is defined as the use of five or more drugs.
- Older adults use more than one-third of all medications, supplements, and over-the-counter remedies sold.

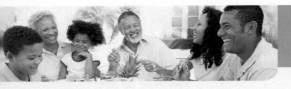

Learning Portfolio (continued)

- Drugs affect appetite, feeding, and nutritional status and vice versa. There are drug–drug interactions and drug–nutrient interactions.
- Adverse events from potentially inappropriate drug prescription and use are very costly to the health-care system.
- A list of medications that should not be prescribed to older people is called the Beers Criteria.
- The use of alcohol and prescription medications is known to cause serious problems and gravely affect nutritional status.

- feeding and hydration, or other potentially invasive treatments.
- There are undesirable consequences to feeding and hydrating someone artificially when that person is close to death.
- The interdisciplinary healthcare team may involve many different kinds of professionals and parapro-fessionals. They are charged with providing EOL care to the dying person.

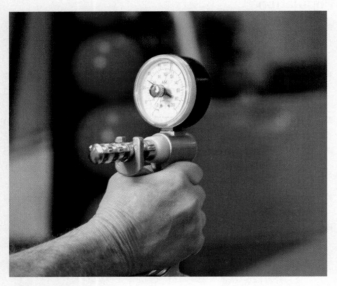

©John Foxx/Stockbyte/Getty Images

End-of-Life Considerations

- End-of-life decision making in health care may occur when there is an emergency and chaotic situation.
- Decision making is influenced by a number of fac-tors, including personal, religious, cultural, or finan-cial factors.
- Decisions should be made based on the person's stated legal wishes when it comes to resuscitation,

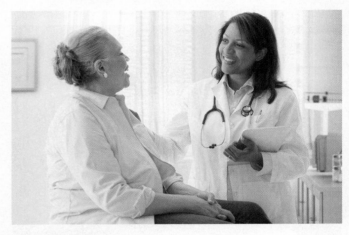

©KidStock/Blend Images/Getty

The Nutrition Care Process

- The Nutrition Care Process provides a standardized format and language for documentation.
- NCP is important for collection, structure, and dis-semination of data to other nutrition profession-als and organizations as well as other healthcare providers.
- The standardized structure and language decreases liability and increases outcomes assessment.
- In geriatrics, this process is particularly important because older adults receiving care often have com-plex situations and require a thorough evaluation, diagnosis, and monitoring plan.

Key Terms

ageusia: Inability to taste that results from damage to or a decrease in taste receptors or pathophysiological neurological changes.

anorexia of aging: Loss of appetite due to advanced degenerative processes, and the pathophysiological effects of aging and disease consequence.

anosmia: Inability to smell. May be genetic from birth or acquired over time.

artificial nutrition and hydration (ANH): The delivery of fluids and food or nutrients via artificial means, such as through a tube or an intravenous line.

ataxia: Inability to walk properly due to pathological changes in the brain and nervous system.

bioavailability: When a nutrient is highly digestible and easily absorbed; it usually refers to proteins with a full complement of needed amino acids.

brain death: Initial requirements for determination include neuroimaging or clinical findings that suggest catastrophic cerebral events where there are no identifiable other conditions that may represent brain death, such as severe metabolic derangement, intoxication, poisoning, or other acute vascular anomaly. There is persistent unresponsiveness, there are no reflexive responses to pain or any brainstem responses, and there is apnea, with cessation of respiration and circulation.

cognitive decline: Decrease in mental acuity, status, and/or memory. Declines are usually due to pathophysiological processes affecting the brain and the central nervous system. Cognitive decline is associated with many different diseases, many of which occur more frequently in older persons.

coma: State of extreme unresponsiveness, with no voluntary movement or behavior, and sometimes normal reflexes may be lost. In coma, there is maintenance of autonomic functions. If coma persists for more than a month, it is called a persistent vegetative state. There are "grades" assigned to comas that delineate severity and type.

comorbid: When one medical condition occurs at the same time, but independently, of another medical condition.

decubitus ulcers: Bedsores or wounds that heal poorly and slowly. A function of being bedridden with fragile skin; decubitus ulcers often occur in very old or very ill persons, who are unable to be moved.

dentition: Having to do with teeth.

drug–drug and drug–nutrient interactions: The impact that drugs have on one another, the system, and the side effects, or the impact that drugs have on nutrients in terms of their intake, absorption, disposition, metabolism, utilization, and excretion, and vice versa.

dysgeusia: Altered sense of taste.

dysosmia: Altered sense of smell.

end-of-life (EOL) care: Persons nearing death have multiple concerns and needs, from provision of adequate nutrition to resuscitation in the event of cardiac failure.

frailty: A syndrome characterized by loss of hand grip strength, slow walking speeds, exhaustion, and loss of lean body mass.

frailty syndrome: A cluster of signs and symptoms that indicate that an older person is at risk for falls, fractures, and other acute health events. Usually characterized by decreased hand grip strength, loss of muscle mass, slower walking speeds, and other measures.

geriatrics: The medical specialty that focuses on managing the care of elderly persons.

healthcare proxy: A legal document in which a competent person makes another person his or her agent for health decisions on their behalf when the individual is no longer able to make or execute healthcare decisions at some future point. The right of a legally named person to execute the wishes for treatment or refusal of treatment when an individual is incapacitated. Usually healthcare organizations, hospitals, and emergency rooms have a generic form of this document that they ask a patient to fill out and that they then keep with the person's chart should another emergency arise.

home health care: Provision of medical services to ill persons in their home by a licensed home health agency using skilled medical professionals and billed to the individuals' insurance. It is overseen by the patient's primary medical provider and includes services deemed appropriate by a medical care plan. Services may include, but are not limited to, the provision of medical equipment, home aides for activities of daily living, nursing, dietetics, speech, occupational and physical therapy, as well as social work and, in some instances, hospice. Curative treatments, life-prolonging measures, and other interventions are used in the person's place of residence. It is usually time limited, and insurance coverage or the person's financial resources determine time for provision of service. Each state has its own budget and procedures, regulations, and stipulations regarding home health care.

hospice care: A multidisciplinary approach to end-of-life care for individuals with a definitive terminal course of illness, usually defined as a 6-month period before death. Treatment of the underlying pathology and curative measures are not attempted but palliative care such as pain control and supportive measures including psychotherapy, social services, religious support, familial support and counseling, grief/anger management, physical/occupational therapy, dietetics, and provision of medical equipment and ancillary services are used as needed.

hydration: The provision of fluids either by mouth or through artificial means, such as an intravenous line or subcutaneous infusion.

immunocompromise: When the immune system does not function correctly or sufficiently.

intensive medical care: Intensive care is performed in critical care medical units to prolong life in patients with potentially reversible critical illnesses, organ-system failure, and traumatic injury or in unstable surgical patients. Life-supportive measures, constant monitoring, and technologically advanced treatments and equipment are used and artificial nutrition and hydration are usually part of this care.

living will: A legal document that can be drawn up and signed that states which medical and other life-sustaining procedures may or may not be done in the event that a person becomes mentally incompetent, comatose, otherwise incapacitated, or

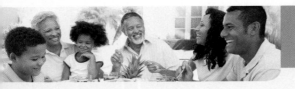

terminally ill. Such documentation should be readily available in the event of an emergent situation and on file with the primary care provider and immediate family members. Included in this documentation should be decisions regarding artificial nutrition and hydration as well as other treatment modalities. Several websites offer a download template for this documentation, and it can be filled out and filed for use at a later date. State and federal regulations govern the language used in these forms of documentation.

Nutrition Care Process: A systematic way to obtain and record patient data that has standard formats and terminology. Instituted by the Academy of Nutrition and Dietetics, it is a means to both collect and disseminate data for outcomes and to other health providers.

oldest old: While the numbers differ across agencies, organizations, and governmental entities, the majority use the cut point for the oldest old at 85 years or greater.

pain management: Management of pain and suffering requires an interdisciplinary approach that uses several branches of medicine and allied health. This may include pharmacotherapy, biofeedback, physical and occupational therapies, as well as psychotherapeutic approaches. Pain medicine employs several different kinds of analgesic medications, including opioids. Opioids at the end of life are common in palliative care but are controversial because of their effects on multiple organ systems and fears regarding their addictive potential. Decrements in respiratory competence and swallowing reflexes, as well as decreases in gastrointestinal motility and hydration status, are common, even with low-dose opioid administration.

palliative care: At any time during illness, the focus of palliative case is on symptom management during assessment and treatment of the underlying pathophysiology. This treatment aims to decrease pain and suffering, using aggressive pain treatments and a holistic approach to provide the best possible quality of life.

percutaneous endoscopic gastrostomy tube: Tube placed laparoscopically and used for feeding directly into the lumen of the stomach.

persistent vegetative state (PVS): A state of extreme unresponsiveness that lasts for more than 1 month, when a person displays no awareness or higher cerebral function. Midbrain and brainstem functions are preserved, with sleep–wake cycling and autonomic control over functions such as breathing and heart rate. There may be some reflexive movement. End-stage dementia often leads to PVS.

polypharmacy: The use of five or more drugs per day.

power of attorney: A durable power of attorney for healthcare decisions is documentation that identifies the person who can make and carry out an individual's wishes in the event

that there is an emergent situation and the individual is incapacitated mentally or physically or is comatose. This responsibility is also known as healthcare proxy, with regard to healthcare matters. Usually, there are two different power of attorney forms, one for financial "gifts" and one for all other estate matters. The gift rider, durable power of attorney, and healthcare proxy documents should all be designed, notarized, and filed prior to an individual becoming sick and incapacitated. It is best to get the advice of a reputable lawyer with estate planning and elder care experience. General durable power of attorney is a legal document that designates another person to act on the individual's behalf concerning legal or business matters. That person can write checks, access bank accounts, and so forth while the individual is incapacitated.

primary aging: Aging as a function of time alone, also sometimes called chronological aging.

resuscitation: The restoration of life or consciousness that involves (usually) cardiopulmonary efforts, such as mouth-to-mouth breathing or cardiac massage. Do Not Resuscitate or DNR orders are medically and legally binding.

secondary aging: Changes that occur on the cellular level as a result of disease processes.

sleep–wake reversal: A pathological change in the brain's sleep–wake circadian rhythm that results in wakefulness at night and drowsiness during the day.

tertiary aging: The social, demographic, and environmental influences over time.

therapeutic index: A ratio of how much drug or specific nutrient is needed to get the desired effect versus how much is toxic.

Uniform Determination of Death Act (UDDA): Adopted by almost all of the states in the United States, the UDDA states: "An individual who has sustained either (1) irreversible cessation of circulation and respiratory functions, or (2) irreversible cessation of all functions of the entire brain, including the brain stem, is dead. A determination of death must be made in accordance with accepted medical standards" and "When an individual is pronounced dead by determining that the individual has sustained an irreversible cessation of all functions of the entire brain, including the brain stem, there shall be independent confirmation by another physician."

vascular dementia: The cumulative loss of brain function due to the changes associated with aging and vascular narrowing of vessels to the brain, leading to loss of oxygen and nutrients and resulting in cell death.

will: A document that is a legal set of directions for what should be done after a person dies.

xerostomia: Dry mouth usually of pathologic origin that occurs more frequently in advanced age.

Discussion Questions

1. Differentiate between the nutritional recommendations and requirements for otherwise healthy older adults with adults in the oldest, most frail geriatric population.

2. Discuss the complexity and implications of declining cognition, polypharmacy, and frailty in older adults.

3. Debate the pros and cons for issues related to end-of-life care including the ethics of artificial hydration and nutrition.

Activities

1. Spend time as a volunteer at a long-term care facility.
2. Observe patients in a dementia unit, especially during mealtimes.
3. Watch the PBS documentary called *Suicide Tourist*.
4. Investigate the right to die movement.
5. Go to webpages for Oregon, Washington, and Montana to view the differences in their legislation on assisted suicide and contrast the information from these states with that from the rest of the United States.

6. Interview clergy representation of different religious groups' observances regarding the feeding and hydration of a dying person.

Study Questions

1. What is apoptosis?
   a. Preprogrammed cell death
   b. Inability to smell
   c. Inability to taste
   d. Inhalation of food particles
2. What is xerostomia?
   a. Preprogrammed cell death
   b. Inability to smell
   c. Dry mouth
   d. Dry skin
3. Dementia patients exhibit sun-downing, which is what?
   a. Agitation that occurs at the end of the day
   b. Alteration in the circadian rhythm
   c. A stimuli overload reaction seen in cognitive decline
   d. All of the above
4. Atrophic gastritis has which of the following effects?
   a. Decreased production of hydrochloric acid
   b. Decreased synthesis of intrinsic factor
   c. Vitamin B_{12} deficiency
   d. All of the above
5. Frailty syndrome has which of the following signs and symptoms?
   a. Dry mouth
   b. Vitamin B_{12} deficiency
   c. Reduced hand grip strength
   d. Both A and B

6. How can sarcopenic obesity be characterized?
   a. As loss of muscle mass
   b. As increase in fat mass
   c. As increase in water retention
   d. Both A and B
7. Protein requirements in general should be based on body weight at which amount?
   a. 0.1–0.5 g/kg
   b. 0.5–1.0 g/kg
   c. 1.0–1.5 g/kg
   d. 1.5–2.0 g/kg
8. Which of the following fats should be decreased in the diet of an older person?
   a. Very long-chain fatty acids
   b. Medium-chain triglycerides
   c. Trans fatty acids
   d. Short-chain fatty acids
9. What might hamper fluid intake in older adults?
   a. Dry mouth
   b. Decreased thirst sensations
   c. Increased hunger sensations
   d. None of the above
10. What is the primary reason why older people are so prone to dehydration?
    a. They have an increased fat mass.
    b. They have a decreased lean body mass.
    c. They have a decrease in bone calcium levels.
    d. They have decreased liver function.

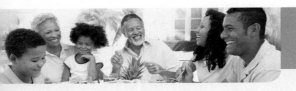

11. Which of the following is activated into a superhormone by the liver?
    a. Calcium
    b. Vitamin D
    c. Vitamin K
    d. Vitamin B_{12}

12. Which trace mineral is directly related to wound healing?
    a. Selenium
    b. Magnesium
    c. Zinc
    d. Chromium

13. What is the chemical compound known as drinking alcohol?
    a. Methanol
    b. Ethanol
    c. Propanol
    d. Isobutyl alcohol

14. What is the definition of major polypharmacy?
    a. The use of two or more drugs/day
    b. The use of three or more drugs/day
    c. The use of four or more drugs/day
    d. The use of five or more drugs/day

15. Some drugs are dangerous to older adults. Which of the following drugs always falls into the "Do Not Prescribe" category?
    a. Tranquilizers
    b. High blood pressure medications
    c. Constipation remedies
    d. Insulin for diabetes

16. Which of the following is the name of the list that has "Do Not Prescribe" categories for medications in older adults?
    a. Beers Criteria
    b. Nutrition Care Process
    c. Assessing Care Criteria
    d. None of the above

17. What percentage of all medications, supplements, herbals, and OTC remedies are consumed by persons older than age 65 in the United States?
    a. 25%
    b. 33%
    c. 50%
    d. 66%

18. Which of the following are consequences of hydrating someone who is near death?
    a. Death rattle
    b. Secretions
    c. Bedsores
    d. All of the above

19. Which is the time period that defines the need for hospice care in someone who is terminally ill?
    a. 2 months
    b. 4 months
    c. 6 months
    d. 8 months

20. What is the name of the document that names an individual legally responsible for making healthcare decisions in the event someone is no longer able to do so for him- or herself?
    a. Healthcare proxy
    b. Power of attorney
    c. Uniform Determination of Death Act
    d. All of the above

21. Which is the most common form of abuse or neglect?
    a. Self-neglect
    b. Resident-to-resident aggression
    c. Caregiver neglect or abuse
    d. Family member neglect or abuse

22. What is the primary "guiding care" principle?
    a. The patient's wishes are the most important.
    b. The family's wishes are the most important.
    c. The doctor's wishes are the most important.
    d. The hospital's wishes are the most important.

23. What does the right to die movement believe in?
    a. A person's right to end his or her own life.
    b. Doctors shouldn't be punished for helping a terminally ill and suffering patient end his or her own life.
    c. The ability to have informed passive or active euthanasia.
    d. All of the above.

24. Which of the following is not a component of the Nutrition Care Process?
    a. Assessment
    b. Monitoring
    c. Scheduling
    d. Intervention

25. Which of the following is not a direct benefit of having standardization in the Nutrition Care Process?
    a. Uniform collection of data
    b. Language that other health professionals can understand
    c. Continuity of care between transfers
    d. Standardized diagnoses specific to nutrition

Weblinks

- **Academy of Nutrition and Dietetics**
  http://www.eatright.org

- **American Society for Parenteral and Enteral Nutrition (ASPEN)**
  https://www.nutritioncare.org/

- **American Speech-Language-Hearing Association**
  http://www.asha.org/

- **Commission for Certification in Geriatric Pharmacy**
  http://www.ccgp.org/

- **Death with Dignity Organization**
  https://www.deathwithdignity.org

- **Dignitas—Worldwide Right to Die Organization**
  http://www.dignitas.ch/?lang=en

- **National Association of Area Agencies on Aging**
  http://www.n4a.org/

- **National Institute on Aging**
  https://www.nia.nih.gov/

References

1. Fulop T, Le Page A, Garneau H, et al. Aging, immunosenescence and membrane rafts; the lipid connection. *Longev Healthspan*. 2012;1:6. doi:10.1186/2046-2395-1-6.

2. Larbi A, Fulop T. From truly naïve to exhausted senescent T-cells. *Cytometry*. 2014;85(1):26–35.

3. Bekhet A, Zauszniewski J. Resourcefulness, positive cognitions, relocation controllability and relocation adjustment among older people. A cross sectional study of older people. *Int J Older People Nurs*. 2013;8(3):244–252.

4. Sole-Aureo E. The oldest old: health in Europe and the United States. *Ann Rev Gerontol Geriatr*. 2013;33(1):3–33.

5. Logemann J, Curro F, Pauloski B, Gensler G. Aging effects on oropharyngeal swallow and the role of dental care in oropharyngeal dysphagia. *Oral Dis*. 2013;19(1):733–737.

6. Lin L, Liv L, Wang Y, et al. The clinical features of foreign body aspiration into the lower airway in geriatric patients. *Clinical Intervent Aging*. 2014;9(1):161–166.

7. Sorensen L, Moller P, Flint A, Martens M, Raben A. Effect of sensory perception of foods on appetite and food intake: a review of studies on humans. *Int J Obes*. 2003;27(10):1152–1159.

8. Weideman T, Heuberger R. The nutritional status of the bariatric patient and its effect on periodontal disease. *Bariatr Surg Prac Patient Care*. 2013; 8(4):161–165.

9. Mann T, Heuberger R, Wong H. The association between chewing and swallowing difficulties and nutritional status in older adults. *Austral Dental J*. 2013;58(1):200–206.

10. Dunlop P, Subashan P, VanSwearingen J, et al. Transitioning a narrow path: the impact of fear of falling in older adults. *Gait Posture*. 2012;35(1):92–95.

11. Rayner C, Horowitz M. Physiology of the aging gut. *Curr Opinion Clinic Nutr Metabol Care*. 2013;16(1):33–38.

12. Millward D. Protein requirements and aging. *Am J Clin Nutr*. 2014;100(4):1210–1212.

13. Pahnke J, Frolich C, Krohn M, et al. Impaired mitochondrial energy production and ABC transporter function—a crucial interconnection in demented proteopathies of the brain. *Mechanism Aging Develop*. 2013;134(10):506–515.

14. Meijers J, Schols J, Halfens R. Malnutrition in care home residents with dementia. *J Nutr Health Aging*. 2014;18(6):595–600.

15. Cimarolli V, Jopp D. Sensory impairments and their associations with functional disability in a sample of the oldest old. *Quality Life Res*. 2014;23(7):1977–1984.

16. Palecek E, Teno J, Casarett D, et al. Comfort feeding only: a proposal to bring clarity to decision making regarding difficulty with eating for persons with advanced dementia. *J Am Geriatr Soc*. 2010;58(3):580–584.

17. Bourdel-Marchasson I. How to improve nutritional support in geriatric institutions. *J Amer Med Dir Assoc*. 2010;11(1):13–20.

18. Maggio M, Colizzi E, Eisichella A, et al. Stress hormones, sleep deprivation and cognition in older adults. *Maturitas*. 2013;76(1):22–44.

19. Heuberger R, Wong H. The association between depression and widowhood and nutritional status in older adults. *Geriatr Nurs*. 2014;35(6):428–433.

20. Duggal N, Upton J, Phillips A, et al. Depressive symptoms post fracture in older adults are associated with phenotypic and functional alterations. *Immunity Aging*. 2013;16(11):25–27.

21. Sirey J, Grenfield A, Depasquale A, et al. Improving engagement in mental health treatment for home meal recipients with depression. *Clin Intervent Aging*. 2013;8:1305–1308.

22. Heuberger R, Caudell K. Profiling users and non-users of senior services. *Advances Aging Res*. 2013;2(4):144–153.

23. Weddle D, Berkshire S, Heuberger R. Evaluating nutrition risk factors of older African Americans in determining use of an urban congregate meals program. *J Nutr Gerontolog Geriatr*. 2012;31(1):38–58.

24. Schnieder A, Ralph N, Olson C, et al. Predictors of senior center use among older adults in NYC public housing. *J Urban Health*. 2014;9(16):1033–1047.

25. Siegel C, Hochgatterer A, Dorner T. Contributions of ambient assisted living for health and quality of life in the elderly and care services. *BMC Geriatrics*. 2014;14:112–126.

26. Heuberger RA. Impact of housing type on nutritional status and oral health of rural older adults. *Seniors Housing Care J*. 2011;19(1):49–64.

27. Fussberg M, Osteling S, Braam A, et al. Functional disability in older Europeans. *Soc Psychiatr Psychiatr Epidemiol*. 2014;49(9):1475–1482.

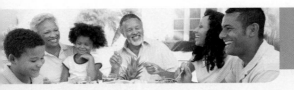

Learning Portfolio (continued)

28. Heuberger R, van Eeden-Moorefield B, Wong H. Perceived versus actual health and nutritional status: results from a cross-sectional survey of rural older adults. *J Gerontol Geriat Res*. 2013;3:141. doi:10.4.4172/2167–7182.1000141.

29. Adelman R, Tmanova L, Delgado D, et al. Caregiver burden: a clinical review. *JAMA*. 2014;311(10):1052–1060.

30. Charlton K, Batterham M, Bowden S, et al. A high prevalence of malnutrition in acute geriatric patients predicts adverse clinical outcomes and mortality within 12 months. *ESPEN J*. 2013;8(3):120–142.

31. Malone Beach E, Franke C, Heuberger R. Electronic access to food and cash benefits. *Soc Work Pub Health*. 2012;27(5):424–440.

32. Heuberger RA. The frailty syndrome: a review. *J Nutr Gerontol Geriatr*. 2011;30(4):315–369.

33. Miller R, Crotty M. Musculoskeletal health, frailty and functional decline. *Best Pract Res Clinic Rheumatol*. 2014;28(3):395–410.

34. Chen X, Maoi G, Leng S. Frailty syndrome: an overview. *Clin Intervent Aging*. 2014;9:433–442.

35. Abellan Van Kan G, Gabor A, Rolland Y, et al. The assessment of frailty in older adults. *Clinic Geriatr Med*. 2010;26(2):275–286.

36. Ng T, Feng L, Nyut M, et al. Frailty in older persons: multi-system risk factors and the frailty risk index. *J Am Med Dir Assoc*. 2014;15(9):635–642.

37. Robertson D, Saava G, Coen R, et al. Cognitive function in the pre-frailty and frailty syndrome. *J Am Geriatr Soc*. 2014;62(11):2118–2124.

38. Kob R, Boltheimer L, Bertsch T, et al. Sarcopenic obesity and molecular clues to a better understanding of its pathogenesis. *Biogerontol*. 2015;16(1):15–29.

39. Bowen M. The relationship between body weight, frailty and the disablement process. *J Gerontol Series B: Psycholog Sci Soc Sci*. 2012;67(5):618–662.

40. Donnini L, Scardella P, Piombo L, et al. Malnutrition in elderly: social and economic determinants. *J Nutr Health Aging*. 2013;17(1):9–15.

41. Vanderwoude M, Michel J, Knight P, et al. Variability of nutritional practice by geriatricians across Europe. *Europ Geriatr Med*. 2011;2(2):67–70.

42. Dorner B. Practice paper of the American Dietetic Association: individualized nutrition approaches for older adults in health care communities. *J Am Diet Assoc*. 2010;110(10):1554–1563.

43. Lachner C, Martin C, John D, et al. Older adult psychiatric inpatients with non-cognitive disorders should be screened for vitamin B-12 deficiency. *J Nutr Health Aging*. 2014;18(2):209–213.

44. Beasley J, Shikany J, Thomson C. The role of dietary protein in the prevention of sarcopenia of aging. *Nutr Clin Pract*. 2013;28(6):684–690.

45. World Health Organization. Nutrition: nutrition for older people. Geneva, Switzerland: World Health Organization. Retrieved from: http://www.who.int/nutrition/topics/ageing/en/index1.html. Accessed June 25, 2015.

46. Ganapathy V, Thangaraju M, Prasad P, et al. Transporters and receptors for short chain fatty acids as the molecular link between colonic bacteria and the host. *Curr Opinion Pharmacol*. 2013;13(6):869–874.

47. Lakshiminarayanan B, Stanton C, O'Toole P. Compositional dynamics of the human intestinal microbiota with aging: implications for health. *J Nutr Health Aging*. 2014;19(9):773–786.

48. Sarri B, Mateos R, Sierra J, et al. Hypotensive, hypoglycemic and antioxidant effects of consuming a cocoa product in moderately hypercholesterolemic humans. *Food Function*. 2012;3(9):857–874.

49. Hsiao P, Mitchell D, Coffman D, et al. Dietary patterns and diet quality among diverse older adults: the University of Alabama at Birmingham Studies on Aging. *J Nutr Health Aging*. 2013;17(1):19–25.

50. Schnelle J, Leung F, Rao S, et al. A controlled trial of an intervention to improve urinary and fecal incontinence and constipation. *J Am Geriatr Soc*. 2010;58(8):1504–1511.

51. Godfrey H, Cloete J, Dymond E, et al. An exploration of the hydration care of older people. *Int J Nurs Studies*. 2012;49(10):1200–1211.

52. Hoope L, Bunn D, Jimi F, et al. Water loss and dehydration in aging. *Mechanism Aging Develop*. 2014;136(137):50–58.

53. Nanas JN, Matsouka C, Karageonrgopoulos D, et al. Etiology of anemia in patients with advanced heart failure. *J Am Coll Cardiol*. 2006;48(12):2485–2489.

54. Deierlein A, Moland K, Scanlin K, et al. Diet quality of urban older adults age 60–99 years. The Cardiovascular Health of Seniors and Built Environment Study. *J Acad Nutr Diet*. 2014;114(2):279–287.

55. Racine E, Lyerly J, Troyer J. The influence of home delivered Dietary Approaches to Stop Hypertension meals on body mass index, energy intake and percent of energy needs consumed among older adults with hypertension and or hyperlipidemia. *J Acad Nutr Diet*. 2012;112(11):1755–1762.

56. Cashman KD, Hayes A, O'Donovan SM, et al. Dietary calcium does not interact with vitamin D in terms of determining the response and catabolism of serum 25-hydroxyvitamin D during winter in older adults. *Am J Clin Nutr*. 2014;99(6):1414–1424.

57. Annweiler C, Rolland Y, Scholt A M, et al. Higher vitamin D intake is associated with lower risk of Alzheimer's disease. *J Gerontol Series A Biol Sci Med Sci*. 2012;67(11):1205–1211.

58. Winzenberg T, Vandermet I, Mason R. Vitamin D and the musculoskeletal health of older adults. *Austral Family Physician*. 2012;41(3):92–99.

59. Oudshoorn C, Hartholt K, Van Leeuwen J, et al. Better knowledge on vitamin D and calcium in older people is associated with a higher serum vitamin D level and a higher daily dietary calcium intake. *Health Educ J*. 2012;71(4):474–482.

60. Truong J, Fu X, Salzman E, et al. Age group and sex do not influence responses to vitamin K biomarkers to changes in dietary vitamin K. *J Nutr*. 2012;142(5):936–942.

61. Macfarlane A, Shi Y, Greene L. High dose compared with low dose vitamin B-12 supplement use is not associated with higher vitamin B-12 status in children, adolescents or older adults. *J Nutr*. 2014;144(6):915–921.

62. Kaplan R. Vascular endothelial function and oxidative stress are related to dietary niacin intake among healthy middle aged and older adults. *J Applied Physiol*. 2014;116(2):156–163.

63. Nazmi A, Weatherall M, Wilkins B, et al. Thiamin concentration in geriatric hospitalized patients using furosemide. *J Nutr Gerontol Geriatr*. 2014;33(1):47–54.

64. De Rocha T, Jacobsen K, Schuch J, et al. SLC30A3 and SEP15 gene polymorphisms influence the serum concentrations of zinc and selenium in mature adults. *Nutr Res*. 2014;34(9):742–748.

65. Bates C, Harner M, Mishra G. Redox modulating vitamins and minerals that prospectively predict mortality in older British people. *Br J Nutr.* 2011;105(1):123–132.

66. Heuberger RA. Alcohol and the older adult: a comprehensive review. *J Nutr Elder.* 2009;28(4):203–235.

67. Breslow R, Faden VB, Smothers B. Alcohol consumption by elderly Americans. *J Stud Alcohol Drug.* 2003;64(3):884–892.

68. Kuerbia A, Sacco P, Blazer D, et al. Substance abuse among older adults. *Clin Geriatr Med.* 2014;30(3):629–654.

69. Moore AA, Whiteman EJ, Ward KT. Risk of combined alcohol and medication use in older adults. *Am J Geriatr Pharmacother.* 2007;5:64–74.

70. Onder G, Landi F, Della C, et al. Moderate alcohol consumption and adverse drug reactions among older adults. *Pharmacoepidemiol Drug Safety.* 2002;11:385–392.

71. Pringle KE, Ahern FM, Heller DA, Gold CH, Brown TV. Potential for alcohol and prescription medication interactions in older people. *J Am Geriatr Soc.* 2005;53:1930–1936.

72. Heuberger RA. Polypharmacy and food drug interactions among older persons. *J Nutr Gerontol Geriatr.* 2012; 31(2):325–403.

73. Heuberger RA, Caudell K. Polypharmacy and nutritional status in older adults: a cross-sectional study. *Drugs Aging.* 2011; 28(4):315–323.

74. Bahat G, Tufan F, Bahat Z, et al. Assessments of functional status, comorbidities, polypharmacy, nutritional status and sarcopenia in Turkish community-dwelling male elderly. *Aging Male.* 2013;16(2):67–72.

75. Hartikainen S, Lönnroos E, Louhivuori K. Medication as a risk factor for falls: critical systematic review. *J Gerontol A Biol Sci Med Sci.* 2007;62(10):1172–1181.

76. Lavikainen P, Leskinen E, Hartikainen S, et al. Impact of missing data mechanism on the estimate of change: a case study on cognitive function and polypharmacy among older persons. *Clin Epidemiol.* 2015;7:169–180.

77. Saad M, Harisingani R, Katinas L. Impact of geriatric consultation on the number of medications in hospitalized older patients. *Consult Pharm.* 2012;27(1):42–48.

78. Toffanello ED, Inelmen EM, Imoscopi A, et al. Taste loss in hospitalized multimorbid elderly subjects. *Clin Interv Aging.* 2013;8:167–174.

79. Bright DR, Calinski DM, Kisor DF. Pharmacogenetic considerations in the elderly patient. *Consult Pharm.* 2015;30(4):228–239.

80. Heintz P, Buchholz M. After rescue: the importance of Beers Criteria for medication assessment in older adults. *Crit Care Nurs Q.* 2015;38(3):312–316.

81. San-José A, Agustí A, Vidal X, et al. Inappropriate prescribing to the oldest old patients admitted to hospital: prevalence, most frequently used medicines, and associated factors. *BMC Geriatr.* 2015;15(1):42–51.

82. Weston C, Weston J. Applying the Beers and STOPP criteria to care of the critically ill older adults. *Crit Care Nurs Q.* 2015;38(3):231–236.

83. Wehling M. Multimorbidity and polypharmacy: how to reduce the harmful drug load and yet add needed drugs in the elderly? Proposal of a new drug classification: fit for the aged. *J Am Geriatr Soc.* 2009; 57(3):560–561.

84. Hanlon JT, Schmader KE. What types of inappropriate prescribing predict adverse drug reactions in older adults? *Ann Pharmacother.* 2010;44(6):1110–1111.

85. Peron EP, Gray SL, Hanlon JT. Medication use and functional status decline in older adults: a narrative review. *Am J Geriatr Pharmacother.* 2011;9(6):378–391.

86. Levy HB, Marcus EL, Christen C. Beyond the Beers Criteria: a comparative overview of explicit criteria. *Ann Pharmacother.* 2010;44(12):1968–1975.

87. Murphy TE, Agostini JV, Van Ness PH, Peduzzi P, Tinetti ME, Allore H. Assessing multiple medication use with probabilities of benefits and harms. *J Aging Health.* 2008;20(6): 694–709.

88. De Smet PA, Denneboom W, Kramers C, Grol R. A composite screening tool for medication reviews of outpatients: general issues with specific examples. *Drugs Aging.* 2007;24(9):733–760.

89. Montalto C, Bhargva V, Hong SG. Use of complementary and alternative medicines by older adults. *J Evidence Based Complement Alternat Med.* 2006;11(17):27–46.

90. Gahche J, Bailey R, Burt V, et al. Dietary supplement use among U.S. adults has increased since NHANES III. *NCHS Data Brief.* 2011;(61):1–8.

91. Stupay S, Siverston L. Herbal and nutritional supplement use in the elderly. *Nurse Pract.* 2000;25(9):56–67.

92. Wade C, Chao M, Kronenberg F, et al. Medical pluralism among American women: results of a national survey. *J Womens Health* (Larchmt). 2008;17(5):829–840.

93. Rolita L, Freedman M. Over-the-counter medication use in older adults. *J Gerontol Nurs.* 2008;34(4):8–17.

94. Tachjian A, Maria V, Jahangir A. Use of herbal products and potential interactions in patients with cardiovascular diseases. *J Am Coll Cardiol.* 2010;55(6):515–525.

95. Heuberger R, Ivanitskaya L. Preferred sources of nutrition information: a comparison between younger and older adults. *J Intergenerat Relat.* 2011;9(2):176–190.

96. Elis JC, Mullan J, Worsley T. Prescription medication hoarding, borrowing or sharing behaviors in older residents in the Illawarra, New South Wales, Australia. *Australas J Ageing.* 2011;30(3):119–123.

97. Ellis JC, Mullan J. Prescription medication borrowing and sharing—risk factors and management. *Austral Fam Physician.* 2009;38(10):816–819.

98. Moen J, Bohm A, Tillenius T, Antonov K, Nilsson JL, Ring L. "I don't know how many of these [medicines] are necessary"—a focus group study among elderly users of multiple medicines. *Patient Educ Couns.* 2009;74(2): 135–141.

99. Schnabel K, Binting S, Witt C. Use of complementary and alternative medicines by older adults. *BMC Geriatr.* 2014;14:38–42.

100. Grief C, Grossman D, Rootenberg M, et al. Attitudes of terminally ill older adults towards complementary treatments and alternative medicine therapies. *J Palliat Care.* 2013;29(4):205–209.

101. Albers G, Van den Block L, Vander Stichele R. The burden of caring for people with dementia at the end of life in nursing homes: a postdeath study among nursing staff. *Int J Older People Nurs.* 2014;9(2):106–117.

102. Barnett MD, Williams BR, Tucker RO. Sudden advanced illness: an emerging concept among palliative care and surgical critical care physicians [published online December 29, 2014]. *Am J Hosp Palliat Care.* 2016;33(4):321–326. doi:10.1177/1049909114565108.

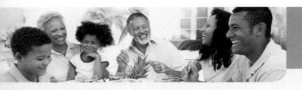

Learning Portfolio (continued)

103. Cartwright CM, White BP, Willmott L, Williams G, Parker MH. Palliative care and other physicians' knowledge, attitudes and practice relating to the law on withholding/withdrawing life-sustaining treatment: survey results [published online May 22, 2015]. *Palliat Med.* 2016;30(2):171–179. doi:10.1177/0269216315587996.

104. Garrido MM, Harrington ST, Prigerson HG. End-of-life treatment preferences: a key to reducing ethnic/racial disparities in advance care planning? *Cancer.* 2014;120(24): 3981–3986.

105. Dillworth J, Dickson VV, Mueller A, Shuluk J, Yoon HW, Capezuti E. Nurses' perspectives: hospitalized older patients and end-of-life decision-making [published online May 22, 2015]. *Nurs Crit Care.* 2016;21(2):e1–e11. doi:10.1111/nicc.12125.

106. Gainey R. Caregiver burden, elder abuse and Alzheimer's disease. *J Health Human Serv Admin.* 2006;29:245–259.

107. Burnett J, Achenbaum W, Murphy K. Prevention and early identification of elder abuse. *Clin Geriatr Med.* 2014;30(4): 743–759.

108. Lachs M, Pillemer K. Elder abuse. *N Engl J Med.* 2015;373:1947–1956.

109. Frazao S, Correia A, Norton P, Magalhaes T. Physical abuse against elderly persons in institutional settings. *J Forensic Legal Med.* 2015;36:54–60.

110. Burnes D, Pillener K, Caccamise P. Prevalence and risk factors for elder abuse and neglect in the community. *J Am Geriatr Soc.* 2015;61:1906–1912.

111. Ayalon L. Reports of elder neglect by older adults, their family caregivers and their home care workers. A test of measurement invariance. *J Gerontol Series B Psycholog Sci Soc Issues.* 2014;70(3):432–442.

112. Wang X, Brisbin S, Loo T, Straus S. Elder abuse: an approach to identification, assessment and intervention. *Canadian Med Assoc J.* 2015;187(8):575–582.

113. Hildebrand C, Taylor M, Bradway C. Elder self-neglect: the failure of coping because of cognitive and functional impairments. *J Am Assoc Nurs Practition.* 2014;26:452–462.

114. Grossman D, Rootenberg M, Perri GA, et al. Enhancing communication in end-of-life care: a clinical tool translating between the Clinical Frailty Scale and the Palliative Performance Scale. *J Am Geriatr Soc.* 2014;62(8):1562–1567.

115. Iijima S, Aida N, Ito H, et al. Position statement from the Japan Geriatrics Society 2012: end-of-life care for the elderly. *Geriatr Gerontol Int.* 2014;14(4):735–739.

116. Lee J, Cheng J, Au KM, et al. Improving the quality of end-of-life care in long-term care institutions. *J Palliat Med.* 2013;16(10):1268–1274.

117. Leheup BF, Piot E, Goetz C, et al. Withdrawal of artificial nutrition: influence of prior experience on the perception of caregivers. *Am J Hosp Palliat Care.* 2015;32(4):401–406.

118. Li Q, Zheng NT, Temkin-Greener H. Quality of end-of-life care of long-term nursing home residents with and without dementia. *J Am Geriatr Soc.* 2013;61(7):1066–1073.

119. Lodhi MK, Cheema UI, Stifter J. Death anxiety in hospitalized end-of-life patients as captured from a structured electronic health record: differences by patient and nurse characteristics. *Res Gerontol Nurs.* 2014;7(5):224–234.

120. Merel SE, Merel S, DeMers S, Vig E. Palliative care in advanced dementia. *Clin Geriatr Med.* 2014;30(3):469–492.

121. Nordin N, Kamaruzzaman SB, Chin AV, Poi PJ, Tan MP. A descriptive study of nasogastric tube feeding among geriatric inpatients in Malaysia: utilization, complications, and caregiver opinions. *J Nutr Gerontol Geriatr.* 2015;34(1):34–49.

122. Parsons C, McCorry N, Murphy K, et al. Assessment of factors that influence physician decision making regarding medication use in patients with dementia at the end of life. *Int J Geriatr Psychiatry.* 2014;29(3):281–290. doi:10.1002/gps.4006.

123. Pasman HR, Kaspers PJ, Deeg DJ, et al. Preferences and actual treatment of older adults at the end of life. A mortality follow-back study. *J Am Geriatr Soc.* 2013;61(10):1722–1729.

124. Plonk WM, Arnold RM. Terminal care: the last weeks of life. *J Palliat Med.* 2005;8(5):1042–1054.

125. Sampson EL, van der Steen JT, Pautex S, et al. European palliative care guidelines: how well do they meet the needs of people with impaired cognition? [published online April 13, 2015]. *BMJ Support Palliat Care.* 2015;5(3):301–305. doi:10.1136/bmjspcare-2014–000813.

126. Sinuff T, Dodek P, You JJ, et al. Improving end-of-life communication and decision making: the development of conceptual framework and quality indicators [published online January 24, 2015]. *J Pain Symptom Manage.* 2015;49(6):1070–1080. doi:10.1016/j.jpainsymman.2014.12.007.

127. Srinonprasert V, Kajornkijaroen A, Bangchang PN, et al. A survey of opinions regarding wishes toward the end-of-life among Thai elderly. *J Med Assoc Thai.* 2014;97(suppl 3):S216–222.

128. Valentini E, Giantin V, Voci A, et al. Artificial nutrition and hydration in terminally ill patients with advanced dementia: opinions and correlates among Italian physicians and nurses. *J Palliat Med.* 2014;17(10):1143–1149.

129. Van der Steen JT, Radbruch L, de Boer ME, et al. Achieving consensus and controversy around applicability of palliative care to dementia. *Int Psychogeriatr.* January 2016;28(1)133–145.

130. Wright I. Gerontology nursing: focus on end-of-life care. *Nurs N Z.* 2014;20(8):37.

131. Zahradnik EK, Grossman H. Palliative care as a primary therapeutic approach in advanced dementia: a narrative review. *Clin Ther.* 2014;36(11):1512–1517.

132. Heuberger R. Artificial nutrition and hydration in persons nearing death. *Clin Nutr Insight.* 2012;38(10):1–3.

133. Heuberger RA. Artificial nutrition and hydration at the end of life. *J Nutr Elder.* 2010;29(4):347–385.

134. Galanos AN, Neff EC, Heuberger RA, Bales CW. What is "optimal nourishment" for older adults at the end of life? A conversation. *J Nutr Elder.* 2010;29(4):386–392.

135. Aita K, Takahashi M, Miyata H, et al. Physicians' attitudes about artificial feeding in older patients with severe cognitive impairment in Japan: a qualitative study. *BMC Geriatr.* 2007;7:22. doi:10.1186/1471-2318-7-22.

136. Costa-Requena G, Espinosa Val M, Cristòfol R. Caregiver burden in end-of-life care: advanced cancer and final stage of dementia. *Palliat Support Care.* 2015;13(3):583–589.

CHAPTER 16

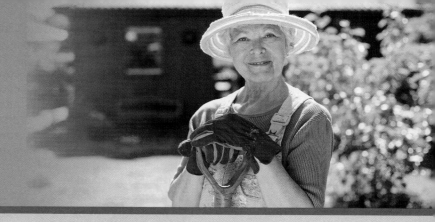

Nutrition for Health and Disease in Older Adults and Geriatrics

Nancy Munoz, DCN, MHA, RDN, FAND

Chapter Outline

Aging Demographics

Cardiovascular, Cerebrovascular, and Respiratory Conditions

Cancer

Cognitive Disorders

Endocrine and Metabolic Conditions

Gastrointestinal Conditions

Obesity and Malnutrition

Skeletal Health

Wound Healing

Renal and Genitourinary Conditions

Learning Objectives

1. Describe cardiovascular disease concepts.

2. Understand the role of nutrition in the care of older adults with cancer.

3. Develop strategies and interventions to encourage adequate nutrition and meal acceptance for older adults with dementia.

4. Comprehend the nutrition recommendations for the care of the older adult with diabetes.

5. Describe nutrition issues that may occur as a result of common gastrointestinal and digestive conditions.

6. Explain the significance of weight management in older adults.

7. Define frequency and management of iron- and folate-deficiency anemias in older adults.

8. List risk factors for developing skeletal disorders.

9. Describe the evidence-based guidelines for treating pressure injuries.

10. List the risk factors associated with impaired kidney function in older adults and the applicable nutrition intervention/prevention strategies.

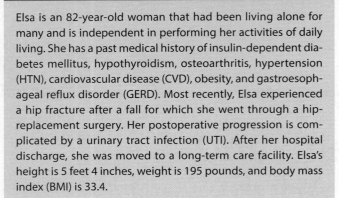

Case Study

Elsa is an 82-year-old woman that had been living alone for many and is independent in performing her activities of daily living. She has a past medical history of insulin-dependent diabetes mellitus, hypothyroidism, osteoarthritis, hypertension (HTN), cardiovascular disease (CVD), obesity, and gastroesophageal reflux disorder (GERD). Most recently, Elsa experienced a hip fracture after a fall for which she went through a hip-replacement surgery. Her postoperative progression is complicated by a urinary tract infection (UTI). After her hospital discharge, she was moved to a long-term care facility. Elsa's height is 5 feet 4 inches, weight is 195 pounds, and body mass index (BMI) is 33.4.

Aging Demographics

Preview Leading causes of death for older adults include heart disease, cancer, stroke, chronic lower respiratory disease, Alzheimer's dementia, and diabetes mellitus.

The aging concerns of healthcare professionals are different from the concerns expressed by older adults themselves.[1] As older Americans age, they express concern with maintaining their physical health, preventing cognitive decline, and promoting mental health.[1] Professionals and healthcare providers are concerned with protecting older adults from financial scams, ensuring access to affordable housing, and promoting brain health to prevent memory loss.[1] Interestingly, both groups agree that healthy eating and maintaining a positive attitude are essential in promoting health and well-being in older adults.[1]

As 10,000 Americans celebrate their 65th birthday every day since 2011, the progression in the number and proportion of older adults is unparalleled in the history of the United States. A longer life span and aging baby boomers will contribute to doubling the population of Americans aged 65 years and older over the next 25 years to about 72 million. By 2030, older adults will account for approximately 20% of the U.S. population.[2]

It is the position of the Academy of Nutrition and Dietetics that all Americans aged 60 years and older receive appropriate nutrition care; have access to coordinated, comprehensive food and nutrition services; and receive the benefits of ongoing research to identify the most effective food and nutrition programs, interventions, and therapies.[3]

Over the last century, there has been a shift in the leading causes of death, from infectious and acute diseases to chronic and degenerative illnesses. Currently, two out of three older adults have numerous chronic conditions. Heart disease and cancer are the leading causes of death in older adults. Other chronic diseases and conditions, such as stroke, chronic lower respiratory diseases, Alzheimer's disease, and diabetes, are also common.[2] (See **FIGURE 16.1** .) Sixty-six percent of all health-care dollars in the United States are spent on managing chronic conditions in older adults.[2]

Cardiovascular, Cerebrovascular, and Respiratory Conditions

Preview Cardiovascular disease (CVD) encompasses a number of conditions such as stroke and heart failure. A cerebrovascular accident is the result of interrupted blood flow to the brain. Chronic obstructive pulmonary disease is a lung disease in which a chronic obstruction of the lung airflow restricts normal breathing.

The term *cerebrovascular disease* encompasses all syndromes in which an area of the brain is briefly or permanently affected by ischemia or hemorrhage, with one or more of the cerebral blood vessels affected by disease. *Stroke* is a broad word denoting a group of illnesses that include cerebral infarction, cerebral hemorrhage, and subarachnoid hemorrhage.[4] Stroke is the third cause of death and second cause of disability and dementia in older adults worldwide.[4] The number of deaths triggered by cerebrovascular diseases increases with age.[5]

Approximately 90% of cerebrovascular disease and its comorbidities are avoidable.[6] Cerebrovascular disease deterrence can occur by encouraging healthy eating habits, being physically active, consuming alcohol in moderation, and avoiding tobacco use. Managing comorbidities such as diabetes mellitus and high cholesterol levels is crucial in decreasing the possibility of acquiring cerebrovascular disease.[7]

Hypertension
Prevalence and Etiology

Hypertension (HTN) is a condition in which the blood pressure (BP) is clinically elevated. Though normally asymptomatic, if left untreated, HTN can have catastrophic outcomes and result in death.[8] HTN is a risk factor for strokes, heart attacks, and arterial aneurysms. Nearly 80 million Americans have a diagnosis of HTN.[8] The kidneys are the main organ system involved in blood pressure regulation. Medical conditions common in older adults related to the renal system can precipitate HTN.[6,7]

The American Heart Association classifies blood pressure as normal, prehypertension, hypertension stage 1, hypertension stage 2, and hypertensive crisis. See **TABLE 16.1** .

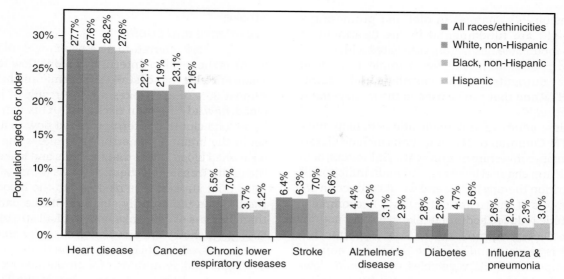

Figure 16.1

Leading causes of death among U.S. adults aged 65 and older in 2007–2009.

Data from: CDC, National Center for Health Statistics. National Vital Statistics Syatem, 2007-2009. National Council on Aging. The United States of Aging Survey 2015 results. Arlington, VA: National Council on Aging; July 2015. Retrieved from: https://www.ncoa.org/news/usoa-survey/2015-results/. Accessed September 29, 2016.

Prevention and Treatment

Signs and symptoms of hypertension involve abnormal (high) blood pressure measurement, severe headaches, anxiety, shortness of breath, and nosebleeds. Treatment goal of HTN is to control (manage) the signs and symptoms present. HTN is treated with medication and lifestyle modifications.[8] Some treatment strategies for older adults with HTN include the following:

- Consuming a healthy diet that includes foods that are low in sodium
- Being physically active
- Promoting a healthy weight
- Managing stress
- Avoiding smoking
- Complying with medication treatment
- Consuming alcoholic beverages in moderation

Research in adults has shown that modest decreases in the range of 20 mm Hg in the systolic and 10 mm Hg in

Let's Discuss

Promoting Community Health

What is the Great American Smokeout? Does your community initiate any activities to participate in this event?

Reference

American Cancer Society. The Great American Smokeout. Atlanta, GA: American Cancer Society. Retrieved from: http://www.cancer.org/healthy/stayawayfromtobacco/greatamericansmokeout/index. Accessed September 29, 2016.

the diastolic blood pressure can have a significant impact in decelerating the development of CVD or cardiac events such as stroke or myocardial infarction (MI).[9,10] Diet and lifestyle are crucial to both the prevention and treatment

Table 16-1

Categories for Blood Pressure Levels in Adults
(in mmHg, or millimeters of mercury)

Category	Systolic (top number)		Diastolic (bottom number)
Normal	Less than 120	And	Less than 80
Prehypertension	120–139	Or	80–89
High blood pressure			
Stage 1	140–159	Or	90–99
Stage 2	160 or higher	Or	100 or higher

Reproduced from Medicine Plus. Blood Pressure Numbers: What They Mean. *Winter 2010 Issue: Volume 5 Number 1 Page 10*. Retrieved from: https://medlineplus.gov/magazine/issues/winter10/articles/winter10pg10a.html

of hypertension.[11,12] Changes in diet and promoting a healthy weight are fundamental in the treatment of many of the modifiable risk factors associated with CVD.[12] Sodium and potassium intake, for example, have been recognized as nutrients that can contribute to the development of HTN and that can be used in the management of the condition.[12]

Many older adults require medications to help manage their HTN. Common HTN medications include diuretics, angiotensin-converting enzyme (ACE) inhibitors, beta blockers, calcium channel blockers, and renin inhibitors.[13] Medical nutrition therapy (MNT) and weight reduction are key components of the treatment.[14–16] MNT recommendations include reduced sodium intake; a dietary pattern such as the Dietary Approaches to Stop Hypertension (DASH) diet is recommended.[17] The DASH diet emphasizes consumption of fruits, vegetables, whole grains, low-fat dairy, seafood, nontropical vegetable oils (such as olive and canola), and nuts and limiting sodium, saturated fat and trans fat. Guidelines from the American Heart Association (AHA) and American College of Cardiology (ACC), published in November 2013, support consumption of 2,300 mg of sodium (or less) per day, with an additional decrease to 1,500 mg/d for individuals with increased risk for HTN.[14,18]

Being physically active has been shown to reduce blood pressure by 4–9 mm Hg.[15] The AHA and ACC endorse engaging in at least 30 minutes of moderate-to vigorous-intensity aerobic physical activity on most days of the week.[14] Guidelines for the management of overweight and obesity in adults support that the loss of approximately 5% to 10% of initial body weight can be effective in improving some of the risk factors associated with CVD, including blood pressure, lipids profiles, and glycemic control.[15]

Stroke

Prevalence and Etiology

A stroke, also referred to as a cerebrovascular accident (CVA), is the result of interrupted blood flow to the brain. There are two types of strokes: ischemic and hemorrhagic. Almost 80% of all strokes are the result of inadequate blood flow to the brain (ischemia). This can be caused by a blood clot that interrupts blood flow to a blood vessel in the brain. A hemorrhagic stroke is the result of a weakened blood vessel that ruptures and leaks blood into the brain. Transient ischemic attacks (TIAs), also referred to as mini strokes, take place when the blood supply to the brain is temporarily stopped. Stroke patients older than 85 years of age make up 17% of all stroke patients.[19] **FIGURE 16.2** shows the prevalence of stroke among noninstitutionalized adults by state in the United States.

Signs and symptoms of a stroke involve an abrupt episode of numbness or weakness of the face, arm, or leg; confusion; difficulty with speech patterns; problems seeing that can affect one or both eyes; inability to walk; dizziness and loss of balance or coordination; and strong headache without apparent cause.[20]

Hypertension is the main contributor for developing a stroke.[21] Other conditions and lifestyles that can contribute to developing a stroke include smoking, overweight and obesity, hyperlipidemia, diabetes mellitus, history of TIA, and atrial fibrillation.[21]

Prevention and Treatment

Managing stroke risk factors is essential to prevent stroke episodes. Uncontrolled HTN contributes to more than 50% of all stroke episodes. Treatment interventions aim to stop a stroke while it is in progress by rapidly dispersing the

Case Study

Upon admission to the long-term facility, Elsa's blood pressure readings are as follows:

Day	BP Reading
1	180/90 mm Hg
2	185/95 mm Hg
3	175/80 mm Hg

Questions

1. After reviewing Elsa's most recent history (s/p surgery, UTI, and just being admitted to a long-term care facility) how should her obesity level be treated?
2. What nutrition interventions and lifestyle changes should be recommended to treat Elsa's stage II blood pressure?

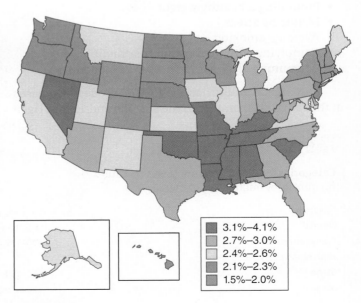

Legend:
- 3.1%–4.1%
- 2.7%–3.0%
- 2.4%–2.6%
- 2.1%–2.3%
- 1.5%–2.0%

Figure 16.2
Stroke prevalence in the United States.

Reproduced from Centers for Disease Control and Prevention. MMWR. Prevalence of Stroke - United States, 2006–2010. Retrieved from: https://www.cdc.gov/mmwr/preview/mmwrhtml/mm6120a5.htm

blood clot or by ending the bleeding. After the stroke, individuals need to participate in rehabilitation to overcome disabilities and damage that remain. The use of blood thinners is the most common drug therapy for stroke treatment.[20] Antihypertensives are used to lower blood pressure by opening the blood vessels, decreasing blood volume, or decreasing the rate or force of heart contraction. When the arteries are affected by plaque buildup, procedures such as carotid endarterectomy, angioplasty, and stents are used.[22]

Heart Failure
Prevalence and Etiology

Heart failure (HF) is caused by the heart's inability to pump adequate amounts of oxygenated blood to support other body organs. HF is a common illness, particularly in older adults.[23,24]

Heart failure is more predominant in some parts of the United States. FIGURE 16.3 shows the death rate in the United States from heart failure from 2011 to 2013.

Laboratory testing can be instrumental in diagnosing the occurrence of heart failure. Blood tests can be helpful for distinguishing heart failure from pulmonary disease. In many instances individuals who smoke suffer from both HF and pulmonary disease. Differentiating between these two disorders to provide a true diagnosis can pose a challenge for the physician.[25]

Prevention and Treatment

History of uncontrolled HTN and history of MI are the two most common risk factors for heart failure.[10,26] Aging contributes to increased risk for this condition. In older adults 75–85 years of age, the risk of developing HF is four times greater than in their younger counterparts.[10] Mortality rate is nearly 50% within 5 years of receiving a diagnosis.[22,23] Research suggests that controlling blood pressure and low-density lipoprotein (LDL) cholesterol can reduce the risk of HF. Prescription medications normally used in the treatment of HF include diuretics, ACE inhibitors, aldosterone antagonists, Angiotensin receptor blockers, beta blockers, Isosorbide dinitrate/hydralazine hydrochloride, and digoxin.[27] Promoting glycemic control, weight reduction, limiting alcohol, and smoking cessation are also keys to preventing this disease.[24]

Lifestyle Changes

Incorporating healthy lifestyle behavior into the older adult's daily routine is an important component in preventing and treating HF. This includes adopting a heart healthy diet, sufficient fluid intake, active lifestyle, promoting a healthy weight, and eluding the use of tobacco and illegal drugs.[23,27]

For older patients with HF, a healthy diet should be low in sodium and saturated fats. High sodium intake may contribute to fluid retention in the body. When there

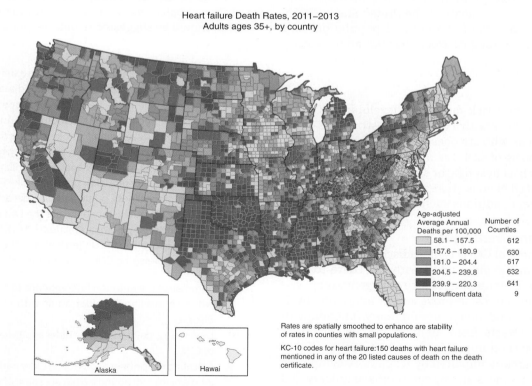

Heart failure Death Rates, 2011–2013
Adults ages 35+, by country

Age-adjusted Average Annual Deaths per 100,000	Number of Counties
58.1 – 157.5	612
157.6 – 180.9	630
181.0 – 204.4	617
204.5 – 239.8	632
239.9 – 220.3	641
Insufficent data	9

Rates are spatially smoothed to enhance are stability of rates in counties with small populations.

KC-10 codes for heart failure:150 deaths with heart failure mentioned in any of the 20 listed causes of death on the death certificate.

Alaska   Hawai

Figure 16.3
Death rates due to heart failure, 2011–2013.

Reproduced from Centers for Disease Control and Prevention Division for Heart Disease and Stroke Prevention. Heart failure fact sheet. Atlanta, GA: Centers for Disease Control and Prevention; last updated June 16, 2016. Retrieved from: http://www.cdc.gov/dhdsp/data_statistics/fact_sheets/fs_heart_failure.htm. Accessed June 26, 2016.

is fluid overload, the heart must work harder to manage greater volume in the body. Consumption of fat and trans fatty acids can promote increased cholesterol levels and increased risks for heart disease. The heart healthy diet is also low in sugar and refined grains.[23,27]

Because some of the medications used to manage HF deplete the body of potassium, potassium-rich foods should be part of a heart healthy diet. Fluid restriction is usually part of the dietary regime of individuals with HF. Fluids are generally limited to 2 liters per day.[23,27]

Older HF patients who are overweight and obese should be encouraged to lose weight to reach a healthy weight in efforts to avert the progression of HF. In HF patients weight is examined every day. Smokers should be encouraged to stop this lifestyle habit.[23,27]

Medications

Prescription medications normally used in the treatment of HF include the following:[27]

- Diuretics aid in controlling fluid accumulation.
- ACE inhibitors support normal blood pressure.
- Aldosterone antagonists help relieve the body of excess fluid and sodium. This action helps to decrease the blood volume that is pushed by the heart.

Chronic Obstructive Pulmonary Disease
Prevalence and Etiology

Chronic obstructive pulmonary disease (COPD) is the fourth leading cause of death in the United States.[28] This condition affects 10% of the general population, and increase in age is strongly associated with an increasing prevalence.[29]

Risk Factors

The most common risk factor for developing COPD is smoking. Individuals with a history of obstructions of the airway and those who are obese are also at risk.[30]

The diagnosis of COPD is difficult to make because symptoms such as dyspnea, or shortness of breath upon exertion, reduced exercise tolerance, and fatigue are also present in other conditions such as HF.[31]

Prevention and Treatment

The management of COPD is multidisciplinary. The goals of treatment in the older adult with COPD are to treat and avert chronic symptoms, reduce emergency room visits and hospitalizations, improve and/or maintain physical activity level, and augment pulmonary function with minimal side effects from medications. Management should also focus on improving health status (quality of life), which is greatly impaired by respiratory symptoms such as breathlessness and by symptoms of anxiety and depression. As the disease advances, the goals of treatment shift to lessen the decline of lung function over time and decrease mortality.[32]

The older adults' nutritional status has an impact on their ability to respond to medical treatment. The presence of malnutrition, particularly protein-calorie malnutrition, can exacerbate the disease development, producing atrophy of the diaphragm and the muscles responsible for the pumping mechanism, which control the expansion and contraction of the diaphragm to move air in and out of the lungs.[33]

A number of factors can affect dietary intake of older adults with COPD and can also contribute to weight loss. Change in taste from chronic sputum production, flattening of the diaphragm leading to early satiety, and fatigue that limits energy for both consuming and preparing meals can interfere with individuals' ability to meet their nutritional needs. As a result of the metabolic changes in COPD produced by a rise in daily expenditure and reduced respiratory muscle efficiency, the caloric needs of these individuals are higher than their non-COPD counterparts.[34–36] For older adults with high protein needs, protein should be provided in sufficient amounts, 1.2–1.7 g/kg of body weight, to promote, maintain, and restore lung and muscle strength as well as promote immune function.[37] Interventions to manage some of the nutrition symptoms associated with COPD include high-calorie/high-protein, nutrient-dense foods to maintain body weight and lean body mass as well as to prevent cachexia.[35] Strategies such as resting before meals to limit fatigue when preparing and consuming meals, eating small and frequent meals to manage dyspnea and early satiety, and consuming high-calorie/high-protein oral nutrition supplements and/or vitamin and mineral supplements should be suggested to older patients with COPD.[35]

Recap Over the last century, there has been a shift in the leading causes of death, from infectious and acute diseases to chronic and degenerative illnesses. Heart disease is one of the leading causes of death in older adults. Conditions and lifestyles that can contribute to developing a stroke include the presence of hypertension, smoking, overweight and obesity, hyperlipidemia, diabetes mellitus, history of TIA, and atrial fibrillation. Managing stroke risk factors is essential to prevent stroke episodes. Heart failure is a common illness, particularly in older adults. History of uncontrolled HTN and history of MI are the two most common risk factors for developing heart failure.[10,26] COPD is the fourth leading cause of death in the United States.[28] The most common risk factor for developing COPD is smoking.

1. Summarize the nutrition interventions to be considered when counseling an older adult with cardiovascular disease.
2. Develop a 2-day menu for an older adult with a diagnosis of CHF.
3. Calculate the protein needs for an older adult with COPD who weighs 190 pounds. What are some of the interventions that can be put in place to meet the protein needs of this individual?

Cancer

> **Preview** Cancer is characterized by an uncontrolled division of abnormal cells in a part of the body. Healthcare providers need to help older adults realize the effect of intensive treatment on their physical, emotional, and social well-being.

It is hard to discern why one individual develops cancer and another goes disease free. Age, alcohol consumption, cancer-causing substances, chronic inflammation, diet, hormones, immunosuppression, infectious agents, obesity, radiation, sunlight exposure, and consumption of tobacco products are the most commonly cited cancer risk factors.[38]

Prevalence and Etiology

Aging is the strongest risk factor for the development of cancer. More than 60% of all episodes of cancer occur in older adults 65 years and older.[39] Cancer is a group of diseases with an abnormal, unregulated cell growth caused by a series of DNA metamorphoses. Abnormal DNA can be inherited or acquired. Damaged DNA can occur as a result of lifestyle activities such as cigarette smoking or environmental causes such as sun exposure.[40] Although genetic and environmental factors have been linked to effected DNA and cell replication abnormalities, the exact causes of cancer-causing transformations are not completely understood.[41] Individuals with cancer need treatment that is intended for the type of cancer with which they have been diagnosed.[40] Older adults with cancer may have additional challenges including other health and medical conditions, social and economic barriers, and physical and functional limitations that make dietary guidance more complex.

Risk Factors

Research suggests that some risk factors increase the probability of anyone developing cancer.[38]

A number of nutrients and food items have been studied in efforts to define their association with increase or decrease in cancer risk with unique considerations for older adults. These include the following:[38]

- *Alcohol:* Alcohol use has been linked to the development of cancer. The association of red wine and reduction of cancer risk has not been scientifically defined.
- *Antioxidants:* Laboratory and animal research has shown that exogenous antioxidants can help avert the free radical injury linked with the development of cancer. Numerous large randomized, placebo-controlled prevention clinical trials, however, did not support this hypothesis, and some of the largest clinical trials had to be abandoned because the patients getting antioxidants had an increased rate of cancer compared with patients who did not receive them.[42]
- *Artificial sweeteners:* Studies have been done on the safety of several artificial sweeteners, such as saccharin, aspartame, acesulfame potassium, sucralose, neotame, and cyclamate. There is no conclusive evidence that the artificial sweeteners available commercially in the United States are associated with cancer risk in humans.
- *Calcium:* Research results examining the association between increased calcium consumption and decreased risk for developing colorectal cancer, while promising, are inconclusive. Whether a relationship exists between higher calcium intakes and reduced risks of other cancers, such as breast and ovarian cancer, is unclear. Some research suggests that a high calcium intake may increase the risk of prostate cancer.
- *Charred meat:* Certain chemicals, called heterocyclic amines (HCAs) and polycyclic aromatic hydrocarbons (PAHs), are formed when muscle meat, including beef, pork, fish, and poultry, is cooked using high-temperature methods. Exposure to high levels of HCAs and PAHs can cause cancer in animals; however, whether such exposure causes cancer in humans is unclear.
- *Cruciferous vegetables:* There is no conclusive evidence demonstrating the association between cruciferous vegetables and reduced risk for developing cancer.
- *Fluoride:* Water fluoridation has been shown to prevent and can even reverse tooth decay. Many studies, in both humans and animals, have shown no association between fluoridated water and cancer risk.
- *Garlic:* Some studies have suggested that garlic consumption may reduce the risk of developing several types of cancer, especially cancers of the gastrointestinal tract. However, the evidence is not definitive.
- *Tea:* Tea contains polyphenol compounds, particularly catechins, which are antioxidants. Results of epidemiologic research exploring the association between tea ingestion and cancer risk have been inconclusive.
- *Vitamin D:* Epidemiologic research in humans has implied that higher intakes of vitamin D or higher levels of vitamin D in the blood may be connected with a decreased risk of colorectal cancer; nonetheless, the results of randomized studies have been inconclusive.

Individuals who are obese may have an added risk of some types of cancer, including cancer of the breast (in women who have been through menopause), colon, rectum, endometrium, esophagus, kidney, pancreas, and gallbladder. Equally, consuming a healthy diet, being physically active, and keeping a healthy weight may help reduce risk of some cancers.[38]

Tobacco use is a leading cause of developing cancer and of death from cancer. Tobacco use should be discouraged at every age.

Prevention and Treatment

Researchers are actively exploring different ways to prevent cancer. These include controlling factors known to cause cancer, changes in diet and lifestyle, identifying precancerous conditions early, and chemoprevention.[43] Interventions to lower cancer risk are being studied in clinical trials.[43] Chemoprevention is the use of drugs, vitamins, or other agents (laboratory made) to try to reduce the risk of, or delay the development or recurrence of, cancer.[44]

When it comes to actual treatment, it is important to note that although cancer treatment for older adults can sometimes be complex and challenging, treatment can be just as useful for them as for younger adults. The goals of cancer treatment for older adults may include the following:[45]

- Getting rid of the cancer
- Helping a person live longer
- Reducing any signs and symptoms related to cancer
- Maintaining physical and emotional abilities and a person's quality of life

Treatment considerations and assessments, made with the healthcare team and the older adult with cancer and their family, should be based on the type of cancer and the level of metastasis (as applicable). Available treatment options, specific for cancer type, including the risks and benefits, should be addressed. The presence of medical conditions other than cancer that may put the older adult with cancer at an increased risk for treatment-related side effects or complications needs to be evaluated. Healthcare providers need to help the older adult realize the effect of intensive treatment on their physical, emotional, and social well-being. Special consideration should be given to quality of life because older adults living with cancer often make treatment choices based on what they value most in their lives and their level of physical, emotional, and social well-being. Older adults are more likely to have limited resources and live on a fixed income; therefore, financial limitations need to be considered. Some older adults might refuse treatment solely based on cost. Spiritual beliefs must be taken into account because many older adults have already come to terms with their mortality as a result of chronic illnesses, the loss of a spouse, or advanced age.[45]

Cancer treatment options for older adults may consist of a single therapy or a combination of therapies. The most common cancer treatment alternatives are surgery, chemotherapy, and radiation therapy. Palliative care is treatment to relieve a person's symptoms, improve a person's quality of life, and provide support to patients and their families. Palliative care is an important component of cancer management for an older adult. Palliative care may be a component of the standard treatment.[45]

Nutrition Recommendations

The Academy of Nutrition and Dietetics Evidence Analysis Library has outlined guidelines for the care of adults with cancer. The goals for nutrition care are to define symptoms that have an impact on the older individual's nutritional status and develop a nutrition plan that helps the person prevent or reverse nutritional deficiencies. Efforts should be made to identify cancer cachexia, help the person preserve lean body mass, and minimize nutrition-related side effects that can interfere with the individual's tolerance to treatment.[46]

Case Study

Elsa's medications include Humalog (insulin lispro), methimazole, nonsteriodal anti-inflammatory drugs (NSAIDs), thiazide diuretic, a calcium channel blocker, an antacid, and antibiotics.

In the past 3 weeks, Elsa has reported changes in bowel habits, abdominal pain, fatigue, decline in appetite, and a 5-pound weight loss in the past week.

Her new weight is 190 pounds. Her BMI is 32.6. The physician ordered laboratory work. Results were significant for low iron level and (+) occult blood in stool.

Question

1. Elsa has had a weight loss with a BMI decline to 32.6. She is showing GI symptoms such as changes in bowel habits, anorexia, and laboratory studies with low iron levels and (+) for occult blood. What additional information would be useful to complete Elsa's nutrition assessment.

Recap Cancer is a group of diseases with an abnormal, unregulated cell growth caused by a series of DNA metamorphoses. The cell changes generate the growth of tumors, which may spread to adjoining tissue or other parts of the body, thus creating metastasis. Healthcare providers need to help older adults realize the effect of intensive treatment on their physical, emotional, and social well-being. Special consideration should be given to quality of life because older adults living with cancer often make treatment choices based on what they value most in their lives and their level of physical, emotional, and social well-being.

1. Which modifiable risk factors should be highlighted for older adults at risk for developing cancer?
2. What are the goals of nutrition recommendations for older adults with cancer?

Cognitive Disorders

> **Preview** In the United States, millions of individuals experience Alzheimer's disease (AD) and other types of dementia. AD is a leading cause of death in the United States. As AD develops, individuals lose the ability to identify food and fail to recognize feelings of thirst and hunger.

Cognitive health is vital to overall health and well-being. As such, it must be treated in older adults with the same perseverance as physical health. More than 16 million people in the United States live with cognitive impairment.[48] The severity of dementia ranges from a mild stage, during which the older adult starts to see changes in functioning, to a severe stage, in which the person becomes fully dependent on caregivers for all activities of daily living. Dementia can also promote variations in mood and personalities, making it impossible for the older adult to solve problems or control emotions.

Prevalence

Every 67 seconds, somebody in the United States acquires Alzheimer's disease. By the year 2050, every 33 seconds an American will develop AD.[47,49] Presently, AD is the sixth leading cause of death in the United States, accounting for about 500,000 deaths every year.[47]

As the overall segment of the adult population continues to increase, so does the percentage of the U.S. population with AD.[47] Unless a cure for this disease is discovered, it is projected that the number of older adults with dementia will triple from around 5 million in 2014 to 16 million by 2050.[49] In the years to come, every U.S. state will see a rise in the number of older adults with a diagnosis of AD. **FIGURE 16.4** portrays the anticipated percentage increase of older adults with AD between the years 2014 and 2025.[47] A national estimate of the incidence of all forms of dementia is approximately 13.9%.[50]

Dementia is frequently defined as cognitive decline that affects a person's ability to clearly think, remember, and reason. Cognitive decline also affects behavioral abilities to the point that it hinders an older adult's capacity to perform activities of daily living (ADLs).[51] The severity of dementia ranges from a mild stage, during which the older adult starts to see changes in functioning, to a severe stage, in which the person becomes fully dependent on caregivers for all ADLs.[51]

Cognition and Memory Loss

Cognition relates to brain-related activities such as attention, memory, learning, executive function, and language. An individual's cognitive performance can define his or her sense of worth and purpose and influence the ability to stay socially engaged, be self-sufficient, recuperate from illness or injury, and handle the physiological changes associated with the aging process.[52] As people age, the confusion or memory loss seen over time can be an indication of decline in cognition.[53]

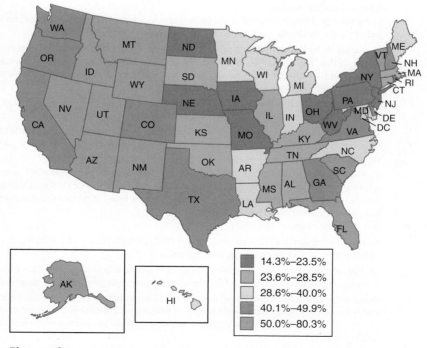

14.3%–23.5%
23.6%–28.5%
28.6%–40.0%
40.1%–49.9%
50.0%–80.3%

Figure 16.4
State prevalence of Alzheimer's disease, 2014–2015.

Reprinted with permission from the Alzheimer's Association. Alzheimer's disease facts and figures. Retrieved from: http://www.alz.org/alzheimers_disease_1973.asp.

Memory loss is classically one of the first warning indications of cognitive decline.[54] Mild cognitive injury is also a possible precursor to AD.[55] Several triggers for cognitive deterioration are modifiable. This includes symptoms such as depression, infections, medication side effects, and nutritional deficiencies such vitamin B_{12} deficiency. All these symptoms should be treated in a timely manner by a healthcare provider.[54]

Dementia

Dementia is a brain condition that interferes with older adults' capacity to remember, obtain and process new information, and communicate. Usual activities, such as clothing oneself or consuming meals, become hard to achieve. These changes in cognitive abilities eventually make it challenging for individuals to care for themselves.

Dementia can also promote variations in mood and personality, making it impossible for the older adult to solve problems or control emotions.[51,56]

Diagnosis

A number of risk factors serve as a precursor for dementia. To determine the specific brain disease that is causing dementia in an individual, different tests must be performed. **TABLE 16.2** offers a list of the different types of dementia and their unique characteristics.

Alzheimer's Disease

Alzheimer's disease (AD) was first identified over a hundred years ago. Research addressing symptoms, causes, risk factors, and treatment has only gained interest in the past 30 years. Through research we have learned a great

---

Table 16.2

Types of Dementia and Their Characteristics

Disease	Description
Alzheimer's disease (AD)	Most common type of dementia; accounts for an estimated 60–80% of cases. About 50% of these cases involve solely Alzheimer's pathology; many have evidence of pathologic changes related to other dementias. This is called mixed dementia (see mixed dementia in this table).
	Difficulty remembering recent conversations, names, or events is often an early clinical symptom; apathy and depression are also often early symptoms. Later symptoms include impaired communication, disorientation, confusion, poor judgment, behavior changes, and, ultimately, difficulty speaking, swallowing, and walking.
	Revised criteria and guidelines for diagnosing AD were proposed and published in 2011. They recommend that AD be considered a slowly progressive brain disease that begins well before clinical symptoms emerge.
	The hallmark pathologies of AD are the progressive accumulation of the protein fragment beta-amyloid (plaques) outside neurons in the brain and twisted strands of the protein tau (tangles) inside neurons. These changes are eventually accompanied by the damage and death of neurons.
Vascular dementia	Previously known as multi-infarct or poststroke dementia, vascular dementia is less common as a sole cause of dementia than AD, accounting for about 10% of dementia cases. However, it is very common in older individuals with dementia, with about 50% having pathologic evidence of vascular dementia (infarcts). In most cases, the infarcts coexist with Alzheimer's pathology.
	Impaired judgment and the inability to make decisions, plan, or organize are more likely to be initial symptoms, as opposed to the memory loss often associated with the initial symptoms of AD.
	Vascular dementia occurs most commonly from blood vessel blockage or damage leading to infarcts (strokes) or bleeding in the brain. The location, number, and size of the brain injuries determine whether dementia will result and how the individual's thinking and physical functioning will be affected.
	In the past, evidence of vascular dementia was used to exclude a diagnosis of AD (and vice versa). That practice is no longer considered consistent with the pathological evidence, which shows that the brain changes of both types of dementia commonly coexist. When two or more types of dementia are present at the same time, the individual is considered to have mixed dementia (see mixed dementia in this table).
Frontotemporal lobar degeneration (FTLD)	Includes dementias such as behavioral-variant FTLD, primary progressive aphasia, Pick's disease, corticobasal degeneration, and progressive supranuclear palsy.
	Typical early symptoms include marked changes in personality and behavior and difficulty with producing or comprehending language. Unlike AD, memory is typically spared in the early stages of disease.
	Nerve cells in the front (frontal lobe) and side regions (temporal lobes) of the brain are especially affected, and these regions become markedly atrophied (shrunken). In addition, the upper layers of the cortex typically become soft and spongy and have protein inclusions (usually tau protein or the transactive response DNA binding protein).
	The brain changes of behavioral-variant FTLD may occur in those age 65 years and older, similar to AD, but most people with this form of dementia develop symptoms at a younger age (at about age 60). In this younger age group, FTLD is the second most common degenerative dementia.

Disease	Description
Mixed dementia	Characterized by the hallmark abnormalities of more than one type of dementia—most commonly AD combined with vascular dementia, followed by AD with dementia with Lewy bodies (DLB), and AD with vascular dementia and DLB. Vascular dementia with DLB is much less common.
	Recent studies suggest that mixed dementia is more common than previously recognized, with about half of those with dementia having mixed pathologies.
Parkinson's disease (PD) dementia	Problems with movement (slowness, rigidity, tremor, and changes in gait) are common symptoms of PD.
	In PD, alpha-synuclein aggregates appear in an area deep in the brain called the substantia nigra. The aggregates are thought to cause degeneration of the nerve cells that produce dopamine.
	The incidence of PD is about one-tenth that of AD.
	As PD progresses, it often results in dementia secondary to the accumulation of Lewy bodies in the cortex (similar to DLB) or the accumulation of beta-amyloid clumps and tau tangles (similar to AD).
Creutzfeldt–Jakob disease	This very rare and rapidly fatal disorder impairs memory and coordination and causes behavior changes.
	Results from a misfolded protein (prion) that causes other proteins throughout the brain to misfold and malfunction.
	May be hereditary (caused by a gene that runs in an individual's family), sporadic (unknown cause), or caused by a known prion infection.
	A specific form called variant Creutzfeldt–Jakob disease is believed to be caused by consumption of products from cattle affected by mad cow disease.
Normal-pressure hydrocephalus	Symptoms include difficulty walking, memory loss, and inability to control urination.
	Caused by impaired reabsorption of cerebrospinal fluid and the consequent buildup of fluid in the brain, increasing pressure in the brain.
	People with a history of brain hemorrhage (particularly subarachnoid hemorrhage) and meningitis are at increased risk.
	Can sometimes be corrected with surgical installation of a shunt in the brain to drain excess fluid.

Modified from Alzheimer's Association. 2014 Alzheimer's disease facts and figures. *Alzheimers Dement.* March 2014;10(2):47–92; Fernando MS, Ince PG. MRC Cognitive Function and Ageing Neuropathology Study Group: vascular pathologies and cognition in a population-based cohort of elderly people. *J Neurol Sci.* 2004;226(1–2):13–17; Schneider JA, Arvanitakis Z, Bang W, Bennett DA. Mixed brain pathologies account for most dementia cases in community-dwelling older persons. *Neurology.* 2007;69:2197–2204; Schneider JA, Arvanitakis Z, Leurgans SE, Bennett DA. The neuropathology of probable Alzheimer disease and mild cognitive impairment. *Ann Neurol.* 2009;66(2):200–208.

deal about this condition, but information addressing the biologic changes that promote the development of AD as well as prevention strategies and the disease's progression need further research.[47]

Risk Factors for Alzheimer's Disease

The true cause of AD is not known. Theories suggest that AD occurs as a result of environmental, lifestyle, and genetic factors congregating to make the pathophysiologic succession of events that over decades progresses to AD. Some of the risk factors that contribute to the development of AD over time include age, genetics, family history, the presence of insulin resistance and vascular factors, dyslipidemia, hypertension, inflammatory markers, Down syndrome, and traumatic brain injury.[47,57] Most cases of AD are identified in those 65 years of age and older. There are instances in which individuals younger than 65 years of age develop AD; however, this is small fraction of the population.[47,57,58]

Researchers have identified two forms of genes that can play a role in determining whether a person develops AD.[56–58] These are the risk genes and opportunistic genes.[56–58] Family history has also been identified as a risk factor in the development of AD. Individuals whose parents, sibling, or child has AD are at increased risk for developing AD. The number of family members and the risk for developing the disease run parallel. As the number

of family members with the disease rises, so does the possibility of developing AD.[47,56,57]

Depression has been identified as a risk factor in the development of AD and other dementias. The Framingham Study revealed a 50% increase in AD and dementia in individuals identified with depression.[59] The study showed that 21.6% of subjects with original history of depression developed dementia, whereas only 16. 6% of participants who had no history of depression developed AD.[59]

A low level of education is being looked at as a risk factor for developing AD as well as other types of dementias.[60] Some researchers report that individuals with more years of formal education build a "cognitive reserve" that protects the brain against some of the changes associated with signs and symptoms of AD.[60]

Diagnosis of Alzheimer's Disease

Individuals with AD show a gradual brain deterioration and atrophy that affects cognition. Signs and symptoms and the rate of advancement through the diverse disease phases are distinctive for each individual.

After almost 30 years, in 2011 the National Institute on Aging and the Alzheimer's Association modified the initial diagnosing criteria/guidelines for AD that were established in 1984.[61] The modified guidelines incorporate scientific and technological trends with the purpose of further defining existing diagnosis techniques, sustaining autopsy studies of brain alterations resulting from the disease process, and ascertaining research priorities. The guidelines emphasize pinpointing the following:[61]

- Dementia as a result of AD
- Mild cognitive impairment (MCI)
- Preclinical expression of AD
- Standards for recording and reporting AD brain alterations assessed through autopsy

Treatment of AD

There is no defined cure for AD. Pharmacological and nonpharmacological interventions are used to control both cognitive and behavioral signs and symptoms. The research agenda for AD ranges from strategies to advance quality of life to dealing with behavioral symptoms, controlling the progression of the disease, and helping individuals maintain cognitive status.[47]

The goal of nonpharmacologic treatment frequently focuses on maintaining cognitive level, helping the brain offset impairments, or increasing quality of life by decreasing behavioral signs and symptoms like depression, indifference, wandering, sleep disturbances, anxiety, and belligerence.

Nutrition Implications and Recommendations

The brain and body changes that take place as a result of AD affect an individual's physical function and make the person susceptible to other health complications. Dysphagia, for example, can make individuals with AD prone to pneumonia and infections, malnutrition, and dehydration.[62]

As AD develops, individuals lose the ability to identify food and fail to recognize feelings of thirst and hunger. In some instances, food and water are declined because of confusion or belligerent conducts linked to AD.[62]

In the initial stages of AD, individuals can continue to shop for food and prepare meals. As the disease progresses, a number of changes that influence food selection and nutritional status occur. As persons with AD start to forget to eat and drink, the risk for weight decrease and dehydration increases. Some individuals react differently in the sense that they forget that they already ate. This results in the consumption of numerous meals during the day, contributing to weight gain and higher BMI.[63] Many of these patients start replacing the consumption of a well-balanced meal with a diet that consists of a small number of items (decreased food selection) that are readily available, such as convenience food items, sweet snacks, and other foods that lack nutrient density. Behaviors such as eating very fast put individuals at increased risk for choking. People who display this behavior usually fail to properly chew their food. The presence of aspiration is very common in the last stages of AD.[64]

As AD advances, patients become poor historians; procuring a diet history and identifying food preferences can be a challenging task for dietitians. Observing individuals at mealtime and obtaining information from family and friends can be helpful strategies in trying to define meal patterns in these individuals.[63]

Eating Strategies

AD can lead to decreased nutrient consumption because of inability to feel hunger and thirst, decreased ability to smell and taste, dysphagia, and incompetence in coordinating the use of eating instruments, diminished ability to feed self, and apraxia. The main nutrition goals when treating individuals with AD and other forms of dementia are to prevent weight loss, malnutrition, pressure injuries and other comorbidities.[57]

Conducting a nutrition assessment in patients with AD involves determining conditions such as poor oral health, capacity to concentrate during mealtime, and swallowing difficulties. Signs of decline, such as rejecting meal substitutes, inability to concentrate on consuming the meal, or wandering away from meals, and leaving 25% or more of meals uneaten, need to be evaluated as part of the nutrition assessment process.[65]

Creating activities to engage patients at mealtime can help stimulate their interest in the meal and promote better meal intake. Activities like getting individuals involved in menu selection and table service can create interest. Strategies such as baking bread and cookies before meals can help to arouse olfactory senses and stimulate appetite. Patients' anxiety level might require mealtimes to be changed to a time when the individual is less confused, unsettled, or restless. AD patients should be encouraged to practice any activities that promote their independence. For example, for patients who are slow eaters, mealtimes need to be prolonged to allow ample time for them to eat at their pace.[65] If patients seem to be overwhelmed by too many food choices, providing one food item at a time might be helpful.

Strategies used during meal service include staff members sitting down next to the patient at eye level while assisting with meals. This promotes trust and helps the patient focus. "Food first" is the preferred approach to ensure adequate nutrient intake. Patients with AD who cannot meet their nutrient needs with food alone might need fortified foods and supplements to boost their intake. On the basis of individuals' wishes and **advance directives**, during the end stage of the disease, the use of enteral nutrition versus comfort measures should be explored. For those near the end of their life, artificial nutrition and hydration may be withdrawn, according to their written/expressed wishes.[65]

Let's Discuss

Repeated nasogastric tube insertions are reported by competent patients to be very unpleasant. Patients with AD may not understand what is being done. They may try to pull their tubes out and potentially have the additional discomfort of being held in restraints. Debate the arguments for and against providing artificial feedings to patients with end-stage AD.

Case Study

During mealtime today, Elsa was staring at her meal without making any effort to pick up the eating utensils to feed herself. When the caregiver approached to encourage intake, Elsa looked the other way.

Question

1. Elsa is easily distracted and makes no effort to feed herself. What mealtime/ eating strategies can be implemented to facilitate meal intake?

Recap Almost every minute, someone in the United States acquires Alzheimer's disease, and this rate is projected to double by the year 2050. The severity of dementia ranges from a mild stage, during which the older adult starts to see changes in functioning, to a severe stage, in which the person becomes fully dependent on caregivers for all ADLs. The true cause of AD is not known.

1. Discuss the nutritional challenges faced by older adults with dementia.
2. What are some of the environmental, behavioral, and physical considerations that need to be considered when assessing patients with a form of dementia?

Endocrine and Metabolic Conditions

Preview There are two main forms of diabetes, type 1 (T1DM) and type 2 (T2DM). T1DM is mainly an autoimmune disorder in which the body's immune system attacks the beta cells of the pancreas where insulin is produced. T2DM occurs as a gradual decline in beta cell function that results in a reduction in insulin production and progresses to insulin resistance and, finally, insulin deficiency. Nearly 50% of adults 50 years and older meet the criteria for metabolic syndrome.

By 2050, one out of every three adults in the United States could have a diagnosis of diabetes. Nearly 50% of adults 50 years and older meet the criteria for metabolic syndrome, with risk factor that include irregular levels of blood lipid, impaired fasting glucose, HTN, and excess abdominal obesity. The American Diabetes Association has created evidence-based guidelines and recommendation that include medical nutrition therapy (MNT) in the treatment of diabetes mellitus (DM). Nutrition therapy is recommended for all people with type 1 and type 2 diabetes as an effective component of the overall treatment plan. Metabolic syndrome is a disease in which the individual suffers from irregular levels of blood lipids (low high-density lipoprotein [HDL] and high triglycerides), impaired fasting glucose, HTN, and excess abdominal obesity.[66]

Diabetes

In the 32 years from 1980–2012, the number of adults with a diagnosis of diabetes mellitus (DM) in the United States has almost quadrupled, from 5.5 million to 21.3 million. On average, approximately 1.7 million new incidents of diabetes are diagnosed every year. At this rate, by 2050 one out of every three adults in the United States could have a diagnosis of DM.[67]

Prevalence and Etiology

The World Health Organization (WHO) estimates that by the year 2030 DM will become the seventh leading cause of death worldwide.[68] In 2012, 29.1 million individuals, accounting for 9.3% of the U.S. population, were classified as having diabetes. This statistic includes 21.3 million people diagnosed and nearly 8 million undiagnosed.[67]

T2DM is more common in older adults. The etiology of T2DM is hereditary and often prompted by lifestyle or environmental elements. T2DM occurs as a gradual decline in beta cell function that results in a reduction in insulin production and progresses to insulin resistance and, finally, insulin deficiency.[69,70] In older adults, changes in body composition accompanied by aging, sarcopenia of aging, vitamin D deficiency, and inflammatory response are believed to contribute to the development of DM.[69,70]

Risk Factors

T2DM typically presents in older adults, and frequency increases with age. It is estimated that approximately one-third of adults age 65 and older have diminished glucose tolerance.[71] Risk factors for development of T2DM include over weight, inactivity, family history, race, age, high blood pressure, and abnormal cholesterol and triglyceride levels.[72]

Screening and Diagnosis

The American Diabetes Association (ADA) advocates that screening for diabetes should be performed in all adults, starting at age 45, and every 1 to 3 years thereafter, depending on the individual's risk factors.[73] Diagnosis of diabetes is characteristically based on the results of one of three blood tests: fasting blood glucose, 2-hour 75-g oral glucose tolerance test (OGTT), or hemoglobin A1c (HbA1c). (See FIGURE 16.5.)

Management
Diabetes Self-Management Education and Support
Older adults can benefit from diabetes self-management education and support (DSME/S). Research supports that DSME is as valuable in the management of older adults with diabetes as it is with their younger counterparts.[74]

Criteria for Diagnosing Diabetes Mellitus

| Adult Hg A1C ≥ 6.5% | or | Fasting plasma Glucose level ≥ 126 mg/dl (7.0 mmol/L) | or | 2h Plasma Glucose level ≥ 200 mg/dl (11.1 mmol/L) during an Oral Glucose Tolerance Test | or | Plasma Glucose ≥ 200 mg/dl (11.1 mmol/L) |

Figure 16.5
Criteria for diagnosing diabetes mellitus.
Data from American Diabetes Association. Classification and Diagnosis. Diabetes Care 2014; 37:515.

The main role of diabetes education is to empower the diabetic patient to acquire the knowledge, skills, and confidence to accomplish self-care behaviors for managing diabetes.[73] The education element emphasizes obtaining the knowledge and skills for managing diabetes. The support component aids individuals with DM to define and implement a plan of action for behavior change to influence care.[73] In older adults, often the plan must consider the presence of multiple medical conditions simultaneously.

Medical Nutrition Therapy

The American Diabetes Association has created evidence-based guidelines and recommendations that include medical nutrition therapy (MNT) in the treatment of DM. Nutrition therapy is recommended for all people with type 1 and type 2 diabetes as an effective component of the overall treatment plan. Older adults who have prediabetes or diabetes should receive individualized MNT as needed to achieve treatment goals, preferably provided by a registered dietitian nutritionist (RDN) familiar with the components of diabetes MNT. Diabetes nutrition therapy can result in improved quality of life for older adults, cost savings, and improved outcomes such as reduction in HbA$_{1c}$. Nutrition plays a significant role in the management of diabetes symptoms and comorbidities. The MNT provided to older adults needs to be individualized and must consider all aspects of care, including comorbid conditions, nutrient needs that might be altered by chronic disease process, and physiologic changes associated with aging such as the ability feed self, difficulty chewing and swallowing, and changes in intake due to anosmia and ageusia.[75]

Diet

It is the position of the American Diabetes Association (ADA) that there is not a one-size-fits-all eating pattern for individuals with diabetes. The ADA also acknowledges the vital role of nutrition therapy in the management of DM and endorses that each person with DM should be actively involved in self-management, education, and treatment planning with a healthcare provider, which includes the creation of a personalized eating plan.[76,77]

As outlined by the ADA, the goals of nutrition therapy for adults with diabetes include encouraging individuals to maintain a healthy eating pattern that accentuates the consumption of nutrient-dense foods and adequate portion sizes in an effort to improve health. Following a healthy diet can help an older adult achieve glycemic, blood pressure, and lipid goals as well as reach and maintain healthy weight, thereby managing risk factors associated with other chromic conditions prevalent in this age group.[73] Evidence-based guidelines suggest there is no ideal percentage of calories from carbohydrate, protein, and fat for all people with diabetes, and macronutrient distribution should be based on individualized assessment of current eating patterns, preferences, and metabolic goals.[73] In older adults, eating patterns must also consider other health and medical conditions, living arrangements, and functional and physical independence.

The use of dietary meal patterns such as a Mediterranean-style eating pattern, the Dietary Approaches to Stop Hypertension (DASH) diet, and low-fat and lower carbohydrate eating patterns has been beneficial in promoting improved metabolic parameters such as glycemic control, lipids, blood pressure, and weight.[71,75,78]

Meal Planning Strategies

Meal planning approaches such as carbohydrate counting have been shown to improve glycemic control.[73,79] In individuals with fixed daily insulin dosage, consistent carbohydrate intake in terms of consistent schedule and consistent meal composition can contribute to improved glycemic response.[77] Recommending meal plans that focus on portion control and healthy eating might be an appropriate intervention for individuals with low health literacy and numeracy.[77] Simple meal planning approaches such as the MyPlate method may be appropriate for some.

Weight Management

Modest weight loss of 7% accompanied by physical activity has produced positive outcomes in terms of improved blood glucose levels and insulin sensitivity.[77] In older adults, BMI alone should not be the sole measurement on which to recommend weight loss. In this population,

BMI is not an accurate indicator of body composition. Body changes that occur as part of the aging process, such as sarcopenia, render this measurement an unreliable indicator of obesity for older adults.[70] Weight loss programs for older adults must be individualized and monitored.[80]

Physical Activity

Being physically active may contribute to improved metabolic control, functional capacity (mobility), and physical fitness.[80] Because muscle strength loss and poor muscle function are linked to aging and diabetes, staying physically active is an important aspect of disease management especially in old age.

Medication Management

When individuals with T2DM are incapable of maintaining stable glycemic control with diet and physical activity, medication must be prescribed. Medication selection is based on treatment goals set for the patient. **TABLE 16.3**

lists medications commonly used in the treatment of DM. Individuals with T1DM require the use of insulin. For those with T2DM, insulin is prescribed after the efficacy of lifestyle changes and oral antihyperglycemic medications are no longer successful.

Metabolic Syndrome
Prevalence, Risk Factors, and Etiology

Metabolic syndrome (MetS) is a disease in which the individual has irregular levels of blood lipids (low HDL and high triglycerides), impaired fasting glucose, HTN, and excess abdominal obesity.[66] Nearly 50% of adults 50 years and older meet the National Cholesterol Education Program (NCEP) Adult Treatment Panel (ATP) III definition of metabolic syndrome.[81] Individuals suffering from MetS are at higher risk for premature death, heart disease, and stroke.[82]

TABLE 16.4 describes the risk factors of MetS. The pathogenesis of MetS is multifaceted, and not fully understood. People with MetS are commonly older, follow a

---

Table 16.3

Diabetic Medications

Drug Name	Class	Reason Prescribed	Action	Risks
Diabinese	Sulfonylurea (first generation)	Insufficient insulin secretion	Stimulates insulin secretion from pancreatic beta cells; basal insulin.	High risk of **hypoglycemia**
Glyburide	Sulfonylurea (second generation)			Weight gain
Amaryl				Monitor cardiovascular risk
Glucotrol				
Glucotrol XL				
Amaryl				
Prandin	Meglitinide	Insufficient insulin secretion at mealtime	Stimulates pancreatic beta cell insulin secretion in response to CHO intake.	Less risk of hypoglycemia
Starlix				
Glucophage	Biguanide	Increased gluconeogenesis; insulin resistance	Decreases hepatic glucose production; increases insulin sensitivity; preserves beta cell function.	May cause gas, bloating, diarrhea, nausea.
				Monitor pts with HF, renal failure, and hepatic failure.
				Decreases folate and vitamin B_{12} absorption.
Actos/ Avandia	Thiazolidinediones	Insulin resistance; hyperinsulinemia	Acts on peripheral cells; increases insulin sensitivity.	Most expensive.
				Slow-acting.
				Weight gain, edema.
				Not for pts with HF.
				Monitor liver function.
Januvia	DPP4-inhibitor	Insufficient insulin secretion in response to meals; elevated glucagon secretion	Increases release of insulin; decreases release of glucagon; decreases stomach emptying; wt loss due to increased satiety.	Long-term side effects are not known.
Onglyza				
Tradjenta				Titrate dose based on renal function.
Precose	α-glucosidase inhibitor	Elevated gluconeogenesis	Delays absorption of glucose in the gut; increases satiety.	Debilitating gas and digestion complaints.
Amylin	Injectable amylin analogs	Postprandial glucagon production	Delays gastric emptying, decreases appetite, decreases glucagon production.	Susceptible to hypoglycemia; GI complaints.
Symlin				Monitor /evaluate renal function.

CHO = carbohydrate; GI, gastrointestinal; HF = heart failure; pt = patient; wt = weight.

Table 16.4

American Heart Association Adult Treatment Panel III Definition of Metabolic Syndrome

Factor	Three or more of the following
Abdominal obesity	Waist circumference: > 40 in. (102 cm) for men > 35 in. (88 cm) for women
Triglycerides, mg/dL	> 150 mg/dL or on drug treatment for high TG
HDL, mg/dL	< 40 mg/dL for men < 50 mg/dL for women, or on drug treatment for low HDL
Blood pressure, mm Hg	Systolic blood pressure (SBP) > 130 mm Hg or diastolic blood pressure > 85 mm Hg, or on drug treatment for HTN
Fasting glucose, mg/dL	FPG > 100 mg/dL

FPG = fasting plasma glucose; HDL = high-density lipoprotein; HTN = hypertension ; TG = triglycerides.

Data from: Grundy SM. Metabolic syndrome scientific statement by the American Heart Association and the National Heart, Lung, and Blood Institute. *Arterioscler Thromb Vasc Biol*. Nov 2005;25(11):2243–2244.

sedentary lifestyle, are overweight or obese, and suffer from insulin sensitivity.[83]

Diagnosis of MetS can be made with the presence of three out of the five factors listed in **TABLE 16.5**.[84]

Prevention and Treatment

The National Heart, Lung and Blood Institute recommends that adopting a healthy lifestyle is the best way to prevent MetS.[85] Changes in diet and exercise that facilitate or preserve a healthy body weight can delay or prevent the onset of MetS.

Weight Management

Treatment plans often focus on promoting weight loss and changes in body composition. The presence of visceral fat is linked to increased production of adipocytokines, leptin, tumor necrosis factor, and angiotension II, which cause the insulin resistance abnormalities of MetS.[86] Weight reduction of 5–10% has been shown to

positively influence the metabolic parameters of MetS, especially insulin sensitivity.[87]

Diet

Research comparing culturally similar population groups exposed to diverse dietary situations support that Westernized diets are connected to an increased possibility of developing MetS.[88] On the contrary, diets containing dairy products, fish, and cereal grains have been connected with a lesser risk of developing MetS.[89] The Mediterranean-style diets seem to contribute to a lower risk for developing this MetS and have a beneficial effect on other chronic disease risk factors common in older adults.[90]

Physical Activity

In addition to dietary adjustments, physical activity plays a key role in the management of MetS. In individuals with MetS, moderate-intensity physical activity, for 135 to 180 minutes per week, considerably decreases waist circumference. Triglyceride levels, blood pressure, and insulin sensitivity are also positively influenced by physical activity.[91]

Case Study

In the past month, Elsa's blood sugar has been running between 195 and 205. The latest HbA$_{1c}$ was 8.9.

Questions

1. What lifestyle changes can be recommended to help her attain her goals?
2. What would be the most appropriate diet for Elsa to follow at this stage?

Table 16.5

Diagnosis of Metabolic Syndrome

1. Abdominal obesity (waist circumference of 40 inches or more in men, and 35 inches or more in women)
2. Triglyceride level of 150 mg/dL of blood or greater
3. HDL cholesterol of less than 40 mg/dL in men or less than 50 mg/dL in women
4. Systolic blood pressure (top number) of 130 mm Hg or greater, or diastolic blood pressure (bottom number) of 85 mm Hg or greater
5. Fasting glucose of 100 mg/dL or greater

Recap   There are two main forms of diabetes, type 1 (T1DM) and type 2 (T2DM). T1DM is mainly an autoimmune disorder in which the body's immune system attacks the beta cells of the pancreas where insulin is produced. T2DM is more common in older adults. T2DM occurs as a gradual decline in beta cell function that results in a reduction in insulin production and progresses to insulin resistance and, finally, insulin deficiency. Nutrition plays a significant role in the management of diabetes symptoms and comorbidities. Metabolic syndrome is a disease in which the individual has irregular levels of blood lipids impaired fasting glucose, HTN, and excess abdominal obesity. A healthy lifestyle is the best way to prevent MetS.

1. Prepare an education pamphlet describing the nutritional needs of an older adult with diabetes mellitus.
2. Outline the nutrition components of older adults with metabolic syndrome.

Gastrointestinal Conditions

Preview The gastrointestinal tract is essential for digesting food and absorbing nutrients. Twenty-three percent of older adults in extended care facilities suffer from gastroesophageal reflux disease. Approximately 50% of older adults suffer from diverticular disease.

The primary function of the gastrointestinal (GI) tract and its accessory organs is to digest food and absorb nutrients. Therefore, diseases and conditions that impair the normal function of the digestive system are likely to affect an individual's nutrition status adversely. Common GI conditions in older adults include gastroesophageal reflux, diverticular disease, lactose intolerance, fructose malabsorption, celiac disease, and constipation. All these conditions rely on specific dietary modifications to control the symptoms associated with the disease.

Gastroesophageal Reflux Disease

Gastroesophageal reflux disease (GERD) is a chronic disorder in which gastric acid and other stomach fluids leak into the esophagus, characteristically producing irritation and damage to the esophageal tissue. GERD escalates the risk for other comorbidities such as **Barrett's esophagus**, a condition characterized by alterations in the mucosa of the esophagus. Individuals with Barrett's esophagus are at higher risk for developing cancer of the esophagus.[92]

Prevalence and Etiology

Approximately 18–28% of adult in the United States suffer from GERD. This number increases to about 23% among older adults living in extended care facilities.[93,94] Older adults account for about 50% of all GERD diagnoses in hospitals.[95] GERD results from a dysfunction of the lower **esophageal sphincter (LES)**. This is a ring of muscle fibers in the lower esophagus that separates the stomach from the esophagus. The LES prevents stomach contents and acids from backing up into the esophagus (reflux).

The most common signs and symptoms of GERD include a burning or painful sensation in the chest (heartburn), feeling that food is "stuck" behind the sternum, and regurgitation of stomach contents (water brash).

Risk Factors

One of the most common risk factors for development of GERD is obesity. The pressure from the visceral fat on the stomach and on the LES serves as a precursor for developing GERD.[96] Other risk factors associated with a decreased LES pressure that can contribute to an exacerbation of GERD include the use of tobacco, alcohol, and some medications.[97]

Prevention

Weight loss and deterrence of weight gain, coupled with smoking cessation and decreased alcohol intake, may be helpful in averting GERD.[97]

Treatment

GERD is normally treated with medications such as **proton pump inhibitors (PPIs)**, which are a form of acid-reducing medication, along with modifications in diet and lifestyle. Weight loss has been identified as a strategy to improve GERD symptoms.[98] Lifestyle interventions to manage symptoms include waiting 3 hours after eating before going to bed (helps to reduce nighttime symptoms); consuming smaller, more frequent meals; elevating the head of the bed (creating an angle at the torso); and eliminating the use of tight, restrictive garments can be effective with older adults in the management of GERD.[97]

Diverticular Disease

Diverticular disease encompasses diverticulosis, or the presence of diverticula projecting through the colonic wall, and diverticulitis, which is an acute inflammation of diverticula usually manifested with symptoms like fever, leukocytosis, and pain. In the United States, the presence of diverticulitis and diverticulosis accounts for approximately 312,000 hospital admissions and 1.5 million days of inpatient care.[99] Annual treatment expenditures in the United States surpass $2.6 billion.[99]

Prevalence

Occurrence of diverticulosis increases with age. Although most cases are asymptomatic and actual disease prevalence is difficult to calculate, it is estimated that 50% of older adults (aged 60 and older) suffer from diverticulosis.[100] It is further estimated that approximately two-thirds of older adults 85 and older have this disease.[100] The diverticulitis form of the disease affects almost 10–25% of individuals with diverticulosis.[100]

Risk Factors

A number of factors can increase the risk for developing diverticulitis. As people age, the incidence of the disorder increases. Being overweight or obese increases the probability of developing diverticulitis and also developing symptoms. Smokers are more likely than nonsmokers to experience diverticulosis. Having a sedentary lifestyle and a diet high in fat and low in fiber have also been identified as risk factors. A number of medications have been associated with an increased risk for the development of diverticulitis. These include opiates and nonsteroidal anti-inflammatory drugs.[101]

Prevention

Choosing a diet high in fiber and low in fat and red meats with adequate fluids and having an active lifestyle have been identified as preventive against diverticular disease.[101–103] Data from the Health Professionals follow-up study did not support the previous belief that consuming nuts, corn, and popcorn contributes to the pathogenesis of diverticulitis.[104]

Treatment

Diverticulitis is normally treated with antibiotics, pain medication, and bowel rest. A small number of cases might require bowel surgery.[101] Diet therapy varies depending on the symptoms and tolerance to intake. Diet restrictions can run the gamut from clear liquids to soft foods to low-residue foods. Once the infection is managed, the patient's diet is advanced to regular as tolerated. In instances in which prolonged bowel rest is needed, parenteral nutrition may be required for nutrition support.

Lactose Intolerance

Lactose intolerance is a common disorder caused by the failure to digest lactose into its components, glucose and galactose, that results from low levels of lactase enzyme in the brush border of the duodenum.[105] Symptoms include loose stools, abdominal pain, bloating, nausea, and flatulence. Condition symptoms are seen after lactose-containing food items are consumed. The severity of the symptoms increases as the amount of lactose consumed increases and the tolerance level of the individual decreases. Symptoms are seen anywhere from 30 to 120 minutes after lactose is consumed. Lactose intolerance diagnosis is assigned based on self-reported symptoms and a hydrogen breath test.[105,106] In the United States, ethnic groups such as African Americans, Hispanics, American Indians, and Asian Indians seem to be more likely to be lactose intolerant than Americans from European background. It is estimated that 30–50 million Americans suffer from lactose intolerance.[107] See TABLE 16.6 for definitions of the different types of lactose intolerance.

Table 16.6

Four Types of Lactase Deficiency that May Lead to Lactose Intolerance

- **Primary lactase deficiency**, also called lactase nonpersistence, is the most common type of lactase deficiency. In people with this condition, lactase production declines over time. This decline often begins at about age 2; however, the decline may begin later. Children who have lactase deficiency may not experience symptoms of lactose intolerance until late adolescence or adulthood. Researchers have discovered that some people inherit genes from their parents that may cause a primary lactase deficiency.
- **Secondary lactase deficiency** results from injury to the small intestine. Infection, diseases, or other problems may injure the small intestine. Treating the underlying cause usually improves the lactose tolerance.
- **Developmental lactase deficiency** may occur in infants born prematurely. This condition usually lasts for only a short time after they are born.
- **Congenital lactase deficiency** is an extremely rare disorder in which the small intestine produces little or no lactase enzyme from birth. Genes inherited from parents cause this disorder.

Reproduced from National Institute of Diabetes and Digestive and Kidney Diseases Lactose intolerance. National Institute of Diabetes and Digestive and Kidney Diseases. June 2014. Retrieved from: http://www.niddk.nih.gov/health-information/health-topics/digestive-diseases/lactose-intolerance/Pages/facts.aspx. Accessed September 30, 2016.

People may find it helpful to talk with a healthcare provider or a registered dietitian nutritionist (RDN) about a dietary plan.

Fructose Malabsorption

Fructose malabsorption is the inability to metabolize free fructose (a 6-carbon monosaccharide) due to decreased expression of fructose-specific GLUT-5 transporters along the brush border membrane of the small intestine.[41] As with lactose intolerance, fructose malabsorption results in abdominal pain, bloating, nausea, and flatulence and loose stools. Symptoms and the severity of the symptoms correlate to the amount of fructose consumed. Fructose malabsorption diagnosis, like lactose intolerance diagnosis, occurs via the use of a breath test and the presence of symptoms.[108]

The nutritional management of fructose intolerance requires decreasing the older adult's intake of foods that have fructose. A fructose-free diet unavoidably means restricting the intake of fruit, particularly those with a high fructose-to-glucose ratio, along with fruit juices, sweeteners such as honey, agave nectar, and high-fructose corn syrup. Because fruit is an important source of vitamin C, supplementation with vitamin C should be recommended along with a diet that restricts fruit consumption.[41]

Celiac Disease

Celiac disease (also known as sprue disease or gluten-sensitive enteropathy) is an immune condition in which the presence of gluten in the diet damages the inner lining of the small intestine and hinders nutrient absorption.[109] Gluten is a protein found in wheat, rye, and barley as well as in other products such as vitamin and nutrient supplements, lip balms, and certain medications. In individuals with celiac disease, gluten causes the immune system to react by damaging or destroying villi on the inner lining of the small intestine. Villi normally absorb nutrients from food and pass the nutrients through the walls of the small intestine and into the bloodstream. Without healthy villi, older adults can become malnourished, regardless of the amount of food consumed.[109]

Celiac disease digestive symptoms include diarrhea; pale, foul-smelling or fatty stools; fatigue; abdominal pain; abdominal distension; constipation; nausea; vomiting; and weight loss. Adults are less likely to have digestive signs and symptoms; instead, they might show symptoms of anemia, bone or joint pain, canker sores in the oral cavity, depression or anxiety, fatigue, headaches, tingling numbness of the hands and feet, and seizures. Skin indications in older adults include dermatitis herpetiformis, an itchy, blistering rash.[109]

The physician diagnoses celiac disease by conducting blood tests for specific antibodies, followed by a biopsy of the small intestine for confirmation.[41] Severity and location of diseased segments of the small intestine can contribute to malabsorption of calcium, iron, folate, and fat-soluble vitamins.[109,110]

Once thought of as a rare condition, celiac disease currently affects approximately 1–2% of the U.S. population.[111] Frequency in the United States has increased considerably from 1.3 new events per 100,000 people in 1999 to 6.5 per 100,000 in 2008.[112]

Following a strict gluten-free diet is a significant intervention in treating celiac disease. Villous atrophy is usually reversed within 6 to 24 months of adopting a gluten-free diet.[113] For individuals suffering from nutrition deficiencies, supplementation should be considered. Common nutrients normally supplemented include calcium, vitamin D, iron, vitamin B$_{12}$, as well as other micronutrients.[109]

Constipation

Constipation is a common condition in older adults. Although constipation is not a normal physiologic change related to aging, decreased mobility and other comorbidities could contribute to its increased frequency in older adults. Limited mobility, medication side effects, and comorbidities can contribute to constipation in older adults.[114]

Prevalence and Etiology

The prevalence of constipation in older adults is not well defined. Prevalence has been reported as 25–50%.[115,116] Laxatives are used on a daily basis by 10–18% of community-dwelling older adults and 74% of nursing home patients.[117]

The etiology of constipation in older adults is frequently multifactorial. Factors that can contribute to constipation include organic conditions related to colorectal cancer; endocrine or metabolic factors such that can be triggered by diabetes mellitus; neurological conditions, as in the case of patients with multiple sclerosis; anorectal disease, as in inflammatory bowel disease; and as a medication side effect, as when opiates and antihypertensive medications are in use.[118] Older adults with limited mobility, poor fluid intake, and insufficient food consumption are at increased risk for constipation.[118]

Treatment

The first step in the treatment of constipation is lifestyle and dietary modification. Common interventions like increased fluid intake and exercise are suggested to treat constipation, but there is little evidence to support this.[119] Bulk-forming laxatives are suggested in patients who do not respond to lifestyle and dietary modification.[119]

Let's Discuss

Drug stores and supermarkets feature arrays of different probiotic supplements, often containing *Lactobacillus* or *Bifidobacterium*, two of the most commonly used species of bacteria. Search the scientific evidence to answer the question: can probiotics ease constipation?

Case Study

In the past month, Elsa has had a 10-pound weight loss. The nursing assistant caring for Elsa reports frequent bowel movements (3+ per day) with foul-smelling stool.

Questions

1. What could be causing the frequent bowel movements and foul-smelling stools?
2. What recommendations can you make to control the symptoms?

Recap Diseases and conditions that impair the normal function of the digestive system are likely to affect an individual's nutrition status adversely. Gastroesophageal reflux disease (GERD) is a chronic disorder in which gastric acid and other stomach fluids leak into the esophagus, characteristically producing irritation and damage to the esophageal tissue. Diverticular disease incorporates diverticulosis, or the presence of diverticula projecting through the colonic wall, and diverticulitis, which is an acute inflammation of diverticula usually manifested with symptoms like fever, leukocytosis, and pain. Lactose intolerance is a common disorder caused by the failure to digest lactose into its components, glucose and galactose, that results from low levels of lactase enzyme in the brush border of the duodenum.[105] Celiac disease (also known as sprue disease or gluten-sensitive enteropathy) is an immune condition in which the presence of gluten in the diet damages the inner lining of the small intestine and hinders nutrient absorption.

1. What nutrition recommendations can be outlined for an older adult suffering from GERD?
2. Develop education materials for patients diagnosed with celiac disease. What topics should be emphasized?

Obesity and Malnutrition

Preview Unintentional and involuntary weight loss has been linked to adverse clinical outcomes and increased mortality. Weight management and maintenance of a healthy weight are encouraged in older adults because of their increased risk for developing chronic diseases associated with obesity.

One of the goals of *Healthy People 2020* is to "Promote health and reduce chronic disease risk through the consumption of healthful diets and achievement and maintenance of healthy body weights."[120] This goal supports that all Americans should prevent unhealthy weight gain and individuals whose weight is too high should consider weight loss.[121]

Underweight/Unintentional Weight Loss

Unintentional or involuntary weight loss is a common occurrence among older adults that is associated with adverse outcomes that include increased mortality.[122] **Unintended weight loss** occurs in approximately 13% of the population.[123] It is estimated that 27% of frail older adults 65 years and older have involuntary and unplanned weight loss.[124] Significant weight loss in older adults is defined as 5% loss in 1 month and 10% in 6 months.[125]

The clinical outcomes of involuntary and unplanned weight loss can involve functional decline, development of infectious diseases, pressure injuries, and exacerbation of cognitive, clinical, and mood disorders.[122,126] Involuntary and unplanned weight loss can occur as a result of decreased food and fluid intake, increased metabolism, and increased caloric needs.[127]

Etiology and Risk Factors

Weight loss in older adults with a BMI below 30 presents a higher mortality risk than not losing weight or having a BMI in the 25–30 range.[128] It is important to note that obesity with a BMI higher than 30 also affects morbidity and mortality in older adults. The benefit of intentional weight loss for older adults with osteoarthritis, limited physical activity, DM, and coronary heart disease (CHD) is becoming progressively evident.[129]

Involuntary weight loss is caused by inadequate food and fluid intake, periods of anorexia, disuse or muscle atrophy resulting in sarcopenia, inflammatory response related to disease process (cachexia), or a combination of any of these factors.

Unplanned weight loss related to inadequate nutrient intake can be influenced by a number of factors. Social factors such as poverty, isolation, psychological conditions such as depression, and dementia and medical conditions like dysphagia and diagnosis of an endocrine condition, as well as the possibility of polypharmacy, can affect intake. The possibility of social isolation at mealtime and financial limitations that influence the quality and quantity of food obtained affects both the enjoyment and the quality of the meals consumed. Research supports that older adults who eat in a asocial setting consume more calories than those who eat alone.[130] Physiologic elements related to unplanned weight loss include changes in taste and smell sensitivity, delayed gastric emptying, early satiety, and impairment in the regulation of food intake that occurs with aging.

Cachexia is a "complex metabolic syndrome associated with underlying illness, and characterized by loss of muscle with or without loss of fat mass."[131] This syndrome is associated with higher morbidity rate. Signs and symptoms of cachexia include anorexia, inflammation, insulin resistance, and increased muscle protein breakdown. The cachexia syndrome includes many dysregulated pathways, which contribute to an imbalance between catabolism and anabolism in the body. Because of the presence of inflammation and catabolism, the cachexia disorder is resistant to nutrition interventions.

Sarcopenia is the progressive loss of skeletal muscle and muscle quality and decreased strength that can occur as part of the aging process. This can be caused by changes in the endocrine system, stimulation of pro-inflammatory cytokines, decreased physical activity, and not meeting protein needs.

Nutrition Management of Unintentional Weight Loss

The Academy of Nutrition and Dietetics Evidence Analysis Library (EAL) has evaluated the literature and provides guidelines for managing unintended weight loss.[132] Medical nutrition therapy (MNT) is strongly recommended for older adults with unintended weight loss. Individualized nutrition care, directed by a registered dietitian nutritionist (RDN) as part of the healthcare team, results in improved outcomes related to increased energy, protein, and nutrient intakes; nutritional status; quality of life; or weight gain. For older adults, the RDN should recommend liberalization of diets with the exception of texture modification. Increased food and beverage intake is associated with liberalized diets. Research has not demonstrated benefits of restricting sodium, cholesterol, fat, and carbohydrate in older adults. Older adults should be encouraged to dine with others rather than dining alone. Improved food intake and nutritional status has been found in older adults who eat in a socially stimulating common dining area. See **FIGURE 16.6** for an algorithm on the steps to manage unintended weight loss in the older adult.

The approach to increase calorie and nutrient intake in older adults should promote real food first. However, when nutritional needs cannot be met with food alone, care guidelines support that medical food supplements should be recommended for older adults who are

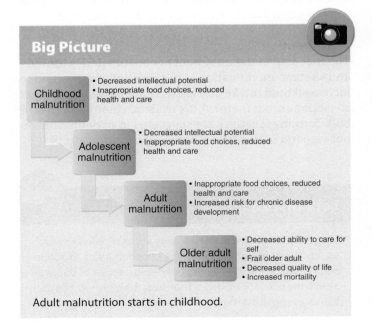

Big Picture

Childhood malnutrition
- Decreased intellectual potential
- Inappropriate food choices, reduced health and care

Adolescent malnutrition
- Decreased intellectual potential
- Inappropriate food choices, reduced health and care

Adult malnutrition
- Inappropriate food choices, reduced health and care
- Increased risk for chronic disease development

Older adult malnutrition
- Decreased ability to care for self
- Frail older adult
- Decreased quality of life
- Increased mortality

Adult malnutrition starts in childhood.

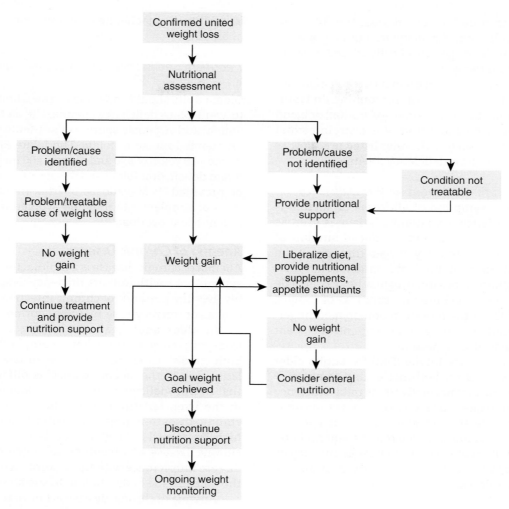

Figure 16.6
Managing unintended weight loss in the older adult.
Modified from Huffman, GB. Evaluating and treating unintentional weight loss in the elderly. Am Fam Physician. 2002; 65(4); 640–651.

undernourished or at risk of undernutrition, for example, for those who are frail and those who have infection, impaired wound healing, pressure injuries, depression, early to moderate dementia, or after hip fracture and orthopedic surgery.[132] Medical food supplementation is a method to provide energy and nutrient intake, promote weight gain, and maintain or improve nutritional status or prevent undernutrition. Care should be taken when evaluating older adults for the use of appetite stimulants.

Anemia

Anemia is a common condition in the older adult population. Although normally mild, it has been linked with significant morbidity and mortality.[133] The World Health Organization (WHO) defines anemia as a level of hemoglobin < 14 g/L in men and < 12.3 g/L in women.[133] Prior to this, in 1968, the WHO had defined anemia as hemoglobin < 13 g/L for men and < 12 g/L for women. Because of the lack of an overall constant definition of anemia,

the prevalence reported in the literature varies greatly. In long-term care facilities, anemia is present in 48–63% of residents.[134] In noninstitutionalized older adults, the National Health and Nutrition Examination Survey (NHANES) III data show that 10.2% of women and 11% of men age 65 and older were categorized with anemia.[135] As the human body ages, the risk of developing anemia also increases. NHANES III data show that 26% of men and 20% of women 85 years of age and older were anemic.[135] Of the older adults with anemia, nearly one-third had iron-, vitamin B_{12}-, or folate-deficiency anemia, another one-third had anemia related to chronic inflammation or renal insufficiency, and the final third had anemia that is unexplained.[134]

Iron-Deficiency Anemia

Iron-deficiency anemia is a disorder in which the body has decreased number of red blood cells (RBCs). A low number of RBCs is symptomatic of a microcytic (small cell) anemia. In iron-deficiency anemia, the RBCs are hypochromic (low in iron). An adequate number of RBCs are needed to provide oxygen to all cells while removing carbon dioxide from the body.[133]

Iron-deficiency anemia can occur as a result of inadequate intake of nutrients such as iron, vitamins, and minerals; long-term infections; impaired absorption; or blood loss from surgery or bleeding from the gastrointestinal tract.[133] Comorbidities such as the ones listed in TABLE 16.7 can also contribute to iron-deficiency anemia.

Treatment and Recommendations for Iron Deficiency

The most common symptom of all forms of anemia is fatigue. With iron-deficiency anemia, fatigue is seen as a result of inadequate RBCs and a reduced amount of hemoglobin in the RBCs to carry oxygen throughout the body. Other signs and symptoms of iron-deficiency anemia include shortness of breath, irregular heartbeat, pale skin and membranes, swelling and soreness of tongue, fissures in the sides of the mouth, spoon-shaped fingernails, cold extremities, enlarged spleen, and recurrent infections. Pica may also be present.

The Dietary Reference Intake (DRI) for adults older than 51 year is 8 mg/d for both males and females.[136] Increasing iron in the diet normally treats mild deficiency anemia that is not related to blood loss. If nutrition strategies are not effective at increasing iron in the body, an iron supplement containing 80–200 mg of elemental iron for 4 weeks should be considered.[136] Older adults may be at increased risk for toxicity from oral iron and may be treated with lower doses.

Folate-Deficiency Anemia

Folate deficiency is the absence (or low levels) of folic acid (one of the B vitamins) in the blood. This can cause a type of anemia known as megaloblastic anemia. Like in iron-deficiency anemia, laboratory profiles will show low hemoglobin and hematocrit and high mean corpuscular volume (MCV).[137]

According to the 2003–2006 NHANES data, most individuals in the United States ingest sufficient amounts of folate. Signs and symptoms of megaloblastic anemia include weakness, fatigue, difficulty concentrating, irritability, headache, heart palpitations, and shortness of breath.[137]

Treatment and Recommendations for Folate-Deficiency Anemia

Older adults should consume fortified breads and cereals to avoid folate-deficiency anemia. The diet should include animal and vegetable sources of nutrients to meet the recommended intake of folate. The folate RDI for men and women 19 years of age and older is 400 mcg/d. To reverse a folate deficit, oral folate at a dosage of 1 to 5 mg/d should be provided.[137] Megadoses of iron and/or folate in the form of supplements must be avoided to avoid toxicity and nutrient overload.

Anemia of Chronic Disease

Anemia of chronic disease is a multifactorial anemia often synchronous with iron insufficiency. Diagnosis normally involves the presence of chronic infection, inflammation, cancer, or microcytic or marginal normocytic anemia.

In older adults, anemia of chronic disease and iron-deficiency anemia have comparable symptoms. Both conditions share symptoms of low levels of circulating iron in the bloodstream. One differential factor is that in iron-deficiency anemia the storage form of iron in the liver, ferritin, is low, whereas when anemia of chronic disease is present, ferritin levels are normal to high. Decreased hemoglobin levels are seen in anemia of chronic disease as a result of inflammatory and chronic disease interference with the absorption of iron from both the diet and the body's failure to use stored iron.[138]

Anemia of chronic disease is linked to increased morbidity involving reduced quality of life, clinical depression, falls, functional impairment, reduced grip strength, decreased mobility, and increased mortality.[138]

Prevention of chronic disease is the best safeguard against anemia of chronic disease. Instructing patients to consume adequate amount of calories, stay physically active, avoid tobacco use, and limit alcohol use should promote healthy aging and may help to decrease the prevalence of anemia of chronic disease.

Anorexia

In older adults, the decrease in appetite termed *anorexia* occurs as a result of many physiological factors. As we age, food intake diminishes and meal patterns change.[139] The intake reduction seen in the early stages of aging seems like a suitable response to the decreased energy needs that occur as an increased sedentary lifestyle, reduced resting energy expenditure, and decrease in lean body mass. This disposes older adults to develop what has been termed *anorexia of aging*. Although anorexia of aging is believed to be a common disorder in older adults, actual prevalence has not been defined. Overall prevalence of anorexia for individuals admitted to an acute rehabilitation facility was reported as 33% in women and 27% in men.[140]

Table 16.7

Conditions that Can Contribute to Iron-Deficiency Anemia

Crohn's disease	Inflammatory bowel disease
Increased or occult blood loss	Malignancy, especially gastrointestinal
NSAIDs therapy	
Intestinal parasites	Gastric or duodenal injury disease
Vitamin A deficiency	Decreased absorption
Gastric surgery	Pernicious anemia with achlorhydria
	Celiac or tropical sprue

Recommendations

To assess the multifactorial causes of anorexia of aging, the use of validated screening tools such as the Simplified Nutritional Assessment Questionnaire (SNAQ) or other supported nutrition screening assessments is recommended. The SNAQ questionnaire contains four questions that ask about appetite and food intake. This tool is easy to use with older adults and has been validated for predictive capability of future weight loss.[141] Other risk factors to screen for that can interfere with proper nutrition in the older adult include depression, chewing and swallowing difficulty, and polypharmacy, to name a few.

The treatment of anorexia of aging involves addressing the root cause of the problem. Nutrition strategies discussed under unintended weight loss are appropriate strategies to treat the anorexia of aging.

Obesity

Centers for Disease Control and Prevention (CDC) data report that more than one-third of adults aged 65 and older were obese in 2007–2010.[142] When compared to older adults 75 years of age and higher, obesity prevalence is higher in older adults between the ages of 65 and 74 years.[142]

News You Can Use

Obesity in the United States (All Ages)

Obesity prevalence in 2013 varied across states and territories:

- No state had a prevalence of obesity less than 20%.
- Seven states and the District of Columbia had a prevalence of obesity between 20% and < 25%.
- Twenty-three states had a prevalence of obesity between 25% and < 30%.
- Eighteen states had a prevalence of obesity between 30% and < 35%.
- Two states (Mississippi and West Virginia) had a prevalence of obesity of 35% or greater.
- The South had the highest prevalence of obesity (30.2%), followed by the Midwest (30.1%), the Northeast (26.5%), and the West (24.9%).
- The prevalence of obesity was 27.0% in Guam and 27.9% in Puerto Rico.[a]

[a] Obesity prevalence in 2013 varied across states and territories. Originally published by the Centers for Disease Control for data available for 2013.

Causal Factors of Obesity in Older Adults

An important factor in securing a healthy weight and body mass index is the association between calories consumed and energy spent. Obesity takes place when individuals consume a greater number of calories than they can process through metabolism and activity level. Researchers suggest that as we age, the amount of calories we consume does not decline.[143] Consequently, the decrease in energy expenditure seen in the 50- to 65-year-old group coupled with no change in intake can be a main contributor to the increase in body weight.

Obesity Comorbidities

A number of chronic conditions are associated with being overweight and obese. The risk for developing diabetes mellitus, hypertension, and dyslipidemia increases with increases in weight. Other comorbidities related to obesity include joint problems such as osteoarthritis, sleep apnea, respiratory problems, some forms of cancers, and psychosocial effects.[144]

Obesity Prevention and Management Strategies

Prevention of obesity in the older adult can contribute to preventing unwanted health outcomes. Recommendations to avoid overweight and obesity include managing caloric intake with calorie expenditure and having an active lifestyle.[144]

Although weight management and maintenance of a healthy weight is advocated in older adults owing to their increased risk for developing chronic diseases related to obesity, it is important to remember that obesity thresholds for BMI, waist circumference, and waist-to-hip ratios for adults may not be appropriate measurements for older adults. Rather than trying to promote weight reduction to meet standard body weight guidelines, sustaining body weight or promoting physical activity as well as increasing functional status may be the best treatment goals for older adults.[145] *Obesity paradox*, also referred to as reverse epidemiology, is a term used for a medical hypothesis that supports that obesity as well as high cholesterol may be protective and linked to increased survival in segments of the population such as older adults. This theory also suggests that normal to low BMI may be disadvantageous and linked with higher mortality.[146] Healthcare providers should direct weight loss interventions on an individual basis, taking into account the benefits of weight loss measured against the risks associated with obesity in older adults.[147]

Case Study

Elsa continues to have unplanned/unintentional weight loss. In the past month Elsa has had another 10-pound weight loss and her meal acceptance continues to decline. Elsa has been feeling exceptionally fatigued and was just diagnosed with iron-deficiency anemia.

Questions

1. What are the physiologic elements related to unplanned, unintentional weight loss?
2. What are the guidelines for the management of unintentional weight loss?
3. List the conditions that can contribute to the development of iron-deficiency anemia

Table 16.8

Academy of Nutrition and Dietetic Guidelines to Promote Weight Loss

1. Weight management program
For weight loss and weight maintenance, the registered dietitian nutritionist (RDN) should include the following components as part of a comprehensive weight management program:

- Reduced calorie diet
- Increased physical activity
- Use of behavioral strategies

Adequate evidence indicates that intensive, multicomponent behavioral interventions for overweight and obese adults can lead to weight loss as well as improved glucose tolerance and other physiologic risk factors for cardiovascular disease.

2. Nutrient adequacy during weight loss
During weight loss, the RDN should prescribe an individualized diet, including patient preferences and health status, to achieve and maintain nutrient adequacy and reduce caloric intake based on one of the following caloric reduction strategies:

- 1,200 kcal to 1,500 kcal per day for women and 1,500 kcal to 1,800 kcal per day for men (kcal levels are usually adjusted for the individual's body weight)
- Energy deficit of approximately 500 kcal per day or 750 kcal per day
- Use of one of the evidence-based diets that restricts certain food types (such as high-carbohydrate foods, low-fiber foods, or high-fat foods) to create an energy deficit by reduced food intake

3. Portion control and meal replacements/structured meal plans
For weight loss and weight maintenance, the RDN should recommend portion control and meal replacements or structured meal plans as part of a comprehensive weight management program. Strong evidence documents a positive relationship between portion size and body weight, and research reports that the use of various types of meal replacements or structured meal plans was helpful in achieving health and food behavior change.

4. Encourage physical activity for weight loss
For weight loss, the RDN should encourage physical activity as part of a comprehensive weight management program, individualized to gradually accumulate 150 to 420 minutes or more of physical activity per week, depending on intensity, unless medically contraindicated. Physical activity less than 150 minutes per week promotes minimal weight loss, physical activity more than 150 minutes per week results in modest weight loss of approximately 2–3 kg, and physical activity of 225 to 420 or more minutes per week results in 5–7.5 kg weight loss, and a dose–response relationship exists.

Data from: Academy of Nutrition and Dietetics. Adult weight managment. Chicago, IL: Academy of Nutrition and Dietetics Evidence Analysis Library; 2014. Retrieved from: https://www.andeal.org/topic.cfm?menu=5276. Accessed August 16, 2015.

The Academy of Nutrition and Dietetics Evidence Analysis Library guidelines to promote weight management in adults are outlined in **TABLE 16.8**.[148]

Recap One of the goals of *Healthy People 2020* is to "Promote health and reduce chronic disease risk through the consumption of healthful diets and achievement and maintenance of healthy body weights."[120] It is estimated that 27% of frail older adults 65 years and older have involuntary and unplanned weight loss.[124] Prevention of obesity in the older adult can contribute to preventing unwanted health outcomes. Recommendations to avoid overweight and obesity include balancing caloric intake with calorie expenditure and having an active lifestyle.[144]

1. Discuss the risk factors for malnutrition in older adults.
2. Go to CDC Obesity Prevalence Maps (http://www.cdc.gov/obesity/data/prevalence-maps.html). What is the obesity rate in your state? What can you do to influence the obesity rate in your community?

Skeletal Health

Preview The presence of osteoporosis increases the risk for fractures. A diet low in calcium and vitamin D, sedentary lifestyle, smoking, and extreme alcohol consumption are modifiable factors that contribute to development of osteoporosis.

The skeletal system is a dynamic body system that includes bones, ligaments, tendons, and cartilage. Bone is a living tissue that is in constant regeneration through **resorption** (removing old bone) and new bone formation. This system gives the body its basic structure, posture, and the ability to move. Development of skeletal diseases impairs bone and joint function, leads to compromised skeletal integrity, and impairs the ability to accomplish activities of daily living.

Osteoporosis

Osteoporosis is a condition in which the bones weaken because of decreased bone mineral density (BMD) and structural changes that increase the risk for fractures. The CDC reports that during 2005–2010, 16.2% of adults aged 65 and older had osteoporosis at the lumbar spine or femur neck. Nonmodifiable risk factors involve age, genetics, small frame, female, Asian or white ethnicity, and the presence of estrogen or testosterone deficiency.[149] Modifiable risk factors include inadequate diet, mainly calcium and vitamin D intake, sedentary lifestyle, smoking, extreme alcohol consumption (because of alcohol's negative effect on balance), and increased risk for falls.

Symptoms

Osteoporosis is referred to as the "silent disease" because bone loss is asymptomatic. Very often the first indication of osteoporosis is fracture of a hip or vertebra resulting from a fall or sudden strain. The first symptoms of collapsed vertebrae include severe back pain, decrease in height, and spinal malformations such as kyphosis.[150]

Prevention

Primary prevention of osteoporosis focuses on halting the disease before it starts by decreasing and removing risk factors. Primary prevention consists of immunoprophylaxis, chemoprophylaxis, and lifestyle modifications. Secondary prevention involves disease diagnosis and treatment in the beginning stages prior to the presence of symptoms and functional loss. In tertiary prevention the signs and symptoms of chronic disease are managed to prevent further functional losses and complications.[151]

To prevent osteoporosis, it is vital to secure optimal peak bone mass to promote new bone tissue generation. Nutrition plays a pivotal role in both preventing and managing osteoporosis. Adequate calcium and vitamin D are essential nutrients throughout the life span for promoting and maintaining bone health. **TABLE 16.9** lists some of the most common food sources of calcium.[150] See **TABLE 16.10** for food sources of vitamin D.[150]

Table 16.9

Food Sources of Calcium

Food Category	Food Items
Low-fat dairy products	Milk, yogurt, cheese, and ice cream
Dark green leafy vegetables	Broccoli, collard greens, bok choy, and spinach
Protein sources	Sardines and salmon with bones, tofu, almonds
Foods fortified with calcium	Orange juice, cereals, breads

Data from National Institutes of Health Osteoporosis and Related Bone Diseases National Resource Center. Osteoporosis overview. Washington, DC: NIH, U.S. Department of Health and Human Services; June 2015. Retrieved from: http://www.niams.nih.gov/Health_Info/Bone/Osteoporosis/overview.asp. Accessed August 18, 2015.

Table 16.10

Food Sources of Vitamin D

Food Category	Food Items
Protein sources	Egg yolks, saltwater fish, and liver
Foods fortified with vitamin D	Milk

Data from NIH Osteoporosis and Related Bone Diseases National Resource Center. Osteoporosis overview. Washington, DC: NIH, U.S. Department of Health and Human Services; June 2015. Retrieved from: http://www.niams.nih.gov/Health_Info/Bone/Osteoporosis/overview.asp. Accessed August 18, 2015.

Weight-bearing exercise such as walking, hiking, and jogging is the best form of exercise to promote bone health.

A number of medications can contribute to increased bone loss. The long-term use of glucocorticoids can contribute to reduced bone density and increased risk for fracture. Bone loss can also occur as a result of long-term therapy with antiseizure drugs, like phenytoin (Dilantin) and barbiturates; excessive use of aluminum-containing antacids; and excessive thyroid hormone.[150]

Treatment

Osteoporosis treatment emphasizes adequate nutrition intake, exercise and an active lifestyle, and safety measures to avert falls that can contribute to fractures. Medication intended to slow or stop bone loss, increase bone density, and reduce the risk for fractures might be indicated.[152]

Osteoarthritis

Osteoarthritis (OA), also known as degenerative joint disease, is an ailment that involves the whole joint, including the cartilage, joint lining, ligaments, and underlying bone. This is the most common form of arthritis. The deterioration of these matters ultimately leads to pain and joint stiffness. The precise causes of OA are not known. However, it is hypothesized that both mechanical and molecular actions affect the joint. Illness onset is slow and typically starts after the age of 40, and currently there is no cure for OA.

Prevalence and Risk Factors

In the United States OA affects 13.9% of adults 25 years and older as well as 33.6% (12.4 million) of older adults (those older than 65 years).[153] Overall, an estimated 30.8 million U.S. older adults suffered from OA. It is more prevalent in older women (13%) than in older men (10%).[154]

Usual risk factors related to OA include aging, overweight and obesity, trauma, repetitive joint use, joint slackness, and muscle weakness. OA characteristically affects the knees, hips, and hand joints.

Prevention and Treatment

The basis for prevention and treatment of OA is weight management and exercise. In individuals who are obese and overweight, the added weight exacerbates the symptoms. Low-caloric diet to produce a fast weight loss for fast symptom relief has been reported to produce the greatest benefits. It is important to remember that weight loss must be sustainable. The macronutrient distribution leading to the weight loss is not as important as the actual weight reduction to promote pain relief and increase mobility.[155] Following a healthy diet to facilitate a slow gradual weight loss of 1–2 lb/wk with the goal of a total 10% weight loss can also be used as an approach to alleviate symptoms and increase mobility.[155] Adding an exercise program to a weight loss or healthy eating program yields a deeper impact to physical function and pain control.[155]

Rheumatoid Arthritis

Rheumatoid arthritis (RA) is a systemic inflammatory illness that shows symptoms in multiple joints of the body. The inflammatory progression mainly affects the synovial membrane lining of the joints, but it is known to attack other organs. The exacerbated synovium causes erosions of the cartilage and bone, which can result in joint deformity. Pain, swelling, and redness are common symptoms. Although the cause for this illness is not known, RA is considered to be the result of a damaged or compromised immune response. RA can manifest at any age and is coupled with fatigue and extended stiffness after rest periods. There is no cure for this condition. New and effective medications are constantly being introduced to treat the disorder and avoid deformed joints. Good self-management that includes being physically active are known to decrease pain and disability.[156]

Prevalence

In 2007, an estimated 1.5 million adults had rheumatoid arthritis.[157,158] This condition is more prevalent in women (9.8/1,000) than in men (4.1/1,000).[157,158]

Nutrition Considerations

A number of diets and diet alterations to reduce inflammation have been used in efforts to treat RA. Vegetarian and plant-based diets with reduced saturated fatty acids have shown to improve pain level, stiffness, and swelling.[159] Omega-3 fatty acids seem to have a protective benefit against RA.[160]

Case Study

Elsa's finger joints are swollen, and she finds it painful to hold utensils when trying to feed herself, which is contributing to her poor intake and recent weight loss.

Questions

1. Describe some of the interventions that can be put in place to relief her symptoms?
2. What are some of the diets proven to be effective in relieving symptoms for patients with OA? RA?

Recap The skeletal system is a dynamic body system that includes bones, ligaments, tendons, and cartilage. Development of skeletal diseases impairs bone and joint function, leads to compromised skeletal integrity, and impairs the ability to accomplish activities of daily living. Nutrition plays a pivotal role in both preventing and managing osteoporosis. Adequate calcium and vitamin D are essential nutrients in promoting and maintaining bone health.

1. When providing nutrition education to an older adult with arthritis, what topics should be highlighted?
2. For older adults with osteoporosis, which are the most important nutrients to monitor?

Wound Healing

Preview A thorough nutrition screening and assessment is vital for the prevention and treatment of pressure injuries. Sufficient macro- and micronutrients are vital for the body to support tissue integrity and prevent breakdown.

The National Pressure Ulcer Advisory Panel (NPUAP) describes a pressure injury (PI) as a "localized injury to the skin and/or underlying tissue usually over a bony prominence, as a result of pressure, or pressure in combination with shear. A number of contributing or confounding factors are also associated with PIs; the significance of these factors is yet to be elucidated."[161]

Prevalence

Because a pressure ulcer (PU) is often referred to as a *bedsore* or *decubitus*, the inconsistency in labeling skin injuries has made it hard to pinpoint the true prevalence of PUs in different care settings.[162] In the United States, approximately 1.3–3.0 million patients have PUs.[163] Prevalence has been estimated at 3–15% of all patients in acute care and 11% of patients in extended care facilities.[163,164]

Nutrition Screening and Assessment

Completing a thorough nutrition screening and assessment is vital for the prevention and treatment of **pressure injuries**. Current literature has identified more than a hundred risk factors for PI development. Some extrinsic (primary/nonphysiological) and intrinsic (secondary/physiological) risk factors that contribute to PU development include diabetes mellitus, peripheral vascular disease, malignancy, prolonged pressure on an area of the body, being 70 years of age and older, smoking, urinary and fecal incontinence, a history of PIs, a low BMI, and malnutrition.[165]

Pathophysiologic and **intrinsic factors** at the core of PU formation include nutrition. Maintaining adequate parameters of nutrition is considered a best practice in both the prevention and treatment of PIs. Older adults with PIs or who are at risk for developing PIs should strive to achieve or maintain adequate nutrition parameters.

Nutrition Screening

There are a number of validated pressure injury risk evaluation tools. These include the Norton Scale, Gosnell Scale, Warlow Scale, and the Braden Scale. In the United States, the Braden Scale for Predicting Pressure Sore Risk is the most frequently used screening instrument. The Braden Scale is composed of six subscales: sensory perception, moisture, activity, mobility, nutrition, and friction/shear. The sensory perception, mobility, and activity subscales help to pinpoint clinical situations that predispose patients to intense and persistent pressure. The moisture, nutrition, and friction/shear subscales identify clinical circumstances that can modify tissue tolerance for pressure. The nutrition subscale can be scored on a 1 to 4 scale to ascertain usual food intake, NPO (nothing by mouth), or enteral and parenteral intake. Patients identified as at risk should be referred to the RDN for assessment. The RDN must evaluate the nutrition subscale as part of conducting a nutrition assessment for pressure injuries. The Braden Scale can be retrieved at http://bradenscale.com/.

Nutrition Assessment

Once the screen is completed, the patients identified as at risk are referred to the RDN for follow-up. A comprehensive nutrition assessment uses the Academy of Nutrition and Dietetics standardized Nutrition Care Process: assessment, diagnosis, intervention, and monitoring/evaluation should be started.[166]

Role of Nutrients in Wound Prevention and Healing

Sufficient macronutrients (carbohydrates, protein, fats, and water) and micronutrients (vitamins and minerals) are vital for the body to support tissue integrity and prevent breakdown. Weight loss and difficulties with eating can increase the incidence of PIs.[166] Other nutrition-related risk factors that can contribute to PI development include a change in appetite, compromised dental health, gastrointestinal and elimination disturbances, decreased self-feeding abilities, drug–nutrient interactions, and alcohol and substance abuse.[125,168,169]

Restrictive diets can contribute to a decreased intake of nutrients.[170] A diet too low in protein lacks the amino acids needed for protein synthesis. Protein plays a major role in the production of enzymes involved in wound healing, cell multiplication, and collagen and connective tissue manufacture. Caloric needs must be met for protein to be spared for buildup and repair.[171] Although the amount of protein needed by patients with PIs can be debated, protein levels higher than the adult recommendation of 0.8 g/kg of body weight per day are generally accepted and recommended. The NPUAP recommends 1.25–1.5 g

of protein per kilogram of body weight per day and 30–35 kcal/kg of body weight per day for wound healing.[172]

Low-fat diets can be deficient in essential fatty acids, which the skin needs to maintain the lipid barrier. Carbohydrates are essential for the cells to carry out basic functions of metabolism and to prevent gluconeogenesis from protein stores.[171]

Water plays an important role in wound-site hydration and oxygen perfusion, is a solvent for nutrients and other small molecules to diffuse in to and out of cells, and removes waste from cells. Dehydration is a risk factor for wound development. Patients with draining wounds need additional fluids to replace losses.

Vitamin A fuels cellular differentiation in fibroblasts and is involved in collagen development. A true vitamin A deficiency, although rare, can result in delayed wound healing and compromised immune function.[173]

Vitamin C is vital for collagen production. Collagen and fibroblasts are the basis for the structure of a healing wound bed. A deficiency in vitamin C has been associated with prolonged wound healing time, decreased wound strength, and decreased immune function.[171,172] For patients with a diagnosed vitamin C deficiency, supplementation is recommended.[171,172]

Zinc is associated with collagen formation, protein metabolism, vitamin A transport, and immune function.[171,172] Zinc deficiency can emerge as a result of severe wound drainage or GI losses, corticosteroid use, or a long-term decreased dietary intake.[171] When considering supplementation, it is important to remember that consumption of increased zinc can interfere with copper metabolism, thus producing copper-induced anemia. The amount of zinc in a multivitamin and mineral supplement is generally adequate. Supplementing to no more than the Tolerable Upper Intake Limit of the Dietary Reference Intake (DRI; 40 mg of elemental zinc) until the deficiency is corrected may be recommended.[174]

Aside from the role of vitamins and minerals, the role of individual amino acids in wound healing has been explored. Arginine is a conditionally essential amino acid that in several studies has been shown to raise concentrations of hydroxyproline, an indicator of collagen

Case Study

Over the past few weeks Elsa has taken less interest in her personal care, bathing, toileting, and dressing requiring increasingly more assistance with her ADLs and IADLs. Upon physical inspection, the nurse discovers a stage 4 pressure injury.

Questions

1. What are her nutritional needs to promote wound healing?
2. What are some of the nutrition factors that contribute to increased risk for developing pressure injuries?

accumulation and protein at the wound site.[171,172] Current research supports the use of arginine to promote PU healing in adults with a pressure injury category/stage 3 or 4 or multiple pressure injuries when nutritional requirements cannot be met with traditional high-calorie and protein supplements.[172]

> **Recap** Current literature has identified more than a hundred risk factors for PU development. Some extrinsic (primary/non-physiological) and intrinsic (secondary/physiological) risk factors that contribute to PU development include diabetes mellitus, peripheral vascular disease, malignancy, prolonged pressure on an area of the body, being 70 years of age and older, smoking, urinary and fecal incontinence, a history of PIs, a low BMI, and malnutrition.[165] Pathophysiologic and intrinsic factors at the core of PI formation include nutrition. Maintaining adequate parameters of nutrition is considered a best practice in both the prevention and treatment of PIs.
>
> 1. For patients with pressure injuries and compromised nutritional status, what are the main nutrition recommendations?
> 2. Which are the most commonly supplemented nutrients in patients with pressure injuries? What is the function of each nutrient?

Renal and Genitourinary Conditions

> **Preview** Nutrition intervention for older adults with renal disease is as individual as every patient. Actual cause, comorbidities, urine output, biochemical data, and the need and use of renal replacement therapy help to determine treatment.

A physiological decrease in kidney function is a normal component of the aging process. As we age, the number of nephrons may decrease, the overall amount of kidney tissue may decrease, and nephrosclerosis can be present, causing the kidneys to filter blood more slowly.[175]

Acute Kidney Injury

Acute kidney injury (AKI) is the sudden loss of kidney function that causes urea nitrogenous waste products retention as well as imbalance of extracellular volume and electrolytes.[175]

Prevalence and Risk Factors

Risk factors contributing to increased episodes of AKI include the presence of comorbidities such as DM and HTN, cardiovascular disease, overweight or obesity, high cholesterol, and autoimmune diseases such as lupus. It is estimated that about one out of three adults with DM and one out of five adults with high blood pressure develops chronic kidney disease (CKD). Changes in the kidney due to normal aging such as nephrosclerosis also contribute to increased risk. Men with CKD are 50% more likely than women to develop kidney failure.[176]

Urinary tract obstructions triggered by benign prostatic hyperplasia (BPH), neurogenic bladder, and cancer are common disorders in older adults and can also contribute to kidney damage.[177]

Prevention and Treatment

AKI prevention strategies in older adults emphasizes categorizing risk factors and making suitable changes. Recommendations to prevent AKI include promoting sufficient fluid consumption to avert dehydration, minimizing polypharmacy, avoiding the use of nephron-damaging substances like contrast dyes, maintaining adequate urine output for the individual, and closely monitoring kidney function (biochemical data: serum creatinine, blood urea nitrogen [BUN]).[177–179]

Treatment for AKI varies depending on the manner of causation, whether it is prerenal azotemia (inadequate renal perfusion), intrarenal (intrinsic kidney damage has occurred), or postrenal azotemia (urinary blockage). Treatment might include restoring fluid and electrolyte balance or the use of catheters to manage urinary tract obstructions.[179] Renal replacement therapy (RRT; dialysis) might be needed for the treatment of some hospitalized patients.[179]

Nutrition Considerations

Nutrition intervention for older adults with AKI is as individual as every patient and differs based on actual cause, comorbidities, urine output, biochemical data, and the need and use of RRT.[180,181] The nutrition treatment goals in AKI center around preventing protein-energy wasting, averting fluid overload/edema, regulating blood pressure and electrolytes, and promoting acid–base balance.[180,181]

For individuals with DM and insulin resistance, episodes of high blood glucose should be prevented and a stable blood glucose level ranging between 110 and 150 mg/dL should be sustained.[182] Protein needs are contingent on the individual's renal function. Protein needs are initially calculated based on 1 g/kg of body weight. For individuals receiving RRT, the protein intake is calculated using 1.2–1.5 g/kg/d range to counterbalance dialysis losses. For individuals with continuous renal replacement therapy (CRRT), protein needs are based on 1.5–2 g/kg per day and could go up to 2.5 g/kg per day depending on the severity of the condition. Caloric needs are calculated using the 20–30 kcal/kg/d range. Care should be taken not to overfeed patients.[181] When oral intake is insufficient, the patient should be evaluated for an enteral/parenteral nutrition feeding alternative.[180,181] Regardless of the feeding mode, the DRIs for vitamins and minerals should be met. For patients receiving RRT, a renal multivitamin formula should be recommended as needed.[181]

To avoid fluid overload and edema, fluid intake is limited to urine output and an additional 500 mL/d.[181] Sodium (Na) is normally restricted to 2–3 g/d. The needs for serum potassium and phosphorus vary with AKI stage and the type of therapy used; thus, the levels for these nutrients need to be carefully monitored and recommendations for intake adjusted as needed.[181]

Chronic Kidney Disease
Prevalence and Symptoms

More than 20 million adults in the United States are assessed as having chronic kidney disease (CKD). This accounts for approximately 10% of the population. NHANES reports that nearly 25% of people aged 60 years and older have CKD.[183] Between 2000 and 2008, the number of older adults diagnosed with CKD doubled.[183]

Staging CKD is about identifying the severity of the disease. CKD can be classified into five stages. See **TABLE 16.11** for a description of CKD stages.[184]

Prevention

Modifiable lifestyle changes to prevent CKD include decreasing sodium consumption to less than 2.3 g/d and promoting a healthy weight.[185] In patients with diabetes, blood glucose levels should be controlled. Decreasing ingestion of cholesterol and saturated fat–rich foods and drinking plenty of fluids to prevent dehydration are also recommended to prevent CKD.

Nutrition Recommendations

The Academy of Nutrition and Dietetics recommends the nutrition prescription guidelines described in **TABLE 16.12** for patients with CKD who are not receiving dialysis and for those receiving hemodialysis treatment.[181]

The goal of the nutrition care treatment is to reduce the effects of the collection of waste products in the blood, delay disease progression, and prevent protein-energy wasting.[181]

Table 16.11

Chronic Kidney Disease Stages

Stage	Description
Stage 1	Normal GFR (≥ 90 mL/min/1.73 m²) plus either persistent **albuminuria** or known structural or hereditary renal disease
Stage 2	GFR 60 to 89 mL/min/1.73 m²
Stage 3	GFR 30–59 mL/min/1.73 m²
Stage 4	GFR 15–29 mL/min/1.73 m²
Stage 5	GFR < 15 mL/min/1.73 m²

GFR = glomerular filtration rate.

From the Merck Manual Professional Version (Known as the Merck Manual in the US and Canada and the MSD Manual in the rest of the world), edited by Robert Porter. Copyright 2016 by Merck Sharp & Dohme Corp., a subsidiary of Merck & Co, Inc, Kenilworth, NJ. Available at http://www.merckmanuals.com/professional. Accessed October 27, 2016.

End-Stage Renal Disease
Prevalence

End-stage renal disease (ESRD), also labeled as stage 5 CKD, takes place when the kidneys stop working to the point that the patient cannot live without dialysis or a kidney transplant. The glomerular filtration rate (GFR) in these patients is < 15 mL/min/1.73 m² (< 15% of kidney function).[186] Patients with ESRD are frequently older adults aged 65 and older.[186]

Prevention

Interventions to avoid ESRD (stage 5 CKD) strive to slow the succession of CKD. These include early diagnosis and referral of individuals at risk, providing MNT commencing in CKD stage 3, modifying the meal plan so that patients consume protein in moderation with adequate amounts of calories, decreasing sodium intake to promote stable blood pressure, maintaining stable blood glucose levels, and controlling serum lipids.

Treatment

There are risks and benefits with all ESRD treatments. A significant consideration for older adults is the potential influence of their treatment choice in their quality of life. Some common treatments include conservative management, hemodialysis, peritoneal dialysis, and kidney transplant.[187]

Conservative Management

Conservative (nondialytic) management of ESRD involves meticulous care of fluid balance, anemia, acidosis, and hyperkalemia management. Lowering dietary potassium intake contributes to hyperkalemia management. Also, specific symptom management and palliative care are critical to sustain an adequate quality of life.[188]

Hemodialysis Treatment

CKD and hemodialysis (HD) are risk factors for negative outcomes in the older adult. Increases in mortality, hospitalizations, frailty syndrome, disability, cognitive dysfunction, falls, and fall-related injuries can occur, and as the disease progresses hemodialysis treatment is needed to sustain life.[189] All risks aside, HD is the treatment of choice of more than 90% of individuals who decide to receive RRT.[190]

Exhaustion is a frequent side effect in patients receiving HD. This affects energy level for meal preparation and possibly reduces intake on treatment days. The use of dietary restrictions should be closely evaluated and monitored because dietary restrictions interfere with the consumption of the individual's favorite foods.

Peritoneal Dialysis

Peritoneal dialysis (PD) can be a valid treatment selection for RRT in older adults.[191] Advantages of selecting PD as the treatment course include the patient's independence

Table 16.12

Nutrition Prescription for Patents with CKD

Nutrient	Patients Not on Dialysis	Patients at Stage 5: Hemodialysis
Protein	• GFR < 50 mL/min/1.73 m^2: kg of body weight × 0.60 g/kg – 0.80 g protein/kg of body weight • If diabetic nephropathy is present: kg of body weight × 0.80–0.90 g protein/kg[a]	• ≥ 1.2 g/kg of body weight, ≥ 50% HBV protein
Energy	• 23–35 kcal/kg[a] • Overweight adults: 1,780–1,823 kcal/d[a]	• < 60 y of age: kg of body weight × 35 kcal; > 60 y of age: kg of body weight × 30–35 kcal/kg
Sodium	• < 2.4 g/d	• < 2.4 g/day
Potassium	• < 2.4 g/d (stages 3–4 CKD)	• < 2.4 g/day
Phosphorus	• 800 to 1,000 mg/d or 10–12 mg phosphorus per gram of protein when serum phosphorus > 4.6 mg/dL or intact PTH is elevated (stages 3–4)	• 800–1,000 mg/d or 10–12 mg phosphorus per gram of protein when serum phosphorus > 5.5 mg/dL or intact PTH is elevated
Calcium	• Total elemental intake (including dietary calcium, calcium supplementation, and calcium-based binders) should not exceed 2 g/d (stages 3–4)	• Total elemental intake (including dietary calcium, calcium supplementation, and calcium-based binders) should not exceed 2 g/d
Fluid	• The need for a fluid restriction is determined by medical status, blood pressure control, physical findings (fluid accumulation), and any alterations in urine output[b]	• Urine output plus 1,000 mL
Vitamins/minerals	• DRI for B-complex vitamins and vitamin C • Vitamin D: supplementation recommended if 25-hydroxyvitamin D level less than 30 ng/mL[a]	• Vitamin C: 60–100 mg/d • Vitamin B$_6$: 2 mg/d • Folate: 1–5 mg/d[b] • Vitamin B$_{12}$: 3 mcg/d • DRI for all other water-soluble vitamins • Vitamin E: 15 IU/d • Zinc: 15 mg/d
Iron	• Oral or intravenous supplementation recommended if serum ferritin below 100 ng/mL and transferrin saturation below 20%	• IV supplementation recommended if serum ferritin below 200 ng/mL and TSAT below 20%[c]
Vitamin D		• It is suggested that 25-hydroxyvitamin D levels be measured, with deficiency or insufficiency being corrected using treatment strategies recommended for general population[a]

CKD = chronic kidney disease; DRI = Dietary Reference Intake; GFR = glomerular filtration rate; HBV = high biological value; PTH = parathyroid hormone; TSAT = transferrin saturation.

[a] Academy of Nutrition and Dietetics. *Chronic Kidney Disease Evidence-Based Nutrition Practice Guidelines*. Chicago, IL: Academy of Nutrition and Dietetics Evidence Analysis Library; 2010.

[b] McCann L, ed. *Pocket Guide to Nutrition Assessment of the Patient with Chronic Kidney Disease*. 4th ed. New York, NY: National Kidney Foundation Council on Renal Nutrition; 2009.

[c] National Kidney Foundation. Clinical practice guidelines for nutrition in chronic renal failure. *Am J Kidney Dis.* 2000;35(suppl 2):S1–S140.

Data from Academy of Nutrition and Dietetics. *Nutrition Care Manual: Renal*. Chicago, IL: AND; 2015. Retrieved from: https://www.nutritioncaremanual.org/topic.cfm?ncm_category_id=1&lv1=5537&ncm_toc_id=5537&ncm_heading=Nutrition%20Care.

in being able to conduct his or her own treatments. Adults 75 years and older using PD as RRT live an average of 19.6 months following treatment.[192]

In individuals who use PD treatment, the absorption of additional calories from the dextrose-containing dialysate increases the risk for undesired weight increase, increased triglycerides, and high blood glucose levels.[193] Educating individuals to control excessive fluid gains that might require the use of greater concentrations of dextrose can help to control these risks.

The risk for hypoalbuminemia and protein-energy wasting is greater in patients utilizing PD (as opposed to HD). These patients should be encouraged to include a source of protein at every meal as well as add high-protein snacks to their meal pattern.

Kidney Transplant

Another RRT to extend the life of individuals with CKD is kidney transplant. It is important to note that a kidney transplant is not a cure for CKD. In older adults, the presence of comorbidities such as CVD can limit their chances of qualifying for a kidney transplant.[194]

Important nutrition interventions to consider after a kidney transplant include ensuring adequate consumption of protein and calories for healing.[193] A diet low in sodium (≤ 2,300 mg/d) and reduced saturated fat and cholesterol should be encouraged to decrease cardiovascular risk. Managing blood pressure (< 130/80 mm Hg), preventing hyperglycemia, and promoting a healthy weight are important components of care status postkidney transplant. Because of the compromised immune system, it is wise for patients to avoid events of foodborne illness.[193]

Urinary Tract Disorders

Three regularly diagnosed urinary tract disorders are **urinary incontinence**, urinary tract infections, and kidney stones. Understanding these ailments can help to improve the health and quality of life for older individuals.[193]

Prevalence, Etiology, and Prevention

Urinary tract infections (UTIs) are one of the most frequently identified infections in hospitalized, institutionalized, and community-dwelling older adults.[195] UTIs in elderly persons are often mistaken as the early stages of dementia or Alzheimer's because of symptoms such as confusion, delirium, and hallucinations. Nutrition interventions for the prevention of UTIs promote the consumption of adequate fluids. The recommended fluid intake is 1½–2 L/d if the kidneys are functioning properly.[195]

Urge incontinence is the inability to control the impulse to urinate. Urinary incontinence is more prevalent in women than in men. Older adults are at increased risk for developing incontinence.[196] Stress incontinence is the most common type of incontinence and often occurs when episodes of sneezing or coughing places a sudden pressure on the bladder.[196] Obesity can exacerbate stress incontinence by delivering abdominal pressure on the bladder.[197]

Case Study

Elsa has had episodes of recurrent UTIs, with episodes of anorexia and confusion. She is refusing to drink the fluids provided with her meals. Her most recent laboratory results reflect mild dehydration.

Questions

1. How much daily fluid should Elsa consume to reduce the risk of recurrent UTI?
2. What suggestions do you have to encourage her to consume more fluids?

Recap A physiological decrease in kidney function is a normal component of the aging process. Acute kidney injury (AKI) is the sudden loss of kidney function that causes the retention of urea nitrogenous waste products as well as imbalance of extracellular volume and electrolytes.[175] Ten percent of the U.S. population suffers from chronic kidney disease (CKD). Modifiable risk factors to prevent CKD include decrease in sodium intake (≤ 2.3 g/d), healthy weight, control of blood glucose levels, a diet low in cholesterol and saturated fats, and adequate consumption of fluids.

1. Prepare a "top 10" list of foods high in protein, phosphorus, sodium, and potassium. How can this list be used when conducting patient education?
2. What are the modifiable risk factors for patients with CKD?

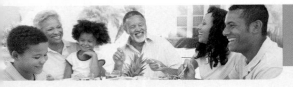

Learning Portfolio

Visual Chapter Summary

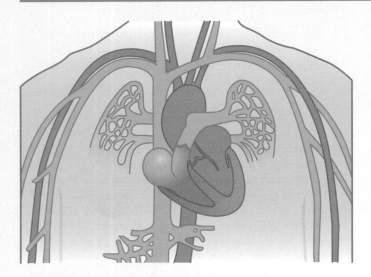

Cardiovascular, Cerebrovascular, and Respiratory Conditions

- The term *cerebrovascular disease* encompasses all syndromes in which an area of the brain is briefly or permanently affected by ischemia or hemorrhage.[4]
- The American Heart Association classifies blood pressure as normal, prehypertension, hypertension stage 1, hypertension stage 2, and hypertensive crisis.
- There are two types of strokes: ischemic and hemorrhagic.
- Heart failure (HF)is caused by the heart's inability to pump adequate amounts of oxygenated blood to support other body organs.

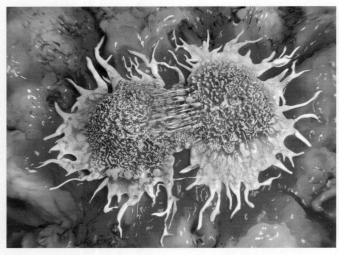

©Juan Gartner/Science Photo Library/Getty

- In chronic obstructive pulmonary disease (COPD), the presence of malnutrition can exacerbate the disease development, producing atrophy of the diaphragm and the muscles that move air in and out of the lungs.[33]

Cancer

- Aging is the strongest risk factor for the development of cancer. More than 60% of all episodes of cancer occur in adults 65 years and older.[39]
- Cancer is a group of diseases that present as abnormal, unregulated cell growth caused by a series of DNA metamorphoses.
- Age, alcohol consumption, cancer-causing substances, chronic inflammation, diet, hormones, immunosuppression, infectious agents, obesity, radiation, sunlight exposure, and consumption of tobacco products are the most commonly cited cancer risk factors.[38]
- The goals for nutrition care are to define symptoms that have an impact on nutritional status and to develop a nutrition plan that helps each older adult prevent or reverse nutritional deficiencies.

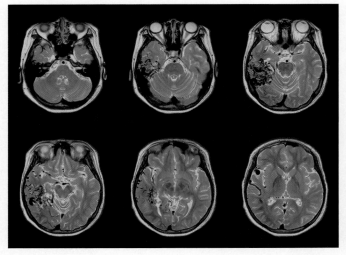

©AkeSak/Shutterstock

Cognitive Disorders

- Dementia is a brain condition that interferes with older adults' ability to remember, obtain and process new information, and communicate.
- The true cause of Alzheimer's disease (AD) is not known. Theories support that AD occurs as a result

of environmental, lifestyle, and genetic factors that combine into the pathophysiologic succession of events that, over decades, progresses to AD.

- Signs and symptoms and the rate of advancement through the diverse disease phases are distinctive for each individual.
- The main nutrition goals when treating individuals with AD and other forms of dementia is to prevent weight loss, malnutrition, pressure injuries, and the presence of other comorbidities.[55]

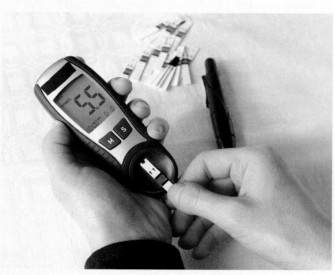

©Bibiphoto/Shutterstock

Endocrine and Metabolic Conditions

- Type 1 diabetes mellitus (T1 DM) is mainly an autoimmune disorder in which the body's immune system attacks the beta cells of the pancreas where insulin is produced. Type 2 DM is more common in older adults.
- T2DM occurs as a gradual decline in beta cell function, which results in a reduction in insulin production that progresses to insulin resistance and finally results in insulin deficiency.[67,68]
- In older adults, changes in body composition accompanied by aging, sarcopenia of aging, vitamin D deficiency, and inflammatory response are believed to contribute to the development of DM.[67,68]
- Metabolic syndrome (MetS) is a disease in which an individual has irregular levels of blood lipids (low HDL and high triglycerides), impaired fasting glucose, hypertension (HTN), and excess abdominal obesity.[64]

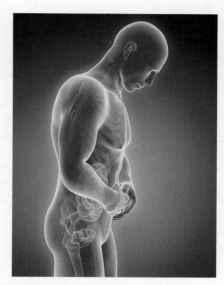

©Science Photo Library/Shutterstock

Gastrointestinal Conditions

- Gastroesophageal reflux disease (GERD) is a chronic disorder in which gastric acid and other stomach fluids leak into the esophagus, characteristically producing irritation and damage to the esophageal tissue.
- Risk factors for development of GERD include obesity. Weight loss and deterrence of weight gain, coupled with smoking cessation and decreased alcohol intake, may be helpful in averting GERD.[95]
- Diverticular disease encompasses diverticulosis, or the presence of diverticula projecting through the colonic wall, and diverticulitis, which is an acute inflammation of diverticula usually manifested with symptoms like fever, leukocytosis, and pain.
- Celiac disease is an immune condition in which the presence of gluten in the diet damages the inner lining of the small intestine and hinders nutrient absorption.[107]

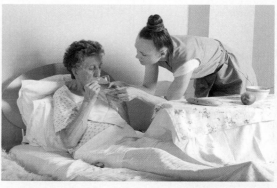

©Tolikoff Photography/Shutterstock

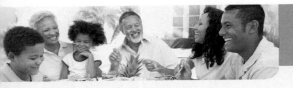

Learning Portfolio (continued)

Obesity and Malnutrition

- Unintentional or involuntary weight loss is a common occurrence among older adults that is associated with adverse outcomes, including increased mortality.[120]
- Significant weight loss in older adults is defined as 5% in 1 month and 10% in 6 months.[123] Weight loss in older adults with a BMI below 30 presents a higher mortality risk than not losing weight or having a BMI in the 25–30 range.[126]
- Cachexia is a "complex metabolic syndrome associated with underlying illness, and characterized by loss of muscle with or without loss of fat mass."[129]
- Sarcopenia is the progressive loss of skeletal muscle, quality, and decreased strength that can occur as part of the aging process.

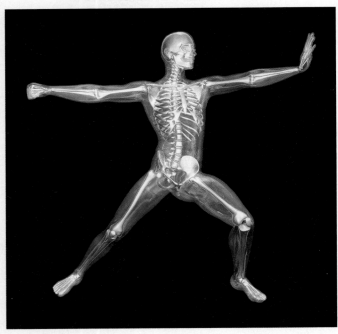

©Spectral-Design/iStock/Getty

Skeletal Health

- Osteoporosis is a condition in which the bones weaken as a result of low bone mineral density (BMD) and structural changes that increase the risk for fractures.
- Osteoporosis treatment emphasizes adequate nutrition intake, exercise to promote an active lifestyle, and safety measures to avert falls that can contribute to fractures.

- Osteoarthritis (OA), also known as degenerative joint disease, is an ailment that involves the whole joint, including the cartilage, joint lining, ligaments, and underlying bone. The basis for prevention and treatment of OA is weight management and exercise.
- Rheumatoid arthritis is a systemic inflammatory illness that shows symptoms in multiple joints of the body. Vegetarian and plant-based diets with reduced saturated fatty acids have shown to improve pain level, stiffness, and swelling.[156]

Wound Healing

- The NPUAP describes a pressure injury (PI) as "localized damage to the skin and/or underlying soft tissue usually over a bony prominence or related to a medical or other device. The injury can present as intact skin or an open ulcer and may be painful. The injury occurs as a result of intense and/or prolonged pressure or pressure in combination with shear. The tolerance of soft tissue for pressure and shear may also be affected by microclimate, nutrition, perfusion, comorbidities and condition of the soft tissue."[158]
- Sufficient macronutrients (carbohydrates, protein, fats, and water) and micronutrients (vitamins and minerals) are vital for the body to support tissue integrity and prevent breakdown.

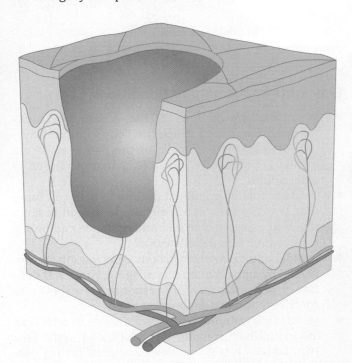

Stage 4 pressure injury

Renal and Genitourinary Conditions

- The NPUAP recommends 1.25–1.5 g of protein/kg of body weight per day and 30–35 kcal/kg of body weight per day for wound healing.[171]
- Acute kidney injury (AKI) is the sudden loss of kidney function that causes retention of urea nitrogenous waste products as well as imbalance of extracellular volume and electrolytes.[176]
- Risk factors contributing to increased episodes of AKI include DM and HTN, cardiovascular disease, overweight or obesity, high cholesterol, and autoimmune diseases such as lupus.
- Treatment might include restoring fluid and electrolyte balance or the use of catheters to manage urinary tract obstructions as well as dialysis.[180]
- The nutrition treatment goals in AKI center around preventing protein-energy wasting, averting fluid overload/edema, regulating blood pressure and electrolytes, and promoting acid–base balance.[181–183]

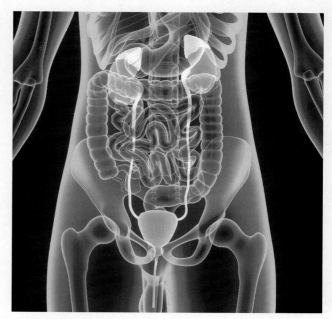

©Sciencepics/Shutterstock

Key Terms

acute kidney injury: A sudden loss of kidney function that results in the accumulation of urea and other nitrogenous waste products as well as the dysregulation of extracellular volume and electrolytes.

advance directives: A written statement of a person's wishes regarding medical treatment , often including a living will, made to ensure those wishes are carried out should the person be unable to communicate them to a doctor.

aerobic physical activity: Physical activity that relies on the presence of oxygen to make ATP. The complete breakdown of glucose, fatty acids, and amino acids to carbon dioxide and water occurs only through aerobic metabolism.

albuminuria: An abnormal excretion rate of albumin.

Alzheimer's disease: A progressive, degenerative disorder that attacks the brain's nerve cells, or neurons, and that results in loss of memory, thinking, and language skills and behavioral changes.

angiotensin: A protein whose presence in the blood promotes aldosterone secretion and tends to raise blood pressure.

atrophy: The deterioration, wasting or decrease in the size of a body organ, tissue, or muscle that results from disease, injury or lack of use.

Barrett's esophagus: A serious condition that results as a side effect of gastroesophageal reflux disease (GERD). The lining of the esophagus changes from its normal lining to a type that is usually found in the intestines.

cachexia: Weight loss, weakness, wasting, and changes in body composition due to emotional disturbance and severe or chronic disease

celiac disease: An autoimmune disorder that occurs in genetically susceptible individuals in which the small intestine is hypersensitive to gluten, leading to difficulty in digesting food and small intestine damage.

diabetes type 1: A form of diabetes in which the body does not produce insulin.

DNA (deoxyribonucleic acid): A self-replicating material present in nearly all living organisms as the main constituent of chromosomes. It is the carrier of genetic information.

fibroblast: A cell in connective tissue that produces collagen and other fibers.

friction: The action of one surface or object rubbing against another.

heart failure: Severe failure of the heart to function properly, especially as a cause of death.

hemoglobin A$_{1c}$: A minor component of hemoglobin to which glucose is bound.

hypoglycemia: Deficiency of glucose in the bloodstream.

insulin: A hormone produced in the pancreas by the islets of Langerhans that regulates the amount of glucose in the blood.

insulin sensitivity: How sensitive the body is to the effects of insulin.

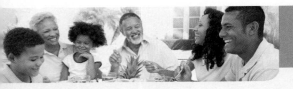

Learning Portfolio (continued)

intrinsic factor: A substance secreted by the stomach that enables the body to absorb vitamin B_{12}. It is a glycoprotein. Deficiency results in pernicious anemia.

lactose intolerance: The inability to digest lactose, a component of milk.

megaloblastic anemia: An anemia (of macrocytic classification) that results from inhibition of DNA synthesis during red blood cell production.

nephron: The functional units in the kidney, consisting of a glomerulus and its associated tubule, through which the glomerular filtrate passes before emerging as urine.

pernicious anemia: A deficiency in the production of red blood cells through a lack of vitamin B_{12}.

pressure injuries: Localized injuries to the skin and/or underlying tissue usually over a bony prominence that results from pressure or pressure in combination with shear.

proton pump inhibitor: Drugs that reduce the activity of proton pumps and that are used to reduce gastric acid secretion in the treatment of ulcers and gastroesophageal reflux disease.

resorption: The process or action by which something is reabsorbed.

shear: A chronic progressive disease that causes inflammation in the joints and that results in painful deformity and immobility, especially in the fingers, wrists, feet, and ankles.

stroke: The sudden death of brain cells due to lack of oxygen that is caused by blockage of blood flow or rupture of an artery to the brain.

unintended weight loss: Decrease in body weight that is not planned or desired.

urinary incontinence: The involuntary leakage of urine.

urinary tract infection: An infection of the kidney, ureter, bladder, or urethra.

Discussion Questions

1. What are the risk factors for CVD?
2. What are common mealtime interventions for patients with exacerbation of COPD?
3. What are the potential causes for cancer in older adults?
4. Discuss common nutrition interventions used in the treatment of cancer.
5. Demonstrate mealtime interventions that can be used to promote adequate intake in older adults with dementia.
6. Do you know any older adults with diabetes? Have you noticed the things they do to manage the disease, like how they eat or medications they take?
7. What are the most common lifestyle modifications associated with the management of GERD symptoms?
8. Describe the nutrition and lifestyle priorities for an overweight older adult with malnutrition?
9. List the different forms of arthritis and discuss how each affects older adults.
10. Discuss the risk factors for developing osteoporosis.
11. Which conditions place older adults at increased risk for developing pressure injuries?
12. Discuss the key features in the dietary management of older adults with acute kidney disease.

Activities

1. Create a blog to promote healthy eating for older adults with chronic diseases. Create an actual blog for free at blogger.com. Each team member is to contribute an article.
2. Select one of the conditions discussed in the chapter and create an informational booklet.

Study Questions

1. What does the term CVD encompass?
   a. All syndromes in which the brain is permanently or briefly affected
   b. Syndromes that affect heart function
   c. Syndromes that affect the cardiovascular system
   d. Syndromes that affect the cardiopulmonary system
2. What is a stroke?
   a. Illnesses related to cerebral infarction
   b. A word denoting cerebral hemorrhage and subarachnoid hemorrhage
   c. A group of illnesses that includes cerebral infarction, hemorrhage, and subarachnoid hemorrhage
   d. A term to denote all diseases of the brain

3. What does treatment for HTN include?
   a. Consuming a healthy diet that is high in sodium and potassium
   b. Consuming a healthy diet that includes foods that are low in sodium
   c. Consuming a diet high in fiber
   d. Consuming a diet high in calories and protein

4. What is a risk factor for developing cancer?
   a. Consuming high amounts of vegetables
   b. Young age
   c. Unlimited alcohol consumption
   d. Active lifestyle

5. What is the role of antioxidants in cancer prevention?
   a. Consuming megadoses of antioxidants can help prevent the development of cancerous cells.
   b. Research supports that consuming antioxidants does not affect the risk of developing cancer.
   c. Laboratory animal research supports the use of antioxidants in the prevention of cancer. This remains to be confirmed in humans.
   d. Consumption of vitamins and natural phenols can help reduce the risk of developing cancer.

6. What are some interventions to lower the risk of developing certain cancers?
   a. Consuming a healthy diet, keeping a healthy weight, taking vitamins and minerals
   b. Consuming a healthy diet, being physically active, and keeping a healthy weight
   c. Being physically active, consuming vitamins and minerals, and adopting a diet low in sodium
   d. Keeping a healthy weight, taking vitamins and minerals, and keeping a sedentary lifestyle

7. In older adults, how can dementia be characterized?
   a. A brain condition that interferes with older adults' ability to stay physically active
   b. A brain condition that requires older adults to be institutionalized to be properly cared for
   c. Cognitive decline that promotes malnutrition
   d. A brain condition that interferers with older adults' ability to remember, obtain and process new information, and communicate

8. Common risk factors that over time serve as precursors for dementia development include?
   a. Age, genetics, family history
   b. Genetics, obesity, sedentary lifestyle
   c. Family history, traumatic brain injury, nutrient-dense diet
   d. Genetics, hypertension, obesity

9. Which AD symptom contributes to decreased nutrient intake?
   a. Increased number of food dislikes
   b. Ability to consume a low-calorie diet
   c. Inability to feel hunger and thirst
   d. Individual's desire to feed self

10. How can T1DM be defined?
    a. Overproduction of insulin
    b. Insufficient insulin production
    c. No insulin is produced in the body
    d. Beta cells are intact

11. How can T2DM be defined?
    a. Increase in beta cell function
    b. Overproduction of insulin
    c. The least common form of DM in older adults
    d. A reduction in insulin production that progresses to insulin resistance

12. What should the meal pattern for an older adult with DM include?
    a. Sixty percent of total calories should come from carbohydrates; the remainder should be divided equally between protein and fat.
    b. There is no ideal percentage of calories from carbohydrate, protein, and fat for all people with diabetes.
    c. The majority of the calories in the diet should come from protein foods.
    d. The highest percentage of calories in the diet should come from fat.

13. How can gastroesophageal reflux disease be defined?
    a. A condition characterized by alterations in the mucosa of the esophagus
    b. A disorder in which bile acids enter the esophagus
    c. A precursor to gastric ulcer
    d. A disorder in which gastric acid and other stomach fluids leak into the esophagus

14. What is a risk factor for developing gastroesophageal reflux?
    a. Obesity
    b. Consuming a high-fat diet
    c. Sedentary lifestyle
    d. Prolonged used of antacids

15. What is a lifestyle intervention to manage gastroesophageal reflux?
    a. Consuming a low-fat diet
    b. Incorporating dietary supplements into the dietary regime
    c. Consuming smaller, more frequent meals
    d. Consuming a high-protein diet

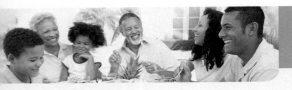

Learning Portfolio (continued)

16. How can the metabolic syndrome cachexia be characterized?
    a. Presence of cancer
    b. Loss of muscle with or without loss of fat mass
    c. Presence of edema
    d. Abnormal weight gain

17. What does *sarcopenia* refer to?
    a. The progressive skeletal muscle loss and strength decrease that occurs as part of the aging process
    b. The increased mortality rate seen in older adults with weight loss
    c. A syndrome that occurs as a result of anorexia, inflammation, and insulin resistance
    d. Increased muscle protein breakdown

18. What does iron-deficiency anemia occur as a result of?
    a. Microcytic red blood cells in the body
    b. Microcytic white blood cells in the body
    c. Hyperchromic red blood cells in the body
    d. Hypochromic red blood cells in the body

19. How can osteoporosis be characterized?
    a. The body produces excessive calcium and decreased bone structure.
    b. The bones are frail as a result of an inactive lifestyle.
    c. The bones are weak owing to decreased bone mineral density.
    d. Inadequate diet contributes to the development of anemia.

20. What does treatment of osteoporosis involve?
    a. Adequate intake, exercise, and fall prevention
    b. High protein intake, active lifestyle, increased ability to perform activities of daily living
    c. Low-impact exercise, medication, high-protein diet
    d. Fall prevention, high-impact exercise, low-protein diet

21. What does treatment for osteoarthritis consist of?
    a. Adequate nutrition intake and fast weight loss
    b. Weight management and exercise
    c. Weight loss and medication
    d. Weight monitoring and diet education

22. Vitamin A is essential in promoting skin integrity. What does this nutrient contribute to?
    a. Increased absorption of other vitamins
    b. The granulation process that occurs during wound healing

    c. Collagen development
    d. Decreased healing time

23. Aside from prolonged healing time, what can vitamin C deficiency in older adults with pressure injuries contribute to?
    a. Anorexia and weight loss
    b. Decreased wound strength and immune function
    c. Decreased collagen and increased fibroblast production
    d. Decreased wound strength and increased fibroblast production

24. When considering supplementation, what is important to remember?
    a. Increased zinc can interfere with copper metabolism and contribute to copper-induced anemia.
    b. Research supports the use of a multivitamin for all older adults with pressure injuries.
    c. Supplementation of vitamin A, vitamin C, zinc, and amino acids is essential for would healing.
    d. Only vitamin A and vitamin C are essential nutrients for wound healing.

25. What does acute kidney injury involve?
    a. Decreased kidney function over time
    b. Increased nutrient elimination
    c. Sudden loss of kidney function that causes retention of urea nitrogenous waste products
    d. Excessive expression of electrolytes

26. To prevent acute kidney injury, what should older adults do?
    a. Reduce the amount of fluids consumed and monitor kidney function via biochemical data.
    b. Consume adequate fluids and monitor kidney function via biochemical data.
    c. Reduce the amount of fluids consumed to promote decreased urine output.
    d. Monitor medications and consume limited amount of fluids.

27. What do treatment goals for patients with AKI center around?
    a. Preventing protein-energy wasting and fluid overload
    b. Preventing weight increase and controlling blood pressure
    c. Promoting weight loss and electrolyte balance
    d. Preventing acid–base balance and weight loss

Weblinks

- **Alz.org**
  http://www.alz.org/alzheimers_disease_what_is
  _alzheimers.asp
- **American Cancer Society**
  http://www.cancer.org
- **American College of Gastroenterology**
  http://gi.org
- **American Diabetes Association**
  http://www.diabetes.org/?referrer=https://www.
  google.com
- *Bulletin of the World Health Organization:* **"Nutritional Surveillance"**
  http://www.ncbi.nlm.nih.gov/pmc/articles/PMC2536157
- **Cancer.net**
  http://www.cancer.net/navigating-cancer-care/
  prevention-and-healthy-living/diet-and-nutrition
- **Celiac Disease Foundation**
  https://celiac.org
- **Centers for Disease Control and Prevention: Heart Disease**
  http://www.cdc.gov/heartdisease
- **Centers for Disease Control and Prevention: Overweight and Obesity**
  http://www.cdc.gov/obesity
- **Medline Plus: Stroke**
  https://www.nlm.nih.gov/medlineplus/stroke.html
- **National Cancer Institute**
  http://www.cancer.gov
- **National Institute of Neurological Disorders and Stroke: NINDS Stroke Information Page**
  http://www.ninds.nih.gov/disorders/stroke/stroke.
  htm
- **National Kidney Foundation**
  https://www.kidney.org/kidneydisease
- **National Pressure Ulcer Advisory Panel**
  http://www.npuap.org
- **National Stroke Association**
  http://www.stroke.org/understand-stroke/what
  -stroke
- **NIH Osteoporosis and Related Bone Diseases National Resource Center: Bone Health for Life**
  http://www.niams.nih.gov/Health_Info/Bone/Bone
  _Health/bone_health_for_life.asp
- **Professional Heart Daily**
  http://my.americanheart.org/professional/index.jsp
- **World Health Organization: Obesity**
  http://www.who.int/topics/obesity/en

References

1. National Council on Aging. The United States of Aging Survey 2015 results. Retrieved from: https://www.ncoa.org/news/usoa-survey/2015-results/. Accessed July 28, 2015.
2. Centers for Disease Control and Prevention. *The Stage of Aging and Health in America 2013.* Atlanta, GA: Centers for Disease Control and Prevention, U.S. Department of Health and Human Services; 2013. Retrieved from: http://www.cdc.gov/aging/pdf/state-aging-health-in-america-2013.pdf. Accessed September 29, 2016.
3. Academy of Nutrition and Dietetics. Position of the Academy of Nutrition and Dietetics: food and nutrition for older adults: promoting health and wellness *J Acad Nutr Diet.* 2012;12(8):1255–1277.
4. Strong K, Mathers C, Bonita R. Preventing stroke: saving lives around the world. *Lancet Neurol.* 2007;6(2):182–187.
5. Administration on Aging. *A Profile of Older Americans 2014.* Washington, DC: U.S. Department of Health and Human Services; 2014. Retrieved from: http://www.aoa.acl.gov/Aging_Statistics/Profile/2014/docs/2014-Profile.pdf. Accessed July 29, 2015.
6. McGill HC, McMahan CA, Gidding SS. Preventing heart disease in the 21st century: implications of the Pathobiological Determinants of Atherosclerosis in Youth (PDAY) study. *Circulation.* 2008;117(9):1216–1227.
7. Mendis S, Puska P, Norrving B. *Global Atlas on Cardiovascular Disease Prevention and Control* Geneva, Switzerland: World Health Organization in collaboration with World Heart Federation and World Stroke Organization; 2011.
8. American Heart Association. The facts about high blood pressure. Dallas, TX: American Heart Association; updated November 2, 2016. Retrieved from: http://www.heart.org/HEARTORG/Conditions/HighBloodPressure/AboutHighBloodPressure/About-High-Blood-Pressure_UCM_002050_Article.jsp. Accessed November 12, 2016.

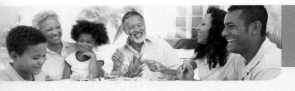

Learning Portfolio (continued)

9. Go AS, Mozaffarian D, Roger VL, et al. Heart disease and stroke statistics—2013 update: a report from the American Heart Association. *Circulation*. 2013;127(1):e6–e245.

10. Yancy CW, Jessup M, Bozkurt B, et al. 2013 ACCF/AHA guideline for the management of heart failure: a report of the American College of Cardiology Foundation/American Heart Association Task Force on Practice Guidelines. *J Am Coll Cardiol*. 2013;62(16):e147–e239.

11. Landsberg L, Aronne LJ, Beilin LJ, et al. Obesity-related hypertension: pathogenesis, cardiovascular risk, and treatment: a position paper of the obesity society and the American Society of Hypertension. *J Clin Hypertens* (Greenwich). 2013;15(1):14–33.

12. Koiaki C, Katsilambros N. Dietary sodium, potassium and alcohol: key players in the pathoghysiology, prevention, and treatment of human hypertension. *Nutr Rev*. 2013;71(6):402–411.

13. Mayo Clinic. High blood pressure (hypertension): choosing blood pressure medications. Retrieved from: http://www.mayoclinic.org/diseases-conditions/high-blood-pressure/in-depth/high-blood-pressure-medication/art-20046280. Accessed September 29, 2016.

14. Jensen MD, Ryan DH, Apovian CM, et al. Guideline for the management of overweight and obesity in adults: a report of the American College of Cardiology/American Heart Association Task Force on Practice Guidelines and the Obesity Society [published online November 12, 2013]. *Circulation*. June 24, 2014;129(25 suppl 2):S102–138.

15. Eckel R, Jakicic JM, Ard JD, et al. 2013 AHA/ACC guideline on lifestyle management to reduce cardiovascular risk: a report of the American College of Cardiology/American Heart Association Task Force on Practice Guidelines [published online November 12, 2013]. *Circulation*. June 24, 2014;129(25 suppl 2):S76–99.

16. Zhu Z, Wang P, Ma S. Metabolic hypertension: concept and practice. *Front Med*. 2013;7(2):201–206.

17. World Health Organization. *Reducing Salt Intake in Populations: Report of a WHO Forum and Technical Meeting, 5–7 October 2006, Paris, France*. Paris, France: World Health Organization; 2007.

18. Appel LJ, Champagne CM, Harsha DW, et al. Effects of comprehensive lifestyle modification on blood pressure control: main results of the PREMIER clinical trial. *JAMA* 2009;289(16):2083–2093.

19. American Heart Association. Older Americans and cardiovascular diseases [statistical fact sheet 2015 update]. American Heart Association. Retrieved from: http://americanheart.biz/idc/groups/heart-public/@wcm/@sop/@smd/documents/downloadable/ucm_472923.pdf. Accessed July 29, 2015.

20. Donnan GA, Fisher M, Macleod M, Davis SM. Stroke. *Lancet* 2008;371(9624):1612–1623.

21. National Heart, Lung, and Blood Institute. Who is at risk for a stroke? Bethesda, MD: National Heart, Lung, and Blood Institute; updated June 22, 2016. Retrieved from: http://www.nhlbi.nih.gov/health/health-topics/topics/stroke/atrisk. Accessed July 5, 2015.

22. American Heart Association. Stroke treatments. Dallas, TX: American Heart Association; May 23, 2013. Retrieved from: http://www.strokeassociation.org/STROKEORG/About Stroke/Treatment/Stroke-Treatments_UCM_310892_Article.jsp. Accessed July 29, 2015.

23. Hobbs R, Boyle A. Heart failure. Cleveland Clinic; March 2014: Figure 1a. Retrieved from: http://www.clevelandclinicmeded.com/medicalpubs/diseasemanagement/cardiology/heart-failure/Default.htm. Accessed September 29, 2016.

24. U.S. National Library of Medicine, U.S. Department of Health and Human Services, National Institutes of Health. Heart failure. Medline Plus. Retrieved from: http://www.nlm.nih.gov/medlineplus/heartfailure.html. Accessed July 5, 2014.

25. National Heart, Lung, and Blood Institute. How is heart failure diagnosed? Bethesda, MD: National Heart, Lung, and Blood Institute. Retrieved from: https://www.nhlbi.nih.gov/health/health-topics/topics/hf/diagnosis. Accessed July 6, 2015.

26. Goff DC Jr, Lloyd-Jones DM, Bennett G, et al. 2013 ACC/AHA guideline on cardiovascular risk: a report of the American College of Cardiology/American Heart Association Task Force on Practice Guidelines [published online November 12, 2013]. *Circulation*. June 24, 2014;129(25 suppl 2):S49–73.

27. National Heart, Lung, and Blood Institute. How is heart failure treated? Bethesda, MD: National Heart, Lung, and Blood Institute. Retrieved from: https://www.nhlbi.nih.gov/health/health-topics/topics/hf/treatment. Accessed July 6, 2015.

28. Centers for Disease Control and Prevention. Chronic obstructive pulmonary disease (COPD) includes: chronic bronchitis and emphysema. Atlanta, GA: Centers for Disease Control and Prevention. Retrieved from: http://www.cdc.gov/nchs/fastats/copd.htm. Accessed July 29, 2015.

29. Rennard SI, Vestbo J. COPD: the dangerous underestimate of 15%. *Lancet*. 2006;367:1216–1219.

30. National Heart, Lung, and Blood Institute. What is COPD? Bethesda, MD: National Heart, Lung, and Blood Institute. Retrieved from: http://www.nhlbi.nih.gov/health/health-topics/topics/copd. Accessed July 29, 2015.

31. Mueller C, Laule-Kilian K, Frana B, et al. Use of B-type natriuretic peptide in the management of acute dyspnea in patients with pulmonary disease. *Am Heart J*. 2006;151:471–477.

32. World Health Organization. COPD managment. Geneva, Switzerland: World Health Organization. Retrieved from: http://www.who.int/respiratory/copd/management/en/. Accessed July 25, 2015.

33. Humphreys K, Cross G, Frith P, Cararella P. Nutritional status of dietary intake of outpatient with chronic obstructive pulmonary disease. *Nutr Diet*. 2008;65(2):168–174.

34. Ahmadi A, Haghighat N, Hakimrabet M, Tolide-ie H. Nutritional evaluation in chronic obstructive pulmonary disease patients. *Pak J Bio*. 2012;15(10):501–505.

35. Academy of Nutrition and Dietetics. Chronic obstructive pulmonary disease. Chicago, IL: Academy of Nutrition and Dietetics Evidence Analysis Library. Retrieved from: https://www.andeal.org/topic.cfm?menu=5301. Accessed August 1, 2015.

36. Vestbo J, Prescott E, Almdal T, et al. Body mass, fat-free body mass, and prognosis in patients with chronic obstructive pulmonary disease from a random population sample: findings from the Copenhagen City Heart Study. *Am J Respir Crit Care*. 2006;173(1):79–83.

37. Agency for Healthcare Research and Quality. Guideline summary: disorders of lipid metabolism. Evidence-based nutrition practice guideline. Rockville, MD: National Guideline Clearinghouse, AHRQ. Retrieved from: https://www.guideline.gov/summaries/summary/32479/disorders-of-lipid-metabolism-evidencebased-nutrition-practice-guideline. Accessed September 29, 2016.

38. National Cancer Institute. Risk factors for cancer. Rockville, MD: National Cancer Institute, National Institutes of Health, U.S. Department of Health and Human Services; updated December 23, 2015. Retrieved from: http://www.cancer.gov/about-cancer/causes-prevention/risk. Accessed July 29, 2015.

39. Ries LAG, Eisner MP, Kosary CL, et al. *Cancer Statistics Review, 1973–1998*. Washington, DC: National Institute of Health; 2000. NIH publication 00-2789.

40. American Cancer Society. What is cancer? Atlanta, GA: American Cancer Society. Retrieved from: http://www.cancer.org/cancer/cancerbasics/what-is-cancer. Accessed July 25, 2015.

41. Bernstein M, Munoz N. *Nutrition for the Older Adult*. 2nd ed. Burlington, MA: Jones & Barltett Learning; 2015.

42. National Cancer Institute. Antioxidants accelerate the growth and invasiveness of tumors in mice. Rockville, MD: National Cancer Institute, National Institutes of Health, U.S. Department of Health and Human Services; November 12, 2015. Retrieved from: http://www.cancer.gov/news-events/cancer-currents-blog/2015/antioxidants-metastasis. Accessed June 22, 2016.

43. National Cancer Institute. Cancer prevention. Rockville, MD: National Cancer Institute, National Institutes of Health, U.S. Department of Health and Human Services https://www.cancer.gov/about-cancer/causes-prevention/patient-prevention-overview-pdq#link/stoc_h2_3. Accessed August 1, 2015.

44. Sestak I. Preventative therapies for healthy women at high risk of breast cancer. *Cancer Manae Res*. October 17, 2014;6:423–430.

45. American Society of Clinical Oncology. *Cancer in Older Adults*. Alexandria, VA: American Society of Clinical Oncology; 2012. http://www.cancer.net/sites/cancer.net/files/cancer_in_older_adults.pdf. Accessed September 29, 2016.

46. Academy of Nutrition and Dietetics Oncology. Chicago, IL: Academy of Nutrition and Dietetics Evidence Analysis Library. Retrieved from: https://www.andeal.org/topic.cfm?menu=5291. Accessed July 30, 2015.

47. Alzheimer's Association. 2014 Alzheimer's disease facts and figures. *J Alzheimer's Assoc*. 2014;10(2):47–92.

48. Family Caregiver Alliance. Incidence and prevalence of the major causes of brain impairment. San Francisco, CA: Family Caregiver Alliance; November 13, 2013. Retrieved from: https://caregiver.org/incidence-and-prevalence-major-causes-brain-impairment. Accessed July 28, 2015.

49. Hebert LE, Weuve J, Scherr PA, Evans DA. Alzheimer disease in the United States (2010–2050) estimated using the 2010 Census. *Neurology*. 2013;80(19):1778–1783.

50. Plassman BL, Langa KM, Fisher GG, et al. Prevalence of dementia in the United States: the Aging, Demographics, and Memory Study. *Neuroepidemiology*. 2007;29(1–2):125–132.

51. National Institute on Aging. About Alzheimer's disease: Alzheimer's basics. Bethesda, MD: National Institute on Aging, National Institutes of Health, U.S. Department of Health and Human Services. Retrieved from: http://www.nia.nih.gov/alzheimers/topics/alzheimers-basics. Accessed August 25, 2014.

52. Hendrie HC, Albert MS, Butters MA, et al. The NIH cognitive and emotional health project: report of the critical evaluation study committee. *Alzheimers Dement*. 2006;2(1):12–32.

53. Wagster MV, King JW, Resnick SM, Rapp PR. The 87%. *J Gerontol A Biol Sci Med*. 2012;67:739–740.

54. National Institute on Aging. Alzheimer's disease fact sheet. Bethesda, MD: U.S. Department of Health and Human Services, National Institutes of Health; 2013. Retrieved from: http://www.nia.nih.gov/alzheimers/publication/alzheimers-disease-fact-sheet. Accessed Juky 29, 2015.

55. Kryscio RJ, Abner EL, Cooper GE, et al. Self-reported memory complaints: implications from a longitudinal cohort with autopsies. *Neurology*. 2014;83:1359–1365.

56. U.S. National Library of Medicine, U.S. Department of Health and Human Services, National Institutes of Health. Dementia. MedlinePlus. Retrieved from: http://www.nlm.nih.gov/medlineplus/dementia.html. Accessed August 28, 2014.

57. Alzheimer's Association. Health care profesionals and Alzheimer's. Chicago, IL: Alzheimer's Association. Retrieved from: http://www.alz.org/health-care-professionals/health-care-clinical-medical-resources.asp. Accessed September 5, 2014.

58. National Institute on Aging. *2011–2012 Alzheimer's Disease Progress Report: Intensifying the Research Effort*. Washington, DC: National Institutes of Health; 2012. Retrieved from: https://www.nia.nih.gov/alzheimers/publication/2011-2012-alzheimers-disease-progress-report/introduction. Accessed September 29, 2016.

59. Saczynski JS, Beiser A, Seshadri S, Auerbach S, Wolf PA. Depressive symptoms and risk of dementia: the Framingham Heart Study. *Neurology*. 2010;75(1):35–41.

60. Stern Y, Gurland B, Tatemichi TK, Tang MX, Wilder D, Mayeux R. Influence of education and occupation on the incidence of Alzheimer's disease. *JAMA*. 1994;271(13):1004–1010.

61. Alzheimer's Association. New diagnostic criteria and guidelines for Alzheimer's disease. Chicago, IL: Alzheimer's Association. Retrieved from: http://www.alz.org/research/diagnostic_criteria/. Accessed October 5, 2014.

62. Alzheimer's Association. Late stage care. Chicago, IL: Alzheimer's Association. Retrieved from: https://www.alz.org/national/documents/brochure_latestage.pdf. Accessed October 6, 2014.

63. Alzheimer's Association. Food, eating and Alzheimer's. Chicago, IL: Alzheimer's Association. Retrieved from: http://www.alz.org/care/alzheimers-food-eating.asp. Accessed October 2, 2014.

64. Alzheimer's Association. Seven stages of Alzheimer's. Chicago, IL: Alzheimer's Association website. Retrieved from: http://www.alz.org/alzheimers_disease_stages_of_alzheimers.asp. Accessed Novemver 2, 2014.

65. Alzheimer's Association. Dementia care practice recommendations for assisted living residences and nursing homes. Chicago, IL: Alzheimer's Association; 2009. Retrieved from: http://www.alz.org/national/documents/brochure_DCPRphases1n2.pdf. Accessed October 15, 2014.

66. Expert Panel on Detection, Evaluation, and Treatment of High Blood Cholesterol in Adults. Executive summary of the third report of the National Cholesterol Education Program (NCEP) Expert Panel on Detection, Evaluation, and Treatment of High Blood Cholesterol in Adults (Adult Treatment Panel III). *JAMA*. 2001;285:2486–2497.

67. Centers for Disease Control and Prevention. *Diabetes Report Card 2014*. Atlanta, GA: Centers for Disease Control and Prevention, U.S. Department of Health and Human Services; 2015. Retrieved from: http://www.cdc.gov/diabetes/pdfs/library/diabetesreportcard2014.pdf. Accessed August 1, 2015.

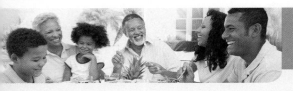

Learning Portfolio (continued)

68. Mathers CD, Loncar D. Projections of global mortality and burden of disease from 2002 to 2030. *PLoS Med.* 2006; 3(11):e442.

69. Gambert SR, Pinkstaff S. Emerging epidemic: diabetes in the older adults: demographic, economic, impact and pathophysiology. *Diabetes Spectrum.* 2006;19:221–228.

70. Kirkman M, Briscoe VJ, Clark N, et al. Diabetes and the older adult: concensus report. *J Am Geriatr Soc.* 2012;60(12):242–256.

71. Kishore P. Diabetes mellitus (DM). Merck Manual Professional Version; reviewed June 2014. Retrieved from: http://www.merckmanuals.com/professional/endocrine-and-metabolic-disorders/diabetes-mellitus-and-disorders-of-carbohydrate-metabolism/diabetes-mellitus-dm. Accessed September 29, 2016.

72. U.S. National Library of Medicine, U.S. Department of Health and Human Services, National Institutes of Health. Diabetes type 2. MedlinePlus. Retrieved from: http://www.nlm.nih.gov/medlineplus/diabetestype2.html. Accessed August 1, 2015.

73. American Diabetes Association. Standards of medical care in diabetes 2015. *Diabetes Care.* 2015;38(S1).

74. Haas L, Maryniuk M, Beck J, et al. on behalf of the National 2012 Standards Revision Task Force. Standards for diabetes self-management education and support. *Diabetes Care.* 2014;37(1):s144–153.

75. Academy of Nutrition and Dietetics. *Nutrition Care Manual: Diabetes* 2015. Retrieved from: http://www.nutritioncaremanual.org. Accessed August 1, 2015.

76. Inzucchi SE, Bergenstal RM, Buse JB, et al. American Diabetes Association (ADA); European Association for the Study of Diabetes (EASD), management of hyperglycemia in type 2 diabetes: a patient-centered approach. Position statement of the American Diabetes Association (ADA) and the European Association for the Study of Diabetes (EASD). *Diabetes Care.* 2012;35:1364–1329.

77. Evert AB, Boucher JL, Cypress M, et al. Nutrition therapy recommendations for the management of adults with diabetes. *Diabetes Care.* 2014;37(s1):s120–s143.

78. Academy of Nutrition and Dietetics. Diabetes type 1 and 2. Chicago, IL: Academy of Nutrition and Dietetics Evidence Analysis Library. Retrieved from: https://www.andeal.org/topic.cfm?menu=5305. Accessed August 1, 2015.

79. McIntyre HD, Knight BA, Harvey DM, Noud MN, Hagger VL, Gilshenan KS. Dose adjustment for normal eating (DAFNE)—an audit of outcomes in Australia. *Med J Aust.* 2010;192:637–640.

80. Jakicic JM, Jaramillo SA, Balasubramanyam A, et al. Look AHEAD Study Group. Effect of a lifestyle intervention on change in cardiorespiratory fitness in adults with type 2 diabetes: results from the Look AHEAD Study. *Int J Obes* (Lond). 2009;33:305–316.

81. Ford ES, Giles WH, Dietz WH. Prevalence of the metabolic syndrome among US adults: findings from the Third National Health and Nutrition Examination Survey. *JAMA.* 2002;287:356–359.

82. Lakka HM, Laaksonen DE, Lakka TA, et al. The metabolic syndrome and total and cardiovascular disease mortality in middle-aged men. *JAMA.* 2002;288:2709–2716.

83. Church TS, Thompson A, Katzmarzyk PT, et al. Metabolic syndrome and diabetes, alone and in combination, as predictors of cardiovascular disease mortality among men. *Diabetis Care.* 2009;32:1289–1294.

84. Grundy SM, Brewer B, Cleeman JI, Smith SC, Lenfant C. Definition of metabolic syndrome: report of the National Heart, Lung, and Blood Institute/American Heart Association Conference on Scientific Issues Related to Definition. *Circulation.* 2004;109:433–438.

85. National Heart, Lung, and Blood Institute. How can metabolic syndrome be prevented? Bethesda, MD: National Heart, Lung, and Blood Institute. Retrieved from: http://www.nhlbi.nih.gov/health/health-topics/topics/ms/prevention. Accessed August 2, 2015.

86. Ilanne-Parikka P, Eriksson JG, Lindstrom J, Peltonen M, et al. Effect of lifestyle intervention on the occurance of metabolic syndrome and its components in the Finnish Diabetes Prevention Study. *Diabetes Care.* 2008;31(3):805–807.

87. Shai I, Schwarzfuchs D, Henkin Y, et al. Weight loss with a low-carbohydrate, Mediterranean, or low-fat diet. *N Engl J Med.* 2008;359:229–241.

88. Yoneda M, Yamane K, Jitsuiki K, et al. Prevalence of metabolic syndrome compared between native Japanese and Japanese Americans. *Diabetes Res Clin Pract.* 2008;79(3):511–522.

89. Ruidavets JB, Bongard V, Dallongeville J, et al. High consumptions of grain, fish, dairy products and combinations of these are associated with a low prevalence of metabolic syndrome. *J Epidemiol Community Health.* 2007;61(9):810–817.

90. Esposito K, Ciotola M, Giugliano D. Mediterranean diet and the metabolic syndrome. *Mol Nutr Food Res.* 2008;51(10):1268–1274.

91. Cohen BE, Chang AA, Grady D, AM. K. Restorative yoga in adults with metabolic syndrome: a randomized, controlled pilot trial. *Metab Syndr Relat Disord.* 2008;6(3):223–229.

92. Spechler S. Barrett esophagus and risk of esophageal cancer: a clinical review. *JAMA.* 2013;31(6):627–636.

93. El-Serag HB, Sweet S, Winchester CC, Dent J. Update on the epidemiology of gastro-oesophageal reflux disease: a systematic review. *Gut.* 2014;63(6):871–880. doi:10.1136/gutjnl-2012–304269.

94. Moore KL, Boscardin WJ, Steinman MA, Schwartz JB. Age and sex variation in prevalence of chronic medical conditions in older residents of U.S. nursing homes. *J Am Geriatr Soc.* 2012;60(4):756–764.

95. Zhao Y, Encinosa W. Gastroesophageal reflux disease (GERD) hospitalizations in 1998 and 2005. Rockville, MD: Agencyfor Healthcare Research and Quality; January 2008. HCUP Statistical Brief No. 44. Retrieved from: http://www.hcup-us.ahrq.gov/reports/statbriefs/sb44.pdf. Accessed August 2, 2015.

96. Kessing BF, Conchillo JM, Bredenoord AJ, Smout AJPM, Masclee AAM. Review article: the clinical relevance of transient lower oesophageal sphincter relaxations in gastro-oesophageal reflux disease. *Aliment Pharmacol Ther.* 2011;33(6):650–666.

97. U.S. National Library of Medicine, U.S. Department of Health and Human Services, National Institutes of Health. GERD. MedlinePlus. Retrieved from: https://medlineplus.gov/gerd.html. Accessed August 2, 2015.

98. Katz PO, Gerson LB, Vela MF. Guidelines for the diagnosis and management of gastroesophageal reflux disease. *Am J Gastroenterol.* 2013;108:308–328.

99. Matrana MR, Margolin DA. Epidemiology and pathophysiology of diverticular disease. *Clin Colon Rectal Surg.* 2009;22(3):141–146.

100. Von Rahden BH, Germer CT. Pathogenesis of colonic diverticular disease. *Langenbecks Arch Surg.* 2012;397(7):1025–1033.

101. National Institute of Diabetes and Digestive and Kidney Diseases Diverticulosis and diverticulitis. Bethesda, MD: National Institute of Diabetes and Digestive and Kidney Diseases, National Institutes of Health, U.S. Department of Health and Human Services. Retrieved from: http://www.niddk.nih.gov/health-information/health-topics/digestive-diseases/diverticular-disease/Pages/facts.aspx. Accessed August 4, 2015.

102. Templeton AW, Strate LL. Updates in diverticular disease. *Curr Gastroenterol Rep.* 2913;15(8):339.

103. Martin ST, Stocchi L. New and emerging treatments for the prevention of recurrent diverticulitis. *Clin Experim Gastroenterol.* 2011;(4):203–212.

104. Strate LL, Liu YL, Syngal S, Aldoori WH, Giovannucci EL. Nut, corn, and popcorn consumption and the incidence of diverticular disease. *JAMA.* 2008;300(8):907–914.

105. Vesa TH, Marteau P, Korpela R. Lactose intolerance. *J Am Coll Nutr.* 2000;19(suppl 2):165S–175S.

106. National Institute of Diabetes and Digestive and Kidney Diseases Lactose intolerance. Bethesda, MD: National Institute of Diabetes and Digestive and Kidney Diseases, National Institutes of Health, U.S. Department of Health and Human Services. Retrieved from: http://www.niddk.nih.gov/health-information/health-topics/digestive-diseases/lactose-intolerance/Pages/facts.aspx. Accessed August 12, 2015.

107. Wilt TJ, Shaukat A, Shamliyan T, et al. Lactose intolerance and health. Rockville, MD: Agency for Healthcare Research and Quality; 2010. AHRQ Publication No. 10-E004.

108. Fernández-Bañares F, Esteve M, Viver JM. Fructose-sorbitol malabsorption. *Curr Gastroenterol Rep.* 2009;5:368–374.

109. National Institute of Diabetes and Digestive and Kidney Diseases Celiac disease. Bethesda, MD: National Institute of Diabetes and Digestive and Kidney Diseases, National Institutes of Health, U.S. Department of Health and Human Services. Retrieved from: http://www.niddk.nih.gov/health-information/health-topics/digestive-diseases/celiac-disease/Pages/facts.aspx. Accessed August 15, 2015.

110. García-Manzanares A, Lucendo AJ. Nutritional and dietary aspects of celiac disease. *Nutr Clin Pract.* 2011;26(2):163–173.

111. Catassi C, Kryszak D, Bhatti B, et al. Natural history of celiac disease autoimmunity in a USA cohort followed since 1974. *Ann Med.* 2010;42(7):530–538.

112. Riddle MS, Murray JA, Porter CK. The incidence and risk of celiac disease in a healthy US adult population. *Am J Gastroenterol.* 2012;107(8):1248–1255.

113. Fasano A, Catassi C. Clinical practice: celiac disease. *N Engl J Med.* 2012;367(25):2419–2426.

114. Rome Foundation. Rome III disorders and criteria for functional gastrointestinal disorders. Retrieved from: http://www.romecriteria.org/criteria/. Accessed August 15, 2015.

115. Alley NJ, Fleming KC, Evans JM, et al. Constipation in an elderly community: a study of prevalence and potential risk factors. *Am J Gastroenterol.* 1996;91(1):19.

116. Choung RS, Locke GR 3rd, Schleck CD, Zinsmeister AR, Talley NJ. Cumulative incidence of chronic constipation: a population-based study 1988–2003. *Aliment Pharmacol Ther.* 2007;26(11):1521.

117. Talley NJ. Definitions, epidemiology, and impact of chronic constipation. *Rev Gastroenterol Disord.* 2004;4(suppl 2):S3.

118. Hsieh C. Treatment of constipation in older adults. *Am Fam Physician.* 2005;72(11):2277–2284.

119. Lindeman RD, Romero LJ, Liang HC, Baumgartner RN, Koehler KM, Garry PJ. Do elderly persons need to be encouraged to drink more fluids? *J Gerontol A Biol Sci Med Sci.* 2000;55(7):M361.

120. U.S. Department of Health and Human Services, Office of Disease Prevention and Health Promotion. *Healthy People 2020: nutrition and weight goals.* Retrieved from: http://www.healthypeople.gov/2020/topics-objectives/topic/nutrition-and-weight-status. Accessed August 12, 2015.

121. NHLBI Obesity Education Initiative Expert Panel on the Identification, Evaluation, and Treatment of Obesity in Adults. *Clinical Guidelines on the Identification, Evaluation, and Treatment of Overweight and Obesity in Adults: The Evidence Report.* Bethesda, MD: National Heart, Lung, and Blood Institute; 1998.

122. Wallace JI, Schwartz RS, LaCroix AZ, Uhlmann RF, Pearlman RA. Involuntary weight loss in older outpatients: incidence and clinical significance. *J Am Geriatr Soc.* 1995;43(4):329–337.

123. Ruscin JM, Page RL 2nd, Yeager BF, Wallace JI. Tumor necrosis factor-alpha and involuntary weight loss in elderly, community-dwelling adults. *Pharmacotherapy.* 2005;25(3):313–319.

124. Alibhai SM, Greenwood C, Payette H. An approach to the management of unintentional weight loss in elderly people. *CMAJ.* 2005;172(6):773–780.

125. Centers for Medicare and Medicaid Services. State operations manual: appendix PP: guidance to surveyors for long-term care facilities. Baltimore, MD: Centers for Medicare and Medicaid Services revised June 10, 2016. Retrieved from: https://www.cms.gov/Regulations-and-Guidance/Guidance/Manuals/downloads/som107ap_pp_guidelines_ltcf.pdf. Accessed September 29, 2016.

126. Stajkovic S, Aitken EM, Holroyd-Leduc J. Unintentional weight loss in older adults. *CMAJ.* 2011;183(4):443–449.

127. Thompson MP, Morris LK. Unexplained weight loss in the ambulatory elderly. *J Am Geriatr Soc.* 1991;39:497–500.

128. Locher JL, Roth DL, Ritchie CS, et al. Body mass index, weight loss, and mortality in community-dwelling older adults. *Gerontol A Biol Sci Med Sci.* 2007;62(12):1389.

129. Villareal DT, Chode S, Parimi N, et al. Weight loss, exercise, or both and physical function in obese older adults. *N Engl J Med.* 2011;3645(13):1218.

130. Locher JL, Robinson CO, Roth DL, Ritchie CS, Burgio KL. The effect of the presence of others on caloric intake in homebound older adults. *Gerontol A Biol Sci Med Sci.* 2005;60(11):1475.

131. Evans WJ, Morley JE, Argilés J, et al. Cachexia: a new definition. *Clin Nutr.* 2008;27(8):793.

132. Academy of Nutrition and Dietetics. Unintended weight loss in older adults. Chicago, IL: Academy of Nutrition and Dietetics Evidence Analysis Library. Retrieved from: https://www.andeal.org/topic.cfm?menu=5294. Accessed August 14, 2015.

133. Price EA, Schrier SL. Anemia in the older adult. UpToDate; September 21, 2015. Retrieved from: http://www.uptodate.com/contents/anemia-in-the-older-adult. Accessed August 15, 2015.

134. Patel KV. Epidemiology of anemia in older adults. *Semin Hematol.* 2008;45(4):210.

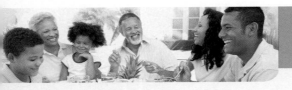

Learning Portfolio (continued)

135. Guralnik JM, Eisenstaedt RS, Ferrucci L, Klein HG, Woodman RC. Prevalence of anemia in persons 65 years and older in the United States: evidence for a high rate of unexplained anemia. *Blood*. 2004;104(8):2263.

136. National Institutes of Health, Office of Dietary Supplements. Iron: dietary supplement fact sheet. Bethesda, MD: National Institutes of Health, Office of Dietary Supplements; February 11, 2016. Retrieved from: https://ods.od.nih.gov/factsheets/Iron-HealthProfessional/. Accessed August 15, 2015.

137. National Institutes of Health, Office of Dietary Supplements. Folate: dietary supplement fact sheet. Bethesda, MD: National Institutes of Health, Office of Dietary Supplements; updated April 20, 2016. Retrieved from: https://ods.od.nih.gov/factsheets/Folate-HealthProfessional/. Accessed August 15, 2015.

138. Lichtin AE. Anemia of chronic disease. Merck Manual Professional Version; May 2013. Retrieved from: http://www.merckmanuals.com/professional/hematology-and-oncology/anemias-caused-by-deficient-erythropoiesis/anemia-of-chronic-disease. Accessed August 14, 2015.

139. Donini LM, Poggiogalle E, Piredda M, et al. Anorexia and eating patterns in the elderly. *PLoS One*. 2013;8(5):463539.

140. Donini LM, Savina C, Piredda M, et al. Senile anorexia in acute-ward and rehabilitations settings. *J Nutr Health Aging*. 2008;12(6):511–517.

141. Rolland Y, Perrin A, Gardette V, Filhol N, Vellas B. Screening older people at risk of malnutrition or malnourished using the Simplified Nutritional Appetite Questionnaire (SNAQ): a comparison with the Mini-Nutritional Assessment (MNA) tool. *J Am Med Dir Assoc*. 2012;13:31.

142. Fakhouri TH, Ogden CL, Carroll MD, Kit BK, Flegal KM. Prevalence of obesity among older adults in the United States, 2007–2010. *NCHS Data Brief*. September 2012;(106):1–8.

143. Gary P, Hunt W, Koehler K, VanderJagt B. Longitudinal study of dietary intakes and plasma lipids in healthy elderly men and women. *Am J Clin Nutr*. 1992;55:682–688.

144. Centers for Disease Control and Prevention. The health effects of overweight and obesity. Atlanta, GA: Centers for Disease Control and Prevention; updated June 5, 2015. Retrieved from: http://www.cdc.gov/healthyweight/effects/index.html. Accessed August 16, 2015.

145. Decaria JE, Sharp C, Petrella RJ. Scoping review report: obesity in older adults. *Int J Obes*. 2012;36(9):1141–1150.

146. Kalantar-Zadeh K, Block G, Horwich T, Fonarow GC. Reverse epidemiology of conventional cardiovascular risk factors in patients with chronic heart failure. *J Am Coll Cardiol*. 2004;43(8):1439–1444.

147. Houston DK, Nicklas BJ, Zizza CA. Weighty concerns: the growing prevalence of obesity among older adults. *J Am Diet Assoc*. 2009;109(11):1886–1895.

148. Academy of Nutrition and Dietetics. Adult weight management. Chicago, IL: Academy of Nutrition and Dietetics Evidence Analysis Library. Retrieved from: https://www.andeal.org/topic.cfm?menu=5276. Accessed August 16, 2015.

149. Leslie WD. Clinical review: ethnic differences in bone mass—clinical implications. *J Clin Endocrinol Metab*. 2012;97(12):4329–4340.

150. National Institutes of Health Osteoporosis and Related Bone Diseases National Resource Center. Osteoporosis overview. Washington, DC: NIH , U.S. Department of Health and Human Services; June 2015. Retrieved from: http://www.niams.nih.gov/Health_Info/Bone/Osteoporosis/overview.asp. Accessed August 18, 2015.

151. Bolster, MB. Osteoporosis. Merck Manual Professional Version; October 2015. Retrieved from: http://www.merckmanuals.com/professional/SearchResults?query=Osteoporosis. Accessed August 20, 2016.

152. Levis S, Lagari VS. The role of diet in osteoporosis prevention and management. *Curr Osteoporos Rep*. 2013;10(4):296–302.

153. Centers for Disease Control and Prevention. Osteoarthritis (OA). Atlanta, GA: Centers for Disease Contol and Prevention; updated October 28, 2015. Retrieved from: http://www.cdc.gov/arthritis/basics/osteoarthritis.htm. Accessed August 21, 2015.

154. Centers for Disease Control and Prevention. Arthritis – related statistics. Atlanta, GA: Centers for Disease Contol and Prevention; updated October 5, 2016. Retrieved from: http://www.cdc.gov/arthritis/data_statistics/arthritis-related-stats.htm. Updated October 5,2016. Accessed November 11, 2016.

155. Messier S, Loeser R, Miller G, et al. Exercise and dietary weight loss in overweight and obese older adults with knee osteoarthritis. The Arthritis, Diet, and Activity Promotion trial. *Arthritis Rheum*. 2004;50(5):1501–1510.

156. Centers for Disease Control and Prevention. Rheumatoid arthritis (RA). Atlanta, GA: Centers for Disease Contol and Prevention; updated July 22, 2016. Retrieved from: http://www.cdc.gov/arthritis/basics/rheumatoid.htm. Accessed August 21, 2015.

157. Centers for Disease Control and Prevention. Arthritis – related statistics. Atlanta, GA: Centers for Disease Contol and Prevention. Website. http://www.cdc.gov/arthritis/data_statistics/arthritis-related-stats.htm. Updated October 5,2016. Accessed 11/11/16.

158. Sacks JJ, Luo YH, Helmick CG. Prevalence of specific types of arthritis and other rheumatic conditions in the ambulatory health care system in the United States, 2001–2005. *Arthritis Care Res (Hoboken)*. 2010;62(4):460–464.

159. Hagen KB, Byfuglien MG, Falzon L, Olsen SU, Smedslund G. Dietary interventions for rheumatoid arthritis. *Cochrane Database Syst Rev*. January 21, 2009;(1):CD006400. doi: 10.1002/14651858.CD006400.pub2.

160. Dawczynski C, Schubert R, Hein G, et al. Long-term moderate intervention with n-3 long-chain PUFA-supplemented dairy products: effects on pathophysiological biomarkers in patients with rheumatoid arthritis. *Br J Nutr*. 2009;101(10):1517–1526.

161. European Pressure Ulcer Advisory Panel and National Pressure Ulcer Advisory Panel. *Prevention and Treatment of Pressure Ulcers: Quick Reference Guide*. Washington, DC: National Pressure Ulcer Advisory Panel; 2009.

162. Brandeis GH, Morris JN, Nash DJ, Lipsitz LA. The epidemiology and natural history of pressure ulcers in elderly nursing home residents. *JAMA*. 1990;264(22):2905–2909.

163. Beers MH, Berkow R. *The Merck Manual of Geriatrics*. 3rd ed. West Point, PA: Merck Research Laboratories; 2000. http://www.merckmanuals.com/professional/geriatrics.html. Accessed August 5, 2012.

164. Park-Lee E, Caffrey C. Pressure ulcers among nursing home residents: United States, 2004. *NCHS Data Brief.* February 2009;(14):1–8. https://www.cdc.gov/nchs/data/databriefs/db14.pdf. Accessed September 29, 2016.

165. Lyder C, Preston, Ahean D, et al. *Medicare Quality Indicator System: Pressure Ulcer Prediction and Prevention Module: Final Report.* Bethesda, MD: Qualidigm/US Healthcare Financing Administration; 1998.

166. Academy of Nutrition and Dietetics. *International Dietetics and Nutrition Terminology (IDNT) Reference Manual: Standardized Language for the Nutrition Care Process.* 4th ed. Chicago, IL: Academy of Nutrition and Dietetics; 2013.

167. Horn SD, Bender SA, Ferguson ML, et al. The National Pressure Ulcer Long-Term Care Study: pressure ulcer development in long-term care residents. *J Am Geriatr Soc.* 2004;52:359–367.

168. Stechmiller JK, Cowan L, Whitney JD, et al. Guidelines for the prevention of pressure ulcers. *Wound Repair Regenerat.* 2008;16:151–168.

169. Academy of Nutrition and Dietetics. Nutrition Care Manual. Chicago, IL: Academy of Nutrition and Dietetics. Retrieved from: http://www.nutritioncaremanual.org. Accessed August 12,2015.

170. Bernstein M, Munoz N. Position of the Academy of Nutrition and Dietetics: food and nutrition for older adults: promoting health and wellness. *J Acad Nutr Diet.* 2012;112(8):1255–1277.

171. Baranoski S, Ayello EA, eds. *Wound Care Essentials: Practice Principles.* 3rd ed. Ambler, PA: Wolter Kluwer/Lippincott Williams & Wilkins; 2012.

172. National Pressure Ulcer Advisory Panel. Haesler E, ed. *Prevention and Treatment of Pressure Ulcers: Quick Reference Guide.* Perth, Australia: Cambridge Media; 2014.

173. MacKay D, Miller A. Nutritional support for wound healing. *Alt Med Rev.* 2003;8:359–377.

174. Dorner B, Posthauer ME, Thomas D. The role of nutrition in pressure ulcer prevention and treatment: National Pressure Ulcer Advisory Panel white paper. *Adv Skin Wound Care.* 2009;22(5):212–221.

175. Rule AD, Glassock RJ. The aging kidney. UpToDate. Retrieved from: http://www.uptodate.com/contents/the-aging-kidney?source=search_result&search=renal+disease+AND+older+adult&selectedTitle=1~150-H9530832. Accessed September 29, 2016.

176. Centers for Disease Contol and Prevention. *National Chronic Kidney Disease Fact Sheet: General Information and National Estimates on Chronic Kidney Disease in the United States, 2014.* Atlanta, GA: U.S. Department of Health and Human Services, Centers for Disease Control and Prevention; 2014.

177. Coca SG. Acute kidney injury in elderly persons. *Am J Kidney Dis.* 2010;56(1):121–131.

178. Anderson S, Eldadah B, Halter JB, et al. Acute kidney injury in older adults. *J Am Soc Nephrol.* 2011;22(1):28–38.

179. Abdel-Kader K, Palevsky P. Acute kidney injury in the elderly. *Clin Geriatr Med.* 2009;25(3):331–358.

180. Fiaccadori E, Maggiore U, Cabassi A, et al. Nutritional evaluation and management of AKI patients. *J Ren Nutr.* 2013;23(3):255–258.

181. Academy of Nutrition and Dietetics. Nutrition Care Manual: Renal. Chicago, IL: Academy of Nutrition and Dietetics. Retrieved from: http://www.nutritioncaremanual.org. Accessed August 1, 2015.

182. National Kidney Foundation. Clinical practice guidelines for nutrition in chronic renal failure. *Am J Kidney Dis.* 2000;35(suppl 2):S1–S140.

183. Kidney Disease: Improving Global Outcomes (KDIGO) Acute Kidney Injury Work Group. KDIGO clinical practice guideline for acute kidney injury. *Kidney Int.* 2012;(suppl 2): S1–S138.

184. National Institute of Diabetes and Digestive and Kidney Diseases. Bethesda, MD: National Institutes of Health, National Institute of Diabetes and Digestive and Kidney Diseases. Retrieved from: http://www.niddk.nih.gov/health-information/health-topics/kidney-disease/Pages/default.aspx. Accessed August 21, 2015.

185. McMillan JI. Chronic kidney disease. Merck Manual Professional Version. Retrieved from: http://www.merckmanuals.com/professional/genitourinary-disorders/chronic-kidney-disease/chronic-kidney-disease. Accessed August 21, 2015.

186. Cheng HT, Huang JW, Chiang CK, et al. Metabolic syndrome and insulin resistance as risk factors for development of chronic kidney disease and rapid decline in renal function in elderly. *J Clin Endocrin Metab.* 2012;97:1268–1276.

187. National Kidney Foundation. K/DOQI clinical practice guidelines for chronic kidney disease: evaluation, classification and stratification. *Am J Kidney Dis.* 2002;39(2 suppl 1): S1–S266.

188. Tamuraa MK. Incidence, management, and outcomes of end-stage renal disease in the elderly. *Curr Opin Nephrol Hypertens.* 2009;18(3):252–257.

189. Fassett RG, Robertson IK, Mace R, Youl L, Challenor S, Bull R. Palliative care in end-stage kidney disease. *Nephrology.* 2011;16:4–12.

190. Go AS, Chertow GM, Fan D, McCulloch CE, Hsu CY. Chronic kidney disease and the risks of death, cardiovascular events, and hospitalization. *N Engl J Med.* 2004;351(13):1296–1305.

191. US Renal Data System. *USRDS 2012 Annual Data Report: Atlas of Chronic Kidney Disease and End-Stage Renal Disease in the United States.* Bethesda, MD: National Institutes of Health, National Institute of Diabetes and Digestive and Kidney Diseases; 2012.

192. Ye X, Rastogi A, Nissenson AR. Renal replacement therapy in the elderly. *Clin Geriatr Med.* 2009;25(3):529–542.

193. Genestier S, Meyer N, Chantrel F, et al. Prognostic survival factors in elderly renal failure patients treated with peritoneal dialysis: a nine-year retrospective study. *Perit Dial Int.* 2010;30(2):218–226.

194. Byham-Gray L, Wiesen K, eds.; Academy of Nutrition and Dietetics. *A Clinical Guide to Nutrition Care in Kidney Disease.* 2nd ed. Chicago, IL: Academy of Nutrition and Dietetics; 2013.

195. Knoll GA. Kidney transplantation in the older adult. *Am J Kidney Dis.* 2013;61(5):790–797.

196. Robichaud S, Blondeau JM. Urinary tract infections in older adults: current issues and new therapeutic options. *Geriatrics Aging.* 2008;11(10):582–588.

197. National Kidney and Urologic Diseases Information Clearinghouse. *Urinary Incontinence in Men.* Bethesda, MD: National Institute of Diabetes and Digestive and Kidney Diseases; June 2007. NIH Publication No. 07-5280. https://www.niddk.nih.gov/health-information/health-topics/urologic-disease/urinary-incontinence-in-men/Documents/uimen_508.pdf. Accessed September 29, 2016.

acculturation: The process whereby a group's or individual's culture is modified while adapting to another culture. Diet acculturation can be seen with immigrants who after years (and generations) of living in a new country begin to adopt food patterns similar to those of the host country.

achlorhydria: The absence of hydrochloric acid in the gastric juice.

activities of daily living (ADLs): Daily activities that people tend to do every day without needing assistance, such as eating, bathing, dressing, toileting, transferring (walking), and continence (holding their bowels and bladder).

acute kidney injury: A sudden loss of kidney function that results in the accumulation of urea and other nitrogenous waste products as well as the dysregulation of extracellular volume and electrolytes.

adequacy As it relates to healthy eating means that the foods you choose to eat provide all of the essential nutrients, fiber, and energy in amounts sufficient to support growth and maintain health.

Adequate Intake (AI): A value based on observed or experimentally determined approximations of nutrient intake by a group of healthy people and used when a Recommended Dietary Allowance (RDA) cannot be determined.

adiposity rebound: A second rise in body mass index that occurs in children between the ages of 3 and 7 years.

advance directives: A written statement of a person's wishes regarding medical treatment, often including a living will, made to ensure those wishes are carried out should the person be unable to communicate them to a doctor.

aerobic physical activity: Physical activity that relies on the presence of oxygen to make ATP. The complete breakdown of glucose, fatty acids, and amino acids to carbon dioxide and water occurs only through aerobic metabolism

ageusia: Inability to taste that results from damage to or a decrease in taste receptors or pathophysiological neurological changes.

acquired immune deficiency syndrome (AIDS): An infectious disease that develops from human immunodeficiency virus (HIV) infection.

albuminuria: An abnormal excretion rate of albumin.

alpha-linolenic acid: A polyunsaturated omega-3 fatty acid essential to the body for the formation of prostaglandins.

Alzheimer's dementia: A progressive, degenerative disorder that attacks the brain's nerve cells, or neurons, and that results in loss of memory, thinking, and language skills and behavioral changes.

amenorrhea: The absence of menstruation.

amylophagia: A form of pica that is often observed in pregnant women. A condition involving the compulsive consumption of excessive amounts of purified starch.

android: Possessing characteristics of the male form; relating to fat deposition around abdomen.

andropause: A gradual but progressive decline in testosterone levels with age.

anemia: A condition in which the blood is deficient in red blood cells, hemoglobin, or total volume. The World Health Organization, the United Nations Children's Fund, and United Nations University define anemia as a hemoglobin (Hb) concentration two standard deviations below the mean Hb concentration for a normal population of the same sex and age range.

angiotensin: A protein whose presence in the blood promotes aldosterone secretion and tends to raise blood pressure.

anorexia nervosa: An eating disorder characterized by self-induced starvation and excessive weight loss.

anorexia of aging: Loss of appetite due to advanced degenerative processes, and the pathophysiological effects of aging and disease consequence.

anosmia: Inability to smell. May be genetic from birth or acquired over time.

anovulation: Failure of the ovary to release an egg over time, usually 3 months or longer.

antagonistic pleiotropy hypothesis: Known as the "pay later" theory, William's theory on aging proposes that some genes are beneficial at earlier ages but harmful at later ages. These genes with age-related opposite effects are called pleiotropic genes. This theory assumes that a particular gene can have an effect on several of an organism's traits (pleiotropy), which can affect the organism in antagonistic ways.

anthropometric measures: Physical measurements of the body, including data on height, weight, body composition, that can be used to help develop a nutrition assessment.

antiepileptic medications: Medication used to treat seizures.

antioxidant: A synthetic or natural substance that inhibits the oxidation of another molecule, especially one used to counteract the deterioration of stored food products.

aphthous stomatitis: common oral mucosal ulcers also known as canker sores.

apnea: When breathing temporarily stops; it usually occurs more frequently in sleep.

apoptosis: Preprogrammed cell death, which occurs when a cell is no longer viable and its mechanisms for fixing errors in DNA, for example, are unable to keep up. This is a naturally occurring phenomenon experienced by all living creatures.

appropriate for gestational age (AGA): Weight, head, and length within normal measurements for gestational age.

areola: The small circular area surrounding the nipple.

artificial nutrition and hydration (ANH): The delivery of fluids and food or nutrients via artificial means, such as through a tube or an intravenous line.

aspiration: Inhalation of food particles or water when the airway is not protected.

assisted reproductive technology (ART): Any treatment or procedure that uses in vitro technology with oocytes (immature ova or egg cells from the female), sperm, or embryos.

ataxia: Inability to walk properly due to pathological changes in the brain and nervous system.

athetosis: A condition in which abnormal muscle contractions cause excessive, involuntary movements.

ATP III: The National Cholesterol Education Program Adult Treatment Panel III Report, which recommends the diagnosis of metabolic syndrome be made when three or more of the following risk determinants are present: abdominal obesity; high levels of triglycerides, high levels of high-density lipoprotein (HDL), high blood pressure, and high fasting plasma glucose.

atrophic gastritis: Also known as type A or type B gastritis; chronic inflammation of the stomach lining (mucosa) that can lead to loss of gastric glandular cells, which produce important substances such as the carrier for vitamin B_{12} known as intrinsic factor or enzymes and hydrochloric acid; that leads to their eventual replacement by intestinal and fibrous tissues. Occurs more frequently in older adults and is often associated with pernicious anemia or gastric carcinoma.

atrophy: The deterioration, wasting or decrease in the size of a body organ, tissue, or muscle that results from disease, injury or lack of use.

autism spectrum disorder (ASD): A diagnosis given to children and adults with pervasive developmental disorders characterized by complex developmental disabilities with severe impairments in social interaction and communication accompanied by behavioral inflexibility, repetitive behaviors, and/or restricted interests.

Barrett's esophagus: A serious condition that results as a side effect of gastroesophageal reflux disease (GERD). The lining of the esophagus changes from its normal lining to a type that is usually found in the intestines.

bifid uvula: A split or cleft uvula that results from incomplete fusion of the palate.

bilateral cleft lip and palate: Split on two sides.

binge eating disorder (BED): An eating disorder characterized as recurring episodes of eating significantly more food in a short period of time than most people would eat under similar circumstances, with episodes marked by feelings of lack of control occurring, on average, at least once a week over 3 months.

binge eating: The consumption of large quantities of food in a short period of time, typically as part of an eating disorder.

bioavailability: When a nutrient is highly digestible and easily absorbed; it usually refers to proteins with a full complement of needed amino acids.

biochemical data: Laboratory measurements obtained through blood, urine, or stool samples as indicators of nutritional status.

body mass index (BMI): A measure of body fat that is the ratio of the weight of the body in kilograms to the square of its height in meters. It is a reliable indicator of body fatness.

body dissatisfaction: Negative subjective assessment of one's weight and body image; may be closely related to onset, severity, and treatment outcomes of eating disorders.

bone-strengthening exercise: Exercises that strengthen the bone structure of the human body.

brain death: Initial requirements for determination include neuroimaging or clinical findings that suggest catastrophic cerebral events where there are no identifiable other conditions that may represent brain death, such as severe metabolic derangement, intoxication, poisoning, or other acute vascular anomaly. There is persistent unresponsiveness, there are no reflexive responses to pain or any brainstem responses, and there is apnea, with cessation of respiration and circulation.

bulimia nervosa: An eating disorder characterized by bingeing (excessive or compulsive consumption of food) and purging (getting rid of food).

cachexia: Weight loss, weakness, wasting, and changes in body composition due to emotional disturbance and severe or chronic disease.

calorie: The energy needed to raise the temperature of 1 g of water 1°C, and the unit used to measure the potential energy in food as it is transferred from its source to the body.

Campylobacter: Bacteria that can spread through unpasteurized milk, that may cause fever and diarrhea, and that may spread to the blood, causing a life-threatening condition.

cancer: A group of more than a hundred diseases. Cancer starts when abnormal cells grow out of control. Instead of dying, cancer cells grow and form new cells that are abnormal, and these cells can also invade other tissues.

carbohydrates: Organic compounds that occur in food that contain carbon, oxygen, and hydrogen and that can be broken down to release energy in the body.

carcinogen: Substance or agent that is known to be or that are strongly suspected to be causes of cancer.

cardiovascular disease (CVD): Any disease or injury of the heart and its blood vessels as well as the blood vessels throughout the body and the brain.

celiac disease: An autoimmune disorder that occurs in genetically susceptible individuals in which the small intestine is hypersensitive to gluten, leading to difficulty in digesting food and small intestine damage.

cerebrovascular disease: Disease of the blood vessels and, especially, the arteries that supply the brain that affects the circulation of blood to the brain, causing limited or no blood flow to certain areas of the brain known as stroke or transient ischemic attacks.

cholesterol: A waxy, fat-like substance found in all of the cells of the body that is a precursor of other steroid compounds; high concentrations of cholesterol in the blood is thought to promote atherosclerosis.

cleft lip and palate (CLP): Congenital split of the lip and palate that varies from a notching to a complete division of the lip or a cleft that may extend through the uvula and soft palate and into the hard palate.

clinical assessment: The component of nutrition assessment that includes a medical history, inventory of currently used medications, vitamins, minerals, and herbal supplements, and a physical examination to identify signs of nutrition status.

cluster feeding: When a baby shifts from feeding every 2 to 3 hours to feeding every hour or feeding in spurts.

Coenzyme: Organic compounds often B-Vitamin derivatives that combine with an inactive enzyme to form an active one. Coenzymes associate closely with these enzymes allowing them to catalyze certain metabolic reactions in a cell.

cognitive decline: Decrease in mental acuity, status, and/or memory. Declines are usually due to pathophysiological processes affecting the brain and the central nervous system. Cognitive decline is associated with many different diseases, many of which occur more frequently in older persons.

cognitive development: Learning that occurs in the mind.

colic: Marked periods of irritability, fussiness, or crying in an infant between 2 weeks and 3 months who is generally healthy.

colostrum: The first secretion from the mammary glands of the mother after giving birth. This fluid is rich in immunologic properties.

coma: State of extreme unresponsiveness, with no voluntary movement or behavior, and sometimes normal reflexes may be lost. In coma, there is maintenance of autonomic functions. If coma persists for more than a month, it is called a persistent vegetative state. There are "grades" assigned to comas that delineate severity and type.

comorbid: When one medical condition occurs at the same time, but independently, of another medical condition.

complex carbohydrates: A form of carbohydrate made up of multiple sugar molecules (polysaccharides) linked together. Examples include starches, glycogen, and most types of fiber.

constipation: Development of hard, dry feces that results in difficulty emptying bowels or abnormally delayed or infrequent passage of hardened feces.

core foods: Foods consumed by particular demographics over many generations.

coronary heart disease (CHD): Disease or injury of the heart that includes myocardial infarction (MI), angina pectoris, heart failure, and coronary death.

Crohn's disease: A subtype of inflammatory bowel disease; chronic ileitis that typically involves the distal portion of the ileum, often spreads to the colon, and is characterized by diarrhea, cramping, and loss of appetite and weight with local abscesses and scarring—also called regional enteritis, regional ileitis. It affects the entire digestive tract and all three intestinal mucosal layers.

cues: Help the parent understand the needs of the baby.

culture: Beliefs and customs that shape the behaviors of a particular group of people.

DASH (Dietary Approaches to Stop Hypertension) diet: A dietary pattern promoted by the U.S.-based National Heart, Lung, and Blood Institute (part of the National Institutes of Health, an agency of the U.S. Department of Health and Human Services) to prevent and control hypertension. It involves decreased sodium intake and increased consumption of fruit and vegetables and low-fat dairy products.

decubitus ulcers: Bedsores or wounds that heal poorly and slowly. A function of being bedridden with fragile skin; decubitus ulcers often occur in very old or very ill persons, who are unable to be moved.

dentition: Having to do with teeth.

developmental milestone: Certain behaviors or physical skills infants gain as they grow and develop.

diabetes mellitus: A disease of the pancreas which inhibits the production and utilization of the hormone insulin. Diabetes is a variable disorder of carbohydrate metabolism caused by a combination of hereditary and environmental factors and usually characterized by inadequate secretion or utilization of insulin, excessive urine production, excessive amounts of sugar in the blood and urine, and thirst, hunger, and loss of weight.

diabetes type 1: A form of diabetes in which the body does not produce insulin.

diabetes type 2: A form of diabetes in which the body does not use insulin properly.

diarrhea: Abnormally frequent intestinal evacuations with more or less fluid stools.

dietary data: The component of nutrition assessment that looks at food intake over time.

Dietary Guidelines for Americans: A set of guidelines published every 5 years and released jointly by the U.S. Department of Health and Human Services and the U.S. Department of Agriculture that provide science-based advice suggesting how nutrition and physical activity can help to promote health across the life span and help to reduce the risk of major chronic diseases among the U.S. population ages 2 years and older.

Dietary Reference Intakes (DRIs): Suggested nutrient intake values intended to serve as a guide for good nutrition for healthy people. These dietary standards include Estimated Average Requirement (EAR), Recommended Dietary Allowance (RDA), Adequate Intake (AI), and Tolerable Upper Intake Limit (UL).

direct calorimetry: Measurement of the heat produced by a reaction, as distinguished from indirect methods, which involve measurement of something other than heat production itself.

disease prevention: The deferral or elimination of medical illnesses and conditions through appropriate interventions for an individual or group with the goal of improving health and quality of life.

diverticular disease: The presence of bulging pockets of tissue or sacs in the walls of the colon.

diverticulitis: Inflammation and/or infection of one or more diverticula, especially in the colon, causing pain and disturbance of bowel function.

diverticulosis: A condition in which diverticula (small, bulging sacs) are present in the intestine without signs of inflammation.

DNA (deoxyribonucleic acid): A self-replicating material present in nearly all living organisms as the main constituent of chromosomes. It is the carrier of genetic information.

drug–drug and drug–nutrient interactions: The impact that drugs have on one another, the system, and the side effects, or the impact that drugs have on nutrients in terms of their intake, absorption, disposition, metabolism, utilization, and excretion, and vice versa.

dysgeusia: Altered sense of taste.

dyslipidemia: A disorder of lipoprotein metabolism, including lipoprotein overproduction or deficiency, marked by abnormal concentrations of lipids or lipoproteins in the blood; dyslipidemias may manifest as elevation of total cholesterol, low-density lipoprotein (LDL) cholesterol, and triglyceride concentrations and a decrease in the high-density lipoprotein (HDL) cholesterol concentration in the blood.

dysosmia: Altered sense of smell.

dysphagia: The inability to swallow properly. Swallowing is a complex cascade of reactions. Dysphagia occurs more frequently in older adults and can result in inhaling food and a lung infection or choking. Dysphagia may result from a neurologic disorder that impairs esophageal motility or a mechanical obstruction of the esophagus.

eclampsia: Convulsions or coma late in pregnancy in an individual affected by preeclampsia.

edema: Excessive extracellular fluid collected usually in the legs and feet, causing swelling.

eicosanoids: Signaling molecules synthesized by fatty acids that exert control over many systems in the body, including inflammation and immunity. They also act as messengers for the central nervous system.

end-of-life (EOL) care: Persons nearing death have multiple concerns and needs, from provision of adequate nutrition to resuscitation in the event of cardiac failure.

energy balance: When calories consumed equal calories burned.

engorgement: Swelling of the breast.

enteral tube feeding (ETF): The delivery of a nutritionally complete feeding, which contains protein or amino acids, carbohydrate, fiber, fat, water, minerals and vitamins, directly into the gut via a tube.

essential nutrients: Nutrients (vitamins, minerals, fatty acids, and amino acids) required for normal physiological function that cannot be synthesized by the body and that, therefore, must be obtained from the diet.

Estimated Average Requirement (EAR): A nutrient intake value that is estimated to meet the requirement of half the healthy individuals in a group.

failure to thrive (FTT): Unexplained deficits in growth in infants and children that require nutrition intervention.

fat: A macronutrient that provides an energy source and that helps the body absorb fat-soluble vitamins, keeps skin and hair healthy, and offers the sensation of satiety after eating. Fat is the source of two essential fatty acids and is used by the body during brain development, for controlling inflammation, and in blood clotting.

fibroblast: A cell in connective tissue that produces collagen and other fibers.

FODMAP diet: A diet consisting of foods containing low fermentable oligosaccharides, disaccharides, monosaccharides, and polyols.

food allergy: An immune system reaction that occurs soon after eating a certain food.

food aversion: A strong feeling of dislike that results in refusal to try or to eat certain foods.

food desert: Geographic neighborhoods and communities that are characterized by limited access to fresh, affordable, healthy, and nutritious foods.

food insecurity: Limited or uncertain availability of nutritionally adequate and safe foods or limited or uncertain ability to acquire acceptable foods in socially acceptable ways, such as when a person lacks the money or the resources to acquire food. Food insecurity manifests as difficulty providing enough food for all family members at some time during the year as a result of a lack of resources.

food intolerance: Any abnormal physical response to a food or food additive.

food jags: When an individual consumes the same food, prepared the same way, on a consistent basis.

food neophobia: Reluctance to try new foods and/or avoidance of certain foods or food groups.

food sensitivity: A condition which occurs when a person has difficulty digesting a particular food.

foodways: Food customs or traditions of a group of people that involve how foods are obtained, prepared, served, and consumed. Foodways encompass beliefs about food, food preferences, and customs and have cultural, social, and economic components.

frailty: A syndrome characterized by loss of hand grip strength, slow walking speeds, exhaustion, and loss of lean body mass.

frailty syndrome: A cluster of signs and symptoms that indicate that an older person is at risk for falls, fractures, and other acute health events. Usually characterized by decreased hand grip strength, loss of muscle mass, slower walking speeds, and other measures.

friction: The action of one surface or object rubbing against another.

full term: Babies born between 37 and 42 weeks of gestation.

functional fibers: Isolated, nondigestible forms of carbohydrate that have been extracted from starchy foods or manufactured from starches or sugars. They may have some of the benefits of naturally occurring dietary fiber, such as helping to prevent constipation or lowering blood glucose levels after meals.

galactagogues: Medications used to increase milk supply.

galactosemia: A genetic disorder that creates an inability to metabolize galactose, a common carbohydrate found in milk and a by-product of lactose metabolism. It results in an inability to use galactose to produce energy.

gallbladder disease: Any impairment of the normal function of the gallbladder that leads to abdominal discomfort and the inability to digest fatty foods.

gastroesophageal reflux (GER): The passage of stomach contents into the esophagus, or throat.

Gastroesophageal Reflux Disease (GERD): A highly variable chronic digestive condition that is characterized by periodic episodes of gastroesophageal reflux, when stomach contents flow back up the esophagus, and usually accompanied by heartburn. It may result in histopathologic changes in the esophagus.

gastroparesis: A condition where the muscles in the stomach do not function normally, limiting stomach motility and leading to delays in gastric emptying. Gastroparesis can interfere with normal digestion and cause symptoms such as nausea, vomiting, blood sugar dysregulation, and altered nutrition.

geophagia: Compulsive consumption of soil-like substances, including soil or clay.

geriatrics: The medical specialty that focuses on managing the care of elderly persons.

gestation: How long an infant is carried in the womb from conception to birth, usually measured in weeks.

gestational diabetes mellitus (GDM): Diabetes diagnosed during pregnancy and that cannot be categorized as overt diabetes.

glossoptosis: Downward displacement (retraction) of the tongue.

gluten: A protein found in the cereal grains wheat, barley, and rye that causes illness when ingested by those with celiac disease. Gluten, which is a is mixture of two proteins, is responsible for the elastic texture of dough.

glycemic control: Achievement and maintenance of an optimal blood glucose level.

gonadarche: First visual sign of puberty. Seen as breast budding in girls and as testicular enlargement in boys.

growth: Anabolic biological function where size of body parts and organs increases.

growth chart: Measurement tool that tracks height, length, weight, head circumference, and body mass index changes over time.

growth faltering: When weight measurements cross three percentiles over 3 months in infancy and over 6 months in the second and third years of life.

growth hormone: A hormone released by the brain that causes the growth process.

growth stunting: A primary manifestation of malnutrition that results in reduced linear growth rate.

growth velocity: Changes in growth measurements that occur over a set period of time.

gynoid: Also called gynecoid. Possessing characteristics of the female form; relating to fat deposition around the hips and thighs.

head circumference: A measurement of a child's head around its largest area. It measures the distance from above the eyebrows and ears and around the back of the head.

healthcare proxy: A legal document in which a competent person makes another person his or her agent for health decisions on their behalf when the individual is no longer able to make or execute healthcare decisions at some future point. The right of a legally named person to execute the wishes for treatment or refusal of treatment when an individual is incapacitated. Usually healthcare organizations, hospitals, and emergency rooms have a generic form of this document that they ask a patient to fill out and that they then keep with the person's chart should another emergency arise.

health disparities: Differences in the health status of different groups of people. For example, some groups of people have higher rates of certain diseases compared to others.

health promotion: Deliberate actions that are taken with the intent of moving an individual to a higher level of wellness.

heart failure: Severe failure of the heart to function properly, especially as a cause of death.

Helicobacter pylori (H. pylori): Bacteria that cause stomach inflammation and injuries in the stomach and duodenum.

hemoglobin A$_{1c}$: A minor component of hemoglobin to which glucose is bound.

high-density lipoprotein (HDL): A blood lipoprotein that contains low levels of triglycerides and high levels of protein. HDL is synthesized primarily in the liver as well as in the small intestine. HDL carries cholesterol out of the bloodstream. HDL is called the good cholesterol.

hind milk: The breastmilk available at the end of a feeding that is higher in fat content than milk provided at the beginning of the feeding.

home health care: Provision of medical services to ill persons in their home by a licensed home health agency using skilled medical professionals and billed to the individuals' insurance. It is overseen by the patient's primary medical provider and includes services deemed appropriate by a medical care plan. Services may include, but are not limited to, the provision of medical equipment, home aides for activities of daily living, nursing, dietetics, speech, occupational and physical therapy, as well as social work and, in some instances, hospice. Curative treatments, life-prolonging measures, and other interventions are used in the person's place of residence. It is usually time limited, and insurance coverage or the person's financial resources determine time for provision of service. Each state has its own budget and procedures, regulations and stipulations regarding home health care.

hospice care: A multidisciplinary approach to end-of-life care, when there is a definitive terminal course of illness, usually defined as a 6-month period before death. A network of professionals and volunteers provides, often in the home, support services that address all the needs of the dying person and their family. The goal is exceptional quality of life in the remaining time while surrounded by family and friends in a familiar environment. Palliative services such as aggressive pain control are employed, but treatment of the underlying pathology is not attempted. Curative measures are not undertaken, but supportive measures are. These include, but are not limited to, psychotherapy, social services, religious support, familial support and counseling, grief/anger management, physical/occupational therapy, dietetics, and provision of medical equipment and ancillary services.

human immunodeficiency virus (HIV): An incurable retrovirus that attacks the immune system, making it difficult for the body to fight off disease.

human milk-based fortifier: Powders or liquids added to breastmilk to increase the amount of calories and protein in the milk.

hydration: The provision of fluids either by mouth or through artificial means, such as an intravenous line or subcutaneous infusion.

hyperemesis gravidarum (HG): Severe persistent vomiting during pregnancy that results in weight loss and dehydration and that often requires hospitalization.

hyperglycemia: High concentration of glucose in the bloodstream.

hypertension: A chronic condition where a person's blood pressure is consistently elevated above the population average. Resting blood pressure exceeds 140 mm Hg systolic or 90 mm Hg diastolic.

hyperuricemia: Chronic elevated serum uric acid levels.

hypoallergenic: Foods that have a low risk of promoting food or other allergies.

hypoglycemia: Deficiency of glucose in the bloodstream.

hypotonia: Also known as "floppy baby syndrome"; a low amount of tension or resistance to stretch in a muscle and often involving reduced muscle strength that causes weight goals to be generally lower than that for a typical child of the same age.

Hypotonic fluids: a solution that contains fewer dissolved particles, such as salt, and potassium, then is found in normal cells and blood.

immunocompromise: When the immune system does not function correctly or sufficiently.

immunosenescence: The gradual deterioration and impairment of the immune system that results from age-related changes in innate and adaptive immunity and an imbalance between them; results in decreased function and ability to respond to infections.

indirect calorimetry: Calculates heat that living organisms produce by measuring either their production of carbon dioxide and nitrogen waste (frequently ammonia in aquatic organisms, or urea in terrestrial ones) or their consumption of oxygen; a way of determining metabolic rate in critically ill patients.

infant mortality: Occurrence of death within the first 5 years of life.

infertility: Inability to get pregnant after 12 or more months of regular unprotected sexual intercourse.

inflammatory bowel disease (IBD): A chronic condition with periodic immune responses combined with inflammation in the gastrointestinal tract. IBD encompasses two inflammatory diseases of the bowel: Crohn's disease or ulcerative colitis.

insoluble fiber: A type of fiber that adds bulk to stool and appears to help food pass more quickly through the stomach and intestines, helping to prevent constipation by increasing stool weight and decreasing gut transit time, which in turn can reduce the risk of diseases and disorders such as diverticular disease and hemorrhoids.

instrumental activities of daily living (IADL): Activities that may not be functional but that enable people to live independently, such as housework, preparing meals, taking medications correctly, and managing finances.

insulin: A hormone produced in the pancreas by the islets of Langerhans that regulates the amount of glucose in the blood.

insulin resistance: A condition characterized by the increasing demand for insulin paired with inadequate insulin secretion and relative insulin deficiency. The diminished ability of cells to respond to the action of insulin in transporting glucose from the bloodstream into muscle and other tissues.

insulin sensitivity: How sensitive the body is to the effects of insulin.

intensive medical care: Intensive care is performed in critical care medical units to prolong life in patients with potentially reversible critical illnesses, organ-system failure, and traumatic injury or in unstable surgical patients. Life-supportive measures, constant monitoring, and technologically advanced treatments and equipment are used and artificial nutrition and hydration are usually part of this care.

intrauterine growth restriction (IUGR): When infant growth is disproportionate in weight, length, or weight-for-length percentiles for gestational age.

intrinsic factor: A substance secreted by the stomach that enables the body to absorb vitamin B_{12}. It is a glycoprotein. Deficiency results in pernicious anemia.

intuitive eating: A nutrition philosophy based on the premise that becoming in tune with the body's natural hunger cues is a more effective way to attain a healthy weight rather than keeping track of calories.

iron deficiency (ID): A state in which there is insufficient iron to maintain normal physiologic functions.

iron-deficiency anemia (IDA): A condition characterized by low hemoglobin levels, paleness, exhaustion, and rapid heart rate. Signs of iron deficiency are also present and include short attention span, poor appetite, irritability, and susceptibility to infection.

irritable bowel syndrome (IBS): A chronic functional disorder of the colon that is of unknown etiology. It is often associated with abnormal intestinal motility and increased sensitivity to visceral pain and characterized by diarrhea or constipation or diarrhea alternating with constipation, abdominal pain or discomfort, abdominal bloating, and passage of mucus in the stool; also called irritable colon, irritable colon syndrome, mucous colitis, and spastic colon.

lactation consultant: Allied health professionals who commonly work in hospitals, physician or midwife practices, public health programs, or private practice and who specialize in the clinical management of breastfeeding. Trained professionals are able to help mothers in overcoming common breastfeeding problems.

lactogenesis I: The initial stage of milk production for a postpartum woman.

lactogenesis II: The stage of lactation that begins 2–5 days after birth and is commonly referred to as transitional milk or the milk "coming in."

lactogenesis III: The stage of lactation that generally occurs 2–5 weeks after birth, producing fluid referred to as "mature milk."

lactose: The sugar present in milk

lactose intolerance: The inability to digest lactose, a component of milk.

large for gestational age (LGA): Weight, head, and length above the 90th percentile for gestational age.

latch: The process whereby the infant creates the right type of contact for positive pressure to initiate the flow of milk from ducts.

laxative: Medication that stimulates and facilitates stooling.

Le Leche League: An organization that helps and supports breastfeeding mothers with advice, ideas, and both legal and medical advocacy.

let-down reflex: An involuntary reflex during the period of time when a woman is breastfeeding that causes the milk to flow freely.

leukemia: A cancer of the white blood cells (WBCs) where the bone marrow produces abnormal WBCs. This leads to an increased accumulation of cancerous cells in the blood, with a variable reduction in normal blood cells, affecting the normal function of blood cells.

linoleic acid: An essential, polyunsaturated, omega-6 fatty acid that is necessary for healthy brain function, skin and hair growth, bone density, energy production, and reproductive health.

lipase: A pancreatic enzyme that catalyzes the breakdown of fats to fatty acids and glycerol or other alcohols.

listeriosis: A serious infection caused by eating foods contaminated with *Listeria monocytogenes*.

living will: A legal document that can be drawn up and signed that states which medical and other life-sustaining procedures may or may not be done in the event that a person becomes mentally incompetent, comatose, otherwise incapacitated, or terminally ill. Such documentation should be readily available in the event of an emergent situation and on file with the primary care provider and immediate family members. Included in this documentation should be decisions regarding artificial nutrition and hydration as well as other treatment modalities. Several websites offer a download template for this documentation, and it can be filled out and filed for use at a later date. State and federal regulations govern the language used in these forms of documentation.

low birth weight (LBW): Less than 2,500 g (5.5 pounds) at birth.

low-density lipoprotein (LDL): Composed primarily of cholesterol transports cholesterol to the cells of the body.

lower esophageal sphincter (LES): A ring of smooth muscle fibers at the junction of the esophagus and stomach.

lymphocyte: A form of small leukocyte (white blood cell) with a single round nucleus that occurs especially in the lymphatic system.

macronutrient: Nutrient the human body needs in relatively large quantities to promote growth.

macrosomia: "Fetal macrosomia" is used to describe a newborn who is significantly larger than average; a baby diagnosed with fetal macrosomia has a birth weight of more than 8 pounds, 13 ounces (4,000 g), regardless of his or her gestational age.

malnutrition: Inadequate intake of protein and/or energy over prolonged periods of time that results in loss of fat stores and/or muscle stores; includes starvation-related malnutrition, chronic disease or condition-related malnutrition, and acute disease or injury-related malnutrition.

mastitis: Inflammation of the mammary gland in the breast, typically due to bacterial infection of a damaged nipple.

megaloblastic anemia: An anemia (of macrocytic classification) that results from inhibition of DNA synthesis during red blood cell production.

menarche: Onset of menses, or the female period.

menopause: A natural biological process in women that involves a decline in estrogen production. It typically occurs 12 months after the last menstrual period and marks the end of menstrual cycles.

mercury: A heavy silvery-white metal that is liquid at ordinary temperatures.

metabolic syndrome: A cluster of at least three biochemical and physiological abnormalities that are risk factors for heart disease and type 2 diabetes: hypertriglyceridemia, low HDL cholesterol, hyperglycemia, hypertension, or excess abdominal fat.

microbiomes: Collective colonies of different microbes that reside in the large intestine.

micronutrient: Chemical element or substances required in small amounts for normal growth and development of all living organisms.

midgrowth spurt: Small increase in the velocity of growth that precedes puberty development.

midparental height: A height calculated using an equation based on parents' height and adjusted for the child's sex; provides an indication of a child's linear growth potential.

minerals: Inorganic and essential nutrients that are needed by the body in small amounts and that play key roles in several body functions.

MyPlate: Federal government's newest health education model that illustrates a healthy diet, including food groups and place setting.

nasopharynx: The space above the soft palate at the back of the nose that connects the mouth with the nose.

National School Breakfast Program (NSBP): A federal program that provides cash assistance to states to operate nonprofit breakfast programs in schools and residential child care facilities.

National School Lunch Program (NSLP): A federally assisted meal program for federal and nonprofit private schools where on a daily basis children receive nutritionally balanced meals either for free or for low cost.

nausea: A stomach distress that manifests as distaste for food and an urge to vomit.

necrotizing enterocolitis: When tissue in the small or large intestine is injured or dies, causing the intestine to become inflamed.

neonatal hypoglycemia: The most common metabolic problem in newborns; defined as a plasma glucose level of less than 30 mg/dL (1.65 mmol/L) in the first 24 hours of life and less than 45 mg/dL (2.5 mmol/L) thereafter.

neonatal jaundice: Presents as a yellow discoloration in the skin and eyes of an affected newborn whose liver is not mature enough to get rid of bilirubin that is in the bloodstream.

neonatal: Classification of infants directly after birth to 28 days.

neophobia: Generally regarded as the reluctance to eat or the avoidance of new foods.

nephron: The functional units in the kidney, consisting of a glomerulus and its associated tubule, through which the glomerular filtrate passes before emerging as urine.

neuroblastoma: An embryonal tumor of the autonomic nervous system that develops from neural crest tissues of the sympathetic nervous system. It can occur in many areas of the body, including the abdomen, adrenal glands, neck, skull, pelvis, spinal column, and bone marrow. Neuroblastoma generally occurs in very young children; the median age at diagnosis is 17 months.

newborn screening: The practice of testing newborn babies for certain treatable disorders and conditions.

nipple confusion: Can occur if an infant has difficulty achieving the correct oral configuration, latching technique, and suckling pattern necessary for successful breastfeeding after bottle feeding or other exposure to an artificial nipple.

nonessential nutrients: Nutrients required by the body for supporting processes. These can be made by the body and therefore do not need to be obtained from the diet.

novel food: Food that does not have a significant history of consumption or that is produced by a method that has not previously been used for food.

nutrient dense: Relatively large amount of nutrients in a small serving of calories.

nutrient density: A characteristic of foods that provide a generous amount of one or more nutrients compared to the number of calories they supply.

Nutrition Care Process: A systematic way to obtain and record patient data that has standard formats and terminology. Instituted by the Academy of Nutrition and Dietetics, it is a means to both collect and disseminate data for outcomes and to other health providers.

nutrition support: The provision of enteral or parenteral nutrients to treat or prevent malnutrition. Nutrition support therapy is part of nutrition therapy, which is a component of medical treatment that can include oral, enteral, and parenteral nutrition to maintain or restore optimal nutrition status and health.

nutritional supplement: Nutrient-dense beverage and food.

obesity: A condition characterized by excessive accumulation and storage of fat in the body. In an adult, obesity is typically indicated by a body mass index of 30 or higher. Obesity may be subdivided into categories: class 1: BMI ≥ 30; class 2: BMI of 35 to < 40; and class 3: BMI of 40 or higher.

obesogenic environment: An environment that promotes gaining weight and that is not conducive to weight loss within the home or workplace.

oldest old: While the numbers differ across agencies, organizations, and governmental entities, the majority use the cut point for the oldest old at 85 years or greater.

omega-3 fatty acids: Polyunsaturated fatty acids that have been shown to be beneficial for the heart as well as play a critical role in brain function and normal growth and development.

omega-6 fatty acids: Polyunsaturated fatty acids that have been shown to play a critical role in brain function and normal growth and development. Omega-6 fatty acids may interfere with the health benefits brought about by omega-3 fatty acids.

oral health: The health and well-being of a person's mouth.

orthorexia nervosa: An obsession with eating foods that one considers healthy and pure; a fixation on righteous eating.

osteoarthritis: A chronic degenerative disease of joint cartilage and the underlying bone, most commonly occurring from middle age onward. It causes pain and stiffness, especially in the hip, knee, and thumb joints.

osteoporosis: A condition of low bone mass, deterioration of bone tissue, disruption of bone structure, compromised bone strength, and increased risk of fracture, typically as a result of hormonal changes or deficiency of calcium or vitamin D.

otitis media: Ear infection.

overweight: Abnormal or excessive fat accumulation in the body with a body mass index ranging between 25 and 29.

ovulation: When the mature egg is released from the ovary into the fallopian tube and becomes available for fertilization.

oxytocin: A hormone associated with contraction of the uterus during labor and that stimulates the ejection of milk into the milk gland.

pagophagia: Compulsive consumption of ice or freezer frost.

pain management: At any time during illness, the focus of palliative case is on symptom management during assessment and treatment of the underlying pathophysiology. This treatment aims to decrease pain and suffering, using aggressive pain treatments and a holistic approach to provide the best possible quality of life.

palate: The top (roof) of the mouth, including the hard palate (front portion, includes bone) and soft palate (back portion, includes muscle).

palliative care: Palliative care may be provided at any time during a person's illness. The focus is on symptom management during assessment and treatment of the underlying pathophysiology. It is not the same as hospice care, although both seek to decrease pain and suffering, often by using aggressive pain treatments and a holistic approach. The intent is to provide the best possible quality of life. It is a branch of internal medicine that is administered either in the healthcare setting or in the home. It is usually done using a team approach, involving palliative care physicians, nurses, dietitians, social workers, clergy, and physical, occupational, and psychotherapists. Many larger institutions have palliative care teams or units affiliated with their intensive medical care division.

paraprofessional: Trained aides who assist fully qualified professionals.

parenteral nutrition (PN): The intravenous administration of nutrients, which include carbohydrate, protein, lipids, electrolytes, vitamins, and minerals.

passive immunity: Immunity that results from the injection of antibodies passed from the mother to the infant through breastmilk, which actively stimulates the infant's immune system.

peak height velocity: The time period of fastest rate of linear (height) growth.

peer counselor: Persons considered equals to another and who provide knowledge, experience, emotional, social, or practical help.

percutaneous endoscopic gastrostomy tube: Tube placed laparoscopically and used for feeding directly into the lumen of the stomach.

perinatal depression: Major and minor depressive episodes during pregnancy (termed antenatal) or within the first 12 months after delivery (termed postpartum or postnatal).

peripheral artery disease (PAD): A narrowing of the peripheral arteries to the legs, stomach, arms, and head.

permanent teeth: Second set of teeth in humans, also known as the adult teeth.

pernicious anemia: A deficiency in the production of red blood cells through a lack of vitamin B_{12}.

persistent vegetative state (PVS): A state of extreme unresponsiveness that lasts for more than 1 month, when a person displays no awareness or higher cerebral function. Midbrain and brainstem functions are preserved, with sleep–wake cycling and autonomic control over functions such as breathing and heart rate. There may be some reflexive movement. End-stage dementia often leads to PVS.

physical activity: Any bodily movement produced by skeletal muscles that requires energy expenditure.

phytochemicals: Substances found in plants that are not considered essential but that play important roles in maintaining health and well-being.

pica: An eating disorder characterized by consuming nonnutritive substances such as clay, paper, starch, chalk, and soil.

placenta: A disk-shaped organ that connects the fetus to the uterine wall, allowing for nutrient and gas interchange.

pneumatosis: Gas cyst in the bowel wall.

polypharmacy: The use of five or more drugs per day.

postnatal: The period after childbirth.

postpartum (or postnatal) depression: Depression suffered by a mother following childbirth, typically arising from the combination of hormonal changes, psychological adjustment to motherhood, and fatigue.

power of attorney: A durable power of attorney for healthcare decisions is documentation that identifies the person who can make and carry out an individual's wishes in the event that there is an emergent situation and the individual is incapacitated mentally or physically or is comatose. This responsibility is also known as healthcare proxy, with regard to healthcare matters. Usually, there are two different power of attorney forms, one for financial "gifts" and one for all other estate matters. The gift rider, durable power of attorney, and health care proxy documents should all be designed, notarized, and filed prior to an individual becoming sick and incapacitated. It is best to get the advice of a reputable lawyer with estate planning and elder care experience. General durable power of attorney is a legal document that designates another person to act on the individual's behalf concerning legal or business matters. That person can write checks, access bank accounts, and so forth while the individual is incapacitated.

prebiotics: A nondigestible food ingredient that promotes the growth of beneficial microorganisms in the intestines.

preconception health care: A type of health care that identifies medical, behavioral, and social risks and modifies them prior to conception.

preconception period: The time prior to or between conceptions.

preeclampsia: Hypertension with onset following 20 weeks of pregnancy that is characterized by a sudden rise in blood pressure, excessive weight gain, generalized edema, proteinuria, severe headache, and visual disturbances and that may result in eclampsia if untreated. It can lead to fetal growth restriction.

preschoolers: Children between the ages of 3 and 5 years.

pressure injuries: Localized injuries to the skin and/or underlying tissue usually over a bony prominence that results from pressure or pressure in combination with shear.

preterm: Babies born before 37 weeks of gestation.

primary aging: Aging as a function of time alone.

primary teeth: The first set of teeth in humans; also known as the baby teeth.

probiotics: Live strains of bacteria and yeasts that are normally found in the digestive system and that contribute to keeping the gut healthy.

prolactin: A hormone that helps to produce breastmilk and that is released by the pituitary gland as the fetus develops, causing enlargement of the mammary glands of the breast, which helps prepare for the production of milk.

protein: Any group of organic molecules that contain carbon, hydrogen, oxygen, and nitrogen, and one or more chains of amino acids. Proteins are in every cell in the body and function to build, repair, and maintain bones, muscles, and skin.

proton pump inhibitor: Drugs that reduce the activity of proton pumps and that are used to reduce gastric acid secretion in the treatment of ulcers and gastroesophageal reflux disease.

puberty: Physical changes that occur as a child attains reproductive capacity.

Recommended Dietary Allowance (RDA): The average dietary intake level that is sufficient to meet the nutrient requirements of nearly all (97% to 98%) healthy individuals in a group.

recumbent length: Measuring an infant's length lying down in a completely stretched out position.

reflexes: Unlearned, automatic responses triggered by some type of stimulus.

resting metabolic rate (RMR): The number of calories needed to support basic functions, including breathing and circulation.

resuscitation: The restoration of life or consciousness that involves (usually) cardiopulmonary efforts, such as mouth-to-mouth breathing or cardiac massage. Do Not Resuscitate or DNR orders are medically and legally binding.

rickets: A bone-softening disease the results from vitamin D deficiency and that causes severe bowing of the legs, poor growth, and sometimes muscle pain and weakness.

Rome III diagnostic criteria: A system developed to classify the functional gastrointestinal disorders (FGIDs) of the digestive system in which symptoms cannot be explained by the presence of structural or tissue abnormality, based on clinical symptoms.

rooting reflex: A reflex that is seen in normal newborn babies who automatically turn the face toward the stimulus and make a sucking or rooting motion with the mouth when the cheek or lip is touched.

sarcopenia: Age-associated loss of skeletal muscle mass (lean body mass) and function. The causes of sarcopenia are multifactorial and can include disuse, altered endocrine function, chronic diseases, inflammation, insulin resistance, and nutritional deficiencies. Sarcopenia is associated with muscle weakness, functional limitations, and disability, as well as impairments in cardiovascular capacity and metabolic health.

sarcopenic obesity: When an obese person has little muscle mass. Sarcopenic obesity is the simultaneous occurrence of sarcopenia and obesity, which results from excess body fat and reduction of muscle mass.

saturated fats: A type of fat where the carbon atoms in the fatty acid component are linked by single bonds. Saturated fats are found in meat and other animal products such as butter, cheese, and milk. This type of fat is associated with increased blood cholesterol levels.

secondary aging: Changes that occur on the cellular level as a result of disease processes.

Surveillance, Epidemiology, and End Results (SEER): Program of the National Cancer Institute to provide information on cancer statistics in an effort to reduce the burden of cancer among the U.S. population.

self-monitoring of blood glucose (SMBG): An empowering technique used by the patient and healthcare team to assess the effectiveness of a treatment plan in maintaining good glycemic control.

senescence: The inevitable decline in organ function and physiological function that occurs over time in the absence of injury, illness, or poor lifestyle choices. The process of growing old; senescence involves the accumulation of deleterious changes in cells that cause them to die more rapidly than they are replaced.

sensorimotor: Learning system where the infant's senses and motor skills provide information to the central nervous system to encourage further development.

sequence: In relation to puberty, the order in which physical changes occur during development. This order does not vary among individuals.

sexual dimorphism: Variation of physical characteristics and body composition between the sexes.

sexual maturity ratings (SMRs): Also called Tanner stages. Stages 1 through 5 of physical developments of puberty, visually assessed by gonadal and pubic hair changes.

shear: A chronic progressive disease that causes inflammation in the joints and that results in painful deformity and immobility, especially in the fingers, wrists, feet, and ankles.

simple carbohydrates: Carbohydrates made up of either one (monosaccharide) or two (disaccharide) simple sugar molecules. Examples include sucrose, maltose, and lactose.

sleep–wake reversal: A pathological change in the brain's sleep–wake circadian rhythm that results in wakefulness at night and drowsiness during the day.

small for gestational age (SGA): Weight below the 10th percentile for gestational age.

soluble fiber: Fiber that attracts water and turns to a gel during digestion, a characteristic that slows down digestion, keeping a person feeling full longer and possibly slowing the digestion and absorption of carbohydrates, which prevents a spike in blood glucose following a meal. Soluble fiber can help lower blood cholesterol and blood glucose levels.

Special Supplemental Nutrition Program for Women, Infants, and Children (WIC): A federal assistance program of the Food and Nutrition Service of the U.S. Department of Agriculture. The service provides health care, nutrition education, and financial support for low-income pregnant women, breastfeeding women, and infants and children younger than 5 years.

spermarche: The first ejaculation of seminal fluid.

strength training: Exercises that strengthen the muscles of the body.

stroke: The sudden death of brain cells due to lack of oxygen that is caused by blockage of blood flow or rupture of an artery to the brain.

stunting: Failure to grow both physically and cognitively; when a child is too short for his or her age. Stunting is the result of chronic or recurrent malnutrition.

subfertility: Diminished fertility but still able to become pregnant; hypofertility.

submucous cleft palate: A split of the muscle layer of the soft palate with an intact layer of mucosa lying over the defect.

sugar-sweetened beverage: Beveragesthat contains caloric sweeteners such as sugar, honey, and high-fructose corn syrup.

Tanner scale: A scale that measures the variability in puberty development.

tempo: In relation to puberty, the pace at which physical changes occur during development. This can vary among individuals.

teratogen: Something in the environment of the embryo that can cause birth defects.

tertiary aging: The social, demographic, and environmental influences over time.

therapeutic index: A ratio of how much drug or specific nutrient is needed to get the desired effect versus how much is toxic

thelarche: Breast budding, a sign of pubertal onset in girls.

theory of mutation accumulation: Medawar's theory of aging that suggests that aging is due to an accumulation of harmful mutations over time.

thermic effect of food (TEF): The increase in energy expenditure in response to the digestion, absorption, and storage of food.

toddlers: Children 2 to 3 years of age.

Tolerable Upper Intake Level (UL): The highest level of daily nutrient intake that is likely to pose no risk of adverse side effects to almost all individuals in the general population. As intake increases above the UL, the risk of adverse effects increases.

total parenteral nutrition (TPN): A method of feeding that bypasses the stomach and gastrointestinal tract. Fluids are administered into a vein and provide nutrients that the body needs.

Toxoplasma gondii: A parasite found in contaminated and undercooked meats and contaminated water that causes the disease toxoplasmosis.

trans fat: A type of unsaturated fat that occurs naturally in some products. The main dietary trans fats are created in an industrial process that adds hydrogen to liquid vegetable oils to make them more solid. Trans fats are used in margarine and many commercial fried products. Like saturated fats, trans fats are associated with increasing blood cholesterol levels. Trans fats on food labels can be referred to as "partially hydrogenated" oils on the ingredient list.

triglycerides: The main constituents of natural fats and oils. They are fats composed of three fatty acid chains linked to a glycerol molecule.

tube feeding: When a medical device is used to provide nutrition to individuals who cannot obtain nutrition by mouth or who are unable to swallow safely.

typhlitis: Inflammation of the cecum.

ulcerative colitis (UC): A subtype of inflammatory bowel disease; a chronic inflammatory disease of the colon that is of unknown cause and that is characterized by diarrhea with discharge of mucus and blood, cramping abdominal pain, and inflammation and edema of the mucous membrane with patches of ulceration.

Uniform Determination of Death Act (UDDA): Adopted by almost all of the states in the United States, the UDDA states: "An individual who has sustained either (1) irreversible cessation of circulation and respiratory functions, or (2) irreversible cessation of all functions of the entire brain, including the brain stem, is dead. A determination of death must be made in accordance with accepted medical standards" and "When an individual is pronounced dead by determining that the individual has sustained an irreversible cessation of all functions of the entire brain, including the brain stem, there shall be independent confirmation by another physician."

unilateral cleft lip and palate: A cleft defect that affects one side of the mouth and that may be present in varying degrees.

unintended weight loss: Decrease in body weight that is not planned or desired.

unsaturated fat: A type of fat that has one or more double bonds between the carbon atoms and that is found in plant foods and in fish. This type of fat is associated with being beneficial to heart health

urinary incontinence: The involuntary leakage of urine.

urinary tract infection: An infection of the kidney, ureter, bladder, or urethra.

vascular dementia: A common form of dementia caused by an impaired supply of blood to the brain, such as may be caused by a series of small strokes. Atherosclerotic changes increase the loss of cognitive function and result in the progressive loss of memory, cognitive skills, and muscle memory. Associated changes are dysphagia (the loss of swallowing ability), frailty (the loss of muscle mass and other pathological changes), and the eventual loss of motor, physical, and mental function.

villous atrophy: Inflammation of the small bowel mucosa and atrophy of the villi, resulting in nutrient malabsorption, wasting, and diarrhea.

vitamins: A group of organic substances that are essential for proper functioning of the body.

vomiting: An act or instance of disgorging the contents of the stomach through the mouth; also called emesis.

wasting: The result of sudden or acute malnutrition, when a child is not getting enough calories and faces an immediate risk of death. A child who is too thin for his or her height is undergoing wasting.

water intoxication: Excessive intake of water that may lead to diluted minerals in the blood, hyponatremia, renal failure, and even death.

xerostomia: Dry mouth usually of pathologic origin that occurs more frequently in advanced age.

Z-scores: Measurements of how far a point is from the mean or average. A Z-score can be a positive or negative number.

INDEX